Introduction for Educators:

Start your students off right!

Your students need to begin thinking like nurses from the moment they walk into your program. Authors Judith Wilkinson and Karen Van Leuven help them with a fresh new approach to teaching *Fundamentals of Nursing* with their innovative 2-volume presentation.

Volume 1: Theory, Concepts and Applications contains the material you'll cover in your classroom. It stresses knowledge mastery, critical thinking, evidence-based practice, and is case based. The content of this volume, as well as the *Electronic Study Guide* on CD-ROM packaged with it, is meticulously cross referenced to

Volume 2: Thinking and Doing in which the critical thinking introduced in *Volume 1* is applied to clinical procedures, and which uses a multi-generational, multi-cultural family as the basis for a case study threaded through *Volume 2*. This approach best suits the way you teach—and no other textbook has it!

The Wilkinson and Van Leuven "think like a nurse" learning suite also includes:

⇒ *Electronic Study Guide* bound into the back of *Volume 1* with
  • Learning Outcomes
  • Answers and suggested responses to the exercises in *Volume 1* and *Volume 2*
  • Additional exercises and suggested supplemental readings
  • Knowledge Maps, Care Plans, and Care Maps
  • Practice test bank for students
  and much more!

⇒ *Instructor's Resource Disk* (for adopters) that includes: a test bank, an instructor's guide, an image bank, and a PowerPoint Presentation.

⇒ *Online Resources at DavisPlus* for instructors and students—see page vi for more information.

⇒ *Procedure Checklists for Fundamentals of Nursing* – a separate print version as a convenience for you and your students. Its content is also available and customizable on the *Electronic Study Guide* and on the *Instructor's Resource Disk*.

⇒ *Fundamentals Packages* – When thinking of resources for your students' coursework, think about saving them money too. You have a choice of packages of essential F.A. Davis texts and references that include:
  • *Taber's Cyclopedic Medical Dictionary*,
  • *Davis's Drug Guide for Nurses*,
  • *Davis's Comprehensive Handbook of Laboratory and Diagnostic Tests with Nursing Implications*,
  and other titles fundamental to your students' success!

The next few pages present an overview to illustrate the key features of this unique text.
A more in-depth description is presented in the authors' *Preface*.

Toward Acting Like a Nurse

Everything your students need for learning procedures in clinical or skills lab is in *Volume 2*. This is incredibly convenient for your students because there is no need to carry the didactic material in *Volume 1* to the lab or to carry the applications-based content in *Volume 2* to lecture-type classes. Nor will your students have to wade through the text-heavy content, boxes, and tables to follow the "think and do" procedures in the lab as presented in other Fundamentals texts.

Urinary Elimination

27 CHAPTER

Overview

The urinary system consists of two kidneys, two ureters, the urinary bladder, and the urethra. The kidneys filter nitrogen and other metabolic wastes, toxins, excess ions, and water from the bloodstream and excrete them as urine. Voiding and control of urination require normal functioning of the bladder and the urethra, as well as an intact brain, spinal cord, and nerves supplying the bladder and urethra.

As an adult ages, the number of functional nephrons gradually decreases, along with the ability to dilute and concentrate urine. An adequately hydrated adult produces clear yellow urine. Concentrated urine is darker in color, but dilute urine can appear colorless. Substances that contain caffeine act as diuretics and increase urine production. Decreased urine production can be caused by a diet high in salt. Medications with anticholinergic effects inhibit the free flow of urine and may also contribute to urinary retention.

empty the bladder, may be caused by obstruction, nerve problems, infection, surgery, medications, or anxiety. To allow drainage of urine, a pliable tube is introduced into the bladder in a procedure called urinary catheterization. Nurses can independently perform the primary interventions to manage urinary incontinence (UI), a lack of voluntary control over urination. Pelvic floor muscle exercises (PFME) are a mainstay of UI treatment for women. PFME strengthen perineal muscles and help to prevent and treat stress, urge, and mixed UI. Kegel exercises are the most commonly used.

Thinking Critically About Urinary Elimination

The exercises in the following section allow you to practice the kind of thinking you will use as a full-spectrum nurse. Because these

Each chapter in *Volume 2* begins with an **Overview** of the *Volume 1* chapter, to refresh your students' memory of the content.

Thinking Critically About is a set of exercises that require students to use the information they learned in *Volume 1*. A summary of critical thinking steps is presented in the back of this volume for easy reference by students.

1 You receive report from a UAP that a patient with no history of urinary elimination problems has had 150 mL of oral liquids in 6 hours and has voided 100 mL of clear, dark amber urine. His vital signs at the start of the shift were as follows: blood pressure, 108/76 mm Hg; pulse, 72 bpm; respirations, 18; temperature, 98.6°F. The most recent check revealed blood pressure, 112/80 mm Hg; pulse, 88 bpm; respirations, 22; and temperature, 100.4°F.

  a What conclusion might you draw about what has caused these symptoms?
  b What actions should you take?

2 As you make rounds, you discover a collection bag for an indwelling catheter placed on the bed above the level of the patient's bladder.

  a What should you do first? What assessments should you make?
  b What teaching would be important in this situation?

3 Unlicensed assistive personnel complain that Mr. Jones, a patient with dementia, keeps urinating in his trash can and in the hallway.

  a What special measures could be taken to assist Mr. Jones in finding the bathroom?
  b What data could be helpful in developing a plan for Mr. Jones?

Knowledge Maps throughout!
☞ See example in Chapter 13, page 146.

Caring for the Garcias

At a recent visit to the Family Health Center, Joe and Flordelisa Garcia confide that Joe's mother, Katherine, has had several "accidents." She has denied the problem but Flordelisa tells you that she helped her mother-in-law with laundry recently and many of the clothes smell of urine. They ask you how to approach Katherine about this problem.

A. How would you respond?

B. What suggestions, if any, could you make to the Garcias about treatment for Katherine?

C. Flordelisa tells you that she has been told that surgery is the best form of treatment. She asks you whether this is true. How would you answer her question?

A unique feature of *Volume 2* is the extended case study, **Caring for the Garcias**, that illustrates and integrates content throughout the whole volume. The Garcia family and their friends and colleagues allow your students to see the human costs and benefits of the procedures they are learning.

PROCEDURE 27–3 — Intermittent Bladder or Catheter Irrigation

For steps to follow in *all* procedures, refer to the inside back cover of this book.

critical aspects
- Establish a sterile field under the specimen removal port or the irrigation port on a three-way catheter.
- Because of the risk of infection, never disconnect the drainage tubing.
- Use sterile irrigation solution, warmed to room temperature.
- Instill the irrigation solution slowly.
- Repeat the process as necessary.

Equipment
For intermittent irrigation through a three-way catheter:
- Bag of sterile irrigation solution
- Connecting tubing (to connect the bag to the irrigation port)
- IV pole
- Antiseptic swabs
- Bath blanket

For intermittent irrigation via the specimen port using a syringe:
- Sterile container
- Sterile 60 mL syringe with large-gauge needle (16 to 18 Fr.)
- 2 pairs of clean procedure gloves

Assessment
- Note the charac[...] color, odor, pres[...]
- Assess for the p[...] tion.
- Note patient co[...]
- Assess the patie[...]

To determine patie[...] tion and the likelih[...]
- Check the chart[...] lution to use.
- Assess the type[...] three-way).

Delegation
Irrigation of an indwelling catheter requires nursing assessment and clinical decision making. Because of the high potential for urinary tract infection, you should not delegate this procedure to the UAP.

Procedural Steps
Note: This is the procedure for the closed methods of irrigation. The "open" method is no longer recommended. Because of the risk for infection, you would never disconnect the drainage tubing from the catheter.

Variation A
Intermittent Irrigation for the Patient with a Three-Way (Triple-Lumen) Indwelling Catheter

Step 1 Prepare the irrigation solution and connecting tubing as directed in Procedure 27-4 (steps 1 thru 5). Once the solution is connected to the irrigation port, complete the following steps.

Step 2 Prior to begi[...] irrigation solution, e[...] may be in the bedsi[...] document the amou[...] record.

Provides a baseline f[...] of true urine output [...]

PROCEDURE 27–3 — Intermittent Bladder or Catheter Irrigation
(continued)

Step 3 Determine whether the irrigant is to remain in the bladder for any length of time. If the irrigant is to remain in the bladder for a certain time period, clamp the drainage tubing for that time.

Clamping the drainage tubing prevents immediate outflow.

Step 4 Slowly open the roller clamp on the irrigation tubing.

Slow instillation prevents patient discomfort.

Step 5 Instill or irrigate with the prescribed amount of irrigant.

Step 6 When the correct amount of irrigant has been used and/or the goals of the irrigation have been [...] roller clamp on the irri[...] [...]ing the tubing con[...]

Step 3 Drape the patient so that only the specimen removal port on the drainage tubing is exposed. Place a sterile waterproof drape beneath the exposed port.

Ensures patient privacy and prevents soiling of the bed linens.

Step 4 Open the sterile irrigation supplies. Pour approximately 100 mL of the irrigating solution into the sterile container, using aseptic technique.

Prevents the contamination of the irrigation solution with microorganisms.

Step 5 Swab the specimen removal port with antiseptic swab.

Cleanses the area of bacteria, preventing [...]

Holding the port above the level of the bladder enhances gravitational flow of irrigant into the bladder. ▼

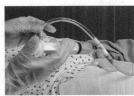

Step 9 When the irrigant has been injected, withdraw the needle. Refill the syringe if necessary. Do NOT recap the needle. If you need to repeat the [...]

PROCEDURE 27–3 — Intermittent Bladder or Cathete[r]
(continued)

Evaluation
- Note the flow rate of irrigant and/or inability to instill irrigant into the catheter.
- Note the characteristics of urine output (e.g., presence of output, color, amount, clots, mucus).
- Note patient complaints of discomfort (e.g., pain, spasms).
- Assess for development of bladder distention accompanied by lack of urine outflow.

Home Care
- A patient who will be irrigating her catheter at home should be aware that the closed method offers the least risk for introducing bacteria into the bladder.
- For the syringe method, the patient will need access to syringes and needles and a process to dispose of them properly.
- Teach the patient and/or caregiver strict aseptic technique.
- Teach the signs and symptoms of urinary retention and urinary tract infection.

Documentation
- Document the time of procedure, the type of irrigant, and the total amount used.
- Document the color of urine and the presence of clots, mucus, sediment, and so on.
- Record evidence of catheter patency (e.g., flow of urine, absence of distention)

Sample documentation:

5/4/07	11:30	Urine cloudy with many mucus shreds noted.
		Catheter irrigated with 60 mL of sterile
		normal saline. ————————— S. Riley, RN

Each **Procedure** is presented step by step, with rationales interspersed so your students better understand real-world practice. Core procedures as well as variants and alternatives are described. Every procedure is appropriately illustrated with photographs, and equipment, delegation, assessments, evaluation, documentation, home care, and patient teaching are all addressed throughout.

Links That Help Your Students Think Like Nurses

The didactic material that you'll cover in your classroom is contained in *Volume 1: Theory, Concepts and Applications*. The content of this volume is systematically linked to *Volume 2: Thinking and Doing* in which the critical thinking introduced in *Volume 1* continues to be applied, this time to a single unifying case study, to chapter content, and to the clinical procedures that are the core of *Volume 2*.

- *Sutures* ("stitches") are the traditional wound closures. Several types of suture materials are available. *Absorbent* sutures are used deep in the tissues, for example, to close an organ or **anastomose** (connect) tissue. Because they are made of material that will gradually dissolve, there is no need to remove absorbent sutures. *Nonabsorbent* sutures are placed in superficial tissues and require removal, often by a nurse. Suturing leads to small puncture wounds along the track of the laceration or incision. For instructions on removing sutures and staples,

Icons meticulously incorporated throughout the text indicate cross references between the "theory, concepts, and applications" in *Volume 1* and the "thinking and doing" in *Volume 2*.

| VOL 2 | Go to Chapter 34, **Technique 34–2: Removing Sutures and Staples,** in Volume 2.

- *Surgical staples* are made of lightweight titanium. They provide a fast, easy way to close a
- *Surgical glue* is a relatively new meth closure. It is safe for use in clean, wounds. It is an ideal wound closure m tears.
- *In vacuum-assisted wound closure,* a in the wound is attached by a tube t pressure pump to remove wound drai subatmospheric pressure to improve h a clean and moist environment, and fo to bacterial infection. The vacuum devi erized and can be programmed for con termittent negative pressure.
- *Compression stockings* are used with ulcers of the lower extremities. They a ous pressure to the veins, which facil return and allows the ulcers to heal.

Critical Thinking questions ask your students to apply what they've just learned to the patient introduced earlier in the chapter, to a new patient, or to their own lives.

TECHNIQUE 34–2   Removing Sutures and Staples

Removing Sutures

1. Obtain a suture removal kit.
2. Use the forceps to pick up one end of the suture.
3. Slide the small scissors around the suture, and cut near the skin. This helps you avoid pulling the exposed portion of the suture through the underlying tissue.
4. With the forceps, gently pull the suture in the direction of the knotted side to remove it.

Removing Staples

1. Obtain a staple remover.
2. Place the staple remover under the center of each staple, and slowly close it. This spreads the ends of the staples apart, freeing them from the skin.
3. Remove every other staple, and check the tension on the wound.
4. If there is no significant pull on the wound, remove the remaining staples. Consider placing a piece of gauze nearby so that you have a place to deposit the staples as you remove them.

Suture types

Plain interrupted

Mattress interrupted

Plain continuous

Mattress continuous

Removal techniques

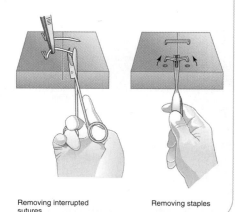
Removing interrupted sutures

Removing staples

CriticalThinking 34–4

Review the Braden and Norton scales. Apply these risk assessment scales to Mr. Harmon ("Meet Your Patient").

- What additional information, if any, do you need to complete these assessments?
- Which scale do you find most useful?

Chapters include **Knowledge Checks**, questions designed to allow your students to check their recall of the material they've just read and that are cross referenced to the corresponding answers on the *Electronic Study Guide* on CD-ROM.

• *Depth of the wound.* **Superficial wounds** involve only the epidermal layer of the skin. The injury is usually the result of friction, shearing, or burning. **Partial-thickness wounds** extend through the epidermis into the dermis. **Full-thickness wounds** extend into the subcutaneous tissue and beyond (Sussmen & Bates-Jensen, 2001). The descriptor **penetrating** is sometimes added to indicate that the wound involves internal organs. Wound depth is a major determinant of healing time: The deeper the wound, the longer the healing time.

KnowledgeCheck 34–3

- Explain the difference between an acute and a chronic wound.
- Describe the wound categorization system based on contamination.
- How does wound depth affect healing?

Go to Chapter 34, **Knowledge Check Response Sheet and Answers,** on the Electronic Study Guide.

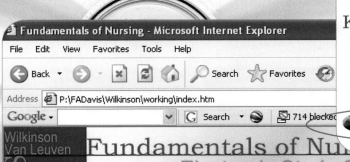

Fundamentals of Nursing - Microsoft Internet Explorer

File   Edit   View   Favorites   Tools   Help

← Back ▾ → ▾ ⊠ ⊠ ⌂ | 🔍 Search ☆ Favorites

Address 🔳 P:\FADavis\Wilkinson\working\index.htm

Google ▾ [   ] ✕ | G Search ▾ ⦿ | ⧄ 714 blocked

Wilkinson
Van Leuven **Fundamentals of Nu** ... alc ⧄ H

Electronic Study Guide

⧉ Chapter & Resources   ⧉ Additional Resources

Knowledge Check 34-3

• Explain the difference between an acute and a chronic wound.

<u>Answer:</u>
Acute and chronic wounds have different durations and causes.
  ○ **Acute** wounds are expected to be of short duration. Acute wounds may be intentional (surgical incisions) or unintentional (trauma).
  ○ Wounds are classified as *chronic* when they exceed the anticipated length of recovery. Chronic wounds include pressure, arterial, venous, and diabetic ulcers. These wounds are frequently colonized with bacteria, and healing is very slow because of the underlying disease process. A chronic wound may linger for months or years.

• Describe the wound categorization system based on contamination.

<u>Answer:</u>
Wounds are categorized based on four levels of contamination:
  ○ **Clean** wounds are uninfected wounds with minimal inflammation. They may be open or closed and do not involve the gastrointestinal, respiratory, or genitourinary tracts (these systems frequently harbor bacteria). There is very little risk of infection for these wounds.
  ○ **Clean-contaminated** wounds are surgical incisions that enter the gastrointestinal, respiratory, or genitourinary tracts. There is an increased risk of infection for these wounds, but there is no obvious infection.
  ○ **Contaminated** wounds include open, traumatic wounds or surgical incisions in which a major break in asepsis occurred. The risk of infection is high for these wounds.
  ○ **Infected** wounds are wounds with evidence of infection, such as purulent drainage or necrotic tissue. Wounds ... 100,000 organisms per gram of

| toward evidence-based practice |

Gibson, M.C., Keast, D., Woodbury, M.G., Black, J., Goettl, L., Campbell, K., et al. (2004). Educational intervention in the management of acute procedure-related wound pain: A pilot study. *Journal of Wound Care, 13*(5), 187–190.

This pilot study investigated the use of an educational intervention to manage acute pain associated with wound care in an outpatient clinic. Five patients aged 65 years or older with a history of pain during wound treatments were included in this pilot study. Each had a chronic wound that required dressing changes or debridement. Before the wound treatment, the nurse gave the patients information about the procedure, discussed strategies

they could use to make it as comfortable as possible, and explained how to use a rating scale to indicate their pain or emotional discomfort. Three out of five patients reported reduced pain and/or distress following the wound treatment.

---

1. How would you apply the findings of this pilot study to your clinical practice?
2. How might these findings be further investigated?

 Go to Chapter 34, **Toward Evidence-Based Practice Suggested Responses,** on the Electronic Study Guide.

Toward Evidence-Based Practice boxes describe important research that applies to the topic at hand and ask your students to consider higher cognitive level questions about the study or studies. Suggested responses appear on the *Electronic Study Guide*.

Online Resources at *DavisPlus*

DavisPlus makes it quick and simple to locate all of F.A. Davis's online resources by serving as an easy-to-navigate centralized hub. Wilkinson and Van Leuven's *Fundamentals of Nursing* offers robust online teaching tools for you and learning tools for your students at http://davisplus.fadavis.com. In addition to the clinically relevant resources presently available, updated content that will keep your students thinking like nurses will be developed and posted as well.

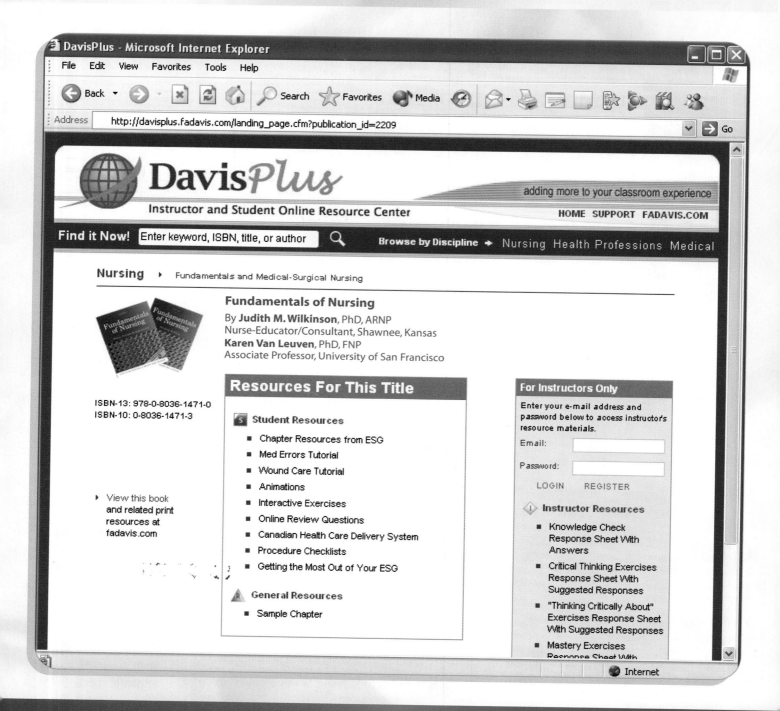

Fundamentals of Nursing

Thinking & Doing

VOLUME 2

JUDITH M. WILKINSON, PHD, ARNP
Nurse Educator/Consultant
Shawnee, Kansas

KAREN VAN LEUVEN, PHD, FNP
Associate Professor
University of San Francisco
San Francisco, California

Family Nurse Practitioner
Oakland, California

 F. A. Davis Company/Publishers   Philadelphia

F. A. Davis Company
1915 Arch Street
Philadelphia, PA 19103
www.fadavis.com

Printed in the United States of America

Last digit indicates print number: 10 9 8 7 6 5 4 3

Acquisitions Editor: Lisa B. Deitch
Content Development Manager: Darlene D. Pedersen
Special Projects Editor: Shirley A. Kuhn
Senior Project Editor: Danielle Barsky

As new scientific information becomes available through basic and clinical research, recommended treatments and drug therapies undergo changes. The author(s) and publisher have done everything possible to make this book accurate, up to date, and in accord with accepted standards at the time of publication. The author(s), editors, and publisher are not responsible for errors or omissions or for consequences from application of the book, and make no warranty, expressed or implied, in regard to the contents of the book. Any practice described in this book should be applied by the reader in accordance with professional standards of care used in regard to the unique circumstances that may apply in each situation. The reader is advised always to check product information (package inserts) for changes and new information regarding dose and contraindications before administering any drug. Caution is especially urged when using new or infrequently ordered drugs.

Library of Congress Cataloging-in-Publication Data

Wilkinson, Judith M., 1939–
    Fundamentals of nursing: thinking & doing/Judith M.
Wilkinson, Karen Van Leuven.
        p. cm.
    Includes bibliographical references and index.
    ISBN 0-8036-1197-8—ISBN 0-8036-1198-6
    1. Nursing.   I. Van Leuven, Karen.   II. Title.
    RT41.W56 2007
    610.73—dc22

                        2006016419

Vol. 2: ISBN 10: 0-8036-1198-6
Vol. 2: ISBN 13: 978-0-8036-1198-6

Set: ISBN 10: 0-8036-1471-3
Set: ISBN 13: 978-0-8036-1471-0

Preface

We chose our book title carefully. We have used the words *theory, concepts, application, thinking,* and *doing* because we believe that excellent nursing requires an equal mix of knowledge, thought and action. It is knowledge and its application—not just the tasks nurses do—that delineate the various levels of nursing. Even so, skillful performance of tasks is essential to full attainment of the nursing role.

We present our material in two volumes to enable students to focus on material suitable for use in specific venues. Volume 2 was designed to be a compact, easy-to-carry reference to use in the skills lab and in clinical. Nevertheless, it includes both thinking and doing—the same as does Volume 1; and it works seamlessly with Volume 1 and the Electronic Study Guide to provide a user-friendly learning experience that will surely stimulate new enthusiasm for learning. For example, throughout Volume 2, students have access to a simulated experience known as "Caring for the Garcias," through which they apply our full-spectrum model of nursing to learn about the nursing role, the healthcare system, and the real-world application of the content in Volume 1.

Other features in each chapter of this volume include critical-thinking activities ("Thinking Critically About . . ."); step-by-step procedures and techniques (with rationales); assessment guidelines and tools; summaries of NANDA/NIC/NOC standardized labels for nursing diagnoses, outcomes, and interventions; a chapter overview; and a summary of the main points that were covered in Volume 1. All of these features will be useful during a student's clinical day.

This volume, like Volume 1, will appeal to non-traditional students of the technology generation, encourage independent learning, promote critical thinking, support a variety of learning styles, and assure students that it is possible to achieve excellent nursing despite today's challenges.

We hope you will read the Preface and other introductory material in the front of Volume 1. It explains the philosophical underpinnings for this text and describes in more detail how to use the various pieces of this highly integrated learning package—which is flexible enough to accommodate a variety of teaching styles and curriculums.

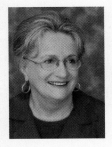

Judith Wilkinson

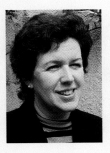

Detailed Contents

UNIT 1

How Nurses Think 5

CHAPTER 1
Evolution of Nursing Thought & Action 6

Caring for the Garcias 7

Thinking Critically About Evolution of Nursing Thought & Action 7

Knowledge Map 11

CHAPTER 2
Critical Thinking & the Nursing Process 12

Caring for the Garcias 13

Thinking Critically About Critical Thinking & the Nursing Process 13

Knowledge Map 19

CHAPTER 3
Nursing Process: Assessment 20

Caring for the Garcias 21

Thinking Critically About Nursing Process: Assessment 21

Knowledge Map 32

CHAPTER 4
Nursing Process: Diagnosis 33

Caring for the Garcias 34

Thinking Critically About Nursing Process: Diagnosis 34

Knowledge Map 43

CHAPTER 5
Nursing Process: Planning Outcomes 44

Caring for the Garcias 45

Thinking Critically About Nursing Process: Planning Outcomes 45

Knowledge Map 52

CHAPTER 6
Nursing Process: Planning Interventions 53

Caring for the Garcias 54

Thinking Critically About Nursing Process: Planning Interventions 54

Knowledge Map 61

CHAPTER 7
Nursing Process: Implementation & Evaluation 62

Caring for the Garcias 63

Thinking Critically About Nursing Process: Implementation & Evaluation 63

Knowledge Map 72

CHAPTER 8
Nursing Theory & Research 73

Caring for the Garcias 74

Thinking Critically About Nursing Theory & Research 74

Knowledge Map 81

UNIT 2

Factors Affecting Health 83

CHAPTER 9
Growth & Development Through the Life Span 84

Caring for the Garcias 85

Thinking Critically About Growth & Development Through the Life Span 85

Procedure 9–1 Assessing for Abuse 89

CHAPTER 10
Experiencing Health & Illness 94

Caring for the Garcias 95

Thinking Critically About Experiencing Health & Illness 95

Procedure 10–1 Admitting a Patient to a Nursing Unit 98

CHAPTER 11
Psychosocial Health & Illness 100

Caring for the Garcias 101

Thinking Critically About Psychosocial Health & Illness 101

Knowledge Map 117

CHAPTER 12
The Family 118

Caring for the Garcias 119

Thinking Critically About the Family 119

Knowledge Map 129

CHAPTER 13
Culture & Ethnicity 130

Caring for the Garcias 131

Thinking Critically About Culture & Ethnicity 131

Knowledge Map 146

CHAPTER 14
Spirituality 147

Caring for the Garcias 148

Thinking Critically About Spirituality 148

Knowledge Map 157

CHAPTER 15
Loss, Grief, & Dying 158

Caring for the Garcias 159

Thinking Critically About Loss, Grief, & Dying 159

Technique 15–1 Communicating with People Who Are Grieving 166

Technique 15–2 Helping Families of Dying Patients 167

Technique 15–3 Caring for the Dying Person 168

Technique 15–4 Providing Postmortem Care 169

Knowledge Map 176

UNIT 3

Essential Nursing Interventions 177

CHAPTER 16
Documenting & Reporting 178

Caring for the Garcias 179

Thinking Critically About Documenting & Reporting 179

Technique 16–1 Giving Oral Reports 182

Technique 16–2 Receiving Telephone and Verbal Orders 182

Technique 16–3 Guidelines for Documentation 183

Knowledge Map 190

CHAPTER 17
Measuring Vital Signs 191

Caring for the Garcias 192

Thinking Critically About Measuring Vital Signs 192

Procedure 17–1   Assessing Body Temperature 198

Procedure 17–1A   Taking an Oral Temperature 199

Procedure 17–1B   Taking a Rectal Temperature 200

Procedure 17–1C   Taking a Chemical Strip Temperature 201

Procedure 17–1D   Taking an Axillary Temperature 201

Procedure 17–1E   Taking a Tympanic Membrane Temperature 202

Procedure 17–2   Assessing Peripheral Pulses 203

Procedure 17–2A   Assessing the Radial Pulse 204

Procedure 17–2B   Assessing the Carotid Pulse 205

Procedure 17–2C   Assessing the Brachial Pulse 205

Procedure 17–2D   Assessing the Temporal Pulse 206

Procedure 17–2E   Assessing the Femoral Pulse 206

Procedure 17–2F   Assessing the Popliteal Pulse 206

Procedure 17–2G   Assessing the Posterior Tibial Pulse 207

Procedure 17–2H   Assessing the Dorsalis Pedis Pulse 207

Procedure 17–3   Assessing the Apical Pulse 208

Procedure 17–4   Assessing for an Apical-Radial Pulse Deficit 210

Procedure 17–5   Assessing Respirations 212

Procedure 17–6   Measuring Blood Pressure 214

Technique 17–1   Taking an Accurate Blood Pressure 217

CHAPTER 18
Communicating & the Therapeutic Relationship 220

Caring for the Garcias 221

Thinking Critically About Communicating & the Therapeutic Relationship 221

Technique 18–1   Enhancing Communication Through Nonverbal Behaviors 225

Technique 18–2   Some Useful Spanish Words and Phrases 225

Technique 18–3   Communicating with Clients Who Have Sensory Deficits 226

Technique 18–4   Communicating with Clients Who Have Impaired Cognition or Consciousness 226

Knowledge Map 229

CHAPTER 19
Health Assessment: Performing a Physical Examination 230

Caring for the Garcias 231

Thinking Critically About Health Assessment: Performing a Physical Examination 231

Procedure 19–1   Performing the General Survey 234

Procedure 19–2   Assessing the Skin 240

Procedure 19–3   Assessing the Hair 248

Procedure 19–4   Assessing the Nails 249

Procedure 19–5   Assessing the Head and Face 251

Procedure 19–6   Assessing the Eyes 253

Procedure 19–7   Assessing the Ears and Hearing 261

Procedure 19–8   Assessing the Nose and Sinuses 266

Procedure 19–9   Assessing the Mouth and Oropharynx 268

Procedure 19–10   Assessing the Neck 272

Procedure 19–11   Assessing the Breasts and Axillae 275

Procedure 19–12   Assessing the Chest and Lungs 280

Procedure 19–13   Assessing the Heart and Vascular System 287

Procedure 19–14   Assessing the Abdomen 293

Procedure 19–15   Assessing the Musculoskeletal System 300

Procedure 19–16   Assessing the Sensory-Neurological System 308

Procedure 19–17   Assessing the Male Genitourinary System 321

Procedure 19–18   Assessing the Female Genitourinary System 325

Procedure 19–19   Assessing the Anus and Rectum 330

Technique 19–1   Performing Percussion 233

Technique 19–2   Performing Auscultation 234

CHAPTER 20
Promoting Asepsis & Preventing Infection 337

Caring for the Garcias 338

Thinking Critically About Promoting Asepsis & Preventing Infection 338

Technique 20–1   Following Standard Precautions 341

Technique 20–2   Following Transmission-Based Precautions 342

Technique 20–3   Maintaining Protective Isolation 342

Technique 20–4   Using Sterile Technique 343

Procedure 20–1   Hand Washing 344

Procedure 20–2   Donning and Removing Personal Protective Equipment (PPE) 346

Procedure 20–3   Surgical Hand Washing 349

Procedure 20–4   Donning Sterile Gown and Gloves (Closed Method) 352

Procedure 20–5   Applying Sterile Gloves (Open Method) 355

Procedure 20–6   Preparing and Maintaining a Sterile Field 357

CHAPTER 21
Promoting Safety 361

Caring for the Garcias 362

Thinking Critically About Promoting Safety 362

Procedure 21–1   Using a Bed Monitoring Device 369

Procedure 21–2   Using Restraints 371

Technique 21–1   Performing the Heimlich Maneuver on an Infant or Child 375

Technique 21–2   Performing the Heimlich Maneuver on an Adult 376

Technique 21–3   Preventing Needlestick Injury 378

CHAPTER 22
Facilitating Hygiene 384

Caring for the Garcias 385

Thinking Critically About Facilitating Hygiene 385

Procedure 22–1 Bathing: Providing a Complete Bed Bath 390

Procedure 22–2 Bathing: Providing a Towel Bath 396

Procedure 22–3 Bathing: Providing a Packaged Bath 397

Procedure 22–4 Providing Perineal Care 399

Procedure 22–5 Providing Foot Care 402

Procedure 22–6 Brushing and Flossing the Teeth 406

Procedure 22–7 Providing Denture Care 409

Procedure 22–8 Providing Oral Care for an Unconscious Patient 411

Procedure 22–9 Shampooing the Hair for a Patient on Bedrest 414

Procedure 22–10 Providing Beard and Mustache Care 418

Procedure 22–11 Shaving a Patient 420

Procedure 22–12 Removing and Caring for Contact Lenses 422

Procedure 22–13 Making an Unoccupied Bed 424

Procedure 22–14 Making an Occupied Bed 427

Technique 22–1 Assisting with a Shower or Tub Bath 429

Technique 22–2 Caring for Artificial Eyes 430

Technique 22–3 Caring for Hearing Aids 431

CHAPTER 23
Administering Medications 438

Caring for the Garcias 439

Thinking Critically About Administering Medications 439

Procedure 23–1   Administering Oral Medications 454

Procedure 23–1A   Administering Medication Through an Enteral Tube 456

Procedure 23–2   Administering Ophthalmic Medications 459

Procedure 23–2A   Irrigating the Eyes 461

Procedure 23–3   Administering Otic Medications 463

Procedure 23–4   Administering Nasal Medications 465

Procedure 23–5   Administering Vaginal Medications 467

Procedure 23–6   Inserting a Rectal Suppository 471

Procedure 23–7   Preparing and Drawing Up Medications 474

Procedure 23–7A   Drawing Up Medications from Ampules 475

Procedure 23–7B   Preparing and Drawing Up Medications from Vials 476

Procedure 23–8   Mixing Medications in One Syringe 479

Procedure 23–9   Recapping Needles Using One-Handed Technique 483

Procedure 23–10   Administering Intradermal Medications 486

Procedure 23–11   Administering Subcutaneous Medications 489

Procedure 23–12   Locating Intramuscular Injection Sites 493

Procedure 23–13   Administering Intramuscular Injections 496

Procedure 23–14   Adding Medications to Intravenous Fluids 500

Procedure 23–14A   Adding Medication to a New IV Bag or Bottle 501

Procedure 23–14B   Adding Medication to a Running IV 502

Procedure 23–15   Administering IV Push Medications 503

Procedure 23–15A   Administering IV Push Through a Running Primary IV Line 504

Procedure 23–15B   Administering IV Push Through an Intermittent Device (IV Lock) When No Extension Tubing Is Attached to the Venous Access Device 505

Procedure 23–15C   Administering IV Push Through an Intermittent Device with IV Extension Tubing 506

Procedure 23–16   Administering Medications by Intermittent Infusion 508

Procedure 23–16A   Using a Volume-Control Administration Set 509

Procedure 23–16B   Using a Piggyback Set 510

Procedure 23–16C   Using a Tandem (Secondary) Set 511

Technique 23–1   Applying Medications to the Skin 513

Technique 23–2   Using Prefilled Unit-Dose Systems 514

Technique 23–3   Reconstituting Medications 515

Technique 23–4   Measuring Dosage When Changing Needles 516

Technique 23–5   Mixing Two Kinds of Insulin in One Syringe 517

Technique 23–6   Administering Heparin Subcutaneously 518

CHAPTER 24
Teaching Clients 527

Caring for the Garcias 528

Thinking Critically About Teaching Clients 528

Knowledge Map 539

UNIT 4
How Nurses Support Physiological Functioning 541

CHAPTER 25
Stress & Adaptation 542

Caring for the Garcias 543

Thinking Critically About Stress & Adaptation 543

Technique 25–1   Dealing with Angry Patients 549

Technique 25–2   Crisis Intervention Guidelines 550

Knowledge Map 556

CHAPTER 26
Nutrition 557

Caring for the Garcias 558

Thinking Critically About Nutrition 558

Procedure 26–1   Checking Fingerstick (Capillary) Blood Glucose Levels 563

Procedure 26–2   Inserting Nasogastric and Nasoenteric Tubes 567

Procedure 26–3   Administering Feedings Through Gastric and Enteric Tubes 572

Procedure 26–4   Removing a Nasogastric or Nasoenteric Tube 577

Technique 26–1   Measuring Triceps Skinfold 579

Technique 26–2   Measuring Circumferences to Evaluate Body Composition 579

Technique 26–3   Interventions for Patients with Impaired Swallowing 580

Technique 26–4   Assisting Patients with Meals 580

Technique 26–5   Checking Feeding Tube Placement 581

Technique 26–6   Monitoring Patients Receiving Enteral Nutrition 582

Technique 26–7   Monitoring Patients Who Are Receiving Total Parenteral Nutrition 582

CHAPTER 27
Urinary Elimination 591

Caring for the Garcias 592

Thinking Critically About Urinary Elimination 592

Procedure 27–1   Collecting a Clean-Catch Urine Specimen 595

Procedure 27–2   Inserting a Urinary Catheter 598

Procedure 27–2A   Inserting a Straight Urinary Catheter 599

Procedure 27–2B   Inserting an Indwelling Urinary Catheter 603

Procedure 27–3   Intermittent Bladder or Catheter Irrigation 610

Procedure 27–4   Continuous Bladder Irrigation 613

Procedure 27–5 Applying an External (Condom) Catheter 616

Technique 27–1 Measuring Voided Urine and Obtaining a Specimen 619

Technique 27–2 Measuring Urine from an Indwelling Catheter 619

Technique 27–3 Obtaining a Sterile Urine Specimen from a Catheter 620

Technique 27–4 Collecting a 24-Hour Urine Specimen 620

Technique 27–5 Dipstick Testing of Urine 621

Technique 27–6 Measuring Specific Gravity of Urine 622

Technique 27–7 Caring for a Patient with an Indwelling Catheter 623

Technique 27–8 Removing an Indwelling Catheter 625

Technique 27–9 Managing Urinary Incontinence 626

Technique 27–10 Caring for Patients with Urinary Diversions 628

CHAPTER 28
Bowel Elimination 636

Caring for the Garcias 637

Thinking Critically About Bowel Elimination 637

Procedure 28–1 Testing Stool for Occult Blood 640

Procedure 28–2 Placing and Removing a Bedpan 643

Procedure 28–3 Administering an Enema 646

Procedure 28–3A Administering a Cleansing Enema 647

Procedure 28–3B Administering a Prepackaged Enema 648

Procedure 28–4 Removing Stool Digitally 650

Procedure 28–5 Changing an Ostomy Appliance 654

Procedure 28–6 Irrigating a Colostomy 659

Technique 28–1 Testing for Pinworms 663

Technique 28–2 Administering an Oil-Retention Enema 663

Technique 28–3 Administering a Return-Flow Enema 663

Technique 28–4 Inserting a Rectal Tube 664

CHAPTER 29
Sensory Perception 672

Caring for the Garcias 673

Thinking Critically About Sensory Perception 673

Procedure 29–1 Performing Otic Irrigation 676

Technique 29–1 Communicating with Visually Impaired Clients 679

Technique 29–2 Communicating with Hearing-Impaired Clients 679

CHAPTER 30
Pain Management 684

Caring for the Garcias 685

Thinking Critically About Pain Management 685

Procedure 30–1 Connecting a Patient-Controlled Analgesia Pump 688

Technique 30–1 Nursing Care of the Patient with an Epidural Catheter 691

CHAPTER 31
Activity & Exercise 696

Caring for the Garcias 697

Thinking Critically About Activity & Exercise 697

Procedure 31–1 Moving and Turning Patients in Bed 699

Procedure 31–1A Moving a Patient Up in Bed 700

Procedure 31–1B Turning a Patient in Bed 702

Procedure 31–1C Logrolling a Patient 703

Procedure 31–2 Transferring Patients 704

Procedure 31–2A Transferring a Patient from Bed to Stretcher 706

Procedure 31–2B Dangling a Patient at the Side of the Bed 709

Procedure 31–2C Transferring a Patient from Bed to Chair 709

Procedure 31–3 Assisting with Ambulation 712

Procedure 31–3A Assisting with Ambulation (One Nurse) 713

Procedure 31–3B Assisting with Ambulation (Two Nurses) 714

Technique 31–1 Applying Principles of Body Mechanics 716

Technique 31–2 Making a Trochanter Roll 717

Technique 31–3 Performing Passive Range-of-Motion Exercises 717

Technique 31–4 Assisting with Physical Conditioning Exercises to Prepare for Walking 718

Technique 31–5   Sizing Walking Aids 718

Technique 31–6   Teaching Patients to Use Canes, Walkers, and Crutches 719

CHAPTER 32
Sexual Health 726

Caring for the Garcias 727

Thinking Critically About Sexual Health 727

Technique 32–1   Taking a Sexual History 733

Knowledge Map 740

CHAPTER 33
Sleep & Rest 741

Caring for the Garcias 742

Thinking Critically About Sleep & Rest 742

Procedure 33–1   Giving a Back Massage 748

CHAPTER 34
Skin Integrity & Wound Healing 754

Caring for the Garcias 755

Thinking Critically About Skin Integrity & Wound Healing 755

Procedure 34–1   Obtaining a Wound Culture by Swab 759

Procedure 34–2   Obtaining a Needle Aspiration Culture from a Wound 762

Procedure 34–3   Performing a Sterile Wound Irrigation 766

Procedure 34–4   Removing and Applying Dry Dressings 770

Procedure 34–5   Removing and Applying Wet-to-Damp Dressings 773

Procedure 34–6   Applying a Transparent Film Dressing 776

Procedure 34–7   Applying a Hydrocolloid Dressing 779

Technique 34–1   Placing Steri-Strips 782

Technique 34–2   Removing Sutures and Staples 783

Technique 34–3   Shortening a Drain 784

Technique 34–4   Emptying a Closed-Wound Drainage System 785

Technique 34–5   Taping a Dressing 786

Technique 34–6   Applying Binders 786

Technique 34–7   Applying Bandages 788

Technique 34–8   Local Application of Heat 791

Technique 34–9   Local Application of Cold 792

CHAPTER 35
Oxygenation 798

Caring for the Garcias 799

Thinking Critically About Oxygenation 800

Procedure 35–1   Collecting a Sputum Specimen 803

Procedure 35–1A   Collecting an Expectorated Specimen 805

Procedure 35–1B   Collecting a Suctioned Specimen 806

Procedure 35–2   Monitoring Pulse Oximetry (Arterial Oxygen Saturation) 809

Procedure 35–3   Applying and Caring for a Patient with a Cardiac Monitor 812

Procedure 35–4   Performing Percussion, Vibration, and Postural Drainage 815

Procedure 35–5   Administering Oxygen by Cannula, Face Mask, or Face Tent 819

Procedure 35–6   Performing Tracheostomy Care 825

Procedure 35–7   Performing Oropharyngeal and Nasopharyngeal Suctioning 831

Procedure 35–8   Performing Orotracheal and Nasotracheal Suctioning 835

Procedure 35–9   Performing Tracheostomy or Endotracheal Suctioning 840

Procedure 35–9A   Performing Tracheostomy or Endotracheal Suctioning Using Inline Suction Equipment 843

Procedure 35–10   Caring for a Patient on a Mechanical Ventilator 846

Procedure 35–11   Caring for a Patient with Chest Tubes (Disposable Water-Seal System) 850

Procedure 35–12   Performing Cardiopulmonary Resuscitation, One- and Two-Person 855

Technique 35–1   Assessing Breathing Patterns 860

Technique 35–2   Tips for Obtaining Accurate Pulse Oximetry Readings 861

Technique 35–3   Guidelines for Preventing Aspiration 861

Technique 35–4   Oxygen Therapy Safety Precautions 862

Technique 35–5   Inserting an Oropharyngeal Airway 862

Technique 35–6   Inserting a Nasopharyngeal Airway 863

Technique 35–7   Caring for Patients with Endotracheal
Airways 863

CHAPTER 36
Fluids, Electrolytes, & Acid-Base Balance 871

Caring for the Garcias 872

Thinking Critically About Fluids, Electrolytes,
& Acid-Base Balance 872

Procedure 36–1   Initiating a Peripheral Intravenous
Infusion 876

Procedure 36–2   Regulating the IV Flow Rate 882

Procedure 36–3   Setting Up and Using IV Pumps 885

Procedure 36–4   Changing IV Solutions, Tubing, and
Dressings 888

Procedure 36–4A   Changing the IV Solution 889

Procedure 36–4B   Changing the IV Administration Tubing
and Solution 890

Procedure 36–4C   Changing the IV Dressing 891

Procedure 36–5   Converting a Primary Line to a Heparin or
Saline Lock 892

Procedure 36–6   Discontinuing an IV Line 895

Procedure 36–7   Administering a Blood Transfusion 898

Technique 36–1   Assessing for Trousseau's and Chvostek's
Signs 903

Technique 36–2   Interpreting Arterial Blood Gases
(ABGs) 904

CHAPTER 37
Perioperative Nursing 914

Caring for the Garcias 915

Thinking Critically About Perioperative Nursing 915

Procedure 37–1   Teaching a Patient to Cough, Deep-
Breathe, Move in Bed, and Perform Leg Exercises 918

Procedure 37–2   Applying Antiembolism Stockings 921

Procedure 37–3   Applying Sequential Compression
Devices 924

Technique 37–1   Preparing a Room for a Patient's Return
from Surgery 927

Technique 37–2   Creating an Operative Field 927

UNIT 5
Nursing Functions 941

CHAPTER 38
Leading & Managing 942

Caring for the Garcias 943

Thinking Critically About Leading & Managing 943

Knowledge Map 948

CHAPTER 39
Nursing Informatics 949

Caring for the Garcias 950

Thinking Critically About Nursing Informatics 950

Knowledge Map 959

CHAPTER 40
Holistic Healing 960

Caring for the Garcias 961

Thinking Critically About Holistic Healing 961

Technique 40–1   Performing Autogenic Training 964

Technique 40–2   Using Calming Technique 964

Technique 40–3   Using Humor 965

Technique 40–4   Facilitating Meditation 965

Technique 40–5   Performing Simple Guided Imagery 966

Technique 40–6   Performing Simple Massage 966

Technique 40–7   Performing Simple Relaxation
Therapy 967

Technique 40–8   Performing Therapeutic Touch 967

Knowledge Map 969

CHAPTER 41
Promoting Health 970

Caring for the Garcias 971

Thinking Critically About Promoting Health 971

Knowledge Map 983

UNIT 6

The Context for Nurses' Work 985

CHAPTER 42
Community Nursing 986

Caring for the Garcias 987

Thinking Critically About Community Nursing 987

Knowledge Map 996

CHAPTER 43
Nursing in Home Care 997

Caring for the Garcias 998

Thinking Critically About Nursing in Home Care 998

Knowledge Map 1004

CHAPTER 44
Ethics & Values 1005

Caring for the Garcias 1006

Thinking Critically About Ethics & Values 1006

Technique 44–1   Using the MORAL Model for Ethical Decision Making 1013

Technique 44–2   Using Guidelines for Advocacy 1013

Knowledge Map 1015

CHAPTER 45
Legal Issues 1016

Caring for the Garcias 1017

Thinking Critically About Legal Issues 1017

Technique 45–1   Using Equipment Safely 1021

Technique 45–2   Tips for Avoiding Malpractice 1021

Technique 45–3   Guidelines for Documenting Care 1022

Knowledge Map 1024

CHAPTER 46
Canadian Healthcare Delivery System
(Refer to the Electronic Study Guide)

Bibliography B-1 (See backmatter)

Index I-1 (See backmatter)

Meet the Garcias

Throughout this text, you will be applying what you have learned as you care for the Garcia family. In this chapter, you will meet Joe Garcia, a construction worker, who arrives at the Family Medicine Center for his first physical exam in 10 years. It is Joe's knee pain that causes him to seek help because it affects his work. But as you will see, Joe will discover that he has other serious health problems that require him to be more vigilant about his health. As you read and work through the exercises in "Caring for the Garcias," you will also get to know Joe's wife Flordelisa, his grandchild Bettina, other members of his extended family, and his friends, as they deal with health issues and life changes.

Your experience in caring for the Garcias will show you that patients come to you with symptoms, but that each person brings unique values, lifestyle, and relationships to the encounter. From the Garcias, you will learn what it means to care for the whole person and how to be a full-spectrum nurse.

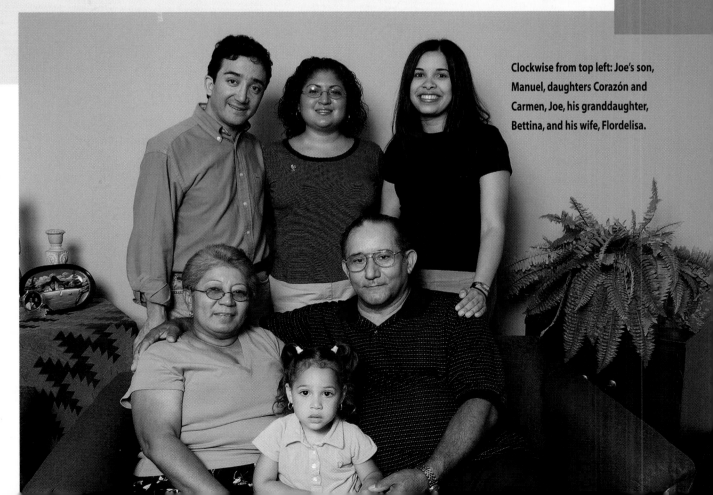

Clockwise from top left: Joe's son, Manuel, daughters Corazón and Carmen, Joe, his granddaughter, Bettina, and his wife, Flordelisa.

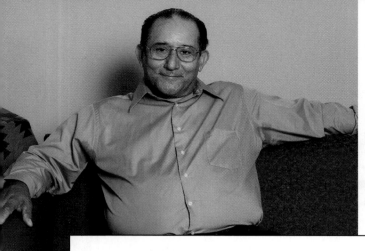

Mr. Joseph Garcia is a new patient at the Family Medicine Center. He arrives at the Center for an appointment for a physical exam and completes the following admission questionnaire.

Name: *Joseph Garcia*   DOB: *7 / 12 / 50*

Marital Status   S   Ⓜ   W   D   Partnered

If applicable, spouse/partner name: *Flordelisa*

Occupation: *Construction worker*   Spouse/partner occupation: *Daycare teacher*

Does your spouse or partner have any health care problems? If so, please list:

High blood pressure

Do you have children? *Yes*   Ages? *30, 27, 22*

Please circle yes or no if you have had the following:

AIDS/HIV +	YES	**NO**	Headaches	YES	**NO**
Allergies	**YES**	NO	Heart Disease	YES	**NO**
Anemia	YES	**NO**	Hernia	**YES**	NO
Anorexia	YES	**NO**	Herpes	YES	**NO**
Anxiety	YES	**NO**	High Cholesterol	YES	**NO**
Arthritis	YES	**NO**	High Blood Pressure	YES	**NO**
Bleeding Disorder	YES	**NO**	Kidney Problems	YES	**NO**
Breast Problems	YES	**NO**	Liver Problems	YES	**NO**
Cancer	YES	**NO**	Abnormal Mammogram	**N/A** YES	NO
Chicken Pox	**YES**	NO	Menopause	**N/A** YES	NO
Colon Disorder	YES	**NO**	Mononucleosis	YES	**NO**
COPD/Emphysema	YES	**NO**	Multiple Sclerosis	YES	**NO**
Depression	YES	**NO**	Osteoporosis	YES	**NO**
Diabetes	YES	**NO**	Pneumonia	YES	**NO**
Epilepsy/Seizures	YES	**NO**	Polio	YES	**NO**
Eye Problems	**YES**	NO	Prostate Problems	YES	**NO**
Gallbladder Disorder	YES	**NO**	Skin Problems	YES	**NO**
Stomach Problems/Ulcer	YES	**NO**	Stroke	YES	**NO**
Gout	YES	**NO**	Suicide Attempt	YES	**NO**
Gynecological Problems	YES	**NO**	Thyroid Problems	YES	**NO**
Sexually Transmitted Disease	YES	**NO**	Other	YES	**NO**

Please List Your Current Medications and Dosages. Also list over-the-counter and herbal products you use regularly.

Tylenol Extra Strength 6 per day   *Ben-Gay Balm on knees*

MultiVitamin 1 per day

Do you have any allergies to any medications? If YES, please list: None

Please list any surgeries or hospitalizations with the dates:

Tonsils   1956

Hernia repair   1985

When was your last Tetanus Vaccine?   ????   unknown

   Have you had the vaccine for Pneumonia? If yes, when? I don't think so

Have you had the Vaccine against Hepatitis B?   No   Hepatitis A?   No

Have you ever had a Sigmoidoscopy or Colonoscopy? If YES, when?   No

Have you ever had a PSA test to screen for prostate cancer?   No

If YES, when?   Has it ever been abnormal?

Any difficulty with achieving or maintaining an erection?   No

Please tell us about yourself.

Do you drink alcohol?   Yes   If yes, what type, how much and how often?

Beer, one or two several times per week

Do you use tobacco?   Yes   If yes, how much do you smoke per day?   1 1/2 packs per day

                                  At what age did you begin smoking? 16

                                  Have you ever tried to quit? yes

                                  Would you like to quit? maybe

Do you drink caffeine?   Yes   How much per day?   2 cups

Do you use recreational drugs?   No   If yes, what type and how often?

Do you exercise?   At work only   Describe the type, frequency, and length of exercise.

Do you have a stressful life? Yes

Is the source of your stress      Family?

Do you use Alternative Medicine (ex. Chiropractic, acupuncture)?   No

Do you have a Living Will or Advance Directive?   No

What are your hobbies?   Watching sports on TV, grandkids

Please tell us about your Family History. For any YES answer please indicate your relationship with the person.

Asthma	YES	**NO**		High Blood Pressure	**YES**	NO
Breast Cancer	YES	**NO**		*both parents*		
Cancer *father, prostate*	**YES**	NO		High Cholesterol *mother*	**YES**	NO
Chemical Dependency	YES	**NO**		Kidney Disease	YES	**NO**
Diabetes *mother*	**YES**	NO		Mental Illness	YES	**NO**
Heart Disease *both parents*	**YES**	NO		Osteoporosis	YES	**NO**
Heart Disease Before 55 yo	YES	**NO**		Unusual Disorders	YES	**NO**
				Other		

The Diagnosis

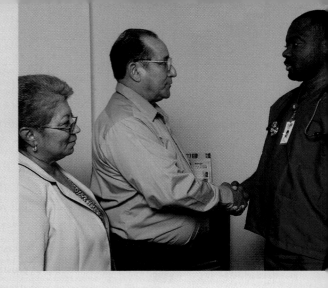

During the visit, the clinic nurse records the following information in Joe's chart.

Height	5' 10"
Weight	225 lbs
BP	162/94
Pulse	84
RR	20
Temp	98.2 oral

Chief Complaint: Patient states he is here to establish at the Center and that he has not had a physical exam in over 10 years. Wife accompanies. He is currently experiencing bilateral knee pain that is affecting his work performance. "I work in construction. I have to climb up and down ladders, lift things, and crawl around a lot." Has not missed any work but has been using increasing amounts of Tylenol and ibuprofen "to get through the day." The medications provide only limited relief. Notes that pain occurs daily even if not at work. Describes the pain as "achy" and "dull." Feels best when he is off his feet. Desires pain relief and check-up. Explains that both parents had heart disease. Wife expressing worry that he may be developing heart problems "because he's so tired after work and he gets short of breath easy."

The nurse explains to Joe that he will be seen by the nurse practitioner shortly. She asks Mr. Garcia if he would like his wife to be present for the exam. Mr. Garcia requests that his wife remain in the room.

Jordan Miller, MSN, FNP is on duty at the Center today. Jordan worked as an RN for over 10 years in the local emergency department and urgent care clinic. He has been an FNP for over 5 years. Jordan enters the room and introduces himself to the Garcia couple. To begin the exam, Jordan reviews the information Mr. Garcia supplied on the admission form, then he asks Joe about his family history.

He begins by talking about family history.

Jordan: "Are your parents still living?"

Joe: "Yes, they're both alive. My father is 80 years old and my mother is 76."

Jordan: "I'd like to hear a little more about your family history. Tell me about your father's cancer. How old was he when he was first diagnosed? Has he had treatment?"

Joe: "He was probably about 60 when he first found out about it. I know he had some kind of surgery and takes medicines but I don't know the details. He seems all right though."

Jordan: "Your father also has high blood pressure and heart disease. Please tell me a little more about that."

Joe: "My father and mother both have high blood pressure and heart disease. They both take medicines for their blood pressure. My father had a small heart attack about 10 years ago. My mother has never had a heart attack that I know of, but she sometimes has chest pain."

Jordan: "Your mother also has diabetes?"

Joe: "She's had that for a long time. My parents joke about that. My father is part Cuban and part Irish. A lot of people in his family, especially on the Cuban side, have diabetes but nobody in my mother's family. Yet my mother is the one with the diabetes!"

Flordelisa: "A lot of people in my family have diabetes too. But so far I'm OK, I think. My family is from Mexico and I know a lot of diabetics back home."

Jordan: "Have you been seen for a health exam lately, Mrs. Garcia?"

Flordelisa: "Not in about a year, but I'm going to schedule an appointment here."

The Garcia couple and Jordan continue to review the health information. After reviewing the history and discussing current complaints, Jordan performs a complete physical exam.

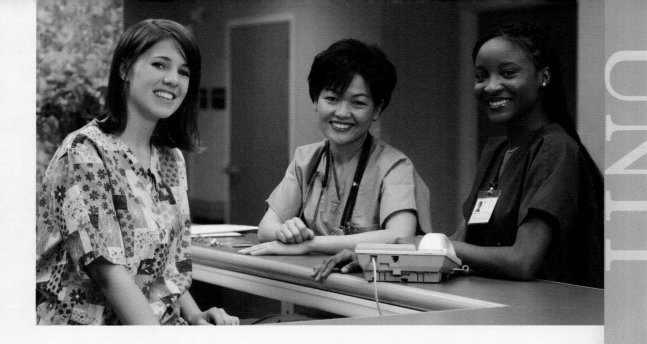

How Nurses
Think

1 EVOLUTION OF NURSING
   THOUGHT & ACTION

2 CRITICAL THINKING & THE
   NURSING PROCESS

3 NURSING PROCESS:
   ASSESSMENT

4 NURSING PROCESS:
   DIAGNOSIS

5 NURSING PROCESS:
   PLANNING OUTCOME

6 NURSING PROCESS:
   PLANNING INTERVENTIONS

7 NURSING PROCESS:
   IMPLEMENTATION
   & EVALUATION

8 NURSING THEORY & RESEARCH

CHAPTER 1

Evolution of Nursing
Thought & Action

Overview

Angel of mercy, handmaiden, battle-ax, naughty nurse—these are just some of the common stereotypes of nurses. Whether flattering, demeaning, or accurate, these images influence how people view the profession.

Religious and military organizations played a major role in the development of nursing and healthcare organizations. At first the nurse's role was limited to bathing, feeding, and supporting the patient, keeping the environment clean and orderly, and supporting the physician.

Nursing has undergone tremendous change from providing only kindness and support to full-spectrum work that is based on science but still focuses on caring. Nurses today collaborate with other members of the healthcare team and work independently.

Only graduates of accredited nursing programs who have passed a licensure exam are legally regarded as nurses. Graduates may enter the profession either as a licensed practical nurse (LPN) or licensed vocational nurse (LVN), or as a registered nurse (RN). In addition, graduate nursing education prepares the RN for advanced practice, expanded roles, or research.

Nursing is regulated by laws at the state (and, in Canada, provincial) level called nurse practice acts. They define nursing practice, establish professional criteria, determine activities within the scope of practice, and enforce the laws that govern nursing.

Nurses focus on health promotion, illness prevention, health restoration, and care of the dying. They work in hospitals, extended care facilities, ambulatory care, and community or home health settings.

Societal trends outside of nursing and health care, particularly the national economy, technology, consumer involvement in health care, the women's movement, and collective bargaining, have strongly affected nursing practice. So have trends within health care, including the development of practice settings outside the hospital, increased autonomy and advanced practice roles, and more use of unlicensed assistive personnel.

Thinking Critically About the Evolution of Nursing Thought and Action

The exercises in the following section allow you to practice the kind of thinking you will use as a full-spectrum nurse. Because these are critical-thinking activities, there is usually no single right answer. Discuss answers with your peers—discussion can stimulate critical thinking. If you have difficulty with any of the questions, consult with your instructor.

Caring for the Garcias

Review the opening scenario in the front of the book on the preliminary visit of Joseph Garcia at the Family Medicine Center. Mr. Garcia is examined by Jordan Miller, MSN, FNP, an African American man.

A. How would you respond to Mr. Garcia's concerns that he was examined by someone who is "just a nurse"?

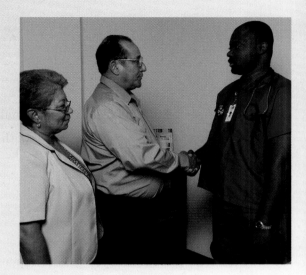

B. What factors might be causing Mr. Garcia to question care by "a male nurse"?

1 At a holiday family gathering, you are at the dinner table with your 60-year-old aunt, your 85-year-old grandmother, and your 15-year-old sister-in-law. Your aunt and grandmother are retired RNs. Your sister-in-law aspires to be a nurse, and you are in school studying to be a nurse.

a What factors will influence how each of you views nursing?

b Your sister-in-law asks you to define nursing. What would you say?

c How could you explain to her how a nurse is different from a nurse's aide or a physician?

2 Review the information on educational pathways into nursing.

a What is your personal opinion on the entry-into-practice debate? (That is, what minimum level of education should be required to practice nursing?)

b What reasons can you give to support your opinion?

3 Review the description of the National Student Nurses Association (NSNA). If your program has a local chapter of NSNA, consider attending a meeting or consulting the association web site for more information. Identify at least three potential benefits of joining this organization.

a

b

c

 For each of the following concepts, use critical thinking to describe how or why it is important to nursing, patient care, or the evolution of nursing thought and action. Note that these are *not* to be merely definitions.

History of nursing

The stereotypes of nurses

The Nightingale era

Definitions of nursing from the International Council of Nursing (ICN), American Nurses Association (ANA), and the Canadian Nurses Association (CNA)

Regulation of nursing practice

Entry into practice debate

Benner's stages of nursing skill

Nursing organizations

The national economy

Better-informed healthcare consumers

Use of unlicensed assistive personnel

Use of life-extending, high-technology equipment

What Are the Main Points in This Chapter?

- Religious organizations and the military have played a major role in the development of nursing and healthcare organizations.
- Initially the role of the nurse was limited to bathing, feeding, and supporting the patient; keeping the patient environment clean and orderly; and providing support for the physician.
- Contemporary nursing care includes activities that are performed in collaboration with other members of the healthcare team and also independently.
- Licensed practical nurses (LPNs or LVNs) are nurses who have successfully completed a practical nursing program and have passed a licensure exam (NCLEX-PN). They are prepared to give direct patient care.
- Registered nurses (RNs) are nurses who have successfully completed a registered nurse education program and have passed a licensure exam (NCLEX-RN). There are several types of RN education programs.

- Graduate nursing education is designed to prepare the RN for advanced practice, expanded roles, or research.
- Benner has identified a five-step progression of skill acquisition in nurses: novice, advanced beginner, competence, proficiency, and expert.
- Nurse practice acts are laws that regulate nursing practice at the state (and, in Canada, provincial) level.
- Nurses engage in health promotion, illness prevention, health restoration, and care of the dying.
- Nurses work in hospitals, extended care facilities, ambulatory care, and community or home health settings.
- The economy, technology, increased consumer involvement in health care, the women's movement, and the change in nursing role are forces that have strongly affected nursing.

Knowledge Map

Factors Affecting the Evolution of Nursing

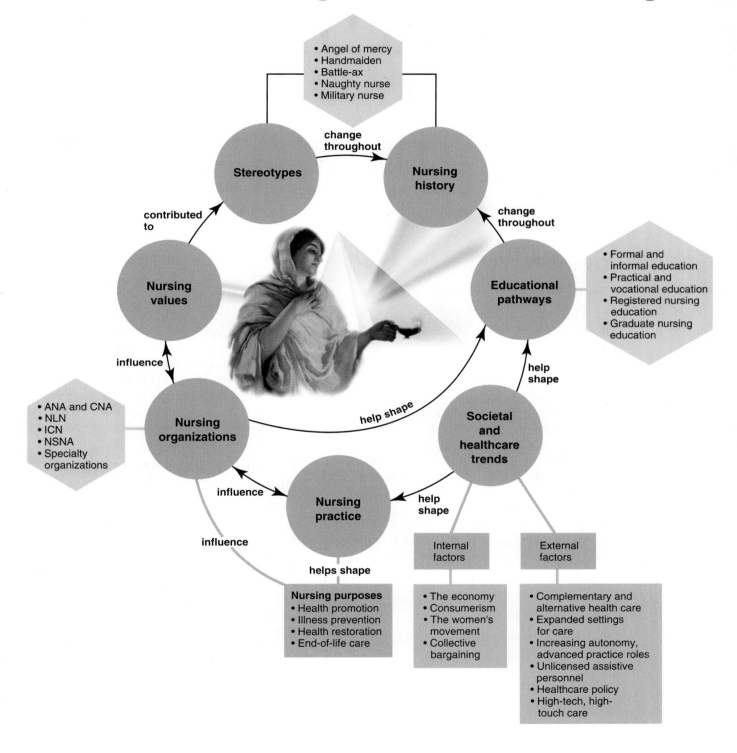

CHAPTER 2

Critical Thinking
& the Nursing Process

Overview

You have been introduced to three concepts:

1. Critical thinking
2. Nursing process
3. Full-spectrum nursing

Critical thinking involves careful consideration of a situation to arrive at a solution based on analysis of data. Critical thinkers need cognitive skills and a mind that is open to alternatives and reflection. Nurses use critical-thinking processes (problem solving, decision making, and clinical reasoning) in all aspects of their work and in each step of the nursing process.

The nursing process is a systematic problem-solving process that guides nurses in the provision of goal-directed, client-centered care. The nursing process consists of six phases:

• Assessment
• Diagnosis
• Planning Outcomes
• Planning Interventions
• Implementation
• Evaluation

The full-spectrum nursing model integrates four components: critical thinking, nursing process, nursing knowledge, and patient situation. Within this model, the nurse uses critical thinking and the nursing process to make decisions about patient care based on nursing knowledge and patient information.

Thinking Critically About Critical Thinking and the Nursing Process

The exercises in the following section allow you to practice the kind of thinking you will use as a full-spectrum nurse. Because these are critical-thinking activities, there is usually no single right answer. Discuss answers with your peers—discussion can stimulate critical thinking. If you have difficulty with any of the questions, consult with your instructor.

Caring for the Garcias

Review the opening scenario of Joseph Garcia in the front of the book. Imagine you are the clinic nurse at the Family Medicine Center. Based on the information presented in the scenario, work through the following questions:

A. Patient Situation

• Why is Mr. Garcia at the clinic?

• What are his wife's concerns?

• Are they similar to or different from his?

B. Critical Thinking

• How do I go about getting the data I need? What sources should I use?

• Are my data congruent?

• What is one possible explanation for what is happening in this situation?

C. Nursing Knowledge. What type of nursing knowledge (theoretical, practical, ethical, or self-knowledge) is needed to answer the following questions?

• What health concerns does Mr. Garcia have that should be addressed by the healthcare team?

• What is the role of Jordan Miller on the health team?

• What role will you play in the care of Mr. Garcia?

D. Nursing Process

• In what phase of the nursing process are you engaged when you are asking Mr. Garcia about the reason for his visit?

• What activities are involved in the diagnosis phase? In planning outcomes? In planning interventions?

• Why would you not, at this point, be using the evaluation phase?

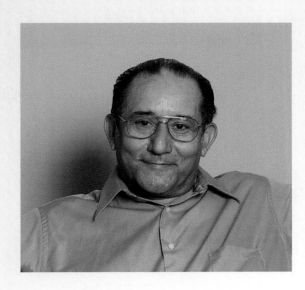

1

At the end of your first nursing class, your instructor gives an overview of a long-term assignment. She informs you that each semester of the program the class is required to complete a project that provides some type of service to the college community or the local community, and that demonstrates the role or importance of nursing. The instructor asks you to begin discussing potential projects and come to class next week prepared to discuss several proposals and their potential benefits to the community. You and several friends gather to talk about the class. "What an odd assignment!" you tell your friends. "How can we possibly do this now? We aren't nurses. We don't have any skills. What could we possibly do?" Your friends echo similar views.

This exercise is designed to help you actually work through the imaginary assignment you have just read. Use the *critical-thinking model* (Figure 2–1 on p. 31 of Volume 1) and the questions in Table 2–2 (p. 30 in Volume 1) to complete the assignment. Also refer to the inside back cover of this volume.

a *Contextual awareness* is one concept in the critical thinking model. Consider the context in which the assignment was given.
- What, exactly, is this assignment?

- Your instructor is perfectly aware of your knowledge and skill level. Why do you think she would make such an assignment to students so early in their studies?

b To complete this assignment you would need to gather information—to find ways to answer the following questions:
- What will I learn this semester?

- What skills will I have by the time this assignment is due?

- What do nurses do?

- How do nurses interact with the community?

- What does my community need?

You would need to *use credible sources* (another point of the critical-thinking model) to address these questions.

c What sources might you use to answer the first two questions in the bulleted list in (b), above?

d What are some ways in which you could answer the third and fourth questions?

e What are some ways in which you could obtain information to answer the fifth question?

f If you had actually gathered the preceding information, you would then need to consider possible solutions. One way would be to develop a list of community needs, a list of activities nurses engage in, and a list of skills and knowledge you will have at the end of the term. Then look at the overlap between the lists. This should help you to get some ideas for projects. Imagine now that you have a list of possible projects similar to the following:
- Take blood pressures at a neighborhood grocery store for a day.

- Hold a health fair at a neighborhood shopping center.

- Create some materials for teaching about a healthy diet; distribute them at a community event.

Now think critically about this list of projects (this involves *reflective skepticism and exploring and imagining alternatives*). What questions could you ask about each project to help you decide which to actually do?

2 Review the following scenarios. Is critical thinking occurring? If so, which part of the critical-thinking model is the student using, or which critical-thinking skill or attitude from Chapter 2 in Volume 1? If there is no evidence of critical thinking, revise the scenario to include it.

a Juan is a first-year nursing student. His clinical rotation is at a skilled nursing facility (SNF). He arrives at the unit at 7:00 A.M. for the start of the day shift. After hearing the shift change report, he prepares to give his client a bedbath per unit policy.

b Lily is instructing her patient, Mr. Johannsen, about the medicines he will be taking when he is discharged from the hospital. When Lily reviews the list with him, he says, "That's too many medicines. It's too confusing." Lily devises a schedule and information sheet about the medicines that she gives to her client. She reviews the medicines with Mr. Johannsen and his wife before discharge.

C   Erin is caring for a young man who has had orthopedic surgery after a skiing accident. She is unable to hear his blood pressure when she attempts to take his vital signs. He is alert and able to converse with her. Since she is unable to hear the blood pressure she records "0" in the client record.

d   As you are walking down the hall on the hospital unit you hear a patient call out, "Nurse!" When you enter the room you notice that the bedside is crowded with equipment. The patient is receiving several fluids intravenously, and a unit of blood is hanging from the IV pole. Since you have limited clinical experience you say to the patient, "I'll get you some help."

3   For each of the following concepts, use critical thinking to describe how or why it is important to nursing, patient care, or critical thinking in the nursing process. Note that these are *not* to be merely definitions.

Critical-thinking skills

Critical-thinking attitudes

Exploring alternatives

The nursing process

Assessment phase

Diagnosis phase

Planning outcomes phase

Planning interventions phase

Implementation phase

Evaluation phase

Theoretical knowledge

Practical knowledge

What Are the Main Points in This Chapter?

- Nursing involves both thinking and doing, and both are important.
- Critical thinking is a combination of reasoned thinking, openness to alternatives, an ability to reflect, and a desire to seek truth.
- Critical thinking involves both attitudes and cognitive skills.
- Nurses use critical thinking in all aspects of their practice.
- Practical knowledge (knowing what to do and how to do it) and theoretical knowledge (knowing why) are equally important in nursing.
- The nursing process is a systematic problem-solving process that guides all nursing actions.

- The nursing process consists of six phases: assessment, diagnosis, planning outcomes, planning interventions, implementation, and evaluation.
- Critical thinking is used in each phase of the nursing process; it is related to, but not the same as, the nursing process.
- Your ability to think critically depends on your theoretical knowledge about critical thinking, your motivation to practice it, and your fund of nursing knowledge.
- In full-spectrum nursing the nurse uses critical thinking to apply nursing process and nursing knowledge to patient situations.
- Full-spectrum nursing involves thinking and doing.

Knowledge Map

Critical Thinking and the Nursing Process

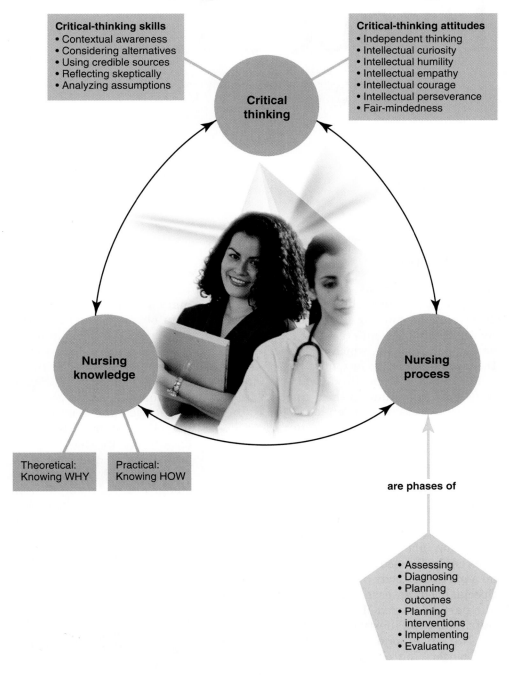

Critical-thinking skills
• Contextual awareness
• Considering alternatives
• Using credible sources
• Reflecting skeptically
• Analyzing assumptions

Critical-thinking attitudes
• Independent thinking
• Intellectual curiosity
• Intellectual humility
• Intellectual empathy
• Intellectual courage
• Intellectual perseverance
• Fair-mindedness

Critical thinking

Nursing knowledge

Nursing process

Theoretical: Knowing WHY

Practical: Knowing HOW

are phases of

• Assessing
• Diagnosing
• Planning outcomes
• Planning interventions
• Implementing
• Evaluating

CHAPTER 3

Nursing Process:
Assessment

Overview

As the first step of the nursing process, assessment provides the foundation for the other steps of nursing care. Nursing assessments focus on a client's *response* to illness, not on detecting disease, which is characteristic of the medical model. In fact, nursing assessment is even used with healthy clients, to identify ways they can maintain their current level of wellness. Assessment is defined as the use of a systematic and ongoing process to:

• Collect data
• Categorize data
• Validate data
• Record data

A comprehensive assessment provides information about a client's overall health, whereas a focused assessment concentrates on a particular body part or functional ability. Special needs assessment looks in more depth at a particular area of client functioning (e.g., nutrition, pain, lifestyle).

Nurses gather data by interviewing clients and performing physical assessments. Data is referred to as either subjective or objective. Information perceived only by the client, family, or community is called subjective data; data that can be observed by the nurse or other healthcare provider (e.g., laboratory tests, vital signs) is considered objective. Primary data is obtained directly from the client; data obtained from a medical record or another person is considered secondary.

A nursing interview is a planned communication in which the nurse talks with the client for the purpose of gathering subjective information. An effective interviewer asks both closed and open-ended questions and is an active listener. The nurse should validate data to ensure that it is accurate, complete, and factual.

Recording (documentation) has professional and legal implications. Record what the client says and what you observe. Do not record conclusions in the assessment step.

Thinking Critically About Nursing Process: Assessment

The exercises in the following section allow you to practice the kind of thinking you will use as a full-spectrum nurse. Because these are critical-thinking activities, there is usually no single right answer. Discuss answers with your peers—discussion can stimulate critical thinking. If you have difficulty with any of the questions, consult with your instructor.

Caring for the Garcias

Review the opening scenario of Joseph Garcia in the front of the book. Imagine you are the clinic nurse at the Family Medicine Center.

A. What type of assessment, comprehensive or focused, is being performed at this clinic visit? Explain your thinking.

B. Identify the types of data (e.g., subjective/objective, primary/secondary) that have been gathered so far. Give an example of each type.

C. How might you verify data that Mr. Garcia provided on the intake sheet?

D. Based on what you know about Mr. Garcia, what follow-up assessments would provide useful data to help with the care of Mr. Garcia? Why would you make these assessments?

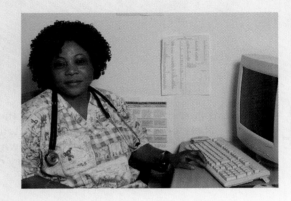

1   Recall the definition of subjective data. Make a list of the kinds of patients from whom you might not be able to get subjective data or who might give unreliable data. One example is a baby who cannot talk yet. How many others can you think of?

thinking critically about nursing process: assessment

21

2 What are some factors that might make it difficult, but not impossible, for a patient to provide you with subjective data? One example is a severely anxious person.

3 For each of the factors in 2, state what you could do to facilitate collection of reliable subjective data from that person.

4 List your current assessment skills and indicate your comfort level using each skill. Include observation, physical assessment, and interviewing skills. Use a scale of 1–5, with 1 = slightly comfortable; 2 = somewhat comfortable; 3 = moderately comfortable; 4 = fairly comfortable; and 5 = very comfortable.

5 For any skill that you score as 3 or less, write a plan describing what you need to do to move to the higher comfort level.

6 The following are criteria from ANA (2004) professional practice Standard 1. For each of the criteria, write an example of what would constitute evidence (proof) that the standard is being followed in a healthcare agency. The first one is done for you.

a Collects data in a systematic and ongoing process.

One example of evidence might be as follows: I would look in the care plan for nursing orders that call for some kind of assessment on a scheduled basis. For example, an order might read, "Temperature q4hrs" or "Check dressing for drainage once per shift." I would also look at the nurses notes, especially for flow sheets (e.g., vital sign flow sheets, input and output records, neurological checks) to see if assessment findings were recorded at regular intervals. The key here is to look for "systematic" and "ongoing" data. To know if nurses were "identifying patterns," I would look for nursing diagnoses or other conclusions they have charted in the nurses notes, such as stating that the medication has effectively relieved pain. Other evidence would be to observe the nurses doing systematic and ongoing data collection.

b Involves the patient, family, other healthcare providers, and environment, as appropriate, in holistic data collection.

c Prioritizes data-collection activities by the patient's immediate condition, or anticipated needs of the patient or situation.

d Uses appropriate evidence-based assessment techniques and instruments in collecting pertinent data.

e Uses analytical models and problem-solving tools.

f Synthesizes available data, information, and knowledge relevant to the situation to identify patterns and variances.

g Documents relevant data in a retrievable format.

thinking critically about nursing process: assessment

7 Your client, Sami ("Meet Your Patient"), is Hispanic. Having worked with many Hispanic clients and being familiar with nursing literature regarding various cultural patterns, you are aware of the following:

- Many Hispanic people who live in Miami are bilingual.
- When communicating, especially with strangers, it is common for Hispanic women not to maintain eye contact. (During the interview, Sami speaks rapidly and does not maintain eye contact with you.)
- Many people of Mexican and South American descent are Catholic and consider birth control to be taboo.
- Many Hispanic women do not obtain annual physical examinations (Purnell & Paulanka, 1998).

a Looking at the four points from the literature, how is Sami's cultural background similar to or different from your own? Remember that you are looking at cultural patterns, not Sami's individual and personal values and behaviors.

b On the basis of your understanding of your own and Sami's culture, what questions might you want to ask Sami to support her reproductive health?

8 What physical examination techniques would you use to:

a Assess for a distended bladder?

b Get information about a patient's headache?

c Obtain data about a patient's ankle edema?

d What subjective data could you obtain by using one of the four physical assessment techniques?

9 For each of the following concepts, use critical thinking to describe how or why it is important to nursing, patient care, or assessment. Note that these are *not* to be merely definitions.

Assessment

ANA standards of practice

JCAHO

Agency policies

Comprehensive assessments

Focused assessments

Specific special needs assessments:
    Pain assessment

      Spiritual health assessment

      Wellness assessment

The nursing health history

Active listening

Nursing frameworks/models

Validating data

Recording data

Reflecting critically about your assessment

Practical Knowledge:
knowing how

In this chapter, practical knowledge involves your skill in using structured and unstructured methods of data collection.

ASSESSMENT FORMS

You can use the forms in this section to make a focused assessment of activities of daily living and to perform a comprehensive patient assessment. You will find other forms on the Electronic Study Guide.

Patient Assessment Tool—Lawton Instrumental Activities of Daily Living (IADL)

Date:_____   Name:_____

Please check the box that most applies for each activity:

Activity	Needs no help (2 pts. each)	Needs some help (1 pt. each)	Unable to do at all (0 pts. each)
1. Using the telephone	___	___	___
2. Getting to places beyond walking distance	___	___	___
3. Grocery shopping	___	___	___
4. Preparing meals	___	___	___
5. Doing housework or handyman work	___	___	___
6. Doing laundry	___	___	___
7. Taking medications	___	___	___
8. Managing money	___	___	___

Total score: ___ = (___ × 2 =) ___ + (___ × 1 =) ___ + 0

A patient is awarded 2 points for each area in which he/she can function totally without help, 1 point in those areas that they need some help, and 0 points for those activities that somebody else must do completely for them. The maximum score is 16; minimum score is 0.

Like other evaluations, the IADL scale provides a baseline of data that can be compared with the results of future evaluations. (Note that some activities may be gender specific. Omit these items if the patient does not usually perform those tasks.)

Permission obtained from M. Powell Lawton, Ph.D., Philadephia Geriatric Center, Philadelphia, PA. May be used freely for patient assessment. Formatted and posted May 25, 1996, to www.acsu.buffalo.edu/~drstall/assessmenttools.html by Robert S. Stall, M.D.

Nursing Admission Data Form

Source: North Broward Hospital District, Ft. Lauderdale, FL.

Name: _Ben J. Ivanos_   Age: _24_   Phone #: _618-445-2300_   Date: _05/20/05_   Time: _10:30_

Primary Physician: _Charles Katz_   Phone #: _618-446-8160_

Chief Complaints/Procedure: _ORIF fx (L) leg, Fx (R) femur + (R) ulna_   Height: _5'10"_   Weight (lbs.): _155_

Historian: _Patient_   Temp: _100°_   Pulse: _90_   Resp: _16_   BP: _140/82_

Religious Affiliation: _Catholic_   Hospitalized within 30 days: Yes ☒   No ☐

UNABLE TO OBTAIN HISTORY .... ☐
Reason: _____

NEUROLOGICAL/SENSORY PERCEPTION
Glaucoma .... ☐
Hearing Loss/Deaf .... Right ☐ Left ☐
Motion Sickness .... ☐
Paresthesia .... Right ☐ Left ☐
Fibromyalgia/Migrane .... ☐
Spina Bifida .... ☐
Stroke/CVA/TIA .... ☐
Altered Mental Status .... ☐
Other: _____

CARDIOVASCULAR/HEMATOLOGY
Bleeding Problems .... ☐
Blood transfusion in the past 3 months ..... ☐
Chest Pain/Angina .... ☐
Heart Attack/Date: .... ☐
Heart Disease .... ☐
High Blood Pressure .... ☐
Irregular Beats/Pacemaker/AICD .... ☐
Mitral Valve Prolapse .... ☐
Murmur .... ☐
Peripheral Vascular Disease .... ☐
Sickle Cell Disease .... ☐
Venous Access Device/Type _____ ☐
Other: _____

RESPIRATORY
Asthma .... ☐
Bronchitis ..._6 months ago_......... ☒
COPD/Emphysema .... ☐
Post Nasal Drip/Rhinitis/Sinusitis ..... ☒
Pneumonia .... ☐
Tracheostomy .... ☐
Other: _____

GASTROINTESTINAL
Dysphagia .... ☐
Hiatal Hernia .... ☐
Liver Disease/Jaundice .... ☐
Pancreatitis .... ☐
Gall Stones .... ☐
Ostomy .... ☐
Last Bowel Movement: _5/19/05_
Other: _____

GENITOURINARY/RENAL
Kidney Disease/Urogenital .... ☐
Prostate Problems .... ☐
Voiding Problems .... ☐
Other: _____

MUSCULOSKELETAL
Arthritis .... ☐
Back/Disc Problem .... ☐
Fractures ...._present admission_.... ☒
Other: _____

ENDOCRINE
Diabetes/type: .... ☐
Thyroid Disease .... ☐
Other: _____

INFECTIOUS DISEASE
Fevers .... ☐
Hepatitis/type/active .... ☐
HIV/AIDS .... ☐
Recent Cold .... ☐
Sexually Transmitted Disease/type .. ☐
Tuberculosis/Active: .... ☐
Other: _____

Pregnant .... ☐
Lactating .... ☐
LMP/Date: _____

VACCINATION/DATE
Flu: _____ Hepatitis B: _____
Pneumonia: _____

BEHAVIORAL HEALTH
Anxiety Disorder .... ☐
Depression .... ☐
Suicide (thoughts/attempts) ...... ☐
Patient is a Baker Act .... ☐
Other: _____

CANCER
Type: _____ ☐
Radioactive Seeds/Implant .... ☐
Date: _____
Other: _____

SOCIAL HISTORY
Tobacco .... ☒
   Number of years: _3_
   # of packs per day: _1/2_
   Year Quit: _2003_
Would you like smoking cessation info?
☒ No ☐ Yes ☐ information provided
Alcohol .... ☒
   Drinks per day: _1_
   Amount: _____
   Type: _____
Recreational Drug .... ☐
   Amount: _____
   Type: _____
   Year Quit: _____
Detoxification Protocol Initiated ..... ☐

ALLERGIES & REACTION   None Known ☒   Allergy Bracelet on ☐

Medications: _none_   Symptoms:

Food/Shellfish/other allergies: _No_   Blood Reaction: ☐
Contrast/Dye: _No_   Latex: ☐   Latex Allergy Protocol Initiated: ☐

PAST HOSPITAL/PROCEDURE (Surgical/Medical/Behavioral Health)
None

CURRENT MEDICATIONS (include ASA/Anticoagulant, over the counter medications, ointments, patches, eye drops, herbal, vitamins and nutritional supplements)

Medication	Dose	Frequency	Last Dose
ASA	"2"	occasionally for HA	

Initiate Social Service Consult

Food/Drug Interaction information provided ☐
(Note: Additional medication can be listed on last page)

ADDRESSOGRAPH

North Broward Hospital District

NURSING ADMISSION DATA

P-10287 - 126005 - (R) 11/02   *Page 1 of 4*   900199

Nursing Admission Data Form *(continued)*

Source: North Broward Hospital District, Ft. Lauderdale, FL.

PAIN HISTORY

Have you been experiencing pain? ☒ Yes
If yes, when ___Now___ Intensity (0-10): __10__ Goal (0-10): __2__
Location: _____Legs and arm, muscles in back_____
Radiation: _____No_____
Duration: _____Constant_____
Quality: _____Sharp, aching_____
Aggravating factors _____Movement_____

What medications/interventions are effective in relieving your pain?
_____Taking PCA Demerol_____

Acute Pain Management - It is Your Right brochure provided ☒

PSYCHOSOCIAL ASSESSMENT

☒ Lives alone ☐ Lives with spouse/SO ☐ Nursing Home/ALF
☐ Homeless ☐ Rehab Facility ☐ Other:_____
Marital Status ☒ Single ☐ Married ☐ Divorced ☐ Widowed ☐ Separated
Next of Kin: _Mother, Clara Ivanos_ **Phone #:** _618-446-3816_
Supportive Adult: _____ - _____ **Phone #:** _____ - _____
Has anybody threatened/hit/abused you within the last year?
☐ Yes (refer to policy RA 004015 mauve manual) ☒ No

EDUCATIONAL LEARNING ASSESSMENT

Learner ☒ Patient ☐ Family ☐ Significant Other
Readiness to learn ☐ Eager to learn ☒ Asks questions
     ☐ Extremely anxious ☐ Denies need for Education
Knowledge of current health status ☐ No knowledge
     ☒ Partial understanding ☐ Full understanding
Barriers to learning ☒ Physical ☐ Emotional
     ☐ Language ☐ Religious ☐ Cultural
     ☐ Reading Ability ☐ Changes in Short Memory
     ☐ None
Preferred Learning Method ☒ Reading ☐ Lecture
     ☒ Video ☒ Demo/Practice
Communication ☒ English ☐ Spanish ☐ Creole
     ☐ Sign Language ☐ Other:_____
Do you have any religious/cultural practices that are important to you or may alter your care or education? ☒ No ☐ Yes _____

☒ Patient Handbook provided   ☒ Patient safety information provided
☒ Patient's Bill of Rights and Responsibilities information provided
Other Educational Materials:_____

PERSONAL EFFECTS: Do you use the following:

	YES	WITH PT.	FAMILY/SO
Wheelchair	☐	☐	☐
Braces	☐	☐	☐
Cane/Crutches	☐	☐	☐
Walker	☐	☐	☐
Prothesis	☐	☐	☐
Medications	☐	☐	☐
Dentures: (Full)	☐	☐	☐
Upper	☐	☐	☐
Lower	☐	☐	☐
Glasses	☐	☐	☐
Contacts	☒	☒	☐
Hearing Aids	☐	☐	☐
Other:			

Initiate Social Service Consult

ADVANCE DIRECTIVES

Do you have an Advance Directive?
(must check one)
☒ **No** Information provided to patient
☐ **No** Patient elects not to receive information
☐ **Yes** (check advance directive patient states he/she has)
☐ **Living Will** ☐ **Health Care Surrogate** ☐ **State DNAR form**
☐ **Durable Power of Attorney** ☐ **Organ Donation**
(If patient has an Advance Directive, inform patient to provide copy within 24 hours or they may complete a new advance directive or verbalize their wishes)
Do you have a guardian? ☐ Yes name_____
(Inform patient to provide guardianship form within 24 hours)
☐ **Patient unable to respond/family not available**

FALL SCREEN: *If any of the following are checked, initiate Safety/Protective Intervention Protocol*

Inability to understand or follow instructions	☐
Impaired mobility, visual impairment, drug therapy, surgical procedure, unsteady gait, incontinence ... _Casts, Traction_	☒
Unable to use call light	☐
Altered mental status ... _Taking Demerol PCA_	☒
Nocturnal/urgency/frequency in elimination	☐
Dizziness	☐
History of falls	☐
No Criteria Met	☐

NUTRITIONAL SCREEN: *If any of the following are checked, enter in the computer request for **Nutritional Consult***

Nausea/vomiting > 5 days	☐
No food/drink for 3 days	☐
Recent unexplained weight loss > 10 lbs.	☐
Difficulty swallowing/dysphagia	☐
Evidence of Stage III - IV pressure ulcer	☐
Feeding tube	☐
New onset diabetes	☐
TPN	☐
Pregnant/lactating	☐
Surgical patients > 70 years of age	☐
Ethnic diet/special needs **(include in diet order and order for Preference consult)**	☐
Difficulty chewing **(include in diet order and order for Preference consult)**	☐
No Criteria Met	☒

FUNCTIONAL SCREEN: *If any of the following are checked, please request physician order for physical therapy consult.*

New onset of paralysis	☐
New onset stroke/CVA	☐
New amputation	☐
Unsteady gait	☐
Decreased mobility _Casts, Tx for Fx_	☒
Dysphagia	☐
No Criteria Met	☐

Nursing Admission Data Form *(continued)*

Source: North Broward Hospital District, Ft. Lauderdale, FL.

MARK LOCATION	WOUND TYPE	COLOR WOUND BED

MARK LOCATION

Anterior View / Posterior View Right Lateral Left Lateral

Left Foot Right Foot

*** Label Wound Type**

WOUND TYPE

P = Pressure ulcer A = Abrasions
ST = Skin tear LU = Leg/Foot ulcers
S = Surgical BR = Bruising
L = Laceration M = Maceration
B = Burns O = Other

STAGE
Pressure ulcer only

I: Reddened area, does not resolve with pressure relief.
II: Blister or superficial break in skin.
III: Full thickness wound into subcutaneous tissue.
IV: Full thickness with muscle, bone or tendon tissue exposed.
U = Unable to stage: Necrotic

COLOR WOUND BED

R = Red (new tissue) Y = Yellow (slough)
P = Pink B = Black (eschar)

EXUDATE

O = None SS = Serosanguinous
S = Serous P = Purulent

ODOR

N = None S = Slight F = Foul

SURROUNDING SKIN

OK = Clean & Intact Ra = Rash
C = Cellulitis (red & tender)
R = Raw & denuded
M = Maceration
I = Induration

Skin Breakdown Present ☐ Consent Obtained ☐ Photograph Taken ☐ Acute/Chronic Wound Flow Sheet Initiated ☐ Swat Consult Initiated ☐

BRADEN SCALE - PRESSURE ULCER RISK ASSESSMENT

	1	2	3	4	Score
SENSORY PERCEPTION Ability to respond meaningfully to pressure-related discomfort	**1. Completely Limited:** Unresponsive (does not moan, flinch, or grasp) to painful stimuli due to diminished level of consciousness or sedation. OR limited ability to feel pain over most of body surface.	**2. Very Limited:** Responds only to painful stimuli. Cannot communicate discomfort except by moaning or restlessness. OR has a sensory impairment which limits the ability to feel pain or discomfort over 1/2 of body.	**3. Slightly Limited:** Responds to verbal commands, but cannot always communicate discomfort or need to be turned. OR has some sensory impairment which limits ability to feel pain or discomfort in 1 or 2 extremities.	**4. No Impairment:** Responds to verbal commands, has no sensory deficit which would limit ability to feel or voice pain or discomfort.	4
MOISTURE Degree to which skin is exposed to moisture	**1. Constantly Moist:** Skin is kept moist almost constantly by perspiration, urine, etc. Dampness is detected every time patient is moved or turned.	**2. Very Moist:** Skin if often, but not always, moist. Linen must be changed at least once a shift.	**3. Occasionally Moist:** Skin is occasionally moist, requiring an extra linen change approximately once a day.	**4. Rarely Moist:** Skin is usually dry, linen only requires changing at routine intervals.	4
ACTIVITY degree of physical activity	**1. Bedfast:** Confined to bed.	**2. Chairfast:** Ability to walk severely limited or non-existent. Cannot bear own weight and/or must be assisted into chair or wheelchair.	**3. Walks Occasionally:** Walks occasionally during day, but for very short distances, with or without assistance. Spends majority of each shift in bed or chair.	**4. Walks Frequently:** Walks outside the room at least twice a day and inside room at least once every 2 hours during waking hours.	1
MOBILITY ability to change and control body position	**1. Completely Immobile:** Does not make even slight changes in body or extremity position without assistance.	**2. Very Limited:** Makes occasional slight changes in body or extremity position but unable to make frequent or significant changes independently.	**3. Slightly Limited:** Makes frequent though slight changes in body or extremity position independently.	**4. No Limitations:** Makes major and frequent changes in position without assistance.	3
NUTRITION usual food intake pattern	**1. Very Poor:** Never eats a complete meal. Rarely eats more than 1/3 of any food offered. Eats 2 servings or less of protein (meat or dairy products) per day. Takes fluids poorly. Does not take a liquid dietary supplement. OR is NPO and/or maintained on clear liquids or IVs for more then 5 days.	**2. Probably Inadequate:** Rarely eats a complete meal and generally eats only about 1/2 of any food offered. Protein intake includes only 3 servings of meat or dairy products per day. Occasionally will take a dietary supplement. OR receives less than optimum amount of liquid diet or tube feeding.	**3. Adequate:** Eats over half of most meals. Eats a total of 4 servings of protein (meat, dairy products) each day. Occasionally will refuse a meal, but will usually take s supplement if offered. OR is on a tube feeding or TPN regimen which probably meets most of nutritionally needs.	**4. Excellent:** Eats most of every meal. Never refuses a meal. Usually eats a total of 4 or more servings of meat and dairy products. Occasionally eats between meals. Does not require supplementation.	4
FRICTION AND SHEAR	**1. Problem:** Requires moderate to maximum assistance in moving. Complete lifting without sliding against sheets is impossible. Frequently slides down in bed or chair, requiring frequent repositioning with maximum assistance. Spasticity contractures or agitation lead to almost constant friction.	**2. Potential Problem:** Moves feebly or requires minimum assistance. During a move skin probably slides to some extent against sheets, chair, restraints, or other devices. Maintains relatively good position in chair or bed most of the time but occasionally slides down.	**3. No Apparent Problem:** Moves in bed and in chair independently and has sufficient muscle strength to lift up completely during move. Maintains good position in bed or chair at all times.		2

RN Signature: _[signature]_ Date: 5/20/05 **TOTAL SCORE:** 18

NOTE: Patients with a total score of 16 or less are considered to be at risk of developing pressure ulcers. Implement Skin Care Protocol. Refer to Surface Bed Decision Tree. (12 or less = high risk)

ANTICIPATED DISCHARGE NEEDS

☒ Transportation ☐ Placement needed

Medical Equipment: ☐ Oxygen ☐ CPAP ☐ Nebulizer ☐ Blood Glucose Meter Other: _Crutches, Wheelchair_

Community Services: (Home Health, Reach to Recovery, Meals On Wheels, etc.): _Home Health for f/u on cast care and pain medication. Transportation to physicians office for return visit._

Nurse Signature: _[signature]_ Unit: 3E Date: 5/20/05 Time: 1045

Nurse Signature: _____ Unit: _____ Date: _____ Time: _____

P-10287 - 126005 - (R) 11/02 **Page 3 of 4**

Nursing Admission Data Form *(continued)*

Source: North Broward Hospital District, Ft. Lauderdale, FL.

OUTPATIENT PRE-ADMISSION NOTE: Date of Call/Visit_____ Date of Surgery:_____ *N/A*

Autologous Blood ☐ Direct Donor ☐ Confirmed with Blood Bank ☐ # of Units Available_____

Parent Present Induction ☐

Pre-op Work Up:
BGMC ☐ NBMC ☐ IPMC ☐ CSMC ☐
Other:_____

ANESTHESIOLOGIST EVALUATION: ASA class I II III IV NPO:_____

Anesthesia Plan Gen ☐ MAC ☐ Regional ☐ Type _____

Airway: _____

Neck_____

Previous Anesthesia ☐

Past anesthesia problems_____

Dentition: Good ☐ Fair ☐ Poor ☐
Natural ☐ Caps ☐
Dentures/Bridges ☐
Malampati score 1 2 3 4
OTHER: _____

EKG _____
CXR *N/A*
H & H _____
Platelets _____

INITIAL EVALUATION EXCEEDING 48 HOURS:
No Change in Assessment ☐
Changes in Assessment ☐
Comments:_____

Comments:_____

Anesthesiologist_____ Date_____ Time_____

Anesthesiologist:_____
Date/Time: _____

NURSING DIAGNOSIS	NURSING INTERVENTIONS	PLANNED OUTCOME/EVALUATION
Potential/actual knowledge deficit Pre-op preparation/ planned surgical intervention.	☐ Patient/family learning needs/level of understanding assessed. ☐ Clear explanation of pre-operative routine given. ☐ Instructions on turning, coughing, deep breathing, leg exercises given. ☐ Procedure specific instructions _____ ☐ Pain management modalities and scale explained. Modality preference_____ Pain scale goal _____	☐ Patient verbalizes understanding of pre-op preparation, pre-op routine and procedure specific information. ☐ Patient copes with anxiety, shows relaxed affect. ☐ Demonstrates understanding of explanations. ☐ Patient verbalizes understanding of pain management and plan of care.
Anxiety *N/A* Psycho/Social	☐ Written copy of pre-op instructions and patient responsibility provided. ☐ Allow to express feelings, ask questions. ☐ Emotional support given. ☐ Sense of wellness promoted. ☐ Cultural/Spiritual Needs: _____ ☐ Discharge planning initiated/home care assessed. ☐ Needs identified/Action:	☐ Needed referrals/arrangements made. ☐ Care individualized to meet patients needs. ☐ Patient verbalizes understanding of discharge plan.
Actual/Potential Individual Needs Self Care/Discharge Planning		Standard of Care/Protocol: ☐ Yes

R.N. Signature:_____ Date:_____

Nurse Signature: _____ Unit: _____ Date: _____ Time: _____
Nurse Signature: _____ Unit: _____ Date: _____ Time: _____

DATE & TIME	INTERDISCIPLINARY NOTES/ADVANCE DIRECTIVES INFORMATION
5/20/05, 11:00	Healthy young adult, on no meds, admitted via E.D. $\bar{p}$ motorcycle accident, and reduction and casting of multiple fx (Ⓛ tibia + fibula, Ⓡ femur, and Ⓡ elbow and ulna). Experiencing severe pain r/t fx, bruises and muscle spasms. Plan:
	① Traction per Rx; check weights $\bar{q}$ 4th
	② Control pain w/PCA Demerol. Assess + instruct prn
	③ Neurovascular + circulatory checks, all extremities, $\bar{q}$ 2h .
	④ Monitor adema of extremities; re-cast after 3 days if edema has subsided.

Nurse Signature: _____ Unit: 3E Date: 5/20/05 Time: 11:00
Nurse Signature: _____ Unit: _____ Date: _____ Time: _____

Current Medications: (Continued)

Medication	Dose	Frequency	Last Dose

P-10287 - 126005 - (R) 11/02 **Page 4 of 4** WHITE - INPATIENT/OUTPATIENT LITE GREEN - OUTPATIENT ONLY DARK GREEN - ANESTHESIA LITE BLUE - INPATIENT ONLY

What Are the Main Points in This Chapter?

- Assessment is a systematic, ongoing process of collecting, categorizing, and recording holistic data about client health status.
- Accurate, complete data is essential to effective nursing diagnosis and care planning.
- Nursing assessments focus on client responses to illness and stressors rather than on identifying disease processes.
- ANA standards of practice state that professional nurses are responsible for assessing clients.
- Comprehensive assessment provides information about the client's overall health, whereas focused assessment provides data about a particular topic, body part, or functional ability.
- Special needs assessments provide in-depth information about a particular area of client functioning (e.g., nutrition, pain, lifestyle).
- Subjective data can be perceived only by the client; objective data is measurable or observable by the nurse or other healthcare providers.
- Nurses obtain data by observing and interviewing patients, and by performing physical assessment.
- The formats and frameworks for the nursing health history vary among agencies; however, all have essentially the same components (e.g., chief complaint, family history, review of body systems).
- Effective interviews require preparation by the nurse and use of both closed and open-ended questions.
- Active listening is one of the most important interviewing techniques.
- Validating data helps to ensure that it is accurate, complete, and factual.
- Documentation of assessment findings is of critical importance and has professional and legal implications.
- When documenting assessments, the nurse should record cues (observations), not inferences (conclusions).

Knowledge Map

Assessment Concepts

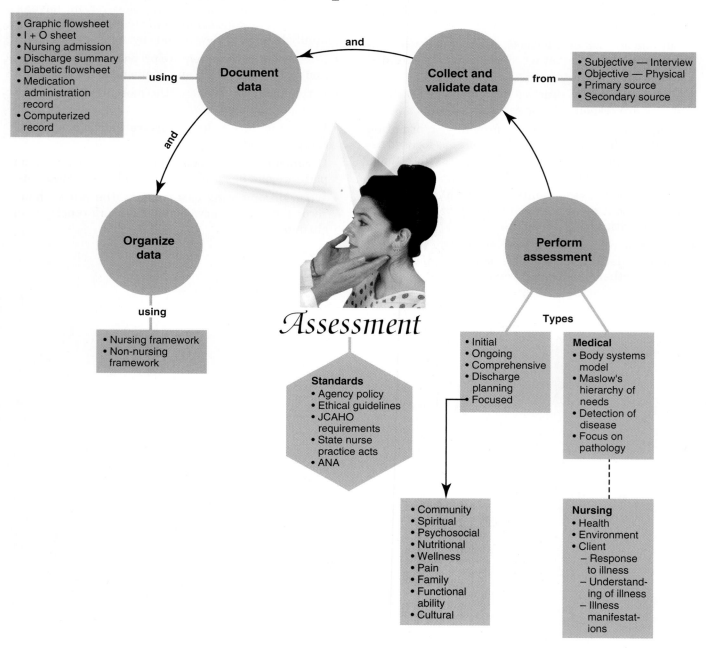

- Graphic flowsheet
- I + O sheet
- Nursing admission
- Discharge summary
- Diabetic flowsheet
- Medication administration record
- Computerized record

using

Document data

and

Collect and validate data

from

- Subjective — Interview
- Objective — Physical
- Primary source
- Secondary source

and

Organize data

using

- Nursing framework
- Non-nursing framework

Assessment

Standards
- Agency policy
- Ethical guidelines
- JCAHO requirements
- State nurse practice acts
- ANA

Perform assessment

Types

- Initial
- Ongoing
- Comprehensive
- Discharge planning
- Focused

Medical
- Body systems model
- Maslow's hierarchy of needs
- Detection of disease
- Focus on pathology

- Community
- Spiritual
- Psychosocial
- Nutritional
- Wellness
- Pain
- Family
- Functional ability
- Cultural

Nursing
- Health
- Environment
- Client
  - Response to illness
  - Understanding of illness
  - Illness manifestations

Nursing Process:
Diagnosis

Overview

Nursing diagnosis is the unique obligation of the professional nurse; it cannot be delegated. Unlike medical diagnoses, which describe a disease or injury, nursing diagnoses describe human responses to changes in health status, such as disease, illness, or injury. An accurate nursing diagnosis directs the choice of client-centered goals and nursing interventions because it identifies health conditions that the nurse can treat independently or help prevent.

Diagnostic reasoning involves analyzing and interpreting data, verifying problems with the patient, and prioritizing the problems. Critical thinking, solid theoretical knowledge, and experience underlie sound diagnostic reasoning.

A NANDA diagnosis includes a diagnostic label, a definition, defining characteristics, and related or risk factors. A diagnostic statement consists basically of a problem and etiology, using any of a variety of formats, to describe a client's health status. The problem side of the diagnostic statement directs the choice of goals; the etiology directs the choice of nursing interventions.

Thinking Critically About Nursing Process: Diagnosis

The exercises in the following section allow you to practice the kind of thinking you will use as a full-spectrum nurse. Because these are critical-thinking activities, there is usually no single right answer. Discuss answers with your peers—discussion can stimulate critical thinking. If you have difficulty with any of the questions, consult your instructor.

Caring for the Garcias

Review the opening scenario of Joseph Garcia in the front of this book. After the nurse practitioner completed his interview and physical examination of Mr. Garcia, he listed the following diagnoses on the problem list:

Hypertension
Obesity
Musculoskeletal pain
Tobacco abuse
Family history of prostate cancer
Family history of cardiovascular disease
Family history of diabetes mellitus (DM)

A. What type of problem list does this represent? How is it similar to or different from a problem list that you might generate?

B. Based on the data in the scenario, identify at least one actual, one potential, and one wellness diagnosis for Mr. Garcia. Identify the NANDA labels, and describe the cues that support your choices.

C. The nurse has identified a problem of Imbalanced Nutrition: More Than Body Requirements for Mr. Garcia.
  • What information do you need in order to determine the etiology of this problem?

• Because you do not have that information, write a two-part diagnostic statement describing Mr. Garcia's nutritional status.

D. Now rewrite the nutrition statement as a three-part statement, including the phrase "as evidenced by."

E. The nurse has identified Acute Pain (knees) for Mr. Garcia. If the pain were caused by a medical condition, osteoarthritis, how would you write a two-part diagnostic statement to describe this health status?

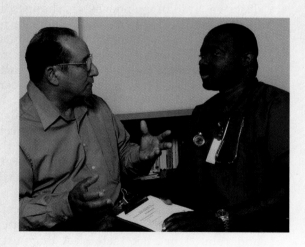

1   Sally Jones, a 45-year-old woman, was admitted to your surgical unit directly from the operating room. She was in a motorcycle accident this evening. In the emergency department, her blood pressure was falling, and she was bleeding profusely from many sites. She was sent directly to the operating room for a splenectomy, internal fixation of a compound fracture of bilateral femurs, and traumatic amputation of the right hand. During surgery she lost 2000 mL of blood and received 3 units of packed red blood cells (volume = 750 mL) along with 1000 mL of fluid administered intravenously.

You receive report on the client at 7:00 P.M. Sally is receiving IV fluid through several peripheral lines and through a central line (a catheter inserted into a major vein leading to the heart). She has a Foley catheter, which is draining 30 mL of concentrated urine each hour. Sally's vital signs are as follows: temperature, 102.8°F (39.3°C) (rectal); heart rate, 120 beats per minute; respirations, 28 per minute, and blood pressure, 160/86 mm Hg. Her skin is flushed, dry, and warm to the touch. On assessment, you find the following: return of skin turgor >3 seconds, dry mucous membranes, and bloodstained dressing on right upper extremity.

She is complaining of thirst, weakness, and pain at a level of 10 on a scale of 1 to 10 (10 highest). Sally is receiving a continuous infusion of morphine. She refuses to cough, deep-breathe, or attempt to turn. She lies very still and rigid. Sally drifts in and out of sleep but remains asleep for less than 30 minutes each time. She is irritable and restless. She communicates with one-word answers only. Frequently, she displays facial grimaces and becomes increasingly stiff. Her eyes appear dull. She complains of severe pain with any passive or active movements. In answering the following questions, use a nursing diagnosis handbook to look up the NANDA defining characteristics, definitions, and so forth, as needed.

a   Based on the data provided, which of the following NANDA labels would you use for Sally? Explain your reasoning.

Deficient Fluid Volume or Risk for Deficient Fluid Volume

b   For Sally's diagnosis of Deficient Fluid Volume, what are the cues? What are her related factors?

c   Using your responses to (a) and (b), write a diagnostic statement that includes problem, etiology, defining characteristics (cues), and the medical condition that the problem is "secondary to."

d   Think of other explanations for these cues: temperature, 102.8°F (39.3°C); heart rate, 120 beats per minute; respirations, 28 per minute; blood pressure, 160/86 mm Hg.

thinking critically about nursing process: diagnosis

e Sally certainly has the defining characteristics for the nursing diagnosis Impaired Physical Mobility. If you use this problem label, what would the etiological factors be?

f Which of those etiological factors could you treat with independent nursing interventions?

g Sally has the following nursing diagnoses (problem labels only are listed) and collaborative problems:

Deficient Fluid Volume
Acute Pain (abdominal incision, amputation site, fractures)
Risk for Disturbed Body Image
Potential Complication of trauma, surgery, and IV lines: infection
Risk for Ineffective Airway Clearance
• From Sally's perspective, which is probably the highest priority problem?

• Using an "urgency" (or threat to life) criterion, name Sally's three most important problems and why you consider them most important.

h Examine your theoretical knowledge. To care for Sally, what additional theoretical knowledge do you need?

i What practical knowledge will you need to use in her care?

2 You have a homebound client with diabetes who has the beginning of a pressure ulcer. You have been treating the client for Impaired Skin Integrity related to decreased circulation and mobility. However, the client's skin continues to break down.

a Your client has diabetes. What type of problem is that (medical, nursing, or collaborative)?

b What is the client's nursing diagnosis?

c The client has Impaired Skin Integrity. The break in the body's first line of defense (intact skin) increases the risk for infection. Write a problem statement reflecting that risk nursing diagnosis.

3 For each of the following concepts, use critical thinking to describe how or why it is important to nursing, patient care, or nursing diagnosis. Note that these are *not* to be merely definitions.

The diagnosis step of the nursing process

NANDA International

Patient strengths

Maslow's hierarchy

Documenting priorities

Nursing diagnoses

Possible nursing diagnoses

Collaborative problems

Wellness nursing diagnosis

Cues

Diagnostic label definition

Defining characteristics

Risk factors

Etiological factors

Standardized nursing languages

Practical Knowledge
knowing how

In this section, you will find the NANDA taxonomy of diagnosis labels and the list of descriptors for NANDA nursing diagnoses. Refer to these lists as you develop nursing diagnoses for your patients.

NANDA Taxonomy II: Domains, Classes, and Diagnoses (Labels)

This taxonomically organized list represents the NANDA-approved nursing diagnoses for clinical use and testing (2003–2004).

DOMAIN 1. HEALTH PROMOTION

The awareness of well-being or normality of function and the strategies used to maintain control of and enhance that well–being or normality of function

Class 1. Health Awareness. Recognition of normal function and well-being

Class 2. Health Management. Identifying, controlling, performing, and integrating activities to maintain health and well-being

Approved Diagnoses

00082	Effective Therapeutic Regimen Management
00078	Ineffective Therapeutic Regimen Management
00080	Ineffective Family Therapeutic Regimen Management
00081	Ineffective Community Therapeutic Regimen Management
00084	Health-Seeking Behaviors (specify)
00099	Ineffective Health Maintenance
00098	Impaired Home Maintenance
00162	Readiness for Enhanced Management of Therapeutic Regimen
00163	Readiness for Enhanced Nutrition

DOMAIN 2. NUTRITION

The activities of taking in, assimilating, and using nutrients for the purposes of tissue maintenance, tissue repair, and the production of energy

Class 1. Ingestion. Taking food or nutrients into the body

Approved Diagnoses

00107	Ineffective Infant Feeding Pattern
00103	Impaired Swallowing
00002	Imbalanced Nutrition: Less Than Body Requirements
00001	Imbalanced Nutrition: More Than Body Requirements
00003	Risk for Imbalanced Nutrition: More Than Body Requirements

Class 2. Digestion. The physical and chemical activities that convert foodstuffs into substances suitable for absorption and assimilation

Class 3. Absorption. The act of taking up nutrients through body tissues

Class 4. Metabolism. The chemical and physical processes occurring in living organisms and cells for the development and use of protoplasm, production of waste and energy, with the release of energy for all vital processes

Class 5. Hydration. The taking in and absorption of fluids and electrolytes

Approved Diagnoses

00027	Deficient Fluid Volume
00028	Risk for Deficient Fluid Volume
00026	Excess Fluid Volume
00025	Risk for Fluid Volume Imbalance
00160	Readiness for Enhanced Fluid Balance

DOMAIN 3. ELIMINATION

Secretion and excretion of waste products from the body

Class 1. Urinary System. The process of secretion and excretion of urine

Approved Diagnoses

00016	Impaired Urinary Elimination
00023	Urinary Retention
00021	Total Urinary Incontinence
00020	Functional Urinary Incontinence
00017	Stress Urinary Incontinence
00019	Urge Urinary Incontinence
00018	Reflex Urinary Incontinence
00022	Risk for Urge Urinary Incontinence
00166	Readiness for Enhanced Urinary Elimination

Class 2. Gastrointestinal System. Excretion and expulsion of waste products from the bowel

Approved Diagnoses

00014	Bowel Incontinence
00013	Diarrhea
00011	Constipation
00015	Risk for Constipation
00012	Perceived Constipation

Class 3. Integumentary System. Process of secretion and excretion through the skin

Class 4. Pulmonary System. Removal of by-products of metabolic products, secretions, and foreign material from the lungs or bronchi

Approved Diagnoses

00030	Impaired Gas Exchange

DOMAIN 4. ACTIVITY/REST

The production, conservation, expenditure, or balance of energy resources

Class 1. Sleep/Rest. Slumber, repose, ease, or inactivity

Approved Diagnoses

00095	Disturbed Sleep Pattern
00096	Sleep Deprivation
00165	Readiness for Enhanced Sleep

Class 2. Activity/Exercise. Moving parts of the body (mobility), doing work, or performing actions often (but not always) against resistance

Approved Diagnoses

00040	Risk for Disuse Syndrome
00085	Impaired Physical Mobility
00091	Impaired Bed Mobility
00089	Impaired Wheelchair Mobility
00090	Impaired Transfer Ability
00088	Impaired Walking
00097	Deficient Diversional Activity
00109	Dressing/Grooming Self-Care Deficit
00108	Bathing/Hygiene Self-Care Deficit
00102	Feeding Self-Care Deficit
00110	Toileting Self-Care Deficit
00100	Delayed Surgical Recovery
00168	Sedentary Lifestyle

Class 3. Energy Balance. A dynamic state of harmony between intake and expenditure of resources

Approved Diagnoses

00050	Disturbed Energy Field
00093	Fatigue

Class 4. Cardiovascular/Pulmonary Responses. Cardiopulmonary mechanisms that support activity/rest

Approved Diagnoses

00029	Decreased Cardiac Output
00033	Impaired Spontaneous Ventilation
00032	Ineffective Breathing Pattern
00092	Activity Intolerance
00094	Risk for Activity Intolerance
00034	Dysfunctional Ventilatory Weaning Response
00024	Ineffective Tissue Perfusion (specify type: Renal, Cerebral, Cardiopulmonary, Gastrointestinal, Peripheral)

DOMAIN 5. PERCEPTION/COGNITION

The human information processing system including attention, orientation, sensation, perception, cognition, and communication

Class 1. Attention. Mental readiness to notice or observe

Approved Diagnoses

00123	Unilateral Neglect

Class 2. Orientation. Awareness of time, place, and person

Approved Diagnoses

00127	Impaired Environmental Interpretation Syndrome
00154	Wandering

Class 3. Sensation/Perception. Receiving information through the senses of touch, taste, smell, vision, hearing, and kinesthesia and the comprehension of sense data resulting in naming, associating, and/or pattern recognition

Approved Diagnoses

00122	Disturbed Sensory Perception (specify: Visual, Auditory, Kinesthetic, Gustatory, Tactile, Olfactory)

Class 4. Cognition. Use of memory, learning, thinking, problem solving, abstraction, judgment, insight, intellectual capacity, calculation, and language

Approved Diagnoses

00126	Deficient Knowledge (specify)
00161	Readiness for Enhanced Knowledge (specify)
00128	Acute Confusion
00129	Chronic Confusion
00131	Impaired Memory
00130	Disturbed Thought Processes

Class 5. Communication. Sending and receiving verbal and nonverbal information

Approved Diagnoses

00051	Impaired Verbal Communication
00157	Readiness for Enhanced Communication

DOMAIN 6. SELF-PERCEPTION

Awareness about the self

Class 1. Self-Concept. The perception(s) about the total self

Approved Diagnoses

00121	Disturbed Personal Identity
00125	Powerlessness
00152	Risk for Powerlessness
00124	Hopelessness
00054	Risk for Loneliness
00167	Readiness for Enhanced Self-Concept

Class 2. Self-Esteem. Assessment of one's own worth, capability, significance, and success

Approved Diagnoses

00119	Chronic Low Self-Esteem
00120	Situational Low Self-Esteem
00153	Risk for Situational Low Self-Esteem

Class 3. Body Image. A mental image of one's own body

Approved Diagnoses

00118	Disturbed Body Image

DOMAIN 7. ROLE RELATIONSHIPS

The positive and negative connections or associations between persons or groups of persons and the means by which those connections are demonstrated

➤

Class 1. Caregiving Roles. Socially expected behavior patterns by persons providing care who are not health care professionals

Approved Diagnoses

00061	Caregiver Role Strain
00062	Risk for Caregiver Role Strain
00056	Impaired Parenting
00057	Risk for Impaired Parenting
00164	Readiness for Enhanced Parenting

Class 2. Family Relationships. Associations of people who are biologically related or related by choice

Approved Diagnoses

00060	Interrupted Family Processes
00159	Readiness for Enhanced Family Processes
00063	Dysfunctional Family Processes: Alcoholism
00058	Risk for Impaired Parent/Infant/Child Attachment

Class 3. Role Performance. Quality of functioning in socially expected behavior patterns

Approved Diagnoses

00106	Effective Breastfeeding
00104	Ineffective Breastfeeding
00105	Interrupted Breastfeeding
00055	Ineffective Role Performance
00064	Parental Role Conflict
00052	Impaired Social Interaction

DOMAIN 8. SEXUALITY

Sexual identity, sexual function, and reproduction

Class 1. Sexual Identity. The state of being a specific person in regard to sexuality and/or gender

Class 2. Sexual Function. The capacity or ability to participate in sexual activities

Approved Diagnoses

00059	Sexual Dysfunction
00065	Ineffective Sexuality Patterns

Class 3. Reproduction. Any process by which new individuals (people) are produced

DOMAIN 9. COPING/STRESS TOLERANCE

Contending with life events/life processes

Class 1. Post-Trauma Responses. Reactions occurring after physical or psychological trauma

Approved Diagnoses

00114	Relocation Stress Syndrome
00149	Risk for Relocation Stress Syndrome
00142	Rape-Trauma Syndrome
00144	Rape-Trauma Syndrome: Silent Reaction
00143	Rape-Trauma Syndrome: Compound Reaction
00141	Post-Trauma Syndrome
00145	Risk for Post-Trauma Syndrome

Class 2. Coping Responses. The process of managing environmental stress

Approved Diagnoses

00148	Fear
00146	Anxiety
00147	Death Anxiety
00137	Chronic Sorrow
00072	Ineffective Denial
00136	Anticipatory Grieving
00135	Dysfunctional Grieving
00172	Risk for Dysfunctional Grieving
00070	Impaired Adjustment
00069	Ineffective Coping
00073	Disabled Family Coping
00074	Compromised Family Coping
00071	Defensive Coping
00077	Ineffective Community Coping
00158	Readiness for Enhanced Coping
00075	Readiness for Enhanced Family Coping
00076	Readiness for Enhanced Community Coping

Class 3. Neurobehavioral Stress. Behavioral responses reflecting nerve and brain function

Approved Diagnoses

00009	Autonomic Dysreflexia
00010	Risk for Autonomic Dysreflexia
00116	Disorganized Infant Behavior
00115	Risk for Disorganized Infant Behavior
00117	Readiness for Enhanced Organized Infant Behavior
00049	Decreased Intracranial Adaptive Capacity

DOMAIN 10. LIFE PRINCIPLES

Principles underlying conduct, thought, and behavior about acts, customs, or institutions viewed as being true or having intrinsic worth

Class 1. Values. The identification and ranking of preferred modes of conduct or end states

Class 2. Beliefs. Opinions, expectations, or judgments about acts, customs, or institutions viewed as being true or having intrinsic worth

Approved Diagnoses

00068	Readiness for Enhanced Spiritual Well-Being

Class 3. Value/Belief/Action Congruence. The correspondence or balance achieved between values, beliefs, and actions

Approved Diagnoses

00066	Spiritual Distress
00067	Risk for Spiritual Distress
00083	Decisional Conflict (specify)
00079	Noncompliance (specify)
00170	Impaired Religiosity
00169	Readiness for Enhanced Religiosity
00171	Risk for Impaired Religiosity

DOMAIN 11. SAFETY/PROTECTION

Freedom from danger, physical injury or immune system damage, preservation from loss, and protection of safety and security

Class 1. Infection. Host responses following pathogenic invasion

Approved Diagnoses

00004	Risk for Infection

Class 2. Physical Injury. Bodily harm or hurt

Approved Diagnoses

00045	Impaired Oral Mucous Membrane
00035	Risk for Injury
00087	Risk for Perioperative Positioning Injury
00155	Risk for Falls
00038	Risk for Trauma
00046	Impaired Skin Integrity
00047	Risk for Impaired Skin Integrity
00044	Impaired Tissue Integrity
00048	Impaired Dentition
00036	Risk for Suffocation
00039	Risk for Aspiration
00031	Ineffective Airway Clearance
00086	Risk for Peripheral Neurovascular Dysfunction
00043	Ineffective Protection
00156	Risk for Sudden Infant Death Syndrome

Class 3. Violence. The exertion of excessive force or power so as to cause injury or abuse

Approved Diagnoses

00139	Risk for Self-Mutilation
00151	Self-Mutilation
00133	Risk for Other-Directed Violence
00140	Risk for Self-Directed Violence
00150	Risk for Suicide

Class 4. Environmental Hazards. Sources of danger in the surroundings

Approved Diagnoses

00037	Risk for Poisoning

Class 5. Defensive Processes. The processes by which the self protects itself from the nonself

Approved Diagnoses

00041	Latex Allergy Response
00042	Risk for Latex Allergy Response

Class 6. Thermoregulation. The physiologic process of regulating heat and energy within the body for the purposes of protecting the organism

Approved Diagnoses

00005	Risk for Imbalanced Body Temperature
00008	Ineffective Thermoregulation
00006	Hypothermia
00007	Hyperthermia

DOMAIN 12. COMFORT

Sense of mental, physical, or social well-being or ease

Class 1. Physical Comfort. Sense of well-being or ease

Approved Diagnoses

00132	Acute Pain
00133	Chronic Pain
00134	Nausea

Class 2. Environmental Comfort. Sense of well-being or ease in/with one's environment

Class 3. Social Comfort. Sense of well-being or ease with one's social situations

Approved Diagnoses

00053	Social Isolation

DOMAIN 13. GROWTH/DEVELOPMENT

Age-appropriate increases in physical dimensions, organ systems, and/or attainment of developmental milestones

Class 1. Growth. Increases in physical dimensions or maturity of organ systems

Approved Diagnoses

00113	Risk for Disproportionate Growth
00101	Adult Failure to Thrive

Class 2. Development. Attainment, lack of attainment, or loss of developmental milestones

Approved Diagnoses

00111	Delayed Growth and Development
00112	Risk for Delayed Development

Source: NANDA International (2003). NANDA Nursing Diagnoses: Definitions and Classification 2003–2004.

Descriptors for NANDA Nursing Diagnoses

Some NANDA labels may include one or more of these descriptors. You may add descriptors to other labels, if necessary, to clarify the diagnostic statement.

Descriptors for Time (Axis 2)

Acute	Less than 6 months
Chronic	More than 6 months
Intermittent	Stopping or starting again at intervals, periodic, cyclic
Continuous	Uninterrupted, going on without stop

Descriptors for Unit of Care (Axis 3)

Individual	A single human being distinct from others, a person
Family	Two or more people having continuous or sustained relationships, perceiving reciprocal obligations, sensing common meaning, and sharing certain obligations toward others; related by blood or choice
Group	Individuals gathered, classified, or acting together
Community	"A group of people living in the same locale under the same government. Examples include neighborhoods, cities, census tracts, and populations at risk" (Craft-Rosenberg, as cited in NANDA, 2001, p. 218).

Descriptors for Age (Axis 4)

Fetus, neonate, infant, toddler, pre-school child, school-age child, adolescent, young adult, middle-age adult, young old adult, middle old adult, old old adult.

Descriptors for Health Status (Axis 5)

Wellness	The quality or state of being healthy especially as a result of deliberate effort
Risk	Vulnerability, especially as a result of exposure to factors that increase the chance of injury or loss
Actual	Existing in fact or reality, existing at the present time.

Miscellaneous Descriptors (Axis 6)

(Suggested; not limited to the following)

Ability	Capacity to do or act
Anticipatory	Realized beforehand, foreseen
Balance	State of equilibrium
Compromised	Made vulnerable to threat
Decreased	Lessened; lesser in size, amount, or degree
Deficient	Inadequate in amount, quality, or degree; defective; not sufficient; incomplete
Delayed	Postponed, impeded, and retarded
Depleted	Emptied wholly or in part; exhausted of
Disproportionate	Not consistent with a standard
Disabling	To make unable or unfit, to incapacitate
Disorganized	To destroy the systematic arrangement
Disturbed	Agitated; interrupted, interfered with
Dysfunctional	Abnormal, incomplete functioning
Excessive	Characterized by an amount or quantity that is greater than necessary, desirable, or useful
Functional	Normal complete functioning
Imbalanced	State of disequilibrium
Impaired	Made worse, weakened; damaged, reduced; deteriorated
Inability	Incapacity to do or act
Increased	Greater in size, amount, or degree
Ineffective	Not producing the desired effect
Interrupted	To break the continuity or uniformity
Organized	To form as into a systematic arrangement
Perceived	To become aware of by means of the senses; assignment of meaning
Readiness for Enhanced	To make greater, to increase in quality, to attain the more desired (for use with wellness diagnoses)

Source: NANDA International. (2003). *NANDA nursing diagnoses: Definitions and classification 2005–2006.* Philadelphia: Author.

What Are the Main Points in This Chapter?

- Nursing diagnosis is the unique obligation of the professional nurse; it cannot be delegated.

- An accurate nursing diagnosis is the foundation for the plan of care because it directs the choice of client-centered goals and nursing interventions.

- A nursing diagnosis is a statement of health status that nurses can identify, prevent, or treat independently.

- A medical diagnosis describes a disease, illness, or injury. A nursing diagnosis, in contrast, more holistically describes human responses to disease, illness, or injury.

- Collaborative problems are potential physiological complications of diseases, treatments, or diagnostic studies that nurses monitor and help to prevent but that cannot be treated primarily by independent nursing interventions.

- You must determine the "status" of each nursing diagnosis—that is, actual, potential, or possible problem; wellness diagnosis; or syndrome—because each status requires (1) different wording and (2) different nursing interventions.

- Diagnostic reasoning involves analyzing and interpreting data, verifying problems with the patient, and prioritizing the problems.

- You can never be certain that an inference is accurate, but you can have more confidence in an inference that is well supported by data.

- A problem etiology consists of the factors causing or contributing to the problem.

- You should involve patients in verifying and prioritizing their problems.

- Sound diagnostic reasoning is based on critical thinking and good theoretical and self knowledge.

- A NANDA nursing diagnosis consists of a diagnostic label, a definition, defining characteristics, and related or risk factors.

- To choose the correct NANDA problem label, match the patient's cue clusters to the definition and defining characteristics.

- A diagnostic statement consists basically of "problem + etiology"; however, a variety of formats is needed to describe client health status.

- In general, the problem side of the diagnostic statement directs the choice of goals; the etiology directs the choice of nursing interventions.

- Diagnostic statements should be descriptive, accurate, clear, concise, and nonjudgmental.

- One criticism of standardized diagnostic language is that it represents a threat to creative, holistic thinking.

Knowledge Map

Nursing Process: Diagnosing

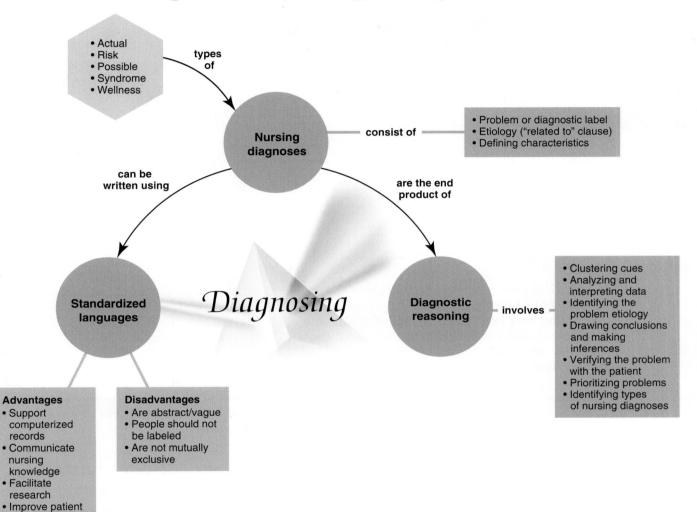

- Actual
- Risk
- Possible
- Syndrome
- Wellness

types of

Nursing diagnoses

consist of

- Problem or diagnostic label
- Etiology ("related to" clause)
- Defining characteristics

can be written using

are the end product of

Diagnosing

Standardized languages

Diagnostic reasoning

involves

- Clustering cues
- Analyzing and interpreting data
- Identifying the problem etiology
- Drawing conclusions and making inferences
- Verifying the problem with the patient
- Prioritizing problems
- Identifying types of nursing diagnoses

Advantages
- Support computerized records
- Communicate nursing knowledge
- Facilitate research
- Improve patient care
- Are rooted in practice

Disadvantages
- Are abstract/vague
- People should not be labeled
- Are not mutually exclusive

CHAPTER 5

Nursing Process:
Planning Outcomes

Overview

Care planning is the responsibility of the registered nurse; it cannot be delegated. A comprehensive care plan consists of a combination of standardized and individualized goals and interventions. It contains information needed to address (1) basic needs and ADLs, (2) medical and collaborative therapies, (3) nursing diagnoses and collaborative problems, and (4) special teaching and/or discharge needs. Computerized care planning saves nursing time and helps ensure that the nurse considers a variety of interventions and does not overlook common and important interventions; it reduces the time spent on paperwork.

Goals guide nursing interventions and serve as criteria for evaluation. They should be concrete, specific, and observable; valued by the patient or family; and not in conflict with the medical treatment plan.

A goal statement should include a subject, an action verb, a performance criterion, a target time, and special conditions if needed. For every nursing diagnosis, you must state one "essential" goal—one that, if achieved, would demonstrate problem resolution or improvement.

Three ANA-recognized standardized vocabularies/taxonomies for describing patient outcomes are NOC (individual patient care), the Omaha System (community health nursing), and the Clinical Classification System (home health nursing).

Thinking Critically About Nursing Process: Planning Outcomes

The exercises in the following section allow you to practice the kind of thinking you will use as a full-spectrum nurse. Because these are critical-thinking activities, there is usually no single right answer. Discuss answers with your peers—discussion can stimulate critical thinking. If you have difficulty with any of the questions, consult your instructor.

Caring for the Garcias

Review the opening scenario of Joseph Garcia in the first pages of this volume. As the clinic nurse, you have written the following nursing diagnostic statement: Imbalanced Nutrition: More Than Body Requirements related to inappropriate food choices and serving size as evidenced by BMI of 32.67.

Write at least two short-term and two long-term goals for Mr. Garcia based on this diagnostic statement. Remember that your goals must be realistic and take into account Mr. Garcia's other health problems.

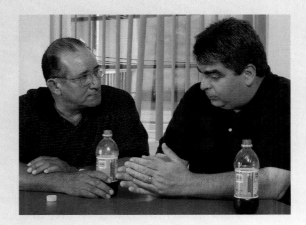

1 Merle Quinn is visiting a family planning clinic, where she has just been informed that she is 6 weeks pregnant. She looks worried and makes the following statements: "This is a shock. I've just started a new business, and I need to work 7 days a week to make it go. . . . I don't know if I am ready to be a mother. . . ." Her husband agrees: "I just don't see how we can afford this. We don't even have any insurance now."

"Still," Mrs. Quinn says, "I don't see how I could deal with having an abortion. My parents would be devastated. I'm sure they'd never speak to me again." Her husband says, "Not to speak of the fact that the Church forbids it. It would be a sin."

A week later Mrs. Quinn calls the clinic in tears. She says she has not been able to eat or sleep and that she doesn't know what to do about her pregnancy. "I don't want this baby, but I can't bring myself to have an abortion." The nurse diagnoses Decisional Conflict related to unexpected/unwanted pregnancy and possibly assuming that abortion is her only alternative; as evidenced by statements of indecision, tearfulness, inability to sleep. She makes an appointment to see Mr. and Mrs. Quinn that same day. Imagine that you are the nurse writing the care plan for the Quinns.

a Analyze your assumptions. What values and beliefs do you have that may influence the goals you write for the Quinns? Specifically, how could your values affect the goals you write?

b Develop a short-term goal to address the problem clause of this nursing diagnosis. The goal should be one you expect the Quinns to be able to achieve during their appointment that same day.

c You also write a goal stating: "By the end of this visit, clients will verbalize and demonstrate decreased anxiety and stress." Which part of the nursing diagnosis does this goal address?

d The NOC standardized outcomes "linked" to the NANDA diagnosis of Decisional Conflict are the following (definitions are given):

Decision Making. Ability to choose between two or more alternatives
Information Processing. Ability to acquire, organize, and use information
Participation: Health Care Decisions. Personal involvement in selecting and evaluating health care options

Which of those outcomes is it most important for the Quinns to achieve *today*? Why?

e Now imagine that you have written the following individualized goals/outcomes for today's visit with the Quinns:

By the end of this visit, clients will:

1. Verbalize and demonstrate decreased anxiety and stress.
2. Verbalize awareness that they have options for coping with whatever decision they make about the pregnancy.
3. Discuss with the nurse options for continuing or terminating the pregnancy.
4. Verbalize intent to discuss their feelings with family (i.e., their parents).
5. Verbalize intent to discuss feelings with a member of the clergy.
6. Decide whether to continue the pregnancy.

• Why is outcome 2 so important?

• What would you have assumed in order to write outcome 4?

• What would you have assumed in order to write outcome 5?

- Which of the outcomes is/are probably *not* appropriate for today's visit? Why?

2 For each of the following concepts, use critical thinking to describe how or why it is important to nursing, patient care, or the process of planning care. Note that these are *not* to be merely definitions.

Discharge planning

A written, individualized nursing care plan

Standardized care-planning documents (e.g., protocols)

Critical pathways

Computerized care planning

Goals (expected outcomes)

Short-term goals

Long-term goals

Action verbs (in goals)

Essential patient goals

The Nursing Outcomes Classification (NOC)

Aggregate goals

Wellness goals

Concrete, specific goal/outcome statements (as opposed to vague statements)

Practical Knowledge
knowing how

Practical knowledge in the planning phase of the nursing process requires you to use a variety of care planning forms. This section includes a discharge planning form, as well as a table of NOC measurement scales.

DISCHARGE PLANNING FORM

<table>
<tr>
<td rowspan="1">FOLLOW UP CARE</td>
<td>
When to call the doctor; symptom management (pain, nausea); plan for meeting outcomes not met during hospitalization:

Call your primary physician to find out if an insurance referral form is needed for follow up appointments.
After discharge, you need to call for an appointment to see physician.
Clinic/Physician   Phone #   Date   Time
_____ _____ _____ _____ or _____days _____weeks ____months
_____ _____ _____ _____ or _____days _____weeks ____months
_____ _____ _____ _____ or _____days _____weeks ____months
Plans for follow up Labs/Tests/Treatments
Date   Time   Test/Treatment   Location   Ordered by
_____ _____ _____ _____ _____
_____ _____ _____ _____ _____
_____ _____ _____ _____ _____
</td>
</tr>
<tr>
<td>PERSONAL CARE</td>
<td>
Bathing: ❑ No restrictions   ❑ Other:

Treatment/Therapy/Wound or Skin Care/ Supplies Needed   2-Day Supply Sent Home ? ❑ Yes
</td>
</tr>
<tr>
<td>ACTIVITY/ REHAB</td>
<td>
❑ No restrictions   ❑ Do not climb stairs   ❑ Drive_____   ❑ Return to Work _____
❑ Do not lift   ❑ May lift up to _____lbs   ❑ Weight Bearing _____# ❑ Other
</td>
</tr>
<tr>
<td>DIET</td>
<td>
❑ No restrictions   ❑ Other:

Food/Drug Interactions: ❑ Coumadin   ❑ MAO Inhibitors   ❑ Other:
</td>
</tr>
<tr>
<td>MEDICAL EQUIPMENT</td>
<td>
❑ 2nd pair of TED hose given
</td>
</tr>
<tr>
<td>COMMUNITY RESOURCES</td>
<td>
Referral Resource   Agency   Phone #   Transportation Arrangements for discharge: ___
Home IV Therapy   _____ _____ _____
Home Health   _____ _____
Home Oxygen   _____ _____ Education/Community Resources:_____
Home PT/OT/Speech _____ _____ _____
Ask-A-Nurse   _____ 816-932-6220
</td>
</tr>
<tr>
<td colspan="2">
Preprinted Discharge Instruction Sheet given to patient ❑ NA ❑ Yes
  List Instruction Sheets:
</td>
</tr>
<tr>
<td colspan="2">
I understand these instructions and agree with this plan of care _____
                                        Patient/SO Signature
</td>
</tr>
</table>

MULTIDISCIPLINARY DISCHARGE INSTRUCTIONS
Shawnee Mission Medical Center
9100 W. 74th Street
Shawnee Mission, Kansas 66204

Form # 60869 Revised: 4/01 PILOT Page 1 of 2

Source: Courtesy of Shawnee Mission Health System, Shawnee Mission, KS

STANDARDIZED LANGUAGE

By combining the following indicators with NOC indicators, you can write observable, concrete, patient outcomes to use in evaluating a patient's response to care.

NOC Measurement Scales

Scale Number	1	2	3	4	5*
a	Severely compromised	Substantially compromised	Moderately compromised	Mildly compromised	Not compromised
b	Severe deviation from normal range	Substantial deviation from normal range	Moderate deviation from normal range	Mild deviation from normal range	No deviation from normal range
f	Not adequate	Slightly adequate	Moderately adequate	Substantially adequate	Totally adequate
g	10 and over	7–9	4–6	1–3	None
h	Extensive	Substantial	Moderate	Limited	None
i	None	Limited	Moderate	Substantial	Extensive
k	Never positive	Rarely positive	Sometimes positive	Often positive	Consistently positive
l	Very weak	Weak	Moderate	Strong	Very strong
m	Never demonstrated	Rarely demonstrated	Sometimes demonstrated	Often demonstrated	Consistently demonstrated
n	Severe	Substantial	Moderate	Mild	None
r	Poor	Fair	Good	Very good	Excellent
s	Not at all satisfied	Somewhat satisfied	Moderately satisfied	Very satisfied	Completely satisfied
t	Consistently demonstrated	Often demonstrated	Sometimes demonstrated	Rarely demonstrated	Never demonstrated

Source: Moorhead, S., Johnson, M., & Maas, M. (Eds). (2004). *Nursing outcomes classification (NOC)* (3rd ed.). St Louis: Mosby, pp. 44–45.

* The scores (1 through 5) are constructed so that 5 is the most desirable, and 1 is the least desirable, condition relative to the outcome.

What Are the Main Points in This Chapter?

- During the planning outcomes phase, you will derive goals/expected outcomes from identified nursing diagnoses.

- Goals/expected outcomes (1) suggest nursing interventions, (2) serve as criteria for use in the evaluation step of the nursing process, and (3) provide motivation for patients and nurses.

- To ensure continuity of care, you should begin discharge planning with the initial patient assessment.

- A holistic, individualized patient care plan contains information needed to address (1) basic needs and ADLs, (2) medical and collaborative therapies, (3) nursing diagnoses and collaborative problems, and (4) special teaching and/or discharge needs.

- Ideally, a care plan consists of a combination of standardized and individualized goals and interventions.

- Standardized approaches to care planning include institutional policies and procedures, protocols, unit standards of care, standardized care plans, critical pathways, and integrated plans of care (IPOCs).

- Computerized care planning helps ensure that the nurse considers a variety of interventions and does not overlook common and important interventions; it reduces the time spent on paperwork.

- Nursing-sensitive goals (expected outcomes, predicted outcomes, desired outcomes) describe the changes in patient health status that are intended to result from and can be influenced by nursing interventions.

- A goal statement should include a subject, an action verb, a performance criterion, a target time, and special conditions if needed.

- For every nursing diagnosis, you must state one "essential" goal—one that, if achieved, would demonstrate problem resolution or improvement.

- Among the ANA-recognized standardized vocabularies/taxonomies for describing patient outcomes are NOC, the Omaha System, and the Clinical Care Classification System.

- Goals should be concrete, specific, and observable; they should be valued by the patient/family; and they should not conflict with the medical treatment plan.

Knowledge Map

Nursing Process: Planning

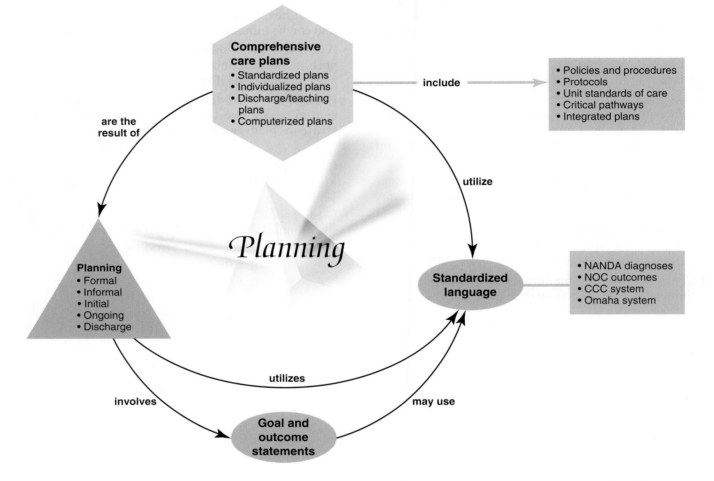

Comprehensive care plans
- Standardized plans
- Individualized plans
- Discharge/teaching plans
- Computerized plans

include →

- Policies and procedures
- Protocols
- Unit standards of care
- Critical pathways
- Integrated plans

are the result of

utilize

Planning

Planning
- Formal
- Informal
- Initial
- Ongoing
- Discharge

Standardized language

- NANDA diagnoses
- NOC outcomes
- CCC system
- Omaha system

utilizes

involves

may use

Goal and outcome statements

Nursing Process:

Planning Interventions

Overview

Nursing interventions are treatments that nurses perform in response to nursing diagnoses. The purposes of nursing interventions are to assess health status, prevent and treat disease or illness, and promote health. Interventions include teaching, counseling, and providing emotional support, physical care, referral services, and environmental management. Ideally, a nursing intervention should have a sound basis in research.

The registered nurse (RN) is responsible for choosing interventions and writing nursing orders; however, the RN can delegate some interventions to unlicensed assistive personnel (UAP) and licensed vocational nurses (LVNs). To generate interventions, nurses use critical-thinking skills such as making interdisciplinary connections, predicting, generalizing, explaining, and making therapeutic judgments. Nursing orders, written on the nursing care plan, consist of the detailed instructions for performing nursing interventions.

The American Nurses Association has approved three standardized vocabularies for nursing interventions: (1) the Nursing Interventions Classification (NIC), (2) the Omaha System (developed for community health nursing), and (3) the Clinical Care Classification (CCC). Standardized vocabularies are especially useful in agencies that have computerized care planning systems. Standardized vocabularies include terminology for describing wellness interventions and spiritual interventions.

Thinking Critically About Nursing Process: Planning Interventions

The exercises in the following section allow you to practice the kind of thinking you will use as a full-spectrum nurse. Because these are critical-thinking activities, there is usually no single right answer. Discuss answers with your peers—discussion can stimulate critical thinking. If you have difficulty with any of the questions, consult with your instructor.

Caring for the Garcias

Recall that you have written the following nursing diagnosis for Mr. Garcia:

Imbalanced Nutrition: More Than Body Requirements related to inappropriate food choices and serving size, as evidenced by BMI of 32.67.

A. Based on the outcomes you wrote in Chapter 5, identify four possible interventions to address the diagnosis and outcomes.

B. Review the interventions, and identify two that would be most appropriate for the patient given all of the information you have about his health status.

C. Write a nursing order for each of the two interventions you identified above.

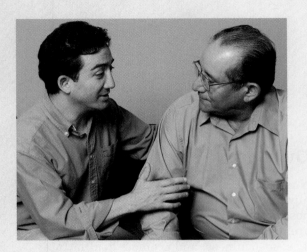

1 Recall the Quinns from Chapter 5. Merle Quinn is visiting a family planning clinic, where she has just been informed that she is 6 weeks pregnant. She looks worried and makes the following statements: "This is a shock. I've just started a new business and I need to work 7 days a week to make it go. . . . I don't know if I am ready to be a mother. . . ." Her husband agrees: "I just don't see how we can afford this. We don't even have any insurance now."

"Still," Mrs. Quinn says, "I don't see how I could deal with having an abortion. My parents would be devastated. I'm sure they'd never speak to me again." Her husband says, "Not to speak of the fact that the Church forbids it. It would be a sin."

A week later Mrs. Quinn calls the clinic in tears. She says she has not been able to eat or sleep and that she doesn't know what to do about her pregnancy. "I don't want this baby, but I can't bring myself to have an abortion." The nurse diagnoses Decisional Conflict related to this unexpected/unwanted pregnancy and inability to accept the only perceived alternative (abortion), as evidenced by statements of indecision, tearfulness, and inability to sleep. The nurse makes an appointment to see Mr. and Mrs. Quinn that same day. Imagine that you are the nurse writing the care plan for the Quinns.

a *Critical thinking: Analyze your assumptions.* To set aside your assumptions and care for the Quinns, you will need to focus on the Quinns' immediate problem, Decisional Conflict, rather than thinking about what they "ought to do." Remember, the nurse's role is not to make decisions for clients, but to provide information, clarification, and support.

- What questions must you ask in this case to analyze your assumptions?

- What are the answers to those questions?

b *Critical thinking (contextual awareness) and knowledge of patient situation.*
- What is going on in the Quinns' lives that may affect your choice of interventions?

- What is going on with Mrs. Quinn's health status that may affect your choice of interventions?

Now imagine that the nurse has written the following care plan for today's visit with the Quinns:

Outcomes	Interventions
NOC Outcomes	*NIC Interventions*
Decision Making	Decision-Making Support
Participation: Health Care Decisions	Family Planning: Contraception
	Family Planning: Unplanned Pregnancy
Individualized Goals	*Computer-Generated Nursing Activities*
By the end of this visit, clients will:	1. Offer emotional support.
1. Verbalize and demonstrate decreased anxiety and stress.	2. Inform client(s) of alternative views or solutions.
2. Verbalize awareness that they have options for coping with whatever decision they make about the pregnancy.	3. Help to identify advantages and disadvantages of each alternative.
3. Discuss with the nurse options for continuing or terminating the pregnancy.	4. Encourage client(s) to explore options, including termination, keeping the infant, or adoption.
	5. Provide information as requested by client(s).

➤

Outcomes (*continued*)

4. Verbalize intent to discuss their feelings with family (i.e., their parents).

5. Verbalize intent to discuss feelings with a member of the clergy.

Interventions (*continued*)

6. Serve as liaison between patient and family.

7. Assist in identifying support system.

8. Refer to community agency for counseling, if needed (e.g., family-planning clinic).

9. Discuss factors related to unplanned pregnancy (e.g., no use or misuse of contraceptives).

10. Teach and clarify misinformation about contraceptive use.

11. Teach regarding preparation and procedures.

12. Monitor for complications of procedure.

c *Nursing process.* Draw a line through the NIC intervention that, based on its label alone, does *not* appear to be relevant to producing the stated goals. (Note that it also does not appear that it would relieve the problem, reduce the etiology, or relieve Mrs. Quinn's symptoms of anxiety and distress.)

d *Nursing process.* Which of the computer-generated activities is/are *not* appropriate for today's visit with the Quinns?

e *Nursing process.* For which individualized outcome is there apparently *not* a computer-generated nursing activity?

f *Critical thinking.* Look at intervention 6 ("Serve as liaison between patient and family"). What critical-thinking questions should you ask about that intervention with regard to:

- Contextual awareness?

- Credible sources?

- Reflecting skeptically?

g Which of the computer-generated interventions will you probably need to do first today?

h Look at computer-generated interventions 2, 3, and 4. Which of these is it most important to do today? Which one could you encourage the Quinns to do during the next week or so? Why?

i What would you need to do to intervention 1 to turn it into a nursing order that another nurse could use to care for the Quinns?

j What questions would you need to ask to individualize intervention 1 for the Quinns' care plan?

2 For each of the following concepts, use critical thinking to describe how or why it is important to nursing, patient care, or the process of planning interventions. Note that these are *not* to be merely definitions.

Nursing interventions/strategies/activities/actions

Individualized interventions

Independent interventions

Collaborative interventions

Dependent interventions

Theories

Research

Evidence-based practice

The patient's problem status

The nursing diagnosis etiology

Client outcomes

Critical thinking (e.g., contextual awareness, reflecting skeptically)

Computerized care planning program

Standardized intervention vocabularies

Nursing Interventions Classification (NIC)

Wellness interventions

Spiritual care interventions

Nursing orders

thinking critically about nursing process: planning interventions

What Are the Main Points in This Chapter?

- Nursing interventions are treatments that nurses perform: (1) in response to nursing diagnoses and (2) for the purpose of achieving client outcomes.

- Nursing interventions include such activities as teaching, counseling and emotional support, referral, physical care, and environmental management.

- Independent interventions are nurse-initiated treatments—those that nurses perform or delegate based on their knowledge and skills.

- Nursing interventions are performed for the purpose of assessing health status, preventing and treating disease/illness, and promoting health.

- The registered nurse (RN) is responsible for choosing interventions and writing nursing orders; however, the RN can delegate actual performance of some interventions to unlicensed assistive personnel (UAP) and licensed vocational nurses (LVNs).

- Theories influence your perspective: What you notice and identify as a problem, as well as how you define a problem, more or less determines your choice of interventions.

- Ideally, a nursing intervention should have a sound basis in research.

- When generating interventions, nurses use critical thinking skills such as making interdisciplinary connections, predicting, generalizing, explaining, and making therapeutic judgments.

- The American Nurses Association has approved the following three standardized vocabularies for nursing interventions: (1) the Nursing Interventions Classification (NIC), (2) the Omaha System (developed for community health nursing), and (3) the Clinical Care Classification (CCC).

- Standardized vocabularies are especially useful in agencies that have computerized care planning systems.

- Standardized vocabularies include terminology for describing wellness interventions and spiritual interventions.

- Nursing orders, written on the nursing care plan, consist of the detailed instructions for performing nursing interventions.

Knowledge Map

Planning Interventions

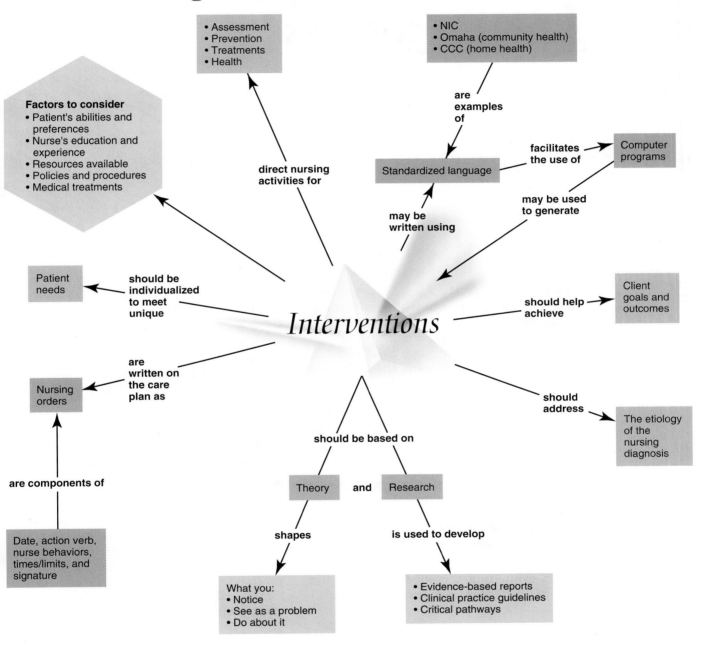

- Assessment
- Prevention
- Treatments
- Health

- NIC
- Omaha (community health)
- CCC (home health)

Factors to consider
- Patient's abilities and preferences
- Nurse's education and experience
- Resources available
- Policies and procedures
- Medical treatments

direct nursing activities for

are examples of

Standardized language

facilitates the use of → Computer programs

may be written using

may be used to generate

Patient needs ← **should be individualized to meet unique**

should help achieve → Client goals and outcomes

Interventions

Nursing orders ← **are written on the care plan as**

should address → The etiology of the nursing diagnosis

are components of

Date, action verb, nurse behaviors, times/limits, and signature

should be based on

Theory   **and**   Research

shapes

is used to develop

What you:
- Notice
- See as a problem
- Do about it

- Evidence-based reports
- Clinical practice guidelines
- Critical pathways

CHAPTER 7

Nursing Process:
Implementation & Evaluation

Overview

Implementation is the step in which the nurse performs or delegates the nursing activities that were planned in preceding steps. Because the nurse delegating a task is held accountable for the outcome, close supervision of the person performing the activity is advisable. During implementation, the nurse continues to make assessments and observe client responses. The final activity in the implementation step is documenting what care was provided.

During the evaluation step, nurses evaluate:

- *Client's progress toward health goals.* When evaluating the client's health status, compare the client's present data or responses to the desired outcomes (goals) set in the planning outcomes phase.
- *The effectiveness of the nursing care plan.* When evaluating the effectiveness of the nursing care plan, remember that not all variables that influence the success of a nursing activity can be controlled.
- *The overall quality of care on a unit, in an organization, or in a geographical area.* Quality assurance programs are specially designed to promote excellence in nursing; they include evaluation of structure, process, and outcomes.

Thinking Critically About Nursing Process: Implementation and Evaluation

The exercises in the following section allow you to practice the kind of thinking you will use as a full-spectrum nurse. Because these are critical-thinking activities, there is usually no single right answer. Discuss answers with your peers—discussion can stimulate critical thinking. If you have difficulty with any of the questions, consult with your instructor.

Caring for the Garcias

Mr. Garcia has the following information recorded on the clinic chart:

> 9/1/06 Imbalanced Nutrition: More Than Body Requirements related to inappropriate food choices and serving size, as evidenced by BMI of 32.67
>
> *Outcome:* Will lose 5 lb by 10/15/06
> *Interventions:*

- Collect 3-day nutrition history 9/2/06–9/4/06.
- Have patient meet with clinic nurse for diet review and nutrition instruction 9/8/06.
- Provide sample meal plans at 9/8/06 instruction.
- Phone patient 9/22/06 to discuss nutrition questions and review progress.
- Have patient return to clinic 10/15/06 for follow-up visit.

A. What must you do before implementing each nursing intervention?

B. Identify at least two strategies that will help promote Mr. Garcia's participation in and adherence to the plan.

C. How will you determine whether Mr. Garcia has met his goal?

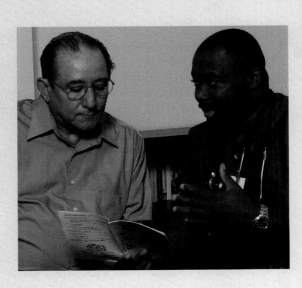

1 You are working a 12-hour shift (7:00 P.M. to 7:00 A.M.) on a medical unit at a local hospital. You will be caring for six adult patients. Make a list of the theoretical and practical knowledge you need about the patients to begin organizing your work for the shift. You may not yet have enough experience to make a complete list, but speculate about the kinds of information you think you might need. For example, to organize your work, you will need to know whether you have a UAP or LVN/LPN to assist you or whether you are providing total care for the patients.

2 Create a form for organizing your work. You will need to use a separate sheet of paper for this. Be sure it has space for at least six patients. You might begin by making a column for each patient's name and age, for example. Be sure to leave enough room to write the necessary information. For example, you will need more room to write the patients' tests and treatments than for writing in age and gender.

3 Alma Newport, who is 80 years old, has diabetes, severe arthritis, and mild dementia secondary to Alzheimer's disease. She lives alone. She refuses to consider an assisted living facility or nursing home, although her physician and children, who live out of town, believe it would be safer for her to do so. On more than one occasion, she has forgotten to turn off a stove burner while cooking, burning the contents of the pan and smoking up the house.

A home health nurse visits Mrs. Newport once a week. The physician wants Mrs. Newport to check and record her blood sugar levels before each meal. When the nurse asks, she says her blood sugar level is "OK" and shows the nurse the record she has kept, on which she has recorded many extremely low readings (e.g., 17, 20, 80, 24, 17 mg/dL). When the nurse checks Mrs. Newport's blood sugar, she obtains a reading of 210. After calibrating the glucose meter, the nurse writes the following care plan:

Nursing diagnosis:
  Deficient Knowledge related to cognitive deficits secondary to dementia

Desired outcomes:
  Mrs. Newport will demonstrate correct method for checking her blood sugar by
    next visit.
  Mrs. Newport will obtain correct readings.

Nursing orders:
  Teach correct method of fingerstick and checking blood glucose.
  Evaluate patient's technique at each visit.

Over the next few weeks, the home health nurse checks Mrs. Newport's log and fingerstick method at each visit. The logs continue to show low readings, and Mrs. Newport remains unable to correctly perform a fingerstick blood glucose test in spite of repeated demonstrations.

a Evaluate Mrs. Newport's progress. Has she met, partially met, or not met the desired outcome?

b What possible reasons may account for your evaluation (of Mrs. Newport's outcome status)? Hints: (1) Use your theoretical knowledge and personal experience with physical changes that occur with aging. (2) Use the data you have about Mrs. Newport. (3) Use your practical knowledge about nursing diagnoses.

4 A nursing assistant (UAP) is helping a patient with a shower when her pager goes off. After ensuring the patient's safety, the UAP goes into the hallway and answers the telephone. You observe that the UAP is still wearing gloves. How would you handle this situation?

5 For each of the following concepts, use critical thinking to describe how or why it is important to nursing, patient care, or the processes of implementing and evaluating. Note that these are *not* to be merely definitions.

Overlapping (of implementation and other nursing process steps)

Preparing for implementation

Client participation and adherence

Coordination of care

Delegation of care

The "five rights" of delegation

Supervision

Reflecting critically about implementation

Evaluation

Outcomes evaluation

Evaluative statements

Quality assurance programs

Practical Knowledge
knowing how

When implementing and evaluating care, you will need to make good decisions about delegating some aspects of care. The two tools in this section will help you delegate wisely.

In addition, you should use the Evaluation Checklist to evaluate patient progress and the effectiveness of the interventions.

DELEGATION AND EVALUATION CHECKLISTS

The Five Rights of Delegation

Right Task *(Can I delegate it?)*

The task is:

—Delegable for a specific patient.

—Within the nurse's scope of practice.

—Permitted by the state's nurse practice act.

—Permitted by the agency's policies.

Right Circumstance *(Should I delegate it?)*

Consider patient safety:

—Is patient setting appropriate?

—Are adequate resources available?

—Other factors to maintain safety?

Right Person *(Who is best prepared to do it?)*

The right person:

—Is delegating the task (the nurse must be competent to delegate).

—Will be performing the task (the UAP must be competent to do the task).

—Will receive the care (i.e., the severity of the patient's illness is considered).

Right Direction/Communication *(What does the UAP need to know?)*

—The task is described clearly, including its objective, limits, and expectations.

—The delegatee (UAP) understands the communication.

Right Supervision *(How will I follow up?)*

—The nurse monitors, evaluates, intervenes as needed.

—The nurse obtains feedback from the patient.

—The nurse obtains feedback from the delegatee.

Source: National Council of State Boards of Nursing. (1995). *Delegation: Concepts and decision-making process.* National Council Position Paper. Chicago: Author.

Delegation Decision-Making Grid

Elements for Review		Client A	Client B	Client C	Client D
Activity/Task	Describe activity/task:				
Level of client stability	Score the client's level of stability: **Client condition:** 0 - Is chronic/stable/predictable 1 - Has minimal potential for change 2 - Has moderate potential for change 3 - Is unstable/acute/strong potential for change				
Level of UAP competence	Score the UAP competence in completing delegated nursing care activities in the defined client population: **UAP is:** 0 - Expert in activities to be delegated, in defined population 1 - Experienced in activities to be delegated, in defined population 2 - Experienced in activities but not in defined population 3 - Novice in performing activities and in defined population				
Level of licensed nurse competence	Score the licensed nurse's competence in relation to both knowledge of providing nursing care to a defined population and competence in implementation of the delegation process: 0 - Expert in the knowledge of nursing needs/activities of defined client population *and* expert in the delegation process 1 - Either expert in knowledge of needs/activities of defined client population and competent in delegation *or* experienced in the needs/activities of defined client population and expert in the delegation process 2 - Experienced in the knowledge of needs/activities of defined client population *and* competent in the delegation process 3 - Either experienced in the knowledge of needs/activities of defined client population *or* competent in the delegation process 4 - Novice in knowledge of defined population *and* novice in delegation				
Potential for harm	Score the potential level of risk the nursing care activity has for the client *(risk is probability of [the client] suffering harm)*: 0 - None 1 - Low 2 - Medium 3 - High				
Frequency	Score based on how often the UAP has performed the specific nursing care activity: 0 - Performed at least daily 1 - Performed at least weekly 2 - Performed at least monthly 3 - Performed less than monthly 4 - Never performed				
Level of decision making	Score the decision-making needed, related to the specific nursing care activity, client (both cognitive and physical status) and client situation: 0 - Does not require decision making 1 - Minimal level of decision making 2 - Moderate level of decision making 3 - High level of decision making				
Ability for self care	Score the client's level of assistance needed for self-care activities: 0 - No assistance 1 - Limited assistance 2 - Extensive assistance 3 - Total care or constant attendance				
TOTAL SCORE					

Scoring: A low score on the grid suggests that an activity can be safely delegated. For example, if a client's stability is ranked 3 (unstable) and the level of UAP competence is also 3 (novice in the activity), then you probably should *not* delegate to that UAP. Each agency should establish a policy regarding the individual and/or total scores to be considered acceptable for delegating.

Source: Used by permission from the National Council of State Boards of Nursing (NCSBN), Chicago, IL (c) 2002. Retrieved September 8, 2002, from the NCSBN web site (www.ncsbn.org)

Evaluation Checklist

Instructions: Check the appropriate response and follow the associated instructions

Assessment Review

1. Were the assessment data complete and accurate?
   ___ YES. No action. ___ NO. Reassess client. Record the new data. Change care plan as indicated.

2. Have all data been validated, as needed?
   ___ YES. No action. ___ NO. Validate with client (by interview and physical examination), significant others, or other professionals. Record validation (or failure to validate). Change care plan as indicated.

3. Have new data become available that require changes in the plan (e.g., a different problem etiology, new goals/outcomes, new medical orders)?
   ___ NO. No action. ___ YES. Record the new data in the progress notes; redefine problem, goals, nursing orders, as needed.

4. Has the patient's condition changed?
   ___ NO. No action. ___ YES. Record data about present health status. Change care plan as indicated.

Move to a review of the diagnosis step.

Diagnosis Review

1. Is the diagnosis relevant and related to the data?
   ___ YES. No action. ___ NO. Revise the diagnosis.

2. Is the diagnosis well supported by the data?
   ___ YES. No action. ___ NO. Collect more data. Support or revise diagnosis.

3. Has the problem status changed (actual, potential, possible)?
   ___ NO. No action. ___ YES. Restate the problem.

4. Is the diagnosis stated clearly?
   ___ YES. No action. ___ NO. Revise the diagnostic statement.

5. Does the etiology correctly reflect the factors contributing to the problem?
   ___ YES. No action. ___ NO. Revise the etiology.

6. Is the problem one that can be treated primarily by nursing actions?
   ___ YES. No action. ___ NO. Label as collaborative and consult appropriate health professional.

7. Is the diagnosis specific and individualized to the patient?
   ___ YES. No action. ___ NO. Revise diagnosis. Revise outcomes and nursing orders as suggested by the new nursing diagnosis.

8. Does the problem (diagnosis) still exist?
   ___ YES. No action. ___ NO. Delete diagnosis and related outcomes and nursing orders.

Proceed to a review of client goals.

Planning Review: Outcomes

1. Have nursing diagnoses been added or revised?
   ___ NO. No action. ___ YES. Write new outcomes.

2. Are the outcomes realistic in terms of patient abilities and agency resources?
   ___ YES. No action. ___ NO. Revise outcomes.

3. Was sufficient time allowed for outcome achievement?
   ___ YES. No action. ___ NO. Revise time frame.

4. Do the outcomes address all aspects of the client's problem?
   ___ YES. No action. ___ NO. Write additional outcomes.

➤

Evaluation Checklist *(continued)*

Planning Review: Outcomes

5. Do the expected outcomes, as written, demonstrate resolution of the problem specified in the nursing diagnosis?
   ___ YES. No action.   ___ NO. Revise outcomes.

6. Have client priorities changed, or has the focus of care changed?
   ___ NO. No action.   ___ YES. Revise outcomes.

7. Is the client in agreement with the goals?
   ___ YES. No action.   ___ NO. Get client input. Write outcomes valued by the client.

Proceed to a review of nursing orders.

Planning Review: Nursing Orders

1. Have nursing diagnoses or outcomes been added or revised in previous review steps?
   ___ NO. No action.   ___ YES. Write new nursing orders.

2. Are the nursing orders clearly related to the stated patient outcomes?
   ___ YES. No action.   ___ NO. Revise or develop new nursing orders.

3. Is the rationale sufficient to justify the use of the nursing order?
   ___ YES. No action.   ___ NO. Revise or develop new nursing orders.

4. Are the nursing orders unclear or vague, so that other staff may have had questions about how to implement them?
   ___ NO. No action.   ___ YES. Revise nursing orders. Add details to make more specific or individualized to the patient.

5. Do the nursing orders include instructions for timing of the activities?
   ___ YES. No action.   ___ NO. Revise nursing orders: add times, schedules.

6. Was an order clearly and obvious ineffective?
   ___ NO. No action.   ___ YES. Delete it.

7. Are the orders realistic in terms of staff and other resources?
   ___ YES. No action.   ___ NO. Revise orders or obtain resources.

8. Have new resources become available that might enable you to change the goals or nursing orders?
   ___ NO. No action.   ___ YES. Write new goals or nursing orders reflecting the new capabilities.

9. Do the nursing orders address all aspects of the client's health goals?
   ___ Yes. No action.   ___ NO. Add new nursing orders.

Proceed to a review of implementation step

Implementation Review

1. Did the nurse [or UAP] get client input at each step in developing and implementing the plan?
   ___ YES. No action.   ___ NO. Obtain client input, revise plan and implementation as needed. [Coach UAP or role model, as needed.]

2. Were the nursing interventions acceptable to the patient?
   ___ YES. No action   ___ NO. Consult patient; change nursing orders or implementation approach.

3. Did the nurse [UAP] prepare the patient for implementation of the nursing order (e.g., explain what the patient should expect or do)?
   ___ YES. No action.   ___ NO. Continue same plan, but prepare patient before implementing. Reevaluate.

4. Did the nurse [UAP] have adequate knowledge and skills to perform techniques and procedures correctly?
   ___ YES. No action.   ___ NO. Continue same plan. Have someone else implement or help the nurse [or UAP] to acquire the needed knowledge or skills. If neither of these is possible, delete nursing order.

(continued)

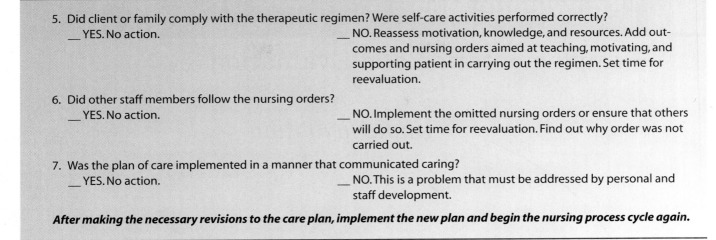

5. Did client or family comply with the therapeutic regimen? Were self-care activities performed correctly?
    ___ YES. No action.   ___ NO. Reassess motivation, knowledge, and resources. Add outcomes and nursing orders aimed at teaching, motivating, and supporting patient in carrying out the regimen. Set time for reevaluation.

6. Did other staff members follow the nursing orders?
    ___ YES. No action.   ___ NO. Implement the omitted nursing orders or ensure that others will do so. Set time for reevaluation. Find out why order was not carried out.

7. Was the plan of care implemented in a manner that communicated caring?
    ___ YES. No action.   ___ NO. This is a problem that must be addressed by personal and staff development.

After making the necessary revisions to the care plan, implement the new plan and begin the nursing process cycle again.

Source: Wilkinson, J. (2001). *Nursing process and critical thinking* (3rd ed.). Upper Saddle River, NJ: Prentice Hall, pp. 409–412.

What Are the Main Points in This Chapter?

- Implementation is the nursing process phase in which you perform or delegate the nursing activities that were planned in preceding steps.

- Before performing interventions, you should organize supplies and equipment and ensure the client's readiness.

- While implementing care, you will continue to make assessments and evaluate client responses.

- Delegation is the transfer of responsibility for an action while retaining the accountability for the outcome—this implies that you must supervise those to whom you delegate care.

- The "five rights" of delegation are: right task, right circumstance, right person, right direction/communication, and right supervision.

- The final activity in the implementation step is documentation of the care provided. Documenting

client responses is actually a part of the evaluation phase; however, you will document both at the same time, often in the same note.

- Nurses evaluate (1) patient progress toward health goals, (2) the effectiveness of the nursing care plan, and (3) the overall quality of care on a unit, in an organization, or in a geographical area.

- When evaluating client health status, you will compare the client's present data/responses to the desired outcomes (goals) set in the planning outcomes phase.

- When evaluating the effectiveness of the nursing care plan, remember that you cannot control all of the variables that influence the success of a nursing activity.

- Quality assurance programs are specially designed to promote excellence in nursing; they include structure, process, and outcomes evaluation.

Knowledge Map

Implementation and Evaluation

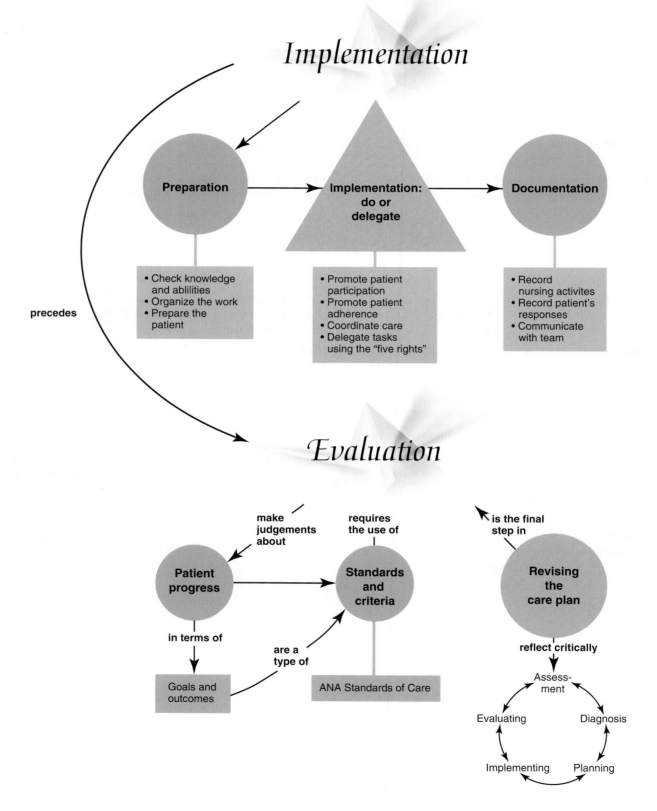

Implementation

Preparation

Implementation:
do or
delegate

Documentation

precedes

- Check knowledge
  and ablilities
- Organize the work
- Prepare the
  patient

- Promote patient
  participation
- Promote patient
  adherence
- Coordinate care
- Delegate tasks
  using the "five rights"

- Record
  nursing activites
- Record patient's
  responses
- Communicate
  with team

Evaluation

**make
judgements
about**

**requires
the use of**

**is the final
step in**

Patient
progress

Standards
and
criteria

Revising
the
care plan

in terms of

**are a
type of**

reflect critically

Goals and
outcomes

ANA Standards of Care

Assess-
ment

Evaluating

Diagnosis

Implementing

Planning

Nursing Theory & Research

Overview

The four basic components of a nursing theory are person, nurse, environment, and health. A theory is developed by recognizing a need in nursing or by having an idea then performing research to see whether the idea makes sense. The validated data are then used to further develop the theory.

Theories help nurses (1) find meaning in their experiences of nursing, (2) organize their thinking around pertinent ideas, and (3) develop new, evidence-based ideas and insights to guide their practice. Three leaders in nursing caring theories are Dr. Jean Watson, Dr. Patricia Benner, and Dr. Madeleine Leininger.

Nursing research is a systematic, objective process of analyzing phenomena of importance in nursing. Quantitative research has tight controls and large numbers of participants, and it is statistically analyzed.

Quantitative data may be generalized to populations similar to the one studied. Qualitative research tells the lived experience of a person or group of people. It is analyzed by examining the words and actions of a small number of participants.

Thinking Critically About Nursing Theory and Research

The exercises in the following section allow you to practice the kind of thinking you will use as a full-spectrum nurse. Because these are critical-thinking activities, there is usually no single right answer. Discuss answers with your peers—discussion can stimulate critical thinking. If you have difficulty with any of the questions, consult with your instructor.

Caring for the Garcias

Mr. Garcia arrives at the clinic for a follow-up visit. As you may recall, he has been diagnosed with hypertension. At a previous visit, you wrote a nursing diagnosis of Imbalanced Nutrition: More Than Body Requirements related to inappropriate food choices and serving size, as evidenced by BMI of 32.67.

Today you have gathered the following intake data:

Blood pressure: 174/96
Heart rate: 88
Respiratory rate: 18 per minute
Temperature: 98.5°F
Weight: 236 lb

A. What observations can you make about today's data in comparison to his initial visit?

B. As part of the treatment plan for Mr. Garcia, you have been asked to educate him about a diet to assist with weight loss and hypertension management. How would you determine the most appropriate diet to include in your treatment plan?

C. A number of sources recommend the DASH (Dietary Approaches to Stop Hypertension) eating plan. Go to the World Wide Web and search for "Dietary Approaches to Stop Hypertension." Is there sufficient research to support incorporating this information into Mr. Garcia's treatment plan? If so, describe the research, and summarize the DASH eating plan.

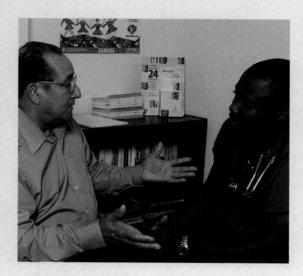

1 Recall the scenario about Mr. Wilkey in Volume 1. Imagine you are the charge nurse on the night shift at a long-term care facility. You hear the certified nursing assistant (CNA) and another voice talking loudly down the hall. You immediately go to see what has happened. You are surprised and shocked by what you see. An older patient, Mr. Wilkey, is naked and in bed with another patient, Mrs. Fredrickson, who is crying and shouting, "Get out! Get out!" Mr. Wilkey is tearful and looks frightened. He keeps repeating, "Where is Momma? Where is Momma?" The CNA is visibly upset and is grabbing at Mr. Wilkey in an effort to get him out of the bed. Use any nursing theory you wish, or your own idea, and describe each of the following concepts as they apply in this scenario:

a Patient (Who is the patient? How do you know?)

b Nurse (Who is the nurse? What is she doing that is "nursing"?)

c Health (Is the patient healthy? What is the patient's state of health?)

d Environment (Where is the nurse-patient encounter occurring?)

2 Recall Maslow's hierarchy of needs. Give one example of a specific nursing intervention a nurse could do to meet each of those needs. If you think the nurse cannot address a need, say why.

a Physiological

b Safety and security (mental and physical protection)

thinking critically about nursing theory & research

c Love and belonging

d Self-esteem (achievement, reputation)

e Cognitive needs (knowledge, self-awareness)

f Aesthetic needs (beauty, balance, form)

g Self-actualization (personal growth, fulfillment)

h Transcendence (helping others to self-actualize)

3 You are an emergency department nurse taking care of a 4-year-old child who has had a bike accident. The child has an open abrasion and a few cuts that will require some minor care. However, he is frightened and crying.

a Using Nightingale's theory, what interventions might you use?

b Using Watson's theory, what might you do?

c Using Henderson's theory, what would be the focus of your interventions?

d Choose one of the following theories. Look it up on the URL listed in Volume 1 [VOL 1] or on the Electronic Study Guide 💿.

Describe how that theory would direct you in this case:
Neuman

Orem

Rogers

4 You are working the night shift, and while making your 2:00 A.M. rounds, you are surprised. As you look into the room of 22-year-old Angela Kindred, you see her mother sitting at her bedside sobbing. Visits are not encouraged at that time of night, and you didn't know Mrs. Kindred was on the floor. Even though Angela's leukemia prognosis is terminal, you understood from the day nurse that the family, as well as Angela, had accepted the inevitable outcome. Explain how you can demonstrate caring to this mother, who will soon lose her beloved daughter. Look at Watson's (1988) ten caring processes below. How can you use them to demonstrate caring to this mother and daughter? Be specific in your answers.

Watson's Ten Caring Processes

1. Forming a humanistic-altruistic system of values
2. Instilling faith and hope
3. Cultivating sensitivity to self and others
4. Forming helping and trusting relationships
5. Conveying and accepting the expression of positive and negative feelings
6. Systematic use of the scientific problem-solving method that involves caring process
7. Promoting transpersonal teaching-learning
8. Providing for supportive, protective, and corrective mental, physical, sociocultural, and spiritual environment
9. Assisting with gratification of human needs
10. Sensitivity to existential-phenomenological forces

thinking critically about nursing theory & research

5 Examine the research priorities from ANA, specialty organizations, and the NINR, all listed below. Then answer the questions following them.

ANA 1980 Commission on Nursing Research
- Health promotion
- Preventive health practices for all age groups
- Health care needs of high-risk groups
- Life satisfaction of individuals and families
- The development of cost-effective healthcare systems

Oncology Nurses Association
- Pain
- Quality of life
- Ethics

Nurse experts in HIV / AIDS
- Pain
- Symptom management

Alzheimer nurses
- Management of physical problems, e.g., incontinence, falls, sleep disturbance, and inadequate nutrition
- Management of disruptive behaviors

Orthopedic nurses
- Preventing confusion in older postoperative client with hip fracture
- Determining safety measures for people with acute confusion

The National Institute of Nursing Research (NINR)
- Changing lifestyle behaviors for better health
- Managing the effects of chronic illness to improve quality of life
- Identifying effective strategies to reduce health disparities
- Harnessing advanced technologies to serve human needs
- Enhancing the end-of-life experience for patients and their families
- Chronic illnesses or conditions (including chronic illness self-management and quality of life)
- Decreasing low birth weight in infants among minority populations
- Enhancing health promotion among minority men
- End-of-life: bridging life and death

a What are some themes shared by all the groups' priorities?

b How are the priorities for the Alzheimer, orthopedic, and HIV/AIDS nurse groups different from the priorities of the 1980 ANA and oncology nurse groups?

c Copy one priority that is very specific and would limit the topic of your research proposal and the number of ideas you might have for a research proposal.

d Copy two priorities that are very broad and that would suggest a wide variety of topics you might develop for a research proposal.

6 For each of the following concepts, use critical thinking to describe how or why it is important to nursing, patient care, or nursing theory and research. Note that these are *not* to be merely definitions.

Nursing theory

The science of human caring

From novice to expert

Culturally competent care

Evidence-based practice

Nursing research

Institutional Review Board

Informed consent

Research utilization

What Are the Main Points in This Chapter?

- According to Florence Nightingale, nursing theories describe "what is" and "what is not" nursing.
- The four basic components of a nursing theory are person, nurse, environment, and health.
- A theory is developed by recognizing a need in nursing or by having an idea, using research to determine whether the idea is effective, and then using the research results to define a theory.
- Theories help nurses (1) find meaning in their experiences of nursing, (2) organize their thinking around pertinent ideas, and (3) develop new, evidence-based ideas and insights into the work they do.
- Nurses use theories as an evidence-based framework for their nursing practice.
- Three leaders in nursing caring theories are Dr. Jean Watson, Dr. Patricia Benner, and Dr. Madeleine Leininger.
- Nursing research is a systematic, objective process of analyzing phenomena of importance in nursing.
- Quantitative research may be generalized to populations similar to the one studied. It has tight controls and large numbers of participants, and the data are statistically analyzed.
- Qualitative research tells the lived experience of a person or group of people. It is analyzed by examining the words and actions of a small number of participants.
- The research process is a systematic way of organizing, preparing, and presenting research.
- Research participants (people in a research study) are protected from harm by specific laws and regulations.
- Research reports are critiqued using preselected criteria.
- Nursing research evolved slowly. The advanced education currently available to nurses is propelling research forward.
- Research is used in evidence-based nursing practice.

Knowledge Map

Theory and Research

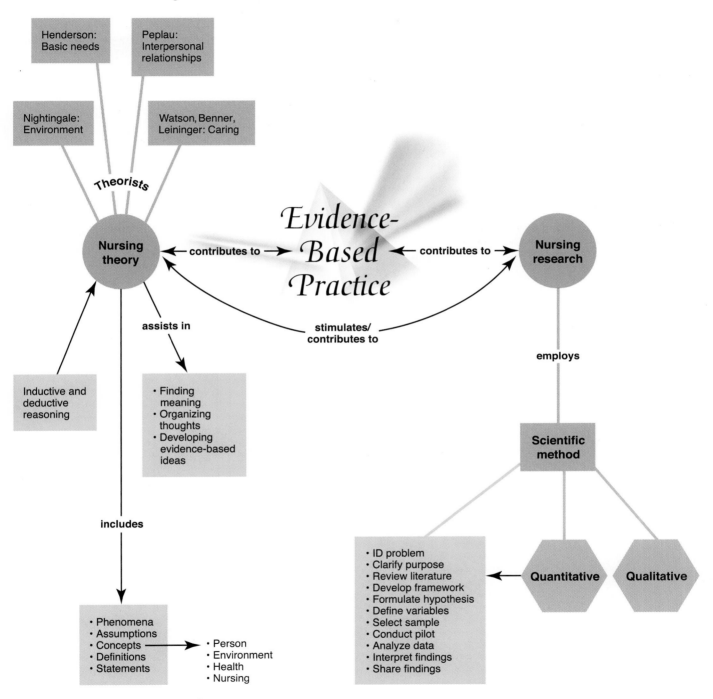

Henderson: Basic needs

Peplau: Interpersonal relationships

Nightingale: Environment

Watson, Benner, Leininger: Caring

Theorists

Nursing theory

← contributes to → **Evidence-Based Practice** ← contributes to → **Nursing research**

stimulates/ contributes to

assists in

Inductive and deductive reasoning

- Finding meaning
- Organizing thoughts
- Developing evidence-based ideas

employs

includes

Scientific method

- Phenomena
- Assumptions
- Concepts
- Definitions
- Statements

→ - Person
- Environment
- Health
- Nursing

- ID problem
- Clarify purpose
- Review literature
- Develop framework
- Formulate hypothesis
- Define variables
- Select sample
- Conduct pilot
- Analyze data
- Interpret findings
- Share findings

← **Quantitative**   **Qualitative**

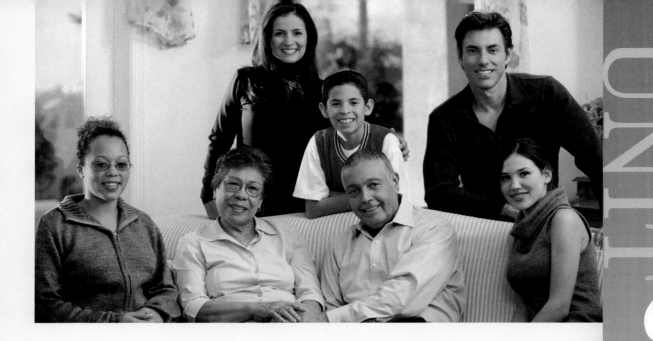

Factors Affecting
Health

9 GROWTH & DEVELOPMENT THROUGH THE LIFE SPAN

10 EXPERIENCING HEALTH & ILLNESS

11 PSYCHOSOCIAL HEALTH & ILLNESS

12 THE FAMILY

13 CULTURE & ETHNICITY

14 SPIRITUALITY

15 LOSS, GRIEF, & DYING

9 Growth
& Development Through the Life Span

Overview

Growth and development occur across the life span in a predictable pattern. Developmental theories identify what to expect behaviorally, cognitively, socially, and morally from patients at various ages. Patients at each stage of development have particular health problems that require specific assessment techniques. Nurses use assessment data to plan and to provide care and developmentally appropriate anticipatory guidance.

Fetal growth begins at the time of conception and continues for 10 lunar months until birth. At birth it is critical that the infant establish respirations, independent circulation, thermoregulation, and urine production.

Between birth and 1 year, infants develop a sense of trust. In the toddler period (12 to 36 months), the child explores the environment. Separating from parents, communicating needs through language, and controlling bodily functions are the developmental milestones of the preschool period (4 to 5 years). School-age children (6 to 12 years) are able to develop relationships outside the home. As they move into adolescence (12 to 18 years), children are working on establishing their own identity.

The young adult (20 to 40 years) leaves home and begins to function as an independent person. In middle adulthood (40 to 64 years), people must balance aspirations with reality and begin to deal with the needs of their aging parents. Older adulthood (age 65 and older) is a time of transition, when people begin dealing with the normal physical and social changes that occur with aging. At this time, chronic health problems can also affect a person's ability to live independently.

Thinking Critically About Growth and Development Through the Life Span

The exercises in the following section allow you to practice the kind of thinking you will use as a full-spectrum nurse. Because these are critical-thinking activities, there is usually no single right answer. Discuss answers with your peers—discussion can stimulate critical thinking. If you have difficulty with any of the questions, consult with your instructor. Before attempting these exercises, you may need to review the complete growth and development chapter.

 Go to **Chapter 9** on the Electronic Study Guide for the expanded chapter.

Caring for the Garcias

Review the scenario of Joseph Garcia. Answer the following questions based on that scenario.

A. Evaluate Mr. Garcia's physical health status in comparison to what is expected for someone in his age group.

B. Mr. Garcia and his wife are raising their 3-year-old granddaughter. What effect might this have on his ability to accomplish his developmental tasks?

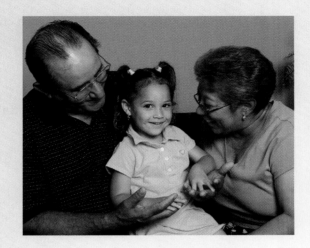

1 Now that you have an understanding of the stages of growth and development, let us return to our three pediatric patients we met at the beginning of Chapter 9–Miguel, Tamika, and Carrie.

VOL 1 Go to Chapter 9, **Meet Your Patients,** in Volume 1.

All three children are diagnosed with pneumonia. You have introduced yourself to Miguel's and Tamika's caregiver and spoken by phone to Carrie's mother. Each is asking you how this hospitalization will affect their child or grandchild. Miguel's mother is 17 years old and is very concerned about her son's condition. Tamika's elderly grandmother appears unconcerned about her granddaughter's health problems and instead asks questions about her husband's multiple medical diagnoses. Carrie's mother, Elaine, a 45-year-old bank vice president, expresses concern about Carrie's condition and asks whether she will need to be hospitalized long. You are wondering whether it would be helpful to schedule a group health teaching session with the parents and caregivers.

a   Based on Erikson's stages of development, contrast the developmental stages of Miguel, Tamika, and Carrie.

b   How will nursing care differ for each child?

c   Analyze each caregiver's developmental stage, and discuss the impact it may have on health teaching.

d   Would it be beneficial to have the caregivers meet for a group health teaching session? Explain.

2   For each of the following concepts, use critical thinking to describe how or why it is important to nursing, patient care, or growth and development. Note these are *not* to be merely definitions.

Ego

Defense mechanisms

Cognitive development

Psychosocial development

Fetal development

Infant development

Reflexes

Toddler development

Preschooler development

School-age development

Puberty

Adolescent development

Young adult development

Middle adult development

Older adult development

Practical Knowledge
knowing how

One important aspect of developmental care is to identify and intervene when patients are being abused.

PROCEDURES

The following flow chart and Procedure 9–1 will aid you in identifying cases of abuse.

Possible Abuse Flow Chart

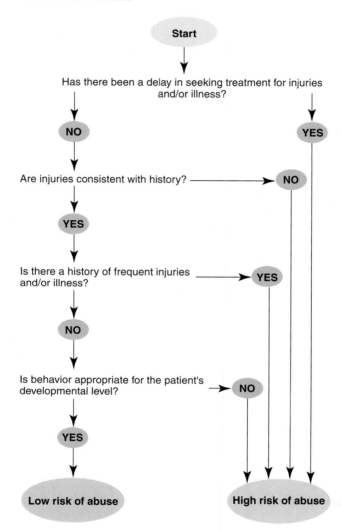

PROCEDURE 9–1　Assessing for Abuse

For steps to follow in *all* procedures, refer to the inside back cover of this book.

critical aspects

- Use a nonjudgmental approach. Do not make assumptions.
- Take a health history, assessing for physical, sexual, and psychological abuse.
- Perform a physical assessment; ensure the integrity of evidence that may be needed for criminal prosecution.
- Assess whether injuries are consistent with history.
- Observe for signs of neglect.
- If appropriate, refer for help in escaping the abusive situation.
- If appropriate, refer parent, caregiver, or partner involved in abuse to hotlines or agencies focused on stopping the abuse.
- Report abuse according to agency and state guidelines.

Procedural Steps

Step 1 Take the health history.

a. Collect information from the patient and parents or caregivers separately.

Allows the patient more freedom to express his concerns. An abused person may be afraid to talk with the abuser present.

b. Consider the patient's developmental and cognitive level in assessing whether the story of how the injury occurred is consistent with the injuries.

The patient must have been able to put himself in the situation in which the injury occurred. For example, an infant is not likely to have opened a medication bottle and taken pills.

c. Determine when the injury occurred or the illness began: "When did this injury happen or when did you first begin to feel ill?" "What have you been doing to treat your symptoms since you first became ill?"

A delay of treatment of 12 to 18 hours may indicate abuse.

d. Obtain a history of past injuries: "Have you ever had similar injuries?" "Have you ever required emergency care in the past?"

Abusive behavior is continual. If an injury is due to abuse, the patient has most likely experienced abuse in the past and may have old injuries.

e. Observe the patient's behavior. Evaluate whether it is inconsistent with the developmental level.

In the presence of the abuser, the patient may appear passive and lethargic, may not make eye contact, may exhibit anxious or fearful behavior, may look at the parent or caregiver before answering questions, or may let the abuser answer the questions for him.

f. Obtain information about the patient's usual diet: "What do you usually eat for breakfast? Lunch? Dinner? What kind of snacks do you have during the day?"

Neglect and/or abuse may be exhibited by an inadequate or inappropriate diet.

g. Ask about the patient's usual level of self-care: "Tell me about your usual day." "Are you able to take care of yourself?" "Who helps you shower and dress?" or "Do you require help with showering or dressing?" "Who is responsible for grocery shopping and cooking in your home?"

h. *To assess for sexual abuse:*
  - Ask whether the patient has been touched inappropriately:
    – *Child older than* 2: Ask about being touched in "private parts."
    – *Older child*: Ask something like, "Sometimes people you know may touch or kiss you in a way that you feel is wrong. Has this ever happened to you?"
    – *Adolescent*: Ask, "Sometimes people touch you in ways you feel are wrong. This can be frightening, and it is wrong for people to do that to you. Has this ever happened to you?"
    – *Adult*: Ask directly about being touched inappropriately or being forced to have sexual relations.

  If a patient is in a potentially abusive situation, the possibility of sexual abuse must be considered. Whenever possible, directly question the patient.

  - Ask whether the patient has genitourinary symptoms. "Have you had any burning or itching when you urinate? How about any vaginal discharge?"

  Genitourinary symptoms may indicate sexual abuse or neglect.

➤

PROCEDURE 9–1   Assessing for Abuse *(continued)*

- For a child, ask the parent or caregiver:
  - "Has the child started wetting the bed?"

  Abuse may result in regression to former behaviors.

  - "Has the child been masturbating or sexually acting out with other children?"

  A child who is sexually abused generally exhibits inappropriate sexual behavior.

  - "Has the child ever run away? If she leaves, does she go to someplace safe?"

  An abused child may consider himself worthless and may demonstrate unsafe behavior, such as running away to places that are unsafe.

i. *To assess for psychological abuse:*
  - For a child, ask the parent or caregiver:
    - "Was the child a result of a planned pregnancy? What were the pregnancy, birth, and postpartum period like?"

    Risk factors for abuse include an unplanned pregnancy, a difficult pregnancy or birth, and lengthy stay in the neonatal intensive care unit.

    - "How would you describe the child now?"

    An abusive parent may describe the child as a "problem child" who is always doing something wrong. The opposite is sometimes seen, where the child is "perfect."

    - "How does the child's behavior compare to others in the family?"

    Determine whether the parent sees the child differently from siblings. This is a risk factor for abuse.

- "Has the child experienced physical or emotional problems in the past?"

A history of physical or emotional problems may indicate abuse.

- "Are there family members or friends who help you with problems?"

Isolation is a risk factor for abuse. The parents or caregivers may not have the support they need.

- "What are your expectations of the child?"

The expectations of parents or caregivers who are more at risk to abuse a child may be that the child will "always be a problem" or will be a "perfect" son or daughter.

- "What form of discipline works best with the child?"

Determine whether the parents or caregivers use physical or emotional punishment that may be abusive.

- For possible spousal or partner abuse, ask the patient:
  - "Who do you talk to when you are having problems?"

  An abuser will try to isolate the victim from family and friends over time. Ask questions to determine whether the patient is becoming more isolated.

  - "Tell me how you feel about yourself."

  An abuser demeans and degrades the victim so that the victim feels worthless and the "punishment" is deserved.

  - "Who manages the family finances, and how are decisions made regarding spending?"

  An abuser frequently controls all the finances, severely limiting the resources of the victim.

- For elder abuse, ask the patient and/or caregiver:
  - "Describe the patient's personal support network. Who visits the patient? How often does the patient have visitors?"

  Like spousal abuse, people who victimize older people often isolate the person from any support network.

  - "Who is the patient's primary healthcare provider?"

  Multiple healthcare providers can be an indication of abuse. The caregiver brings the patient to a different physician with each injury or illness to avoid discovery.

  - Ask the patient, "Do you feel safe in your home?"

  The patient who is being abused does not feel safe.

  - "Has the patient ever received the wrong dose of medication?"

  Getting the wrong medication or dosage of medication (especially oversedation) may indicate abuse or inability to provide safe care.

  - "Who manages the patient's finances?"

  Financial abuse may be occurring. Determine who has control of the older person's finances and makes the decisions regarding spending.

Step 2   Perform a physical assessment.
a. If sexual abuse is suspected, have a forensic nurse or sexual assault nurse examiner (SANE) present if possible.

A forensic nurse and SANE are specially trained to identify findings that indicate abuse and how to handle the evidence to ensure validity in a court of law.

PROCEDURE 9–1   Assessing for Abuse *(continued)*

b. Assess the current injury and look for evidence of previous injuries. Look for the following:
- Bruises that form an outline of a hand, cord loop, buckle, or belt.

Observe for signs of physical abuse, especially injuries of different ages, because multiple injuries may show a pattern of abuse. Be careful to accurately assess the bruise. Some home treatments may cause what looks like bruising. For example, moxibustion (includes such things as firmly rubbing a warm spoon down the affected area) is used in some Asian cultures.

- Bruises on head, face, ears, buttocks, and lower back that are inconsistent with the history of the injury and are of varying ages (different colors).

Bruising may occur in different patterns. One pattern is the "swimsuit zone" on the trunk, breast, abdomen, genitalia, and buttocks.

- Obvious nonaccidental burns, such as burns to both feet and lower legs from immersion in hot water.

One method of abuse is to immerse the victim's hands or feet into scalding water. The resulting injury is very regular on both extremities.

- Circular burns, possibly from cigarettes.

Observe for burns all over the body, which will indicate abuse.

- Bite marks.

Bite marks in different areas of the body indicate abuse.

- Oral ecchymosis or injury from forced oral sex.

Forced oral sex will cause injuries to the mouth.

- Hyphema, subconjunctival hemorrhage, detached retina, ruptured tympanic membrane.

Injuries to the head are common in abuse. The shaken-baby syndrome will cause detached retinas and hemorrhages and subdural hematomas.

- Bleeding or bruising of genitalia, poor sphincter tone, and bruises on inner thighs.

These signs are indications of sexual abuse.

- Bruises on wrists and ankles from being restrained.

Abused individuals may be tied or locked in a closet or other small space.

c. Assess whether injuries are consistent with history.

If injuries are not consistent with the history, abuse must be assumed.

d. *Observe for signs of neglect:*
- Malnutrition, such as a distended abdomen, or weight markedly below ideal body weight
- Poor hygiene, including oral hygiene

- Ingrown nails
- Untreated sores or pressure sores
- Matted hair
- Dehydration

Signs of neglect occur because of long-term starvation or underfeeding, poor personal care, untreated sores or injuries, and inadequate fluid intake.

e. Provide referrals, if appropriate, for the abused person, partner, parent, or caregiver to obtain assistance in escaping the abusive situation and/or stopping the abuse.

Resources are available to assist the abused individual and to assist the parent or caregiver to stop the abuse. Be aware of local and national resources regarding abuse.

Step 3 If abuse has occurred, follow all legal procedures to ensure that all evidence is secured. If possible, have a forensic nurse work with the patient.

In situations where violation of the law has occurred, strict procedures need to be followed to ensure that your findings can be used in a court of law and to protect yourself against legal liability.

Step 4 Report concerns regarding abuse according to agency and state guidelines.

Child and elder abuse must be reported to the appropriate agency. Spousal abuse may be mandatory to report, depending on state law.

Evaluation

- Determine whether abuse may have occurred.
- Ensure that appropriate agencies have been notified of the possible abuse.
- Evaluate whether it is safe to let the patient leave the facility.

Documentation

- Chart all findings factually—do not add any interpretations. For example:

   Don't Chart:
   4-yr-old boy admitted with immersion burns to both feet extending to midpoint of shins.

➤

PROCEDURE 9–1 Assessing for Abuse *(continued)*

Do Chart:
4-yr-old boy admitted with first-degree burns to both feet extending to midpoint of shins. Father says, "I put him in the bathtub and didn't realize how hot the water was."

- Follow legal requirements for documenting possible abuse, including disposition of potential evidence.
- If possible, include pictures of the injuries in the charting.

Patient Teaching

- Inform patient, parent, partner, and/or caregiver of local resources for prevention or intervention in situations of child, spousal, or elder abuse.
- Inform patient that abuse is suspected. Ask for her perceptions of the situation.
- Emphasize to the patient that her safety is the primary concern.

Home Care

- If potential abuse is identified in the home, follow agency and state legal guidelines.
- If the patient's safety is at risk, immediate intervention is required. You may need to notify the police or call an ambulance.
- If you believe you are at risk for harm (common in abusive situations), leave the setting before notifying the police.

What Are the Main Points in This Chapter?

- Growth and development occur across the life span in a predictable pattern.
- Developmental theories help nurses identify what to expect behaviorally, cognitively, socially, and morally from patients at various ages.
- Fetal growth begins at the time of conception and continues for 10 lunar months until birth.
- Critical adaptations at birth include the establishment of respirations and independent circulation, thermoregulation, and the production of urine.
- Between birth and 1 year, infants develop a sense of trust when the caregiver provides the child with love, warmth, and food.
- The toddler period (12 to 36 months) is the time when the child explores the environment and attempts to become autonomous.
- In the preschool period (4 to 5 years) children are able to separate from their parents, communicate needs through language, and control bodily functions.
- The school-age child (6 to 12 years) begins to develop relationships outside the home. This leads to increasing confidence and independence.

- In the adolescent period (12 to 18 years) children establish their own identity and begin to make decisions that will affect their future.
- The young adult (20 to 40 years) leaves home and begins to function as an independent person.
- Middle adulthood (40 to 65 years) is a time when people balance aspirations with reality. It is often a time when the needs of children diminish whereas the needs of aging parents increase.
- The number of older adults (age 65 and older) has risen significantly because of increasing life expectancy.
- Older adulthood is a time of transition. Most health problems experienced by older adults are chronic in nature and often affect the person's ability to live independently.
- Growth and developmental differences result in each age group's having specific health problems requiring specific assessment techniques. Data from these assessments are used to plan and provide care and anticipatory guidance that are developmentally appropriate.
- Abuse of both children and adults is common. Assess all patients for signs of abuse.

10 Experiencing
Health & Illness

Overview

Health is a complex phenomenon that involves physical, mental, and spiritual aspects. Wellness is a way of life oriented toward optimal health and well-being.

People with an illness often describe the experience in terms of how it makes them feel—pain, sadness, loss, fatigue, or feelings of being overwhelmed. Those with life-threatening illness have to figure out how to live while they are dying.

Clients cope with illness by trying to maintain a sense of normalcy. The way a person responds to disruptions in life is influenced by such factors as age, family patterns, culture, hardiness, support, access to health care resources, the nature and stage of the illness, and the intensity, duration, and multiplicity of the disruption. People who are suffering often feel lonely because of actual physical separation, a sense of the world going on without them, and a sense of no one really being in their world.

A healing presence may be your most meaningful contribution to patients.

Part of the art of nursing is to envision strengths and potential in patients and families too overwhelmed to identify them on their own. You can provide a healing presence by listening, being attentive and willing to learn from patients, and recognizing and respecting others' ways of coping.

Thinking Critically About Experiencing Health and Illness

The exercises in the following section allow you to practice the kind of thinking you will use as a full-spectrum nurse. Because these are critical-thinking activities, there is usually no single right answer. Discuss answers with your peers—discussion can stimulate critical thinking. If you have difficulty with any of the questions, consult with your instructor.

Caring for the Garcias

Mr. Garcia has recently been diagnosed with hypertension, obesity, and degenerative joint disease (DJD). He is struggling with these diagnoses. He tells his wife, Flordelisa, "I feel so old now. These are the kind of things my parents are dealing with."

At a clinic visit Mr. Garcia tells you, "It's hard to think of myself as sick. I've been depressed ever since Jordan told me about his findings. Now he's asked me to get some lab work. I'm afraid he may find even more problems."

A. Identify the disruptions that Mr. Garcia must deal with based on these diagnoses. Explain your reasons for choosing these disruptions.

B. How would you evaluate Mr. Garcia's health status? To review the concepts of health status,

VOL 1 Go to Chapter 10, **The Health-Illness Continuum** and **Dunn's Health Grid,** in Volume 1.

C. What kinds of activities could you suggest to Mr. Garcia to improve his health status?

D. What stage of illness behavior is Mr. Garcia exhibiting in regard to his recent medical diagnoses?

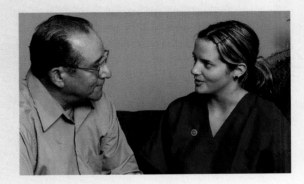

1 Describe your personal view of health.

2   Identify an individual in your life, personally or professionally, who personifies health. What characteristics do you identify in this individual that represent health? What factors do you think contribute to this individual's health status?

3   Use the nursing process to develop a plan to improve your personal health.

4   What attributes, resources, or life experiences do you have as an individual to offer in your role as a nurse?

5   For each of the following concepts, use critical thinking to describe how or why it is important to nursing, patient care, or experiencing health and illness. Note that these are *not* to be merely definitions.

Health

Wellness

Illness

Disruptions

Hardiness

Responses to illness

Health-illness continuum

Practical Knowledge
knowing how

Practical knowledge in this chapter means using the nursing process to apply what you have learned about how people experience health, wellness, and illness.

PROCEDURES

There is only one procedure in this chapter. It is designed to help you admit patients to the nursing unit in such a way that you can begin, at first contact, to establish trust.

PROCEDURE 10–1   Admitting a Patient to a Nursing Unit

 For steps to follow in *all* procedures, refer to inside back cover of this book.

critical aspects
- Orient patient and family to hospital environment.
- Answer patient's and family's questions.
- Complete nursing admission paperwork according to agency policy.
- Institute nursing care plan or clinical pathway.

Equipment
- Patient's chart, including physician's orders and nursing admission record
- Thermometer, blood pressure cuff, and stethoscope
- Nursing care plan or clinical pathway, if one has already been made

Assessments
- Assess patient for signs of emotional and/or physical distress.
- Assess patient's ability to ambulate and/or move.
- Assess patient's understanding of what is occurring.

Procedural Steps

Step 1 Introduce yourself to the patient and family.

Talking to the patient and family reassures them and provides information about the patient's level of consciousness and awareness, social relationships, and so on.

Step 2 Assist patient into hospital gown.

If the patient is able to stand, assist her into a gown prior to weighing her to obtain the most accurate weight.

Step 3 If possible, measure weight while the patient stands on a scale.

If the patient is able to stand, use a floor scale. If she is unable to stand, transfer her into the bed and measure her weight using a bed scale. Weigh in the same manner each time to ensure accuracy.

Step 4 Transfer the patient to the bed.

Get the patient comfortable prior to continuing the admission to prevent overtiring her.

Step 5 Check patient's identification band to ensure that the information, including allergies, is correct. Verify this information with the patient or family.

Questioning the patient about allergies will ensure that the information is accurate and documented on the wristband and the chart.

Step 6 Measure patient's vital signs.

Measuring the vital signs before completing the rest of the admission ensures that you will be aware of the patient's status. If the vital signs are abnormal, further assess the patient's condition before continuing. Report your findings to the primary care provider.

Step 7 Explain equipment, including how to use the call system and point out location of personal care items.

These actions ensure that the patient and family will be able to call for assistance if needed and increase the patient's and family's level of comfort and ability to function in the hospital setting.

Step 8 Explain hospital routines, including use of side rails, meal times, and so on. Answer the patient's and family's questions.

Hospitalization takes away control of basic decisions. Knowing the routines and available choices increases patient and family comfort.

Step 9 Obtain nursing admission assessment, including health history and physical assessment.

These are needed to identify problems and establish a baseline.

Step 10 Document all findings.

Identification of trends in the patient data is essential. A comparison of patient data against baseline information provides trend data.

Step 11 Complete inventory of patient's belongings. Encourage family to take home valuable items. If that is not possible, arrange to have valuables placed in the hospital safe.

Patient belongings, including valuables, are frequently lost during hospitalization. If possible, have the family take the patient's belongings home. Documenting the disposition of everything ensures being able to return the belongings to the patient upon discharge.

Step 12 Ensure that all admission orders have been completed.

Some orders need to be done immediately, while others can be delayed. Make sure the orders are completed in the most appropriate time frame.

Step 13 Initiate care plan or clinical pathway.

Identifying the patient's priority problems enables the nurse to develop the most appropriate nursing orders.

What Are the Main Points in This Chapter?

- Health is a complex phenomenon that involves physical, mental, and spiritual aspects. Having good health is an almost universal desire.
- Wellness is a way of life oriented toward optimal health and well-being.
- Life and wellness require nourishment. Nourishment comes in the form of food, exercise, sleep, relationships, meaningful work, the environment, and memories.
- The person with an illness rarely perceives the experience as a medical diagnosis. Instead, illness is usually described in terms of how it makes the person feel—such as pain, sadness, loss, fatigue, or being overwhelmed.
- People dealing with life-threatening illness have to figure out how to live and still be dying. Dealing with death is one of the most difficult experiences you will face as a nurse.
- One aspect of persevering in illness and life disruption is maintaining some semblance of "normalcy." Normalcy helps clients cope with illness.
- Nurses deal with people who have been thrust into new life situations, situations for which they did not ask and for which they were not prepared.
- People who are suffering experience loneliness. Part of aloneness can be related to the actual physical separation, part of it from a sense of the world going on without them, and part of it from a sense of no one really being in their world.
- Several factors influence a person's responses to disruptions. These factors include age, family patterns, culture, hardiness, support, access to healthcare resources, the stage and nature of the illness, and the intensity, duration, and multiplicity of the disruption.
- As a nurse, you will need to cultivate a healing presence. Listening, being attentive, being willing to learn from those in your care, and recognizing and respecting others' ways of coping are behaviors associated with a healing presence.
- Most people experience health, illness, and wellness as an ever-changing continuum on which they move.
- Communicating genuine care, concern, and sensitivity comes from who you are as a person, not from assuming a professional persona that you "put on" to fulfill a role.
- Patients and families may not recognize the strengths and creative abilities that they bring to a situation. Part of the art of nursing is to envision strengths and potential in patients and families who may be too overwhelmed to identify them on their own.
- Your healing presence may be the most memorable aspect of nursing care that you have to offer.

CHAPTER 11

Psychosocial
Health & Illness

Overview

Health and well-being are influenced by psychological, social, and spiritual development. Erikson's theory of psychosocial development and Maslow's hierarchy of human needs illustrate the interaction of psychological and social factors throughout the life span.

Self-concept is developed throughout the life span. Four dimensions contribute to self concept: body image, role performance, personal identity, and self-esteem. Not surprisingly, each can be threatened by illness and hospitalization.

Anxiety is a common emotional response to a (usually unknown) stressor; it results from psychological conflicts and is accompanied by physical symptoms (e.g., trembling). Anxiety can be mild, moderate, severe, or disabling (panic). Assessment should identify the presence, level, and cause of anxiety. Interventions for anxiety should help the patient become aware that he is anxious, identify the source of anxiety, and deal with the symptoms it produces.

Depression is characterized by diminished interest or pleasure in previously enjoyed activities, sadness, emptiness, a flat or hollow feeling (absence of feeling), tearfulness, difficulty concentrating, feelings of worthlessness, and some physical symptoms (e.g., insomnia, constipation). Assessment of depression includes a comprehensive history of mood, thoughts, behavior, and physical status. If you suspect severe depression, you should refer the patient to a mental health specialist; if there is a risk of suicide, referral should be immediate.

Thinking Critically About Psychosocial Health and Illness

The exercises in the following section allow you to practice the kind of thinking you will use as a full-spectrum nurse. Because these are critical-thinking activities, there is usually no single right answer. Discuss answers with your peers—discussion can stimulate critical thinking. If you have difficulty with any of the questions, consult with your instructor.

Caring for the Garcias

Recall the case of Joseph Garcia. Mr. Garcia has been diagnosed with hypertension, obesity, and degenerative joint disease. At clinic visits he has made the following comments: "Every time I come in here, I get some new diagnosis. I guess it's amazing I'm not dead yet. I thought I had a lot more time left, but I'm not so sure anymore." When you ask him what his main concerns are, he tells you, "Just take a look at me! I'm a mess. Nothing is turning out the way I planned. I might as well just die now. It would save my family a lot of grief."

A. What information do you need in order to respond to Mr. Garcia? How should you respond to Mr. Garcia? What actions should you take?

B. What conclusions can you make about Mr. Garcia's self concept (body image, role performance, personal identity, and self-esteem)? What additional information do you need about his self-concept?

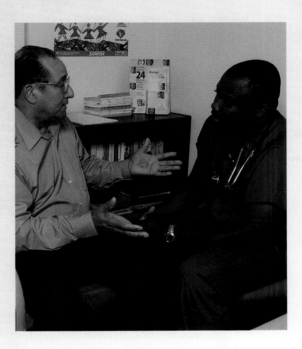

1 Review the scenario about Karli ("Meet Your Patient" from Volume 1):

You are caring for a 16-year-old patient named Karli who is suffering from fractures to both arms and several ribs, as well as extensive first- and second-degree burns to 30% of her body, following a motor vehicle accident. Karli had recently received her driver's license. She was driving her parents' car home from her part-time job when she lost control of the car and crashed into a containment wall. The car exploded into flames. A passerby quickly reported the accident, and fast action by the emergency response team saved Karli's life.

Karli is suffering from a moderate amount of shock and pain. She alternates between outbursts of anger, self-directed sarcasm, and despondence. She tells you that she cannot understand how the accident happened, that one moment she was adjusting the car radio, and the next moment she awoke in the hospital. Then suddenly she explodes. "It's not fair! I just took my eyes off the road for a second, that's all!" She bursts into tears. Picking at her bandages, she sobs that no one will love her looking as she will, that her life is over, and that she hates herself. You take her hand. "I used to be pretty," she says, "but now I'll look like a freak! What did I do to deserve this? I know plenty of kids who drive drunk or high all the time. I wasn't doing anything wrong! Why did this happen to me?"

a Now that you have completed the chapter in Volume 1, make a list of the multiple physical, psychological, and social issues that you would need to consider in developing a comprehensive care plan for Karli.

b Compare your list with the one you made when you first began reading the chapter. How is it different? Or is it the same?

2 In the "Meet Your Patient" scenario, Karli perceives herself as unlovable "looking this way." Which of the following nursing activities do you think might be helpful in *exploring and changing her perception*? For those you *do not* choose, explain why.

Role Enhancement
- Help the patient distinguish ideal and actual self. Help her describe realistic roles and expectations tailored to specific health changes.
- Compare realistic roles to previous and less functional roles.

Conflict Mediation
- Provide a quiet, private, neutral setting for mediation to take place.
- Maintain your own neutrality in the process; do not "take sides."

Promoting Family Integrity
- Encourage and facilitate communication among family members.
- Encourage family members to care for the patient as much as possible.

Family Mobilization
- Help family to identify strengths they can use to support the patient.
- Teach family members how to provide home care for the patient.

- Help the family identify community resources and/or support groups.
- Keep the family informed about the patient's progress, with the patient's permission.

Enhancing Socialization
- Explore and reinforce the individual's established relationships.
- Provide opportunities to rehearse relationship-building skills.
- Investigate, assist, and promote any developing relationships with persons of similar interests and goals.
- Provide information and links to community activities that relate to the person's past, current, and future interests.
- Promote access to education in social skills development.
- Encourage the patient to communicate and engage in interpersonal relationship activities by providing ongoing positive feedback.
- Organize small, cohesive group activities.
- Provide or act as role model where appropriate.

3 Mrs. King is being admitted into the orthopedics unit for a scheduled total knee replacement. Even though she appears to be in good health for a 72-year-old woman, you are concerned about her excessive weight, which can be described as moderate to severe obesity. You are troubled by how the obesity may negatively affect post-surgical recovery, wound healing, and mobility.

a What theoretical knowledge will you draw on to plan care to meet her biopsychosocial needs?

b What assumptions are you making? What stereotypes do you have that might affect your understanding of Mrs. King's situation?

c What do you think is contributing to Mrs. King's obesity?

thinking critically about psychosocial health & illness

d What facts do you have to support those ideas?

e How could you find out for sure what is contributing to Mrs. King's obesity?

4 Day by day you notice that your patient is eating less and complaining about constipation and tiredness. You carefully review her nutritional requirements against the food menu, as well as check nursing records for bowel movements. You have exhausted your initial search for obvious reasons why your client's appetite has changed. After sitting down next to your client, you cannot help noticing how tired she looks.

a What psychosocial problem do you suspect (low self-esteem, depression, anxiety, or disturbed personal identity)?

b What data do you have to support your inference in (a)?

c Objective data in her chart indicate that the patient has been eating very little and that she has been having bowel movements only every 3 or 4 days—and even then only with a laxative or enema. What other symptom do you need to investigate further?

d How could you obtain more information about that symptom?

e Think of depressed people you have known or depressed patients you have cared for. What have you found to be difficult about dealing with them?

5 Edna Jackson is 42 years old. She has had a hysterectomy (removal of her uterus). Her surgery was uncomplicated, her overall health is good, and she is expected to make a full and rapid physical recovery.

Her husband was not present when she was admitted and has not been to see her since the surgery. He did not want her to have the surgery. He told Edna that he doesn't know whether he will want to have sex with her when she is no longer "a whole woman." He has had casual affairs during their marriage, which Edna has tolerated because she feels that difficulty is balanced by the many positive benefits of their relationship, which include a "good sex life."

Edna has seven brothers and sisters, and she has five children of her own, ages 23, 21, 18, 6, and 4. She comes from a culture and a religion that value children and motherhood. She believes she is a good mother, although she must work full time outside the home.

Edna is an office manager—respected by her boss and by those who work for her. She has an internal locus of control and evaluates her job performance as "better than most people would do."

a Look at the context. What aspects of this situation may negatively impact Mrs. Jackson's recovery?

b Based on your answers in (a), what nursing diagnoses might be useful in describing the psychosocial aspects of Mrs. Jackson's health? (State both the problem and the etiology.)

c What strengths does Mrs. Jackson have that may help her to avoid and/or overcome those problems?

thinking critically about psychosocial health & illness

6

Matthew has been admitted to the emergency department with extensive wounds to both forearms, including tendon and vascular damage, from an attempted suicide. Matthew seems very quiet, almost withdrawn, and answers most of your questions in monosyllables.

Matthew reports that he is the third child in a family of five. Matthew's middle-class white parents are now retired, and his brothers and sisters are scattered across the country in various large cities. Although Matthew claims his schooling years were unremarkable, he reminisces about several occasions when he was bullied and physically beaten by gangs of older adolescents.

Matthew graduated from Harvard Law School and became vice president of an influential law firm. Despite his apparent success in life, he has continued to question his self-worth from early childhood. Plagued by worries and depression that have increased over the past few years, Matthew wrote a note indicating that he now realizes what a failure he is and proceeded to slash both his forearms with a sharp razor.

During the nursing assessment, Matthew reports that he has not been eating much, feels tired all the time, and has no interest in getting outside the house. He says, "I just don't feel like doing anything; I just want to sleep all the time."

a After Matthew's tendon and vascular repair, Matthew is admitted to your medical-surgical unit. What, broadly speaking, are your first two priorities for Matthew's care?

b Which of the following nursing diagnoses would you use, and why? (Consult a NANDA handbook, if necessary.)

Risk for Suicide or Risk for Self-Mutilation

c Prioritize the following interventions for Matthew. Rank them (1 = highest rank, 4 = lowest rank). Explain your thinking.

Refer to a mental health professional for help with his depression.
Examine Matthew's belongings and the room for anything he might use to harm himself.
Encourage Matthew to tell you if he begins having thoughts of suicide.
Begin establishing a therapeutic relationship and gaining his trust.

d Evaluate your self-knowledge. To plan comprehensive care for Matthew, in what areas do you need to increase your theoretical and practical knowledge? How will you do that?

7 For each of the following concepts, use critical thinking to describe how or why it is important to nursing, patient care, or psychosocial health and illness. Note that these are *not* to be merely definitions.

Self-concept

Self-esteem

Body image

Biopsychosocial well-being

Anxiety

Defense mechanisms

Depression

Therapeutic relationships

Hopelessness

Practical Knowledge
knowing how

This section provides guidelines and forms for assessing self-concept, self-esteem, anxiety, and depression. In addition, you will find tables of selected standardized outcomes and interventions to consider when planning care for patients with problems related to self-concept, anxiety, or depression.

TECHNIQUES

TECHNIQUE 11–1	Assessing Self-Concept Problems

Area of Assessment	Examples of Assessment Questions
Body image	• When you look in the mirror, what do you see? • How do you think others see you? • How does your current ability to engage in work and leisure activities compare to how you would like to be?
Role performance	• What are your three or four major roles (e.g., daughter, student)? • How successful are you in each of these roles? • How important is it to you to be successful in each of these roles? • What is interfering with your ability to perform any of these roles? What can you do about it?
Personal identity	• How did you see yourself before your illness/injury/loss? • How do you see yourself now? • How would you describe yourself to others? • What special abilities do you have? • How do you think others see you?
Self-esteem (also refer to Technique 11–2)	• How do you feel about yourself? • What do you like about yourself? • To what extent do you feel you are in control of your life? • If you could change one thing about yourself, what would it be? • Where would you like to be 5 years from now? • How realistic are your expectations of yourself? • How do you see your illness/injury/loss in relation to yourself?

TECHNIQUE 11–2   Performing a Self-Esteem Inventory

Place a check mark in the column that most closely describes the client's answer to each statement. Each check is worth the number of points listed.

	3 Often or a great deal	2 Some times	1 Seldom or occasionally	0 Never or not at all
1. I become angry or hurt when criticized.				
2. I am afraid to try new things.				
3. I feel stupid when I make a mistake.				
4. I have difficulty looking people in the eye.				
5 I have difficulty making small talk.				
6. I feel uncomfortable in the presence of strangers.				
7. I am embarrassed when people compliment me.				
8. I am dissatisfied with the way I look.				
9. I am afraid to express my opinions in a group.				
10. I prefer staying home alone rather than participating in group social situations.				
11. I have trouble accepting teasing.				
12. I feel guilty when I say no to people.				
13. I am afraid to make a commitment to a relationship for fear of rejection.				
14. I believe that most people are more competent than I am.				
15. I feel resentment toward people who are attractive and successful.				
16. I have trouble thinking of any positive aspects about my life.				
17. I feel inadequate in the presence of authority figures.				
18. I have trouble making decisions.				
19. I fear the disapproval of others.				
20. I feel tense, stressed out, or "uptight."				

Problems with low self-esteem are indicated by items scored with a 3 or by a total score higher than 46.

Source: Townsend, M. C. (2003). *Psychiatric mental health nursing: Concepts of care* (4th ed.). Philadelphia: F. A. Davis Company, p. 238.

TECHNIQUE 11–3   Identifying Depressed Patients Who Should Be Referred for Evaluation

One way to identify depression that is more than simple, situational depression is to ask the following two questions. A yes merits a referral.

1. "Over the past 2 weeks, have you felt down, depressed, or hopeless?"
2. "Over the past 2 weeks, have you felt little interest or pleasure in doing things?"

Source: U.S. Preventive Services Task Force. (2002). Screening for depression: Recommendations and rationale. *Annals of Internal Medicine, 136*(10), 760–764.

Another method is to use the mnemonic SIGECAPS, a concise version of the *DSM-IV-TR* diagnostic criteria. Ask the patient if he has experienced, for 2 or more weeks:

Sleep increase/decrease
Interest in formerly compelling or pleasurable activities diminished
Guilt, low self-esteem
Energy poor
Concentration poor
Appetite increase/decrease
Psychomotor agitation or retardation
Suicidal ideation

Both of the following require referral for evaluation and treatment:

Major depression = depressed mood or interest *plus* 4 SIGECAPS for 2 or more weeks
Mild depression (mood disorder) = depressed mood or interest *plus* 3 SIGECAPS most days for 2 or more years

Source: Brigham and Women's Hospital, 2001.

Some people prefer a mnemonic from an older source, IN SAD CAGES, which you would use in essentially the same way. Ask the patient if he has experienced, for 2 or more weeks:

Interest reduced
Negative thoughts
Sleep disturbance
Appetite change
Decreased confidence or self-esteem
Concentration reduced
Affect blunt or flat
Guilt
Energy reduced
Suicidal ideas

The original reference does not include a suggested total that requires referral. However, you can assume that more symptoms, the more severe the depression. We would suggest the following:

IN (reduced interest and negative thoughts or depressed mood) *plus* 4 of the other **SAD CAGES** requires referral.

Do not try to differentiate mild and major depression with this method.

Source: Adapted from Rund, D. A., & Hutzler, J. C. (1983). *Emergency psychiatry,* St Louis: Mosby, p. 144.

ASSESSMENT GUIDELINES AND TOOLS

Anxiety Assessment Guide

Rating Scale: None = 0, Mild = 1, Moderate = 2, Severe = 3, Disabling (Panic) = 4

Physiological Effects		**Psychological Effects**	
Shortness of breath (dyspnea)	____	Depersonalization (unreal)	____
Choking sensation	____	Feeling "on edge"	____
Dry mouth	____	Poor concentration	____
Pounding heart, increased heart rate	____	Poor memory	____
Chest pain	____	Depressed mood	____
Increased sweating and clammy	____	Loss of interest	____
Feeling faint, dizzy, unsteady	____	Restlessness	____
Nausea and abdominal upsets	____	Sense of panic	____
Numbness (pins and needles)	____	Worry, anticipation of the worst	____
Hot/cold flashes	____	Irritability	____
Trembling, shaking	____	Nightmares	____
Muscle tension and aches	____	Feeling of fear and foreboding	____
Exaggerated startle response	____	Excessive apprehension	____
Difficulties in falling asleep and staying asleep	____	Feeling lack of control	____

Assessing Overall Scores
0–28   Mild anxiety
29–56   Moderate anxiety
57–84   Severe anxiety
85–112   Disabling anxiety

Creating a total score from this table can help you assess whether overall anxiety is mild, moderate, severe, or disabling. However, individual physiological or psychological symptoms that are rated as severe (3) or disabling (4) may be more important and relevant to your nursing assessment. For example, your patient's overall or total assessment may be 26 (in the mild range, 0–27) but she has rated "Excessive apprehension" as 4 (disabling).

TABLES: STANDARDIZED OUTCOMES AND INTERVENTIONS FOR SELECTED PSYCHOSOCIAL NURSING DIAGNOSES

You can use the tables in this section when planning care for patients with problems of self-concept, anxiety, or depression. The tables provide standardized wording for nursing diagnoses, outcomes, and interventions. You can use the NOC indicators with the outcomes to write goals. Non-NOC outcomes are also suggested. In addition to the broad NIC interventions, the tables also provide specific nursing activities suggested by NIC.

Selected Standardized and Individualized Outcomes for Self-Concept Diagnoses

Nursing Diagnosis	NOC Outcomes	NOC Outcome Indicators and Scale Letter	Individualized Outcomes (not NOC)
Chronic Low Self-Esteem	Depression Level Quality of Life Self-Esteem	Crying spells mild (n) Satisfaction with economic status, completely satisfied (s) Verbalizations of self-acceptance often positive (k)	Participates and expresses pleasure in activities. Incidence of expressions of worthlessness decreases. Reports improved libido. Reports satisfaction with close relationships. Makes frequent eye contact. Maintains erect posture.
Situational Low Self-Esteem	Decision Making Grief Resolution Psychosocial Adjust-ment: Life Change Self-Esteem	Identifies alternatives, not compromised (a) Expresses feelings about loss, often demonstrated (m) Expressions of feeling socially engaged, consistently demonstrated (m) Maintenance of eye contact, often positive (k)	Expresses appropriate self-worth and self-acceptance. Maintains and improves social interaction. Verbalizes positive self-description. Asks for and accepts help from others. Makes frequent eye contact. Maintains erect posture.
Disturbed Personal Identity	Distorted Thought Self-Control Identity Self-Mutilation Restraint	Refrains from responding to hallucina-tions or delusions, sometimes demon-strated (m) Verbalizes clear sense of personal identity, consistently demonstrated (m) Does not injure self, consistently demonstrated (m)	Reports when experiencing hallucinations or delusions; describes their content. Verbal and nonverbal behaviors are congruent. Accurately differentiates self from environment and other people. Maintains control of urges; does not injure self. Reports to nurse when feeling the urge to harm self.
Ineffective Role Performance	Caregiver Lifestyle Disruption Coping Depression Level Psychosocial Adjust-ment: Life Change Psychomotor Energy Role Performance	Financial burden to caregiver, moderate (n) Identifies effective coping patterns, often demonstrated (m) Impaired concentration, none (n) Maintains productivity, consistently demonstrated (m) Exhibits ability to accomplish daily tasks, consistently demonstrated (t) Ability to meet role expectations, totally adequate (f)	Demonstrates ability to meet role expectations. Identifies strategies for role change(s). Reports comfort with role expectation. Verbalizes feeling in control of his life. Identifies and uses effective coping strategies.
Body Image Disturbance	Body Image Child Development (2 to 17 years) Grief Resolution Psychosocial Adjust-ment: Life Change Self-Esteem	Internal picture of self, often positive (k) Balances on one foot, consistently demonstrated (m) Progresses through stages of grief, consistently demonstrated (m) (see Situational Low Self-Esteem diagnosis)	Congruence between body reality, body ideal, and body perception. Openly expresses signs of grief over loss of body function. Expresses satisfaction with body appearance and function. Demonstrates willingness to use strategies to enhance appearance and function. Verbalizes positive aspects of body.
Impaired Adjusment	Acceptance: Health Status Compliance Behavior Coping Grief Resolution Health-Seeking Behavior Participation in Health Care Decisions Psychosocial Adjust-ment: Life Change Treatment Behavior: Illness or Injury	Performs self-care tasks, consistently demonstrated (m) Performs treatment regimen as prescribed, often demonstrated (m) Reports increase in psychological comfort, consistently demonstrated (m) (see Body Image Disturbance diagnosis) Asks health-related questions when indicated, consistently demonstrated (m) Seeks relevant information, consistently demonstrated (m) Sets realistic goals, sometimes demonstrated (m) Follows prescribed activities, consistently demonstrated (m)	Expresses feelings about illness. Verbalizes acceptance of losses due to illness. Accurately perceives the reality of health status. Keeps appointments with health provider. Follows prescribed regimen for medications and other therapies. Maintains usual hygiene and grooming measures. Requests information about physical condition and measures to maximize health. Participates in social activities. Sets realistic goals for self. Participates in making decisions about health care. Identifies barriers to achieving health goals. Performs self-care to the level of ability. Monitors for changes in disease symptoms. Alters lifestyle to meet treatment requirements.

Sources: Johnson, M., Bulechek, G., Dochterman, J., Maas, M., & Moorhead, S. (2001). Nursing diagnoses, outcomes, and interventions: NANDA, NOC, and NIC linkages. St. Louis: Mosby; and Moorhead, S., Johnson, M., & Maas, M. (Eds.). (2004). Nursing outcomes classification (NOC) (3rd ed.). St. Louis: Mosby, pp. 48–60. Used with permission.

* See NOC Measurement Scales in Chapter 5, Volume 2, for scales to use in describing desired outcomes or goals.

NIC Standardized Interventions and Selected Nursing Activities for Self-Concept Problems

NIC Intervention	Selected Nursing Activities (NIC)
Anticipatory Guidance	Help the patient adapt to anticipated role changes. Suggest books/literature for the patient to read, as appropriate. Schedule visits at strategic developmental/situational points.
Behavior Modification	Determine patient's motivation to change. Maintain consistent staff behavior. Reinforce constructive decisions concerning health needs.
Body Image Enhancement	Use anticipatory guidance to prepare patient for changes in body image that are predictable. Monitor frequency of statements of self-criticism. Assist patient to separate physical appearance from feelings of personal worth, as appropriate.
Coping Enhancement	Use a calm, reassuring approach. Assist the patient in developing an objective appraisal of the event. Encourage the acceptance of the limitations of others.
Decision-Making Support	Inform patient of alternative views or solutions. Help patient identify the advantages and disadvantages of each alternative. Obtain informed consent, when appropriate.
Delusion Management	Establish a trusting, interpersonal relationship with patient. Avoid arguing about false beliefs; state doubt matter-of-factly. Avoid reinforcing delusional ideas.
Developmental Enhancement: Child and Adolescent	(depends on developmental stage) Assist each child to become aware he/she is important as an individual. Facilitate a sense of responsibility for self and others.
Grief Work Facilitation	Identify the loss. Encourage expression of feelings about the loss. Instruct in phases of the grieving process, as appropriate.
Hallucination Management	Maintain a safe environment. Provide patient with opportunities to discuss hallucinations. Provide antipsychotic and antianxiety medications on a routine and PRN (as-needed) basis.
Hope Instillation	Assist patient or family to identify areas of hope in life. Inform the patient about whether the current situation is a temporary state.
Mood Management	Assist patient to identify thoughts and feelings underlying the dysfunctional mood. Determine whether patient presents safety risk to self or others. Provide opportunity for physical activity (e.g., walking or riding the exercise bike).
Parent Education: Childrearing Family	Facilitate parents' discussion of methods of discipline available, selection, and results obtained. Give parents a variety of strategies to use in managing a child's behavior.
Reality Orientation	Inform patient of person, place, and time, as needed. Provide a consistent physical environment and daily routine. Dress patient in personal clothing.
Role Enhancement	Assist patient to identify usual role in family. Assist patient to identify role insufficiency. Assist patient to identify positive strategies for managing role changes.
Risk Identification	Institute routine risk assessment, using reliable and valid instruments. Determine presence and quality of family support. Determine financial resources.
Self-Esteem Enhancement	Monitor patient's statements of self worth. Convey confidence in patient's ability to handle situation. Refrain from teasing.
Values Clarification	Pose reflective, clarifying questions that give the patient something to think about. Encourage patient to make a list of what is important and not important in life and the time spent on each. Avoid use of cross-examining questions.

Source: Dochterman, J. M., & Bulechek, G. M. (Eds). (2004) *Nursing interventions classification (NIC)* (4th ed.). St Louis: Mosby. Used with permission.

Selected Standardized Outcomes and Interventions for Anxiety-Related Diagnoses

Cue Cluster	NANDA Diagnosis*	NOC Outcomes[†]	Selected Indicators	NIC Interventions and Specific Activities[‡]
Susan is pacing the floor and does not make eye contact when she speaks to you. Her hands are shaking. Her BP is 140/88, P is 100, and R are 24. She says she is worried.	Anxiety	Anxiety Self-Control *Other Outcomes* Aggression Self-Control Coping Impulse Self-Control Self-Mutilation Restraint Social Interaction Skills	(Often demonstrated) • Maintains concentration. • Controls anxiety response.	Anxiety Reduction • Use a calm, reassuring approach. • Explain all procedures, including sensations the patient is likely to experience during the procedure. • Help the patient identify situations that precipitate anxiety. *Other Interventions* Anger Control Assistance Anticipatory Guidance Behavior Management: Self-Harm Behavior Modification: Social Skills Complex Relationship Building Coping Enhancement Impulse Control Training
Martin has a terminal illness. He looks very sad. He states that he is worried that his dying will be prolonged and difficult for his family and that he is afraid of dying.	Death Anxiety	Acceptance: Health Status *Other Outcomes* Anxiety Control Depression Level Dignified Dying Fear Control Hope	(Often demonstrated) • Appears peaceful. • Demonstrates positive self regard. • Clarifies personal values.	Emotional Support • Listen to and encourage expressions of feelings and beliefs. • Provide support during denial, anger, bargaining, and acceptance phases of grieving. *Other Interventions* Anxiety Reduction Coping Enhancement Dying Care Hope Instillation Spiritual Support
Ms Eng says,"I just don't know whether to have this chemotherapy or not. I know I could live a little longer, but the side effects …" She has decided twice to do it and each time has changed her mind. She says,"I just can't focus on anything else."	Decisional Conflict	Decision Making *Other Outcomes* Anxiety Control Information Processing Participation: Health Care Decisions	(Not compromised) • Identifies alternatives. • Identifies resources necessary to support each alternative.	Decision-Making Support • Determine whether there are differences between the patient's view of own condition and the view of healthcare providers. • Serve as a liaison between patient and family. • Serve as a liaison between patient and other healthcare providers. *Other Interventions* Health System Guidance Learning Facilitation Mutual Goal Setting
Bryan is to have his burns debrided today. He is crying. He says,"I wish my mom was here. It hurts so bad when they do that. I'm so scared."	Fear	Fear Self-Control *Other Outcomes* Anxiety Self-Control Coping	(Often demonstrated) • Uses relaxation techniques to reduce fear. • Maintains concentration. • Controls fear response.	Security Enhancement • Spend time with patient. • Answer questions about health status in an honest manner. • Hold a young child or infant, as appropriate. *Other Interventions* Anxiety Reduction Coping Enhancement
Mr. Paul's blood pressure remains dangerously high, yet he does not make the changes in diet and exercise that are needed, and he often fails to take his pills."I feel OK. This is a bunch of mumbo jumbo. My folks ate fried foods, and they lived to be over 80."	Ineffective Denial	Health Beliefs: Perceived Threat *Other Outcomes* Acceptance: Health Status Anxiety Self-Control Fear Self-Control Symptom Control	(Strong) • Perceives threat to health. • Perceives vulnerability to progressive health problems. • Perceives impact on functional status.	Self-Awareness Enhancement • Assist patient to identify the values that contribute to self-concept. • Assist patient to identify the impact of illness on self-concept. • Verbalize patient's denial of reality, as appropriate. *Other Interventions* Anxiety Reduction Coping Enhancement Counseling Emotional Support Health Education Security Enhancement Self-Modification Assistance Self-Responsibility Facilitation Teaching: Disease Process

* NANDA International. (2005). *Nursing diagnoses: Definitions and classification 2005–2006*. Philadelphia: Author.

† Johnson, M., Bulechek, G., Dochterman, J., Maas, M., & Moorhead, S. (2001). *Nursing diagnoses, outcomes, & interventions: NANDA, NOC, and NIC linkages*. St Louis: Mosby; and Moorhead, S. Johnson, M., & Maas, M. (Eds.). (2004). *Nursing outcomes classification (NOC)* (3rd ed.). St Louis: Mosby.

‡ Johnson, M., Bulechek, G., Dochterman, J., Maas, M., & Moorhead, S. (2001). *Nursing diagnoses, outcomes, & interventions: NANDA, NOC, and NIC linkages*. St Louis: Mosby; and Dochterman, J. M., & Bulechek, G. M. (Eds.). (2004). *Nursing interventions classification (NIC)* (4th ed.). St Louis: Mosby.

Selected Standardized Outcomes and Interventions for Depression-Related Nursing Diagnoses

Cue Cluster	NANDA Diagnosis*	NOC Outcomes†	Selected Indicators	NIC Interventions and Specific Activities‡
John is dying of HIV. He sleeps most of the time. During care activities (e.g., bath), he closes his eyes and remains passive. When asked to move or participate, he sighs and says, "I can't." When friends visit, he turns away from them; when they talk to him, he just shrugs. He has quit eating. He says, "It doesn't matter what I do. Nothing can change the way this turns out."	Hopelessness	Hope *Other Outcomes* Decision Making Depression Level Depression Self-Control Mood Equilibrium Quality of Life	(Often demonstrated) Expresses meaning in life. Expresses inner peace. Expresses belief in self. Expresses belief in others. Expresses sense of self-control.	Hope Instillation • Demonstrate hope by recognizing the patient's intrinsic worth and viewing the patient's illness as only one facet of the individual. • Help the patient expand spiritual self. • Create an environment that facilitates patient practicing religion, as appropriate. • Facilitate the patient or family's reliving and savoring past achievements and experiences. • Teach family about the positive aspects of hope (e.g., develop meaningful conversational themes that reflect love and need for the patient). • Avoid masking the truth. *Other Interventions* Decision-Making Support Mood Management Resiliency Promotion Self-Modification Assistance Spiritual Growth Facilitation Values Clarification
Jennifer is 16 and pregnant. She does not follow good health practices. She angrily says, "It's *my* body, and I don't want this baby. But my parents say abortion is a sin. I should honor my parents, but I hate them. I hate having to depend on them, and I hate being pregnant."	Powerlessness	Health Beliefs: Perceived Control *Other Outcomes* Depression Self-Control Health Beliefs Health Beliefs: Perceived Ability to Perform Participation in Health Care Decisions	(Strong) Requests involvement in health decisions. Makes efforts to gather information. Believes that own actions control health outcomes. Is willing to designate surrogate decision maker.	Self-Responsibility Facilitation • Discuss with patient the extent of responsibility for present health status. • Determine whether patient has adequate knowledge about healthcare condition. • Encourage verbalizations of feelings, perceptions, and fears about assuming responsibility. • Discuss consequences of not dealing with own responsibilities. • Encourage patient to take as much responsibility for own self-care, as possible. • Provide positive feedback for accepting additional responsibility and/or behavior change. *Other Interventions* Cognitive Restructuring Decision-Making Support Family Involvement Promotion Financial Resource Assistance Health Education Health System Guidance Mood Management
Tim has attempted suicide twice. He now says, "I will get it right this time. I know where I can get a gun."	Risk for Suicide	Suicide Self-Restraint *Other Outcomes* Impulse Self-Control	(Often demonstrated) Seeks help when feeling self-destructive. Controls impulses. Refrains from gathering means for suicide. Refrains from giving away possessions. Upholds suicide contract. Expresses feelings.	Suicide Prevention • Refer patient to mental healthcare provider . . . for evaluation and treatment. . . . • Administer medications to decrease anxiety, agitation, or psychosis and to stabilize mood, as appropriate. • Conduct mouth checks following medication administration to ensure that patient is not "cheeking" the medications for later overdose attempt. • Assist patient to identify network of supportive persons and resources (e.g., clergy, family, providers). • Initiate suicide precautions (e.g., ongoing observation and monitoring of the patient, provision of a protective environment) . . . • Limit access to windows, unless locked and shatter-proof, as appropriate. • Monitor patient during use of potential weapons (e.g., razor).

* NANDA International. (2005). *Nursing diagnoses: Definitions and classification 2005–2006.* Philadelphia: Author.

† Johnson, M., Bulechek, G., Dochterman, J., Maas, M., & Moorhead, S. (2001). *Nursing diagnoses, outcomes, & interventions: NANDA, NOC, and NIC linkages.* St Louis: Mosby; and Moorhead, S. Johnson, M., & Maas, M. (Eds.). (2004). Nursing outcomes classification (NOC) (3rd ed.). St Louis: Mosby.

‡ Johnson, M., Bulechek, G., Dochterman, J., Maas, M., & Moorhead, S. (2001). *Nursing diagnoses, outcomes, & interventions: NANDA, NOC, and NIC linkages.* St Louis: Mosby; and Dochterman, J. M., & Bulechek, G. M. (Eds.). (2004). *Nursing interventions classification (NIC)* (4th ed.). St Louis: Mosby.

What Are the Main Points in This Chapter?

- Health and well-being are influenced by psychological, social, and spiritual development.
- Psychosocial theory provides a way to understand people as the interaction of psychological and social events.
- Self-concept is one's overall view of oneself; it answers the question, "Who do you think you are?"
- Self-concept is developed throughout the life span and is influenced by multiple factors. Four dimensions contribute to self-concept: body image, role performance, personal identity, and self-esteem.
- Body image is a person's mental image of his physical self.
- Role performance consists of the actions a person takes and the behaviors she demonstrates in fulfilling a role, such as the role of a student.
- Personal identity is a person's view of himself as a unique human being, different and separate from all others.
- Self-esteem evaluations arise from the differences between ideal self and actual self.
- Communication skills are important because psychosocial information is personal and sometimes sensitive.
- When you formulate psychosocial diagnoses it is difficult, but important, to determine what is cause and what is effect.
- Many of the NOC standardized psychosocial outcomes are found in the domains of Psychosocial Health and Family Health.

- Many of the NIC standardized psychosocial interventions are found in the Behavioral and Family domains.
- Anxiety is a common emotional response to a (usually unknown) stressor; it results from psychological conflicts, and it is accompanied by physical symptoms (e.g., trembling).
- Assessment should identify the presence, level, and cause of anxiety.
- Interventions for anxiety should help the patient become aware that he is anxious, identify the source of anxiety, and deal with the symptoms it produces.
- Depression is characterized by diminished interest or pleasure in previously enjoyed activities, sadness, emptiness, a flat or hollow feeling (absence of feeling), tearfulness, difficulty concentrating, feelings of worthlessness, and some physical symptoms (e.g., constipation).
- Assessment of depression includes a comprehensive history of mood, thoughts, behavior, and physical status.
- If you suspect severe depression, you should refer the patient to a mental health specialist; if there is a risk of suicide, referral should be immediate.
- In communicating with depressed persons, it is important to not be overly cheerful and to avoid phrases such as, "Cheer up."

Knowledge Map

Psychosocial Health and Self-Concept

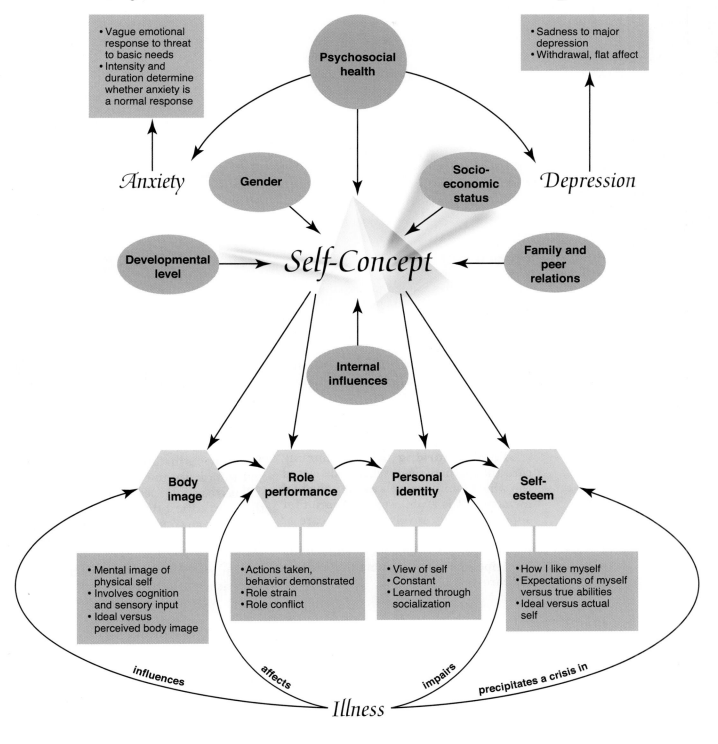

Psychosocial health

• Vague emotional response to threat to basic needs
• Intensity and duration determine whether anxiety is a normal response

Anxiety

Gender

• Sadness to major depression
• Withdrawal, flat affect

Depression

Socio-economic status

Developmental level

Self-Concept

Family and peer relations

Internal influences

Body image

Role performance

Personal identity

Self-esteem

• Mental image of physical self
• Involves cognition and sensory input
• Ideal versus perceived body image

• Actions taken, behavior demonstrated
• Role strain
• Role conflict

• View of self
• Constant
• Learned through socialization

• How I like myself
• Expectations of myself versus true abilities
• Ideal versus actual self

influences   affects   impairs   precipitates a crisis in

Illness

CHAPTER 12

The Family

Overview

The definition of family has expanded beyond the traditional nuclear family to include a group of individuals who provide physical, emotional, and economic support and assistance to each other. The *traditional nuclear family* represents only 13% of all married-couple families in the United States; *dual-earner families* with children represent 31%. *Single-parent families* make up about 25% of all families with children.

Family nursing refers to nursing care that is holistically directed toward the whole family as well as to individual members. It is a philosophy of care that supports family involvement in care of the ill client by encouraging family visiting, liberal visiting hours, and family participation in decision making regarding care.

The way families cope with everyday life and hospitalization can influence the care they receive. To assess family communication patterns, interview the family as well as the patient. You can promote family wellness by addressing both individual and family concerns.

Thinking Critically About the Family

The exercises in the following section allow you to practice the kind of thinking you will use as a full-spectrum nurse. Because these are critical-thinking activities, there is usually no single right answer. Discuss answers with your peers—discussion can stimulate critical thinking. If you have difficulty with any of the questions, consult with your instructor.

Caring for the Garcias

Bettina Sanford, 3 years old, is the first grandchild for Joseph and Flordelisa Garcia. Until recently, Bettina lived with her mother, Corazón, the Garcia's daughter. Corazón was diagnosed with schizophrenia at age 18, but was functioning adequately on her medications initially. However, her condition has been worsening and for the past year she has not been taking her medications. When Corazón became unable to care for herself and Bettina, Joe and Flordelisa assumed the child's care. Corazón rarely visits Bettina. Joe and Flordelisa have convinced Corazón to admit herself to a psychiatric hospital. Joe tells you at a clinic visit that he wishes his family were "normal."

A. What do you need to clarify about Joe's statement about his family?

B. What do *you* think Joe means by a "normal" family?

C. How would you respond to Joe's comments?

D. What effect might this new family structure have on Joe's and Flordelisa's health?

E. How might you promote family functioning for the Garcias? What assessments should you make? What interventions should you consider?

F. What personal values or biases do you have that may affect your ability to care for the Garcias?

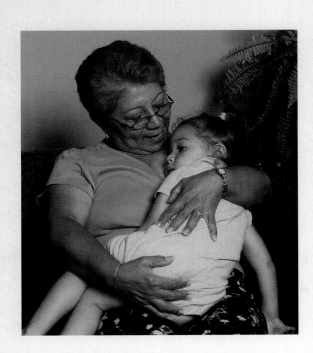

1 You are the nurse caring for a 58-year-old woman who was admitted for surgery of the foot. Today is the second day you have cared for the patient. You notice that the family seems quiet and subdued. You ask the client whether something is wrong. She reveals that her 29-year-old niece just lost her job as a TV programming assistant because her employer found out she is HIV positive. Apparently the diagnosis was revealed on her health insurance claim forms when they were processed.

a Name two things in this scenario that you, as a nurse, *cannot* change.

b Do the client and family have a problem that you *can* help them with? How could you find out?

c Imagine you were your client (the aunt). What concerns would you have?

d Try to depict this situation by using systems theory. Draw circles for each system involved and show where they interact.

e Draw on your self-knowledge. What biases or values do you have that might affect your thinking in this case, either positively or negatively?

2 You are the nurse in the ICU who is caring for a 45-year-old man who was involved in a serious car accident. He suffered severe head trauma and, if he lives, probably will have serious deficits. He was admitted 24 hours ago and has not made significant improvements. The family is aware of his status and likely outcome.

a What are some of the concerns this family might have?

b Using structural-functional theories, describe how this family might be affected.

c How could you help this family?

3 You are the nurse in the emergency department caring for a child who experienced a fall. The 3-year-old child will be OK and is being discharged. As you are reviewing the discharge instructions, the mother reveals that she and the child spent last night in a hotel because of violence in the home. She tells you that her husband (the child's stepfather) drinks excessively and at times has become violent, hitting her but not the child. She did not call him when they went to the emergency room, and she is afraid to go home.

a What do you think this woman's main concerns might be?

b Do you think this is a common or an unusual problem?

c What is the developmental stage of this family?

d What theoretical knowledge do you need to help this family?

e What kinds of help do you think this woman might need if she decides to escape from her husband?

f How could you help her at this moment?

4 For each of the following concepts, use critical thinking to describe how or why it is important to nursing, patient care, or the family. Note that these are *not* to be merely definitions.

Family relationships

Blended families

Communication

Systems theory

Structural-functional theory

Developmental theory

Family as the unit of care

Family health risk factors

The national economy

Health beliefs

Family coping mechanisms

Unexpected illness

Practical Knowledge
knowing how

Material in this section will help you to assess and plan care for families.

TECHNIQUES

TECHNIQUE 12–1	Conducting a Family Assessment

In general, a family assessment should include the following:

Identifying data	Include such information as name, address, phone number, cultural/ethnic background, religious identification, social class
Family composition	For each member of the family, include gender, age, relationship, date and place of birth, occupation, and education
Family history and developmental stage	This refers to the stages and developmental tasks in the following table, "Family Development"
Environmental data	Include a description of the home, neighborhood, and larger community, as well as the family's social supports and transactions with the community.
Family structure	In addition to identifying the structural type (e.g., traditional nuclear, single-parent, etc.), assess: —*communication patterns:* functional and dysfunctional patterns; the manner in which emotions are expressed, and contextual variables that affect communication —*power and role structures* (e.g., How are family decisions made? What are the roles of each member? Have there been changes in these?) —*family values* (What are their values? What are their priorities? How do they compare to the values of their cultural group? Are there value conflicts in the family?)
Family functions	Assess the effectiveness of the family's: —nurturing (e.g., Are the members close? Are they separate or connected?) —socialization and child-rearing (e.g., Who is the socializing agent(s) for the children? What are their child-rearing practices? Are needs for play being met?)
Health beliefs, values, and behaviors	For example, how do they define health and illness? What are their dietary, sleep, physical, and drug habits? What are their dental and medical health practices, including physicals, eye exams, immunizations, etc.? Do they have access to health services?)
Family stressors and coping	What are their stressors (e.g., financial, family communication or relationships, neighbors, holidays, children's behavior)? What successful coping strategies have they used? What dysfunctional strategies?
Abuse and violence within the family	Because of the prevalence of abuse and because families are likely to be secretive about it, you should assess every family to see if any abuse or neglect are occurring. For detailed guidelines, go to Procedure 9–1, Assessing for Abuse.

TABLES

Family Development

Stages	Tasks	Children's Age (Approximate)
Beginning family	• Making marriage work • Deciding whether to have children	None
Childbearing family	• Achieving pregnancy and birth • Adjusting to life changes following birth and to the infant's needs • Determining ways to meet all members needs • Renegotiating marriage • Increasing contact with extended family	Newborn to 2 years
Family with preschool children	• Adjusting to increased costs associated with family life • Socializing the preschoolers • Coping with loss of parental energy and privacy	3–5 years
Family with school-age children	• Adjusting to the needs and demands of growing children • Promoting joint decision making among parents and children • Encouraging and supporting educational and school-related activities	6–12 years
Family with teenagers and young adults	• Maintaining open communication among family members • Reinforcing ethical and moral values • For teens, balancing independence with parental rules	13–20 years
Family launching young adults	• Maintaining support to young adults as they leave the security of family • Rediscovering marriage	21–30 years
Postparental family	• Preparing for retirement • Adjusting to children's moving into new phases of adulthood, marriage, and childbearing and to becoming a grandparent	Adult
Aging family	• Adjusting to retirement and changes associated with aging • Adjusting to the loss of a spouse and friendships	Adult

Sources: Friedman, M. M. (1992). *Family nursing: Theory and practice* (3rd ed.). Norwalk, CT: Appleton & Lange; Friedman, M. M., Bowden, V. R., & Jones, E. G. (2003). *Family nursing: Research, theory, and practice* (5th ed.). Upper Saddle River, NJ: Prentice Hall; Hanson, S. M. (2001). *Family health care nursing: Theory, practice, and research* (2nd ed). Philadelphia: F. A. Davis Company; Leahy, J. M., & Kizilay, P. A. (Eds.). (1998). *Foundations of nursing practice: A nursing process approach.* Philadelphia: W. B. Saunders; and McGoldrick, M., & Carter, E. (1985). The stages of the family life cycle. In J. Henslin (Ed.), *Marriage and family in a changing society.* New York: Free Press.

STANDARDIZED OUTCOMES AND INTERVENTIONS

NOC Family Health Outcomes

Class	Outcome Labels
Family Caregiver Status: Outcomes that describe the adaptation and performance of a family member caring for a dependent child or adult	Caregiver Adaptation to Patient Institutionalization Caregiver Home Care Readiness Caregiver Lifestyle Disruption Caregiver-Patient Relationship Caregiver Performance: Direct Care Caregiver Performance: Indirect Care Caregiver Stressors Caregiving Endurance Potential
Family Member Health Status: Outcomes that describe the physical and emotional health of an individual family member	Abuse Cessation Abuse Protection Abuse Recovery: Emotional Abuse Recovery: Financial Abuse Recovery: Physical Abuse Recovery: Sexual Caregiver Emotional Health Caregiver Physical Health Caregiver Well-Being Maternal Status: Antepartum Maternal Status: Intrapartum Maternal Status: Postpartum Neglect Recovery
Family Well-Being: Outcomes that describe the physical, emotional, and social health of a family as a unit	Family Coping Family Functioning Family Health Status Family Integrity Family Normalization Family Participation in Professional Care Family Physical Environment
Parenting: Outcomes that describe behaviors of parents that promote optimum growth and development	Parenting: Adolescent Physical Safety Parenting: Early/Middle Childhood Physical Safety Parenting: Infant/Toddler Physical Safety Parenting Performance Parenting: Psychosocial Safety

Source: Moorhead, S., Johnson, M., & Maas, M. (Eds.). (2004). *Nursing outcomes classification (NOC)* (3rd ed.). St. Louis: Mosby.

NIC Family Interventions

Class	Examples of Interventions
Childbearing Care: Interventions to assist in the preparation for childbirth and management of the psychological and physiological changes before, during, and immediately following childbirth	Birthing Breastfeeding Assistance Childbirth Preparation Family Integrity Promotion: Childbearing Family Family Planning: Contraception Family Planning: Infertility Family Planning: Unplanned Pregnancy Intrapartal Care Labor Induction Postpartal Care Prenatal Care Risk Identification: Childbearing Family
Childrearing Care: Interventions to assist in raising children	Abuse Protection Support: Child Attachment Promotion Developmental Care Lactation Counseling Parent Education: Childrearing Family Parenting Promotion Sibling Support Teaching: Infant Nutrition Teaching: Toddler Safety
Life Span Care: Interventions to facilitate family unit functioning and promote the health and welfare of family members throughout the life span	Caregiver Support Family Integrity Promotion Family Involvement Promotion Family Mobilization Family Process Maintenance Family Support Family Therapy Home Maintenance Assistance Respite Care Risk Identification: Genetic Role Enhancement

Source: Dochterman, J. M., & Bulechek, G. M. (Eds.). (2004). *Nursing interventions classification (NIC)* (4th ed.). St. Louis: Mosby.

What Are the Main Points in This Chapter?

- *Family* is not limited to the traditional definition of husband, wife, and their children; defined more broadly, it is a group of individuals who provide physical, emotional, and economic support and assistance to each other.
- Families are structured in a variety of ways. Three examples are the traditional nuclear family, dual-earner families, and single-parent families, which make up about 25% of all families with children.
- Family nursing views the family from three perspectives: as the context for care of an individual, as the unit of care, and as a system.
- Wellness of each member is critical to health of the family unit.
- Under general systems theory, the family is viewed as a system in interaction with other systems (e.g., other families, groups, communities, and individuals).
- Under structural-functional theories, families are viewed as social systems, with a focus on outcomes.

- Developmental theories focus on family stages: beginning family, childbearing family, family with preschool children, family with school-age children, family with teenagers and young adults, family launching young adults, postparental family, and aging family.
- The family teaches health beliefs, values, and behaviors to its individual members.
- Assessment of family communication patterns consists of interviewing the family and the individual seeking care, as well as astute observation by the nurse.
- How families cope with everyday life situations and hospitalization can influence the effectiveness of care rendered.
- Nurses can promote family wellness by addressing both individual and family concerns.
- The family can be a source of support or a source of difficulties for the ill person.

Knowledge Map

Family Health Concepts

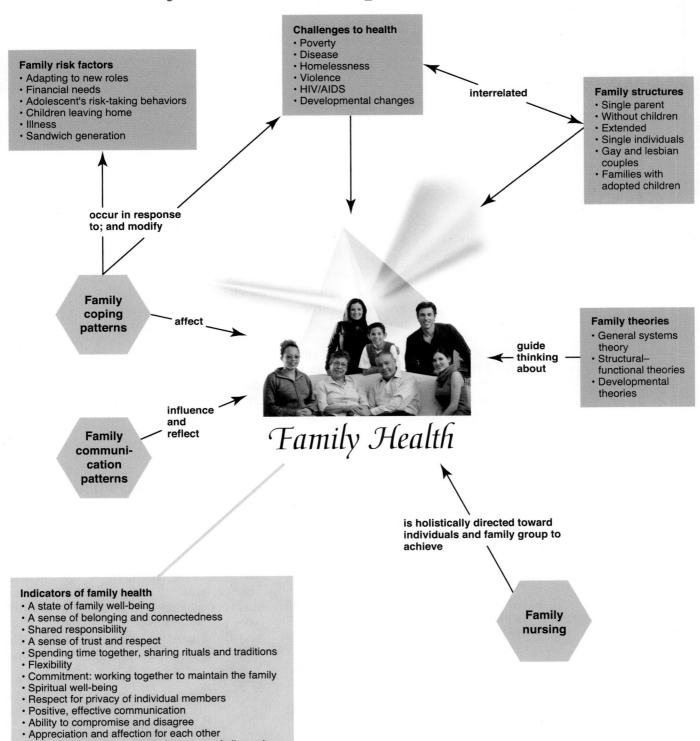

Challenges to health
- Poverty
- Disease
- Homelessness
- Violence
- HIV/AIDS
- Developmental changes

Family risk factors
- Adapting to new roles
- Financial needs
- Adolescent's risk-taking behaviors
- Children leaving home
- Illness
- Sandwich generation

interrelated

Family structures
- Single parent
- Without children
- Extended
- Single individuals
- Gay and lesbian couples
- Families with adopted children

occur in response to; and modify

Family coping patterns — *affect*

Family theories
- General systems theory
- Structural–functional theories
- Developmental theories

guide thinking about

Family communication patterns — *influence and reflect*

Family Health

is holistically directed toward individuals and family group to achieve

Family nursing

Indicators of family health
- A state of family well-being
- A sense of belonging and connectedness
- Shared responsibility
- A sense of trust and respect
- Spending time together, sharing rituals and traditions
- Flexibility
- Commitment: working together to maintain the family
- Spiritual well-being
- Respect for privacy of individual members
- Positive, effective communication
- Ability to compromise and disagree
- Appreciation and affection for each other
- Responding to the needs and interests of all members
- Egalitarian distribution of power
- Health-promoting lifestyle of individual members

13 CHAPTER

Culture
& Ethnicity

Overview

Culture refers to the shared values, beliefs, norms, and practices that guide thinking, decision making, and actions. Acknowledging that there are commonalities within a group is not the same as saying that *all* people in the group have those characteristics. Each person must be seen as unique—as *influenced* by his heritage, but not *defined* by it.

Consider each client's cultural values, beliefs, and practices regarding health as an important part of your assessment. Your understanding of cultural concepts, theories, and models will help you develop cultural competence.

Conventional Western medicine advocates the treatment of symptoms with pharmaceutical agents and/or surgery. In contrast, a variety of "alternative" healing systems, including folk medicine, attempt to treat the whole person, including the psyche and spirit, with therapies and rituals that have been passed down from generation to generation. Health providers with a Western frame of reference may find some of these therapeutic practices hard to accept. Culturally competent care, however, requires a nonjudgmental attitude, self-awareness, sensitivity, and respect for differences. In addition to building your theoretical knowledge of different cultures, you need to incorporate the client's cultural beliefs into the nursing care and to support the use of traditional therapies, provided that they are not harmful.

Thinking Critically About Culture and Ethnicity

The exercises in the following section allow you to practice the kind of thinking you will use as a full-spectrum nurse. Because these are critical-thinking activities, there is usually no single right answer; so answers may vary. Discuss answers with your peers—discussion can stimulate critical thinking. If you have difficulty with any of the questions, consult with your instructor.

Caring for the Garcias

Review the initial assessment of Joseph Garcia. Recall that Mrs. Garcia is from Mexico, whereas Mr. Garcia is of Cuban and Irish heritage.

A. How might the Garcias' cultural heritage affect their health beliefs?

B. What factors would you want to consider when performing a cultural assessment of the Garcia family?

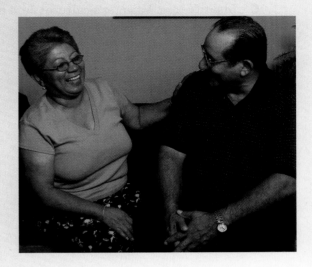

1 Mrs. Vasquez, a 70-year-old Mexican American woman, has diabetes mellitus and has come to the hospital because of a sore on her lower leg that will not heal. Mrs. Vasquez, a widow, cares for herself at home. She speaks only broken English and has some difficulty understanding your questions. After great effort on your part, you determine that she has missed her last appointment with her diabetes specialist because she has no transportation, so she has just been putting a dressing on the sore. Mrs. Vasquez tells you that she loves to see her grandchildren, who visit often, and that she enjoys cooking and eating Mexican food. She also says that she believes she is sick because she has not pleased God. However, God is a source of comfort and assurance to her. She prays a lot and has rosary beads in her hand.

a What are some pertinent cultural data that you should assess for Mrs. Vasquez?

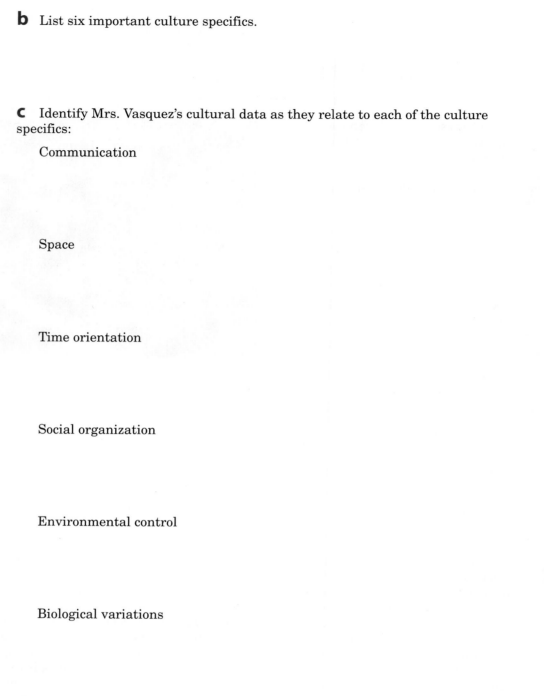

b List six important culture specifics.

c Identify Mrs. Vasquez's cultural data as they relate to each of the culture specifics:

Communication

Space

Time orientation

Social organization

Environmental control

Biological variations

d Using your theoretical knowledge, identify your expectations about communicating with Mrs. Vasquez. Compare your expectations to the actual data you have about her ability to communicate.

e   What does your theoretical knowledge lead you to expect about her personal space? What, if any, actual patient data do you have about that?

f   What does your theoretical knowledge lead you to expect about her time orientation, social organization, and environmental control? Compare your expectations to the actual patient data that you have.

g   What theoretical knowledge do you have regarding biological variations among Hispanic people? How does this compare to the actual data, if any, that you have for Mrs. Vasquez?

h   You have learned that cultural data can have implications for nursing care. Answer each of the following:

   • What additional information should you assess for in this situation?

   • What biases do you have that affect your thinking in this situation?

2   An Asian woman comes to your clinic for assessment of her blood pressure. In casual conversation, she tells you that her oldest daughter is about to be married. She reveals that her daughter has some type of anemia for which she needs medication. She tells you that she has recently heard terrible stories about sickle-cell anemia and is afraid that this is what her daughter has.

a   What additional data do you need to collect in order to answer this client's questions?

thinking critically about culture & ethnicity

b What are the biological variations that normally affect this cultural group?

c What assurances, if any, can you give this client about her daughter?

3 At times we must care for clients who do not speak our language. This poses a challenge to the nurse who strives to provide culturally competent care to all clients. Even with the assistance of interpreters, this can be difficult because of such barriers as differing dialects, street talk, and jargon. Keeping these facts in mind, answer the following questions:

a What options do you have when you encounter an individual who cannot speak English?

b How do you communicate with such a client if no interpreter is available?

c What biases do you have about such a situation? Why?

4 Alma is of European descent; she is white. She is a Roman Catholic and believes abortion is wrong. She believes that it should be illegal to own a gun. She is a nursing student.

Violetta's parents came to the United States from Europe. They were born in France. Before that, her great-grandparents lived in Africa. Violetta is black. She is Roman Catholic, and she believes that abortion is wrong. She believes that it should be illegal to own a gun. She is a nursing student.

Darcy is of European descent. She is white. She laughs at the idea of religion, saying "Nobody's 'up there' looking out for me; and when you're dead, you're dead."

Darcy is a gang member and carries a gun in her purse or her pocket at all times. She did not finish high school, and by the age of 19 she had had two abortions.

All of the women live in the United States. Which two women do you think share the most cultural commonalities? Explain your thinking.

5 Helen is 52 years old and African American. She is divorced. Her only child, Tamika, is incarcerated for prostitution and possession of narcotics. Helen is now raising her two grandchildren, Calvin, age 13 years, and Jevetta, age 2. Helen is a nursing assistant at the local hospital. It's hard for her to make ends meet because she has hypertension and diabetes, for which she takes a number of medications and insulin—that is, when she can afford them. She has not applied for medical assistance because she believes she should be able to take care of herself, but she does receive assistance for Jevetta's day-care costs. In addition to her grandchildren, Helen has a large group of friends, many of whom attend her church. She has little time to spend with her friends since she took custody of the children. Jevetta has been admitted to the hospital for asthma. You are Jevetta's student nurse.

a Using your data collection skills, identify NANDA diagnostic labels that you could apply to Jevetta and to Helen as Jevetta's caregiver.

b What resources may be helpful to Helen?

6 **a** Examine the following nursing diagnosis labels. For this set of labels, write an etiology that might be caused by cultural differences. The first one is completed for you as an example.

- Imbalanced Nutrition: Less than (or More Than) Body Requirements *r/t patient's lack of knowledge about how to adapt his preferred ethnic foods to his prescribed low-fat diet.*

- Ineffective Health Maintenance

- Ineffective Role Performance

- Anxiety

- Powerlessness

- Deficient Knowledge

b For the following set of labels, explain or give an example of how the nurse might misdiagnose or misperceive the data because of cultural differences. The first one is done for you.

- Decisional Conflict

  The nurse might ask a woman to make some decision about her care. The woman may seem very indecisive and unable to reach a conclusion. The reason may be that the husband is the decision maker in the family. When the husband arrives, the Decisional Conflict ("problem") may disappear.

- Disturbed Thought Processes

- Effective or Ineffective Breastfeeding

- Impaired Social Interaction

- Social Isolation

- Noncompliance

- Pain (Acute or Chronic)

7 For each of the following concepts, use critical thinking to describe how or why it is important to nursing, patient care, or cultural competence. Note that these are *not* to be merely definitions.

Culture

Subculture

Ethnicity

Race

Religion

Acculturation

Health and illness belief

Health and illness practice

Phenomena of culture

Ethnocentric

Folk medicine

Cultural competence

Trancultural nursing

Giger and Davidhizar assessment model

Biological variations among cultures

Prejudice and racism

Professional (e.g., nursing) subculture

Cultural sensitivity

Cultural awareness

Culture universals

Culture specifics

Practical Knowledge
knowing how

Information in this section may be useful for assessing and communicating with clients of cultures different from your own.

TECHNIQUES

TECHNIQUE 13–1	Assessing for Biological Variations

People differ genetically and physiologically. Some biological variations create susceptibility to certain diseases and injuries. The following are examples (Spector, 2004, p. 23; Andrews & Boyle, 2003):

Body Build and Structure

- 12% of Native Americans have 25 vertebrae instead of 24, which relates to an increased number of back problems.
- The lower a person's socioeconomic class, the more likely he is to be obese.
- African American and Caucasian men are on average about 3.5 inches taller than Asian American men and 2 inches taller than Mexican American men.

Skin Color

- Darker skin challenges the nurse to be more observant when assessing skin color changes (e.g., when assessing oxygenation or skin rashes).

Vital Signs

- The average systolic blood pressure of African American men between the ages of 35 and 65 is 5-mm Hg higher than European American men of the same age.

Laboratory Tests

- Native Americans, Hispanic Americans, and Japanese Americans, on average, have higher blood glucose levels than whites.

Susceptibility to Disease

- African Americans have a higher incidence of hypertension and sickle cell anemia, while Native Americans have a higher incidence of tuberculosis than other groups.

Nutritional Variations

- All groups demonstrate food preferences.
- Soy sauce, used in many Asian foods, is high in sodium.
- There is a high incidence of diabetes mellitus in areas where sugar cane is a major crop.

Enzymatic and Genetic Variations and Body Secretions

- Lactose intolerance, caused by a deficiency of the enzyme lactase, is more commonly seen in African Americans, Native Americans, and Asians.

Drug Metabolism

- Native Americans and Asians are more likely to experience facial flushing and palpitations after ingesting alcohol.
- African Americans metabolize alcohol, antihypertensives, and beta blockers differently from European Americans and they are more susceptible to side effects of haloperidol and tricyclic antidepressants.
- Asian Americans tend to experience more gastrointestinal side effects from opiates, even though the analgesic effect is less.
- Recall that most drug studies in the past were normed on European Americans, so "variations" refers to differences from those norms.

TECHNIQUE 13–2 Obtaining Minimum Cultural Information

Begin the interview with open-ended questions, such as the following:
- I would like to know more about your family.
- Who will be able to help you when you go home?
- What do you do to help keep yourself well?

You will not need to perform an in-depth cultural assessment on every patient, but you will need to recognize situations in which this is needed. Lipson and Meleis (1985) suggest that the following minimum information is important:

Language(s) spoken; proficiency in the language of the host country	• What language(s) do you speak? • Are you comfortable speaking [English], or would you like to have an interpreter?
Length of time client has been here; where client was raised	• Where were you raised? • How long have you lived here?
Ethnic affiliation and identity	• With what racial and ethnic group(s) do you identify? • How closely do you identify with the values of those groups?
Usual religious practices	• What religion do you practice? • Are there any special rituals or practices you want us to be aware of?
Nonverbal communication style	• You will need to observe the patient and draw on your theoretical knowledge of the patient's cultural group for this information.
Family roles, primary decision-maker	• Who is in your family? • Who makes most of the decisions? • How are decisions made in your family? • Who should I talk to for decisions about your health care?
Social support in the new country	• Do you have family and friends here? • Who can you go to when you need help? • Where do you work? • Will you need any help with your health care expenses?

TECHNIQUE 13–3 Assessing Pain Perception in Selected Cultural Groups

The following are some general cultural beliefs about and responses to pain. Remember that these are only a starting point and that you must never stereotype a person on the basis of culture. Assess each person individually.

Cultural Group	Pain Perception and Responses
African American heritage	Depending on the religion, may believe that pain is inevitable and must be endured; therefore, may tolerate a great deal of pain. Depending on the religion, may seek prayers and the laying on of hands for pain relief. May see pain as a test of faith. May see pain as the only sign of illness or disease, so may not follow medical treatments or therapies (e.g., for hypertension) if pain is absent.
Arab heritage	View pain as unpleasant and something to be controlled. Expect medical science to be able to relieve their suffering. Express pain openly with family members, less so with health professionals. This may cause the nurse to evaluate pain relief as adequate even though the family may be demanding more medication for the patient.
Chinese heritage	Pain expression similar to traditional U.S. culture, but description of pain may be different.
Filipino heritage	View pain as a part of living an honorable life or as an opportunity to atone for sins. Commonly tolerate severe pain, with stoic acceptance. May not complain of pain or ask for interventions.
Irish heritage	Value stoic response to pain. Ignore, deny, or minimize pain. Delay seeking treatment.
Italian heritage	Verbalization of pain is common and acceptable, even with chronic pain. Women are especially likely to report and express pain. Expect immediate treatment for pain.
Japanese heritage	It is a virtue, and a matter of family honor, to bear pain without expressing it. There may be taboos against use of narcotics for pain relief. May be more accepting of analgesics if reassured that pain control enhances healing.
Jewish heritage	Verbalization of pain is common and acceptable. Knowing the reason for pain is as important as obtaining relief.
Mexican heritage	View pain as the will of God or a part of life. May view pain as punishment for immoral behavior. May view enduring pain as a sign of strength. May endure pain longer and report it less frequently than other groups. May delay seeking help for pain, hoping it will go away.
Navajo Indian heritage	View pain as a part of life. Do not express pain openly. May hide the intensity of their pain. May not request pain medication. May prefer herbal medications for pain.
Puerto Rican heritage	Loud and outspoken expression of pain is not an exaggeration, but a socially learned coping mechanism. Older or rural people may not be able to interpret pain-rating scales. Most prefer oral or intravenous analgesics to intramuscular or rectal routes. Many use herbal teas, heat, and prayer to manage pain.

Sources: Andrews, M. M., & Boyle, J. S. (2003). *Transcultural concepts in nursing care* (4th ed.). Philadelphia: Lippincott; Giger, J., & Davidhizar, R. (2004). *Transcultural nursing: Assessment and intervention* (4th ed.). St Louis: Mosby; Purnell, L., & Paulanka, B. (2003). *Transcultural health care: A culturally competent approach* (2nd ed.). Philadelphia: F. A. Davis Company; and Spector, R. (2004). *Cultural diversity in health and illness* (6th ed.). Upper Saddle River, NJ: Prentice Hall.

TECHNIQUE 13–4   Performing a Cultural Assessment Using Giger and Davidhizar's Transcultural Assessment Model

Assess information listed in the following categories.

Cultural Uniqueness

- Cultural and ethnic identification
- Place of birth
- Time in country

Communication

- Voice quality
- Pronunciation and enunciation
- Use of silence
- Use of nonverbal communication
- Touch
- Spoken language

Space

- Degree of comfort
- Distance in conversations
- Definition of space
- Body movement

Social Organization

- Normal state of health
- Marital status
- Number of children
- Parents living or deceased
- Friends
- Work
- Leisure

Time

- Orientation to time
- View of time
- Physiochemical reaction to time

Environmental Control

- Locus of control
- Value orientation
- Health and illness beliefs

Biological Variations

- Physical assessment (including body structure, skin color, skin discoloration, hair color and distribution, other visible physical characteristics, weight, height, lab variances)
- Susceptibility to illness
- Nutritional preferences
- Psychological characteristics

In addition to the Giger and Davidhizar categories, obtain information about the following:
- Educational experiences (formal and informal)
- Family patterns of health care
- Family role and function
- Healthcare beliefs and practices (folk and professional)
- Religious practices
- Social networks
- Values orientation

Source: Adapted from Giger, J. N., & Davidhizar, R. E. (2004). *Transcultural nursing: Assessment and intervention* (4th ed.). St Louis: Mosby.

TECHNIQUE 13–5   Communicating with Clients Who Speak a Different Language

I. **When possible, use an interpreter or a translator.** An *interpreter* is specially trained to provide the meaning behind the words, whereas a *translator* just restates the words from one language to another. An interpreter can serve as a cultural broker by conveying the client's responses to questions, and by providing general information about the client's culture (Luckmann, 2000).

II. **When using any type of interpreter, it is important to do the following:**
   - Have the interpreter spend some time alone with the patient.
   - Address your questions to the client, not the interpreter.
   - Ask the interpreter to interpret the words used by the health care provider as closely as possible, except where literal translation might be offensive or misunderstood. In such cases, an interpreter (as compared to a translator) would provide the meaning of your words in terms acceptable to the client.
   - Because of confidentiality issues, avoid asking a family member, especially a child or spouse, to act as an interpreter.
   - Avoid using an interpreter who is socially or politically incompatible with client (e.g., you would not ask an Israeli to interpret for a Palestinian).
   - Be aware of gender and age differences. (It usually is preferable to have an interpreter of the same gender as the client.)
   - Do not use metaphors (pain "stabbing like a knife") or medical jargon.
   - Observe nonverbal communication (e.g., body language) when the client is listening and talking to the interpreter.
   - Maintain eye contact with both the client and interpreter.

   - Speak slowly and distinctly, facing the client; do not speak loudly.
   - Ask one question at a time; allow time for interpretation and response from the client before asking another question.
   - Use active rather than passive voice (e.g., say, "The doctor will see you tomorrow" rather than "You will be seen by the doctor tomorrow.")
   - Be aware that many clients can understand more English words than they can express.
   - Have health education materials translated into the clients' language, or have an interpreter audiotape or videotape instructions.

III. **If there is no one available to interpret for you,** in addition to the strategies listed above, Luckmann (2000, pp. 163–164) suggests the following:
   - Greet the client with respect. Greet the person formally, using Mr., Ms., and so forth, until given permission to do otherwise. People in some groups consider it disrespectful to use a person's first name.
   - Identify the client's primary language, and use any words that you are familiar with in her language to show that you are trying to communicate.
   - If appropriate, use a third language that both of you speak. For example, some Vietnamese and some Cambodians speak French.
   - Speak slowly and clearly, using simple sentences to talk about one question or need at a time.
   - Use gestures to help convey meaning.
   - Restate in different words, if needed.
   - Use pictures or diagrams.
   - Be aware that some clients may answer yes even if they don't understand what you have said.

What Are the Main Points in This Chapter?

- The cultural and ethnic composition of North America has changed dramatically over the past several decades, making it essential that nurses understand the healthcare beliefs and practices of diverse populations.

- Culture includes shared values, beliefs, norms, and practices that guide a particular group's thinking, decision making, and actions in a patterned way.

- Through acculturation, most ethnic and cultural groups modify some of their traditional cultural characteristics, values, beliefs, and practices.

- You should be familiar with the common characteristics of different cultural groups in your community.

- The U.S. Census Bureau has identified the following six racial categories: (1) American Indian or Alaska Native, (2) Asian, (3) Black or African American, (4) Native Hawaiian or Other Pacific Islander, and (5) White, (6) Other. The two Census Bureau ethnicity categories are (1) Hispanic or Latino and (2) Not Hispanic or Latino.

- Six organizing phenomena of culture that influence health include communication patterns, space, social organization, time, environmental control, and biological variations.

- Healthcare providers cannot understand the health beliefs and practices of diverse populations if they view them through the lens of the conventional (Western, U.S.) culture of health care.

- A variety of "alternative" healing systems, such as folk medicine, exists. These remedies have been passed down from generation to generation and include the use of herbs, customs, and rituals.

- An understanding of cultural concepts, theories, and models can help you develop cultural competence.

- Some barriers to culturally competent care include ethnocentrism, stereotyping, prejudice, and racism.

- When assessing a client, you must consider the client's cultural values, beliefs, and practices related to health and health care.

- Culturally competent care requires a nonjudgmental attitude, self-awareness, sensitivity, respect for differences, and theoretical knowledge.

Knowledge Map

Culture and Ethnicity

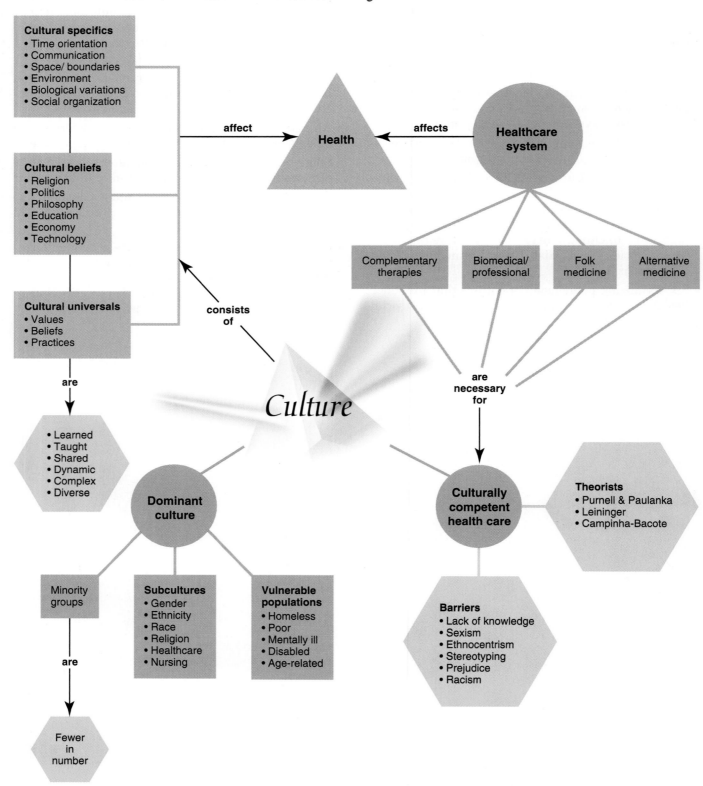

Cultural specifics
• Time orientation
• Communication
• Space/ boundaries
• Environment
• Biological variations
• Social organization

Cultural beliefs
• Religion
• Politics
• Philosophy
• Education
• Economy
• Technology

Cultural universals
• Values
• Beliefs
• Practices

are

• Learned
• Taught
• Shared
• Dynamic
• Complex
• Diverse

affect → **Health** ← affects **Healthcare system**

consists of

Culture

Complementary therapies   Biomedical/ professional   Folk medicine   Alternative medicine

are necessary for

Dominant culture

Culturally competent health care

Theorists
• Purnell & Paulanka
• Leininger
• Campinha-Bacote

Minority groups

Subcultures
• Gender
• Ethnicity
• Race
• Religion
• Healthcare
• Nursing

Vulnerable populations
• Homeless
• Poor
• Mentally ill
• Disabled
• Age-related

Barriers
• Lack of knowledge
• Sexism
• Ethnocentrism
• Stereotyping
• Prejudice
• Racism

are

Fewer in number

Spirituality

Overview

Nursing has historical roots in religion and spirituality, and research now suggests that religion and spirituality have the potential to affect people's health and well-being. Nurses who are open to diversity, including different forms of spiritual expression, are comfortable in the spiritual care domain. Currently, nurses work with other disciplines to provide spiritual care.

Religion is a sort of "map" that outlines and integrates essential beliefs and values. Within any religion, people vary in the degree to which they follow the rituals and practices. In contrast, spirituality can be seen as a more personal "journey"—an attempt to find meaning, value, and purpose in life.

Spiritual assessment tools can help you gather spiritual data about your client, and other such tools can help you clarify your spiritual values. In addition, your understanding of the world's major religions will help you provide comprehensive, compassionate care to patients. The three NANDA labels that describe spiritual needs are Spiritual Distress, Risk for Spiritual Distress, and Readiness for Enhanced Spiritual Well-Being.

Thinking Critically About Spirituality

The exercises in the following section allow you to practice the kind of thinking you will use as a full-spectrum nurse. Because these are critical-thinking activities, there is usually no single right answer. Discuss answers with your peers—discussion can stimulate critical thinking. If you have difficulty with any of the questions, consult with your instructor.

Caring for the Garcias

Bettina Sanford is the 3-year-old grandchild of Joseph and Flordelisa Garcia. The Garcias are both practicing Catholics. Bettina's mother, Corazón, is the Garcia's daughter. Corazón feels that Catholicism is "a waste of time" and does not attend church. Bettina has had no formal religious experiences or training.

A. At a clinic visit, Joe asks you what you think about keeping religion away from a child. How would you respond?

B. Joe explains his views on the situation: "If anything were to happen to her, she would go straight to hell. I think we should take her to Church and get her baptized right away. I don't know how anyone can live like that. She has no connection to God." Do you agree with this statement? Explain your views.

C. Joe asks you to pray for Bettina and her mother. How would you feel about this situation? What would you say to Joe?

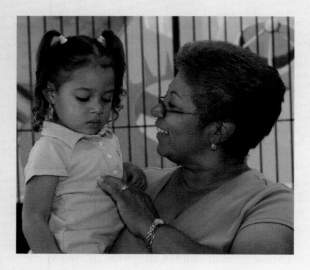

---

1   A 5-year-old boy was admitted to the hospital last night with a fever of 103°F (39.4°C). He was diagnosed with a serious infection that is easily treated with intravenous (IV) antibiotics. However, his parents are Christian Scientists, and they do not want the boy to be given antibiotics. They have called their Christian Science practitioner to visit as soon as possible.

   a What practical knowledge do you have that will give you some insight into this situation?

b What essential piece of knowledge do you need that is *not* given in this scenario?

c If the parents do not agree to accepting IV antibiotics for their child, what can you do to (1) ensure that the child receives treatment and (2) to support their spiritual needs?

2 A woman is admitted to the emergency department and gives birth to a premature baby boy who is in severe respiratory distress. The woman is a devout Roman Catholic. What interventions could you use to provide holistic spiritual care in such an emergency situation?

3 Interview nurses in the area where you have your clinical experiences. Discuss the interviews with classmates.

a Ask them to describe spiritual problems their patients have had.

b Ask them to tell you of any spiritual interventions they have used with patients and how effective they believe them to be.

c Ask them how comfortable they are in using spiritual interventions, especially prayer.

4

For each of the following concepts, use critical thinking to describe how or why it is important to nursing, patient care, or spirituality. Note that these are *not* to be merely definitions.

Spirituality and religion

Nursing research in religion and health care

Major religions and health care

The nurse and spirituality

Assessment of the spiritual domain of care

Spiritual care nursing interventions

Spiritual well-being

Practical Knowledge
knowing how

In this section you will find guidelines for performing spiritual assessments and interventions, including guidelines for prayer.

ASSESSMENT GUIDELINES AND TOOLS

Spiritual Assessment

(based on Highfield, 2000)

- Obtain information from the patient when possible.
- For an emergency admission or if the patient cannot give information, consult the next of kin or a designated power of attorney (DPOA) as soon as possible for information.
- Assess the following key areas.

S—Spiritual/religious belief system
Religion, tradition, sect, or denominational affiliation
Text/writing(s) that provide source of authority and codes for behavior
Name and phone number of supporting or affiliated church, synagogue, temple, or other place of worship
Past experience with belief system (positive or negative)
Beliefs related to health, illness, health care, healthcare providers, Western medicine, adjuvant therapies, herbal or natural healing methods or techniques
Beliefs about suffering, terminal or chronic illness, advanced directives, autopsy, organ donation
Pertinent stigmas related to illness, if applicable

P—Personal spirituality
Individual beliefs and practices of affiliation that patient or family accepts and attempts to follow (may be directly or indirectly related to above assessment areas)
Individual beliefs that may differ or even be contrary to affiliation beliefs
Whether spirituality is a part of personal experience of religion or a separate entity
Level of comfort discussing spirituality
Whether personal spirituality is viewed positively or negatively at the present time

I—Integration with a spiritual community
Name and title of religious or spirtual leader or authority figure(s)
Names and titles of religious groups that may need to be contacted: Stephen Ministry, prayer group leader, prayer chain support person, shaman, medicine man or woman, men's or women's group within denomination

Role of patient or individual in any of above named groups

R—Ritualized practices and restrictions
Activities that patient or family's faith encourages or forbids
Needs for modesty and covering of body parts or appendages
Any special beliefs or needs in relation to drawing blood or to laboratory tests or procedures
Dietary needs and restrictions: food preferences, preparation of foods, and location of food preparation areas
Gender-specific roles and responsibilities of care providers
Prayer needs and restrictions: Who delivers and offers such practices?
Articles or other materials needed for worship, devotion, or prayer (rosaries, prayer beads, prayer books, religious tracts, Bibles, crosses, prayer shawls or cloths)

I—Implications for medical care
Beliefs and practices that healthcare providers should remember while providing care
Specific medications that may not be administered and withheld; implications for pain-control
Specific medical procedures or products that may not be administered (abortion, blood products)
Communication patterns and needs for effective care delivery: Who makes decisions? What is the role of parents or guardians when children or other vulnerable populations are the recipients of care? Does the guardian reflect the beliefs of patient, if these are known?

T—Terminal events planning
Wishes for advance directives (cardiopulmonary resuscitation, intubation, ventilator assist, feeding tubes)
Wishes for transplantation or organ donation
Need for religious services (last rites, ministries of healing, baptism, initiation, communion, confession)
Clergy or ministry groups to be contacted and when
Ideas of afterlife
Treatment of body at time of death
Funeral planning

Other Assessments

You can acquire information about a patient's spirituality from a variety of sources other than interviews.

- *Patient's environment.* Observe the patient's environment for hints about her spirituality (e.g., pictures of family and or pets, the presence of sacred texts or reading materials, articles used in worship [a crucifix, rosary beads], or copies of church bulletins/sermon tapes).

- *Patient's questions.* The patient may ask questions that are indicative of spiritual comfort, longing, or distress. For example, the patient may ask if you attend church and if so, does it provide you with a sense of comfort and meaning.

- *Patient's behaviors, moods, and feelings.* Multiple behaviors/moods/feelings give clear and certain indication that the patient is struggling with issues that have spiritual overtones. These warrant further assessment and nursing intervention. For example, a patient may ask you if you have ever really felt guilty about something you did as a child.

- *Nonverbal communication.* Body language may indicate hopeful or distressing times. For example, you may observe a patient praying; or when asking about spirituality, you may see the patient rolling his eyes, shaking his head, and demonstrating muscle tension.

TECHNIQUES

| TECHNIQUE 14–1 | Using Selected NIC Interventions and Activities for Spiritual Diagnoses |

Dying Care

Facilitate obtaining spiritual support for patient and family.

Support patient and family through stages of grief.

Facilitate discussion of funeral arrangements.

Forgiveness Facilitation

Listen empathetically without moralizing or offering platitudes.

Explore forgiveness as a process.

Assist client to seek out arbitrator (objective party) to facilitate process of individual or group concern.

Explore possibilities of making amends and reconciliation with self, others, and/or higher power.

Hope Instillation

Assist patient/family to identify areas of hope in life.

Help the patient expand spiritual self.

Facilitate the patient/family's reliving and savoring past achievements and experiences.

Create an environment that facilitates patient practicing religion, as appropriate.

Presence

Be physically available as a helper.

Remain physically present without expecting interactional responses.

Offer to remain with patient during initial interaction with others in the unit.

Listen to the patient's concerns.

Stay with the patient to promote safety and reduce fear.

Self-Awareness Enhancement

Assist patient to realize that everyone is unique.

Assist patient to identify life priorities.

Assist patient to identify guilty feelings.

Assist patient to identify source of motivation.

Spiritual Growth Facilitation

Encourage conversation that assists the patient in sorting out spiritual concerns.

Assist patient with identifying barriers and attitudes that hinder growth or self-discovery.

Offer individual and group prayer support, as appropriate.

Encourage participation in devotional services, retreats, and special prayer/study programs.

Assist the patient to explore beliefs as related to healing of body, mind, and spirit.

Refer for pastoral care or primary spiritual caregiver as issues warrant.

Spiritual Support

Be open to patient's expressions of loneliness and powerlessness.

Encourage chapel service attendance, if desired.

Provide desired spiritual articles, according to individual preferences.

Be available to listen to individual's feelings.

Listen carefully to individual's communication, and develop a sense of timing for prayer or spiritual rituals.

Be open to individual's feelings about illness and death.

Values Clarification

Think through the ethical and legal aspects of free choice, given the particular situation, before beginning the intervention.

Pose reflective, clarifying questions that give the patient something to think about.

Encourage patient to make a list of what is important and not important in life and the time spent on each.

Encourage patient to list values that guide behavior in various settings and types of situations.

Avoid use of this intervention with persons with serious emotional problems.

Other NIC Spiritual Care Interventions

Active Listening	Crisis Intervention
Anticipatory Guidance	Decision-Making Support
Anxiety Reduction	Emotional Support
Bibliotherapy	Grief Work Facilitation
Coping Enhancement	Guilt Work Facilitation
Counseling	Humor

►

TECHNIQUE 14–1 Using Selected NIC Interventions and Activities for Spiritual Interventions *(continued)*

Meditation Facilitation	Religious Addiction	Resiliency Promotion	Self-Responsibility
Mood Management	Prevention	Role Enhancement	Facilitation
Music Therapy	Religious Ritual	Self-Esteem Enhancement	Support Group
Referral	Enhancement	Self-Modification Assistance	Touch

Source: Dochterman, J. M., & Bulechek, G. M. (Eds.). (2004). *Nursing interventions classification (NIC)* (4th ed.). St Louis: Mosby, pp. 880–881.

TECHNIQUE 14–2 Praying with Patients

Because there is a rich diversity in religious expression, keep the following guidelines in mind when you pray for or with patients:

1. ***Ask how the patient prefers to address the divine.*** Some people prefer the use of parental language in their prayers, for example, *Father God* or *Divine Mother*. Some use the word *Jehovah, Yahweh,* or *Allah.* Hindus may address one or more of multiple gods, each of whom has several names. So don't be afraid to seek direction from the patient in these matters: most people are honored to be able to explain their beliefs and practices to someone who is open to the experience.

2. ***Before the prayer begins, ask the patient whether any rituals or religious items are necessary.*** Muslims may want water to wash the mouth, nostrils, and hands before beginning prayer. Roman Catholics may want to hold their rosary beads while praying, and some Buddhists and Hindus meditate with a set of beads called a *mala.* Others may have a prayer cloth or other item that needs to be accessible.

3. ***Always feel free to pray or not to.*** Never feel that you are being forced to do or say something that makes you uncomfortable.

4. ***Do not be a compulsive "pray-er" or a compulsive avoider of prayer.*** Always make sure that the patient (and/or family) is comfortable with prayer if they have not yet requested it.

5. ***Know that there are appropriate times and places for the offering of prayer.*** Although it may be most appropriate at the bedside, prayer may make people uncomfortable in a crowded waiting room. Perhaps the statement "I will be praying for you and

your family" might be more appropriate than actually praying aloud at that moment.

6. ***When a patient asks for prayer, consider using this reply:*** "I would be honored to offer prayer. What would you like me to *especially* address in the prayer?" Knowing what the patient hopes for in prayer gives you an idea of the type of prayer the person is requesting.

7. ***When the patient tells you what he wants you to pray for, be sure to focus your prayer around the request.*** It is always good to summarize the results of previous conversations with the patient and his needs in the course of your prayer. For example, imagine that a patient with cancer who has been treated with chemotherapy now finds his blood counts are coming back to normal levels. The chemotherapy treatment seems successful at this point, but the patient is afraid of a relapse and asks you to pray for the cancer to be cured. There is a lot going on in this situation and it is easy to get lost in the complexity of need. Analyze the situation in terms of what has happened in the past, what is happening now, and what the patient is requesting. This will help you organize your thoughts and then put them into the form of a prayer. Perhaps you would want to take the patient's hand in yours (if appropriate, based on your intuition and the nature of your nurse-patient relationship) and compose a prayer in the following manner: Dear [Lord], I give you thanks that [John] has done so well with his treatments. Please continue to help him be to be strong and open to your healing presence. We pray for his family, doctors, and nurses that all may be a part of [John's] continued healing and sense of

TECHNIQUE 14–2   Praying with Patients *(continued)*

comfort. I pray that the treatments that he is receiving, together with the prayers that we are offering, may all be effective in his care and in the treatment of his cancer. Watch over [John], and visit us all at this time with your healing presence. [Amen.]

8. ***When a terminally ill patient requests a prayer for a cure, total healing, or a miracle,*** you may be challenged. Knowing how to pray prayers that are "realistic" allows for the occurrence of miracles and healings of all types while also keeping in perspective the physical realities of the nature of disease and the reality of death.

9. ***If composing a prayer is difficult for you,*** you may want to explore the use of the Psalms in The Hebrew Bible (Old Testament) or some New Testament scriptures, if appropriate for the patient. (See especially Psalms 43, 51, 67, 121). In terms of larger themes, the following sources for patients who profess Christianity may be helpful:

> *Forgiveness and guilt:* Psalm 51, Isaiah 55:7, and Matthew 6:9-15
> *Comfort:* Psalm 23, John 14

> *Hope:* Psalm 42, Romans 15:4
> *Love and acceptance:* Matthew 5:11
> *Caring:* I Corinthians 12

For exact quotations of these passages,

 Go to Chapter 14, **Psalms for Prayers,** on the Electronic Study Guide.

For patients of other religions, ask whether they have examples of their sacred writings from which you might be allowed to read. Perhaps the patient has a favorite prayer or a text from an authoritative source that brings comfort and hope.

10. ***It is always good to include in the course of your prayer a request for God's help and direction with the patient's healthcare team,*** doctors, surgeons, and family members. This expresses the reality that we are all working together for a common good and purpose and that we depend on God and others for our welfare and place in life.

11. ***Once the prayer is over, thank the patient for asking you to participate*** in that way and ask whether you can be of any further assistance.

What Are the Main Points in This Chapter?

- Spirituality is a powerful force in the lives of many patients—a force that has the potential to affect their health and perception of well-being.
- Nursing has historical roots in religion and spirituality.
- Nurses work with other disciplines to provide spiritual care.
- Religion is a sort of "map" that outlines and integrates essential beliefs, values, and codes of conduct into a manner of living.
- Spirituality, like a journey, takes place over time and involves the accumulation of life experiences and understandings. It is the attempt to find meaning, value, and purpose in life.
- Spiritual development involves struggles with faith, hope, and love.
- Religion and spirituality affect health and well-being; and in turn, health and well-being affect a person's religion and spirituality.

- Research suggests that religion and spirituality are important to healthcare outcomes; however, it does not explain *how* or *why* this is so.
- The more you know about similarities in and differences among the world's major religions, the more you will be able to offer comprehensive, compassionate care to patients.
- People, even within the same religion, vary greatly in the degree to which they follow the rituals and practices of their religion.
- Self knowledge helps you to avoid abuses of spiritual care (e.g., imposing your religion on a patient).
- Barriers to spiritual care include (1) lack of awareness of spirituality in general and of your own spiritual belief system, (2) differences in spirituality between you (the nurse) and the patient, (3) fear that your spiritual knowledge is insufficient, and (4) fear of where spiritual discussions might lead.

- Various ready-made tools are available for performing an in-depth spiritual assessment.
- Three NANDA labels to describe spiritual needs are Spiritual Distress, Risk for Spiritual Distress, and Readiness for Enhanced Spiritual Well-Being.
- Nursing interventions related to spiritual care require you to be self-aware, fully present, supportive, empathetic, and nonjudgmental and to have a wish to benefit the patient.
- When a patient asks you to pray, you must determine whether he wishes you to pray *for* or *with* him, and you should ask what he would like you to *especially* address in the prayer.
- A miracle does not necessarily involve the notion of a cure; miracles are more often events that proceed according to natural law but still have a powerful impact upon the person's expectations.
- Nurses who are open to diversity, who exhibit multiple understandings of religion, and who fashion for themselves different means of spiritual expression are comfortable in the spiritual care domain.

Knowledge Map

Spirituality

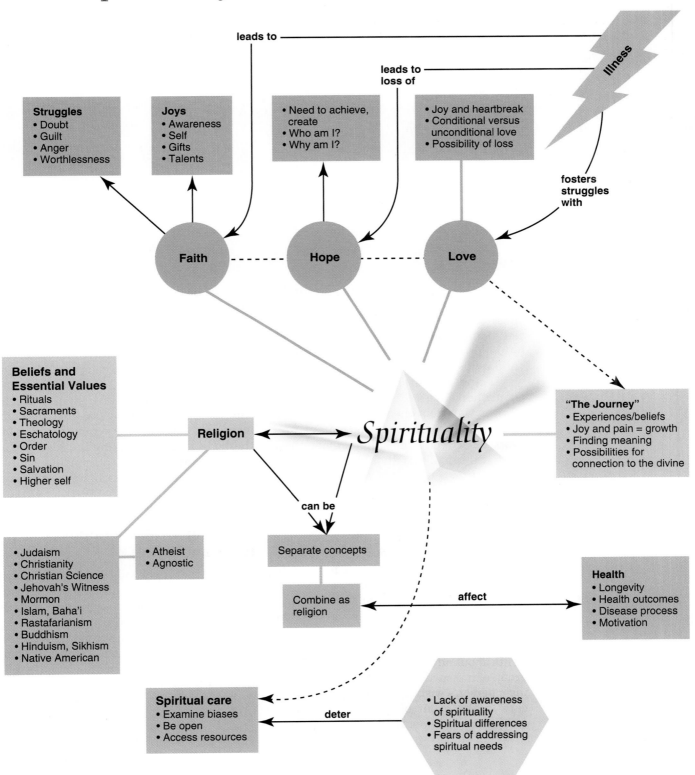

leads to

leads to
loss of

Illness

Struggles
• Doubt
• Guilt
• Anger
• Worthlessness

Joys
• Awareness
• Self
• Gifts
• Talents

• Need to achieve, create
• Who am I?
• Why am I?

• Joy and heartbreak
• Conditional versus unconditional love
• Possibility of loss

fosters struggles with

Faith

Hope

Love

Beliefs and Essential Values
• Rituals
• Sacraments
• Theology
• Eschatology
• Order
• Sin
• Salvation
• Higher self

Religion

Spirituality

"The Journey"
• Experiences/beliefs
• Joy and pain = growth
• Finding meaning
• Possibilities for connection to the divine

can be

• Judaism
• Christianity
• Christian Science
• Jehovah's Witness
• Mormon
• Islam, Baha'i
• Rastafarianism
• Buddhism
• Hinduism, Sikhism
• Native American

• Atheist
• Agnostic

Separate concepts

Combine as religion

affect

Health
• Longevity
• Health outcomes
• Disease process
• Motivation

Spiritual care
• Examine biases
• Be open
• Access resources

deter

• Lack of awareness of spirituality
• Spiritual differences
• Fears of addressing spiritual needs

15 CHAPTER

Loss, Grief, & Dying

Overview

How people cope with loss (e.g., of independence, self-esteem, body image, loved ones) directly affects their healing and well-being. You can facilitate grief work by using therapeutic communication to validate feelings ("It's normal to feel that way") and encouraging people to talk about their losses. People do not move in a linear way from one stage of grief to the next; there is constant movement and overlap between stages. Remember, most grief is normal; you should not diagnose Dysfunctional Grieving for every person who is grieving a loss.

In palliative care, comfort and symptom relief are provided, but no further efforts are made to stop the disease process or prevent death. The purpose of hospice care is to allow terminally ill persons to experience death with dignity.

The Uniform Determination of Death Act states the conditions determining that death has occurred. Healthcare providers are responsible for educating staff and patients about advance directives, which is a group of instructions (written or oral) stating a person's wishes concerning his health care in the event of mental or physical incapacity. A *do not attempt resuscitation* (DNAR) order is a specific order *not* to do cardiopulmonary resuscitation.

When the patient is near death, focus on relieving physical symptoms and emotional distress. If he can communicate, ask about immediate concerns. At the moment of death, do not interrupt or intrude upon the family; give them as much time as they need to say good-bye to their loved one; express your sympathy. Care of the body includes making it presentable for the family, carefully placing identification tags, and arranging to have the body sent to the morgue.

Thinking Critically About Loss, Grief, and Dying

The exercises in the following section allow you to practice the kind of thinking you will use as a full-spectrum nurse. Because these are critical-thinking activities, there is usually no single right answer. Discuss answers with your peers—discussion can stimulate critical thinking. If you have difficulty with any of the questions, consult with your instructor.

Caring for the Garcias

At a clinic visit, Joe Garcia tells you that his father's health is declining rapidly. Joe tells you, "I thought he was doing ok. I knew he had surgery for his prostate, so I thought it was all over. Lately he's been having lots of low back and hip pain. So my mom begged him to go to the doctor, and they told him he has cancer all over." Joe shakes his head and looks away from you. You notice tears in his eyes.

As you talk with him, he tells you that his family has avoided discussions about serious illness and death. "It just never got discussed. The whole idea made my parents uncomfortable. When my father got sick the first time, he refused to discuss it. 'I'm going to get better. Don't even think about it,' he would say." Now Joe feels the need to discuss this situation with his parents but doesn't know how to bring up the topic. He asks for your advice.

A. What would you think and feel when you see Joe's tears and when Joe asks for this advice?

B. What would you advise Joe?

C. What type of grief is Joe experiencing?

D. Examine the factors that affect grief. Apply these factors to Joe's situation. You will need to review the family history included in the introduction to the Garcias (in the front of this book) to fully answer this question. Indicate whether the information for any of the factors to be evaluated is insufficient.

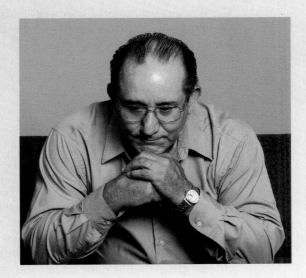

1 Jessie McCarthy is a 69-year-old woman who is terminally ill with multiple myeloma. She is currently hospitalized for a week of chemotherapy. Her husband of 49 years is recuperating from recent hip surgery and has difficulty getting around. Her daughter and son-in-law are very close to them, and her granddaughter, 14 years old, has a very special relationship with her "Gammie." The side effects of Mrs. McCarthy's chemotherapy include nausea and headaches. She doesn't like to have people around when she feels this way. Jessie's pastor comes to visit every other day and seems to bring her comfort. Her 50th wedding anniversary will occur when she is in the hospital. She verbalizes fear of "not making it home this time." You are her nurse in a hospital where palliative care is provided. Begin developing a holistic plan of care for Mrs. McCarthy, addressing the main issues noted.

a What immediate physical problems does Mrs. McCarthy have? Do not use her medical diagnosis as an answer.

b What might you do to meet her physical needs?

c What psychological needs does Mrs. McCarthy have: (1) what are her fears? (2) what social and emotional issues is she facing? (3) how might you help meet her needs?

2 You are caring for Jack Wirtz, a 37-year-old male who was admitted to the hospital for a lumbar laminectomy. As you are doing Jack's pre-op assessments, he tells you that his 12-year-old son died 6 months ago in an automobile accident in which Jack was the driver. He is a builder and has been out of work since the accident. His wife has gone back to work to help support them. Jack's affect is flat, and he talks in a monotone.

a What losses has Jack experienced?

b What further assessments need to be made for Jack, and why?

3 Marie is 84 years old and has sustained a right-sided cerebrovascular accident (CVA, or stroke). Doctors say she is unlikely to regain much physical function, if she even awakens from the coma. She was alert and active prior to her stroke and was able to maintain her independence with the help of a home health aide, who assisted her with ADLs and meal preparation three times a week. Kelly and Dan, her children, have met with the physician, who wants to put a feeding tube into Marie and has asked about resuscitation orders. Kelly wants to do what is best for her mother, but she feels that Marie would not want to be kept alive in the condition she is in. She is also concerned about putting her through uncomfortable procedures if there is no chance of recovery. Her brother, Dan, thinks Marie should have the feeding tube. Kelly asks to speak with you and wants to know the best thing to do for her mother.

a Write a possible nursing diagnosis to describe Kelly's situation.

b How do you think the situation came to this? What might Kelly, Dan, and Marie have done prior to the stroke to prevent this confusion and indecision?

c What are your responsibilities? What might you do to help Kelly and Dan?

4 A patient requests your participation in a plan for assisted suicide or seeks passive euthanasia. What are your options as a nurse? Use the Internet to get information about this.

a List the URLs for the pages you found to be helpful in answering the question. Beside each URL, state the name of the organization, person, or agency to whom the web site belongs.

b For each URL, state what you believe to be the *purpose* of the web site.

thinking critically about loss, grief, & dying

5 Find a partner. Take 5 minutes to describe to her a personal loss you have had (e.g., a person, a pet, an object, an aspect of health). The partner must listen silently and not speak at all during this 5 minutes. When you have finished, answer the following questions.

a What did you feel when describing your loss?

b Did you feel that the listener was really listening to you?

c How did the listener respond to you?

6 Now reverse the process; you become the listener. When you have finished, answer the following questions:

a What did you feel while you were listening?

b Did the time go quickly or seem long?

c What did you learn from this listening experience?

7 John is 17 years old and volunteers at the hospital. He has just moved from another state because of his father's work, so he is a new senior in high school. As you chat with him, he reveals that his mother is getting radiation and chemotherapy treatments for breast cancer and has been very ill. What are some loss issues this young man is facing?

8 Sharon is a 48-year-old woman who is in the hospital for a hysterectomy (removal of her uterus) due to fibroids and heavy bleeding. With teary eyes, she shares with you, her nurse for the evening, that she is feeling "down" and doesn't want any visitors this evening. She says, "I really thought I would feel better after having this surgery done."

a Why do you think Sharon is teary and feeling "down"?

b What should you do to begin helping Sharon cope with her loss?

9 You are having lunch with a nursing colleague, who reveals to you that her mother has Alzheimer's disease. Her mother has been placed in a nursing home because she is losing her memory and is not safe at home. Your friend tells you that lately she (the nurse) has been feeling distracted, angry for no reason, and can't seem to shake her feelings of sadness. How would you respond?

a What might be causing your colleague to feel distracted and angry?

b How would you respond to her?

10

You are caring for Mr. Bishop, a 57-year-old man who is terminally ill with metastatic bone cancer. He wants to donate his organs for research after his death, but his wife is totally against this.

a What do you do or say to him to help resolve this issue? Go to the following URL, and download the organ donor brochure for information to use in this situation: *http://www.organdonor.gov/signup1.html*

b Now go to the bottom of the page and look at the logo and other information. Who do you think provides and maintains the content for this web site? What else would give you a clue about the source of the site?

c Now go to *http://www.organdonor.gov* (the home page), and click on "HHS." What department of the U.S. government "owns" this page?

d In the lower right-hand corner of the HHS page is an item called "Features." Under that is a link called "Gift of Life: Organ Donation Initiative." (If the web page has been updated, the link may be in another place. Look for it. If you cannot find it, then search for "organ donation initiative.") Where does that link take you?

e From what you discovered in (d), can you conclude which branch of the federal government is responsible for the organ donation initiative?

11

For each of the following concepts, use critical thinking to describe how or why it is important to nursing, patient care, or loss, grief, and dying. Note that these are *not* to be merely definitions.

Physical loss

Actual loss

Complicated grief

Disenfranchised grief

Significance of the loss

Stages of grief

Advanced directives

Assisted suicide

Palliative care

Practical Knowledge
knowing how

TECHNIQUES

This section provides guidelines for communicating with people who are grieving, caring for dying patients and their families, and providing postmortem care.

TECHNIQUE 15–1   Communicating with People Who Are Grieving

- *Perfect your listening skills.*
  - Listen to what is *not* said as well as what is said.
  - Be alert for nonverbal cues.
- *Respond to nonverbal cues with appropriate touch and eye contact.* A smile, a gentle touch, sitting with a patient, and eye contact all relay a message of genuine care and concern. You may not need to say very much at all.
- *Encourage and accept expression of feelings.*
  - Receiving expression of intense feelings (e.g., anger and guilt) may be painful for you. It may help to remember that it is therapeutic for people to express their feelings.
  - You don't need to change the person's feelings or "make them better." As much as we would like to do this, it is not possible.
  - You do need to validate the person's feelings (e.g., "It is normal to feel that way; it is OK")
- *Reassure the person that it is not "wrong" to feel anger, guilt, relief, or other feelings she may believe to be unacceptable.*
  - A dying patient might say, "I know it's awful, but I feel so angry with God for giving me this

disease." Or a bereaved spouse might admit, "I shouldn't feel this way, but I'm relieved that it's finally over."
  - Patients need to hear you say their feelings are not "wrong" or "bad" and that they are going through a normal process.
- *Increase your self awareness.* Become more aware of your own attitudes and feelings regarding death and dying. If you are comfortable with these phenomena, you will be able to hear patients' expressions of anger, guilt, frustration, fear, and loneliness more comfortably.
- *Continue to communicate with dying patients even if they are in a coma. Encourage family members to do so as well.*
  - Talk to the patient. Tell him what is going on around him, what care you are providing, and when you or others enter or are about to leave the room. Research indicates that patients continue to hear even though they cannot respond, sometimes up to the moment of death.
  - Avoid discussing the dying person as though he were not present.

TECHNIQUE 15–2 Helping Families of Dying Patients

- View the family as your unit of care.
- Provide education, support, and a listening ear.
- Encourage family members to help with care if they are able. This helps meet their need to be useful as well as promoting family ties and making the patient more comfortable. Provide instruction and supervision as appropriate. If family members are not physically or emotionally able to provide care, accept that.
- Encourage family members to ask questions, listen actively to the patient's and family's concerns, and help them solve problems when needed.
- Follow up with other healthcare team members promptly if the family has questions that are outside your scope of practice.
- Encourage the family to visit the hospital chapel and to talk with a chaplain or to speak with their own spiritual adviser.
- Provide anticipatory guidance to the family regarding the stages of loss and grief, so that they will know what to expect after their loved one dies.
- Acknowledge the family's feelings and the loss they are experiencing. Many times family members begin the grieving process before the loved one dies.
- Help the family members explore past coping mechanisms and reinforce successful past coping mechanisms.

- Remind family members and significant others to take care of themselves. Watching a loved one die is a very difficult experience. A sensitive, caring nurse can make it a little easier.
  - Many times they need "permission" to go eat or to go home and rest.
  - If the patient is near death and family and friends do not want to leave the patient's side, make them as comfortable as possible.
  - Provide comfortable chairs, coffee, and snacks (according to organizational policy), and be alert for other needs they may have.
- Teach the family what to expect with regard to medications, treatments, and signs of approaching death. If family members know what is normal, they will be less likely to panic or fear the inevitable.
- As physical signs of death become apparent, keep the family informed. You may say something like, "Her blood pressure is becoming difficult to hear. That is one of the signs that she is closer to death."
- Reassure families of patients who become withdrawn near the time of death that this does not mean the patient is rejecting them, but only that his body is conserving energy and that he has come to terms with dying.
- When approaching death is apparent, ask family members directly, "Do you want to be present while he is dying?" Tell them what to expect, if they do not know.

TECHNIQUE 15–3 Caring for the Dying Person

Meeting Physiological Needs

Active dying usually occurs over a period of 10 to 14 days (although it can take as little as 24 hours). The "final hours" refers to the last 4 to 48 hours of life, in which failure of body systems results in death (Pitorak, 2003). Physiological needs during this time include mobility, oxygenation, safety, nutrition, fluids, elimination, personal hygiene, and pain and control of symptoms (nausea, vomiting).

- Encourage the patient to be as independent as possible, so that she will maintain a sense of control.
- Monitor the patient's energy level. If she tires easily or lacks the energy to care for herself, you should provide this care.
- Maintain skin integrity.
  - Turn the patient frequently.
  - Provide massage to increase circulation.
  - Assess for increased diaphoresis and/or incontinence.
  - Maintain adequate nutrition.
  - During the final hours of life, the goal of these activities changes from preserving skin integrity to providing comfort. Realize that during this time even excellent care may not prevent skin breakdown.
- If the patient is comatose or unconscious, provide special care for the eyes so they do not become too dry. Many agencies use a form of artificial tears for this purpose.
- If the patient is not able to take fluids, wet the lips and mouth frequently with cool water or with a prepared product to prevent dryness and cracking of lips and mucous membranes. There is some evidence that glycerin swabs dry the mucous membranes and should not be used.
  - You may provide artificial hydration unless the patient has an advance directive requesting no artificial hydration per nasogastric or intravenous route. However, IV fluids can cause edema, nausea, and even pain in a patient who is actively dying.
- Assess for and provide interventions for constipation, urinary retention, and incontinence. Pads are helpful, but change them frequently to prevent skin breakdown and, near the end, to promote comfort.
- Administer laxatives for constipation.
- Catheterize the patient if he is unable to void and the bladder becomes distended.
- Intervene for "death rattle" if it occurs and if it is distressing to the family.
  - Turn the patient on his side, and elevate the head of the bed.
  - Administer antispasmodic and anticholinergic medications if necessary.
- Provide adequate pain control. This can be a major issue for patients and caregivers. In fact, dying patients are often more concerned about pain and loss of control than about dying itself. See Chapter 30 for more information about pain management.
  - Provide education as necessary to dispel the myths about pain medication (e.g., addiction, overdose). Effective pain control medications exist and can be administered by various routes.
  - Assure the patient and family that analgesics will not be addictive in this situation.
  - Respect the patient's informed decision to refuse pain medications. For example, a patient may prefer to endure pain rather than to be sleepy and not alert when his family is at the bedside.
  - Follow one of the common pain protocols to ensure that pain is controlled.
  - To ensure pain control, administer pain medication on a regular schedule instead of waiting until the patient asks (prn).
  - Teach and perform nonpharmacological pain-relief measures when you judge they may be helpful. These might include meditation, heat/cold therapies, massage, distraction, imagery, deep breathing, and herbal-scented lotions. It may be soothing to play soft music, add "white noise," or turn off the television.
  - Patients who are near death may moan or grunt as they breathe; this does not necessarily indicate pain. Be sure that families understand this.
- Provide medication for other symptoms, such as nausea.
- Continue to talk to the patient as if he can hear. Do not talk about him to others in his presence. The patient is usually able to hear even after he can no longer respond to sounds and other stimuli.

Meeting Psychological Needs

Patients experience many emotions at end of life, including anger, sadness, depression, fear, relief, loneliness, and grief. At this time communication and support are most helpful. Discussing concerns and issues is a viable means of coping. The following interventions are important:

- Answer all questions honestly.
- Explain procedures that are being done.
- Realize that the patient may feel he is losing control.
  - Help the person acknowledge what she does have control over.

TECHNIQUE 15–3 *(continued)*

- Include the patient in care decisions as much as she is able to participate.
- Attend to social needs. Relationships are a priority at this time. Some patients may simply need to keep the bonds with family members and friends intact. For other patients, this may be a time to reestablish or mend relationships.
- Early in the dying process, assess the sources of financial support for the patient and family.
  - Finances may be a concern and may place an additional burden on the family.
  - The patient may feel she is a burden to care for.
- Be aware of sexual needs, and suggest ways a couple can be close and affectionate at this time. Some people may feel it is not right to have sexual feelings when the person they love is dying. Others may be afraid of harming the patient if they are sexually intimate.
  - Provide realistic information about these issues.
  - Be aware that expressions of sexuality may change as a person becomes closer to death.

- When the patient is very near death, focus on relieving symptoms (e.g., pain, nausea) and emotional distress.
- If the person can communicate, ask about immediate concerns (Pitorak, 2003):
  - "Are you in pain?" "Are you comfortable?"
  - "What are you afraid of now?"
  - "What can we do to help you go peacefully?"
  - "Who do you want in the room with you right now?"
  - If the patient asks whether he is dying, be honest.
  - If the patient cannot communicate, ask the family, who may know what the patient would want.
- When the patient is very near death, it may be helpful to say something like, "Your family will be fine" rather than, "It is OK for you to go now."
- Be aware that some people seem to wait to die until after a significant date (birthday, anniversary, and so on) has passed. Others wait for family to gather, whereas others wait until loved ones leave so they will not upset the family by dying in their presence.

TECHNIQUE 15–4   Providing Postmortem Care

Supporting the Family

- At the moment of death, do not interrupt or intrude on the family. Wait quietly and observe. Give them as much time as they need. When they move away from the body, or have said last good-byes, then it is time to assess and report the lack of vital signs.
- Immediately after death, express sympathy to the family. This is very important. Make a simple statement, such as, "I am sorry for your loss." Avoid statements that interpret the situation for the family, such as, "It's God's will." Also avoid attempts to mitigate the family member's grief, for example, "It will get better in time," or "You still have your son."
- If the family wishes to be alone with the body, straighten the bedcovers and make the patient look as natural as possible.
- Be accepting of family members' behavior at this time, no matter how strange it may seem to you. A

family might want to take a picture, or the spouse may lie down beside the deceased person.
- For family members who arrive after the death, offer to take them to the bedside.
- Viewing the body is useful to many individuals. Take care to present the client's body in a way that is appropriate for the family (remove any tubes, IV lines, and so on, according to the institution's policy) and have the client positioned in a way that appears comforting (e.g., bed covers pulled up, hands at the side).
- Ask whether each family member wishes to spend time alone with the deceased person, and arrange for them to do so. Never remove the body until the family is ready.
- Ask, "How can I help?" "What do you need?" "What would you like for me to do?"

TECHNIQUE 15–4 Providing Postmortem Care *(continued)*

Legal Responsibilities

- Usually the physician must pronounce death; however, in some areas a coroner or a nurse may also perform this task.
- The person who pronounces death must sign the death certificate. In some agencies the nurse is responsible for checking to see that it has been signed.
- If the patient is donating organs, review and make any necessary arrangements.
- As a rule, the physician (or other person designated by the institution) is responsible for obtaining signed permission from the next of kin if an autopsy is to be performed.

Care of the Body

- Follow agency policies, and respect cultural and spiritual preferences.
- Wash the body if there has been any incontinence or drainage. In some cultures, the body is not washed, or family members arrange to have someone special do it; so you should ask the family before performing this task.
- Dress the body in a clean gown, comb the hair, and straighten the bed linens.
- Be sure to place the body in a natural position, place the dentures in the mouth, and close the eyes and mouth before rigor mortis occurs. Place a pillow under the head and shoulders to prevent blood from settling there and causing discoloration.

- Be sure that dressings are clean, and unless an autopsy is to be done, remove all tubes and drains. Be careful when removing tape or dressings because the skin loses its elasticity and can be torn easily.
- Some institutions require that you close the patient's mouth and tie a strip of soft gauze (e.g., Kling) under the chin and around the head. This keeps the mouth set in a natural position in case there is a viewing later.
- If the family asks about the coldness and color of the body, explain to them that **algor mortis** occurs when the blood stops circulating. The body temperature drops about 1.8°F (1°C) per hour until it reaches room temperature. The dependent parts of the body appear bluish and mottled because when the blood stops circulating, the red blood cells break down, releasing hemoglobin. This is called **livor mortis.**
- After the family has spent time with the body, arrange to have it sent to the morgue, where it will either be autopsied or, if no autopsy is performed, picked up by the funeral home in charge of arrangements.
- Make sure there are identification tags on the body, on the shroud or body bag, and on the patient's possessions. Misidentification can create legal problems, for example, if the body is prepared incorrectly for a funeral.
- Follow institution policy if the patient has died of a communicable disease. By law, there are special preparations to perform in such cases.
- Handle the body with dignity.

ASSESSMENT GUIDELINES

You can use these guidelines for assessing dying patients as well as for other types of loss.

Assess the patient and significant others for common grief reactions.

Physical	Emotional	Behaviors	Cognitions
Loss of appetite	Anger	Forgetfulness	Decreased concentration
Weight loss/gain	Sadness	Withdrawal	Forgetfulness
Fatigue	Guilt	Insomnia or too much	Impaired judgment
Decreased libido	Relief	sleep	Obsessive thoughts of the
Decrease in immune	Shock	Dreaming of deceased	deceased or lost object
system	Numbness	Verbalizing the loss	Preoccupation
Decreased energy	Loneliness	Crying	Confusion
Possibly physical symptoms,	Fear	Loss of productivity at	Questioning spiritual beliefs
such as headache or	Anxiety	work or school	Searching to understand
stomach pain	Powerlessness		Searching for purpose and
	Helplessness		meaning

Assess Knowledge Base

- Do the patient and family have the information they need to make informed decisions about healthcare choices? For example, you might ask the following questions:
  - "Tell me what you understand about your illness."
  - "Are there any questions about your illness that you'd like me to answer?"
  - "What are your options for treatment?"
  - "Do you know how to reach your provider if you do have questions about your care?"
- Also determine what and how much the patient and family *want* to know. Some people wish to have all the details of their condition and care. For others, the details cause anxiety.

Assess History of Loss

Determine whether the patient or family has sustained recent losses or major changes (e.g. death, moving, divorce, retirement). Ask such questions as:

- "Have you had any recent changes in your life?"
- "Tell me about your family."
- "Are your parents still living?" (as appropriate)
- "What previous experiences have you had with the loss of someone you loved (or with this condition)?"

Assess Coping Abilities and Support Systems

The way individuals have coped in the past will affect how they cope with dying or with their current loss. It may also be therapeutic for them to identify their resources and supports. Some coping assessment questions include the following:

- "What do you do to help you reduce stress?"
- "Do you have family/friends you can talk with?"
- "What would you say is your greatest support when going through difficult times?"
- "Tell me about a previous loss and what you did to cope with it."
- "Are you using any community resources to help you get through this? Do you know what they are?"

ASSESSMENT GUIDELINES *(continued)*

Assess Meaning of the Loss or Illness

In trying to "make sense" of their loss or their dying, people try to attach a meaning to their suffering. Be alert for statements such as the following, which may indicate the patient or family is struggling to find meaning:

- "I'm being punished."
- "She doesn't deserve this."

Physical Assessment

A thorough physical examination adds data to help you determine how well the patient is coping with the loss or illness. Look for signs of increased stress, such as tension, forgetfulness, distraction, increased or decreased appetite and sleep, weight gain or loss, fatigue, and decreased self-care (e.g., deficient hygiene).

Cultural and Spiritual Assessment

Assess the patient's and family's religious beliefs, any spiritual needs they may have (e.g., forgiveness, hope, meaning, love), and cultural influences that may affect the way they cope. You cannot assume that a person adheres closely to the dominant values of his religious or cultural group. Always assess. For example, ask:

- "To what religious and ethnic groups do you belong?"
- "How closely do you identify with those groups?" See Chapter 13 for details of cultural assessment and Chapter 14 for details of spiritual assessment.

Specific Assessments for Dying Patients

For dying patients, in addition to the other assessments in this guideline, you should also assess the following:

- When the client and family are ready, encourage them to talk about what wishes the client might have for burial or cremation or whether there are tasks that the client would like taken care of (e.g., giving away valuables, calling family members).
- Determine whether the dying client has a living will or advance directives.
- Discuss with client and family the possibility of organ donation if appropriate for the client's circumstances.
- Observe for physical changes indicating the approach of death:
  1 to 3 months prior to death: increased sleep, decreased appetite, difficulty digesting food
  1 to 2 weeks prior to death: Decreased blood pressure, pulse and respiration changes (decreased or increased), a yellowish pallor to the skin, extreme pallor of extremities; temperature fluctuations, increased perspiration, brief periods of apnea during sleep, rattling breathing sounds, nonproductive cough
  Days to hours prior to death: A brief surge of energy and mental clarity, with a desire to eat and talk with family members.
  – Dehydration, difficulty swallowing, decreasing blood pressure, weak pulse
  – Sagging of tongue and soft palate, diminished gag reflex, secretions accumulating in the oropharynx and/or bronchi
  – Shallow, rapid, or irregular breathing; Cheyne-Stokes respirations; apnea of 10 to 30 seconds; "death rattle"
  – Decreased peripheral circulation, "clammy" skin; extremities cool and mottled; dependent body parts darker than the rest of the body
  – Decreased urinary output secondary to decreased kidney function
  – Slack facial muscles
  – Retained feces; bowel and bladder incontinence
  – Blurred vision; eyes open but unseeing
  – Restlessness or agitation (check for impacted stool, distended bladder, pain)
  – Decreased communication, quiet, withdrawal
  Moments prior to death: Does not respond to touch or sound; cannot be awakened. There may be a short series of long-spaced breaths before breathing stops entirely and the heart stops beating. Auscultate to determine whether apical pulse and respirations are absent.

STANDARDIZED OUTCOMES AND INTERVENTIONS FOR LOSS AND GRIEVING DIAGNOSES

Nursing Diagnoses	Selected NOC Outcomes	Selected NIC Interventions

Anticipatory Grieving
 	
Defining characteristics: Anger, potential loss of significant object (e.g., job. status, body function), denial of potential loss, sorrow, guilt, bargaining, altered eating and sleep patterns, changes in activity level or libido, difficulty taking on new roles
	Coping
	Family Coping
	Grief Resolution
	Psychosocial Adjustment:
	  Life Change
		Anticipatory Guidance
		Coping Enhancement
		Family Integrity Promotion
		Family Support
		Grief Work Facilitation
		Grief Work Facilitation:
		  Perinatal Death

- For Thomas Manning ("Meet Your Patient") in Volume 1, do you see any symptoms of Anticipatory Grieving?

Dysfunctional Grieving
 	
Defining characteristics: Repetitive use of ineffective coping behaviors, reliving of past experiences with little or no reduction in intensity of grief, prolonged interference with functioning, psychosomatic responses, expressions of grief (e.g., anger, sadness, crying), idealization of lost object or person, labile affect, developmental regression, denial of loss, expression of unresolved issues or guilt
	Coping
	Family Coping
	Grief Resolution
	Psychosocial Adjustment:
	  Life Change
		Coping Enhancement
		Counseling
		Family Integrity
		  Promotion
		Family Therapy
		Grief Work Facilitation
		Grief Work Facilitation:
		  Perinatal Death

- Notice that the outcomes are the same for Anticipatory and Dysfunctional Grieving.
- How do the interventions differ? Do you understand why? (If not, review the "Theoretical Knowledge" section of this chapter.)
- Notice that for both diagnoses, many of the defining characteristics include normal grief reactions. But for Anticipatory Grieving, the symptoms occur before the loss. For Dysfunctional Grieving, they continue to occur for a long time after the loss, and/or they are more intense than normal.

Ineffective Denial *Defining characteristics:* Does not admit fear of death, makes dismissive comments when speaking of death/loss, minimizes the grief/pain, displaces feelings to body (i.e., somatic and psychosomatic symptoms)	Acceptance: Health Status Anxiety Self-Control Fear Self-Control Health Beliefs: Perceived Threat Symptom Control	Anxiety Reduction Calming Technique Coping Enhancement Counseling Emotional Support Security Enhancement Self-Awareness Enhancement Teaching: Disease Process

- Does Mr. Manning exhibit any of the defining characteristics for Ineffective Denial?

Hopelessness *Defining characteristics:* Verbal cues (e.g., "I can't" or "Why go on"), sighing, closing eyes, shrugging, decreased appetite, lack of emotion, increased or decreased sleep, little or no involvement in care, passivity, lack of initiative, seeing no solution or way out	Decision Making Depression Level Depression Self-Control Hope Mood Equilibrium Quality of Life	Decision-Making Support Hope Instillation Mood Management Resiliency Promotion Spiritual Growth Facilitation

- Does Mr. Manning exhibit any of the defining characteristics for Hopelessness?
- Which outcome and intervention seem *most directly* related to Hopelessness?

STANDARDIZED OUTCOMES AND INTERVENTIONS FOR LOSS AND GRIEVING DIAGNOSES *(continued)*

Nursing Diagnoses	Selected NOC Outcomes	Selected NIC Interventions
Powerlessness		
Defining characteristics: Sees that the situation could be changed but does not think it is within his power to change it; expresses helplessness, anger, frustration over inability to perform previous tasks; does not seek information or participate in care or decisions about care	Depression Self-Control Family Participation in Professional Care Health Beliefs Health beliefs: 　Perceived Ability to Perform, Perceived Control, Perceived Resources Participation in Health Care Decisions	Cognitive Restructuring Decision-Making Support Family Involvement Promotion Financial Resource Assistance Health Education Mood Management Mutual Goal Setting Self-Esteem Enhancement Self-Responsibility Facilitation Values Clarification

- Why do you think that Self-Esteem Enhancement is an intervention for Powerlessness but not for Hopelessness?

Nursing Diagnoses	Selected NOC Outcomes	Selected NIC Interventions
Caregiver Role Strain		
Defining characteristics: Fear that loved one may need to be institutionalized; alterations in caregiver's health, ability to give care, or complete caregiving tasks; apprehension about the future	Caregiver Lifestyle Disruption Caregiver Well-Being Role Performance	Caregiver Support Coping Enhancement Respite Care Role Enhancement Teaching: Individual

- Do you know what Respite Care is? If not, look it up on the Internet or in the *NIC* manual.

Nursing Diagnoses	Selected NOC Outcomes	Selected NIC Interventions
Chronic Sorrow		
Defining characteristics: Periodic, recurrent sadness; feelings of varying intensity that interfere with high-level well being; expresses one or more of the following feelings: anger, being misunderstood, confusion, depression, disappointment, emptiness, fear, frustration, guilt, helplessness, hopelessness, loneliness, low self-esteem, being overwhelmed	Acceptance: Health Status Depression Level Depression Self-Control Grief Resolution Hope Mood Equilibrium	Coping Enhancement Grief Work Facilitation Hope Instillation Mood Management Spiritual Support
Spiritual Distress		
Defining characteristics: Nightmares or other sleep disturbances, concern over the meaning of life/death/suffering/existence, gallows humor, questions moral implications of therapeutic regimen, anger at God, desires but unable to participate in usual religious practices	Dignified Life Closure Hope Spiritual Health	Dying Care Hope Instillation Spiritual Growth Facilitation Spiritual Support

Sources: Moorhead, S., Johnson, M., & Mass, M. (Eds.). (2004). *Nursing outcomes classification (NOC)* (3rd ed.). St. Louis: Mosby
Dochterman, J. M., & Bulechek, G. M. (Eds.). (2004). *Nursing interventions classification (NIC)* (4th ed). St. Louis: Mosby.
Johnson, M., Bulechek, G., Dochterman, J., Mass., & Moorhead, S. (2001). *Nursing diagnoses, outcomes, and interventions: NANDA, NOC, and NIC linkages.* St. Louis: Mosby.
NANDA International. (2005). *Nursing diagnoses: Definitions and classification 2005–2006.* Philadelphia: Author.

What Are the Main Points in This Chapter?

- The manner in which people cope with loss directly affects their healing and well-being.
- Loss may be actual or perceived, physical or psychological, external or internal.
- Grief is the physical, psychological, and spiritual response to loss.
- People do not move neatly from one stage of grief to the next; there is constant movement and overlap between and among them. The same is true for the stages of dying.
- The grieving process is affected by the significance and circumstance of the loss, the timeliness of the death, the amount of support for the bereaved, spiritual beliefs, cultural values, the person's developmental stage, and conflicts existing at the time of death.
- It is important for nurses to understand loss. Patients go through the grieving process when they are ill and/or hospitalized (loss of independence, body image, self-esteem, and so on). Recognizing these as losses, you can assist the patient with the grieving process, thus promoting physical, emotional, and spiritual healing.
- The Uniform Determination of Death Act states that death has occurred when "An individual . . . has sustained either (1) irreversible cessation of circulatory and respiratory functions, or (2) irreversible cessation of all functions of the entire brain, including the brain stem. . . ."
- Palliative care means providing comfort care and symptom relief but without further efforts to stop the disease process or prevent death.
- Hospice care is a movement to allow terminally ill persons to face death with dignity and surrounded by the comfort of their home and family.
- Healthcare providers are responsible for educating staff and patients about advance directives.
- A *do not attempt resuscitation (DNAR)* order is a specific order to *not* do cardiopulmonary resuscitation. DNAR orders must be written and reviewed frequently.
- Nurses should be aware of what is involved with assisted suicide and euthanasia. Patients are much more aware than they have ever been about their options for care and treatment, so you should think ahead about what your response might be if a patient wants to discuss these topics. You may find the ANA position statement on assisted suicide and euthanasia helpful.
- An autopsy is a medical examination of the body to determine cause of death.
- When a patient is dying or has experienced a loss, you should assess his knowledge of his situation, the history of past losses, coping abilities, support systems, the meaning he attaches to the loss or illness, physical status, cultural beliefs, and spiritual needs.
- Most grief is normal, not dysfunctional; you should not diagnose Dysfunctional Grieving for every person who is grieving a loss.
- Therapeutic communication is extremely important when caring for dying or grieving persons.
- You can facilitate grief work by validating feelings ("It's normal to feel that way") and providing opportunity and encouragement to talk about the lost person or object.
- At the moment of death, do not interrupt or intrude upon the family; give them as much time as they need to say good-bye to their loved one. Express your sympathy.
- Active dying usually occurs over a 10- to 14-day period, although it can take as little as 24 hours. During the final 4 to 48 hours, failure of body systems results in death.
- When the patient is very near death, focus on relieving physical symptoms (e.g., pain) and emotional distress. If he can communicate, ask about immediate concerns, such as, "Who do you want in the room right now?"
- Care of the body includes making it presentable for the family, carefully placing identification tags, and arranging to have the body sent to the morgue.
- The death certificate must be signed by the person who legally pronounced the death (usually a physician).
- It is normal for the nurse to feel grief when a patient dies.

Knowledge Map

Loss, Grief, and Dying

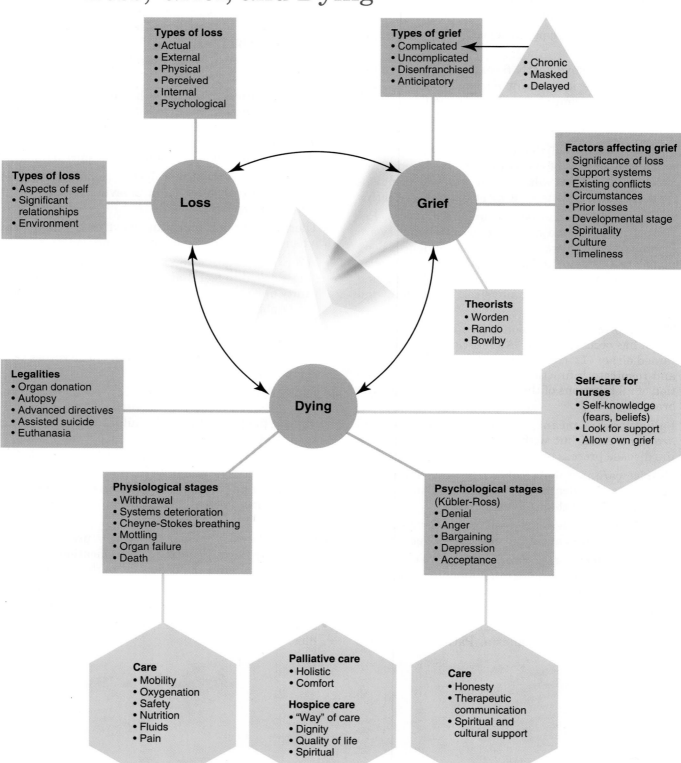

Types of loss
- Actual
- External
- Physical
- Perceived
- Internal
- Psychological

Types of grief
- Complicated
- Uncomplicated
- Disenfranchised
- Anticipatory

- Chronic
- Masked
- Delayed

Types of loss
- Aspects of self
- Significant relationships
- Environment

Loss

Grief

Factors affecting grief
- Significance of loss
- Support systems
- Existing conflicts
- Circumstances
- Prior losses
- Developmental stage
- Spirituality
- Culture
- Timeliness

Theorists
- Worden
- Rando
- Bowlby

Legalities
- Organ donation
- Autopsy
- Advanced directives
- Assisted suicide
- Euthanasia

Dying

Self-care for nurses
- Self-knowledge (fears, beliefs)
- Look for support
- Allow own grief

Physiological stages
- Withdrawal
- Systems deterioration
- Cheyne-Stokes breathing
- Mottling
- Organ failure
- Death

Psychological stages
(Kübler-Ross)
- Denial
- Anger
- Bargaining
- Depression
- Acceptance

Care
- Mobility
- Oxygenation
- Safety
- Nutrition
- Fluids
- Pain

Palliative care
- Holistic
- Comfort

Hospice care
- "Way" of care
- Dignity
- Quality of life
- Spiritual

Care
- Honesty
- Therapeutic communication
- Spiritual and cultural support

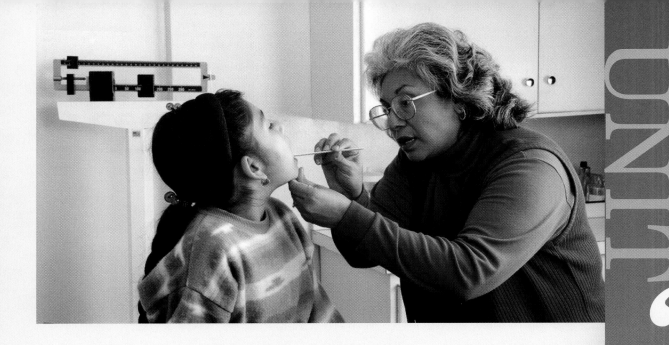

Essential Nursing
Interventions

16 DOCUMENTING & REPORTING

17 MEASURING VITAL SIGNS

18 COMMUNICATING & THE THERAPEUTIC RELATIONSHIP

19 ASSESSING HEALTH: PHYSICAL EXAMINATION

20 PROMOTING ASEPSIS & PREVENTING INFECTION

21 PROMOTING SAFETY

22 FACILITATING HYGIENE

23 ADMINISTERING MEDICATIONS

24 TEACHING CLIENTS

16 Documenting & Reporting

CHAPTER

Overview

The client record is a collection of printed materials that form a legal record of the client's healthcare experience. Documentation can take many forms, for example, SOAP. SOAP is an acronym for *subjective data, objective data, assessment,* and *plan.* This format may be used to address single problems or to write summative notes on a patient. In Focus Charting, data is entered in a DAR format. DAR is an acronym for *data, action,* and *response.* Preprinted flowsheets document most aspects of care used in charting by exception (CBE). CBE assumes that unless a separate entry is made—an exception—all standards have been met with a normal response. The most commonly used home health documentation form is OASIS, a federally required form that includes history, assessment, demographics, and information about the client's and caregiver's abilities.

You are responsible for documenting the care you provide. Charting should be accurate and nonjudgmental, and you should perform it as soon as possible after you make an observation or provide care. Document any significant events, changes in condition, client teaching, the use of restraints, and refusals of treatment or medications. Never chart the actions of others as though you had performed them. If you believe a physician's order is inappropriate or unsafe, you are legally and ethically required to question the order.

Thinking Critically About Documenting and Reporting

The exercises in the following section allow you to practice the kind of thinking you will use as a full-spectrum nurse. Because these are critical-thinking activities, there is usually no single right answer. Discuss answers with your peers—discussion can stimulate critical thinking. If you have difficulty with any of the questions, consult with your instructor.

Caring for the Garcias

Flordelisa Garcia arrives at the Family Medicine Clinic complaining of pain and drainage from her right eye. She requests an appointment. As part of your clinical experience, you are working as a triage nurse at the clinic. As the triage nurse, you must evaluate the patient's status and determine whether she needs to be seen today. Below is your conversation with Mrs. Garcia.

Mrs. Garcia: I don't have an appointment, but I need to see someone today. My husband is a patient here. I have an appointment in 2 weeks for a physical, but I've never been here before. I just can't wait 2 weeks.

You: What seems to be the problem?

Mrs. Garcia: My eye is killing me. My right one. It burns and stings, and there's all this nasty gunk coming out. I need some medicine for it.

You: Tell me a little about this problem. When did this start?

Mrs. Garcia: I woke up with a painful, itchy eye yesterday. I used some Visine, but the eye seems to be worse. I work at a preschool, and they won't let me go to work unless I take care of this. I also think I need to be checked for other things. I haven't had an appointment in a long time. I suppose I need some tests. My husband just found out he has high blood pressure, but I don't think I do. I guess I'm not old enough. I'm 50, but my mother got high blood pressure when she was 70.

As she is talking, you notice a large amount of thick, yellow-green drainage in the corners of her right eye. She is rubbing the eye vigorously. The lashes are matted together, and the skin is puffy around the eye. Her left eye is slightly red, but there is no drainage.

Her vital signs are as follows: blood pressure, 132/76 mm Hg; heart rate, 88; respirations, 18 per minute; and temperature, 98.9°F (37.2°C).

Based on your brief assessment, you ask the receptionist to give Mrs. Garcia an urgent appointment.

A. Make two charting entries to describe the above events. First, make a brief narrative note.

B. Next, construct a SOAP note. Be sure to follow charting guidelines when you prepare your note.

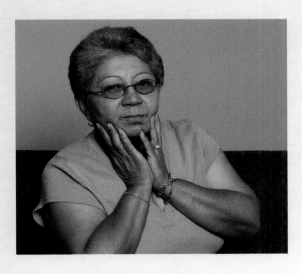

1

You are caring for a 96-year-old patient, James Wilson. Mr. Wilson has been admitted to the hospital for pneumonia. He is normally alert and oriented to place, time, and person. However, during this admission he has been confused and agitated. He frequently yells at staff and resists care by kicking and punching. While you are providing morning care, Mr. Wilson becomes very agitated and yells and curses at you. When you attempt to provide oral hygiene, he hits you and throws his dentures at you. The dentures break when they hit the floor.

a Construct a charting note about this situation using the format you prefer.

b You will need to complete an occurrence report regarding the broken dentures. The report asks you to identify actions that you might have taken to prevent this incident. Brainstorm this question with your peers. Identify one or two actions that might have prevented this incident.

2

The physician has written an order on your patient's chart that you find illegible. A veteran nurse states that she can read it, and she translates it for you. What factors should you consider before determining how to proceed?

3

For each of the following concepts, use critical thinking to describe how or why it is important to nursing, patient care, or documenting and reporting. Note that these are *not* to be merely definitions.

Narrative charting

SOAP charting

Nursing admission database

Medication administration record

Occurrence report

Flowsheets

Charting by exception

Computerized records

Change-of-shift report

Late entry

thinking critically about documenting & reporting

Practical Knowledge
knowing how

TECHNIQUES

TECHNIQUE 16–1 | Giving Oral Reports

For all reports, remember the acronym CUBAN (Currie, 2002):

C onfidential
U ninterrupted
B rief
A ccurate
N amed nurse

Include the following in a *change-of-shift report*:

- Patient's name, age, and room number
- Patient's admitting diagnosis—one or several may exist
- Patient's relevant past medical history
- Treatments the patient has received at this admission (e.g., surgery, line placements, breathing treatments)
- Upcoming diagnostic tests, surgeries, or treatments
- Restrictions on the patient (e.g., diet, bed rest, isolation)
- Plan of care for the patient (e.g., IV therapy, pain management, medications, wound care, and patient or family concerns)
- Significant assessment findings from the previous shifts

Include the following in a *transfer report*:

- Your name, facility, and phone number
- Patient's name, age, gender, and admitting and current diagnoses
- Patient's physician(s), if still following patient
- Procedures or surgeries performed
- Medications
- Patient status at present as well as progression since admission
- Vital signs
- Tubes in the patient (IV tubes, catheters, drainage tubes, and so on), as well as the input and output of the tubes
- Presence of wounds or open areas of the skin
- Names and contact numbers of family or significant others
- Special directives, such as code status (resuscitation requests), preferred intensity of care, or isolation required
- Reason the patient is being transferred (e.g., special procedure or insurance reasons)
- Always ask the receiving nurse whether she has any questions. Get the nurse's name; record it in your final note ("Oral report given to N. Smith, RN").

TECHNIQUE 16–2 | Receiving Telephone and Verbal Orders

- Write the order only if you heard it yourself; no third-party involvement is acceptable.
- Repeat the order even if you believe you have understood it entirely. Spell unfamiliar names, saying, for example, "B as in boy," to make sure the spelling is correct.
- Pronounce digits of numbers separately; for example, instead of "seventeen," say "one, seven." As another example, "fifty" sounds much like "fifteen," and mishearing it could lead to a serious error in medication dosage.
- Make sure the verbal orders make sense in light of the patient's status.
- If possible, have a second nurse listen to the order to verify its accuracy.
- Directly transcribe the order onto the chart. Transcribing it onto a piece of paper and then copying it again introduces another chance of error.
- When writing the order, first document the date and time. Then write the text of the order. Following the text of the order, write "TO" (telephone order), followed by the ordering provider's name and then your name.
- Be sure you have the phone number of the provider so that you can reach her if future questions arise.
- The physician must countersign all verbal and phone orders within 24 hours.

TECHNIQUE 16–3   Guidelines for Documentation

General Guidelines

- Use accurate, nonjudgmental language; avoid labeling patients (e.g., as uncooperative).
- Provide details about the patient's condition; give examples.
- Remember that the patient's record is permanent and that the information in it is confidential.
- Never allow anyone to chart your nursing actions, and never document the actions of others as though you had performed them (e.g., if the UAP helps the patient ambulate, do not chart, "Helped patient to ambulate to the bathroom." Instead, chart, "Assisted to the bathroom by J. Scott, UAP."

Timing

- Chart as soon as possible after you give care or make an observation, but never chart ahead.
- Begin charting at the beginning of your shift. Document specific times in chronological order. Do not chart in blocks of time.
- Add late entries to the first available line. Record the time and date you are charting, but in the body of the entry clearly designate that this is a late entry.

Aspects of Care to Chart

- *Your interventions and the patient's responses.* Also chart your evaluation of progress toward goals.
- *Any significant events or changes in condition.* When possible, quote the patient to document his response.
- *Informed consent.* If you are asked to obtain informed consent for a procedure, you should document your actions in the nurse's notes. In most states, your signature confirms only that the patient signed the consent. The physician conducting the procedure is legally responsible for discussing the procedure and its risks and benefits. For further discussion on informed consent, see Chapters 44 and 45.
- *Occurrences such as falls and medication errors.* Chart your findings accurately and objectively, and fill out a separate occurrence form. Do not make reference to the occurrence form in your narrative charting.
- *Any attempts you have made to contact the primary care provider about the patient's condition or attempts to clarify orders.* If you are unable to make contact with the primary care provider, include in your notes any contact with your supervisor or the medical director.

- *Any teaching performed,* including medication instruction, instruction on the patient's diagnoses, or discharge teaching. Documenting patient teaching can positively affect reimbursement. If the patient's physical or cognitive condition prevents teaching, explain in your documentation.
- *Any use of restraints.* Most facilities have a separate form that allows you to document the reason for restraint use, type of restraint, and frequent checks of the patient. The primary care provider must place a signed order for restraints in the chart.
- *The patient's refusal of treatment.* Quote the patient whenever possible.
- *If the patient leaves the facility against medical advice (AMA),* chart the patient's condition, any explanations of risks and consequences given to the patient, the patient's destination (if known), and your notification of the patient's providers. Many facilities have specific forms for AMA departures. If possible, use the designated form, and have the patient sign this form before she leaves.
- *Complete data about medications,* including the date, time given, medication given, and your initials. In most cases, you will chart routine medicines on a medication administration record (MAR). PRN, stat, or one-time orders may also appear on the MAR, and you should always document them in your narrative charting. State the reason the medication was given and the patient's response.
- *Chart on the MAR and your narrative notes any medications that the patient refuses or that are omitted.* If the patient states a reason for refusing the medication, quote him in your narrative notes. If you hold or omit a medication, chart your rationale in the narrative notes.
- *Any spiritual concerns expressed by the patient, and your interventions.*

The "Mechanics" of Charting

- *Write neatly and legibly.* Sloppy or illegible handwriting creates errors or, at least, leads to poor communication.
- Before you start documenting, *check that the chart and documentation forms are clearly marked with the patient's name and identification number.*
- *Always use black or blue ink* for handwritten notes. Inks other than black or blue are not legible when a chart is photocopied. Remember the chart is a legal document.

➤

TECHNIQUE 16–3   Guidelines for Documentation *(continued)*

- **Date and time all of your notes.** To avoid confusion between A.M. and P.M., many institutions use a 24-hour clock or military time.

 Go to Chapter 16, **Figure 16–5,** in Volume 1.

The day begins at 0001, which is equivalent to 12:01 A.M., and ends at 2400 (12 midnight). After 12 noon, just add 12 to the P.M. time (e.g., 1:30 P.M. + 12 = 1330 P.M. in military time).

- **Avoid words such as good, average, or normal.** These are vague, subjective terms that do not clearly define the status of the client.
- **Use proper spelling and grammar.** Incorrect spelling may raise questions about what you are attempting to communicate. Incorrect grammar implies carelessness on your part and makes a poor impression if your chart is reviewed.

- **Use only those abbreviations authorized by your institution.** See "Abbreviations Commonly Used in Health Care," on p. 185 of this chapter.
- **Do not leave blank lines in the narrative notes.** If you need to leave space for clarity, draw a straight line through the area and begin on the next line. Open areas leave an opportunity for tampering.
- **Never use correction tape, an eraser, "white-out,"** or other products that cover up notes.
- **Never scribble out an entry.** If you make a mistake, draw a single line through the entry, and place your initials next to the change. In some institutions you may be advised to chart "error" or "mistaken entry" above the lined-out entry. Check with your facility to determine which method is preferred.
- **Sign all your charting entries.** Use your first initial and last name. Clearly designate your professional status (e.g., J. Long, RN).

ABBREVIATIONS COMMONLY USED IN HEALTH CARE

*Abbreviations should *not* be used (JCAHO, 2004)

Abbreviation	Meaning	Abbreviation	Meaning
ADL	activities of daily living	LPN	licensed practical nurse
ad lib	as desired, if the patient desires	LMP	last menstrual period
AKA	above-knee amputation	LVN	licensed vocational nurse
amb	ambulation, ambulatory	MD	medical doctor
amt	amount	med	medication
@	at	mL	milliliter
ASAP	as soon as possible	MN	midnight
bid	twice a day	NAS	no added salt
BM	bowel movement	N/V/D	nausea, vomiting, diarrhea
BR	bedrest	NKA or NKDA	no known allergies or no known drug allergies
BRP	bathroom privileges		
BSC	bedside commode	NG	nasogastric
c̄	with	NGT	nasogastric tube
cal	calories	noc	at night
cath	catheter	NPO	nothing by mouth
CBC	complete blood count	O₂	oxygen
CCU	critical care unit or coronary care unit	OB	obstetrics
c/o	complaint of	OOB	out of bed
CO₂	carbon dioxide	OPD	outpatient department
CPR	cardiopulmonary resuscitation	ortho	orthopedics
CVA	cerebrovascular accident (stroke)	OR	operating room
*d/c	discharge	os	mouth, opening
D&C	dilatation and curretage	OT	occupational therapy
DM	diabetes mellitus	oz	ounce
dsg or drsg	dressing	pc	after meals
DX or Dx	diagnosis	PCA	patient-controlled analgesia
EBL	estimated blood loss	PO	by mouth
EKG/ECG	electrocardiogram	P, p̄	after
ED/ER	emergency department, emergency room	PPBS	postprandial blood sugar
EEG	electroencephalogram	PRN	as needed
EENT	eyes, ears, nose, throat	pt	patient
ETOH	alcohol	PT	physical therapy
F	female	q	every
FBS	fasting blood sugar	qam	every morning
ft	foot	*qd	every day
fx	fracture	qh	every hour
GI	gastrointestinal	*qhs	every night/at bedtime
gtt(s)	drop(s)	qid	four times a day
GU	genitourinary	*qod	every other day
GYN	gynecology	RN	registered nurse
HA	headache	R/O	rule out
HMO	health maintenance organization	RX or Rx	treatment or prescription
h/o	history of	s̄	without
hob	head of bed	SCD	sequential compression device
HOH	hard of hearing	SOB	short of breath
H&P	history and physical	s̄s̄	one-half
hr	hour	SSE	soapsuds enema
*HS or hs	hour of sleep/bedtime	stat	immediately
ht	height	STD or STI	sexually transmitted disease or sexually transmitted infection
HTN	hypertension		
hyper	above or high	TB	tuberculosis
hypo	below or low	TO	telephone order
ICU	intensive care unit	TPR	temperature, pulse, respirations
I&O	intake and output	tid	three times a day
isol	isolation	VO	verbal order
IV	intravenous	vs	vital signs
IVP	intravenous push (caution: do not use to mean "IV piggyback")	WBC	white blood count
		w/c	wheelchair
L	liter	WNL	within normal limits
lb	pound	wt	weight

CHARTING FORMS

A flowsheet used in long-term care.

C.N.A. SIGNATURE	INITIALS

PHYSICAL MOB./TRANSF.		SAFETY DEVICE/RESTRAINT	
AMB.	Ambulatory	N	NON-RELEASE
AA	Amb. With Assist	S	SELF-RELEASE BELT
W/C	Wheelchair bound	M	MITTEN
B	Bedfast	W	WRIST
I	Ind. Transfers	GC	GERI-CHAIR/TABLE
A	1 person A with trans	R	RECLINER
D	Dependent transf.	A	ALARM
H	Hoyer Lift transf.	N/A	NONE

MONTH: YEAR:

NIGHT SHIFT	16	17	18	19	20	21	22	23	24	25	26	27	28	29	30	31
Mental Status (Oriented or Confused)																
Quality of Sleep (Slept well or Restless)																
Turn/Reposition(Ind,Assist or Total)																
Safety Device/Restraint (see legend)																
Siderails (Up or Down)																
Behavior(Resists care,Combative or N/A)																
Bladder Function (Inc.,Cont. or Foley)																
Bowel Function (Inc or Continent)																
Bowel Movement (Lrg or Med or Small)																
Certified Nurse Assitant Initials																

DAY SHIFT																
Mental Status (Oriented or Confused)																
Breakfast (percentage eaten)	%	%	%	%	%	%	%	%	%	%	%	%	%	%	%	%
Amt. of assist. (Ind. or Assist or Fed)																
Lunch (percentage eaten)	%	%	%	%	%	%	%	%	%	%	%	%	%	%	%	%
Amt. of assist. (Ind. or Assist or Fed)																
10am Nourishment (% ,Refused or N/A)																
Bathing (Shower, Bedbath or Tub bath)																
Personal Hygiene (Ind., Assist or Total)																
Dressing (Ind or Assist or Total)																
Physical Mobility (see legend)																
Transfer Ability (see legend)																
Toileting (Ind., Assist or Total)																
Safety Device/Restraint (see legend)																
Siderails (Up or Down)																
Turn/Reposition(Ind,Assist or Total)																
Behavior(Resists care,Combative or N/A)																
Bladder Function (Inc. or Cont. or Foley)																
Bowel Function (Inc or Continent)																
Bowel Movement (Lrg or Med or Small)																
Certified Nurse Assistant Initials																

P.M. SHIFT																
Mental Status (Oriented or Confused)																
Dinner (percentage eaten)	%	%	%	%	%	%	%	%	%	%	%	%	%	%	%	%
Amt. of assist. (Ind. or Assist or Fed)																
2pm Nourishment (% or Refused or N/A)																
HS Nourishment (% or Refused or N/A)																
Bathing(Shower or Bedbath or Tub bath)																
Physical Mobility (see legend)																
Transfer Ability (see legend)																
Safety Device/Restraint (see legend)																
Siderails (Up or Down)																
Turn/Reposition(Ind,Assist or Total)																
Behavior(Resists care,Combative or N/A)																
Bladder Function (Inc., Cont. or Foley)																
Bowel Function (Inc or Continent)																
Bowel Movement (Lrg or Med or Small)																
Certified Nurse Assistant Initials																

RT. NAME:	MEDICAL REC. #	RM#	PHYSICIAN

Nursing assessment flowsheets are comprehensive charting documents.

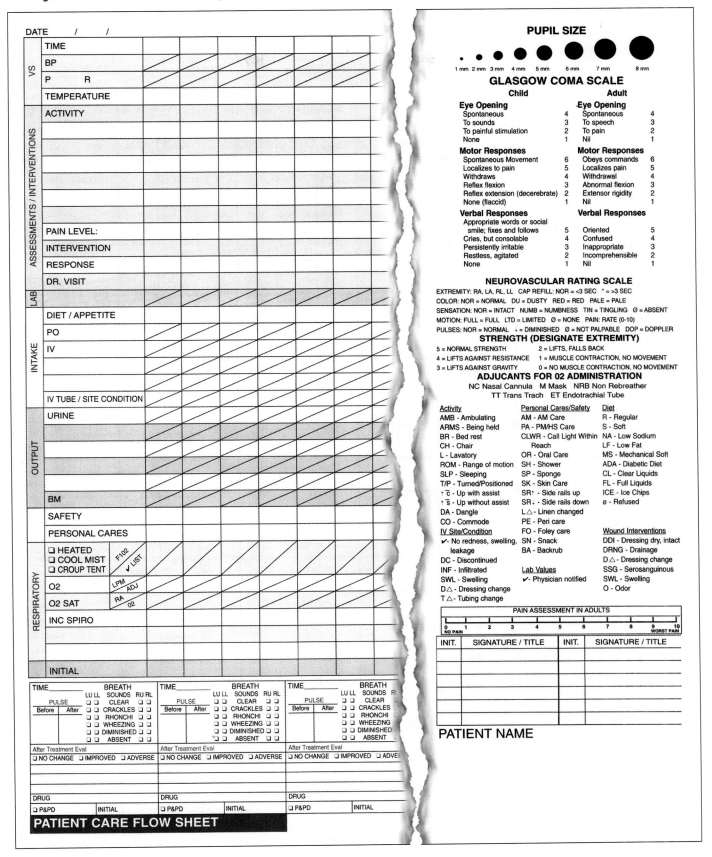

Courtesy of Teton Valley Hospital, Driggs, ID

Nurses use intake and output (I&O) records to record data about the patient's fluid status.

INTAKE AND OUTPUT SHEET

DATE	Time	INTAKE						OUTPUT						SIGNATURE OF NURSE
		ORAL	IV	IV MED	BLOOD PRODUCT	OTHER	TOTAL	URINE	EMESIS	STOOL	SUCTION	OTHER	TOTAL	
	6 A.M.-2 P.M.													
	2 P.M.-10 P.M.													
	10 P.M.-6 A.M.													
	TOTAL													
	6 A.M.-2 P.M.													
	2 P.M.-10 P.M.													
	10 P.M.-6 A.M.													
	TOTAL													
	6 A.M.-2 P.M.													
	2 P.M.-10 P.M.													
	10 P.M.-6 A.M.													
	TOTAL													
	6 A.M.-2 P.M.													
	2 P.M.-10 P.M.													
	10 P.M.-6 A.M.													
	TOTAL													
	6 A.M.-2 P.M.													
	2 P.M.-10 P.M.													
	10 P.M.-6 A.M.													
	TOTAL													

What Are the Main Points in This Chapter?

- The client record is a collection of printed materials that form a legal record of the client's healthcare experience.
- The client record is used by health professionals to communicate about the client's care, to legally document the care delivered to the client, to educate students, to determine whether care is adequate, as a data source for health research, and as the basis for determining the cost of care.
- In source-oriented records, members of each discipline record findings in a separately labeled section.
- In problem-oriented records, members of each discipline chart on shared notes, and the record is organized around a problem list.
- In narrative charting, the writer tells the story of what has occurred in a chronological format.
- SOAP is an acronym for *subjective data, objective data, assessment,* and *plan.* This format may be used to address single problems or to write summative notes on a patient.
- In Focus Charting®, data is entered in a DAR format. DAR is an acronym for *data, action,* and *response.*
- Charting by exception (CBE) utilizes preprinted flowsheets to document most aspects of care. CBE assumes that unless a separate entry is made—an exception—all standards have been met and the patient has responded as expected.
- Flowsheets and graphic records are used to record recurring assessments such as vital signs, intake and output, weight, hygiene, and ADLs.
- Progress notes are used to document the patient's response to care. They may be in the form of narrative, SOAP, PIE, or DAR notes.
- A discharge summary should be completed on the patient's discharge from or transfer within the facility.

- An occurrence report, or incident report, is a formal record of an unusual occurrence or accident (e.g., a patient fall) that is not part of the patient's chart.
- The most commonly used home health documentation form is OASIS, a federally required form that includes history, assessment, demographics, and information about the client's and caregiver's abilities.
- Federal law requires that a resident in long-term care must be evaluated using the Minimum Data Set for Resident Assessment and Care Screening (MDS) within 14 days of admission. The MDS must be updated every 3 months and with any significant change in client condition
- Change-of-shift report is designed to alert the next nurse about the client's status, changes in the client condition, planned activities, tests or procedures, or concerns that require follow-up.
- Telephone orders offer more room for error because of differences in pronunciation, dialect, or accent; background noise; and unfamiliar terminology.
- Charting should be accurate and nonjudgmental.
- You should document as soon as possible after you make an observation or provide care.
- Document any significant events or changes in condition, teaching performed, the use of restraints, and patient refusal of treatment or medications.
- You are responsible for documenting the care you provided. Never chart the actions of others as though you had performed them.
- If you believe a physician order is inappropriate or unsafe, you are legally and ethically required to question the order.

Knowledge Map

Documenting and Reporting

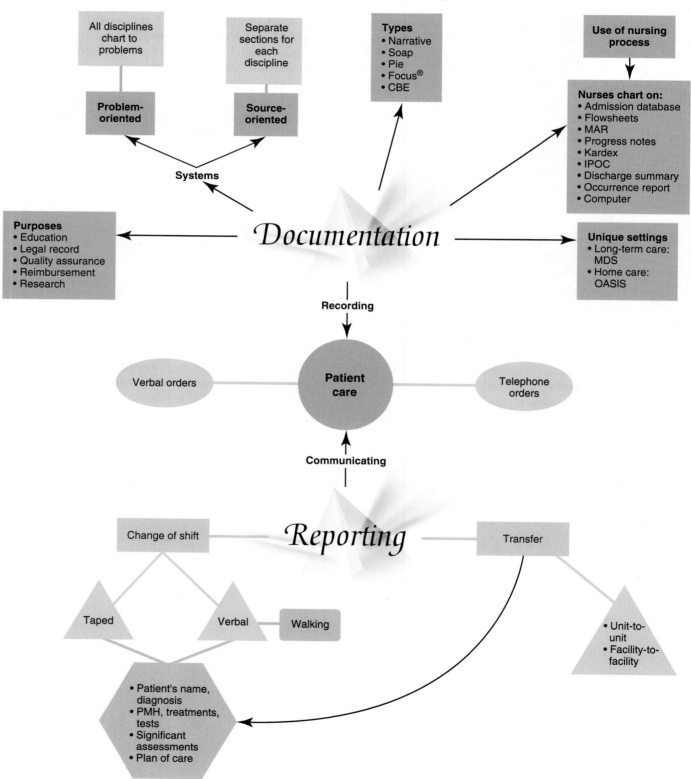

All disciplines chart to problems

Separate sections for each discipline

Problem-oriented

Source-oriented

Systems

Types
• Narrative
• Soap
• Pie
• Focus®
• CBE

Use of nursing process

Nurses chart on:
• Admission database
• Flowsheets
• MAR
• Progress notes
• Kardex
• IPOC
• Discharge summary
• Occurrence report
• Computer

Purposes
• Education
• Legal record
• Quality assurance
• Reimbursement
• Research

Documentation

Unique settings
• Long-term care: MDS
• Home care: OASIS

Recording

Verbal orders

Patient care

Telephone orders

Communicating

Reporting

Change of shift

Transfer

Taped

Verbal

Walking

• Unit-to-unit
• Facility-to-facility

• Patient's name, diagnosis
• PMH, treatments, tests
• Significant assessments
• Plan of care

Measuring
Vital Signs

Overview

Vital signs (temperature, pulse, respirations, and blood pressure) indicate a client's health status by measuring the functioning of the body systems. Age, activity, smoking, and gender are among the elements that cause variations in vital signs.

Body temperature is the balance between heat production and heat loss. Although fever (temperature above normal) is a symptom of infection, it is a beneficial part of the body's immune response.

A normal pulse rate varies widely according to age. Assess the pulse for quality, bilateral equality, volume, and rate.

Respiration is the process of supplying the body with oxygen and disposing of carbon dioxide. Assess respirations for rate, depth, rhythm, and associated clinical signs (e.g., breath sounds, chest movement, cough, pallor, and cyanosis).

Blood pressure (BP) is the pressure of the blood as it is forced against arterial walls during cardiac contraction. Hypertension is persistent elevated blood pressure (above 140 mm Hg systolic or above 90 mm Hg diastolic) on more than two separate occasions. Clients can prevent or modify hypertension by certain lifestyle changes (e.g., exercise, weight control, and stress management).

Although they can delegate the activity of taking vital signs, nurses are responsible for evaluating the meaning of the data.

Thinking Critically About Vital Signs

The exercises in the following section allow you to practice the kind of thinking you will use as a full-spectrum nurse. Because these are critical thinking activities, there is usually no single right answer. Discuss answers with your peers—discussion can stimulate critical thinking. If you have difficulty with any of the questions, consult with your instructor.

Caring for the Garcias

Recall that on the preliminary visit of Joseph Garcia at the family medicine center, his BP was 162/94. On subsequent visits, his BP was 168/100 and 174/98. Mr. Garcia was diagnosed with hypertension and placed on Lisinopril 20 mg every A.M. This A.M. Mr. Garcia presents at the clinic for follow-up. The following information is gathered as he checks in for his visit.

VS: BP, 168/92; pulse, 80; respirations, 20; temperature, 98. 4°F (36.9°C)
Weight: 231 lb (105 kg)

Review the preliminary data and the preceding information to answer the following questions:

A. What patterns do you see in the data?

B. Do you have enough information to draw any conclusions? If not, what other information should you gather?

C. Identify three alternatives that may explain what is happening with his vital signs.

D. How could you determine which of these alternatives provides the best explanation of what is happening?

E. Why is it important to intervene in this situation?

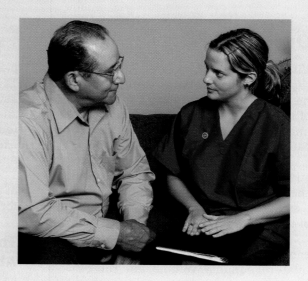

1 Recall the clients you encountered at the community health fair (Meet Your Patient, Volume 1). Two-year-old Jason's oral temperature was 102°F (38.9°C); his skin was warm, dry, and flushed. His mother told you that he had been eating poorly and was very irritable. What changes in behavior alert you to know that something is wrong?

2 You have already determined (in Volume 1) what, if any, additional information you need in order to determine the meaning of Jason's temperature elevation.

a What theoretical knowledge may account for Jason's temperature?

b Are there any actions you should take while meeting with Jason and his mother? If so what?

c What biases do you have that affect your thinking about this situation? (This requires self-knowledge.)

3 Suppose you have the following (imaginary) data:
In a long-term-care center, where most patients are older, the average normal oral temperature of the patients is 97.6°F (36.4°C). In a local well-baby nursery, the average skin temperature of the newborns ranges from 97.7 to 98.6°F (36.5 to 37.0°C), but it fluctuates during the first 24 hours after birth. At a walk-in surgery center, the average oral temperature of the healthy clients is 98.6°F (37.0°C).

a What conclusion might you draw about what is causing the differences in average body temperature among these three groups? (*Clue:* First list the average temperatures in order, from highest to lowest.)

thinking critically about measuring vital signs

b What theoretical knowledge did you use to answer that question?

4 Suppose you have the following data about patients' temperatures:

Patient A, 58 years old: 6 A.M., 97.7°F (36.5°C); 12 noon, 98.8°F (37.1°C); 9 P.M., 99.0°F (37.2°C)

Patient B, 14 years old: 6 A.M., 97.5°F (36.4°C); 12 noon, 97.9°F (36.6°C); 9 P.M., 98.4°F (36.9°C)

Patient C, 80 years old: 6 A.M., 98.4°F (36.9°C); 12 noon, 98.8°F (37.1°C); 9 P.M., 99.4°F (37.4°C)

What conclusion can you draw about what is probably affecting the patients' temperatures? (*Clue:* Look at the pattern for each patient. How are the patterns similar?)

5 Organize a small group of classmates. Obtain several different sizes of blood pressure cuffs for each member of the group. Practice checking blood pressures on each other. Vary the size of the cuffs used, and note the variation generated by the change in cuff size. List your findings here (for at least three different people and at least two cuff sizes).

	Cuff Size		
	Large	Medium	Small
Person:			
Person:			
Person:			

6 A patient in the critical care unit has a weak pulse and blood pressure and is receiving intravenous fluids in both arms. Use your practical knowledge to decide how to assess blood pressure on this client. Do you need to validate your findings? If so, how will you do so?

7 Analyze the following scenario.
A 46-year-old man is hospitalized for multiple trauma after a mountain bike accident.
Vital signs on admission: BP, 138/90; pulse, 108; respirations, 24; temperature, 37.2°C (98.9°F)
8 hours later: BP, 162/100; pulse, 122; respirations, 26; temperature, 37.9°C (100.2°F)
He is restless, agitated, and in pain.

a What is going on in this situation that may be influencing the VS?

b Do you have enough patient information to determine what is happening?

c What nursing actions should you consider?

d Should you involve others in your discussion of possible actions? If so, who?

e What can you delegate in this situation?

f Should you report this change in vital signs to the primary care provider? Why or why not?

thinking critically about measuring vital signs

8 Ms. Alvin is an 80-year-old patient in a long-term care facility. Her blood pressures have been in the range of 120/70 to 130/80 for the past month. When she is newly assigned to your care, you see that according to her chart, she has a history of hypertension. She is taking an antihypertensive medication. You observe that she is very thin, especially her extremities. She weighs only 90 lb (40.8 kg) although she is of average height.

a Do you think the charted BPs are probably accurate? Why or why not?

b How could you make sure that the recorded BP readings are accurate?

c After looking for a small BP cuff, you discover that there is only one size available in the agency: a standard adult size. What should you do?

9 For each of the following concepts, use critical thinking to describe how or why it is important to nursing, patient care, and measuring vital signs. Note that these are not to be merely definitions.

Vital signs

Circadian rhythm

Metabolism

Shivering

Fever

Pulse

Stethoscope

Radial artery

Brachial artery

Apical pulse

Diaphragm

Oxygen saturation and pulse oximetry

Blood pressure

Peripheral resistance

thinking critically about measuring vital signs

Practical Knowledge
knowing how

PROCEDURES

| PROCEDURE 17–1 | **Assessing Body Temperature** |

 For steps to follow in *all* procedures, refer to the inside back cover of this book.

Note: Glass thermometers are rarely used in healthcare settings, but because many people still use them at home, we include them in this procedure. Glass-and-mercury thermometers should not be used in any healthcare setting. Teach patients the hazards associated with their use.

critical aspects
- Select the appropriate site and thermometer type.
- "Zero" or shake down the thermometer as needed.
- Insert the thermometer in its sheath, or use a thermometer designated only for the patient.
- Insert the thermometer in the chosen site.
- Leave a glass thermometer in the site for the recommended time (oral, 3 to 5 minutes; rectal, 2 minutes; axillary, 6 to 8 minutes).
- Leave an electronic thermometer in place until it beeps.
- Read the temperature. Hold a glass thermometer at eye level to read.
- Shake down a glass thermometer, and clean or store it.
- For an oral temperature, obtain a reading 15 to 30 minutes after the patient consumes hot or cold food or fluids or smokes.
- Hold a rectal thermometer securely in place, and never leave it unattended.

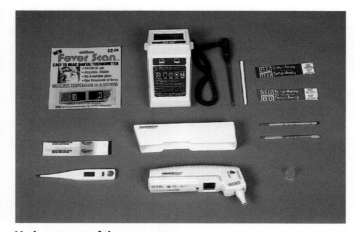

Various types of thermometers.

Equipment
- Thermometer (glass, electronic, chemical strip, or tympanic)
  - An oral thermometer generally has a blue tip
  - A rectal thermometer generally has a red tip

- Thermometer cover, if needed
- Procedure gloves, if taking a rectal temperature or if there is risk of contact with body secretions (e.g., saliva)
- Water-soluble lubricant, if taking a rectal temperature
- Towel, if needed, for taking an axillary temperature (*to dry the axillae*)
- Tissues

Delegation
You can delegate temperature measurement to the UAP if you conclude that the patient's condition and the UAP's skills allow. Perform the following assessments, and inform the UAP of the route (e.g., oral, rectal) and type of thermometer (e.g., glass, electronic) to use. Inform the UAP of any special considerations; for example, tell the UAP to be sure the patient has not had anything to eat or drink in the last 15 to 30 minutes; or inform the UAP that the patient is confused. Ask the UAP to record and report the temperature to you, and to report immediately if the temperature is elevated (e.g., over 101°F [38.3°C]).

PROCEDURE 17–1   **Assessing Body Temperature** *(continued)*

Assessments

• What site is most appropriate for the patient? Consider patient comfort, safety, and accuracy.

The oral route is contraindicated if the patient is unable to hold the thermometer properly or if there is a risk that the client may bite the thermometer. Do not use the oral route for children or other patients who cannot follow instructions (e.g., unconscious patients).

• What were the previous recordings, if any?

Noting changes over time is important in all patient assessments.

• Has the patient had anything to eat or drink, smoked, or exercised within the last 15 to 30 minutes? If yes, wait 20 to 30 minutes to obtain an accurate reading.

• Assess for clinical signs and symptoms of temperature alterations.

PROCEDURE 17–1A   **Taking an Oral Temperature**

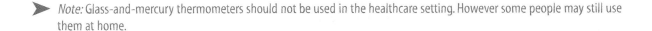

➤ *Note:* Glass-and-mercury thermometers should not be used in the healthcare setting. However some people may still use them at home.

Procedural Steps

Step 1 For a glass thermometer, shake down the mercury if necessary.

a. Stand in an open area away from tables and other objects.

Prevents breaking the thermometer.

b. Hold the end opposite the bulb between your thumb and forefinger, and snap your wrist downward.

c. Shake the thermometer until the reading is less than 96° F (35.6°C).

The reading must be below the anticipated temperature measurement.

Step 2 Slide the thermometer into a protective sheath.

The protective sheath provides a barrier to prevent transmission of organisms.

Step 3 Place the thermometer tip under the tongue in the posterior sublingual pocket (right or left of frenulum). ▼

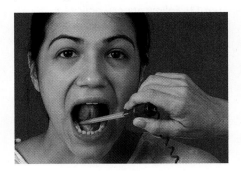

Puts the tip in close proximity to the major blood vessels under the tongue, allowing the thermometer to reflect the core temperature.

Step 4 Have the patient close the lips around the thermometer, cautioning the patient not to bite down on it.

Protects the thermometer from exposure to the air, which could alter the reading. Biting may cause a glass thermometer to break, injuring the mouth.

Step 5 Leave the thermometer in place for the recommended time.

a. Glass thermometer: 3 to 5 minutes
b. Electronic thermometer: until it beeps

An electronic thermometer will beep when a constant temperature is reached.

c. According to agency policy

Research findings differ on the optimal time for measuring an oral temperature, so follow agency policy.

Step 6 Remove the thermometer.

a. Discard the thermometer cover.
b. For a glass thermometer: If there is no cover, wipe the thermometer with a tissue to remove any mucus.

Step 7 Read the temperature.

a. For a glass thermometer: Position the thermometer at eye level, and rotate it until the markings are clear.

Ensures an accurate reading. ▼

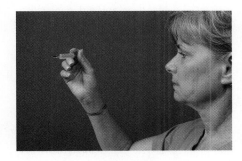

b. For an electronic thermometer: read the digital display.

Step 8 Clean and replace the thermometer. Follow agency policy.

a. For a glass thermometer: Clean with soap, rinse with cool water, shake it down, and place it in the appropriate storage container.

Prevents microbial growth.

b. For an electronic thermometer: Place the thermometer in its charging base.

PROCEDURE 17–1B   Taking a Rectal Temperature

Procedural Steps

Step 1 If necessary, shake down the glass thermometer so that the reading is less than 96°F (35.6° C).
a. Hold the end opposite the bulb between your thumb and forefinger, and snap your wrist downward.
b. Shake the thermometer until the reading is less than 96°F (35.6° C).

The reading must be below the anticipated temperature measurement.

Step 2 Slide the thermometer into a protective sheath.

A protective sheath provides a barrier to prevent transmission of organisms.

Step 3 Position an adult patient on the side with the knees flexed (Sims' position); place a child in the prone position. Drape the patient so that only the anal area is exposed.

Flexing the knees helps relax the muscles to ease insertion and aid in visualization. Draping provides privacy and decreases embarrassment. ▼

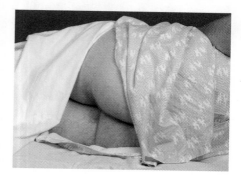

Step 4 Lubricate the tip of the thermometer by squeezing water soluble lubricant onto a tissue and then applying it to the thermometer.

Prevents injury to the rectal mucosa and eases insertion. Inserting the thermometer into the lubricant container would contaminate contents of the container.

Step 5 With your nondominant hand, separate the patient's buttocks to visualize the anus.

Step 6 Gently insert the thermometer approximately 1 to 1.5 inches (2.5 to 3.7 cm) in an adult; 0.9 inch (2.5 cm) for a child, and 0.5 inch (1.5 cm) for an infant.

The thermometer needs to be placed past the rectal sphincter. ▼

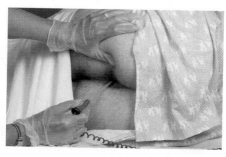

a. Have the patient take a deep breath. Insert the thermometer as he exhales.

Taking a deep breath helps the patient relax the anal sphincter.

b. If you feel resistance, do not use force.

Inserting the thermometer too far or forcing against resistance may cause injury to the rectal mucosa.

Step 7 Hold the thermometer in place the recommended amount of time.

The thermometer must be held in place to prevent inadvertent injury to the patient.

a. For a glass thermometer, hold the thermometer 2 to 3 minutes.
b. For an electronic thermometer, hold the thermometer in place until it beeps.

Research findings differ on the optimal time for measuring a rectal temperature, so follow agency policy. An electronic thermometer will beep when a constant temperature is reached.

Step 8 Remove the thermometer.
a. Discard the thermometer cover.
b. For a glass thermometer: If there is no cover, wipe the thermometer with a tissue to remove any stool.

Step 9 Read the temperature.
a. For a glass thermometer: Position the thermometer at eye level, and rotate it until the markings are clear.

Ensures an accurate reading.

b. For an electronic thermometer: Read the digital display.

Step 10 Clean and replace the thermometer.
a. For a glass thermometer: Clean the thermometer with soap, rinse with cool water, and place it in the appropriate storage container.
b. For an electronic thermometer: Place the thermometer in its charging base.

Prevents microbial growth on glass thermometers.

Step 11 Follow agency policy for cleaning and storing thermometers.

PROCEDURE 17–1C Taking an Axillary Temperature

Procedural Steps

Step 1 If necessary, shake down the thermometer.
a. Hold the end opposite the bulb between your thumb and forefinger, and snap your wrist downward.
b. Shake the thermometer until it reads below 96°F (35.6° C).

The reading must be below the anticipated temperature measurement.

Step 2 Slide the thermometer into a protective sheath.

A protective sheath provides a barrier to prevent transmission of organisms.

Step 3 Position the patient.
a. Assist the patient to a supine or sitting position.
b. Place the thermometer tip in the middle of the axilla. ➤
c. Position the patient's upper arm down, with the lower arm across the chest.

Puts the thermometer in close proximity to the axillary blood vessels, allowing it to better reflect the core temperature.

Step 4 Hold the thermometer in place the recommended time.
a. Leave a glass thermometer in place 6 to 8 minutes, according to agency policy (usually 5 minutes for children).
b. Leave an electronic probe in place until it beeps.

Study findings differ for accuracy of temperature measurements at the axillary site. Follow agency policy.

Step 5 Remove the thermometer.
a. Discard the thermometer cover.
b. For a glass thermometer: If there is no cover, wipe the thermometer with a tissue.

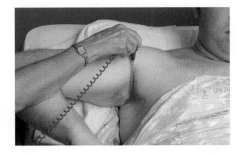

Step 6 Read the temperature.
a. For a glass thermometer, position the thermometer at eye level, and rotate it until the markings are clear.

Ensures an accurate reading.

b. For an electronic thermometer, read the digital display.

Step 7 Clean and replace the thermometer.
a. For a glass thermometer: Clean the thermometer with soap, rinse with cool water, and place it in the appropriate storage container.
b. For an electronic thermometer: Place the thermometer in its charging base.

Prevents microbial growth on glass thermometers.

Step 8 Follow agency policy for cleaning and storing thermometers.

PROCEDURE 17–1D Taking a Chemical Strip Temperature

Procedural Steps

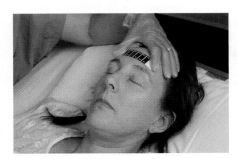

Step 1 Place the thermometer strip to the patient's skin, generally on the forehead or abdomen. ◄

The thermometer strip must be in contact with the skin.

Step 2 Leave the thermometer strip in place 15 to 60 seconds.
a. Follow the manufacturer's directions.
b. Observe for color changes.

Chemical strips have indicators that change colors to indicate temperature changes.

Step 3 Read the temperature before removing the strip from the patient.

Ensures the most accurate reading. Note that chemical strip thermometers are not very accurate. If temperature is not within normal range, retake it with an electronic or other thermometer.

Step 4 Remove and discard the thermometer strip.

PROCEDURE 17–1E   Taking a Tympanic Membrane Temperature

Procedural Steps

Step 1 Attach a probe cover to the tympanic thermometer.

Step 2 Position the patient's head to one side, and straighten the ear canal.
a. For an adult, pull the pinna up and back. ▼

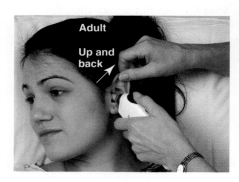

b. For a child, pull the pinna down and back.

Straightens the ear canal. The external auditory canal is curved upward in children under 3 years of age. In an adult, it is an S-shaped structure. ▼

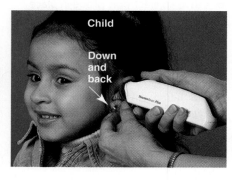

Step 3 Insert probe into ear canal gently and firmly, directing it toward the tympanic membrane, rotating probe handle toward jaw and making a firm seal around the probe.

Creates a seal to obtain an accurate reading without causing trauma to the ear canal.

Step 4 Take the measurement.
a. Depress the button to obtain the reading.
b. Follow the instructions for the specific tympanic thermometer being used.

Some tympanic thermometers immediately record the reading, and some require you to wait for approximately 3 seconds.

Step 5 Remove the thermometer.
a. Note the reading.
b. Discard the probe cover.

Step 6 Replace the thermometer in its charging base.

Evaluation

- Identify whether the temperature reading indicates hypothermia or hyperthermia.
- If the temperature is abnormal, perform other assessments to determine the cause or severity of the findings.
- Compare to normal range for developmental stage and to client's baseline data.
- Look for trends to identify potential concerns.

Patient Teaching

- Inform the patient of the temperature reading.
- Explain the significance of the temperature reading and any interventions that may be needed.
- Teach the hazards of using a glass-and-mercury thermometer.

Home Care

Reinforce the following points with your patient:
- If you use the same thermometer for more than one person, clean it well between uses.
- Clean the thermometer after each use, even if it is used for only one person. Wash with soap and water, rinse with cold water, dry well, and store in a clean, dry container.
- If the person has an infection or communicable illness, soak the thermometer in 70% isopropyl alcohol between uses.
- If you store the thermometer in alcohol, rinse it with cold water before taking the person's temperature.
- Do not use the same glass thermometer for both oral and rectal temperatures.
- Do not use an oral thermometer for taking a rectal temperature; use a specially shaped rectal thermometer to avoid injury.
- Chemical strip thermometers are not accurate. If you obtain a high or low reading, retake the person's temperature using a glass or other type of thermometer.

Documentation

You will usually record temperature on a flowsheet. In some situations (e.g., a fever), you may need to write a nurse's note. If so, follow these suggestions:

- Chart the temperature, indicating the route of measurement.

- Document the temperature according to agency policy.
- Notify the appropriate person of abnormal findings.
- Document supporting findings, such as "Skin is hot and dry" and state whether temperature reading is consistent with client's condition.

<table>
<tr><td>PROCEDURE 17–2</td><td>**Assessing Peripheral Pulses**</td></tr>
</table>

 For steps to follow in *all* procedures, refer to the inside back cover of this book.

critical aspects

- Make sure the client is resting while you assess a peripheral pulse.
- Select and palpate the appropriate site.
- Count for 30 seconds if pulse is regular; for 60 seconds if it is irregular.
- Note pulse rate, rhythm, and quality.
- Compare pulses bilaterally.
- Palpate the carotid pulse on only one side at a time.

Equipment

- Watch with a second hand or second readout
- Stethoscope
- Alcohol wipes (to wipe stethoscope, if used)
- Pen, pencil, and flowsheet or record form

Delegation

You can delegate measurement of pulses to the UAP if you conclude that the patient's condition and the UAP's skills allow. For example, if pedal circulation is critical and you suspect it may be difficult to palpate, you should not delegate assessment of the pedal pulse. If you do delegate, perform the following assessments, and inform the UAP of the site (e.g., radial, brachial) to use. Inform the UAP of any special considerations (e.g., to note what the patient's activity has been just before taking the pulse). Ask the UAP to record and report the pulse to you and to report immediately if it is outside normal limits (you must specify what is "normal" for each patient).

Assessments

- Determine why assessment of pulses is indicated.

Conditions that require an assessment of pulses include blood loss, cardiac or respiratory disease, diabetes mellitus, and other conditions that affect oxygenation.

- Assess factors that may alter the pulse, such as activity and medications. If the client has been recently active, wait 5 to 10 minutes before measuring.

Activity increases the pulse; increased intracranial pressure decreases the pulse; medications such as digoxin decrease the pulse; other medications, such as albuterol, increase the pulse.

PROCEDURE 17–2A   Assessing the Radial Pulse

Procedural Steps

Step 1 With patient sitting or supine, flex the patient's arm, and place the patient's forearm across chest.

Exposes radial artery for palpation. Placing the patient's forearm across the patient's chest aids in counting the patient's respiratory rate.

Step 2 Palpate radial artery.

The radial site is the most frequently used to calculate the patient's heart rate because it is generally the easiest site to use.

a. Place the pads of your index and middle fingers in the groove on the thumb side of the patient's wrist, over the radial artery. ➤
b. Press lightly but firmly until you are able to feel the radial pulse. Start with light pressure to prevent occluding the pulse, and gradually increase the pressure until you feel the pulse.

The fingertips are the most sensitive parts of the hand to palpate arterial pulsations. Avoid using the thumb, because it has its own pulsation and may interfere with the accuracy of your count.

Step 3 Note the rhythm and quality of the pulse. Note whether the thrust of the pulse against your fingertips is bounding, strong, weak, or thready.

The rhythm and quality of the pulse is a reflection of the patient's cardiac output. The strength of the pulse reflects the volume of the blood that is ejected against the arterial wall with each contraction of the heart. An irregular or weak pulse indicates decreased cardiac output. A bounding pulse indicates increased cardiac output.

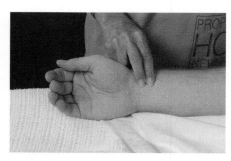

Step 4 Count the pulse:
a. Count a regular pulse for 30 seconds; then multiply by 2 to get the beats per minute.
b. Begin timing with the count of 1— the first beat that you feel.
c. Count an irregular pulse for a full minute (60 seconds).

Thirty seconds are sufficient to determine heart rate with a regular rhythm. An irregular pulse must be counted for a full minute to be accurate.

Step 5 For an admission assessment or peripheral vascular check, palpate the radial pulses on both wrists simultaneously.
a. Note any difference in the quality of the pulse between arms. Is the pulse on one side weaker than the other?

Palpating simultaneously enables the recognition of small differences in peripheral circulation.

PROCEDURE 17–2B   Assessing the Brachial Pulse

Procedural Steps

Step 1 Palpate the brachial artery.

a. Using firm pressure, press in the inner aspect of the antecubital fossa until you palpate the brachial artery. ➤

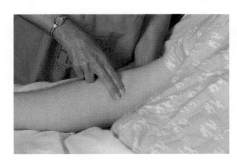

Step 2 Assess pulse rate, rhythm, and quality, and assess bilaterally as for the radial pulse (see Procedure 17–2A).

The brachial pulse is used most frequently to assess blood pressure and to identify the presence of a pulse during CPR in an infant.

PROCEDURE 17–2C   Assessing the Carotid Pulse

Procedural Steps

Step 1 Palpate the carotid artery.

a. Place your fingers on the patient's trachea, and slide them to the side into the groove between the trachea and the sternocleidomastoid muscle.

Palpate the carotid artery carefully to prevent complications of using this site. Compressing the carotid arteries can stimulate the carotid bodies and may significantly decrease the patient's heart rate. ➤

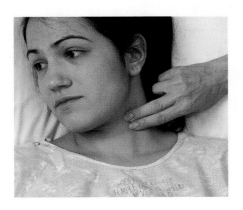

b. NEVER compress the carotid artery on both sides of the neck at the same time.

Compressing the carotid artery can decrease circulation to the head.

Step 2 Assess the rate, rhythm, and quality, and compare bilaterally as for the radial pulse (see Procedure 17–2A).

The carotid pulse is used to identify the presence of a pulse during cardiopulmonary resuscitation in an adult, and to assess circulation to the head.

PROCEDURE 17–2D — Assessing the Temporal Pulse

Procedural Steps

Step 1 Palpate the temporal pulse by pressing lightly lateral and superior to the eye. ➤

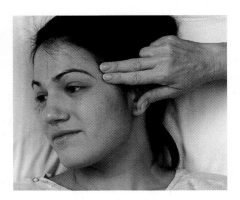

Step 2 Assess pulse rate, rhythm, and quality, and assess bilaterally as for the radial pulse (see Procedure 17–2A).

The temporal pulse is easily accessible and is used frequently in infants.

PROCEDURE 17–2E — Assessing the Femoral Pulse

Procedural Steps

Step 1 Palpate the femoral pulse by pressing deeply in the groin midway between the anterosuperior iliac spine and the symphysis pubis. ➤

The femoral artery is very deep and requires significant pressure to palpate. You may need to use both hands to feel the artery on an adult.

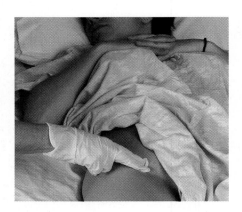

Step 2 Assess pulse rate, rhythm, and quality, and assess bilaterally as for the radial pulse (see Procedure 17–2A).

The femoral pulse is used to determine the presence of a pulse during cardiopulmonary resuscitation and to assess circulation to the leg.

PROCEDURE 17–2F — Assessing the Popliteal Pulse

Procedural Steps

Step 1 Palpate the popliteal pulse by pressing behind the knee in the middle of the popliteal fossa. ➤

The popliteal pulse can be difficult to feel. It is not used unless specifically indicated because of absence of pedal pulses or for taking a thigh blood pressure.

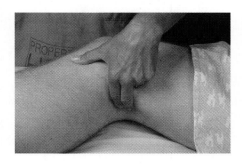

Step 2 Assess pulse rate, rhythm, and quality and assess bilaterally as for the radial pulse (see Procedure 17–2A).

The popliteal pulse is used to assess circulation of the lower leg and auscultate a thigh blood pressure.

PROCEDURE 17–2G   Assessing the Posterior Tibial Pulse

Procedural Steps

Step 1 Palpate the posterior tibial pulse by pressing on the inner (medial) side of the ankle below the medial malleolus. ➤

The posterior tibial pulse is usually palpated easily, but it may be deeper in some people. So, press down moderately and then increase pressure until you feel the pulse.

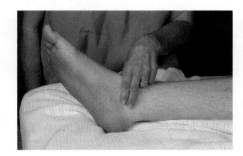

Step 2 Assess pulse rate, rhythm, and quality, and assess bilaterally as for the radial pulse (Procedure 17–2A).

The posterior tibial pulse is used to assess circulation to the lower extremity; it is assessed with the dorsalis pedis pulse.

PROCEDURE 17–2H   Assessing the Dorsalis Pedis Pulse

Procedural Steps

Step 1 Palpate the dorsalis pedis pulse.

The dorsalis pedis pulse is used to access circulation of the foot.

a. Run your fingers up the groove between the great and first toes to the top of the foot. ➤
b. Palpate very lightly.

The dorsalis pedis pulse is easily obliterated, so use very light pressure.

Step 2 Assess pulse rate, rhythm, and quality, and assess bilaterally as for the radial pulse (see Procedure 17–2A).

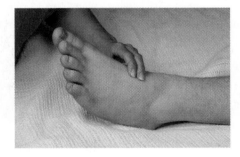

Step 3 If you are unable to palpate the dorsalis pedis pulse, use a Doppler ultrasound device to listen for the pulse.

Lack of pulses indicates inadequate circulation to the lower extremities. If you cannot feel the pulse, you must determine whether the pulse is absent or whether you are having difficulty feeling. To draw the conclusion that the pulse is "absent," you must use a Doppler.

Evaluation

Especially if pedal pulses are decreased, observe for other indications of inadequate circulation, such as cool skin, decreased capillary refill, and bluish or ashen skin tone. You must always provide supporting evidence if you chart that pedal pulses are decreased or absent. Complete absence of pulse requires immediate intervention.

Patient Teaching

• Teach the patient about the significance of any abnormalities in pulse rate or rhythm.
• Explain any interventions that may be needed.

Home Care

Assess the skill level of the person who will be assessing the patient's peripheral pulses in the home, and provide instruction if necessary.

Documentation

Usually you will document routine VS, including pulse, on a flowsheet. If you record it in a nurse's note, document the pulse rate, rhythm, and quality (e.g., *radial pulse at 64, regular, and strong bilaterally*).

PROCEDURE 17–3   **Assessing the Apical Pulse**

> For steps to follow in *all* procedures, refer to the inside back cover of this book.

critical aspects
- Palpate the 5th intercostal space at the midclavicular line for stethoscope placement.
- Count for 60 seconds.
- Note pulse rate, rhythm, and quality and the S_1 and S_2 heart sounds.

Equipment
- Watch with a second hand or second readout
- Stethoscope
- Alcohol wipes (to wipe stethoscope between patients)

Delegation

You can delegate measurement of the apical pulse to the UAP if you conclude that the patient's condition and the UAP's skills allow. Perform the following assessments. Inform the UAP of any special considerations (e.g., to note what the patient's activity has been just before taking the pulse, or to mark the time exactly so you can compare it to the patient's ECG). Ask the UAP to record and report the pulse to you, and to report immediately if it is outside normal limits (you must specify what is "normal" for each patient).

Assessments
- Determine why assessment of the apical pulse is indicated.

Conditions that require assessment of the apical pulse include digitalis therapy, blood loss, cardiac or respiratory disease, or other conditions that affect oxygenation status.

- Assess factors that may alter the pulse, such as activity and medications. If the client has been recently active, wait 10 to 15 minutes before obtaining measurement.

Procedural Steps

Step 1 With the client supine or sitting, lift the gown to expose the left side of the chest, but only as much as necessary.

Prevents distortion of sound from the patient's gown rubbing on the stethoscope while also protecting the patient's privacy.

Step 2 Palpate the 5th intercostal space at the midclavicular line for the apical pulse. ➤
a. To locate the 5th intercostal space, slide your finger down from the sternal notch to the angle of Louis (the bump where the manubrium and sternum meet).
b. Slide your finger over to the left sternal border to the 2nd intercostal space.
c. Now place your index or ring finger (depending on which hand you use) in the 2nd intercostal space, and count down to the 5th intercostal space by placing a finger in each of the spaces.
d. Slide over to the midclavicular line, keeping your finger in the 5th intercostal space.

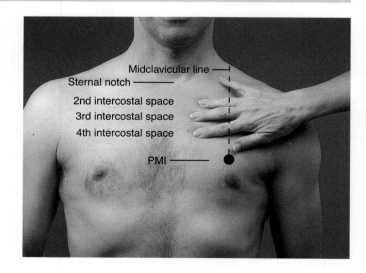

The apical pulse is generally best heard at the point of maximum impulse (PMI) in the 5th intercostal space at the midclavicular line. The PMI is located over the apex of the heart.

PROCEDURE 17–3   **Assessing the Apical Pulse** *(continued)*

Step 3 Palpate the apical pulse.
a. The palpated apical pulse is also called the point of maximal impulse (PMI).
b. The pulse area should be about the size of a quarter, without lifts or heaves.

A larger than normal pulsation may indicate ventricular hypertrophy.

Step 4 Warm the stethoscope in your hand for 10 seconds. Then place the diaphragm over the PMI, and listen to the normal S_1 and S_2 heart sounds (lub dup).

 Go to **Sound Files, Heart Sounds,** on the Electronic Study Guide.

Heart sounds result when blood moves through the valves of the heart. The first heart sound is louder at the apical area and should be audible when the pulse is auscultated.

Step 5 Count the apical heart rate for 1 full minute.

Ensures accuracy. Because the apical heart rate is needed as an assessment measure for the administration of some medications (e.g., digoxin), accuracy is essential. Some cardiac conditions cause either slow or irregular rates, both of which must be counted for a full minute to ensure accuracy.

Evaluation

- Are the findings within normal limits?
- Are there other factors supporting the findings?
- Look for trends.
- Compare pulses bilaterally.
- Is the skin pink, warm, and dry?
- Any cyanosis?

Patient Teaching

- Teach the patient about the significance of any abnormalities in the pulse rate or rhythm.
- Explain any interventions that may be necessary.

Home Care

- Assess the skill level of the person who will be assessing the patient's apical pulse in the home, and provide instruction if necessary.
- Teach the home caregiver when to hold medications and/or to call primary care provider (e.g., to hold the digitalis if the rate is <60).

Documentation

Document the pulse rate and rhythm.

Example

9/05/06	0900	*Apical pulse regular and strong, rate 64.* ———
		S. Jonas, RN

| PROCEDURE 17–4 | **Assessing for an Apical-Radial Pulse Deficit** |

> For steps to follow in *all* procedures, refer to the inside back cover of this book.

critical aspects
- Palpate 5th intercostal space at the midclavicular line for stethoscope placement.
- Palpate the radial pulse.
- When possible, have two nurses carry out the procedure. (This is ideal; can be done by one person skilled in the procedure.)
- Count for 60 seconds.
- Compare the pulse rate at both sites.

Equipment
- Watch with a second hand or second readout
- Procedure gloves, if indicated
- Stethoscope
- Alcohol wipes (to clean stethoscope between patients)

Delegation
Instead of delegating measurement of an apical-radial pulse to the UAP, you would most likely ask the UAP to assist you in this procedure because it is best performed by two persons working together.

Assessments
- Determine why assessment of pulse deficit is indicated.

Conditions that require assessment of pulse deficit include digitalis therapy, blood loss, cardiac or respiratory disease, and other conditions that affect oxygenation status.

- Assess factors that may alter the pulse, such as activity and medications.

Procedural Steps

Step 1 Lift the patient's gown to expose the left side of the chest, minimizing patient exposure.

Prevents distortion of sound from the patient's gown rubbing on the stethoscope and protects privacy.

Step 2 If two nurses are performing the procedure, place the watch so that the second hand is visible to both nurses.

Using one watch increases accuracy of counts.

Step 3 Palpate the 5th intercostal space at the midclavicular line for the apical pulse, and firmly hold the diaphragm of the stethoscope in place.

Use firm pressure to ensure good contact between the diaphragm of the stethoscope and the skin, which aids in hearing high-pitched sounds.

Step 4 The second nurse palpates the radial pulse. ➤

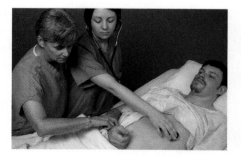

PROCEDURE 17–4 **Assessing for an Apical-Radial Pulse Deficit**
(continued)

Step 5 The nurse taking the radial pulse says "Start" when ready to begin, and "Stop" when finished. Both nurses count the pulse for 1 full minute.

Count simultaneously to ensure accuracy. Counting for 1 full minute is necessary for an accurate assessment of any discrepancies that may exist between the two sites.

Step 6 To obtain pulse deficit, subtract the radial rate from the apical rate.

Apical Rate − Radial Rate = Pulse Deficit

Atrial and ventricular dysrhythmias may cause beats that do not perfuse, so although you hear an apical heart beat, you do not feel a peripheral pulse. The pulse deficit is the number of heart beats that do not perfuse.

Step 7 Note any changes from previous recordings.

An increase in pulse deficit means that the patient's cardiac output is decreased. Assess other measures of cardiopulmonary status to identify a decline in the patient's condition.

Evaluation

Identify the presence of an apical-pulse deficit, and compare to previous findings.

Look for trends. The presence of any apical-pulse deficit is abnormal.

Patient Teaching

- Teach the patient about the significance of an apical-pulse deficit.
- Explain any interventions that may be necessary.

Home Care

Assess the skill level of the person who will be measuring the patient's apical-pulse deficit in the home, and provide instruction if necessary.

Documentation

Document the apical-pulse deficit.

Example

> 9/6/06   1030   Apical-pulse deficit is 4 beats/minute.
>   S. Albertson, RN

| PROCEDURE 17–5 | **Assessing Respirations** |

For steps to follow in *all* procedures, refer to the inside back cover of this book.

critical aspects
- Count unobtrusively (e.g., while palpating the radial pulse).
- Count for 30 seconds if respirations are regular; for 60 seconds if they are irregular.
- Observe the rate, rhythm, and depth of respirations.

Equipment
- Watch with a second hand

Delegation

You can delegate the counting of respirations to the UAP if you conclude that the patient's condition and the UAP's skills allow. Perform the following assessments, and inform the UAP of any special considerations (e.g., the need to keep the patient in a certain position). Ask the UAP to record and report the respirations to you, and to report immediately if they are not within the normal range for this patient (specify the range).

Assessments

- Observe for signs of respiratory distress—breathing faster or slower than normal, gasping breaths, confusion, circumoral (around the month) cyanosis

Signs of hypoxemia may indicate that the patient is not adequately oxygenated.

- Determine the baseline respiratory rate and character of respirations.
- Assess for factors that may affect the respiratory rate (e.g., pain, activity, fever, respiratory disorders).

Procedural Steps

Step 1 With the patient in a sitting position (preferably), flex the patient's arm, and place the patient's forearm across the chest. ➤

Aids in counting the patient's pulse rate by making the rise and fall of the chest more discernible and by making the patient less aware of the measurement of the respiratory rate. The patient's awareness might alter the patient's respiratory rate and/or pattern because respirations are partially under voluntary control.

a. For infants and children, placing your hand on the abdomen to assess the respiratory rate may be helpful.

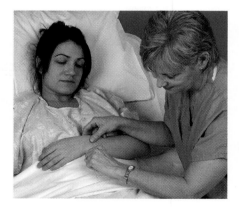

Infants and children are diaphragmatic breathers.

b. Another method for counting respirations unobtrusively is to palpate and count the radial pulse; remember that number; then,

keeping your hand on the patient's wrist, count the respirations.

Step 2 Observe the respiratory rate, rhythm, and depth.
a. Rate: normal for patient's age, fast (tachypnea), or slow (bradypnea).
b. Rhythm: regular or irregular.
c. Depth: normal, shallow, or deep (e.g., Kussmaul's).

All of these characteristics are necessary to evaluate respiratory status. Different pathologies affect each of these characteristics differently.

PROCEDURE 17–5 **Assessing Respirations** *(continued)*

Step 3 Count the number of breaths per minute. Begin timing the respirations with a count of 1, not 0, the same as with measurement of the pulse.

a. If the respiratory rhythm is regular, count the rate (one inhalation and one exhalation is one respiration) for 30 seconds, and multiply by 2.

b. If the rhythm is irregular, count the rate for 1 full minute (60 seconds).

c. For infants and young children, count for 1 full minute.

Variations in rhythm may cause an inaccurate rate when counted for less than 1 minute.

Evaluation

• Compare the respiratory rate and rhythm with previous readings.
• Note other vital signs, especially temperature.
• Look for trends, and note whether the respiratory rate and rhythm are changing in conjunction with changes in the other vital signs.

If the patient has an elevated temperature, the respiratory rate will increase. Corresponding elevation in pulse with respiratory rate may indicate hypoxemia.

Patient Teaching

Teach the patient about factors that affect respiratory status, such as smoking and activity.

Home Care

Assess the skill level of the person who will be measuring the patient's respiratory rate in the home, and provide instruction if necessary.

Documentation

You will document routine VS (including respirations) on a flowsheet. When a nurse's note is needed, follow these guidelines.
• Document the respiratory rate and rhythm.
• Document any pertinent information regarding respiratory status, such as intercostal retractions.

Example

10/14/06	1415	*Respirations are 12 per minute, regular, and deep. Skin is pale, but patient states he is having no more shortness of breath.* ———— N. Pearce, RN

PROCEDURE 17–6   Measuring Blood Pressure

For steps to follow in *all* procedures, refer to the inside back cover of this book.

critical aspects

- If possible, place the patient in a sitting position, with the feet on the floor and the legs uncrossed.
- Measure BP after the patient has been inactive for 5 minutes.
- Support the patient's arm at the level of the heart.
- Use cuff of the appropriate size.
- Position the cuff correctly, and wrap it snugly.
- Inflate the cuff while palpating the radial artery. Inflate to 30 mm Hg above the point at which you can no longer feel the radial artery.
- Place the stethoscope on the brachial artery, and release pressure at 2 to 3 mm Hg per second.
- Read the mercury manometer at eye level.
- Record systolic/diastolic pressures (first and last sounds heard—e.g., 110/80).
- Wait at least 2 minutes before remeasuring.

Equipment

- Stethoscope
- Sphygmomanometer with a cuff of the appropriate size
  To select the correct size, make sure that the inflatable portion of the cuff (bladder) is as follows:
  a. As shown in Figure 17–11 (in Volume 1), the *width* of the bladder of a properly fitting cuff will cover approximately two-thirds of the length of the upper arm (or other extremity) for an adult, and the entire upper arm for a child (National Institutes of Health, 1996).
  b. Alternatively, you can check that (1) the cuff *width* is 20% greater than the diameter of the midpoint of the limb or (2) the *length* of the bladder encircles 80% to 100% of the arm in adults (Joint National Committee, 1997; Perloff et al., 1993).

Using a cuff that is too small will result in a false-high reading; using a cuff that is too large will result in a lower reading.

Delegation

You can delegate measurement of BP to the UAP if you conclude that the patient's condition and the UAP's skills allow. Perform the following assessments, and inform the UAP of the site (e.g., radial, brachial) to use. Inform the UAP of any special considerations (e.g., not to place a BP cuff on the same side as the site of a mastectomy, or to use a larger cuff). Ask the UAP to record and report the BP to you, and to report immediately if it is outside normal limits (you must specify

what is "normal" for each patient). Tell the UAP that if BP is elevated, to note which arm, the patient's position during measurement, and activity immediately preceding the measurement.

Assessments

- Check for factors or activities that may alter the readings.

Caffeine, smoking, exercise, and stress can all elevate the blood pressure.

- What were the previous recordings, if any?

Noting changes over time is important with all patient assessments.

- Determine which arm to use.

Do not use an arm with an arteriovenous fistula, on the side of a radical mastectomy, or with an infusing intravenous therapy solution. Consider factors that might affect circulation to the extremity and alter the blood pressure reading.

PROCEDURE 17–6   Measuring Blood Pressure *(continued)*

Procedural Steps

Step 1 Position the patient comfortably, ensuring that:

a. Legs are uncrossed.

Crossing the legs may elevate the blood pressure reading.

b. Feet are resting on the floor (if the patient is sitting in a chair).

This position allows for the most accurate reading.

c. The arm being used to measure the blood pressure is at heart level, slightly flexed, with the palm facing upward.

The blood pressure will decrease if the arm is above the heart and increase if the arm is below the heart.

Step 2 Fully expose the arm, being careful that clothing is not tight.

Clothing that is tight enough to restrict blood flow will alter the reading.

Step 3 Wrap the cuff snugly around the upper arm. ▼

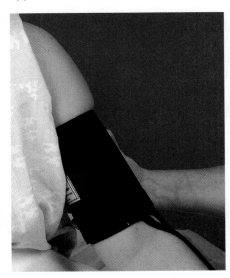

a. Ensure that the cuff is totally deflated, and palpate the brachial artery.

b. Place the bottom edge of the cuff approximately 1 inch (2.5 cm) above the antecubital space.

c. Place the center of the cuff bladder directly over the brachial artery (the center is often indicated with an arrow on the blood pressure cuff).

The center of the cuff bladder needs to be directly over the brachial artery so that you obtain an accurate reading when the cuff is inflated. Loose application of the cuff results in overestimation of the pressure.

Step 4 Place the stethoscope ear pieces in your ears so that the ear pieces are pointing slightly forward.

When the ear pieces point slightly forward, they direct sound into the ear canal, making the sounds more audible.

Step 5 Palpate the artery on the arm with the cuff.

Palpating the radial artery while inflating the cuff ensures that that the cuff is inflated higher than the systolic blood pressure. If the patient has an auscultatory gap, the systolic pressure can be mistakenly identified as lower than it actually is. Palpation is particularly important if the baseline systolic blood pressure is unknown.

Step 6 Close the sphygmomanometer valve.

Step 7 Pump up the cuff while continuing to palpate the radial pulse. When you can no longer feel the pulse, continue inflating the cuff an additional 30 mm Hg.

Inflating the cuff an additional 30 mm Hg beyond the point where the radial pulse can be palpated helps ensure an accurate systolic reading because it identifies the client's approximate systolic pressure and determines the maximal inflation point for an accurate reading. It also prevents an auscultatory gap.

Step 8 Place the bell (or diaphragm) of the stethoscope over the brachial artery, ensuring that the stethoscope tubing is not touching anything.

The American Heart Association recommends using the bell of the stethoscope for measuring blood pressure. The bell is better for lower-pitched sounds and must be lightly placed on the skin. A diaphragm is better for higher-pitched sounds and is held firmly on the skin. The diaphragm is often used in blood pressure measurement because of ease of use. If the stethoscope tubing contacts anything during blood pressure measurement, the artifact may be misinterpreted as part of the blood pressure reading. ▼

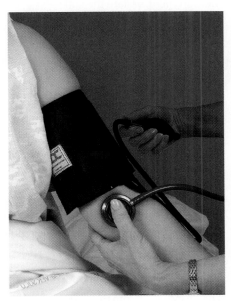

Step 9 Slowly release the sphygmomanometer valve, so that the cuff is deflated at a rate of 2 to 3 mm Hg per second.

Deflating the cuff more slowly increases patient discomfort and may alter the reading. Deflating the cuff faster may cause errors in hearing the Korotkoff sounds.

Step 10 Note the point on the manometer at which you hear the first sound. This is the systolic blood pressure.

The 1st Korotkoff sound is the systolic pressure.   ➤

PROCEDURE 17–6   **Measuring Blood Pressure** *(continued)*

Step 11   Continue deflating the cuff, and note the level at which the sounds become muffled and disappear. The diastolic pressure is the point at which the sound disappears.

The 5th Korotkoff sound (the disappearance of sound) is the diastolic blood pressure in adults. The 4th Korotkoff sound (the muffling of sounds) is the diastolic blood pressure in children. The AHA recommends recording the first sound, muffling, and last sound in children younger than 13 years, pregnant women, and people with high cardiac output or peripheral vasoconstriction.

Step 12   If you need to repeat the measurement, deflate the cuff completely, and wait 2 minutes before reinflating it.

Prevents venous congestion and false high readings.

Procedure Variation

Measuring Thigh Blood Pressure

Note: The thigh systolic measure may be 20 to 30 mm Hg higher than an arm blood pressure reading. The diastolic is generally comparable.

Follow the same steps as preceding, with these variations:

Step 1   Ensure that the cuff is completely deflated, and wrap the cuff snugly around the thigh so that the:
a. Bottom edge of the cuff is approximately 1 inch (2.5 cm) above the popliteal fossa.

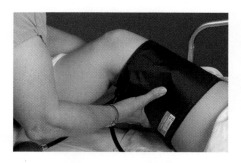

b. Center of the cuff bladder is positioned directly over the popliteal artery (often indicated with an arrow on the blood pressure cuff).▲

Step 2   Palpate the dorsalis pedis or posterior tibial artery on the leg with the cuff.

Step 3   Place the bell (or diaphragm) of the stethoscope over the popliteal artery.

Evaluation

- Compare the blood pressure reading with previous readings.
- Look for trends. Is the blood pressure slowly decreasing (e.g., impending shock) or slowly increasing (e.g., hypervolemia)?
- Look for a corresponding change in pulse rate, indicating potential hypoxemia.
- If this is the first blood pressure measurement for the client, check readings in both arms.

A difference of 10 mm Hg or less is normal.

- Report any significant changes in the blood pressure reading.

Patient Teaching

Teach the patient about:
- Normal blood pressure values (keep in mind that prehypertension occurs at a lower level when using self-monitored readings).
- Significance of the blood pressure reading.
- Further follow-up that may be necessary.

PROCEDURE 17–6 **Measuring Blood Pressure** *(continued)*

Home Care

- If possible, use the same equipment to prevent false changes in measurement.
- Explain the need for frequent recalibration of the home-monitoring device.
- Assess the skill level of the person who will be measuring the patient's blood pressure in the home, and provide instruction if necessary.

Documentation

- Document the blood pressure systolic/diastolic readings (e.g., 130/80).
- If you hear the 4th Korotkoff sound or muffling, document systolic/muffling/ diastolic (e.g., 130/80/70).
- Follow agency policy regarding the recording of muffled sounds.
- You will usually document routine BP readings on a flowsheet.

TECHNIQUES

TECHNIQUE 17–1 **Taking an Accurate Blood Pressure**

- Select the proper cuff size for the client (bladder should encircle at least 80% of arm).
- Use a mercury sphygmanometer if possible; otherwise, use a *recently calibrated* aneroid manometer or a *validated* electronic device.
- When using a mercury manometer, position the meniscus at eye level.
- Seat the client in a chair, with the feet on the floor, the back supported, and the arms bared and supported at heart level. BP reading may increase by up to 20 mm Hg if taken with the arm unsupported ("Vital Signs," 1999).
- Be sure the client has been at rest for at least 5 minutes before measuring BP. If the client has exercised strenuously, wait at least 20 minutes before assessing BP.
- Wrap the cuff snugly and evenly; do not apply over clothing.
- Do not deflate the cuff too slowly or too quickly (2 mm Hg per second, or 2 mm Hg per beat).
- Listen for a possible auscultatory gap.

- Do not be influenced by the client's previous BP measurements.
- Keep environmental noise and client movement to a minimum.
- Use the same limb for each measurement, unless you are comparing arms or averaging readings from both arms.
- Wait 30 minutes before assessing BP after client has ingested caffeine or smoked.
- Do not assess BP while the client is in pain.
- If you need to retake the BP (e.g., because you did not hear it clearly), wait at least 30 to 60 seconds before measuring again (Perloff et al., 1993). A 2-minute wait is recommended.
- Do not draw conclusions based on one reading. Take two or more readings, at least 6 minutes apart, and average them. If the readings differ by more than 5 mm Hg, obtain and average additional readings.
- When you take more than one reading on the same occasion, take one reading from each arm. For serial readings, perform the measurement on the same arm each time for consistency.

STANDARDIZED LANGUAGE

NOC Outcomes and NIC Interventions Associated with Abnormal Vital Signs

Selected Nursing Diagnoses	Selected NOC Outcomes	Selected NIC Interventions
	Temperature	
Hyperthermia	Neglect Recovery	Fever Treatment
Hypothermia	Risk Control	Hypothermia Treatment
Ineffective Thermoregulation	Risk Detection	Malignant Hyperthermia Precautions
Risk for Imbalanced Body Temperature	Thermoregulation	Temperature Regulation
	Thermoregulation: Newborn	Temperature Regulation: Intraoperative
	Vital Signs	Vital Signs Monitoring
	Pulse	
Decreased Cardiac Output	Vital Signs Status	Dysrhythmia Management
Ineffective Peripheral Tissue Perfusion		Vital Signs Monitoring
Risk for Impaired Tissue Integrity		
	Respirations	
Ineffective Breathing Pattern	Respiratory Status: Airway Patency	Airway Management
	Respiratory Status: Ventilation	Asthma Management
	Tissue Perfusion: Pulmonary	Anxiety Reduction
	Vital Signs	Mechanical Ventilation
		Oxygen Therapy
		Respiratory Monitoring
		Ventilation Assistance
	Blood Pressure	
Risk for Falls secondary to hypotension	Falls Occurrence	Fall Prevention
	Vital Signs Status	Self-Care Assistance: Transfer
Risk for Decreased Cardiac Output secondary to hypertension		Surveillance: Safety
		Vital Signs Monitoring
		Hemodynamic Regulation

Sources: NANDA International (2005). *Nursing diagnoses: Definitions and classification 2005–2006.* Philadelphia: Author; Moorhead, S., Johnson, M., & Maas, M. (Eds.). *Nursing outcomes classification (NOC)* (3rd ed.). St Louis: Mosby; Johnson, M., Bulechek, G., McCloskey Dochterman, J., Maas, M., & Moorhead, S. (2001). *Nursing diagnoses, outcomes, and interventions: NANDA, NIC, and NOC linkages.* St Louis: Mosby.

CONVERSION TABLE

Converting Between Fahrenheit and Centigrade

Centigrade	Fahrenheit		Centigrade	Fahrenheit
34.0	93.2		38.8	101.8
34.2	93.6		39.0	102.2
34.4	93.9		39.2	102.5
34.6	94.3		39.4	102.9
34.8	94.6		39.6	103.2
35.0	95.0		39.8	103.6
35.2	95.4		40.0	104.0
35.4	95.7		40.2	104.3
35.6	96.1		40.4	104.7
35.8	96.4		40.6	105.1
36.0	96.8		40.8	105.4
36.2	97.1		41.0	105.8
36.4	97.5		41.2	106.1
36.6	97.8		41.4	106.5
36.8	98.2		41.6	106.8
37.0	**98.6**		41.8	107.2
37.2	98.9		42.0	107.6
37.4	99.3		42.2	108.0
37.6	99.6		42.4	108.3
37.8	100.0		42.6	108.7
38.0	100.4		42.8	109.0
38.2	100.7		43.0	109.4
38.4	101.1		44.0	111.2
38.6	101.4			

What Are the Main Points in This Chapter?

- Vital signs (temperature, pulse, respirations, and blood pressure) are indicators of a person's state of health and functioning of the body systems.
- Many factors, such as, age, activity, smoking, and gender, cause normal variations in vital signs.
- Body temperature is the balance between heat production and heat loss.
- Fever is a symptom, but it is also beneficial to the immune response.
- A normal pulse rate varies widely according to age, from an average of 120 bpm for newborns to less than 80 bpm for adults over age 70.
- Assess the pulse for quality, bilateral equality, volume, and rate.
- Respiration is the process of supplying the body with oxygen and disposing of carbon dioxide.
- Assess respirations for rate, depth, rhythm, and associated clinical signs (e.g., breath sounds, chest movement, cough, pallor, and cyanosis)
- Blood pressure is the pressure of the blood as it is forced against arterial walls during cardiac contraction.
- Prehypertension is blood pressure ranging between 120 and 139 systolic and between 80 and 89 diastolic.
- Hypertension is persistent elevated blood pressure (>140 systolic or >90 diastolic) on more than two separate occasions.
- Clients can prevent or modify hypertension by certain lifestyle changes (e.g., exercise, weight control, and stress management).
- Nurses can delegate the activity of taking vital signs, but the nurse is responsible for evaluating the meaning of the data.

18 CHAPTER Communicating & the Therapeutic Relationship

Overview

Communication is a dynamic process of sending and receiving messages that can occur on three levels:

1. Intrapersonal, or self-talk
2. Interpersonal (between two or more people)
3. Group communication

People communicate verbally and nonverbally. Verbal communication refers to the use of spoken and written words and can be influenced by educational background, culture, language, age, and past experiences. Nonverbal communication, sometimes called body language, is a more accurate indicator of how someone is feeling than is verbal communication.

Therapeutic communication is the foundation of professional nursing practice. To enhance communication, listen actively, establish trust, be assertive, restate messages, clarify and validate messages, interpret body language, share observations, explore issues, use silence, and summarize the conversation.

Language barriers, sensory perceptual alterations, impaired cognitive skills, and physiological barriers make therapeutic communication with some clients challenging, but the nursing activities identified above can enhance communication.

Thinking Critically About Communicating and the Therapeutic Relationship

The exercises in the following section allow you to practice the kind of thinking you will use as a full-spectrum nurse. Because these are critical thinking activities, there is usually no single right answer. Discuss answers with your peers—discussion can stimulate critical thinking. If you have difficulty with any of the questions, consult with your instructor.

Caring for the Garcias

Below is a transcript of an interaction that occurred during Mr. Joseph Garcia's first visit to the family medical center. As you may recall, Jordan Miller is a family nurse practitioner who is examining Mr. Garcia. Analyze the interaction. Identify open-ended and closed questions and therapeutic communication techniques. Comment on responses that Jordan might have improved on.

Jordan: Are your parents still living?

Mr. Garcia: Yes, they're both alive. My father is 80 years old, and my mother is 76.

Jordan: I'd like to hear a little more about your family history. Tell me about your father's cancer. How old was he when he was first diagnosed? Has he had treatment?

Mr. Garcia: He was probably about 60 when he first found out about it. I know he had some kind of surgery and takes medicines, but I don't know the details. He seems all right, though.

Jordan: Your father also has high blood pressure and heart disease. Please give me a little more history about that.

Mr. Garcia: My father and mother both have high blood pressure and heart disease. They both take medicines for their blood pressure. My father had a small heart attack about 10 years ago. My mother has never had a heart attack that I know of, but she sometimes has chest pain.

Jordan: Your mother also has diabetes?

Mr. Garcia: She's had that for a long time. My parents joke about that. My father is part Cuban and part Irish. A lot of people in his family, especially on the Latin side, have diabetes, but nobody in my mother's family. Yet my mother is the one with the diabetes!

Mrs. Garcia: A lot of people in my family have diabetes, too. But so far I'm OK, I think. My family is from Mexico, and I know a lot of diabetics back home.

Jordan: Have you been seen for a health exam lately, Mrs. Garcia?

Mrs. Garcia: Not in about a year, but I'm going to schedule an appointment here.

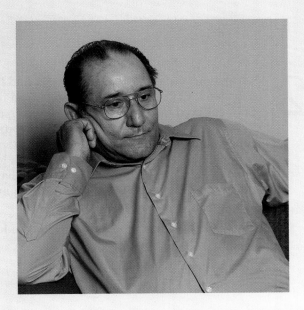

1   Mrs. Washington presents to the clinic complaining of a painful lump in her left breast. She is 40 years old and appears very nervous. She tells you, "I was afraid to come in, but I guess I have to find out what this is."

a   How might you acknowledge the client's feelings? Give examples.

b   What might you say to clarify and validate the client's messages?

c   Write a hypothetical conversation with Mrs. Washington that:
- Acknowledges her feelings
- Establishes trust
- Explores the issue
- Clarifies and validates the client's messages
- Uses silence
- Summarizes the conversation

2   Paramedics bring a 35-year-old man and his 14-year-old son to the emergency department (ED). Both have been involved in a recreational vehicle gas explosion and have suffered burns. The son is placed in one of the trauma rooms adjacent to his father. He has partial and full-thickness burns over his face, neck, chest, arms, and hands, and he is unresponsive. The father has partial-thickness burns on his right hand and forearm. He appears to be in a lot of pain and is screaming for his son in Spanish. He speaks limited English. Thirty minutes later, his wife (and the boy's mother) arrives at the ED. She is crying and asking whether her husband and son will be OK. Her English is fluent.

a   Identify at least two interventions to help you communicate with the father.

b   What kind of body language would you expect from the father?

c How could you show acceptance of and establish trust with the father?

d Identify at least two factors that will influence communication with the son.

e Identify at least two communication strategies to use with the son.

f Explain or give an example of how to use the following techniques as you communicate with the anxious wife and mother.

- Establishing trust

- Using silence

- Offering nonverbal support

3 For each of the following concepts, use critical thinking to describe how or why it is important to nursing, patient care, or communication. Note that these are *not* to be merely definitions.

Verbal communication

Nonverbal communication

thinking critically about communicating & the therapeutic relationship

Intrapersonal communication

Interpersonal communication

Group communication

Therapeutic communication

Therapeutic relationship

Barriers to therapeutic communication

Distance between sender and receiver

Communication strategies

Practical knowledge
knowing how

This section provides guidelines, outcomes, and interventions for communicating with patients.

TECHNIQUES

TECHNIQUE 18–1	Enhancing Communication Through Nonverbal Behaviors

Nonverbal Behaviors	Interpretation
Direct eye contact	Demonstrates interest and attention. The nurse must consider the client's cultural heritage when determining how much eye contact is appropriate.
Concerned facial expression	Lends credibility, if congruent with conversation.
Leaning forward	Shows interest in the conversation.
Personal space	Maintaining a distance of 18 inches to 4 feet allows most clients to feel comfortable during the interaction. Adjust the distance within that range based on the client's preference.
Professional appearance	Gives people an impression of how you may act in your role as a healthcare provider.
Sitting down to talk with the client	Communicates willingness to listen and a sense of not wanting to rush the client.
Touch	Conveys caring and concern when used appropriately.

TECHNIQUE 18–2	Some Useful Spanish Words and Phrases

English	Spanish	English	Spanish
How do you feel?	¿Como se siente?	Cough	Tosa
Good	Bien	Open your mouth	Abra la boca
Bad	Mal	Take a deep breath	Respire profundamente
Have you any difficulty in breathing?	¿Tiene dificultad al respirar?	You may eat	Puede comer
		Tea	Té
Are you thirsty?	¿Tiene sed?	Coffee	Café
Have you any pain?	¿Tiene dolor?	I will give you something for that	Le daré algo para eso
Show me where	Enséñeme dónde		
Is it worse now?	¿Está peor ahora?	A pill	Una píldora

Some medical dictionaries (e.g. *Taber's Cyclopedic Medical Dictionary,* 2005) have a comprehensive list of English-Spanish phrases. If you wish to purchase software to provide quick English-Spanish translation of healthcare phrases,

Go to **http://mobilearn.net/English_Spanish_health_care_translator.htm**

TECHNIQUE 18–3 Communicating with Clients Who Have Sensory Deficits

Clients Who Have Impaired Hearing

- Use touch to get the client's attention.
- Face the client directly. Speak slowly, clearly, and concisely.
- Do not shout; shouting distorts your voice.
- Speak in short sentences.
- Confirm that the client understood you by asking her to repeat what you said.
- If the hearing deficit is predominantly in one ear, move closer to the less affected ear.
- Use paper, pencil, or computer communication when necessary.
- If possible, arrange a hearing evaluation for the client and construction of any required hearing aids.

Clients Who Have Impaired Speech

- Nonverbal communication is the key to communication with clients with impaired speech.
- Have the patient use hand gestures and a picture board, as appropriate.
- Solicit family assistance in understanding the client's speech.
- Provide a comfortable environment for the client to practice speaking.
- Be positive and patient.
- Although the client may have difficulty speaking, you should continue to speak and explain all procedures.
- A referral to a speech pathologist may be necessary.

TECHNIQUE 18–4 Communicating with Clients Who Have Impaired Cognition or Consciousness

Clients Who Are Cognitively Impaired

- Make every effort to communicate, even if you think that the client cannot understand you.
- Provide adequate time to allow the client to communicate. Do not rush the client. Give the client time to respond to your questions or commands.
- Use multiple communication modalities. For example, you may want to provide verbal and written discharge instructions. Review the instructions several times with the client before discharge, and include family members in the teaching.
- Use memory aids, schedules, and reminder notices to reinforce information.
- Verbally orient to time, person, and place, and provide visual orientation materials, such as a calendar or schedule.
- If the client loses his place in conversation, stimulate memory by repeating his last expressed thought (e.g., "We were talking about your back pain. Tell me more about your back pain").
- Use short sentences, containing a single thought (e.g., "Are you hungry?"). Avoid complex statements (e.g., "You look hungry. Would you like a sandwich or a milk shake? Or can you hold off until dinner?")

- Do not use vague comments to indicate that you are listening. The client may be unable to interpret comments such as, "I see." Instead, repeat the client's words and directly state your response (e.g., "You are cold. I will bring you a blanket").
- Bear in mind that the client cannot behave differently and that he is confused about reality. When the person is talking about superficial, routine matters, he may seem more competent than he is.

Clients Who Are Unconscious

- Speak to unconscious or sedated clients, and advise them of care you are providing. Although the client may not be able to respond, she may be able to hear your comments.
- Consult with previous caregivers or the family to determine what the client responds to.
- Begin each interaction by identifying yourself and calling the client by name.
- Speak calmly and slowly.
- Explain all healthcare procedures.
- Provide soothing music and periods of rest.

STANDARDIZED LANGUAGE

Selected NOC Outcomes and NIC Interventions for Impaired Verbal Communication

NOC Outcomes	Selected Outcome Indicators	NIC Interventions	Selected NIC Activities
Communication	Acknowledgment of messages received Exchanges messages accurately with others	Active Listening	Be aware of the tone, tempo, volume, pitch, and inflection of the voice. Use questions or statements to encourage expression of thoughts, feelings, and concerns.
Communication: Expressive	Use of written language Use of pictures and drawings to communicate	Assertiveness Training	Promote expression of thoughts and feelings, both positive and negative.
Communication: Receptive	Interpretation of spoken language Interpretation of sign language	Communication Enhancement (Hearing Deficit, Speech Deficit, Visual Deficit)	(Hearing) Move close to less affected ear. (Speech) Give one simple direction at a time, as appropriate. (Vision) Identify yourself when you enter the patient's space.
		Presence	Be physically available as a helper.
		Touch	Give a reassuring hug, as appropriate. Hold patient's hand to provide emotional support.

Sources: Moorhead, S., Johnson, M., & Maas, M. (Eds.). (2004). *Nursing outcomes classification (NOC)* (3rd ed.). St Louis: Mosby; Dochterman, J. M., & Bulechek, G. (Eds.) (2004). *Nursing interventions classification (NIC)* (4th ed.). St Louis: Mosby; Johnson, M., Bulechek, G., Dochterman, J., Maas., M., & Moorhead, S. (Eds.). (2001). *Nursing diagnoses, outcomes, and interventions: NANDA, NOC, and NIC linkages.* St Louis: Mosby; and NANDA International. (2005). *Nursing diagnoses: Definitions and classification 2005–2006.* Philadelphia: Author.

What Are the Main Points in This Chapter?

- Communication is a dynamic, reciprocal process of sending and receiving messages.

- Communication occurs on three levels: intrapersonal, or self-talk; interpersonal (between two or more people); and group communication.

- The sender delivers a message to the receiver via verbal and/or nonverbal communication. The receiver provides feedback to the sender.

- Verbal communication is the use of spoken and written words. It is influenced by factors such as educational background, culture, language, age, and past experiences.

- Nonverbal communication, sometimes called body language, communicates how someone is feeling and gives a more accurate account of an individual's true sentiment.

- Communication is most successful in a comfortable environment. A favorable environment is quiet, private, free of noxious smells, and a comfortable temperature.

- Physical development, language skills, intellectual abilities, culture, gender, and maturity influence the communication process.

- The distance between individuals engaged in communication is affected by the relationship of the individuals, the nature of the conversation, the setting, and cultural influences.

- Relationships affect the choice of vocabulary, tone of voice, use of gestures, and distance associated with the communication.

- Therapeutic communication is the use of communication skills that result in a positive effect on client care; it is the foundation of professional nursing practice.

- Therapeutic communication occurs in the context of a helping relationship. The helping relationship has four phases: pre-interaction, orientation, working phase, and termination.

- Group communication occurs when you are interacting with a family, a community, or a committee. Groups may be focused on a task, self-improvement, coping skills, or work-related issues.

- To enhance communication, listen actively, establish trust, be assertive, restate messages, clarify and validate messages, interpret body language, share observations, explore issues, use silence, and summarize the conversation.

- Barriers to communication include asking too many questions, asking why, changing the subject inappropriately, failing to listen, failing to probe, expressing approval or disapproval, offering an opinion, providing false reassurance, stereotyping, and using patronizing language.

- Language barriers, sensory perceptual alterations, impaired cognitive skills, and physiological barriers make therapeutic communication challenging, but nursing activities can enhance communication with these clients.

Knowledge Map

Communicating

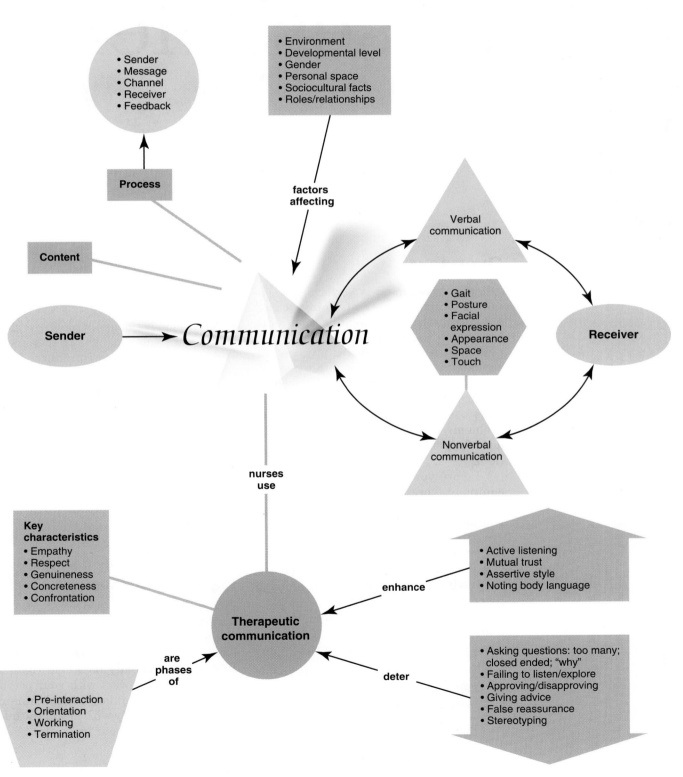

Process
- Sender
- Message
- Channel
- Receiver
- Feedback

factors affecting
- Environment
- Developmental level
- Gender
- Personal space
- Sociocultural facts
- Roles/relationships

Content

Sender → *Communication*

Verbal communication

- Gait
- Posture
- Facial expression
- Appearance
- Space
- Touch

Receiver

Nonverbal communication

nurses use

Therapeutic communication

Key characteristics
- Empathy
- Respect
- Genuineness
- Concreteness
- Confrontation

are phases of
- Pre-interaction
- Orientation
- Working
- Termination

enhance
- Active listening
- Mutual trust
- Assertive style
- Noting body language

deter
- Asking questions: too many; closed ended; "why"
- Failing to listen/explore
- Approving/disapproving
- Giving advice
- False reassurance
- Stereotyping

CHAPTER 19

Health Assessment:

Performing a Physical Examination

Overview

A health assessment is performed to obtain data about a patient, to investigate a health problem, to monitor a patient's health status, or to screen for health problems. A comprehensive physical assessment is a complete head-to-toe examination of every body system. A focused physical assessment is confined to systems associated with a specific patient problem. Ongoing assessment may be done for periodic reassessment of the patient.

Before you assess a patient, gather equipment, prepare the environment, review the skills you will use, familiarize yourself with the patient situation, go over the nursing plan of care, and explain the examination to the patient. Attempt to develop rapport with the patient to improve his comfort and promote relaxation.

Sharpen your senses. You will use them as you employ the four techniques you use to examine your patient.

- Inspection is the use of sight. It begins the moment you meet the patient.
- Palpation is the use of touch to assess temperature, skin texture, moisture, anatomical landmarks, and abnormalities such as edema, masses, or areas of tenderness.
- Percussion is the use of touch to tap the skin with short strokes from your fingers. The vibrations produced allow you to determine location, size, and density of underlying structures.
- Auscultation is the use of hearing. Direct auscultation is unassisted listening. Indirect auscultation is listening to the sounds produced by the body with the help of a stethoscope.

Throughout your assessment compare data from side to side in each system (bilaterally).

Thinking Critically About Physical Assessment

The exercises in the following section allow you to practice the kind of thinking you will use as a full-spectrum nurse. Because these are critical-thinking activities, there is usually no single right answer. Discuss answers with your peers—discussion can stimulate critical thinking. If you have difficulty with any of the questions, consult with your instructor.

Caring for the Garcias

Joe Garcia has had a comprehensive physical examination with Jordan Miller, the nurse practitioner at the clinic. To review the note written by Jordan,

 VOL 1 Go to Chapter 19, **Documenting Physical Assessment Findings,** in Volume 1.

A. Discuss how each of the following would differ from the examination Jordan Miller conducted and what would be expected if:

- A registered nurse conducted the exam.

- A nursing student performed the exam.

B. Review Jordan's charting of the exam. Identify the abnormal findings.

C. Review the lab work. Identify the abnormal findings.

D. What conclusions, if any, can you draw from these findings? What actions should you consider based on these conclusions?

E. Identify at least two nursing diagnoses based on these findings.

F. Jordan Miller has identified a problem of Imbalanced Nutrition: More than Body Requirements for Mr. Garcia.

- What information do you need to determine the etiology of this problem?

- Because you do not have that information, write a two-part diagnostic statement describing Mr. Garcia's nutritional status.

G. Now rewrite the nutrition statement as a three-part statement, using "as evidenced by."

H. Jordan Miller has identified the diagnosis Acute Pain (knees) for Mr. Garcia. If the pain is caused by a medical condition, osteoarthritis, how would you write a two-part diagnostic statement to describe this health status?

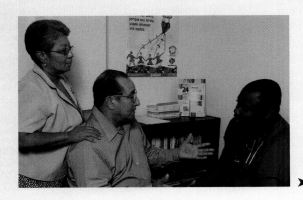

I. How would the examination of Flordelisa Garcia differ from the exam Joe experienced?

J. How would the examination of Bettina Sanford, Joe's 3-year-old granddaughter, differ?

K. If you were responsible for examining Joe Garcia, what aspects of the exam would you find most challenging? Explain why.

Practical Knowledge
knowing how

The registered nurse is responsible for patient assessment. You should (1) perform the initial assessment to establish a baseline, and (2) perform follow-up assessments for any changes. You can instruct unlicensed assistive personnel (UAPs) to report any additional changes to you.

You can delegate assessment of height, weight, and vital signs to the UAP; however, you should perform the initial admission general survey. You may also want to obtain the first set of vital signs yourself, because they will serve as a baseline.

PROCEDURES

In this section, you will find all the procedures necessary for a complete physical examination (Procedures 19–1 through 19–19). In addition you will find two techniques to assist you with your physical examination, and an Abnormal Atlas at the end of the chapter.

When examining each body system be sure to compare findings on both sides of the body.

TECHNIQUE 19–1   Performing Percussion

Direct Percussion

Tap lightly with the pads of the fingers directly on the skin.

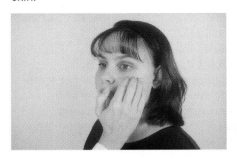

Direct percussion over the sinuses

Indirect Percussion

- Keep your fingernails short.
- Strive for a quiet environment: Turn off the television and radio, shut the door, and so on. This allows you to better perceive the subtle differences in percussion notes.
- One hand is considered the stationary hand; the other is the striking hand.
- Hyperextend the middle finger of your stationary hand, and place its distal portion firmly against the client's skin over the area you wish to percuss.
- Lift the rest of your fingers off the patient's skin so you don't dampen the sounds produced.

- Be sure both of your hands are relaxed.
- Use the middle finger of your dominant hand as the striking finger **(plexor),** and tap the distal portion of the middle finger of the stationary hand using a quick motion from your wrist.
- Use enough force to elicit a clear sound.
- Percuss two times over each location, then move to a new body location and repeat.

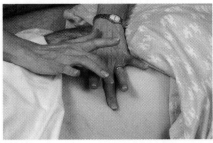

Indirect percussion

Use the terms in the following table to describe the sounds you hear. The terms are based on the following components of the sounds produced by percussion:

- *Amplitude:* the loudness or softness of a sound
- *Pitch:* the number of vibrations per second; either high or low in nature
- *Quality:* a distinctiveness about the sound produced
- *Duration*: how long the sound lingers

Percussion Notes

Sound	Amplitude	Pitch	Quality	Duration	Example
Resonant	Medium-loud	Low	Hollow	Medium	Normal lung
Hyperresonant	Louder	Lower	Booming	Longer	Hyperinflated lung (as in emphysema)
Dull	Soft	High	Muffled thud	Short	Liver/spleen
Flat	Very soft	High	Absolute dullness	Very short	Thigh or tumor
Tympany	Loud	High	Musical	Longest	Gastric air bubble, intestinal air

TECHNIQUE 19–2   Performing Auscultation

- Provide a quiet environment to facilitate auscultation.
- Use the diaphragm to listen to high-pitched sounds that normally occur in the heart, lungs, and abdomen. Press the diaphragm hard enough to produce an obvious ring on the patient's skin.
- Use the bell to hear low-pitched sounds, such as extra heart sounds (murmurs) or turbulent blood flow, known as bruits. Always apply the bell lightly with just enough pressure to produce an air seal with its full rim.
- Place the earpieces facing forward to seal the ear canal and improve detection of sounds.

- Warm the stethoscope before you place it on the client's skin.
- Place the stethoscope directly on the client's skin. Do not listen through clothing.
- If hair prevents good contact with the skin, wet the hair before you listen.
- Close your eyes as you listen through the stethoscope. This helps improve your focus.
- Concentrate on one sound at a time. Do not try to evaluate breath and heart sounds at the same time. Although this increases the length of time required for assessment, it improves the quality of the data.

PROCEDURE 19–1   Performing the General Survey

 For steps to follow in *all* procedures, refer to the inside back cover of this book.

critical aspects

- Observe the patient's apparent age, gender, race, facial expression, body size and type, posture, movements, speech, grooming, dress, hygiene, mental state, and affect.
- Identify any signs of distress.
- Measure vital signs.
- Measure height and weight, and calculate BMI.
- Consider the client's cultural/ethnic background, gender, and developmental stage.
- Review history data that may influence general survey findings, including usual state of health, current health problem, allergies, and unexplained changes in weight.
- Note verbal and nonverbal responses throughout exam.

Equipment

Refer to the accompanying table.

Positioning

- Have the client seated as you begin the examination (on an exam table or on the side of the bed).
- If the client is unable to sit, use Fowler's or semi-Fowler's position.

Focused History Questions

- How are you feeling today?
- (If the client is an outpatient) What brings you to the clinic today?

- Are you in any discomfort or pain?
- Have you had any hospitalizations or surgeries?
- What medicines do you take?
- Do you use any herbal products, natural remedies, or over-the-counter medicines?

Developmental Modifications

- Infants and toddlers usually feel most secure if a parent is present for the examination. Position an infant on a padded examination table or held against the parent's chest.
- Offer toddlers choices. Involve the parent in the exam. Praise the toddler for cooperation.

Text continues on page 237.

Equipment Needed for Physical Examination

Usual Equipment for Ongoing Assessment

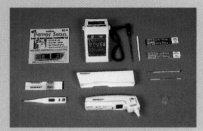
Thermometer (for measuring temperature)

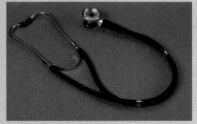
Stethoscope (for measuring blood pressure and listening to heart, lung, and bowel sounds)

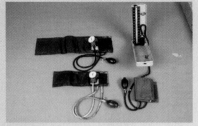
Sphygmomanometer (for measuring blood pressure)

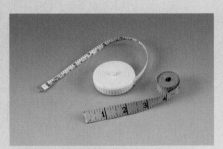
Tape measure (to measure circumference and length)

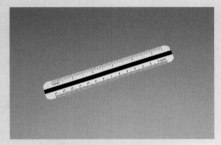
Pocket ruler (to measure size or distance)

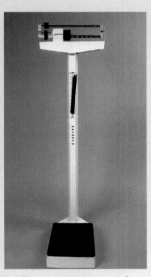
Scale (to measure weight and height)

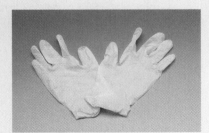
Gloves (to wear if there is any possible exposure to blood or body fluids)

Equipment Needed for Physical Examination *(continued)*

Additional Equipment for a Comprehensive Assessment

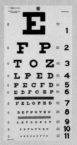

Snellen acuity chart (for screening vision)

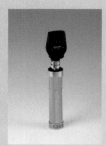

Ophthalmoscope (for inspection of the internal structures of the eye)

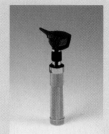

Otoscope (for examining the external auditory canal and tympanic membrane)

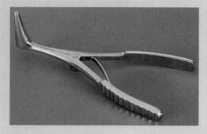

Nasal speculum (for examining the nasal turbinates)

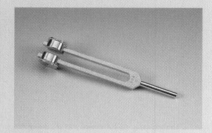

Tuning fork (for auditory screening and assessment of vibratory sensation during the neurological exam)

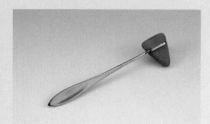

Percussion hammer (for eliciting deep tendon reflexes)

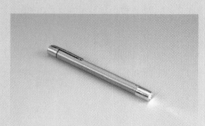

Penlight (for visualizing the eyes and inside of mouth, or highlighting a skin lesion)

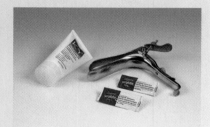

Vaginal speculum and lubricant (for examining the female pelvis; lubricant is also used for rectal exams)

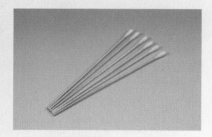

Cotton-tipped applicators (for obtaining specimens)

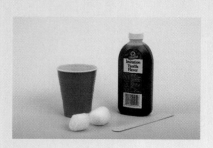

Cotton balls, tongue depressor, strong-smelling substance, a glass of water (for testing various cranical nerves)

- Preschoolers often are fearful of body injury and invasive procedures. Allow the preschool child to sit in the parent's lap if she wishes. Let the child help with the exam. Give reassurance as you proceed. Compliment the child on her cooperation.
- Support the school-age child's independence. Develop rapport by asking the child about his teacher or favorite school and play activities. Allow the child to undress himself and get up and down from the exam table. Demonstrate your equipment before you use it.
- Adolescents are self-conscious and introspective and should be examined without parents or siblings

present unless they request otherwise. Provide privacy.
- Observe the older adult's energy level during the physical examination, and provide rest periods if needed. If the client tires easily, arrange the exam sequence to limit position changes.
- Allow extra time to interview and examine older adults.
- Be aware that stiff muscles and arthritic joints may make it impossible for older adults to assume certain positions.
- Be alert for hearing and vision deficits in older adults, and adapt your interview techniques accordingly (e.g., elicit feedback to be sure the client has heard you correctly).

Procedural Steps	Expected Findings
Performing the General Survey	
1. Identify signs of distress.	Client is in no apparent distress.
If signs of distress are present, perform a focused assessment, and address the immediate problem.	**Abnormal findings:** pain, grimacing, breathing problems, skin color changes.
2. Observe apparent age, gender, and race. Ask the patient, "What racial or ethnic group do you identify with?" Ask yourself, • Is apparent age consistent with biological age? • Are there cultural or gender-related factors that influence the exam or findings?	Client appears his stated age. Makes eye contact consistent with his cultural norms. Is reasonably comfortable with being examined.
3. Note facial characteristics, including facial expression, symmetry of facial features, and the condition and color of the skin. Ask yourself, • What is the client's face telling me? • Is there evidence of pain, fear, or anxiety? • Is the facial expression appropriate to the situation? • Are facial features symmetrical (palpebral fissure and nasolabial folds)? • Are there any changes in condition or color of skin? • Does the client maintain eye contact?	Client appears relaxed, with no evidence of pain, fear, or anxiety. Face is symmetrical; visible skin is intact without excessive wrinkling, discoloration, or deformity.
4. Note body type and posture. Greet the client with a handshake to assess muscle strength and surface skin characteristics while at the same time conveying that you care. (Be aware that shaking hands is not acceptable in all cultures.) Ask yourself, • Is the body build stocky, slender, average, obese or cachectic? • Are the body parts proportional to the client's overall size? • Does the client have abnormal fat distribution? • Does the client assume a specific position for comfort (e.g., sitting versus supine)?	Posture is upright, and body appears proportionate.

Procedural Steps

Expected Findings

Performing the General Survey *(continued)*

5. Observe gait, and note any abnormal movements. If the client is bedridden, determine her ability to move and the amount of assistance needed. Ask yourself,

- Does the client move in a coordinated manner?
- Are there any obvious gait problems?
- Does the client walk with a wide base of support or short stride length?
- Does the client use assistive devices?
- Are there any abnormal or spastic movements?

Movements are coordinated; gait is steady; does not use assistive devices.

Abnormal findings: unstable or shuffling gait; spastic movements, stiff movements.

---

6. Listen to your client's speech pattern, pace, quality, tone, vocabulary, and sentence structure. Ask yourself,

- Are the responses appropriate?
- Is there any difficulty with speech?
- Does the client's tone of voice match her statements?

Special Consideration

If there is an apparent language barrier, obtain an interpreter.

Client responds appropriately to questions. Tone of voice matches responses. Speech is clear, evenly paced, and rises and falls based on content.

Abnormal findings: rapid speech, slow speech, slurred speech.

---

7. Assess mental state and affect.

a. Determine level of consciousness.

b. Determine orientation to time, place, and person. Ask yourself,

- If the client is disoriented, does he reorient easily?
- What is the client's mood? Is it appropriate for the situation?

Many medical conditions and medications can affect mental status.

Awake, alert, and oriented to time, place, person, and self. Mood is appropriate for the situation.

Abnormal findings: confusion and irritability, inability to recall information or provide history, lethargy and somnolence.

---

8. Observe dress, grooming, and hygiene. Ask yourself,

- Is the client appropriately and neatly dressed?
- Is the client well groomed?
- Are there any unusual odors?

Client is dressed appropriately for the climate. Skin is clean, and clothing is in good repair. No noticeable odor.

Abnormal findings: poor hygiene, dirty skin or nails, uncombed hair, visible soiling of clothing, mismatched or wrinkled clothing, objectionable odor.

---

9. Measure vital signs: blood pressure, temperature, radial pulse, respiratory rate.

BP: <130/85
Temperature: 98–98.6°F (36.7–37°C) oral
Pulse: 60–100 bpm, regular, and easily palpated
Respiratory rate: 12–20, regular and even

Abnormal findings: See Chapter 17.

Procedural Steps

(continued)

10. Measure height and weight.

a. For adults: Calculate BMI, or use the accompanying table.

b. For children: Plot height and weight on growth chart.

Developmental Modifications: Infants and Children

- Weigh infants without clothing; weigh older children in their underwear.
- For infants and children under 2 years, position supine to measure height; be sure knees are extended.
- For infants and children under age 2, also measure head circumference.

Expected Findings

For adults: BMI is 20–25.

For children: Height and weight are consistent with previous trend on growth chart.

Abnormal findings:

BMI < 20 = underweight

BMI 25–29.9 = overweight

BMI > 30 = obese

Body Mass Index

Weight (lb)

Height (ft/in)	120	130	140	150	160	170	180	190	200	210	220	230	240	250	260	270	280	290	300	310	320	330
4'5"	30	33	35	38	40	43	45	48	50	53	55	58	60	63	65	68	70	73	75	78	80	83
4'6"	29	31	34	36	39	41	43	46	48	51	53	56	58	60	63	65	68	70	72	75	77	80
4'7"	28	30	33	35	37	40	42	44	47	49	51	54	56	58	61	63	65	68	70	72	75	77
4'8"	27	29	31	34	36	38	40	43	45	47	49	52	54	56	58	61	63	65	67	70	72	74
4'9"	26	28	30	33	35	37	39	41	43	46	48	50	52	54	56	59	61	63	65	67	69	72
4'10"	25	27	29	31	34	36	38	40	42	44	46	48	50	52	54	57	59	61	63	65	67	69
4'11"	24	26	28	30	32	34	36	38	40	43	45	47	49	51	53	55	57	59	61	63	65	67
5'0"	23	25	27	29	31	33	35	37	39	41	43	45	47	49	51	53	55	57	59	61	63	65
5'1"	23	25	27	28	30	32	34	36	38	40	42	44	45	47	49	51	53	55	57	59	61	62
5'2"	22	24	26	27	29	31	33	35	37	38	40	42	44	46	48	49	51	53	55	57	59	60
5'3"	21	23	25	27	28	30	32	34	36	37	39	41	43	44	46	48	50	51	53	55	57	59
5'4"	21	22	24	26	28	29	31	33	34	36	38	40	41	43	45	46	48	50	52	53	55	57
5'5"	20	22	23	25	27	28	30	32	33	35	38	38	40	42	43	45	47	48	50	52	53	55
5'6"	19	21	23	24	26	27	29	31	32	34	36	37	39	40	42	44	45	47	49	50	52	53
5'7"	19	20	22	24	25	27	28	30	31	33	35	36	38	39	41	42	44	46	47	49	50	52
5'8"	18	20	21	23	24	26	27	29	30	32	34	35	37	38	40	41	43	44	46	47	49	50
5'9"	18	19	21	22	24	25	27	28	30	31	33	34	36	37	38	40	41	43	44	46	47	49
5'10"	17	19	20	22	23	24	26	27	29	30	32	33	35	36	37	39	40	42	43	45	46	47
5'11"	17	18	20	21	22	24	25	27	28	29	31	32	34	35	36	38	39	41	42	43	45	46
6'	16	18	19	20	22	23	24	26	27	29	30	31	33	34	35	37	38	39	41	42	43	45
6'1"	16	17	19	20	21	22	24	25	26	28	29	30	32	33	34	36	37	38	40	41	42	44
6'2"	15	17	18	19	21	22	23	24	26	27	28	30	31	32	33	35	36	37	39	40	41	42
6'3"	15	16	18	19	20	21	23	24	25	26	28	29	30	31	33	34	35	36	38	39	40	41
6'4"	15	16	17	18	20	21	22	23	24	26	27	28	29	30	32	33	34	35	37	38	39	40
6'5"	14	15	17	18	19	20	21	23	24	25	26	27	29	30	31	32	33	34	36	37	38	39
6'6"	14	15	16	17	19	20	21	22	23	24	25	27	28	29	30	31	32	34	35	36	37	38
6'7"	14	15	16	17	18	19	20	21	23	24	25	26	27	28	29	30	32	33	34	35	36	37
6'8"	13	14	15	17	18	19	20	21	22	23	24	25	26	28	29	30	31	32	33	34	35	36
6'9"	13	14	15	16	17	18	19	20	21	23	24	25	26	27	28	29	30	31	32	33	34	35
6'10"	13	14	15	16	17	18	19	20	21	22	23	24	25	26	27	28	29	30	31	32	34	35

Less risk   More risk

Documentation

- Document BP as right or left arm, and note the patient's position: sitting, standing, or lying.
- Document temperature measurement route: oral, rectal, or tympanic membrane.
- For more information,

 VOL 1 Go to Chapter 19, **Documenting Physical Assessment Findings,** in Volume 1.

See also Chapter 17.

| PROCEDURE 19–2 | **Assessing the Skin** |

 For steps to follow in *all* procedures, refer to the inside back cover of this book.

critical aspects

- Techniques: inspection, palpation, and olfaction.
- Assess both exposed and unexposed areas.
- Inspect skin color; note any unusual odors.
- Inspect and palpate any lesions. Describe their size, shape, color, distribution, texture, surface relationship, and exudate. Note the presence of tenderness or pain.
- Evaluate the lesions for the possibility of malignancy, remembering the mnemonic ABCDE.
- Palpate skin for temperature with the dorsal aspect of your hand.
- Palpate skin for turgor by gently pulling up skin, noting its return when you release it.
- Palpate skin for texture, moisture, and hydration.
- In interpreting data, consider the client's cultural/ethnic background, gender, and developmental stage.
- Review history that may influence skin findings, including usual state of health, current health problem, allergies, and occupation.

Equipment

- Nonlatex gloves (if exposure to body fluids is a possibility)
- Flexible transparent ruler (to measure any lesions)
- Penlight (to provide adequate lighting to unexposed areas)
- Magnifier (for better visualization of lesions)
- Pen and record form

Focused History Questions

Ask the patient about the history or presence of any:
- Rashes
- History of allergies
- Areas of skin that have changed color
- Skin lesions
- Skin with rough or unusual texture
- Skin that is always warm or cool, regardless of room temperature

---

Procedural Steps

1. Inspect skin color.

   a. Provide good lighting to assess color changes of exposed and unexposed areas.

   b. In dark-skinned clients, look for color changes in the conjunctiva or oral mucosa.

   c. Note any unusual odors.

Expected Findings

Skin color is uniform, with darker exposed areas. Mucous membranes and conjunctiva are pink and moist. No unusual odors.

Newborns—may be jaundiced for a few weeks. Blue-black Mongolian spots and pink-red capillary hemangiomas are common and fade with time.

Older adults— may have thin, translucent skin and wrinkles due to loss of elasticity.

Procedural Steps

(continued)

Skin color varies widely among individuals by age, culture, and ethnicity, but in each individual skin color is fairly uniform over his body.

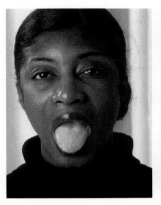 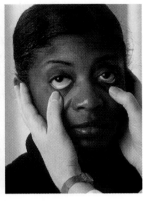

Step 1

2. Palpate skin for temperature.

    a. Wear procedure gloves if there are potentially open areas of the skin.

    b. Use dorsal aspect of hand or fingers.

    c. Compare bilaterally.

The dorsum of the hands and the fingers are most sensitive to temperature variations.

3. Palpate skin for turgor.

    a. Test an unexposed area, such as the area below the clavicle, by gently pinching up the skin, noting its return when you release it.

Developmental Modifications

- *Infants*—Check skin turgor on the abdomen.
- *Older adults*—Check skin turgor over the sternum or clavicle.

4. Palpate skin for texture.

Texture varies, depending on the area being assessed and the age of the client.

Expected Findings

Abnormal findings: pallor, jaundice, cyanosis, erythema, hyperpigmentation, hypopigmentation. Refer to the Abnormal Atlas: Skin Color Changes on page 333 for examples of color changes. Color changes and odors may indicate underlying disease and should be fully investigated.

Skin is warm; temperature is the same bilaterally

Abnormal findings: local area(s) that are warmer or cooler than the rest of the skin; generalized temperature increase or decrease.

Skin returns immediately to its original position.
Older adults—have decreased skin turgor due to decreased elasticity.

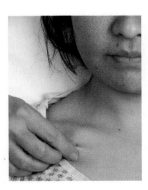

Abnormal findings: Tenting (decreased turgor): skin takes > 3 seconds to return to original position. Increased turgor: skin tension does not allow the skin to be pinched up. Decreased turgor or tenting is seen with dehydration or normal aging.

Step 3

Skin is smooth and soft. Exposed areas and extensor surfaces (e.g., elbows and knees) are drier and coarser than other areas.

Infants and young children—have very smooth skin.

Abnormal findings: coarse, thick, rough, or dry skin; very smooth, thin, fine-textured, shiny skin.

Procedural Steps

Expected Findings

Assessing the Skin *(continued)*

5. Palpate skin for moisture/hydration.

a. Use the dorsum of your hand.

Skin is warm and dry.

Older adults—skin may be dry and flaky because of decreased activity of sebaceous and sweat glands.

Adolescents—may have skin that is oilier than normal.

Abnormal findings: increased moisture (skin feels damp, visible diaphoresis); decreased moisture (skin feels dry).

---

6. Inspect for edema.

a. Press firmly with your fingertip for 5 seconds over a bony area, such as the tibia.

b. Release your finger, and observe the skin for the reaction. Normally there will be no evidence of the pressure once you remove your finger. If pitting edema is present, you will see a depression in the skin.

c. If edema is present, note the location, degree, and type of swelling. For example, if you observe edema in the lower leg, how far up the leg does it extend?

Edema is an abnormal finding.

Grading system:

Trace: Minimal depression.

+1—2 mm depression; rapid return of skin to position.

+2—4 mm depression, which disappears in 10–15 seconds.

+3—6 mm depression that lasts 1–2 minutes. Area appears swollen.

+4—8 mm depression that persists for 2–3 minutes. Area is grossly edematous.

---

7. Identify any skin lesions.

a. Inspect and palpate lesions.

b. When you notice bruises, be alert for signs of abuse (see Chapter 9).

c. Ask the client: "Do you have any new moles or other lesions? Has there been any change in existing moles/lesions?"

d. Assess for malignant lesions using ABCDE:

- A (asymmetry)
- B (irregular borders)
- C (color variations)
- D (diameter > 0.5 cm)
- E (elevation)

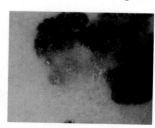

Malignant melanoma

No lesions are present.

Normal variations include moles, freckles, birthmarks, striae (in pregnant women or clients who have lost much weight), and wrinkles.

Newborns—Milia, tiny collections of sebum, usually on the face, are common.

Adults—Acrochordons (skin tags) may be seen around the neck, axillae, skinfolds, or areas where clothing rubs.

Older adults—flat beige or brown macules are common on exposed skin areas.

Abnormal findings: See the accompanying Abnormal Atlas: Skin Lesions on page 333. Also see the table on pages 244 to 247.

Adolescents—Acne is a common abnormal finding among adolescents.

Describing Lesions

When you observe a lesion, evaluate and describe the following:

- *Size.* Measure the length, width, and depth of the lesion.
- *Shape and pattern.* Describe the *shape* of individual lesions. If there are clusters or groups, describe the *pattern*. Is it linear or circular? Are the *borders*

Abnormal Findings: See the accompanying Abnormal Atlas: Skin Lesions on page 333, and the tables on pages 244–247.

Procedural Steps

Expected Findings

(continued)

distinct, or do they run together? Is the border smooth or irregular?

- *Color.* Describe the color of the lesion, and determine whether there is any variation of color within the lesion.
- *Distribution.* Examine the body to determine the distribution. Are the lesions distributed over the entire body? Are they confined to a specific region? What parts of the body are affected?
- *Texture.* The texture (e.g., smooth, rough, scaly) of a lesion helps with classification.
- *Surface relationship.* To assess surface relationship, you will need to palpate the lesion. Is it flat, raised, or depressed? Is it firmly attached to the surrounding skin or mobile?
- *Exudate.* Examine the lesion(s) for signs of drainage. Describe the color, appearance, amount, and odor of drainage, if present.
- *Tenderness, pain, or itching.* Press on the lesion, and determine the patient's reaction. Does touching the lesion cause pain or discomfort?

Patient Teaching

Teach the client the signs and symptoms of skin cancer, the importance of the skin exam, and preventive measures.

Home Care

- Assess the skill level of the caregiver. Instruct the caregiver in the importance of skin assessment and measures to prevent skin breakdown.
- Be alert for lesions (e.g., burns, bruises) that may signal physical abuse. For more signs of abuse, refer to Procedure 9–1.

Documentation

 Go to Chapter 19, **Documenting Physical Assessment Findings,** in Volume 1.

Sketch the location of skin lesions on body diagrams, if available (see example below); or sketch a body if necessary.

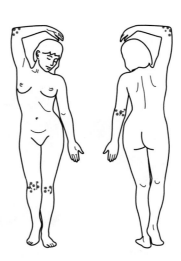

Describing Skin Lesions

Types	Description
Primary Lesions	

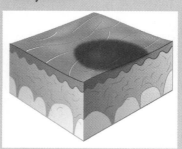

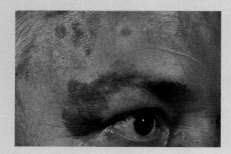

Macule (nonpalpable, <1cm)   Macule (nonpalpable, <1cm)   Flat and colored. Examples: freckle, petechiae, birthmark, Mongolian spot.

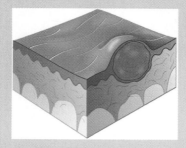

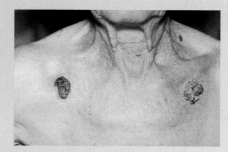

Papule (palpable), <1cm; plaque, >1 cm   Papules (seborrheic keratosis)   Elevated and: raised, but superficial. Examples: mole, psoriasis

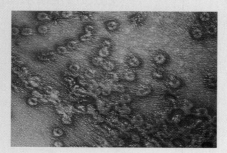

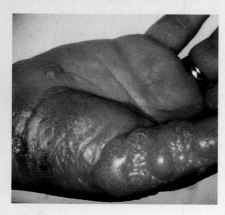

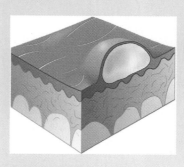

Vesicle (palpable), <1cm; bulla, >1 cm   Vesicles (blisters)   Elevated and filled with serous fluid. Examples: blister, herpes simplex.

Describing Skin Lesions (*continued*)

Types		Description
Primary Lesions		
Cyst (palpable), <2cm	Keratogenous cyst	Palpable, fluid-filled, and encapsulated.
Pustule (palpable)	Pustules (acne)	Elevated and filled with pus. Examples: acne, folliculitis, impetigo.
	Nodule (palpable) <2 cm	Elevated, solid, and firm, with depth into dermis. Examples: wart, lipoma (fatty cyst).
Wheal	Hive	Elevated, superficial, with localized edema. Examples: insect bites, hives.

Describing Skin Lesions *(continued)*

Types		Description
Secondary Lesions		
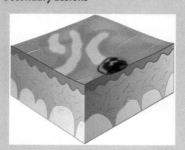 Excoriation	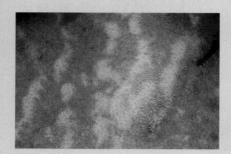 Excoriation from pruritus	Abrasion or loss of skin that does not extend beyond the superficial epidermis. Examples: scratches, stasis dermatitis, atopic dermatitis
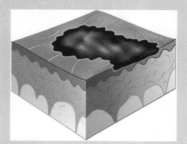 Erosion	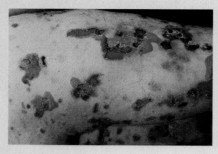 Erosions	Loss of superficial epidermis, usually secondary to rupture of a blister. Examples: abrasions and impetigo.
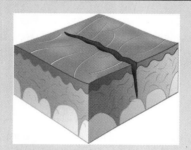 Fissure	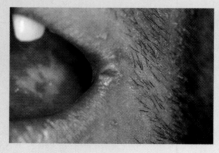 Cheilitis	Linear break in the skin ("crack"); may extend to the dermis. Examples: athlete's foot, cheilitis.
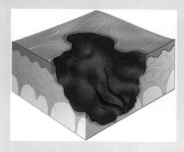 Ulcer	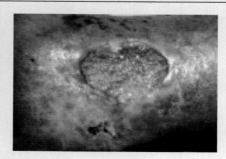 Stasis ulcer	Irregularly shaped with loss of tissue. Graded based on depth and tissue involvement. Examples: pressure ulcers, stasis ulcers.

Describing Skin Lesions (*continued*)

Types		Description
Secondary Lesions		
Crust	Crust	Elevated, rough texture with dried exudate. Examples: impetigo, herpes simplex.
Scales	Psoriasis	White to tan flaking, dead skin cells; may be adherent or loose. Examples: psoriasis and dandruff.
Scar		Fibrous tissue at site of injury, trauma, or surgery. Examples: surgical site, trauma site.
Keloid	Keloids	Raised and irregular scar due to excess collagen formation. Examples: surgical scars, ear piercing.

PROCEDURE 19–3   Assessing the Hair

 For steps to follow in *all* procedures, refer to the inside back cover of this book.

critical aspects
- Techniques: inspection and palpation.
- Assess both scalp hair and body hair.
- Consider the client's cultural/ethnic background, gender, and developmental stage.
- Inspect hair for color, quantity, distribution, condition of scalp, and presence of lesions or pediculosis.
- Palpate the texture of the hair.
- Palpate the scalp for mobility and tenderness.

Equipment
- Nonlatex gloves (if exposure to body fluids is a possibility)
- Pen and record form

Focused History Questions
- Have you had any changes in hair texture?
- Have you had any loss of hair?
- Do you use dyes or chemical treatments for curling or straightening?

Procedural Steps

1. Inspect the hair and scalp.

  a. Check the color, quantity, and distribution of the hair and the condition of the scalp. Note the presence of lesions or pediculosis.

Gender, genetics, and age affect hair distribution. Puberty marks the onset of pubic hair growth and increased hair growth on the legs and axillae.

2. Palpate the texture of the hair.

3. Palpate the scalp for mobility and tenderness.

Tenderness may indicate a localized infection, lesion, or trauma.

Expected Findings

The hair is evenly distributed on the scalp, and fine body hair is present over the body. The hair is clean and free of debris or pediculosis.

Infants—may have very little scalp hair.
Adolescents—may have oily hair.
Older adults—may have thin scalp, axillary, and pubic hair; hair of the ears, nostrils, and eyebrows may become coarse.

Abnormal findings: generalized hair loss not attributed to genetics or aging; patchy hair loss; **hirsutism** (excess facial or trunk hair). Also see Abnormal Atlas: Hair on page 334.

Hair texture varies (fine, medium, coarse) depending on genetics and treatments.

Abnormal findings: very dry, coarse hair; very fine, silky hair.

Scalp is smooth, firm, symmetrical, nontender, and without lesions.

Abnormal findings: tenderness, lesions.

Patient Teaching
If indicated, teach the client to check for head lice, and provide preventive measures.

Documentation

 Go to Chapter 19, **Documenting Physical Assessment Findings,** in Volume 1.

| PROCEDURE 19–4 | **Assessing the Nails** |

> For steps to follow in *all* procedures, refer to the inside back cover of this book.

critical aspects

- Techniques: inspection and palpation.
- Inspect the nails for color, condition, and shape.
- Palpate the texture of the nails.
- Assess capillary refill by pressing on the nails and releasing.
- Assess factors that may alter nail assessment findings (e.g., a cold environment may cause peripheral cyanosis).
- Examine nails on both hands and feet. However, you may defer examination of the toenails until the assessment of peripheral circulation.

Equipment

- Nonlatex gloves (if exposure to body fluids is a possibility)
- Pen and record form

Focused History Questions

- Have you had any recent changes in the way your nails grow or look?
- Have you had any recent trauma to your nails?
- Do you use acrylic nails?
- Do you have any medical problems, such as peripheral vascular disease or diabetes?

Procedural Steps

1. Inspect nails.

- Check nails for color, condition, and shape.
- Examine nails on both hands and feet. However, you may defer examination of the toenails until the assessment of peripheral circulation.

Expected Findings

Healthy nail beds are level, firm, and similar to the color of the skin. The shape is convex, with a nail plate angle of about 160°.

About 160°

Newborns—have very thin nails.

Children—may bite their nails. Most children outgrow this habit.

Older adults—nails grow more slowly, become thicker, and tend to split.

Abnormal findings: yellow, blue, or black discoloration. White spots may indicate zinc deficiency. Spoon-shaped (concave) nails are associated with iron deficiency. Also see Abnormal Atlas: Nail Appearance, on page 334.

Procedural Steps

Expected Findings

Assessing the Nails (continued)

2. Inspect and palpate for texture.

Grooves or lines in the nails provide information about nutrition and health problems.

Nails are smooth and uniform in texture, with a nail plate angle of 160°.

Abnormal findings: thickened, brittle, or soft nails; nails with deep vertical grooves.

---

3. Assess capillary refill.

   a. Briefly press the tip of the nail with firm, steady pressure; then release and observe for changes in color.

This test assesses circulatory adequacy rather than the nails themselves. However, circulatory insufficiency affects the nails and nailbeds; also, it is convenient to perform the assessment at this point in the exam.

Normal capillary refill is < 3 seconds.

Abnormal findings: delayed capillary refill.

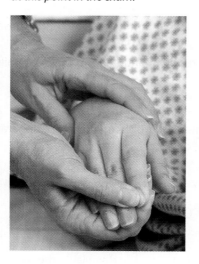

Step 3

Documentation

 Go to Chapter 19, **Documenting Physical Assessment Findings,** in Volume 1.

PROCEDURE 19–5 Assessing the Head and Face

 For steps to follow in *all* procedures, refer to the inside back cover of this book.

critical aspects
- Techniques: inspection, palpation, auscultation.
- Inspect the head for size, shape, symmetry, and position.
- Inspect the face for expression and symmetry.
- Palpate the head for masses, tenderness, and scalp mobility.
- Palpate the face for symmetry, tenderness, muscle tone, and TMJ function.

Equipment
- Nonlatex gloves (if exposure to body fluids is a possibility)
- Penlight (to transilluminate the sinuses)
- Pen and record form

Position
Preferably, the client should be sitting.

Focused History Questions
- Have you had any recent headaches?
- Have you ever had a head injury or loss of consciousness?
- Have you ever had a seizure?
- Do you have jaw or facial pain?

Procedural Steps

1. Inspect the head.

   a. Check for size, shape, symmetry, and position.

Developmental Modification:

Newborns and infants—assess and transilluminate fontanelles, and measure head circumference.

2. Inspect the face.

   a. Note the client's facial expression.

Expected Findings

There is wide variation in head size and shape, although the shape should be symmetrical and rounded. The head should be erect, midline, and proportional to the body size based on age.

Newborns and infants— cranial bones are not fused at birth, and head shape may reflect normal pressure or trauma during vaginal birth for several weeks. The anterior fontanelle ("soft spot") fuses at about 18 months; the posterior, at about 8 weeks. Infants normally cannot hold their head up until about 6 months of age.

Abnormal findings: larger or smaller than expected size for age, asymmetry of skull.

Facial expression is appropriate for the situation. No visible lesions. Facial features and movement are symmetrical.

Procedural Steps

Expected Findings

Assessing the Head and Face *(continued)*

b. Ask yourself,

- Are the facial features symmetrical?

- Are there any abnormal facial movements?

- Are there any visible lesions of abnormal hair distribution?

! Helpful hint: Look for symmetry in the palpebral fissures and the nasolabial folds.

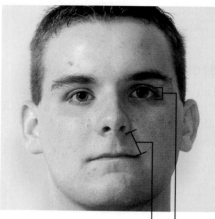

Step 2

Nasolabial fold

Palpebral fissure

3. Palpate the head.

a. Check for masses, tenderness, and scalp mobility.

Developmental Modification: Newborns and infants—palpate anterior and posterior fontanelles.

Abnormal findings: facial appearance inconsistent with gender, age, or racial/ethnic group; asymmetry of facial features or facial movement.

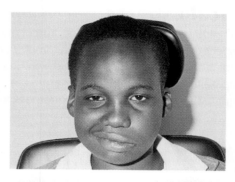

Bell's palsy

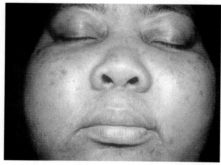

Cushing's syndrome

The head should be relatively smooth, with no tenderness or lesions.

Abnormal findings: contour abnormalities (e.g., indentations, "bumps").

4. Palpate the face for symmetry, tenderness, muscle tone, and TMJ function.

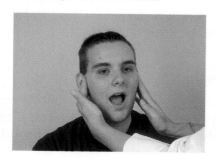

Palpating the TMJ

There should be smooth, symmetrical movement with no pain, crepitus, or clicking of the jaw.

Abnormal findings: irregular or uneven movement of the jaw; pain or popping with movement.

Documentation

 Go to Chapter 19, **Documenting Physical Assessment Findings,** in Volume 1.

PROCEDURE 19–6   Assessing the Eyes

 For steps to follow in *all* procedures, refer to the inside back cover of this book.

critical aspects

- Techniques: inspection and palpation.
- Assess distance vision using a Snellen chart.
- Test near vision by measuring the client's ability to read newsprint at a distance of 14 inches (35.5 cm).
- Test color vision by using color plates or the color bars on the Snellen chart.
- Assess peripheral vision by determining when an object comes into sight.
- Assess EOMs by examining the corneal light reflex, assessing the ability to move through the six cardinal gaze positions, and performing the cover/uncover test.
- Inspect the external eye structures.
- Test the corneal reflex with a cotton wisp.
- Check pupil reaction for direct and consensual response.
- Assess accommodation by having the patient focus on an approaching object.
- Palpate the external eye structures.

Equipment

- Nonlatex gloves (if exposure to body fluids is a possibility)
- Visual acuity chart with color bars (Snellen)
- A card (to cover one eye during the acuity exam)
- Penlight
- Cotton ball and cotton-tipped applicator
- Ophthalmoscope
- Pen and form

Position

Preferably, the client should be sitting.

Focused History Questions

- Have you noticed any changes in your vision?
- Do you wear glasses or contact lenses?
- Have you ever had an eye injury?
- Have you ever had an eye infection or stye?
- Do you have problems with excessive tearing or dry eyes?
- Have you ever had eye surgery?
- Have you ever experienced blurred vision?
- Do you have difficulty with nighttime vision?
- Do you ever see halos of light, spots or floaters, or flashes of light?
- Do you have a history of eye problems, such as glaucoma, or medical problems, such as diabetes or hypertension?
- When was your last eye exam?
- Do you use any prescription or over-the-counter eye medications?

Procedural Steps

1. Test distance vision

- Depending on patient's age and literacy level, use the Snellen standard eye chart or Snellen E chart (for those who cannot read). Picture charts are available for preschoolers.
- If the client wears corrective lenses, they should be worn during a test.

Expected Findings

Expect 20/20 vision in the right eye, left eye, and both eyes. The top number of the fraction indicates the distance the person was standing from the chart; the bottom number is the distance from which a person with normal vision would be able to read the chart.

Children—distance vision does not reach 20/20 until around 6 or 7 years of age.

Procedural Steps

Expected Findings

Assessing the Eyes *(continued)*

a. Have the patient stand 6 m (20 ft) from the chart. With a card, cover the eye not being tested; ask the patient to read the smallest line of print that he can distinguish.

   Consider a line to be read correctly if the client makes no more than 2 mistakes in that line.

b. Test the opposite eye.

c. Test both eyes together.

d. At the end of each line of the Snellen chart is a fraction—the top line is 20/200. After each test, record the resulting fraction: the number at the end of the smallest line the patient could read with no more than 2 errors.

Middle adults—At about middle age, the lens of the eye begins to lose some ability to accommodate to near objects.

Abnormal findings: A smaller fraction (e.g., 20/100) indicates diminished distant vision or myopia.

A larger fraction (e.g., 20/15) indicates diminished near vision, called hyperopia.

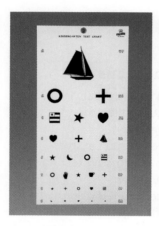

Preliterate chart

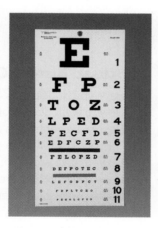

Snellen standard chart

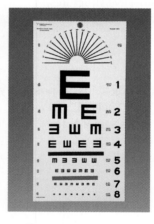

Snellen E chart

---

2. Test near vision.

Test the client's ability to read newsprint at a distance of 35.5 cm (14 in.) from the eyes. Use print-sized pictures if the patient is unable to read.

The client reads newsprint at a distance of 35.5 cm (14 in.).

Abnormal findings: The need to hold the print at a greater distance indicates hyperopia or presbyopia.

---

3. Test color vision.

• Have the patient differentiate patterns of colors on color cards or identify the color bars on the Snellen eye chart.

Color vision is intact.

Older adults—experience some decline in color vision, especially in the ability to see purples and pastels.

Procedural Steps

(continued)

- Inability to distinguish colors requires a thorough evaluation using the Ishihara cards to determine the scope of the color deficit.

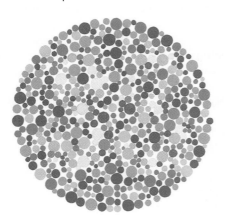

Ishihara card

Expected Findings

Abnormal findings: inability to distinguish colors.

---

4. Test peripheral vision.

a. Seat the client 60 to 90 cm (2 to 3 ft) from you.

b. Have her cover one eye and fix her gaze straight ahead while you bring an object in from the periphery to the center of the visual fields. Be sure to begin by holding the object well outside the range of normal peripheral vision. Instruct the patient to identify when the object becomes visible.

c. Repeat this in each of the four visual fields, moving clockwise.

Expect no deficits in the visual fields.

Abnormal findings: loss of peripheral vision. Report gross deficits to an ophthalmologist for further assessment.

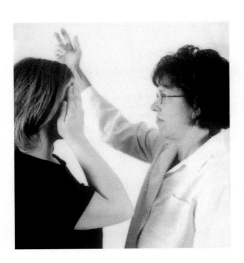

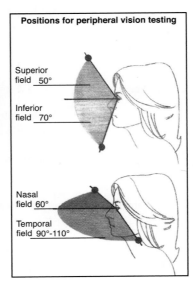

Positions for peripheral vision testing

Superior field __50°__

Inferior field __70°__

Nasal field __60°__

Temporal field __90°-110°__

Step 4

Procedural Steps

Expected Findings

Assessing the Eyes *(continued)*

5. Assess extraocular movements.

a. Inspect the eyes for parallel alignment.

b. Test the corneal light reflex by shining a penlight at the bridge of the nose. Note where the light reflects on the cornea of each eye.

c. Test the six cardinal fields of gaze. Stand in front of the patient, and have the patient follow an object through the six cardinal fields without moving her head.

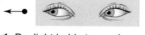
1. Penlight held at nurse's extreme left.

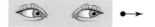
4. Penlight held at nurse's extreme right.

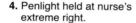
2. Penlight moved left and up.

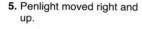
5. Penlight moved right and up.

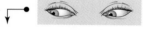
3. Penlight moved left and down.

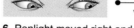
6. Penlight moved right and down.

Step 5c

d. Perform the cover/uncover test. Cover one eye and have the patient gaze at a distant object. Uncover the eye. Repeat on the opposite side.

a. The eyes should be in parallel alignment.

b. Corneal light reflex appears at the same position in each eye.

Abnormal findings: An asymmetrical corneal light reflex may indicate weak extraocular muscles or strabismus.

c. The eyes move through all six gaze positions.

Abnormal findings: inability to move through all gaze positions.

d. The gaze should be steady when the eye is covered and uncovered.

Abnormal findings: A shift in gaze indicates weak eye muscles.

---

6. Inspect the external structures.

a. General appearance: Check the color and alignment of the eyes.

b. Inspect the eyelids. Note the presence of any lesions, edema, or lid lag.

a. Eyes are clear and bright and in parallel alignment.

Older adults—a decrease in periorbital fat may give the eyeballs a sunken appearance.

Abnormal findings: Glazed eyes may indicate a febrile state.

b. No lesions are present, and the lids move freely. The upper eyelid covers half of the upper iris.

Older adults—the lower lids may sag; skinfolds are prominent in the upper lids.

Procedural Steps

(continued)

c. Inspect the eyelashes. Note symmetry and distribution.

d. Inspect the lacrimal ducts and glands. Note any edema, excessive tearing, or drainage.

e. Inspect the conjunctivae.

1) Note the color, moisture, and contour of the conjunctivae.

2) The palpebral conjunctivae cover the lids. To assess, have the patient look up as you place a cotton-tipped applicator on the upper lid, gently grasp the upper lid and lashes, and evert the lid over the cotton-tipped applicator.

3) The bulbar conjunctiva covers the eyeball. To assess, pull the lower lid down.

Expected Findings

Abnormal findings: Asymmetry of lids may result from CN III damage or from a stroke.

Lesions may be benign (e.g., a stye) or pathological (e.g., basal cell carcinoma).

c. Eyelashes are evenly distributed and curve outward. No crustations or infestations are present.

Abnormal findings: inflammation of the eyelids, which may be caused by infection; inverted eyelashes (entropion); everted eyelashes (ectropion); visible sclera between the iris and upper lid.

d. No periorbital edema or lesions are present. No drainage.

Abnormal findings: swelling, redness, drainage, or tenderness.

e. The palpebral conjunctivae are smooth, glistening, and peach in color. Minimal blood vessels are present. The bulbar conjunctivae are clear with few underlying blood vessels and white sclera visible.

Older adults—the conjunctivae may be pale or have a slightly yellow tint due to fat deposits.

Abnormal findings: pallor, dryness, edema; pterygium; subconjunctival hemorrhage.

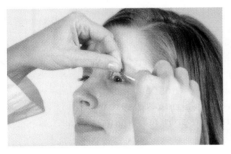

Step 6e(2): Examining the palpebral conjunctiva

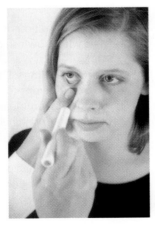

Step 6e(3): Examining the bulbar conjunctiva

Procedural Steps

Expected Findings

Assessing the Eyes *(continued)*

f. Inspect the sclera.
- Note the color of the sclera and whether lesions are present.

f. The sclera should be smooth, white, and glistening. Dark-skinned patients may have a yellowish cast to the peripheral sclera or small brown spots more centrally.

Abnormal findings: yellow (icteric) sclera.

g. Inspect the cornea and lens.
- As the client looks straight ahead, shine a penlight at an angle to the eye, and move it across the corneal surface. Note the color and whether any lesions are present.

g. The cornea and lens are clear, smooth, and glistening.

Older adults—arcus senilis is a normal variant.

Abnormal findings: lens opacities (cataracts); roughness or irregularity of the cornea.

h. Test the corneal reflex.
- Touch the cornea with a wisp of cotton, or use a needleless syringe to shoot a small amount of air over the cornea.

h. Blink reflex is prompt.

Abnormal findings: Failure to blink may result from neurosensory deficits.

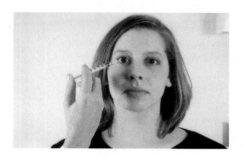

Step 6h

i. Inspect the iris and pupils.
- Note the color, size, shape, and symmetry.

i. The iris is blue, green, brown, or a combination of these colors; its shape is circular. The pupils are round and of equal size. Unequal pupils (anisocoria) can be a normal variation if the difference is less than 0.5 mm.

Older adults—pigment degeneration may cause the iris to be pale with brownish discolorations.

Abnormal findings: Damage to one eye may cause the iris to be a different color. Absence of part or all of the iris is a congenital problem. Unequal pupils may result from CN III damage, brain herniation, or increased intracranial pressure.

j. Test pupillary reaction.
- In a dimly lighted room, have the patient look straight ahead. Bring a penlight in from the side, and shine the light onto one eye. Note the reaction, equality, and speed of response of both eyes. For example, when you shine a light onto the right eye, the right pupil reaction is direct; the left eye is consensual. Repeat the test on the opposite eye.

j. Normal direct and consensual response to light is brisk, with equal constriction of both pupils.

Older adults—Pupil reaction may be slower but should be symmetrical.

Abnormal findings: Sluggish or fixed pupils may result from CN II damage or brain injury. Absence of consensual response may result from nerve compression or anoxia.

Procedural Steps

Expected Findings

(continued)

k. Test pupil accommodation.

- Have the patient look straight ahead and focus on an object about 30 cm (12 in.) from his face. Slowly bring the object in toward the patient's eyes. Note pupil size and location.

l. Inspect the anterior chamber for color, size, shape, and symmetry.

- To assess, shine a penlight across the eye from the side as the patient looks straight ahead.

k. The pupils constrict and the eyes cross as a person attempts to focus on a near object.

Older adults—accommodation may be slow.

Abnormal findings: One or both pupils fail to accommodate, or they accommodate slowly.

l. The chamber should be clear and symmetrically curved.

Abnormal findings: blood or pus in the chamber. Also see Abnormal Atlas: Eyes on page 334.

---

7. Palpate the external structures.

a. Gently palpate the globe with your fingertips on the upper lids over the sclera. Note the consistency and any tenderness.

b. Palpate the lacrimal glands and ducts by palpating below the eyebrow and below the inner canthus of the eye. Note tenderness and excessive tearing or discharge.

The globe is firm and nontender. Lacrimal glands are nonpalpable; no tenderness is present.

Abnormal findings: firm or tender globe; swelling and tenderness over the lacrimal glands.

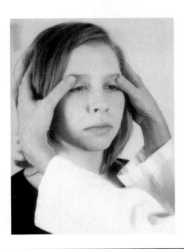

Step 7

---

8. Assess the internal structures via ophthalmoscopy. This is an advanced physical assessment technique.

a. Darken the room.

b. Stand about 1 foot from the patient at a 15° lateral angle.

c. Dial the lens wheel to zero with your index finger. Hold the ophthalmoscope to your brow.

Expect a positive red light reflex. On internal examination, the optic disk is round with sharp margins. There are no opacities and the cup:disk ratio is 1:2. The disk is yellow with a white cup.

Abnormal findings: Any findings not consistent with above should be promptly reported.

Procedural Steps

Expected Findings

Assessing the Eyes *(continued)*

d. Have the patient look straight ahead while you shine the light on one pupil and identify the red light reflex.

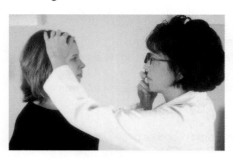

Step 8d: Checking red reflex

e. Once you identify the red light reflex, move in closer to within a few inches of the eye and observe the internal structures of the eye. Adjust the lens wheel to focus as needed. Use your right eye to examine the patient's right eye, and your left eye to examine the patient's left eye.

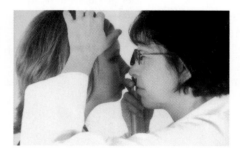

Step 8e

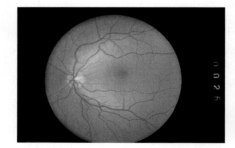

f. Repeat for the opposite eye.

Patient Teaching

Teach the client the importance of routine eye examinations.

Documentation

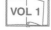 Go to Chapter 19, **Documenting Physical Assessment Findings,** in Volume 1.

PROCEDURE 19–7   Assessing the Ears and Hearing

For steps to follow in *all* procedures, refer to the inside back cover of this book.

critical aspects
- Techniques: inspection and palpation.
- Inspect the external ear for placement, size, shape, symmetry, and the condition of the skin.
- Palpate the external structures of the ear for the condition of the skin and for tenderness.
- Inspect the tympanic membrane and bony landmarks.
- Assess gross hearing with the whisper and watch-tick tests.
- Perform the Weber test to assess hearing loss.
- Perform the Rinne test to identify whether hearing loss is conductive or sensorineural.
- Perform the Romberg test to assess balance.

Equipment
- Nonlatex gloves (if exposure to body fluids is a possibility)
- Tuning fork
- Watch
- Otoscope with pneumatic tube
- Pen and record form

Position
Have the patient seated, if possible.

Focused History Questions
- Do you have any hearing problems?
- Have you ever had ringing in your ears?
- Have you had any changes in your hearing?
- Do you have any ear drainage? If yes, how much and what color?
- Do you have any ear pain?
- Do you have any balance problems, dizziness, or vertigo?
- Do you have a history of head trauma?
- Are you exposed to noise pollution at work or in your home environment?

Procedural Steps

1. Inspect the external ear

a. Check the placement and angle of attachment of the ear.

Expected Findings

a. The normal angle of attachment is < 10°.

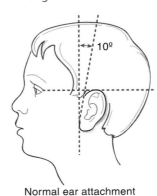

10°

Normal ear attachment

Abnormal findings: High or low placement of the ear may be a sign of hearing deficit or genetic problems.

Procedural Steps

Expected Findings

Assessing the Ears and Hearing *(continued)*

b. Note the shape, size, and symmetry of the ears.

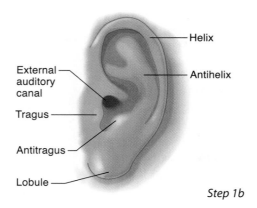

Helix

External auditory canal

Antihelix

Tragus

Antitragus

Lobule

Step 1b

c. Observe the color of the ear.

d. Observe the condition of the skin; observe for drainage and visible lesions.

b. The helix, antihelix, antitragus, tragus, and lobule are present. The ears are 4–10 cm in length and symmetrical in size and shape.

Older adults—the ear changes shape as the lobe elongates.

Abnormal findings: Absence of any of the landmarks may indicate a hearing deficit. Ears that are < 4 cm long or > 10 cm long may indicate a genetic disorder.

c. Color is consistent with skin color.

Abnormal findings: Redness may indicate inflammation or infection.

d. Skin is intact with no drainage or lesions. Piercings may be present.

Older adults—may have coarse hair on the helix, antihelix, and tragus; skin may be dry.

Abnormal findings: bloody or purulent drainage; lesions. The ears are a common location for skin cancer.

---

2. Palpate the external structures of the ear.

a. Note the consistency of the skin, the presence of lesions, and any signs of tenderness.

Skin is soft, pliable, and nontender. No nodules or lesions are present.

Abnormal findings: Tenderness is often associated with infection.

---

3. Perform an otoscopic exam. This is an advanced physical assessment technique.

a. Use a speculum with the largest diameter and shortest length that the ear canal can accommodate.

This enables you to see the entire ear canal and tympanic membrane (TM).

b. Have the patient tilt his head to the side not being examined.

c. Look into the canal before inserting the scope.

Ensures that a foreign object is not present.

The ear canal is light in color and patent, with a small amount of yellow cerumen (color may vary). TM is pearly gray and intact. Bony landmarks are visible. The TM is mobile. No bulging or retraction of the TM.

Older adults—may have dry ear wax. The TM is translucent, and the light reflex may be diminished.

Abnormal findings: Excessive wax may occlude the canal. TM that is red, with a distorted light reflex, suggests otitis media. A change in the position or shape of the cone of light reflex indicates an imbalance in middle ear pressure.

Procedural Steps

Expected Findings

(continued)

    d. To straighten the external ear canal, pull the helix.

- *For an adult*: up and back.
- *For a preschool child*: down and back.

Enables you to see the TM.

    e. Slowly insert the speculum. Avoid contact with the inner two-thirds of the canal.

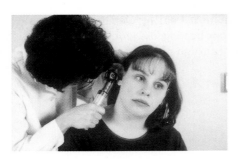

Step 3e

    f. Observe the ear canal.

    g. Observe the tympanic membrane.

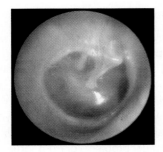

Step 3g

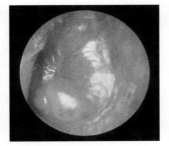

Otitis media

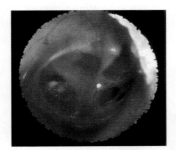

Perforated TM

    h. Test the mobility of the tympanic membrane by using the pneumatic tube to gently "puff" air into the external ear canal while observing movement of the cone of light.

Note: The ears are mirror images, with the cone of light at 7 o'clock in the left ear and 5 o'clock in the right ear.

Developmental Modification

Children—Many young children fear the otoscopic examination. Demonstrating the procedure on a parent or a doll may relieve their anxiety.

Procedural Steps

Expected Findings

Assessing the Ears and Hearing (continued)

4. Test gross hearing.

   a. Stand 1 to 2 feet behind the patient. Have the patient cover one ear as you whisper some words. Repeat on the other side. Have the patient repeat the words she heard.

   b. Have the patient occlude one ear. Hold a ticking watch next to the patient's unobstructed ear. Slowly move it away until the patient says she can no longer hear the sound. Repeat for the opposite ear.

Developmental Modification

Infants—For infants under 3 months of age, clap your hands behind the infant and observe whether he startles. After 3 months of age, the infant should turn his head or eyes toward the sound, for example, when the parent stands behind the infant and calls his name.

The patient is able to hear you whisper on both sides. The patient hears the watch at a distance of about 12 to 13 cm (5 in.).

Older adults—often have a generalized loss of hearing. It first occurs in the high-frequency sounds (*f, s, sh,* and *ph*) and then progresses to include all frequencies.

Abnormal findings: Problems with the whisper test indicate low-tone hearing loss. Problems with the watch-tick test indicate a high-pitch deficit.

---

5. Perform the Weber test.

   • Place a vibrating tuning fork on top of the patient's head. Ask the patient whether the sound is the same in both ears or louder in one ear.

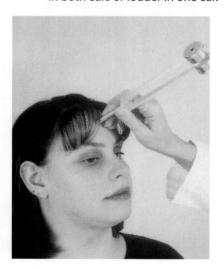

Step 5

The patient hears the sound equally in both ears.

Abnormal findings: sound louder in one ear.

   • If there is a *conductive hearing loss,* the vibration will be louder in the impaired ear. Conductive hearing loss may be caused by external or middle ear problems, such as infection, blockage of the canal by cerumen, or trauma to the TM.

   • If there is a *sensorineural hearing loss,* the sound will be louder in the unaffected ear. Sensorineural loss may result from inner ear problems or from some medications.

   • Perform the Rinne test to further identify the type of hearing loss.

---

6. Perform the Rinne test (if the Weber test is positive).

   a. Strike a tuning fork on the table. While it is still vibrating, place it on the patient's mastoid process.

   b. Measure the elapsed time in seconds that the patient hears the vibration.

Normally, sound transmission through air (step 6c) is twice as long as transmission through bone (step 6b); that is, $AC = 2 \times BC$.

The ratio of AC to BC is similar in both ears.

Procedural Steps

Expected Findings

(continued)

c. Move the tuning fork to 2.5 cm (1 in.) in front of the ear, and measure the elapsed time until the patient can no longer hear the vibration.

d. Repeat for the opposite ear.

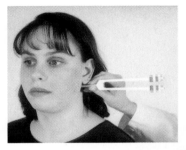

Step 6a

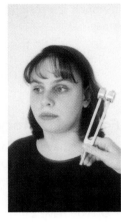

Step 6c

Abnormal findings:

- Conductive loss: AC is less than 2 $\times$ BC
- Sensorineural loss: AC is greater than BC but not 2$\times$ longer; or the client is unable to hear the tuning fork through BC.
- A difference between ears indicates unilateral hearing loss.
- Inability to hear the tuning fork through BC indicates sensorineural hearing loss.

A difference between ears indicates unilateral hearing loss.

---

7. Perform the Romberg test.

- Have the client stand with feet together, hands at side, with eyes opened and then with eyes closed. Note the client's ability to maintain balance.

The client maintains balance with minimal sway.

Abnormal findings: Positive Romberg (swaying) is seen with vestibular disorders.

Patient Teaching

Teach the client the importance of routine hearing examinations.

Documentation

 Go to Chapter 19, **Documenting Physical Assessment Findings,** in Volume 1.

PROCEDURE 19–8 Assessing the Nose and Sinuses

For steps to follow in *all* procedures, refer to the inside back cover of this book.

critical aspects
- Techniques: inspection and palpation.
- Insert the speculum about 1 cm, and then open it as much as possible.
- Inspect the external and internal structures of the nose.
- Transilluminate and palpate the sinuses.
- Palpate the external structures of the nose.

Equipment
- Nonlatex gloves (if exposure to body fluids is a possibility)
- Penlight
- Nasal speculum or otoscope with a wide-tipped speculum
- Pen and record form

Position
Have the client seated, if possible.

Focused History Questions
- Do you have any nasal congestion?
- Do you have a history of nose or sinus problems?
- Do you have problems with seasonal or environmental allergies?
- Do you have a history of sinus headaches?
- Do you experience nose bleeds (epistaxis)?
- Have you ever broken your nose?
- Have you had any changes in your sense of smell?
- Do you use any nasal sprays or allergy medications?

Procedural Steps

1. Have the client sitting, if possible.

---

2. Inspect the external nose.

   a. Note the position, shape, and size. Observe for discharge and flaring.

Expected Findings

The nose is midline and symmetrical. No discharge or flaring.

Abnormal findings: Asymmetry suggests congenital deformity or trauma. Flaring suggests respiratory distress (especially in infants, who cannot breathe through the mouth). Clear drainage suggests allergy; yellow or green drainage suggests upper respiratory infection; bloody drainage may result from trauma, hypertension, or a bleeding disorder.

---

3. Check for patency of the nasal passages.

   a. Ask the client to close his mouth, hold one naris closed, and breathe through the other naris. Repeat with the opposite naris.

The client breathes freely through both nares.

Procedural Steps

Expected Findings

(continued)

4. Inspect the internal structures.

   a. Use a nasal speculum or an otoscope with a large speculum (or a penlight with a speculum) to assess the internal structures.

   b. Tilt the client's head back to facilitate speculum insertion and visualization.

   c. Brace your index finger against the client's nose as you insert the speculum.

   d. Insert the speculum about 1 cm into the nares. Use the other hand to position the client's head and to hold the penlight if you do not have a lighted scope.

Nasal mucosa is pink and moist. Septum is intact and midline. No lesions.

Abnormal findings: deviated septum; polyps. Pale boggy mucosa is seen with allergies; bright red mucosa is associated with rhinitis, sinusitis, and cocaine use. Clustered vesicles suggest herpes infection.

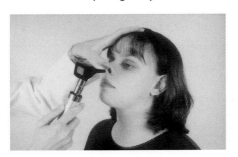

Step 4d

   e. Observe the nasal mucosa for color, edema, lesions, and discharge. Inspect the septum for position and intactness.

Developmental Modification

Infants and children—you will not need a speculum to examine internal structures. Push the tip of the nose upward with your thumb, and direct a penlight into the nares.

---

5. Transilluminate the frontal and maxillary sinuses.

   a. Darken the room.

   b. Frontal sinuses: Shine a penlight or the otoscope with speculum below the eyebrow on each side.

A red glow is seen above the eyebrow, indicating that the frontal sinus is patent.

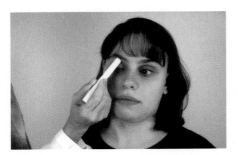

Step 5b

Procedural Steps

Expected Findings

Assessing the Nose and Sinuses *(continued)*

c. Maxillary sinuses: Place the light source below the eyes and above the cheeks. Look for a glow of red light at the roof of the mouth through the client's open mouth.

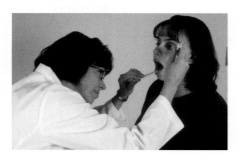

Step 5c

A red glow is seen in the roof of the mouth, indicating that the maxillary sinus is patent.

Abnormal findings: Absence of transillumination may result from mucosal thickening or sinusitis.

---

6. Palpate the external structures.

No tenderness, lesions, or deformity.

---

7. Palpate the frontal and maxillary sinuses.

There is no tenderness.

Abnormal findings: Tenderness may indicate infectious or allergic sinusitis.

Documentation

 Go to Chapter 19, **Documenting Physical Assessment Findings,** in Volume 1.

PROCEDURE 19–9   Assessing the Mouth and Oropharynx

▶ For steps to follow in *all* procedures, refer to the inside back cover of this book.

critical aspects
- Techniques: inspection and palpation.
- Inspect the lips, oral mucosa, gums, teeth, and bite.
- Inspect the hard/soft palate, tonsils, and uvula.
- Inspect the tongue and frenulum; inspect under the tongue.
- Palpate the lips and tongue for tenderness and muscle tone.
- Test the gag reflex by touching the back of the soft palate with a tongue blade.

Equipment

- Nonlatex gloves (if exposure to body fluids is a possibility)
- Penlight
- Tongue blade
- Small gauze pad
- Pen and record form

Position

Have the client seated, if possible.

Focused History Questions

- Do you have any problems with your mouth or teeth?
- When was your last dental exam?
- Do you have any discomfort in your mouth or throat?
- Have you had any recent changes in your mouth or teeth?
- How often do you brush your teeth? Floss?
- Do you smoke or chew tobacco?
- Do you have any sores or irritation in your mouth? If so, when did you first notice this?

Procedural Steps	Expected Findings
1. Inspect the mouth externally. a. Note the placement of the lips and their color and condition. Ask the client to purse his lips.	The lips are midline, symmetrical, moist, and intact with no lesions. Coloring is consistent with ethnic group/race. Client can purse lips. **Abnormal findings:** asymmetry (may be due to congenital deformity, trauma, paralysis, or surgical alteration); pallor; cyanosis; redness; inability to purse lips (may indicate facial nerve damage); lesions (may be caused by bacteria, viruses, or trauma).

2. Note the color and condition of the oral mucosa and gums.
 	
   a. Inspect and palpate the lower lip. Pull the lower lip away from the teeth, and inspect the inner side of the lip. Palpate any lesions for size, mobility, and tenderness.
 	
   b. Inspect the buccal mucosa, top to bottom and back to front.
 	
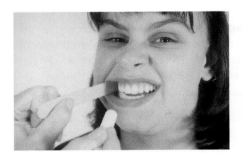
Step 2b
	Oral mucosa is pink, moist, and intact; no lesions. Gingiva is consistent in color with the other mucosae and is intact, with no bleeding. Buccal mucosa is pink and moist, with no lesions. (Mucosa is darker in dark-skinned clients.)
	
	Older adults—mucosa is drier than in young adults (because of decreased salivary gland activity); brownish pigmentation of gums may be seen, especially in dark-skinned people.
	
	Abnormal findings: receding gums, sponginess, bleeding, inflammatory changes, gingival hyperplasia, ulcerations, or other lesions.

Procedural Steps

Expected Findings

Assessing the Mouth *(continued)*

- Ask the client to open his mouth. Use a tongue depressor to retract the cheek, then shine a penlight onto the mucosa.

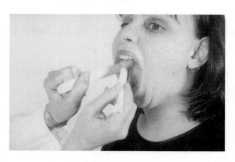

Step 2b

- Using a tongue blade and penlight, inspect the Stensen's duct openings to the parotid glands.
- Finally, palpate inside each cheek by placing a finger inside and thumb outside. Grasping the cheek between them, move the finger about. Repeat on both sides.

c. As you are inspecting the buccal mucosa, also examine the gums. Check for color, bleeding, edema, retraction, and lesions. Press gum tissue gently with gloved finger or tongue blade to assess firmness.

---

3. Inspect the teeth. You can do this while you are inspecting the oral mucosa and gums, in Step 2.

a. Observe the number, color, and condition of the teeth. Note the occlusion ("bite").

b. If the client wears dentures, ask her to remove them. Inspect for cracked or worn areas; assess the fit.

Most adults have 28 teeth, or 32 if the wisdom teeth have erupted. Children have 20 teeth. The teeth should be white, in good repair, with no caries and good occlusion. The top front teeth should slightly override the lower ones.

Older adults—may have receding gums, so teeth appear longer. Teeth may be chipped, eroded, or stained.

Abnormal findings: missing or poorly anchored teeth, misalignment, and brown or black enamel (indicative of dental caries or staining, e.g., from taking tetracycline). White spots may indicate excessive fluoride intake.

---

4. Inspect the tongue and the floor of the mouth.

a. Ask the client to "stick out" his tongue. Examine the upper surface for its color, texture, position, and mobility.

b. Ask the client to roll his tongue upward and move it side to side.

c. Have the client place the tip of his tongue on the roof of his mouth, as far back as possible. Using the penlight, inspect the underside of the tongue, the **frenulum** (which fastens the tongue to the floor of the mouth, in the center), and the floor of the mouth.

Tongue is moist, and the coloring is consistent with the client's ethnic group/race. Mucosa has no lesions or discoloration. Papillae are intact. Tongue is midline with full mobility. The base of the tongue is smooth with prominent veins. No tenderness; no palpable nodules.

Older adults—may have varicosities under the tongue.

Abnormal findings: red, smooth, or painful tongue;. inflamed mucosa or ducts; tongue that is not midline or has restricted mobility; ulcerations of the tongue or the floor of the mouth (e.g., from trauma, viral infection, or cancerous changes).

Procedural Steps	Expected Findings

(continued)

d. Inspect the two Wharton's duct openings to the sub-maxillary glands, on either side of the frenulum.

e. Use a tongue blade or gloved finger to move the tongue aside and examine the lateral aspects of the tongue and the floor of the mouth bilaterally. Use caution when placing your finger into the mouth of a noncompliant client.

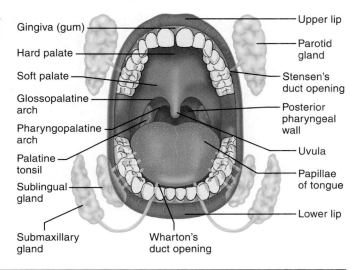

5. Palpate the tongue and floor of the mouth. Stabilize the tongue by grasping it with a gauze pad. Palpate top, bottom, and sides with your other index finger.

6. Inspect the oropharynx (hard/soft palate, tonsils, and uvula). Note the color, shape, texture, and condition.

a. Have the client tilt his head back and open his mouth as widely as possible. Depress the tongue with a tongue blade, and shine a penlight on the areas to be inspected.

b. To inspect the uvula, ask the client to say "ah," and watch the uvula as the soft palate rises.

c. Inspect the oropharynx by depressing one side of the tongue at a time, about halfway back on the tongue.

d. Note the size and color of the tonsils; note any discharge.

e. Look for cleft palate, especially in infants.

Hard and soft palate are pink and smooth. Uvula is midline and rises symmetrically. Tonsils are pink, symmetrical, and without lesions or exudate.

Children—Until about age 12, the tonsils may extend beyond the palatine arch.

Abnormal findings: redness, edema, lesions, plaques, drainage; yellow or greenish streaks on the posterior wall of pharynx (indicate postnasal drainage); tonsils that are red, edematous, or enlarged or have white or pale patches of exudates. Asymmetrical rise of the uvula may indicate a problem with CN IX or X.

7. Test the gag reflex by touching the back of the soft palate with a tongue blade.

Positive gag reflex is present.

Older adults—may have a slightly slower gag response.

Abnormal findings: Absence of a gag reflex is seen with extreme sedation, head injury, or damage to CN IX and X. Also see Abnormal Atlas: Mouth and Oropharynx, page 334.

Patient Teaching

Instruct the client in the importance of dental care and the need for regular checkups.

Documentation

 Go to Chapter 19, **Documenting Physical Assessment Findings,** in Volume 1.

PROCEDURE 19–10   **Assessing the Neck**

 For steps to follow in *all* procedures, refer to the inside back cover of this book.

critical aspects
- Techniques: inspection and palpation (auscultation as needed).
- Inspect the neck. Note symmetry, range of motion (ROM), and the condition of the skin.
- Palpate the cervical lymph nodes. Note the size, shape, symmetry, consistency, mobility, tenderness, and temperature of any palpable nodes.
- Palpate the thyroid. If it is enlarged or if there is a mass, follow up with auscultation of the gland.

Equipment
- Stethoscope
- Pen and record form

Position
- Have the client seated, if possible.
- For infants and children, position supine.

Focused History Questions
- Do you have any difficulty swallowing?
- Do you have any neck pain or stiffness?
- Do you have any neck masses or lumps?
- Do you have any history of thyroid disease?
- Do you have any difficulty swallowing?

Procedural Steps

1. Inspect the neck. Note symmetry, range of motion (ROM), and the condition of the skin.

- Inspect the neck in a neutral position.
- Inspect the neck when it is hyperextended.
- Inspect the neck when the patient swallows water.

2. Palpate the cervical lymph nodes. Note the size, shape, symmetry, consistency, mobility, tenderness, and temperature of any palpable nodes.

a. Use light palpation with one or two fingerpads in a circular movement.

b. Palpate the cervical nodes in the following order:
- Preauricular: in front of the ear
- Posterior auricular: behind the ear
- Tonsilar: at the angle of the jaw
- Submandibular: halfway up the lower jaw
- Submental: under the tip of the chin
- Occipital: at the base of the skull in the occipital area

Expected Findings

Neck is erect, midline, and symmetrical with full ROM. No masses are present; skin is intact. Larynx and trachea rise with swallowing. Thyroid is not visible.

Abnormal findings: Swollen lymph nodes may be visible. An enlarged thyroid may be visible in the lower half of the neck.

Lymph nodes are supple and nontender; no masses are palpable.

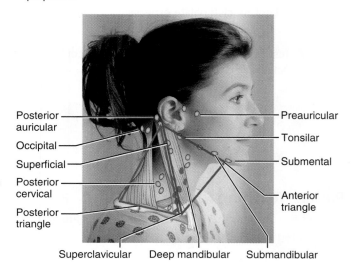

Procedural Steps

Expected Findings

(continued)

- Superficial cervical: below the tonsilar node over the sternocleidomastoid muscle
- Deep cervical: under the sternocleidomastoid muscle
- Posterior cervical: in posterior triangle along trapezius muscle
- Supraclavicular: above the clavicle

Use the same sequence every time so that the steps will become automatic and you will not omit any area.

Abnormal findings: lymphadenopathy (palpable nodes 1 cm or greater). Immobile nodes may indicate malignancy, inflammation, or infection in the area they drain.

---

3. Palpate the thyroid.

To use the posterior approach:

a. Stand behind the client, and ask her to flex her neck slightly forward and to the left.

b. Position your thumbs on the nape of the client's neck.

c. Using the fingers of your left hand, locate the cricoid cartilage, which is located below the thyroid cartilage. Push the trachea slightly to the left with your right hand as you palpate just below the cricoid cartilage and between the trachea and sternocleidomastoid muscle. Ask your client to swallow (give her small sips of water if necessary), and feel for the thyroid gland as it rises up.

d. Reverse and repeat the same steps to palpate the right thyroid lobe (use the fingers of your left hand to displace the trachea to the right, while using the fingers of your right hand to palpate the thyroid to the right of the trachea).

The thyroid is generally nonpalpable. If some tissue is palpable, the consistency is firm and smooth. There is no nodularity, enlargement, or tenderness.

Abnormal findings: An enlarged thyroid may signify a tumor or goiter. A tender thyroid is associated with inflammation.

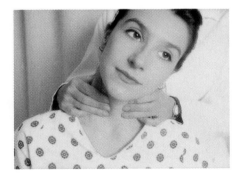

Step 3a–d

Procedural Steps

Expected Findings

Assessing the Neck *(continued)*

To use the anterior approach:

   e. Stand in front of the client, and ask her to flex her neck slightly forward and in the direction you intend to palpate.

   f. Place your hands on the neck, and apply gentle pressure to one side of the trachea while palpating the opposite side of the neck for the thyroid as the client swallows.

   g. Reverse and repeat the same steps on the opposite side.

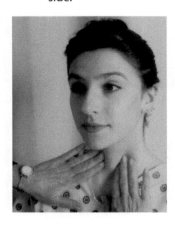

Steps 3e-3g

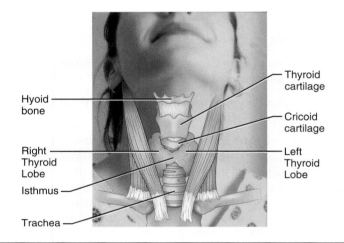

4. If the thyroid gland is palpable, auscultate it for bruits using the bell portion of the stethoscope. Ask the client to hold her breath as you auscultate.

No bruit is present.

Documentation

 VOL 1   Go to Chapter 19, **Documenting Physical Assessment Findings,** in Volume 1.

PROCEDURE 19–11   Assessing the Breasts and Axillae

> For steps to follow in *all* procedures, refer to the inside back cover of this book.

critical aspects
- Techniques: inspection and palpation.
- Inspect the breasts and axillae for skin condition, size, shape, symmetry, and color.
- If you notice an open lesion or nipple discharge, wear procedure gloves to palpate the breasts.
- Inspect the nipples for discharge. Culture any discharge, if present.
- Palpate the breasts using the vertical strip method, pie wedge method, or concentric circles method.
- Palpate the nipples, areolae, and lymph nodes.

Equipment
- Nonlatex gloves (for possible exposure to body fluids)
- Glass slide
- Culturette
- Pen and record form

Position
There are several positions the patient must assume during breast examination:
- Sitting, arms at side
- Sitting, arms over head (aids in detecting dimpling or retraction of breast tissue)
- Sitting, hands on hips (aids in detecting dimpling or retraction of breast tissue)
- Sitting, leaning forward (helpful when examining large, pendulous breasts)
- Supine with a small pillow under shoulder of breast being examined (helps spread the breast tissue over the chest wall)

Focused History Questions
- Do you have a lump or thickening in your underarm or breasts that persists throughout your menstrual cycle?
- Do you have any breast pain or discharge?
- Have you noticed any changes in the skin on your breasts, nipples, or underarms?
- Have you had any changes in your nipples?
- Have your breasts changed in size, shape, or contour?
- Do you perform breast self-examination (BSE)?
- Are you taking any medications or hormones?
- If you are premenopausal, when was your last period?

Procedural Steps

1. Inspect the breasts

Note size, shape, symmetry, and color.
   a. Inspect the breasts with the client in a sitting position with arms at her side.

   b. Inspect the breasts with the client sitting with her arms raised overhead.

Expected Findings

The breasts are symmetrical; however, the dominant side may be more developed, resulting in a slightly asymmetrical appearance. Skin color is lighter than exposed areas, and there are no lesions, redness, or edema. Texture is smooth, with no dimpling or retraction. Striae are a normal variation.

Procedural Steps

Expected Findings

Assessing the Breasts and Axillae *(continued)*

c. Inspect the breasts with the client seated and her hands pressed on her hips.

d. Inspect the breasts as the client leans forward.

e. Inspect the breasts with the client supine with a pillow under her shoulder.

Newborns—You may see breast enlargement and watery, white discharge from the nipples during the first 2 weeks of life.

Children—Breasts typically begin to develop at about 13 years of age; the breasts may not develop at equal rates.

Pregnancy—Breast size increases; areolae and nipples darken; superficial veins become prominent; stretch marks may be present; **colostrum** (a thick, yellow precursor to breast milk) can sometimes be expressed as early as the second trimester.

Older adults—Breasts lose firmness and become flaccid and pendulous.

Abnormal findings:

- Asymmetry warrants further investigation.
- Swelling or erythema may be seen in infection (**mastitis**).
- **Peau d'orange** (dimpled skin texture) skin changes may be seen with lymphatic obstruction that is present in some forms of breast cancer.
- Puckering, lesions, and retraction may also be seen with breast cancer.
- **Gynecomastia** (enlargement of breasts in males) is an abnormal finding.

---

2. Inspect the nipples and areolae. Note color, shape, and symmetry.

The areolae and nipples are darker in color than breast tissue. Nipples are everted and point in the same direction. No discharge is present, except in newborns and during pregnancy and lactation. No lesions or erosion is present.

Abnormal findings:

- Nipple discoloration that is not associated with pregnancy.
- Nipples pointing in different directions. Such findings warrant follow-up as a potential sign of an underlying mass.
- Flat or inverted nipples, which are caused by shortening of the mammary ducts. May make breastfeeding difficult.
- Any nipple discharge not associated with newborns, pregnancy, or breastfeeding requires a thorough evaluation.
- Cracks and nipple redness, which may occur with breastfeeding.

Procedural Steps	Expected Findings

(continued)

a. If there is nipple discharge in a woman who is not pregnant or breastfeeding, obtain a specimen by placing a glass slide up to the breast to capture a drop of discharge. Transport the slide to the lab as soon as possible. If there is ample discharge, obtain a swab of the discharge with a culturette.

No discharge is expected except in pregnancy and lactation.

---

3. Inspect the axillae. Note the color, condition of the skin, and hair distribution.

Skin is intact with no lesions or rashes. Presence of hair depends on the age of the client and personal preference. Axillary hair develops with puberty. Some women may choose to shave the hair, whereas others will allow it to grow.

Abnormal findings: Rashes, redness, or unusual pigmentation may indicate infection or allergy to deodorants. Dark-pigmented, velvety skin may be seen with *acanthous nigricans,* a condition associated with obesity and type II diabetes mellitus.

---

4. Palpate the breasts using the fingerpads of your three middle fingers, making small circles with light, medium, and deep pressure. Choose one of the following three techniques.

a. *Vertical strip method:* Start at the sternal edge, and palpate the breast in parallel lines until you reach the midaxillary line. Go up one area and down the adjacent strip (like "mowing the grass").

Breasts are soft and nontender with no lesions or masses. Consistency depends on age; premenopausal women have firm and elastic tissue, whereas postmenopausal women have softer tissue that may be stringy or cordlike.

Abnormal findings: Breast lumps or masses may be benign or malignant and require follow-up.

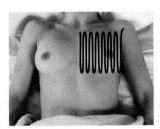

Step 4a

b. *Pie wedge method:* This method examines the breast in wedges. Move from one wedge to the next.

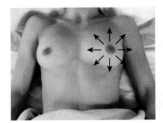

Step 4b

Procedural Steps

Expected Findings

Assessing the Breasts and Axillae *(continued)*

c. *Concentric circles method:* Start at the outermost area of the breast at the 12 o'clock position. Move clockwise in concentric, ever smaller, circles.

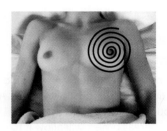

Step 4c

Technique Hints

- Do not remove your fingers from the skin surface once you have begun palpating. Move from area to area by sliding the fingers along the skin.
- Most breast lesions in women are found in the upper outer quadrant.
- Most breast cancer in men occurs in the areola.

---

5. Palpate the nipples and areolae.

a. If the woman is supine, place a small pillow or folded towel under the shoulder of the breast you are examining.

b. Squeeze the nipple gently between your thumb and finger to check for discharge.

c. Note tissue elasticity and tenderness.

Nipples are elastic and nontender. No discharge is present.

Abnormal findings: Loss of elasticity may indicate underlying malignancy. Bloody, purulent discharge may indicate infection. Other forms of drainage may indicate malignancy.

---

6. Palpate the axillae and clavicular lymph nodes.

a. Have the woman sitting with her arms at her sides or supine.

b. Using your fingerpads, move your fingers in circular fashion.

- *Central nodes:* located high in the midaxillary region
- *Anterior pectoral nodes:* located on the lower border of the pectoralis major in the anterior axillary fold
- *Lateral brachial nodes:* located high in the axilla on the inner aspect of the humerus
- *Posterior subscapular nodes:* located high in the axilla on the lateral scapular border

Nodes are nonpalpable.

Abnormal findings: Palpable nodes may be seen with infection or malignancy. Enlarged lymph nodes caused by infection are tender.

Procedural Steps	Expected Findings

(continued)

- *Epitrochlear nodes:* located above the elbow
- *Infraclavicular nodes:* located below the clavicle
- *Supraclavicular nodes:* located above the clavicle

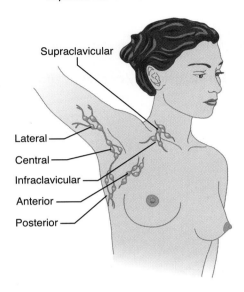

Step 6

Patient Teaching

Instruct patient in BSE.

Documentation

 Go to Chapter 19, **Documenting Physical Assessment Findings**, in Volume 1.

- If you palpate a mass or lump, document its size, shape, symmetry, mobility, tenderness, and skin color changes. To document the location, divide the breast into four quadrants by intersecting vertical and horizontal lines. With the nipple as the center, locate the mass or lump as though the breast were a clock; state the distance in cm from the nipple (e.g., 4 o'clock, 2.5 cm from nipple).

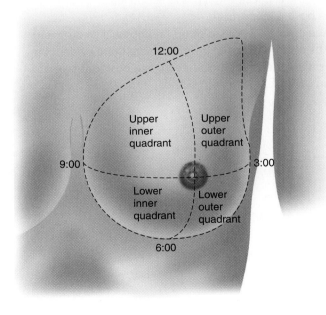

PROCEDURE 19–12   Assessing the Chest and Lungs

 For steps to follow in *all* procedures, refer to the inside back cover of this book.

critical aspects

- Techniques: inspection, palpation, percussion, auscultation.
- Assess respirations by counting the respiratory rate and observing the rhythm, depth, and symmetry of chest movement.
- Inspect the chest for anteroposterior (AP):lateral ratio, costal angle, spinal deformity, respiratory effort, and skin condition.
- Palpate the trachea.
- Palpate the chest for tenderness, masses, or crepitus.
- Palpate chest excursion.
- Palpate the chest for tactile fremitus.
- Percuss the chest.
- Percuss diaphragmatic excursion.
- Auscultate the chest.

Equipment

- Stethoscope
- Felt-tipped marker and ruler
- Pen and record form

Position

- Have the client sitting, if possible, and leaning forward for the posterior approach.
- If the client is unable to sit up, findings will be distorted.
- If the client is lying down, findings are more evident on the dependent side; help her change positions so that you can assess with each side dependent.

Focused History Questions

- Do you have fatigue or activity intolerance?
- Do you have any current respiratory problems?
- Have you had any recent respiratory problems?
- Do you have a cough?
- Do you have any difficulty breathing?
- What, if anything, causes you to be short of breath?
- Have you had any chest pain?
- Do you have a history of allergies or asthma?
- Do you smoke? If so, how much and for how long?
- If you smoke, have you tried to quit? Would you like to quit?
- Are you exposed to air pollutants at home or at work?

Procedural Steps

Expected Findings

1. Count the respiratory rate, and observe the rhythm and depth; observe the symmetry of chest and respiratory movements.

- The normal respiratory rate varies by age. A newborn may have a respiratory rate of 40 to 90. The rate gradually declines as the child matures. For an adult, a rate of 12–20 is normal. (See Chapter 17 for more information about counting respirations.)
- Respirations are quiet with a regular rhythm and depth.
- Chest movement is symmetrical.

Infants and children—breathe abdominally, so you will see little chest movement.

Older adults—rate changes very little; however, respirations decrease in depth as muscles become weakened.

Abnormal findings:

- Chest asymmetry may be seen with musculoskeletal disorders of the spine, such as kyphosis or scoliosis.
- Asymmetrical chest movement during breathing is seen in rib fractures, pneumothrax, and atelectasis; affected chest area may not move at all with respiration.
- Sternal and intercostal retractions are seen with hypoxia, respiratory distress, and airway obstruction.
- Respiratory rate may be increased with activity, smoking, fever, pain or anemia.

2. Inspect the chest.

a. Inspect the anteroposterior (AP):lateral ratio.

a. The normal adult AP:lateral ratio is 1:2.

Infants—AP is equal to the lateral diameter

Older adults—Kyphosis and osteoporosis change the size and shape of the chest; weakening thoracic and diaphragm muscles allow the chest to widen and become more barrel-shaped.

Abnormal findings: AP:lateral ratio is increased in COPD (barrel chest).

b. Inspect the costal angle.

b. The costal angle is < 90°.

Abnormal findings: Costal angle is > 90° in COPD.

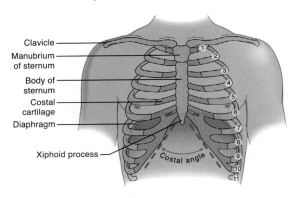

Clavicle
Manubrium of sternum
Body of sternum
Costal cartilage
Diaphragm
Xiphoid process
Costal angle

Step 2b

Procedural Steps

Expected Findings

Assessing the Chest and Lungs (continued)

c. Identify any spinal deformities.

c. The spine is straight without lateral curvatures or deformity.

Abnormal findings: Scoliosis is a lateral curvature of the spine. Kyphosis is excessive thoracic curvature.

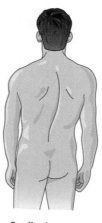 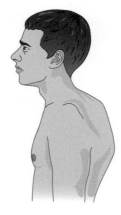

Scoliosis   *Kyphosis*

d. Observe the effort required to breathe.

d. Respirations appear effortless. There is no retraction or use of accessory muscles.

Abnormal findings: Sternal and intercostal retractions are seen in severe hypoxia or respiratory distress.

e. Note the color and condition of skin.

e. Skin color and hair distribution are consistent with the client's gender, ethnicity, and exposure to the sun. The skin is intact with no scars.

Abnormal findings: cyanosis of the chest wall (due to extreme hypoxia or cold temperature).

3. Palpate the trachea.

a. Place your fingers and thumb on either side of the trachea and note its position.

Trachea is in the midline.

Abnormal findings: Tracheal deviation may occur from a mass in the neck (e.g., thyroid enlargement) or from excess pressure in the lungs (e.g., tension pneumothorax).

Developmental Modification:

Infants—have a short neck, so it may not be possible to palpate the trachea.

4. Palpate the chest for tenderness, masses, or **crepitus** (crackling skin due to air in the subcutaneous tissue).

a. Palpate the anterior, posterior, and lateral chest by placing your hands on the chest wall.

The chest is nontender. No masses or crepitus is present.

Abnormal findings: Pain in the chest wall may be due to fracture, inflammation, or trauma. Crepitus results from air leaking into the subcutaneous tissue. It is most likely to occur around wounds, central IV line sites, chest tubes, or a tracheostomy.

Procedural Steps

Expected Findings

(continued)

5. Palpate chest **excursion** (expandability).

a. Place your hands at the base of the client's chest with fingers spread and thumbs about 5 cm (2 in.) apart (at the costal margin anteriorly and at the 8th to 10th rib posteriorly).

b. Press your thumbs toward the client's spine to create a small skinfold between them.

c. Have the client take a deep breath, and feel for chest expansion.

This may be performed on the anterior or posterior portion of the chest, or both.

Chest excursion is symmetrical on the anterior and posterior aspect of the chest (you should feel equal pressure on your hands; thumbs should move apart equal distances).

Abnormal findings: Limited chest excursion may occur with shallow breathing, restrictive clothing, or restrictive airway disease. Asymmetrical excursion may result from airway obstruction, pleural effusion, or pneumothorax.

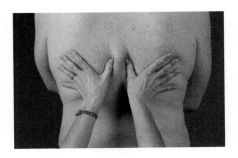

Step 5

6. Follow the same pattern and sequence for palpating fremitus, percussing, and auscultating the chest. See the accompanying diagram.

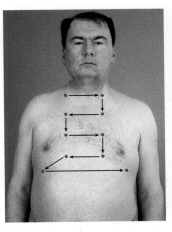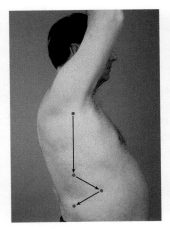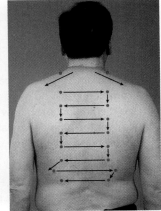

Percussion and auscultation sites

7. Palpate the chest for tactile fremitus.

a. Use the palmar surface of your hands, but raise the fingers off the client's chest so that you palpate with the bony metacarpophalangeal joints of your hands.

Tactile fremitus is equal bilaterally on the anterior and posterior chest; it is diminished at midthorax. Fremitus is normally diminished if the chest wall is very thick or the voice very soft.

Procedural Steps

Expected Findings

Assessing the Chest and Lungs *(continued)*

Bony prominences are best for detecting vibrations.

  b. Palpate for vibrations as the client says, "99."

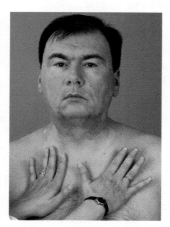

Step 7

Developmental Modification

Infants—place your hand over the chest while the infant is crying.

Children and thin adults—may have increased fremitus.

Abnormal findings: Increased fremitus occurs with conditions that cause fluid in the lungs (e.g., pulmonary edema). Decreased or absent fremitus occurs when there is decreased air movement or tissue consolidation (e.g., emphysema, asthma).

---

8. Percuss the chest. Percuss over the intercostal spaces rather than over the ribs.

Percussion over bone produces less resonance.

Use the indirect percussion method on the anterior, posterior, and lateral chest, following the diagram in step 6. Compare the right side to the left side.

- The anterior chest is resonant to the 2nd ICS on the left and to the 4th ICS on the right.
- The lateral chest is resonant to the 8th ICS.
- The posterior chest is resonant to T12.

Abnormal findings: Dullness is heard with fluid or masses in the lungs. Hyperresonance is heard with air trapping that occurs with emphysema.

---

9. Percuss the posterior chest for diaphragmatic excursion.

  a. Percuss the level of the diaphragm on full expiration. Have the client exhale completely and hold his breath while you percuss (beginning just below the scapula) from resonance over the lung downward toward the diaphragm. The sound will become dull at the diaphragm. Mark the area with a pen.

  b. Percuss the diaphragm level on full inspiration. Have the client take a deep breath and hold it as you percuss again. Mark the location.

Diaphragmatic excursion is normally 3–6 cm (the distance between the two marks).

Abnormal findings: Decreased excursion may indicate paralysis, atelectasis, or COPD with overinflated lungs.

Procedural Steps

Expected Findings

(continued)

    c. Measure the distance between the two marks.

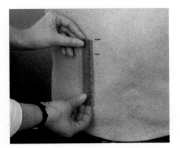

Step 9

---

10. Auscultate the chest.

    a. Follow the pattern in Step 6.

    b. Use the diaphragm of the stethoscope.

    c. Have the client take slow, deep breaths through his mouth as you listen at each site through one full respiratory cycle. Refer to the table at the end of this procedure.

Lung fields are clear to auscultation. Bronchial breath sounds are heard over the trachea. Bronchovesicular breath sounds are heard over the sternum anteriorly and between the scapulae posteriorly. Vesicular breath sounds are heard over most of the lung fields. No abnormal or adventitious sounds are heard.

Infants—breath sounds are louder than in adults.

Abnormal findings: Crackles or rales are heard with atelectasis, pneumonia, or pulmonary edema. Rhonchi result from mucus secretions in the large airways. Wheezing is a high-pitched sound produced by narrowing of an airway by spasm, inflammation, mucus, or tumor.

---

11. Auscultate for abnormal voice sounds if there is evidence of lung congestion. Follow the pattern in Step 6.

    a. Assess for bronchophony by having the client say, "1, 2, 3," as you listen over the lung fields.

    b. Assess for egophony by having your client say, "eee," as you listen over the lung fields.

    c. Assess for whispered pectoriloquy by having your client whisper, "1, 2, 3," as you listen over the lung fields.

No abnormal voice sounds are heard.

Abnormal findings

    a. Bronchophony is present if the words are clearly heard over the lungs.

    b. Egophony is present if the sound you hear is "ay."

    c. Whispered pectoriloquy is present if you hear, "One, two, three" clearly.

Patient Teaching

Instruct patient about the dangers of smoking; exposure to air pollutants and environmental pollutants, such as radon or asbestos; and the signs and symptoms of lung cancer.

Home Care

- Instruct caregivers to identify any pollutant within the home that may cause respiratory problems, such as radon, dirty heating/air conditioning systems, or mold.
- Instruct caregivers of patients with allergies and/or asthma to eliminate potential allergens, such as cigarette smoke, dust, feathers, and pet dander.

Documentation

Document chest and lung assessment findings on the client's record. Identify exact locations using the chest landmarks (vertical lines and ICS).

 Go to Chapter 19, **Documenting Physical Assessment Findings**, in Volume 1.

Abnormal Lung Sounds

Abnormal Lung Sound	Cause	Characteristics	Examples
Crackles (sometimes called rales)	Air bubbling through moisture in the alveoli	Soft, high-pitched, and very brief sounds, usually heard during inspiration	Pneumonia Congestive heart failure (CHF) Bronchitis Emphysema
Rhonchi	Mucus secretions in the large airways	Snoring, low-pitched sounds heard during inspiration and expiration	Bronchitis Emphysema Narrowed airways Fibrotic lungs
Wheezes	Narrowing of an airway by spasm, inflammation, mucus, or tumor	High-pitched musical sounds heard during inspiration and expiration	Acute asthma Emphysema
Stridor*	Partial upper airway obstruction or tracheal or laryngeal spasm	High-pitched, continuous honking sounds heard throughout the respiratory cycle but most prominent on inspiration	Acute respiratory distress Foreign body in airway Epiglottitis
Friction rub	Rubbing together of inflamed pleural layers	A high-pitched grating or squeaking sound that may be heard throughout the respiratory cycle	Pleuritis
Grunting	Retention of air in the lungs	A high-pitched tubular sound heard on expiration	Emphysema

*Clients with stridor need immediate medical evaluation.

PROCEDURE 19–13 Assessing the Heart and Vascular System

 For steps to follow in *all* procedures, refer to the inside back cover of this book.

critical aspects

- Techniques: inspection, palpation, auscultation.
- If possible, work from your patient's right side.
- Inspect the neck for pulsations.
- Measure jugular venous pressure (JVP).
- Inspect the precordium for pulsations.
- Palpate the carotid arteries.
- Palpate the precordium for pulsations, lifts, heaves, or thrills.
- Auscultate the carotid arteries with the bell of the stethoscope.
- Auscultate the jugular veins with the bell of the stethoscope.
- Auscultate the precordium at the apex, left lower sternal border, base left, and base right. Use the bell and then the diaphragm of the stethoscope.
- Palpate the peripheral pulses. Any abnormalities require further evaluation.

Equipment

- Combination stethoscope with bell and diaphragm
- Two rulers
- Pen and record form

Position

Place the client in three positions: sitting, supine, and left lateral (to facilitate hearing specific sounds).

Focused History Questions

- Have you experienced any fatigue or activity intolerance?
- Do you have a history of high blood pressure or stroke?
- Have you ever passed out or felt light-headed?
- Do you have any problems with your heart or circulation?
- Do you ever experience chest pain? If so, describe the circumstances that triggered the pain.
- What was the pain like? What did you do to relieve it?
- Do you ever experience palpitations or a rapid heart beat?
- Do you ever feel short of breath?
- Do you ever get swelling in your feet?
- What medications are you taking?

Procedural Steps

Expected Findings

Assessing the Heart and Vascular System *(continued)*

1. Inspect the neck.

a. With the patient supine, inspect the carotid and jugular venous system in the neck for pulsations.

b. Assess jugular flow: Compress the jugular vein below the jaw. The vein collapses, and the jugular wave is more prominent at the supraclavicular area.

c. Assess jugular filling: Compress the jugular above the clavicle. The vein distends and the jugular wave disappears.

Carotid pulsation is easily visible. A slight pulsation in the supraclavicular area or suprasternal notch indicates jugular venous pressure. The pulsation should be easily obliterated when you apply pressure to the area.

Abnormal findings: Significant jugular vein distention suggests right-sided heart failure.

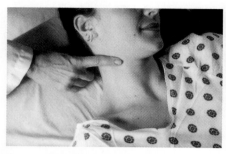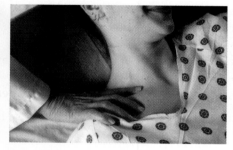

Step 1: B, Assessing jugular flow;   *C, Assessing jugular fill*

2. Measure jugular venous pressure (JVP).

a. Elevate the head of the bed to a 45° angle.

b. Identify the highest point of visible internal jugular filling.

c. Place a ruler vertically at the sternal angle (where the clavicles meet).

d. Place another ruler horizontally at the highest point of the venous wave.

e. Measure the distance in centimeters vertically from the chest wall.

Normal jugular venous pressure is < 3 cm.

Abnormal findings: elevated JVP (in CHF or constricted flow into the right side of the heart); low JVP (in hypovolemia).

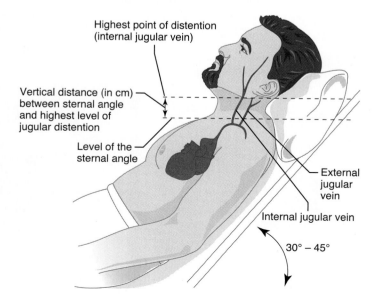

Highest point of distention (internal jugular vein)

Vertical distance (in cm) between sternal angle and highest level of jugular distention

Level of the sternal angle

External jugular vein

Internal jugular vein

30° – 45°

Step 2

Procedural Steps

Expected Findings

(continued)

3. Inspect the precordium for pulsations. (Have the patient supine with tangential lighting.)

Developmental Modification

Children—Look for the PMI more medially and at about the 4th ICS in children under age 8.

Visible pulsation at the point of maximal impulse (PMI, the 5th ICS in the midclavicular line). In thin adults and children, a pulsation may also be visible over the base of the heart.

Abnormal findings: A pulsation (a heave or lift) displaced toward the axillary line indicates left ventricular hypertrophy. Pulsations to the right of the sternum may indicate an aortic aneurysm.

---

4. Palpate the carotid arteries.

a. Palpate each side separately.

Bilateral pressure may impair cerebral blood flow.

b. Avoid massaging the carotid artery as you palpate.

Increased pressure on the carotid will lead to a drop in the pulse rate.

c. Note the rate, rhythm, amplitude, and symmetry of the pulse; note the contour, symmetry, and elasticity of the arteries; note any thrills.

- *Pulse rate* is age dependent.
- *Rhythm* is regular with +2 amplitude.
- *Contour:* There should be a smooth upstroke with less acute descent.
- *Symmetry:* Pulses are equal bilaterally.
- *Elasticity:* Carotids are soft and pliable.

Older adults—the carotids may be stiff and cordlike.

Abnormal findings: A thrill indicates turbulent flow.

---

5. Palpate the precordium.

a. Palpate in all five areas: apex, left lateral sternal border, epigastric area, base left, and base right.

b. For this part of the examination, have the patient sit up and lean forward. If lying down, have him turn to the left side.

Brings the apex of the heart closer to the chest wall.

NOTE: Perform cardiac auscultation from the right side, whenever possible. *This allows you to stretch the stethoscope during auscultation so that you minimize interference and "static."*

PMI is palpable at the apex over a 1–2 cm area. Slight pulsation from the abdominal aorta may be felt at the epigastric area. No pulsations, lifts, heaves, or thrills are palpable.

Abnormal findings: A pulsation, lift, or heave may be seen with left ventricular hypertrophy. A thrill indicates turbulent flow.

---

6. Auscultate the carotids.

a. Place the bell portion of the stethoscope over the carotid artery to listen for bruits.

b. Have the patient hold his breath as you listen.

No audible bruit is present.

Children—bruit may be heard because of a high output state.

Abnormal findings: In adults, a bruit suggests carotid stenosis.

Procedural Steps

Expected Findings

Assessing the Heart and Vascular System *(continued)*

7. Auscultate the jugular veins.

No venous hum is audible.

   a. Place the bell portion of the stethoscope over the jugular veins to listen for a venous hum.

Children—A venous hum may be heard.

   b. Have the patient hold his breath as you listen.

---

8. Auscultate the precordium.

No extra sounds are heard. No murmurs, clicks, or rubs are present.

To review heart sounds,

Infants—You may hear a split S_2 when the child takes a deep breath.

 Go to **Sound Files,** on the Electronic Study Guide.

Children—The chest wall is thinner, so heart sounds are louder than in adults.

- Listen for the S_1, S_2, S_3, and S_4 sounds.
- Listen for murmurs.
- Listen with both the bell and the diaphragm at the following sites:

Older adults—An S_4 sound is considered normal; extra systoles per minute are considered normal.

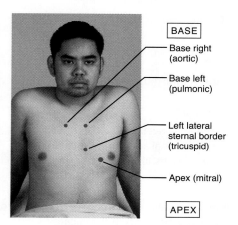

BASE

Base right (aortic)

Base left (pulmonic)

Left lateral sternal border (tricuspid)

Apex (mitral)

APEX

   a. *Base right (aortic valve).* Locate the angle of Louis. (It is the prominence on the sternum, 2 to 3 finger-breadths below the suprasternal notch.) Slide your fingers laterally until you feel the 2nd ICS on either side. The right 2nd ICS is the best place to palpate the aortic valve.

   a. $S_1 < S_2$

   b. *Base left (pulmonic valve).* Locate the angle of Louis (the prominence on the sternum, 2 to 3 finger-breadths below the clavicular notch). Slide your fingers laterally until you feel the 2nd ICS on either side. The left 2nd ICS is the best place to palpate the pulmonic valve.

   b. $S_1 < S_2$

   c. *Apex (mitral valve).* You may be able to locate the apex by observing the pulsation at the PMI. It is at the 5th ICS in the midclavicular line.

   c. $S_1 > S_2$

Children—You will hear S_3 at the apex in about 30% of children.

   d. *Left lateral sternal border (LLSB) (tricuspid valve).* From the apex, slide your finger up to the 4th ICS, then move close to the sternum.

   d. $S_1 >$ or $= S_2$. You may hear a split S_1.

Procedural Steps

Expected Findings

(continued)

Murmurs Auscultating murmurs is an advanced technique that requires practice and experience. However, if you hear a murmur, assess its:

- Location
- Quality
- Frequency (high, medium, or low pitch)
- Intensity (loudness)
- Timing (in relation to S_1 and S_2)
- Duration
- Configuration (constant or crescendo/decrescendo)
- Radiation (can you hear this in other locations?)
- Respiratory variation (does it change with breathing?)

Classifying Murmurs

Grade

1/6 Very faint, comes and goes
2/6 Quiet, but heard immediately
3/6 Moderately loud
4/6 Loud, associated with a thrill
5/6 Heard with stethoscope half off the chest wall; thrill present
6/6 Heard with stethoscope entirely off the chest wall; thrill present

Abnormal findings: extra sounds (S_3 or S_4), murmurs, clicks, or rubs. *Note:* A diastolic murmur or a murmur greater than grade 3/6 is never innocent. For a description of murmurs,

 Go to Chapter 19, **Tables, Boxes, Figures: ESG Table 19–1,** on the Electronic Study Guide.

Infants—A split S_2 sound during normal respirations may indicate an atrial-septal defect.

---

9. Inspect the periphery for color, temperature, and edema. (You will probably already have done this when examining the integumentary system.)

Skin is warm. No edema is present. Color is appropriate for race.

Abnormal findings: pallor, cyanosis, coolness, shininess, sparse hair growth, and clubbing of the nails (may indicate pulmonary oxygenation problems or impaired central or peripheral circulation).

---

10. Palpate the peripheral pulses: radial, brachial, femoral, popliteal, dorsalis pedis, and posterior tibial.

a. Using the distal pads of your second and third fingers, firmly palpate pulses.

b. Palpate firmly but not so hard that you occlude the artery.

c. If you have trouble finding a pulse, vary your pressure, feeling carefully at the correct anatomical location.

d. Assess pulses for rate, rhythm, equality, amplitude, and elasticity.

e. Describe pulse amplitude on a scale of 0 to 4:
   0 = absent, not palpable
   1 = diminished, barely palpable
   2 = normal, expected
   3 = full, increased
   4 = bounding

All pulses are regular, strong, and equal bilaterally. Pulse amplitude is +2.

Abnormal findings: Weak, absent, or asymmetrical pulses may indicate partial or complete occlusion of the artery. Other signs of arterial occlusion include pain, pallor, cool temperature, paresthesia, or paralysis.

Procedural Steps

Expected Findings

Assessing the Heart and Vascular System *(continued)*

Developmental Modification

Older adults—arterial pulses may be difficult to palpate because of decreased arterial perfusion.

Note: If inspection or palpation findings are abnormal, perform the following more extensive tests.

a. *Perform the capillary refill test* anywhere you note signs of diminished blood flow.
- Press the skin with sufficient pressure to produce blanching.
- Release the pressure and observe the return of color.

a. Color returns in less than 3 seconds

b. *Perform Allen's test* to assess abnormal pulse findings and arterial flow in the hands.
- Have the client form a tight fist with one hand.
- With her fist still clenched, compress her radial and ulnar arteries.
- Ask the client to open her hand; observe for pallor.
- Release the ulnar artery and watch for natural color to return. Normally pallor resolves in 3 to 5 seconds.
- Then repeat the process, but release the radial artery.

b. In a healthy individual skin color returns rapidly with each maneuver. Failure to return to normal color indicates impaired flow through the open artery.

c. *Check the ankle-brachial index (ABI)* to assess circulatory impairment of the feet.
- Use a Doppler (hand-held ultrasonic device) to measure blood pressure at the posterior tibialis or dorsalis pedis pulse sites.
- Compare that pressure with blood pressure obtained over the brachial artery.
- To calculate the ABI, divide the systolic pressure at the ankle by the systolic pressure at the brachial site.

c. Normally ankle pressure is higher than brachial pressure. The following is a summary of ABI findings.

Normal:	1 or greater
Minimal disease:	0.8 – 0.95
Moderate disease:	0.8 – 0.4
Severe disease:	0.4 – 0

Example: If the systolic pressure at the ankle is 75 and at the brachial artery is 100, the ABI is 75/100, or 0.75. This indicates moderate peripheral vascular disease.

d. *Perform the color change test* to assess arterial circulation in the legs.
- While the client is lying supine, elevate the legs to increase venous return.
- Have the client quickly move to a sitting position with the feet dangling.

d. Normal color should return to the feet in less than 10 seconds. Pallor with the legs elevated and dependent rubor (reddish-purple color) are signs of arterial insufficiency.

---

11. Inspect the venous system. If a client has varicosities, assess for valve competence with the manual compression test.
- With the client standing, compress the distal portion of the vein.
- Still holding the distal portion, compress the proximal portion.

Veins are not distended. Superficial spiderlike veins, especially on the lower extremities, may occur with normal aging.

If the valves are competent, you will not feel backflow. If the valves are incompetent, you will feel a wave pulsation with your lower hand as a result of backflow when you press on the proximal segment of the veins.

Procedural Steps

(continued)

Expected Findings

Older adults—often have peripheral edema as a result of chronic venous insufficiency.

Abnormal findings: ropelike, distended, tortuous, or painful veins **(varicosities).**

Patient Teaching

Instruct the patient in the risk factors of heart disease and stroke and in the signs and symptoms of heart disease.

Documentation

 VOL 1 Go to Chapter 19, **Documenting Physical Assessment Findings,** in Volume 1.

PROCEDURE 19–14   Assessing the Abdomen

➤ For steps to follow in *all* procedures, refer to the inside back cover of this book.

critical aspects
- Techniques: inspection, auscultation, percussion, palpation (in that order).
- Have the client void prior to the exam.
- Position the client supine with the knees slightly flexed.
- Inspect the abdomen.
- Auscultate the abdomen for bowel sounds and bruits.
- Use indirect percussion to assess at multiple sites in all four quadrants.
- Using your fist or blunt percussion, percuss the costovertebral angle bilaterally to assess for kidney tenderness.
- Lightly palpate throughout the abdomen by pressing down 1 to 2 cm in a rotating motion. Identify surface characteristics, tenderness, muscle resistance, and turgor.
- Use deep palpation to palpate organs and masses.

Equipment
- Stethoscope
- Felt-tipped marker
- Tape measure and ruler
- Penlight or examination light
- Pen and record form

Position

Begin with client supine, arms at sides, with small pillows under the head and knees.

Relaxes the abdominal muscles.

Focused History Questions
- What types of foods do you typically eat?
- Are there any foods that you cannot eat? If so, why?
- How many cups of coffee, tea, cola, or caffeinated beverages do you drink per day?
- Do you smoke? If so, how much and at what age did you start?
- Do you drink alcohol? If so, how many drinks per day? Per week?
- Do you use recreational drugs?
- Do you have any abdominal pain?

- Have you ever been diagnosed with an ulcer, hemorrhoids, hernia, bowel problem, cancer, hepatitis, liver problems, cirrhosis, or appendicitis?
- Have you ever had abdominal surgery? If so, when, what type, and what if any follow-up was done for the problem?
- Do you have any family history of abdominal problems, such as ulcers, gallbladder disease, bowel disease, or cancer?
- Do you ever have trouble with:

Swallowing?

Heartburn?

Nausea?

Vomiting?

Diarrhea?

Bloating?

Excess gas?

Yellowing of the skin?

- How often do you have a bowel movement (BM)?
- Have you noticed any changes in your BMs?
- Are you having any problems with constipation, diarrhea, or getting to the bathroom in time to use the toilet?
- Have you ever seen blood in your stool or noticed blood when you wipe after a BM?
- Have you ever had black, tarry BMs?
- How often do you use antacids, laxatives, enemas, aspirin, or anti-inflammatory medicines such as Anaprox or Motrin?
- What home remedy, herbal, or over-the-counter medicines do you use?
- What prescription medicines do you use?
- Have you ever been immunized for hepatitis?
- Have you ever had a blood transfusion?
- What is your occupation?

Procedural Steps

Expected Findings

1. Have the client void prior to the exam.

Empties the bladder so that you do not mistake a full bladder for a mass.

---

2. Position the client supine with the knees slightly flexed.

Relaxes the abdominal muscles.

---

3. Inspect the abdomen.

   a. Observe the size, symmetry, and contour of the abdomen.
   - Stand at the client's side and view across the abdomen.
   - If distention is present, use a tape measure to measure girth at the level of the umbilicus.
   - Have the client raise his head and check for bulges.

Accentuates hernia, if present.

   b. Observe the condition of skin and skin color. Look for lesions, scars, striae, superficial veins, and hair distribution (if you have not already done this in your examination of the integumentary system).

   a. Abdomen is flat, slightly rounded, scaphoid (concave), or slightly protuberant; sides are symmetrical. No visible masses or distention are present.

Infants and toddlers—protruberant abdomen is normal.

Abnormal findings: Tumors, cysts, bowel obstruction, or scoliosis may cause asymmetry.

   b. Skin color is consistent with ethnicity but is usually lighter in color than exposed areas. No lesions are present. Hair distribution is appropriate for age and gender. Striae, superficial veins, and scars are common variations.

Abnormal findings:

- Skin color changes may be associated with bruising, internal bleeding, or jaundice.
- Striae occur after periods of rapid growth. Pink striae are new. Older striae are silver-white in color.
- Dilated veins are associated with liver disease and obstruction of the vena cava.

Procedural Steps

Expected Findings

(continued)

    c. Note abdominal movements.

    c. On a thin client, peristalsis and aortic pulsations may be visible. Men tend to use their abdominal muscles for breathing.

Infants and children—Peristaltic waves are often visible.
Older adults—Abdomen may be more rounded because of decreased muscle tone.

Abnormal findings:

- Persitaltic waves may be seen if there is intestinal obstruction.
- Abnormal respiratory movements may be seen with respiratory distress.
- Pulsations (in other than a thin client) may indicate an aortic aneurysm.

    d. Note the position, contour, and color of the umbilicus.

    d. Umbilicus is inverted and in the midline. No discoloration or discharge is present.

Abnormal findings:

Protrusion of the umbilicus may result from a hernia or underlying mass.

---

4. Auscultate the abdomen.

    a. Ask the client when he last ate.

Bowel sounds are loudest 5 or 6 hours after the person eats, when the small intestine contents empty through the ileocecal valve into the large intestine. They also increase immediately after eating.

    b. Listen for bowel sounds.
- Using the stethescope diaphragm, listen in several areas in all four quadrants (see the figure).

The diaphragm of the stethoscope is used because bowel sounds are high-pitched.
- If bowel sounds are infrequent or difficult to hear, listen to the right of the umbilicus over the ileocecal valve.
- Listen for 5 minutes before concluding that bowel sounds are absent.

    b. Audible bowel sounds, occuring every 5 to 15 seconds or 5 to 30 times per minute in a healthy adult.

Abnormal findings:

- *Hyperperistalsis* (hyperactive bowel sounds): > 2 or 3 sounds per second or > 30 bowel sounds/minute; loud, rushing sounds
- *Hypoperistalsis:* < 5 sounds per minute; faint sounds
- *Absent* bowel sounds: none after listening for 5 minutes.

Procedural Steps

Expected Findings

Assessing the Abdomen *(continued)*

c. Use the stethoscope bell to listen for bruits over the aorta and the renal, femoral, and iliac arteries.

c. No audible bruits are present.

Abnormal findings: A bruit is abnormal and may indicate an aneurysm or altered blood flow.

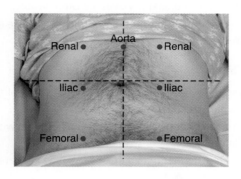

Step 4c

---

5. Percuss the abdomen. (See Technique 19–1 on page 233.)

- Use indirect percussion to assess at multiple sites in all four quadrants.
- Estimate organ size by noting the change in sounds as you percuss over the liver, spleen, and bladder.

Tympany, with dullness over organs or fluid, is present. No tenderness.

Abnormal findings: Extremely high-pitched tympanic sounds are heard with distention. Extensive dullness indicates organ enlargement or underlying mass.

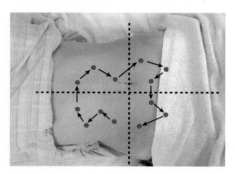

Step 5

---

6. Using fist or blunt percussion, percuss the costovertebral angle (where the end of the rib cage meets the spine) bilaterally to assess for kidney tenderness.

No costovertebral angle tenderness is present.

Abnormal findings: Pain or tenderness is associated with kidney infection or musculoskeletal problems.

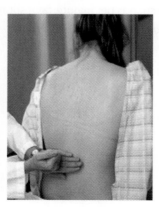

Step 6

Procedural Steps

Expected Findings

(continued)

7. Palpate the abdomen.

- For patients who are ticklish or guarding, distract them by giving them a task, such as "Count aloud to 10" or, "Count backwards from 100."

  Alternatively, have the client place her hand on her abdomen; place your hand on hers and begin light palpation. When she begins to feel more relaxed, slip your hand underneath hers.

- Encourage children to place their hand lightly over yours as you palpate.

a. Begin with light palpation throughout the abdomen. Identify surface characteristics, tenderness, muscular resistance, and turgor.

- Using your fingertips, press down 1 to 2 cm in a rotating motion.
- Lift your fingers and move to the next site.
- Palpate the entire abdomen if possible.
- Proceed in an organized fashion through all quadrants, using the same sequence in every examination.
- Observe for grimacing, guarding, or verbal statements of tenderness or pain.

Caution: Do not palpate the abdomen if the client has a Wilm's tumor, a large diffuse pulsation, or a history of organ transplant

b. Use deep palpation to palpate organs and masses.

a. The abdomen is soft and nontender, with no masses. Muscles are easily palpated; no guarding is present.

Abnormal findings: Guarding and rigidity may indicate peritonitis. Tenderness on light palpation indicates the need for further evaluation.

b. Tenderness may be noted in a normal adult near the xiphoid process and over the cecum and sigmoid colon.

Older adults—have a higher pain threshold, so they may not react even if there is a problem in the abdomen.

Abnormal findings: A mass indicates the need for further evaluation.

Procedural Steps

Expected Findings

Assessing the Abdomen *(continued)*

b. *(continued)*

Deep Palpation: One-Handed Technique

- Using your fingertips, press down 4 to 6 cm in a dipping motion.
- Proceed in an organized fashion through all four quadrants.

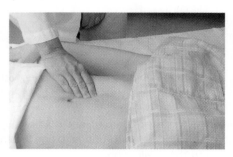

Deep Palpation: Bimanual Technique

- This technique is useful when palpating a large abdomen.
- Place your nondominant hand on your dominant hand.
- Depress your hands 4 to 6 cm in a dipping motion.
- Proceed in an organized fashion through all four quadrants.

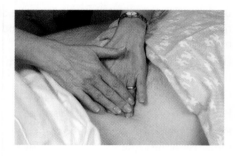

Note: If you palpate a mass, have the client tighten her abdominal muscles. If the mass is in the abdominal wall, it will become easier to palpate. If it is deep in the abdomen, it will be difficult to palpate.

c. Palpate the Liver

- Stand at the client's right side.
- Place your right hand at the client's right midclavicular line under the costal margin, parallel to the right costal.
- Place your left hand under the client's back at the lower (11th to 12th) ribs, and press upward. This elevates the liver toward the abdominal wall.
- Ask the client to inhale and deeply exhale while you press in and up, gently but deeply, with your right fingers.
- *Alternative approach: Hooking technique.* Place your hands over the right costal margin, and hook your fingers over the edge. Have the client take a deep breath, and feel for the liver's edge as the liver drops down on inspiration and then rises up over your fingers during expiration.

c. The liver is not normally palpable unless the client is very thin. If it is palpable, the edge should be smooth and nontender.

Children—Liver is relatively large and can be palpated 1 to 2 cm (0.5 to 1 in.) below the right costal margin.

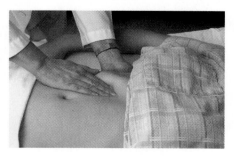

Abnormal findings: Palpation below the costal margin indicates enlargement.

Procedural Steps

Expected Findings

(continued)

d. Palpate the Spleen

- Stand at the client's right side.
- Reach across the client to place your left hand under the costovertebral angle, and pull upward to move the spleen anteriorly.
- Place your right hand under the left anterior costal margin, and have the client take a deep breath.
- During exhalation, press your hands together (inward) to try to palpate the spleen.

d. The spleen is not normally palpable.

Abnormal findings: Splenic enlargement or tenderness may result from infection, enlargement, trauma, or cancer.

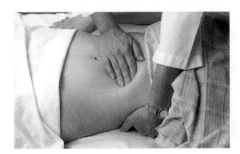

Patient Teaching

Instruct the patient in the importance of proper diet, the signs and symptoms of colorectal cancer, and the importance of screening colonoscopy.

Documentation

VOL 1 Go to Chapter 19, **Documenting Physical Assessment Findings,** in Volume 1.

PROCEDURE 19–15   Assessing the Musculoskeletal System

> For steps to follow in *all* procedures, refer to the inside back cover of this book.

critical aspects
- Techniques: inspection and palpation.
- Assess posture, body alignment, and symmetry.
- Assess the spinal curvature.
- Examine the gait by assessing the base of support (distance between the feet), stride length (distance between each step), and phases of the gait.
- Assess balance through tandem walking, heel-and-toe walking, deep knee bends, hopping, and the Romberg test.
- Assess coordination by testing finger-thumb opposition, rhythmic movements of lower and upper extremities, and rapid alternating movements.
- Test the accuracy of movements by having the client touch his finger to his nose with his eyes closed.
- Measure limb length and circumference. Compare limbs on both sides of the body.
- Inspect muscle symmetry.
- Perform ROM at all joints.
- Assess muscle strength by having the client perform ROM against resistance.

Equipment
- Tape measure
- Goniometer
- Pen and record form

Focused History Questions
- Do you have any difficulty with coordination (e.g., folding clothes, brushing your teeth)?
- Do you now have, or have you ever had, musculoskeletal problems, pain, or disease? If so, what medications or treatments are you using?
- Have you ever injured your bones or joints?
- Do your joints, muscles, or bones limit your activities?
- Do you lose your balance or fall?
- Do you have any occupational hazards that could affect your muscles and joints?

Procedural Steps	Expected Findings
1. Assess posture.	
a. Note the body and head position.	a. Posture is erect, with the head in the midline.
b. Check the alignment and symmetry of the shoulders, scapula, and iliac crests. Inspect from the front, back, and side.	b. The shoulders, scapula, and iliac crests are symmetrical.

Procedural Steps

Expected Findings

(continued)

Developmental Modification

Newborns—Palpate clavicles for fractures that may have occurred at birth. Check for congenital hip dysplasia (dislocation) by examining for asymmetry of the gluteal folds or shortening of the femur.

c. Assess the spinal curvature by:
 • Observing the client's profile while he is standing erect.
 • Having the client bend forward at the waist with arms hanging free at the sides.

c. Cervical and lumbar curves are concave; thoracic and sacral curves are convex.

Children—**Lordosis** (exaggerated lumbar curve) is normal before age 5.

Abnormal findings: kyphosis, scoliosis, lordosis. Also see Abnormal Atlas: Musculoskeletal System on page 335.

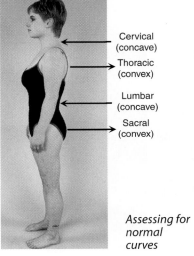

Cervical (concave)

Thoracic (convex)

Lumbar (concave)

Sacral (convex)

Assessing for normal curves

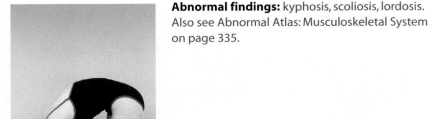

Assessing for kyphosis and scoliosis

d. Have the client stand erect with the feet together. Note the position of the knees.

d. Patella is in the midline on an imaginary line drawn from the anterior superior iliac crest to the feet.

Children—**Genu varum** (bowlegs) is normal for 1 year after a child begins to walk.

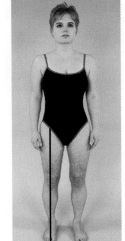

Step 1d

Procedural Steps

Expected Findings

Assessing the Musculoskeletal System *(continued)*

2. Assess gait by observing the client walking.

Children—observe them at play.

    a. Pay attention to the base of support (distance between the feet) and stride length (distance between each step).

    a. Average base of support for an adult is 5–10 cm (2–4 in.). Average stride length is 30–35 cm (12–14 in.); the longer the legs, the longer the stride length.

    Abnormal findings: A wide base of support and shortened stride length reflect a balance problem.

    b. Observe the phases of the gait.

    b. Movements are smooth and coordinated, weight is evenly distributed, arms swing in opposition, and toes point forward.

Stance Phase

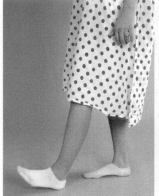 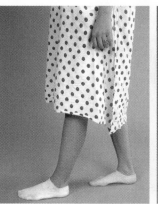 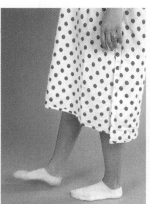 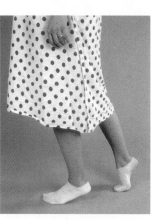

    Heel Strike   Foot Flat   Midstance   *Push-off*

Swing Phase

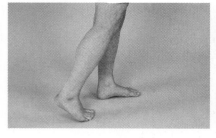 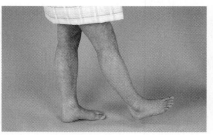 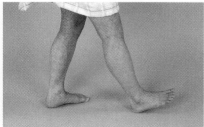

    Accelerate   Swing-thru   Decelerate

---

3. Assess balance.

If the client's gait is steady, you may proceed. If the client was unsteady when walking, do not complete this portion of the exam.

    a. Have the client tandem walk heel-to-toe.

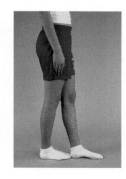

Step 3a

The client is able to perform each of these maneuvers smoothly. The Romberg test (see Procedure 19-7) is negative—the client is able to maintain balance with minimal sway.

Infants—should be able to sit alone by age 8 months.

Abnormal findings: Balance problems may indicate a cerebellar disorder, an inner ear problem, or muscle weakness.

Procedural Steps	Expected Findings

(continued)

b. Have the client walk alternately on heels and toes.

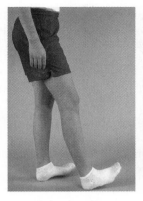 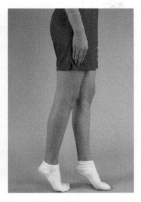

Step 3b, heel-and-toe walking   *Step 3b, walking on toes*

c. Ask the client to do a deep knee bend.

d. Ask the client to hop in place on each foot several times.

e. Perform the Romberg test (if you did not already do so when examining the ears): Have the client stand with feet together and eyes open. Then have him close his eyes.

Developmental Modification

Children—Often, the best way to assess a child's movement, coordination, range-of-motion, and so on, is to watch the child at normal play.

---

4. Assess coordination while the client is seated.

a. Test upper extremity coordination by having the client perform finger-thumb opposition. Test one side and then the other.

b. Test rapid alternating movements by having the client alternate between supinating and pronating her hands.

The client is able to perform these movements smoothly and in a coordinated fashion. The dominant side (usually the right) may be slightly more coordinated.

Older adults—Decreased coordination and reaction time may result from slower nerve conduction and loss of muscle tone.

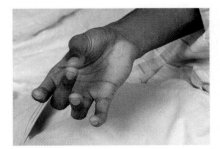

Step 4a

Procedural Steps

Expected Findings

Assessing the Musculoskeletal System *(continued)*

c. Test lower extremity coordination by having the client perform rhythmic toe-tapping, one side at a time.

d. Have the client run the heel of one foot down the shin of the other leg. Repeat on the opposite side.

Abnormal findings: Slowness or awkwardness with movement may indicate a cerebellar disorder or muscle weakness.

---

5. Test accuracy of movements. Have the client touch his finger to his nose with his eyes open. Repeat with his eyes closed.

The movement is accurate.

Abnormal findings: Inaccurate movements indicate cerebellar dysfunction.

---

6. Measure the limbs.

a. Measure arm length from the acromion process to the tip of the middle finger.

b. Measure leg length from the anterior superior iliac crest to the medial malleolus.

a. and b. The differences in length between the right and left arm and leg are 1 cm or less.

Abnormal findings: Leg length discrepancies may cause back and hip pain and gait problems.

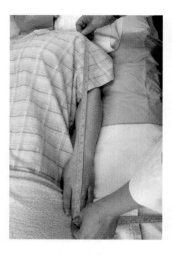 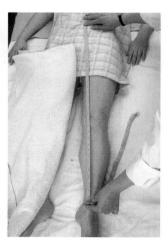

Steps 6a and 6b

c. Measure the circumference of the forearms, upper arms, thighs, and calves.

c. The differences in circumference between the right and left arm and leg are 1 cm or less.

Abnormal findings: Circumference differences > 1 cm may reflect atrophy or hypertrophy.

---

7. Inspect muscles and joints bilaterally for symmetry and shape.

Developmental Modification

Older adults—Observe for surgical scars indicating joint replacement or joint surgeries.

Size and shape are symmetrical. Muscles and joints are smooth, nontender, and similar in color and temperature to surrounding tissue.

Older adults—Muscle mass and tone decrease.

Procedural Steps

Expected Findings

(continued)

Abnormal findings:

- Hot, red, swollen, stiff, or painful joints may indicate injuries, arthritis, gout, bursitis, or other inflammatory diseases.
- Heberden's nodes are hard, painless nodules over the distal interphalangeal joints—usually seen with degenerative joint disease (DJD), but they may be seen with rheumatoid arthritis (RA).
- Severe misalignment and deformity are more often a result of DJD than of RA.
- Crepitus may be heard in DJD.

---

8. Test active ROM by asking the client to move the following joints through ROM:

- Temporomandibular joint

The client is able to flex, extend, move side to side, protrude, and retract the jaw.

- Neck

The neck flexes, extends, hyperextends, bends laterally, and rotates side to side.

- Thoracic and lumbar spine

The client is able to bend at the waist, stand upright, hyperextend (bend backward), bend laterally, and rotate side to side.

- Shoulder

The client is able to move the arm forward and backward, abduct, adduct, and rotate internally and externally.

- Upper arm and elbow

The client is able to bend, extend, supinate, and pronate the elbow.

- Wrist

The wrist flexes, extends, hyperextends, and moves side to side.

- Hands and fingers

The client is able to spread the fingers (*abduct*), bring them together (*adduct*), make a fist (*flex*), extend the hand (*extend*), bend fingers back (*hyperextend*), and bring thumb to index finger (*palmar adduction*).

- Hip

The client is able to extend the leg straight, flex the knee to the chest, abduct and adduct the leg, rotate the hip internally and externally, and hyperextend the leg.

- Knee

The client is able to flex and extend the knee.

- Ankles and feet

The client is able to dorsiflex, plantar flex, evert, invert, abduct, and adduct the feet and ankles.

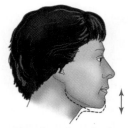
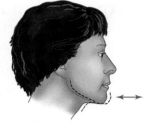

Depression: lowering a body part
Elevation: raising a body part

Retraction: moving backward
Protraction: moving forward

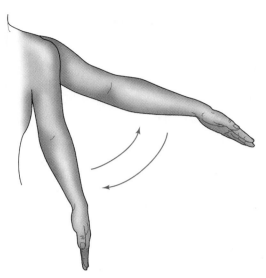

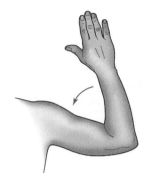

Flexion: bending, decreasing joint angle

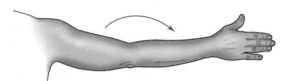

Extension: straightening, increasing joint angle

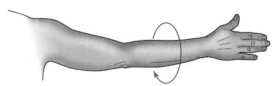

Circumduction: moving in a circular fashion

Abduction: moving away from midline
Adduction: moving toward midline

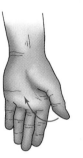
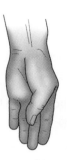

Resposition

Opposition

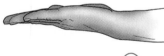

Supination: turning upward

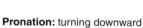

Pronation: turning downward

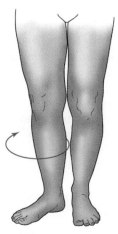
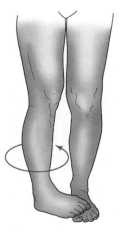

External rotation:
turning away from midline

Internal rotation:
turning toward midline

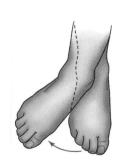
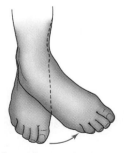

Eversion: turning outward

Inversion: turning inward

Procedural Steps

Expected Findings

(continued)

9. Test muscle strength by repeating ROM against resistance. Use the accompanying rating scale.

Expect active motion against full resistance. There should be no crepitus (clicking) or pain with joint movement.

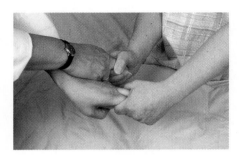

Step 9

Muscle Strength Rating Scale

Rating	Criteria	Classification
5	Active motion against full resistance	Normal
4	Active motion against some resistance	Slight weakness
3	Active motion against gravity	Weakness
2	Passive ROM	Poor ROM
1	Slight flicker of contraction	Severe weakness
0	No muscular contraction	Paralysis

Documentation

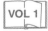 VOL 1 Go to Chapter 19, **Documenting Physical Assessment Findings,** in Volume 1.

PROCEDURE 19–16 Assessing the Sensory-Neurological System

> For steps to follow in *all* procedures, refer to the inside back cover of this book.
>
> *Note:* This procedure provides guidelines for performing a comprehensive neurological exam. A simple mental status screen that is useful for screening cognitive status (Steps 1–10) follows at the end of the procedure.

critical aspects

- Assess behavior.
- Determine level of arousal.
- Determine level of orientation.
- Assess memory.
- Assess mathematical and calculation skills.
- Assess general knowledge.
- Evaluate thought processes.
- Assess abstract thinking.
- Assess judgment.
- Assess communication ability.
- Test cranial nerves.
- Test superficial sensations.
- Test deep sensations.
- Test discriminatory sensations.
- Test deep tendon reflexes.
- Test superficial reflexes.

Equipment

- Pen and record form
- Wisp of cotton
- Sharp object, such as a toothpick or sterile needle
- Objects to touch, such as a coin, button, or key
- Something fragrant, such as coffee or rubbing alcohol
- Something to taste, such as sugar, salt, or lemon
- Tongue blade
- Two test tubes
- Reflex hammer
- Ophthalmoscope

Focused History Questions

- Do you have any neurological ("nerve") problems?
- Have you ever had head trauma, loss of consciousness, dizziness, headaches, or seizures?
- Do you have memory problems, forgetfulness, or inability to concentrate?
- Have you noticed any changes in your ability to see, smell, taste, hear, feel, or maintain balance?
- Do you have any weakness, numbness, or paralysis?
- Do you have any problems performing activities of daily living (ADLs)?
- Do you have any problems walking?
- Do you have mood problems or depression?
- Do you use alcohol or drugs?
- Have you ever been treated for neurological or psychiatric problems?
- Do you have a history of hypertension, diabetes, stroke, or circulation problems?

Developmental Modifications: Children

- For children under age 5 years, use the Denver Developmental Screening Test II to assess neurological and motor function.
- Check the child's ability to understand and follow instructions.

Developmental Modification: Older Adults

- You may need to perform the sensory-neurological exam over several sessions. The full exam is lengthy, and older adults fatigue easily. If the client seems to be getting tired, stop the test and finish at a later time.

Procedural Steps

Expected Findings

1. Assess behavior. Note the client's facial expression, posture, affect, and grooming.

The client is well groomed, with an erect posture, pleasant facial expression, and appropriate affect.

Abnormal findings: Inappropriate behavior may result from neurological or psychological problems, as well as from a variety of medications, alcohol, and street drugs.

2. Determine level of arousal:

a. Note the client's response to verbal stimuli.

b. If the client does not respond to verbal stimuli, try tactile stimulation: Gently shake the client's shoulder.

c. If the client does not respond to tactile stimuli, try painful stimuli: Squeeze the trapezius muscle, rub the sternum, apply pressure on the mandible at the angle of the jaw, or apply pressure over the moon of the nail.

The patient is awake and alert and readily responds to verbal stimuli.

Abnormal findings: Lethargy, stupor, or coma may result from trauma, neurological disorder, hypoxia, or chemical substances.

Eye response	Score	Motor response	Score	Verbal response	Score
Opens spontaneously	4	Reacts to verbal commands	6	Oriented and converses	5
Opens to verbal commands	3	Reacts to localized pain	5	Disoriented but converses	4
		Flexes and withdraws (general body response)	4	Uses inappropriate words	3
Opens to pain	2	Assumes flexor posture (decorticate posturing— arms flexed to chest, hands clenched and internally rotated); indicates problem is at or above the brainstem	3	Makes incomprehensible sounds	2
No response	1	Assumes extensor posture (decerebrate posturing— arms extended, hands clenched and hyperpronated); indicates problem at the brainstem level	2	No response	1
		No response	1		

3. Determine level of orientation.

a. Orientation to time: Ask the client to state the year, date, and time of day.

b. To assess orientation to place, ask the client to state where he is (i.e., city, state, where he lives).

c. To assess orientation to person, ask the names of family members. Ask, "Do you know who I am?" If the client cannot answer these questions, ask him to state his name.

Self-identity remains intact the longest.

The client is awake, alert (see Step 2), and oriented to time, place, and person (AAO×3).

a. Hospitalized patients commonly lose track of date and time of day, but they easily reorient. As a rule, they should at least know the year.

b. Interpret data carefully. In some situations (e.g., after an automobile accident away from home), the patient may know he is in the hospital but not know which hospital or which city.

c. Patient should know you are a healthcare worker, but not necessarily your name.

Older adults—Be aware that the stress of an unfamiliar situation can create confusion in an older adult.

Abnormal findings: Disorientation may result from physical or psychological problems. Bizarre responses are usually associated with psychiatric problems.

Procedural Steps

Expected Findings

Assessing the Sensory-Neurological System (continued)

4. Assess memory.

   a. Assess immediate memory by asking the client to repeat a series of three numbers that you speak slowly (e.g., 1, 5, 8). Gradually increase the length of the series until the client cannot repeat the series correctly. Record the length of the last correct series (e.g., "Able to repeat a series of 7 numbers correctly.")

   b. Repeat the test, beginning with a series of three numbers, but ask the client to repeat them back to you in reverse order.

   c. Assess recent memory by naming three items (e.g., "mirror, truck," and "the letter X") and asking the client to recall them later during the exam. Alternatively, you can ask questions such as, "How did you get to the hospital? What did you have for breakfast?" However, you will need to verify the patient's answers.

   d. Assess remote memory by asking the client his birth date or the date of a major historical event.

Developmental Modification

Children—Assess memory by using names of toys (e.g., truck, ball, puzzle), names of people in his family, or names of familiar cartoon characters.

Immediate, recent, and remote memory is intact. Average series recall is 5 to 8 numbers in sequence and 4 to 6 numbers in reverse order.

Children—Number of objects recalled is usually fewer than the child's age in years.

Older adults—Loss of immediate and recent memory is common; long-term memory is usually unimpaired.

Abnormal findings: Memory problems may be benign or may signal underlying neurological problems. Temporary memory loss may occur after trauma.

---

5. Assess mathematical and calculation skills.

   a. Have the client solve a simple mathematical problem, such as 3+3.

   b. If he is able to solve that problem, present a more complex example, such as, "If you have $3 and you buy an item for $2, how much money will you have left?"

   c. To assess both calculation skills and attention span, ask the client to count backwards from 100.

   d. A more difficult test is to have the client perform serial threes or serial sevens. Ask him to begin at 100 and keep subtracting 3 (or 7).

Consider the person's language, education, and culture in deciding whether this test is appropriate for him.

Mathematical and calculation ability is appropriate for the patient's age, education level, and language ability. The average adult can solve simple mathematical problems and can complete serial sevens in about 90 seconds with 3 errors or fewer.

Abnormal findings: Inability to calculate at a level appropriate for age and educational level may indicate neurological impairment or developmental delay.

---

6. Assess general knowledge by asking the client how many days in the week or months in the year.

Vocabulary and general knowledge are intact.

---

7. Evaluate thought processes. Assess throughout the exam. Notice attention span, logic of speech, ability to stay focused, and appropriateness of responses.

Thought processes are clear, client responds appropriately, and speech is coherent and logical.

Procedural Steps	Expected Findings
(continued)	**Abnormal findings:** Alteration in thought processes may be due to physical disorders, such as dementia; psychiatric disorders, such as psychosis; or alcohol and drugs.
8. Assess abstract thinking.	Abstract thinking is intact.
Ask the client to interpret a proverb, such as "A penny saved is a penny earned."	**Abnormal findings:** Inability to think abstractly is associated with dementia, delirium, mental retardation, and psychoses.
Developmental Modification	
Children—The ability to think abstractly does not develop until the late school-age years or adolescence. To assess a child under the age of 12, ask her to describe things that are like and unlike a named object (e.g., "Tell me something that is like a cup").	
9. Assess judgment.	Judgment is intact.
Ask the client to respond to a hypothetical situation, such as, "If you were walking down the street and saw smoke and flame coming from a house, what would you do?"	**Abnormal findings:** Impaired judgment may be associated with dementia, psychosis, or substance abuse.
10. Assess communication ability.	
a. Listen to the client's speech. Note the rate, flow, choice of vocabulary, and enunciation.	a. Speech flows easily, and patient enunciates clearly. Vocabulary is consistent with the client's age, education, and language fluency.
	Abnormal findings: Problems with flow (e.g., halting speech, stuttering, very rapid speech, slurred words) may be due to language problems, nervousness, anxiety, or neurological problems.
b. Test spontaneous speech: Show the client a picture, and have him describe it.	b. Spontaneous speech is intact.
	Abnormal findings: Impaired spontaneous speech is associated with cognitive impairment.
c. Test motor speech by having the client say, "Do, re, mi, fa, sol, la, ti, do."	c. Motor speech is intact.
	Abnormal findings: Impaired motor speech is associated with problems with CN XII or with coordination of speech muscles.
d. Test automatic speech by having the client recite the days of the week.	d. Automatic speech is intact.
	Abnormal findings: Cognitive impairment or memory problems cause difficulty with automatic speech.
e. Test sound recognition by having the client identify a familiar sound, such as clapping hands.	e. Sound recognition is intact.
	Abnormal findings: Temporal lobe problems may be the cause of impaired sound recognition.

Procedural Steps

Expected Findings

Assessing the Sensory-Neurological System *(continued)*

f. Test auditory-verbal comprehension by asking the client to follow simple directions (e.g., "Point to your nose; rub your left elbow").

g. Test visual recognition by pointing to objects and asking the client to identify them.

h. Test visual-verbal comprehension by having the client read a sentence and explain its meaning.

i. Test writing by having the client write her name and address.

j. Test ability to copy figures by having the client copy a circle, x, square, triangle, and star.

f. Auditory-verbal comprehension is intact.

Abnormal findings: Temporal lobe problems affect reception. Frontal lobe problems affect expression.

g. Visual recognition is intact.

Abnormal findings: Impaired visual recognition indicates parieto-occipital lobe problems.

h. Visual-verbal comprehension is intact.

Abnormal findings: Impaired visual-verbal comprehension indicates cognitive impairment.

i. Writing ability is intact.

j. The client is able to copy figures.

---

11. Test cranial nerve I—olfactory nerve.

Note: You can assess CN I with your examination of the nose and sinuses (see Procedure 19–8).

a. Before testing, check the patency of the nostrils by gently occluding each nostril and having the patient sniff.

b. Have the patient occlude one nostril and hold an aromatic substance (e.g., lemon, coffee, vanilla, alcohol) under the nostril.

c. Repeat with a different substance under the other nostril.

The client can identify the substances.

Older adults—May have a decreased sense of smell.

Abnormal findings: Anosmia is the loss of the sense of smell. It may be genetic, related to chronic nose or sinus problems, heavy smoking, snorting cocaine, or zinc deficiency.

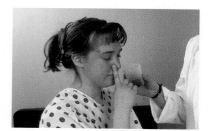

Developmental Modification

Children—select a substance that you are certain the child is familiar with (e.g., peanut butter).

---

12. Test cranial nerve II—optic nerve.

Note: You can assess CN II with your examination of the eyes.

a. Test visual acuity by asking the patient to identify the smallest print readable on the Snellen chart (use picture chart for small children, Snellen E for school-age children).

a. Visual acuity is 20/20 in the right eye, left eye, and both eyes.

Procedural Steps	Expected Findings
(continued)	**Abnormal findings:** Many visual deficits are correctable by eyeglasses or contact lenses. They are not necessarily caused by optic nerve damage.
b. Identify visual field by having the client describe the boundaries of the visual field while her eye is in a fixed position.	b. Peripheral vision range is approximately 50° in the superior field, 70° in the inferior field, 60° in the nasal field, and 90–110° in the temporal field.
c. Perform a fundoscopic exam.	c. Disc margins are sharply demarcated. The cup is half the size of the disc or less.
	Abnormal findings: CN II deficits may be due to tumor or CVA.

---

13. Test cranial nerves III, IV, and VI—oculomotor, trochlear, and abducens nerves.

a. Test EOMs by having the client move the eyes through the six cardinal fields of gaze while holding her head steady.

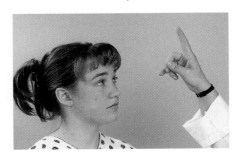

Step 13a

b. Test pupillary reaction to light and accommodation.

See Procedure 19–6 for further details on each of these tests.

Client can move her eyes through the six cardinal fields of gaze. Pupils are equal in size and react to light and accommodation.

Abnormal findings: Changes in intracranial pressure (ICP) may affect EOMs and pupillary reaction.

---

14. Test cranial nerve V—trigeminal nerve.

a. Test motor function by having the client move his jaw from side to side, clenching his jaw, and biting down on a tongue blade.

Note: You can assess this function in your examination of the mouth and oropharynx (see Procedure 19–9).

b. Test sensory function by having the client close her eyes and identify when you are touching her face at the forehead, cheeks, and chin bilaterally—first with your finger and then repeat with a toothpick.

c. Test the corneal reflex by touching the cornea with a wisp of cotton or puffing air from a syringe over the cornea.

Note: You can assess this function in your examination of the eyes (see Procedure 19–6).

The client is able to perform all motor functions and can perceive light touch and superficial pain bilaterally; corneal reflex is intact.

Abnormal findings: Inability to perceive light touch and superficial pain may indicate peripheral nerve damage. An absent corneal reflex is an ominous neurological sign.

Procedural Steps

Expected Findings

Assessing the Sensory-Neurological System *(continued)*

15. Test cranial nerve VII—facial nerve.

    a. Test motor function by having the client make faces, such as smile, frown, or whistle.

Note: You can assess this function in your examination of the head and face (see Procedure 19–5).

    b. Test taste on the anterior portion of the tongue by placing sweet (sugar), salty (salt), or sour (lemon) substance on the tip of the tongue.

Note: You can assess this function in your examination of the mouth and oropharynx (see Procedure 19–9).

The client is able to perform all movements and can distinguish sweet, salty, and sour tastes.

Older adults—have decreased taste sensation, especially sweet and salty, due to taste bud atrophy and diminished sense of smell.

Abnormal findings: Asymmetrical movement may be seen with nerve damage from a CVA or Bell's palsy. Impaired taste may be associated with nerve damage, chemotherapy, or radiation to the face or neck.

---

16. Test Cranial Nerve VIII—acoustic nerve.

Note: You can assess this function in your examination of the ears (see Procedure 19–7).

    a. Perform watch-tick test for hearing by holding a watch close to the patient's ear.

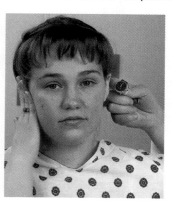

    b. Perform Weber and Rinne tests to assess air and bone conduction.

    c. Test balance with the Romberg test, if it has not already been performed.

See Procedure 19–7 for further details on each of these tests.

Developmental Modification

Children: Romberg test is appropriate only after age 3.

Hearing is intact.

Romberg test is negative.

Abnormal findings: Hearing loss, loss of balance, or vertigo may result from acoustic nerve damage.

---

17. Test cranial nerves IX and X—glossopharyngeal and vagus nerves.

    a. Observe ability to talk, swallow, and cough.

    b. Test motor function by asking the client to say "ah" while you depress a tongue blade and observe the soft palate and uvula.

Swallow and cough reflex are intact. Speech is clear. The uvula and soft palate rise symmetrically, and the gag reflex is intact. Taste on the posterior tongue is intact.

Older adults—have decreased taste sensation, especially sweet and salty, due to atrophy of the taste buds and a decreased sense of smell.

Abnormal findings: Damage to CN IX and X impairs swallowing. Damage to CN X changes voice quality.

Procedural Steps

Expected Findings

(continued)

   c. Test sensory function by taking a tongue blade and gently touching the back of the pharynx to induce a gag reflex.

   d. Test taste (sweet, salty, and sour) on the posterior portion of the tongue.

---

18. Test Cranial Nerve XI—accessory nerve.

Note: You can assess this motor nerve function with your examination of the musculoskeletal system (see Procedure 19–5).

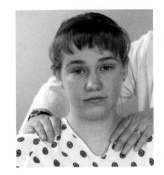

   a. Place your hands on the client's shoulder, and have the client shrug his shoulders against resistance.

Step 18a

   b. Have the client turn his head from side to side against resistance.

Movement is symmetrical and pain-free. Full ROM of the neck with +5 strength.

Abnormal findings: Asymmetrical movement, pain, or absent movement indicates CN XI disorders.

---

19. Test cranial nerve XII—hypoglossal nerve.

   a. Have the client say "d, l, n, t."

   b. Have the client protrude the tongue and move it from side to side.

The client can articulate the sounds and move the tongue easily.

Abnormal findings: tongue paralysis.

---

20. Test superficial sensations.

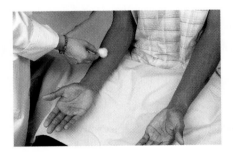

  • Begin with the most peripheral part when testing the limbs (e.g., test the foot before the leg).

If the client can feel sensation in the most peripheral part, you can assume the sensory nerve is intact to that point.

  • If the client does not perceive the touch in an area, determine the boundaries of the dysfunction by testing at about every inch (2.5 cm). Sketch the area of sensory loss.

  • Wait about 2 seconds before moving to each site.

Procedural Steps

Expected Findings

Assessing the Sensory-Neurological System *(continued)*

Wait so that you can be sure that the patient is perceiving each stimulus separately.

a. With the patient's eyes closed, test light touch by brushing a cotton wisp on various areas of the body, comparing sides. Ask the client to say, "Now," when he feels your touch and to point to the spot you are touching.

b. With the patient's eyes closed, test pain using a toothpick (or sterile needle) with dull and sharp ends. Touch various areas of the body (except the face), and have the patient identify whether the sensation is dull or sharp. Alternate the dull and sharp ends as you move from spot to spot. Compare sides of the body.

c. Test temperature sensation only if the patient's perception of pain is abnormal. Use test tubes filled with hot and cold water. Touch the tube to various areas of the body, comparing sides; have the client say "Hot," "Cold," or "Don't know."

a. Able to identify areas of light touch.

Abnormal findings: diminished sensation or areas of absent perception.

b. The client is able to identify the areas stimulated and the type of sensation.

Abnormal findings:

- **Hyperalgia**—increased pain sensation
- **Analgesia**—no pain sensation
- **Paresthesia**—numbness and tingling

Older adults—may have a decreased perception of temperature and deep pain.

---

21. Test deep sensations.

a. Assess vibratory sensation by placing a vibrating tuning fork on a metatarsal joint and distal interphalangeal joint. Have the patient identify when she feels the vibration and when it stops.

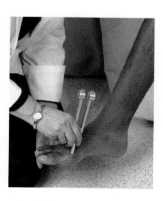

Step 21a

a. Vibratory sense is intact bilaterally in the upper and lower extremities.

Abnormal findings: Diminished or absent vibration sense is seen with peripheral nerve damage from vascular disease, diabetes, alcoholism, or damage to the posterior column of the spinal cord.

b. Test kinesthetic sensation (position sense) by holding the client's finger or toe on the sides and moving it up or down. Keeping her eyes closed, have the client identify the direction of the movement.

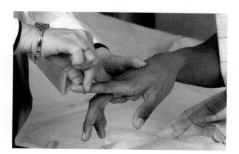

Step 21b

b. Position sense is intact bilaterally in the upper and lower extremities.

Older adults—may lose position sense in the great toes.

Abnormal findings: Diminished or absent position sense indicates nerve or spinal cord damage.

Procedural Steps	Expected Findings

(continued)

22. Test discriminatory sensations.

    a. Assess stereognosis by placing a familiar object (e.g., a coin or a button) in the palm of the client's hand and having her identify it.

    a. Stereognosis is intact bilaterally.

    b. Assess graphesthesia by drawing a number or letter in the palm of your patient's hand and having the patient identify what was drawn.

    b. Graphesthesia is intact bilaterally.

    c. Test two-point discrimination with toothpicks. Have the patient close her eyes. Touch her on the finger with two toothpicks simultaneously. Gradually move the points together, and have the patient say, "One," or "Two," each time you move the toothpicks. Document distance and location at which she can no longer feel two separate points.

    c. Discriminates between two points on fingertips no more than 0.5 cm apart.

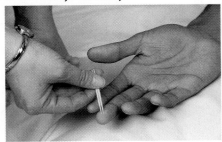

Step 22c

    d. Test point localization by having the patient close her eyes while you touch her. Have her point to the area you touched. Repeat on both sides and the upper and lower extremities.

    d. Point localization is intact bilaterally in the upper and lower extremities.

    e. Test sensory extinction by simultaneously touching the patient on both sides (e.g., on both hands, both knees, both arms). Have the patient identify where she was touched.

    e. Extinction is intact: Client should feel the sensation on both sides of his body.

Abnormal findings: Abnormalities in any of the discriminatory sensation tests may indicate a lesion or disorder of the sensory cortex or disorder of the posterior column of the spinal cord.

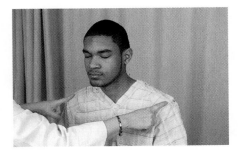

Step 22e

Developmental Modification

Older adults—may need more time to respond to a stimulus, as reaction time may be slower.

---

23. Test deep tendon reflexes. (See the accompanying scale to grade responses.)

    a. Biceps reflex (spinal cord level C5 and C6). Rest the patient's elbow in your nondominant hand, with

Older adults—Reflex responses may not be as strong as in young adults. Reaction time is slower as well.

    a. +2 response: You can feel the biceps contract with your thumb; slight flexion of the elbow.

Procedural Steps

Expected Findings

Assessing the Sensory-Neurological System *(continued)*

your thumb over the biceps tendon. Strike the percussion hammer to your thumb.

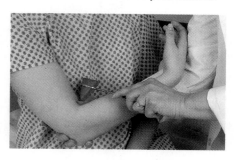

Step 23a

b. Triceps reflex (spinal cord level C7 and C8). Abduct the patient's arm at the shoulder, and flex it at the elbow. Support the upper arm with your nondominant hand, letting the forearm hang loosely. Strike the triceps tendon about 2.5–5 cm (1–2 in.) above the olecranon process.

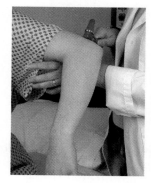

Step 23b

c. Brachioradialis reflex (spinal cord level C3 and C6). Rest the patient's arm on her leg. Strike with the percussion hammer 2.5–5 cm (1–2 in.) above the bony prominence of the wrist on the thumb side.

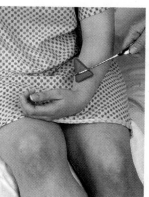
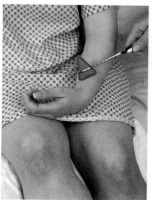

Step 23c

d. Patellar reflex (spinal cord level L2, L3, and L4). Have the patient sit with her legs dangling. Strike the tendon directly below the patella.

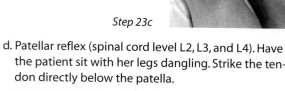
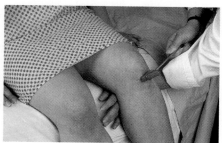

Step 23d

Deep Tendon Reflex Grading Scale

0	No response detected
+1	Diminished response
+2	Response normal
+3	Response somewhat stronger than normal
+4	Response hyperactive with **clonus** (involuntary contractions that continue after the first contraction is elicited by the hammer)

b. +2 response: Contraction of triceps with slight extension at elbow.

c. +2 response: Flexion at elbow and supination of forearm.

d. +2 response: Contraction of quadriceps with extension of leg.

Procedural Steps

Expected Findings

(continued)

    e. Achilles reflex (spinal cord level S1, S2). Have the patient lie supine or sit with her legs dangling. Hold the patient's foot slightly dorsiflexed, and strike the Achilles tendon about 5 cm (2 in.) above the heel with the percussion hammer.

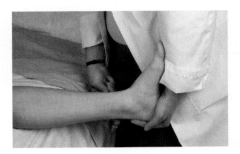

Step 23e

Developmental Modification

Newborns—test the following reflexes:

- Rooting reflex—Stroke the cheek; the head should turn to the side you touched.
- Palmar grasp—Place one finger in the baby's hand; his fingers should curl around your finger.
- Tonic neck reflex—Position the baby supine; turn his head to one side. The arm and leg on that side should extend, and those on the other side will flex.

Note: These reflexes should not be present after about 6 months of age.

e. +2 response: Plantar flexion of foot.

Older adults—may lose this reflex.

Abnormal findings:

- Absent or diminished responses are seen with degenerative disease, nerve damage, or lower motor neuron disease.
- Hyperactive reflexes are seen with spinal cord injuries and upper motor neuron disease.

---

24. Test superficial reflexes.

Plantar reflex (Babinski response): With your thumbnail or pointed object, stroke the sole of the client's foot in an arc from the lateral heel to medially across the ball of the foot. Record a normal response if all the toes curl downward or if there is no response. Record a positive response if there is dorsiflexion of the great toe and fanning of the other toes.

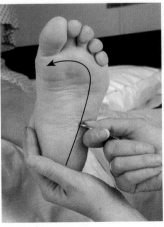

Developmental Modification

Older adults—this reflex may be difficult to elicit.

Step 24a

Babinski response is negative.

Infants and children—Positive Babinski is normal until age 2 or until the child begins walking.

Abnormal findings: A positive Babinski response is seen with drug or alcohol intoxification or upper motor neuron disease.

Procedural Steps

Expected Findings

Assessing the Sensory-Neurological System *(continued)*

25. Mental status screening.

These questions may be used for a rapid evaluation of
cognitive status.

Mental Status Screening

Question	Function Assessed
"What is today's date?"	Orientation to time
"What time is it?"	Orientation to time
"Where are you?"	Orientation to Place
"What is the reason for your visit?" If the patient is hospitalized, modify the question as: "Why are you in the hospital?"	Communication, vocabulary, thought processes, recent memory
Ask the client to "Count backwards from 100."	Word comprehension, abstract reasoning
Ask the patient to name several objects that you point to. Be sure to use common objects such as a pen, shoe, or window.	Vocabulary, general knowledge, and word comprehension
Write a brief command, such as "Clap your hands" on a slip of paper. Hand the paper to the patient and ask him to follow the instructions.	Reading comprehension
Ask the patient to write down the names of his family members along with their relationship to him.	Writing, thought processes, memory, sound recognition
Ask the patient to name three things that begin with the letter "D."	Auditory comprehension, thought processes
Ask the patient to draw a circle, square, and triangle next to each other on a sheet of paper.	Word comprehension, mathematical and calculation skills communication (naming)

Difficulty with any of these questions requires further evaluation.

Home Care

Instruct caregivers in home safety if the client has cerebral function deficits or sensory or motor
deficits.

Documentation

 Go to Chapter 19, **Documenting Physical Assessment Findings,** in Volume 1.

PROCEDURE 19–17   Assessing the Male Genitourinary System

For steps to follow in *all* procedures, refer to the inside back cover of this book.

critical aspects
- Techniques: inspection and palpation.
- Inspect the external genitalia, including the pattern of hair distribution.
- Palpate for lumps, masses, hernias, or enlarged lymph nodes.

Equipment
- Nonlatex procedure gloves
- Penlight
- Pen and record form

Focused History Questions
- Have you noticed any redness, swelling, discharge, or odor in your genital area?
- Have you noticed asymmetry, lumps, or masses in your genitals? If so, describe them, and show me where they are.
- Have you ever been told you have a hernia?
- Have you ever had trauma to your genitals?
- Are you having any problems urinating?
- Are you sexually active? If not, have you ever been?
- Do you have sex with men, women, or both?
- What types of sexual activity do you engage in? Oral, anal, genital?
- Do you have more than one partner? How many partners have you had in the last 6 months?
- Do you use birth control? If so, what type and how often?
- Have you ever been treated for a sexually transmitted infection (STI)? If so, what type?
- Are you concerned about STIs or HIV?
- Do you take any precautions to avoid infections?
- Do you have any concerns about your sexual function?
- Do you have any difficulty achieving or maintaining an erection?
- Have you been taught to examine your testicles?
- How often do you do testicular self-examination?
- Have you had any surgery of your reproductive tract?

Developmental Modification: Children
- Obtain the parent's permission to perform this assessment.
- Explain to the child what you are going to do, and expect some resistance or embarrassment.

Children are taught to not let strangers touch their genitals, and many children are extremely modest.

Procedural Steps

1. Instruct the client to empty his bladder and undress to expose the groin area.

2. Have the patient stand while you sit at eye level to the genitalia; alternatively, the patient can lie supine on the exam table with his legs slightly apart.

3. Inspect the external genitalia.

    a. Note the hair distribution pattern and condition of pubic hair. See the table discussing Tanner staging, at the end of this procedure.

Expected Findings

a. Hair distribution is triangular and appropriate for age. No pediculosis is present.

Abnormal findings: Sparse or absent hair may result from genetic factors, aging, or local or systemic disease.

Procedural Steps

Expected Findings

Assessing the Male Genitourinary System (continued)

b. Inspect the condition of the skin of the penis. Observe for the presence or absence of the foreskin. Note the position of the urethral meatus and any lesions or discharge.

b. Skin is intact with no lesions or discharge. Color is consistent with ethnicity. The urethral meatus is midline. The foreskin may be absent (circumcised); if present, it covers the glans and easily retracts.

Infants—foreskin is difficult to retract until about age 3 months.

Older adults—penis and testes decrease in size.

Abnormal findings: ulcerations or lesions (may be seen with a number of sexually transmitted infections, such as genital warts and genital herpes); **phimosis** (foreskin cannot be retracted and becomes swollen).

c. Observe the condition, size, position, and symmetry of the scrotal skin.

c. The skin should be free of lesions, nodules, swelling, rash, and erythema. The skin is rugated and deeper in color than the rest of the body. Size and shape vary greatly. The left scrotal sac is usually lower than the right.

Abnormal findings: A rash may be caused by **tinea cruris,** a fungal infection often called "jock itch." Swelling may indicate hernia, tumor, or infection.

d. Note the condition of the inguinal areas. Look for swelling or bulges. The best way to do this is to have the client bear down while you palpate the inguinal canal.

d. The inguinal area should be free of swelling or bulges.

Abnormal findings: A bulge may indicate a hernia or enlarged lymph node.

---

4. Palpate the penis.

a. With a gloved hand, use your thumb and fingers to palpate the shaft of the penis. Note consistency, tenderness, masses, or nodules.

b. Retract the foreskin if present.

The penis is nontender with no masses or nodules. Pulsations are present on the dorsal side. The foreskin, if present, easily retracts.

Abnormal findings: Inability to palpate a pulse may indicate vascular insufficiency; difficulty retracting the foreskin or problems with its return to position need further evaluation.

---

5. Palpate the scrotum, testes, and epididymis.

a. With a gloved hand, use your thumb and fingers to palpate the scrotum, testes, and epididymis. Note size, shape, consistency, mobility, masses, nodules, or tenderness.

The scrotal skin is rough but without lesions. Each testicular sac contains a testicle and epididymis. The testes are rubbery, round, movable, and smooth. They are sensitive to pressure but nontender. The epididymis is comma shaped. The spermatic cord is smooth and round. There is no swelling or nodules. The left scrotal sac is usually lower than the right.

Procedural Steps

Expected Findings

(continued)

    b. Transilluminate any lumps, nodules, or edematous areas by shining a penlight over the area in a darkened room.

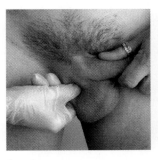 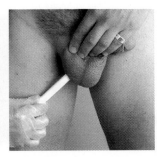

Step 5a   *Step 5b*

Abnormal findings:

- A unilateral mass is abnormal.
- Painless intratesticular masses may represent testicular cancer.
- A testicle that is swollen or tender may indicate infection or torsion.

---

6. Palpate the inguinal and femoral area for hernias.

    a. Assess for inguinal hernias with a gloved hand. Have the patient hold his penis to one side. Place your index finger in the client's scrotal sac above the testicle, and invaginate the skin. Follow the spermatic cord until you reach a slitlike opening **(Hesselbach's triangle).** Ask the client to cough or bear down as you feel for bulges.

    b. Palpate for femoral hernias by palpating below the femoral artery while having the client cough or bear down.

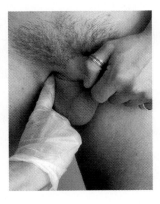

Step 6

No bulges or palpable masses are present in the inguinal or femoral area.

Abnormal findings: A bulge or mass often represents a hernia.

---

7. Palpate the lymph nodes in the groin area and the vertical chain over the inner aspect of the thigh.

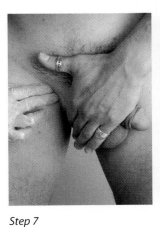 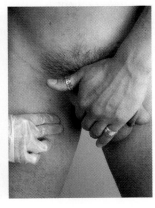

Step 7   *Step 7*

Nodes should be less than 1 cm in size and freely mobile.

Abnormal findings: Enlarged or tender lymph nodes may indicate local or systemic disease. Also see Abnormal Atlas: Male Genitourinary System on page 336.

Procedural Steps	Expected Findings

Assessing the Male Genitourinary System *(continued)*

Documentation

VOL 1 | Go to Chapter 19, **Documenting Physical Assessment Findings,** in Volume 1.

Tanner Staging

Stage	Pubic Hair	Penis	Testes and Scrotum
Stage 1: Preadolescent	No pubic hair except for fine body hair similar to that on abdomen.	Same size and proportions as in childhood.	Same size and proportions as in childhood.
Stage 2	Sparse growth of long, slightly pigmented, downy hair, straight or only slightly curled, chiefly at base of penis.	Slight or no enlargement.	Testes larger, scrotum larger, somewhat reddened and altered in texture.
Stage 3	Darker, coarser, curlier hair spreading sparsely over pubic symphysis.	Larger, especially in length	Further enlarged
Stage 4	Coarse and curly hair, as in adult; area covered greater than in stage 3 but not as great as in adult.	Further enlarged in length and breadth, with development of glans.	Further enlarged; scrotal skin darkened.
Stage 5: Adult	Hair same as adult in quantity and quality, spreading to medial surfaces of thighs but not up over abdomen.	Adult in size and shape.	Adult in size and shape.

PROCEDURE 19–18	Assessing the Female Genitourinary System

> For steps to follow in *all* procedures, refer to the inside back cover of this book.

critical aspects

- Techniques: inspection and palpation.
- Inspect the external genitalia.
- Palpate lymph nodes and possible hernia sites.

Equipment

- Patient drape
- Additional light source
- Nonlatex procedure gloves (if exposure to body fluids is a possibility)
- Pen and record form

Focused History Questions

- Have you noticed any redness, swelling, discharge, or odor in your genital area?
- Have you ever been told you have a hernia?
- Have you ever had trauma to your genitals?
- Are you sexually active? If not, have you ever been?
- Do you have sex with men, women, or both?
- What types of sexual activity do you engage in? Oral, anal, or genital?
- How many partners do you currently have?
- How many partners have you had in the last 6 months?
- Do you use birth control? If so, what kind and how often?
- Have you ever been treated for a sexually transmitted infection (STI)? If so, what type?
- Are you concerned about STIs or HIV?
- Do you take any precautions to avoid infection?
- Do you have any concerns about your sexual function?
- Have you had any surgery of your reproductive tract?
- When was your last menstrual period?

- How often are your periods?
- Do you have any problems with your periods, such as cramping, breast pain, or heavy flow?
- When was your last Pap smear?
- Have you ever had an abnormal Pap smear? If so, how was it treated?
- How many times have you been pregnant?
- How many children do you have?
- Have you ever had a miscarriage? An abortion?

Developmental Modifications: Children

- Obtain parental permission for this examination.
- Explain to the child what you are going to do, and expect some resistance or embarrassment.

Children are taught to not let strangers touch their genitals, and many children are extremely modest.

- Do not perform internal assessment of an adolescent unless the girl is sexually active.

Developmental Modifications: Older Adults

Older women may have arthritis, which, along with muscle weakness, may make it difficult for them to assume the lithotomy position. You may need to use Sims' position and/or provide support for them to maintain a position.

Procedural Steps

1. Inspect the external genitalia.

   a. Note the hair distribution pattern and the condition of pubic hair. See the box entitled Maturation Status in Females at the end of this procedure.

Expected Findings

   a. Hair distribution in the pubic region is inverse triangular. Some hair may extend onto her abdomen and upper thighs. Hair distribution is appropriate for age. No **pediculosis pubis** (pubic lice).

Procedural Steps

Expected Findings

Assessing the Female Genitourinary System *(continued)*

Abnormal findings: sparse or absent hair (may result from genetic factors, aging, or local or systemic disease); lice, **nits** (white lice eggs), or flecks of dried blood on the skin.

   b. Inspect the condition of the skin of the mons pubis and labia. Observe for color, condition, lesions, and discharge.

   b. Skin is intact with no lesions or discharge. Labia majora and minora are symmetrical, with smooth to moderate wrinkling. Skin color is consistent with ethnicity. No ecchymosis, excoriation, nodules, edema, rash, or lesions are present.

Older adults—Labia and vulva are atrophied.

Abnormal findings: Ulcerations or lesions may be seen with a number of sexually transmitted infections.

2. Inspect the clitoris, urethral meatus, and vaginal introitus.

   a. Wearing gloves, use your thumb and index finger to separate the labia and expose the clitoris. Observe the clitoris for size and position.

   a. The clitoris is about 2 cm long and 0.5 cm in diameter. No redness or lesions are present.

Abnormal findings: Enlargement of the clitoris may result from androgen excess. Absence of the clitoris, along with parts of the labia, is seen with female circumcision.

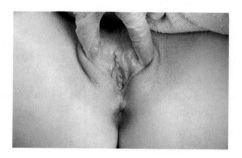

Step 2a

   b. With the labia separated, observe the urethral meatus and vaginal introitus. Observe for color, size, and presence of discharge or lesions.

   b. The urethral meatus is slitlike, midline, and free of discharge, lesions, swelling, or erythema. The mucosa of the introitus is pink and moist. Some clear to white discharge may be present and is odor-free.

   c. Have the client bear down while you observe the introitus.

   c. The introitus is patent, and there is no bulging or discomfort with bearing down.

Abnormal findings: Discharge, redness, or swelling may result from infection. Pale and dry mucosa may result from aging or use of topical steroids. Bulging may indicate prolapse of the uterus, bladder, or rectum.

3. Palpate Bartholin's glands, the urethral glands, and Skene's ducts.

   a. Lubricate the index and middle fingers of your dominant hand with water-soluble lubricant.

No swelling, masses, or tenderness of the glands is present. There is no urethral discharge. The labia are uniform in texture, and there is no discharge or pain with palpation. The perineum is smooth and firm in **nulliparous** women (women who have had no children), thinner in **parous** women (women who have had children).

Procedural Steps

(continued)

b. To palpate Bartholin's glands, insert your lubricated fingers into the vaginal introitus, and palpate the lower portion of the labia bilaterally between your thumb and fingers.

c. To palpate Skene's ducts, rotate your internal fingers upward, and paplate the labium bilaterally.

d. To milk the urethra, apply pressure with your index finger on the anterior vaginal wall, and observe for urethral discharge. Culture any discharge you see.

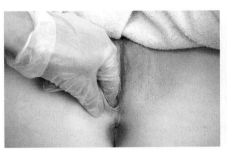

Step 3b

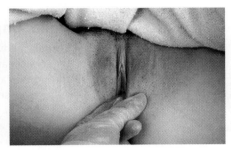

Step 3c

Expected Findings

Abnormal findings: Pain or discharge from the glands may indicate infection. Fissures or tears in the perineum are painful and require treatment.

---

4. Assess vaginal muscle tone and pelvic musculature.

a. Insert two gloved fingers into the vagina.

b. Ask the woman to constrict her vaginal muscles and then to bear down as though she were having a bowel movement.

Muscle tone should be strong in women who have never given birth. With increasing **parity** (number of births), pelvic muscle tone diminishes. Diminished tone may also result from injury, age, or medication. No bulges should be noted.

---

5. Palpate the inguinal and femoral area for hernias.

No bulges or palpable masses are present in the inguinal or femoral area.

---

6. Palpate the lymph nodes in the groin area and the vertical chain over the inner aspect of the thigh.

Nodes should be less than 1 cm in size and freely mobile.

Abnormal findings: Enlarged or tender lymph nodes may indicate local or systemic disease. Also see Abnormal Atlas: Female Genitourinary System on page 336.

Assisting with a Speculum Exam

Equipment

- Patient drape
- Nonsterile gloves
- Vaginal speculum (see accompanying figure)
  May be plastic or metal
  The size of the speculum depends on the patient's history. Use a small speculum for a woman who has never been sexually active or an older woman who is not sexually active.
  If a culture or a Pap smear is to be obtained, lubricate the speculum with warm water. Otherwise, use a water-soluble lubricant.

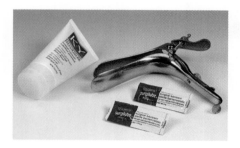

A vaginal speculum

- Lubricant
- Pap smear slide, spatula, brush, or specimen broom and container with solution
- Fixative, if the smear technique is used
- Genital culture supplies
- Additional light source

Preparing the Patient

- Explain to the patient that an internal examination of her vagina and pelvic organs will be performed. The examination usually takes only a few minutes and is not painful. Reassure her that you will provide privacy and keep her warm for the procedure.
- Have the woman urinate prior to the examination if needed.
- Assist the woman to the lithotomy position, and cover her with a drape.

Inserting the Speculum

The speculum is inserted into the vagina to visualize the cervix (see accompanying figure). Once the speculum is inserted, you may need to adjust the light source for the examiner.

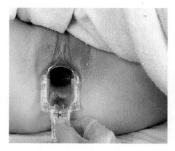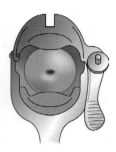

A vaginal speculum examination: A, Placement of the speculum in the vagina; B, View through the speculum

Collecting Specimens

Sexually active women should be screened annually for cervical and uterine cancer. This is detected through a Papanicolaou test (Pap smear). Additional cultures or screens may be required if there is unusual discharge or risk of sexually transmitted infection. Genital cultures are endocervical smears.

- Pap smear procedure
  Most commonly, the examiner inserts a small brush through the cervical os and rotates it to obtain cells from within the cervical canal (**endocervical smear**). The brush is then rolled onto the slide.
  A second specimen may be obtained by lightly scraping the cervix with a wooden spatula to obtain cells from the **ectocervix** (the lowest portion of the cervix that protrudes into the vagina). The spatula is then smeared on the slide. Some examiners use both specimen sources and then apply a fixative, usually a spray or liquid on top of the specimen to preserve it for examination.

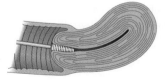

Using a specimen broom to obtain endocervical cells

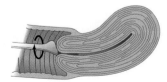

Using a spatula to obtain ecto-cervical cells

(continued)

• Pap smear, alternative method
The examiner inserts a specimen broom into the cervical os and rotates it. The broom is then inserted into a fixative solution and rotated to disperse cells into the solution. This technique is gaining popularity because it is considered more sensitive for detection of cervical changes.
• After the samples are obtained, the speculum is removed.

Bimanual Exam

After removing the speculum, the examiner then inserts lubricated gloved fingers into the vagina while pressing down on the lower abdomen and suprapubic area. This is known as a **bimanual exam.** It is used to assess the consistency of the cervix, the size of the uterus, and to detect tenderness over the ovaries, fallopian tubes, or with movement of the cervix.

Post-procedure

• Assist the woman to a sitting position at the end of the exam.
• You may need to assist the woman with perineal care.
• If there is any bleeding or discharge, provide a perineal pad.
• Document the date and time of the procedure, the name of the examiner, the patient's tolerance of the procedure, and any nursing assessments or interventions performed.

Documentation

VOL 1 | Go to Chapter 19, **Documenting Physical Assessment Findings,** in Volume 1.

Maturation Status in Females

Stage 1

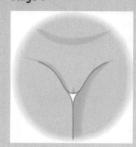

Preadolescent: No pubic hair except for fine body hair similar to hair on abdomen.

Stage 2

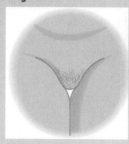

Sparse growth of long, slightly pigmented, downy hair, straight or only slightly curled, mostly along labia.

Stage 3

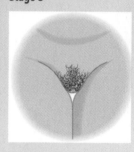

Hair becomes darker, coarser, and curlier and spreads sparsely over pubic symphysis.

Stage 4

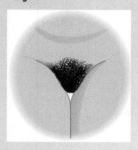

Pubic hair is coarse and curly as in adults. It covers more area than in Stage 3 but not as great as in adults.

Stage 5: Adult

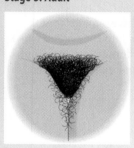

Quality and quantity are consistent with adult pubic hair distribution and spread over medial surfaces of thighs but not over abdomen.

| PROCEDURE 19–19 | **Assessing the Anus and Rectum** |

 For steps to follow in *all* procedures, refer to the inside back cover of this book.

critical aspects

- Inspect the external anal area, sphincter tone, and stool for occult blood.
- Palpate the anus and rectum for muscle tone and masses.
- For females, assessment of the anus and rectum is usually performed at the end of the internal pelvic exam; for males, it is done after the genitourinary exam.

Equipment

- Water-soluble lubricant
- Hemoccult test
- Nonlatex procedure gloves
- Pen and record form

Focused History Questions

- Do you have any pain or discomfort around your anus?
- Do you ever have difficulty passing stool?
- Have you ever noticed blood on your stool or when you wipe?
- Have you ever been told you have hemorrhoids?

- For men, have you ever had a prostate exam or a prostate-specific antigen (PSA) blood test? If so, what were the results?

Developmental Modification: Infants and Children

You will not usually perform a rectal exam on infants and children.

Procedural Steps

1. Inspect the anus. Note the condition of the skin and the presence of any lesions.

2. Palpate the anus and rectum.

   a. For women, change gloves to prevent cross-contamination. Insert a lubricated index finger gently into the rectum. Palpate the rectal wall, noting masses or tenderness.

   b. For males, have the client bend over the exam table or turn on his left side if recumbent. Insert a lubricated index finger gently into the rectum. Palpate the rectal wall, noting, masses or evidence of tenderness.

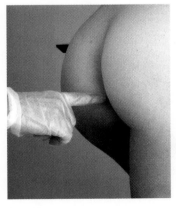 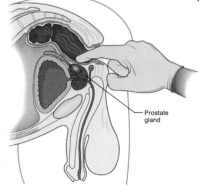

Prostate gland

Step 2b   *Step 2b*

   c. Test any stool on the gloved finger for occult blood. See Procedure 28–1.

Expected Findings

Anal area is intact, with no inflammation or lesions. Anus is a darker color than surrounding tissue.

Abnormal findings:

- A fissure or tear may be due to trauma, severe constipation, or an abscess.
- External hemorrhoids or skin tags may be visible.

Good sphincter tone. Rectum is nontender. No palpable masses or hard stool.

The stool is brown and negative for occult blood.

Abnormal findings:

- Hard stool in the rectum indicates impaction.
- Positive occult blood indicates bleeding in the GI tract.
- A palpable mass or enlarged prostate gland requires further evaluation.
- Internal hemorrhoids may be present.

Patient Teaching

Instruct the client in the importance of colonoscopy and prostate exam.

Documentation

 Go to Chapter 19, **Documenting Physical Assessment Findings,** in Volume 1.

What Are the Main Points in This Chapter?

- A physical examination may be conducted to obtain data about the patient, to further investigate an identified health problem, to monitor a client's health status, or to screen for health problems.

- A comprehensive physical assessment includes a complete head-to-toe examination of every body system. Data from a comprehensive physical assessment provide guidance for care and determine the need for further assessment.

- A focused physical assessment is performed to obtain data about an actual, potential, or possible problem that has been identified. A focused exam adds to the database created from the comprehensive assessment.

- An ongoing assessment is appropriate for periodic reassessment of the client and reflects the dynamic state of the client.

- Prior to a physical assessment, you will need to gather equipment, prepare the environment, review the skills you will use, familiarize yourself with the patient situation, review the nursing plan of care, and assist the patient to relax by taking the time to develop a rapport.

- Inspection is the use of sight to gather data. Inspection begins the moment you meet the client.

- Palpation is the use of touch to gather data. Use palpation to assess temperature, skin texture, moisture, anatomical landmarks, and abnormalities such as edema, masses, or areas of tenderness.

- Percussion, tapping on the skin with short strokes from your fingers, produces vibrations that allow you to determine the location, size, and density of underlying structures.

- Auscultation is the use of hearing to gather data. Direct auscultation is unassisted listening. Indirect auscultation is listening to the sounds produced by the body with the help of a stethoscope.

 Go to Chapter 19, **Resources for Caregivers and Health Professionals,** on the Electronic Study Guide.

 Suggested Readings: Go to Chapter 19, **Reading More About Health Assessment: Performing a Physical Examination,** on the Electronic Study Guide.

Abnormal ATLAS

Skin Color Changes

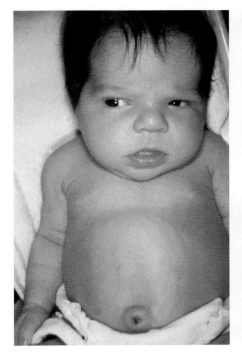

Jaundice

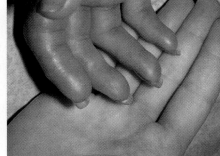

Cyanosis

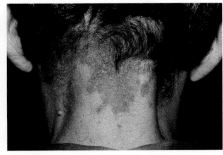

Port-wine stain (nevus flammeus)

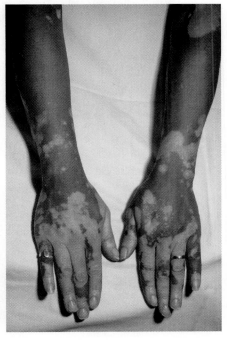

Vitiligo

Skin Lesions

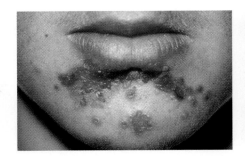

Herpes simplex

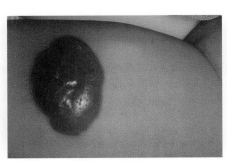

Capillary hemangioma

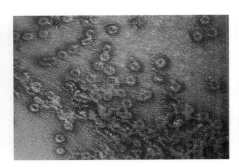

Vescicles (blisters)

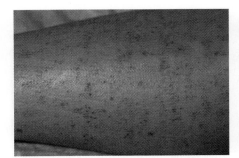

Petechiae

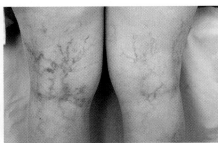

Venous star

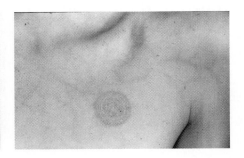

Ringworm

Hair

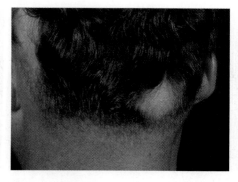

Alopecia areata

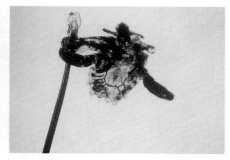

Pediculosis (lice)

Nail Appearance

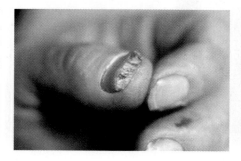

Fungal infection

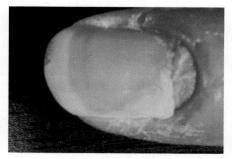

Paronychia

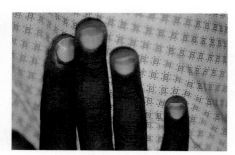

Half-and-half nails

Eyes

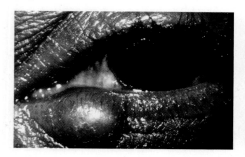

Hordeolum

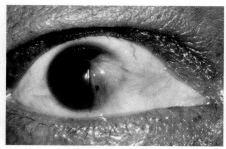

Pterygium

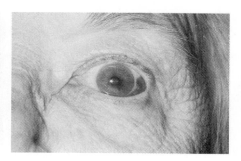

Subconjunctival hemorrhage

Mouth and Oropharynx

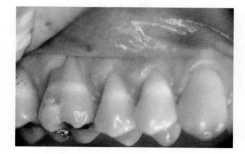

Gingival recession

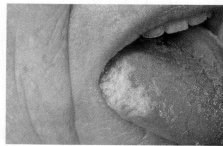

Leukoplakia

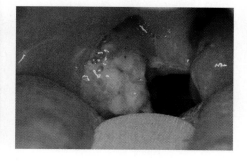

Enlarged tonsils with exudates

Musculoskeletal System

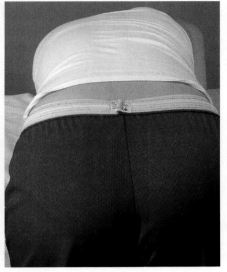

Scoliosis

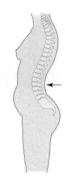

Lordosis

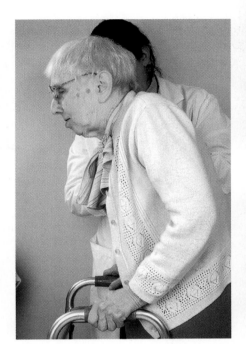

Kyphosis

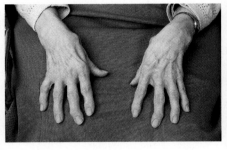

Degenerative joint disease (Heberden's nodes)

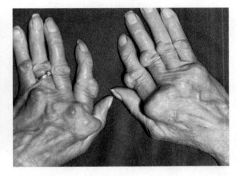

Rheumatoid arthritis

Abnormal Gaits

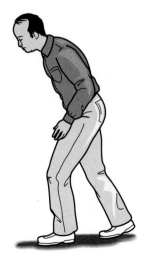

Propulsive gait

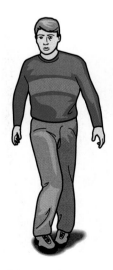

Scissors gait

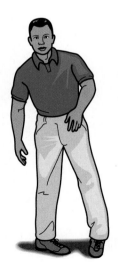

Spastic gait

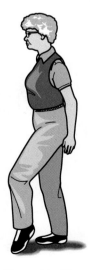

Steppage gait

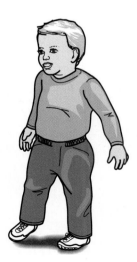

Waddling gait

Male Genitourinary System

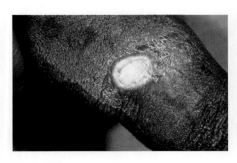

Syphilitic chancre

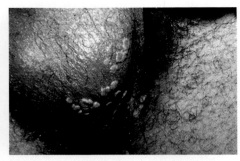

Genital warts

Female Genitourinary System

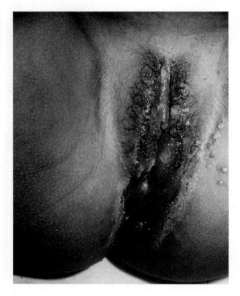

Herpes vulvovaginitis

Promoting Asepsis

& Preventing Infection

Overview

Nosocomial infections (infections acquired in healthcare facilities) are a major health problem worldwide. All nurses can help prevent infections in the healthcare facility. However, it is the infection control nurse who has the specific task of minimizing the number of infections in the healthcare facility.

Six links must be present to transmit infection: infectious agent, reservoir, portal of exit, mode of transmission, portal of entry, and susceptible host. The body is protected by primary defenses that block entry of pathogens, such as intact skin and mucous membranes. Secondary defenses, which are triggered by the invading microorganisms, include phagocytosis, the complement cascade, the inflammatory response, and fever.

Nutrition, hygiene, rest, exercise, stress reduction, and immunization protect the body against infection. Illness, injury, medical treatment, infancy or old age, frequent public contact, and various lifestyle factors can make the body more susceptible to infection.

The most important aspect of medical asepsis is scrupulous hand washing, either with soap and water or with solutions, rubs, and sprays containing at least 60% alcohol to decontaminate your hands. These products significantly decrease the transmission of infection. Standard precautions are used with all clients whenever there is a possibility of coming in contact with body fluids (except sweat). If exposure occurs, contact the infection control or employee health nurse as soon as possible after the exposure, and complete an injury report.

Surgical asepsis requires creating a sterile environment and using sterile equipment. You will use sterile technique (in addition to general principles of asepsis) when administering an injection, starting an IV line, or performing a sterile dressing change.

Thinking Critically About Promoting Asepsis and Preventing Infection

The exercises in the following section allow you to practice the kind of thinking you will use as a full-spectrum nurse. Because these are critical-thinking activities, there is usually no single right answer. Discuss answers with your peers—discussion can stimulate critical thinking. If you have difficulty with any of the questions, consult with your instructor.

Caring for the Garcias

Ms Garcia works as a preschool teacher in her community. Bettina, her grandchild, has been attending the preschool since she came to live with her grandparents. Ms Garcia tells you at a recent visit to the clinic that Bettina has had a lot of problems with colds and runny nose since she started preschool.

A. Based on your theoretical knowledge of asepsis and immunity, what is the most likely explanation for Bettina's symptoms?

B. Do you have enough patient data to make any conclusions? If not, what other information should you gather?

C. Identify three alternatives that may explain what is happening.

D. What strategies could you recommend that Ms Garcia implement at the preschool to help limit the number of infections? Identify at least two strategies.

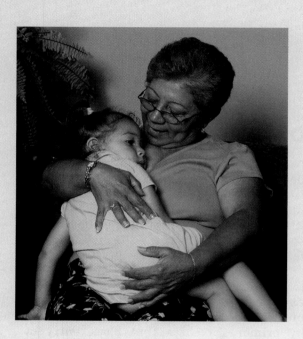

1 You notice that your clinical instructor is not washing his hands between patients. What should you do?

2 As you are gowning and gloving for your first experience in the operating room, you become nervous and forget the proper procedure for applying sterile surgical garb. How should you handle this situation?

3 What action should you take if you contaminate yourself while gowning and gloving?

4 For each of the following concepts, use critical thinking to describe how or why it is important to nursing, patient care, or promoting asepsis and preventing infection. Note that these are *not* to be merely definitions.

Chain of infection

Pathogens

thinking critically about promoting asepsis & preventing infection

Asepsis

Nosocomial infections

Contamination

Standard precautions

Transmission-based precautions

Protective isolation

Sterile

Medical asepsis

Surgical asepsis

Practical Knowledge
knowing how

As a nurse, you play a vital role in preventing the transmission of infection. Most infection control measures are independent nursing activities. You do not need an order for them; you do need theoretical knowledge and scrupulous medical and surgical asepsis technique. The techniques in this section and the procedures in the next section provide the guidance you will need to perform this important role.

TECHNIQUES

TECHNIQUE 20–1   Following Standard Precautions

- Immediately wash your hands with soap and water after contact with blood, body fluids (except sweat), excretions and secretions, mucous membranes, any break in the skin, or contaminated objects, REGARD-LESS of whether you have been wearing gloves.
- Wear clean gloves whenever there is potential for contact with blood, body fluids, secretions, excretions, nonintact skin, or contaminated materials.
- Remove gloves immediately after use. Avoid touching clean items, environmental surfaces, or another patient.
- Change gloves between tasks or procedures on the same patient if you have made contact with material that may contain a high concentration of microorganisms.
- Wash your hands with soap and water after removing gloves, between patient contacts, and between procedures on the same patient to prevent cross-contamination of different body sites.
- Wear a mask and eye protection or a face shield to protect mucous membranes of the eyes, nose, and mouth during patient care activities that are likely to generate splashes or sprays of blood, body fluids, secretions, and excretions.
- Wear a clean, nonsterile gown to protect skin and prevent soiling of clothing whenever there is a risk of spray or splash onto clothing. Promptly remove the gown once it is soiled. Avoid contaminating clothing when removing the gown. Wash hands after removing the gown.
- Clean reusable equipment that is soiled with blood or body fluids according to agency policy.
- Do not reuse equipment to care for another patient until it has been cleaned and reprocessed appropriately.
- Dispose of single-use equipment that is soiled with blood or body fluids in appropriate biohazard containers.
- Carefully handle contaminated linens to prevent skin and mucous membrane exposures, contamination of clothing, and transfer of microorganisms to other patients or the environment.
- Never recap used needles, or otherwise manipulate them using both hands, or use any other technique that involves directing the point of a needle toward any part of the body; rather, use either a one-handed "scoop" technique or a mechanical device designed for holding the needle sheath.
- Use puncture-resistant containers for disposal of "sharps"—scalpels, needles, and so on.
- Use mouthpieces, resuscitation bags, or other ventilation devices as an alternative to mouth-to-mouth resuscitation methods in situations when the need for resuscitation is predictable.

TECHNIQUE 20–2   Following Transmission-Based Precautions

Contact Precautions

- Follow all standard precautions.
- Place the patient in a private room or in a room with a patient with an active infection caused by the same organism and no other infections.
- Wear a clean gown and gloves when you anticipate any contact with the patient or with any contaminated items in the room.
- Either dispose of all items entering the room within the room, or disinfect them per institution policy prior to removing them from the room.
- Double bag all linen and trash, and clearly mark them contaminated.
- Follow any additional precautions specific to the microorganism.

Droplet Precautions

- Follow all standard precautions.
- Place the patient in a private room or in a room with a patient with an active infection caused by the same organism and no other infections.
- Wear a clean gown and gloves when you anticipate any contact with the patient or with any contaminated items in the room.
- Wear a mask and eye protection when working within 3 feet of the patient.
- Either dispose of all items entering the room within the room, or disinfect them per institution policy prior to removing them from the room.

- Double bag all linen and trash, and clearly mark them contaminated.
- Follow any additional precautions specific to the microorganism.

Airborne Precautions

- Follow all standard precautions.
- Place the patient in a private room or in a room with a patient with an active infection caused by the same organism and no other infections. Make sure that the room has negative air pressure and that the air is discharged through a filtration system.
- Wear a clean gown and gloves when you anticipate any contact with the patient or with any items in the room.
- Wear a special mask (N95 respirator) if the patient is suspected of having pulmonary tuberculosis.
- If the patient is known to have or is suspected of having measles (rubeola) or varicella (chickenpox), only immune caregivers should provide care. Immune caregivers do not need to wear masks.
- Either dispose of all items entering the patient's room within the room, or disinfect them per institution policy prior to removing them from the room.
- Double bag all linen and trash on exit from the room, and clearly mark them contaminated.
- Follow any additional precautions specific to the microorganism.

TECHNIQUE 20–3   Maintaining Protective Isolation

- Follow all standard precautions.
- Healthcare workers caring for patients in protective isolation should not also be providing care for other patients with active infections.
- When patients in protective isolation need to leave the room, they should wear a mask and have minimal contact with others.
- All persons entering the patient's room should wear a mask and wash their hands thoroughly with soap and water.

- After hand washing, caregivers and visitors should put on a clean or sterile gown over clothing and take care to keep the outside of the gown from any contact with surfaces outside the room.
- Once the gown is placed, don gloves.
- If the mask or gown becomes wet while you provide care, change it.
- On exiting the room, remove the mask, gloves, and gown. Do not use them again.

TECHNIQUE 20–4 Using Sterile Technique

- Close doors and limit foot traffic when setting up a sterile field. Air currents can carry dust and microorganisms.
- A sterile field is sterile only on a horizontal plane. Consider nonsterile any material that drapes over the horizontal plane.
- The border of a sterile drape is considered unsterile even if it remains on a horizontal surface. Consider a 1-inch margin around the drape unsterile because it is in contact with contaminated surfaces.
- Remain at least 1 foot away from a sterile field if you are not wearing sterile garb.
- Remain at least 1 foot away from nonsterile areas if you are wearing sterile garb.
- Avoid reaching over a sterile field even if you are in sterile garb.
- Handle sterile equipment only if you are wearing sterile gloves.

- If you are wearing sterile attire, you are considered sterile only in the front of your body from shoulders to waist.
- Never turn your back to a sterile field.
- Only sterile items can be placed on a sterile field.
- Liquids can act as wicks and contaminate a field. Sterile liquids must be contained in sterile bowls on the field or a drape must be non-permeable in order to avoid wicking.
- Never assume an item is sterile. If there is any doubt about its sterility, consider it contaminated.
- All items applied to a sterile field must be sterilized in an approved manner.
- A sterile field or open sterile items must be kept in constant view.
- Limit the amount of time a sterile field remains set up in advance of a procedure.

PROCEDURES

| PROCEDURE 20–1 | **Hand Washing** |

For standard steps to follow in *all* procedures, refer to the inside back cover of this book.

critical aspects
- Remove your jewelry and watch.
- Wet your hands and wrists under running water.
- Apply 3 to 5 mL of liquid soap.
- Wash hands for at least 15 seconds, lathering all surfaces of the hands and fingers.
- Clean under your fingernails if they are dirty.
- Rinse and dry your hands thoroughly.
- Turn off the faucet with a dry paper towel.
- Apply non-petroleum-based hand lotion or skin protectant at least twice per day to prevent skin breakdown.

Equipment
- Liquid soap
- Paper towels
- Warm, running water
- Non-petroleum-based hand moisturizer (optional)

Assessments
- Check your hands for breaks in the skin.

Breaks in the skin provide a route for microbial entry. Wear gloves if the potential of microbial contamination may occur.

Procedural Steps

Step 1 Bare your hands and forearms. Push your sleeves and wristwatch above wrists, and remove rings.

Moist clothing facilitates transfer of microorganisms; rings can harbor bacteria.

Step 2 Turn on the water. Adjust the water temperature to warm.

Warm running water aids in removing microorganisms without removing excess skin oils.

Step 3 Wet your hands and wrists. Keep your hands below your wrists and forearms. ▼

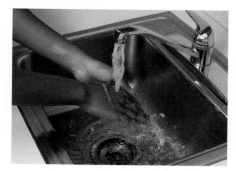

The hands are considered more contaminated than the wrists and arms, so prevent water from running from your hands onto your wrists and forearms.
a. Avoid splashing water onto clothing.
b. Avoid touching the inside of the sink.

The inside of the sink is considered contaminated.

Step 4 Apply 3 to 5 mL of liquid soap; rub the soap over all surfaces of your hands.

Using 3 to 5 mL of antimicrobial soap is recommended by the "APIC Guideline for Handwashing and Hand Antisepsis in Health-Care Settings." Soap removes microbes.

PROCEDURE 20–1   Hand Washing *(continued)*

Step 5 Vigorously rub your hands together for at least 15 seconds, lathering all surfaces of the hands and fingers.

Washing for at least 15 seconds is required for mechanical removal of microorganisms and to give antimicrobial products adequate contact with the skin surfaces to be effective; parts of the hands and fingers are often missed. ▼

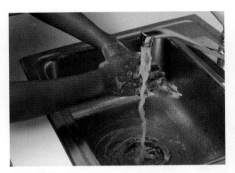

Step 6 Clean under your fingernails if they are dirty.

Debris under the nails can promote microbial growth, especially in the warm, moist environment inside the gloves.

Step 7 Rinse your hands thoroughly. Keep your hands below your wrists and forearms.

Washes away microorganisms and removes any residual soap. Keeping hands lower prevents soap, debris, or rinse water from flowing down your arms or wetting your uniform.

Step 8 Dry your hands thoroughly, moving from your fingers up to your forearms and blotting with paper towel.

Move from the cleaner area (hands) to less clean areas. Blotting decreases skin irritation.

Step 9 Turn off the faucet with a dry paper towel.

Prevents contamination of hands from faucet. ▼

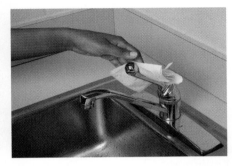

Step 10 Apply non-petroleum-based hand lotion or skin protectant at least twice daily.

Petroleum-based lotions facilitate absorption of latex proteins through the skin, increasing the incidence of latex allergies. The use of non-petroleum-based hand lotion is recommended to prevent skin from drying and becoming chafed.

Variation Using Alcohol-Based Handrubs

Step 1 Use alcohol-based handrubs when hands are not soiled.

Antiseptic solutions are not effective when organic material or dirt from hands is present.

Step 2 Apply a sufficient quantity of antiseptic solution to cover the hands and wrists.

All surfaces must be covered to remove microorganisms.

Step 3 Rub antiseptic solution on all surfaces of your fingers and hands until they are dry.

Ensures the effectiveness of the solution; usually takes 10 to 15 seconds. ▼

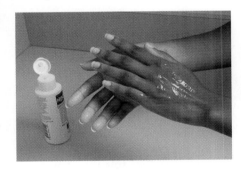

Evaluation

Hands are free of soap and dry.

Documentation

Hand washing is a responsibility of all healthcare providers. It does not require documentation.

| PROCEDURE 20–2 | **Donning and Removing Personal Protective Equipment (PPE)** |

> For steps to follow in *all* procedures, refer to the inside back cover of this book.

critical aspects

- Prior to exposure, don appropriate personal protective equipment according to standard precautions or transmission guidelines.
- Avoid contaminating self or others when removing equipment.
- Remove the most soiled item first.

Equipment

- Disposable gloves of the proper size
- Disposable isolation gown
- Face mask
- Face shield or goggles

Procedural Steps

Step 1 Assess the need for personal protective equipment.
a. Gloves: when you may be exposed to potentially infective secretions or materials
b. Gowns: when your uniform may become exposed to potentially infective secretions
c. Face mask: when splashing may occur and potentially contaminate your mouth or nose
d. Face shield or eye goggles: when splashing may occur and potentially contaminate your eyes

Step 2 Determine the availability of appropriate personal protective equipment.

Ensure that the correct equipment is available. A patient gown is not a substitute for a disposable isolation gown, because the isolation gown is made to prevent fluid strike-through and contamination of underlying clothing.

Donning Personal Protective Equipment

Step 3 Don the isolation gown.
a. Pick up gown by the shoulders, allowing the gown to fall open without touching the floor or other surfaces.

Touching the floor or other surfaces will contaminate the gown. ▼

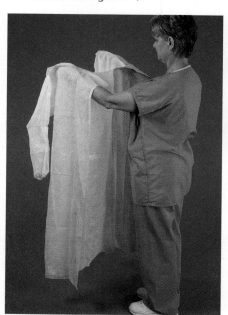

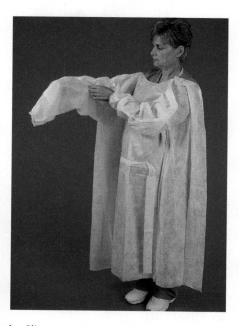

b. Slip your arms into the sleeves. ▲
c. Fasten ties at the neck.
d. If the gown does not completely cover your clothing, wear two gowns. Put on the first gown so that the opening is in the front, and then place the second gown over the first, so that the opening is in the back

Clothing must be covered to prevent contamination.

PROCEDURE 20-2

Donning and Removing Personal Protective Equipment (PPE) *(continued)*

Step 4 Don the face mask.

a. Identify the top edge of the mask by locating the thin metal strip that goes over the bridge of the nose.

b. Pick up the mask with the top ties or ear loops.

Securing the top of the mask first prevents the mask from accidentally falling down onto the gown.

c. Place the metal strip over the bridge of your nose, and tie the upper ties or slip loops around your ears.

d. Place the lower edge of the mask below your chin, and tie the lower ties.

Covering the nose and mouth offers the best protection from airborne pathogens and splashing.

e. Press the thin metal strip so that it conforms to the bridge of your nose.

The metal strip helps contour the mask to the face and helps keep the mask from falling down. ▼

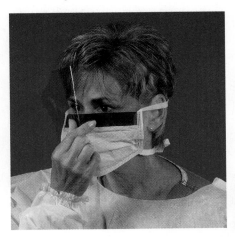

Step 5 Don the face shield or goggles.

a. Don the face shield by placing the shield over your eyes, adjusting the metal strip over the bridge of your nose, and tucking the lower edge below your chin.

b. Secure the straps behind your head.

Eyes are a potential entry point for pathogens. Protect them from potential splashes.

c. Don safety glasses or goggles by setting them over the top edge of the mask.

Placing the glasses or goggles on top of the face mask helps decrease fogging of the glasses.

Step 6 Don gloves.

a. Select gloves of the appropriate size.

No special application technique is required for clean disposable gloves.

b. If you are wearing a gown, make sure that the glove cuff extends over the cuff of the gown.

c. Tape the glove cuff to the gown if coverage is not complete.

Provides complete protection of hands and wrists.

Removing Personal Protective Equipment

Step 7 If your gown is tied in front, untie the waist ties before removing your gloves. If the gown is tied in back, remove your gloves before untying the waist ties.

Step 8 Remove one glove by grasping the cuff of the glove and pulling downward so that the glove turns inside out. Hold the glove you removed in the remaining gloved hand. ▼

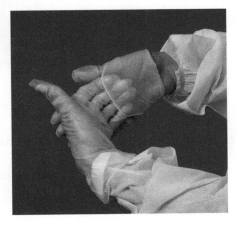

Allows you to dispose of both gloves at once by enclosing one glove within the other.

Step 9 Slip your fingers of the ungloved hand inside the cuff of the other glove. Pull the glove off, inside out. You can at the same time turn it over to enclose the first glove.

The inside of the glove is considered cleaner than the outside. ▼

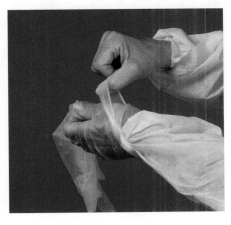

Step 10 Hold contaminated gloves away from your body. Dispose of them in a designated waste receptacle.

Step 11 Release the neck ties of the gown, allowing the gown to fall forward.

➤

PROCEDURE 20–2

Donning and Removing Personal Protective Equipment (PPE) *(continued)*

Step 12   Grasp the gown inside of the neck, and peel it down off your arms so that the inside of the gown faces outward.

The inside of the gown is considered cleaner. ▼

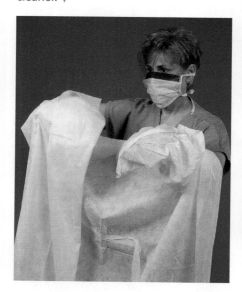

Step 13   Hold the gown away from your uniform, and discard it. Do not contaminate your clothing with the dirty gown. ▼

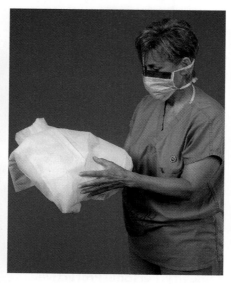

Step 14   If wearing a mask and goggles, remove the mask first and then the goggles.

Step 15   Remove the mask or face shield by untying lower ties first. Untie upper ties next, being careful not to let go of the mask. Dispose of the mask in a designated waste receptacle.

Prevents the mask from falling down onto your clothing.

Patient Teaching

Answer questions the patient may have about the need for personal protective equipment or his disease process.

Home Care

- Identify the type of personal protective equipment needed, and ensure that the necessary supplies are available.
- Develop a plan with the patient and family for using and disposing of personal protective equipment and contaminated items.

Documentation

The use of personal protective equipment is generally assumed and does not require documentation.

PROCEDURE 20–3 Surgical Hand Washing

 For steps to follow in *all* procedures, refer to the inside back cover of this book.

critical aspects
- Apply surgical shoe covers, cap, and face mask before the scrub.
- Use warm water.
- Perform an initial hand wash, and lather up to 2 inches above your elbows.
- Clean under your nails.
- Wet the scrub brush, and apply a generous amount of antimicrobial soap.
- Using a circular motion, scrub all surfaces of nails, hands, and forearms at least 10 times.
- Rinse hands and arms by keeping your fingertips higher than your elbow.
- Grasp a sterile towel, and back away from the sterile field.
- Thoroughly dry your hands before donning sterile gloves.

Equipment
- Antimicrobial soap
- Surgical scrub brush
- Plastic disposable nail file

- Deep sink with foot or knee controls
- Surgical shoe covers, cap, and face mask
- Sterile gloves of the correct size
- Surgical pack containing a sterile towel

Procedural Steps

Step 1 Determine agency policy for duration of the surgical scrub and the type of cleansing agent used.

The type of cleansing agent determines how long to scrub. Typically, an antimicrobial soap requires 2 to 6 minutes, whereas an alcohol-based handrub is rubbed onto hands and arms until dry.

Step 2 Avoid chipped polish or artificial nails.

Chipped nail polish harbors pathogens, and artificial nails are more likely to harbor gram-negative pathogens.

Step 3 Put on surgical shoe covers, cap, and face mask prior to the surgical scrub.

Step 4 Determine that sterile gloves, gown, and towel are set up for use after the scrub.

To maintain sterility, the sterile towel, gown, and gloves must be ready for use immediately after you scrub. If you need to gather supplies after the scrub, you will need to start the scrub procedure over again.

Step 5 Turn on the water, using the knee or foot controls. Adjust the temperature so that the water is warm.

Hot water removes too many of the skin's protective oils. Knee and foot controls avoid contamination of the hands. ▼

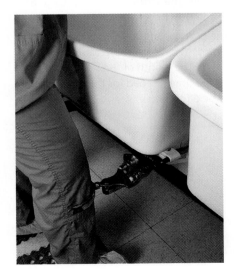

Step 6 Wet your hands and forearms from elbows to fingertips, keeping hands above elbows and away from your body.

Prevents water running down from your elbows and forearm over rinsed hands.

Step 7 Apply a liberal amount of soap onto your hands, and lather well to 2 inches above the elbow. Rinse your hands and arms, keeping your hands above elbows. Do not touch the inside of the sink with your fingers, hand, or elbow. (*Note:* Some facilities use an antibacterial gel for the initial handwash. Apply the gel liberally and let dry. Do not rinse the gel.)

This is a hand wash prior to the scrub. The purpose is to reduce the number of microorganisms. The inside of the sink is considered contaminated. If you touch it, you will need to repeat the handwash.

➤

PROCEDURE 20–3 **Surgical Hand Washing** (continued)

Step 8 Remove debris from underneath your fingernails using a nail file under running water.

Decreases the number of microorganisms. ▼

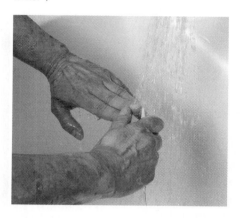

Step 9 If you are using an alcohol-based surgical hand-scrub product:

a. Using the indicated amount of handrub, rub all surfaces of the hands, including the nails, and up the arm to 2 inches above the elbow.

b. Allow the handrub to dry completely before you don sterile gloves.

Many different products are being developed. Be careful to follow manufacturer's guidelines for use. ▼

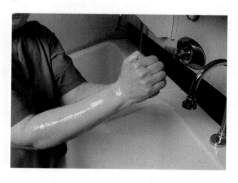

Step 10 If you are using an antimicrobial soap:

a. Wet the scrub brush, and apply a generous amount of antimicrobial soap.

Scrub brushes can be harsh on the skin. Using plenty of water and soap helps decrease the skin irritation. Antimicrobial soap reduces the number of microorganisms.

b. Using a circular motion, scrub all the surfaces of one hand and arm. Start at the fingers. Scrub at least 10 strokes each on nail, all sides of fingers, and both sides of hand. When scrubbing the arm, use 10 strokes each for the lower, middle, and upper areas of the forearm. Keep your hands higher than your elbows. ▼

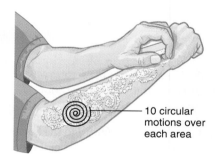

10 circular motions over each area

c. Rinse the brush, and reapply antimicrobial soap. Repeat the scrub on the second hand and arm. Normally the scrub takes at least 2 to 6 minutes.

The purpose of the scrub is to decrease the number of microorganisms on the hands. The length of the scrub depends on the time needed for the scrub agent to be effective.

Step 11 Rinse your hands and arms, keeping your fingertips higher than your elbow.

Prevents contamination of hands from water running from the upper arm down onto hands. ▼

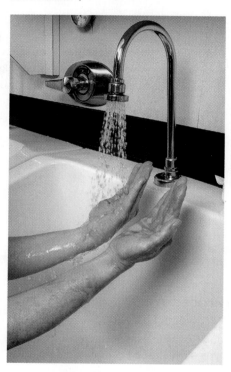

Step 12 With your arms flexed and your hands held higher than your elbows, move to the area with sterile towel and gown.

Avoids contamination of hands from water runoff.

PROCEDURE 20–3   Surgical Hand Washing *(continued)*

Step 13 Grasp the sterile towel, and move away from sterile field.

Moving away keeps the sterile field dry and prevents you from inadvertently brushing against the table, which would contaminate the field. ▼

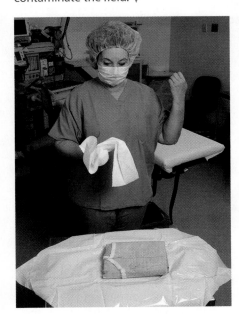

Step 14 Lean forward slightly, and allow the towel to fall open, being careful not to let it touch your uniform.

The towel would be contaminated if it brushed against your uniform.

Step 15 Use one end of the towel to dry one hand and arm. Use the opposite end to dry the other hand and arm. Be

certain that your skin is thoroughly dry before donning sterile gloves.

Dry skin prevents maceration and allows gloves to go on much more easily. Use a separate section of the towel to prevent rewetting the skin.

Patient Teaching

If the patient is awake for the procedure, explain the purpose of the surgical scrub and sterility.

Documentation

A surgical hand scrub does not require documentation. Instead, chart the procedure (or surgery) and how the patient tolerated it.

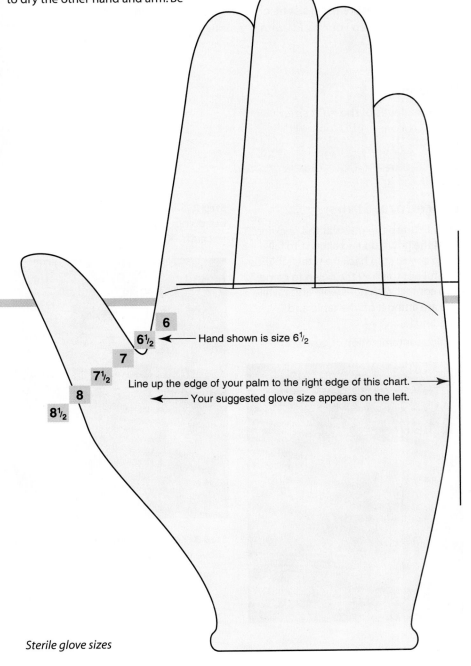

6
6½   ← Hand shown is size 6½
7
7½
8   Line up the edge of your palm to the right edge of this chart. ⟶
8½   ← Your suggested glove size appears on the left.

Sterile glove sizes

PROCEDURE 20–4 Donning Sterile Gown and Gloves (Closed Method)

For steps to follow in *all* procedures, refer to the inside back cover of this book.

critical aspects

- Grasp the gown at the neckline, and slide your arms into the sleeves without extending your hands through the cuffs.
- Have a co-worker pull the shoulders of the gown up and tie the neck tie.
- Don gloves using the closed method by keeping your hands covered at all times, first with the gown cuffs, and then with the sterile gloves.
- Secure the waist tie on your gown by handing it to a co-worker.
- Keep your hands within your field of vision at all times.

Equipment

- Sterile gloves of the right size
- Sterile gown

Procedural Steps

Step 1 Grasp the gown at the neckline. Hold the gown up and allow it to fall open as you step back from the table. Be careful not to allow the gown to come into contact with nonsterile areas while you are lifting it off the table and opening it.

Avoids contamination of gown. ▼

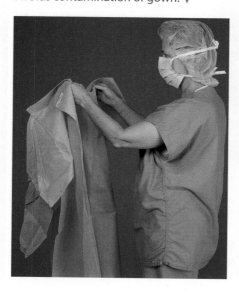

Step 2 Slide both arms into the sleeves, but do not extend your hands through the cuffs. ▼

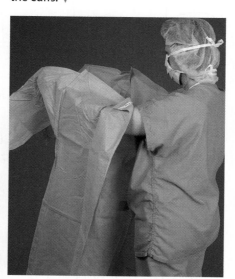

Step 3 Keep the sleeves of the gown above waist level.

Ensures sterility.

Step 4 Have a co-worker (or the circulating nurse, if you are in the operating room) stand behind you and pull the shoulders of the gown up and tie the neck tie. The co-worker touches only the inside of the gown while pulling it up.

Touching only the inside prevents contamination of the gown with the nurse's hands.

Step 5 Don sterile gloves using the closed method.

a. Open the sterile glove wrapper, keeping your fingers inside the sleeve of the gown. The outer wrapper has already been discarded.

PROCEDURE 20–4

Donning Sterile Gown and Gloves (Closed Method) *(continued)*

b. Keeping your hands inside the gown sleeves, grasp the cuff of the glove for the dominant hand.

Keeping the hand inside the cuff ensures that you are making contact with the sterile gown; sterile is touching sterile. ▼

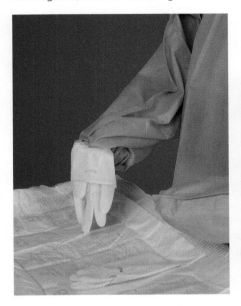

c. Lay the glove on the forearm of the dominant hand with the palm of the glove facing down, the fingers pointed toward the elbow, and the thumb of the glove positioned on the thumb side. ▼

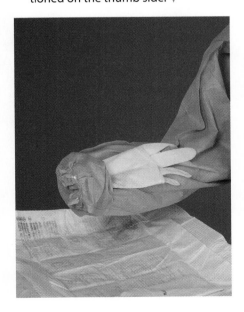

d. Grasp the inside glove cuff with your dominant hand through the gown, being careful to keep fingers inside the gown.

Bare fingers would contaminate the sterile glove.

e. With your nondominant hand encased in the gown sleeve, pull the glove cuff over the cuff of the gown. ▼

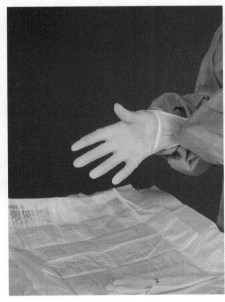

f. Grasping the sleeve of your gown (with your nondominant hand) and the cuff of glove, pull the glove onto your dominant hand.

g. Place the second glove on the forearm of your nondominant hand with the palm of the glove down, fingers pointed toward the elbow, and glove thumb on thumb-side of the hand.

h. Grasp the inside glove cuff with your nondominant hand through the gown, being careful to keep fingers inside the gown.

i. With your dominant hand, pull the glove cuff over the cuff of the gown.

j. Grasp the sleeve of your gown and the cuff of the glove, and pull the glove onto your nondominant hand. ▼

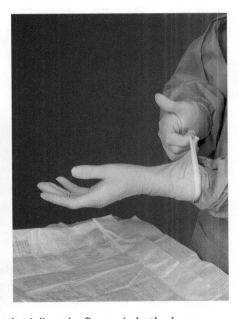

k. Adjust the fingers in both gloves.

Maintains sterility of the gown and gloves by maintaining a closed system. Final adjustment of the gloves is done when both gloves are in place to prevent contaminating the gloves.

➤

PROCEDURE 20–4

Donning Sterile Gown and Gloves (Closed Method) *(continued)*

Step 6 Grasp the waist tie on the gown, and hand the tie to the circulating nurse or a co-worker who is wearing a hair cover and mask. Your co-worker will grab the tie with sterile forceps. Make a three-quarter turn, and receive the tie from your co-worker.

Because only areas within your field of vision are considered sterile, a co-worker must pull the waist tie around you. ➤

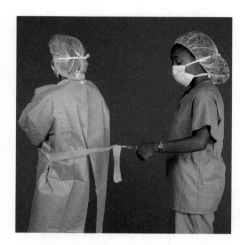

Step 7 Secure the waist tie.

Ensures that the gown is secured.

Patient Teaching

- If the patient is alert during the procedure, explain the need for the sterile procedure.
- Explain any special precautions during the procedure, such as the need to hold still.

Documentation

- Donning sterile gown and gloves does not require documentation.
- You will need to chart the procedure performed and how the patient tolerated it.
- In the operating room, the circulating nurse charts about the surgery and the patient's response.

PROCEDURE 20–5 | Applying Sterile Gloves (Open Method)

For steps to follow in *all* procedures, refer to the inside back cover of this book.

critical aspects

- Place the glove package on a clean, dry surface.
- Open the inner package so that the cuffs are closest to you.
- Apply the glove of your dominant hand first by touching only the inside of the glove (the folded-over cuff) with your nondominant hand.
- Apply the second glove by touching only the outer part of the glove with your already-gloved hand.

Equipment

- Sterile gloves of the correct size.

Procedural Steps

Step 1 Determine the correct size of sterile gloves (see page 351). The gloves should be snug, but not tight.

Gloves that are too loose are more easily contaminated and make handling equipment or supplies difficult. Gloves that are too tight are uncomfortable.

Step 2 Assess the glove package for intactness and expiration date. Do not use the package if it is torn, has become moist, or is past the expiration date.

Torn packaging may allow the gloves to become contaminated. Moisture allows wicking and may cause contamination. Expired gloves are not considered sterile. ▼

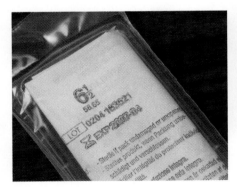

Step 3 Assess the patient environment for a space that is clean and has adequate space to allow you to open the glove package and don the gloves without touching a nonsterile item.

Step 4 Open the outer wrapper, and place the inner glove package on a clean, dry surface.

Prevents contamination of the gloves.

Step 5 Open the inner glove package so that the glove cuffs are closest to you. Be careful to fully open the flaps of the package so that they do not fold back over and contaminate the gloves.

Makes donning gloves easier. ▼

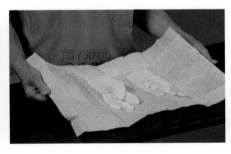

Step 6 Taking care to not touch anything else on the sterile field, with your nondominant hand, grasp the inner surface of the glove for the dominant hand. Lift the glove up and away from the table, keeping it away from your body.

The inside of the glove is not considered sterile because it is in contact with your skin. Lifting the glove up and away from the table prevents you from accidentally touching the table while donning the glove and thereby contaminating the glove.

Step 7 Slide your dominant hand into the glove, keeping your hand and fingers above your waist and away from your body.

Reaching down when donning the glove may result in unrecognized contamination. ▼

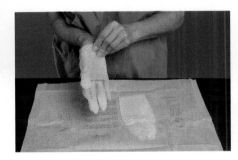

▶

PROCEDURE 20–5   Applying Sterile Gloves (Open Method)
(continued)

Step 8 Slide your gloved fingers under the cuff of the glove for the nondominant hand. Lift the glove up and away from the table and away from your body.

The outside of the glove is sterile and may be touched with your sterile gloved hand. ▼

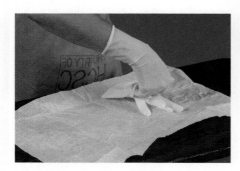

Step 9 Slide your nondominant hand into the glove, being careful to avoid contact with your gloved hand. ▼

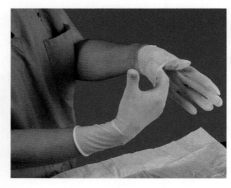

Step 10 Adjust both gloves to fit your fingers. If necessary, pull the fingers of the gloves down so that no excess is at the fingertips.

Adjusting your gloves after both have been donned decreases the risk of contamination.

Step 11 Keep your hands between shoulder and waist level in front of you.

Keeps the gloves within your field of vision.

Patient Teaching

Explain the reason sterile gloves are needed for the procedure.

Home Care

• Many home care procedures are clean rather than sterile. The patient is in his own environment and not surrounded by other patients who may serve as hosts for infection.
• You may need to teach caregivers how to apply sterile gloves for some procedures. No modifications are required. Demonstrate the procedure, and have the caregiver do a return demonstration.

Documentation

• No special documentation is needed for sterile gloving.
• Chart the procedure you performed and the patient's response to the procedure.

PROCEDURE 20–6 | Preparing and Maintaining a Sterile Field

 For steps to follow in *all* procedures, refer to the inside back cover of this book.

critical aspects

- Check to ensure that all supplies are ready for the procedure.
- Clear the area for the sterile field.
- Position the patient appropriately for the procedure.
- Establish the sterile field with a sterile drape or sterile package wrapper.
- Add items to the sterile field by gently dropping them onto the sterile field.
- Pour sterile solutions into a sterile bowl or receptacle without touching the bowl or splashing onto the sterile field.
- Don sterile gloves and perform procedure.

Equipment

- Package of sterile supplies required for the procedure
- Sterile gloves of the correct size

Procedural Steps for Setting Up a Sterile Field

Step 1 Assess the sterility of all packages and equipment. Check to make sure the packaging is intact and the expiration dates have not passed.

Only sterile items enter a sterile field. Any compromise in packaging means that the item is assumed not to be sterile.

Step 2 Arrange the environment for performing the sterile procedure.
a. Clean off the surface you will use to set up the sterile field.

Inadequate space causes inadvertent contamination during sterile procedures.

b. Position the patient as needed for the procedure.

Allows you to immediately proceed with the planned procedure. Once the sterile field is established, air movement can create contamination of the sterile items.

Step 3 Establish a sterile field.
a. Using sterile packaged equipment:
1) Place the sterile package on a clean, dry surface.

Prevents contamination of the sterile item. If a surface is damp, strike-through may occur, making the item unsterile. ▼

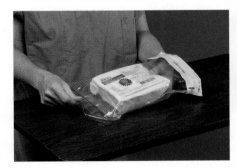

2) Open the flap away from you first.

If you move an unsterile item over a sterile field, the field is no longer considered to be sterile. ▼

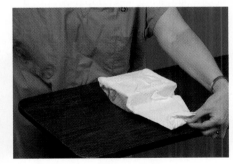

3) Open the side flaps. ▼

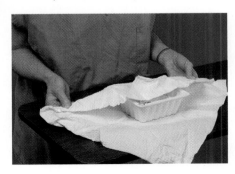

▶

PROCEDURE 20–6

Preparing and Maintaining a Sterile Field
(continued)

4) Pull the final flap toward you. The wrapper is now the sterile field. The area 1 inch from the edge of the wrapper and 1 inch from the table edge is considered unsterile. Do not readjust the sterile area after the package has been opened.

Only the horizontal surface of the draped area is considered sterile. Any part of the sterile wrapper that falls below the level of the sterile area (e.g., top of the table) is considered unsterile. If you move the field after opening, the field shifts and places unsterile areas of the wrapper on the surface. ▼

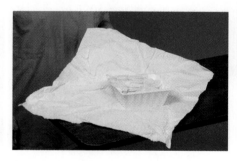

b. Opening a fabric- or paper-wrapped sterile package:
1) Check and remove the chemical indicator strip.

The indicator tape confirms sterility. The pack usually is also dated.

2) Remove the outer wrapper, and place the inner package on a clean, dry surface.

The outer wrapper is not considered sterile and is discarded.

3) Open the inner wrapper following the same technique described in Step 3a.

c. Using a sterile drape:
1) Place the package on a clean, dry surface. Hold the edge of the package flap down toward the table, grasp the top edge of the package, and peel back.

Opens the package without contaminating the contents. ▼

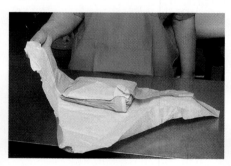

2) Pick up the sterile drape by the corner. Allow the drape to fall open. Place it on a clean, dry surface by touching only the edge of the drape. Avoid fanning the drape.

A 1-inch border around the sterile drape is considered unsterile.

Procedural Steps for Adding Supplies to a Sterile Field

Step 4 Using your nondominant hand, peel back the wrapper.

The inside of the wrapper is sterile and will be used as a barrier when placing the sterile item onto a sterile field.

Step 5 Holding the contents several inches above the field, allow the supplies to drop onto the field inside the 1-inch border of the sterile field. Do not let your arms pass over the sterile field.

By holding the package upside down, you ensure that the sterile part of the package is facing the sterile field and that you deposit the item onto the sterile field. ▼

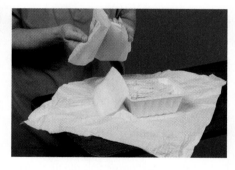

Step 6 Dispose of the wrapper, and continue opening any needed supplies for the procedure.

Once sterile gloves are on, you will not be able to add items without contaminating the gloves.

PROCEDURE 20–6

Preparing and Maintaining a Sterile Field
(continued)

Procedural Steps for Adding Sterile Solutions to a Sterile Field

Step 7 Use a sterile bowl or receptacle if the sterile field is fabric or at risk for strike-through. You may add a sterile bowl to the field by unwrapping (as discussed above) and holding the bowl through the sterile wrapper as you place it near the edge of the sterile field. The sterile bowl may also be placed next to the sterile field.

If you place the sterile bowl on the field, place it near the edge so that you can pour the sterile solution from the back of the sterile field. This prevents you from reaching over and thereby contaminating the field.

Step 8 Check that the sterile solution is correct, and confirm that the expiration date has not passed.

Check the solution as you would a medication. Validate that the solution and concentration are correct and have not expired. ▼

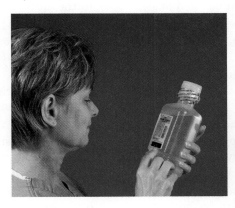

Step 9 Remove the cap off the solution bottle by lifting it directly up. If cap will be reused, set it upside down on a clean area.

Avoids contamination of bottle cap. For repeating procedures, the solution is dated, timed, and left in the patient's room for reuse according to agency policies.

Step 10 Holding the bottle of solution 4 to 6 inches above the bowl to prevent inadvertent contamination, pour the needed amount into the bowl.

Prevents you from touching the sterile bowl with the bottle and thereby contaminating the bowl. Limited height reduces risk of splashing, which strikes through and contaminates a cloth or permeable sterile field. A disposable sterile drape generally has a plastic membrane in the middle to prevent strike-through. ▼

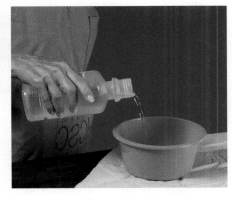

Step 11 Before donning sterile gloves to perform the procedure, double-check that all supplies have been added to the field. Do not leave the sterile field unattended.

If a sterile item is out of your field of vision, it is no longer considered sterile because airborne particles, insects, or liquids could contaminate the field.

Home Care

- Most sterile procedures in the home are done by visiting nurses.
- Procedures performed by patients or family members are usually clean as opposed to sterile.

Documentation

- You will not document the actual setting up of the sterile field.
- Document the procedure, your assessment of the patient's tolerance for the procedure, and your assessment of the area being treated by the procedure.

What Are the Main Points in This Chapter?

- Nosocomial infections (infections that are acquired in healthcare facilities) are a major health problem worldwide.

- The chain of infection consists of six links that must all be present for infection to be transmitted from one individual to another: infectious agent, reservoir, portal of exit, mode of transmission, portal of entry, and susceptible host.

- Pathogens are strains of bacteria, viruses, fungi, protozoa, helminths, and prions that cause disease.

- Infectious illnesses typically follow five predictable stages: incubation, prodromal stage, illness, decline, and convalescence.

- Primary body defenses, such as intact skin and mucous membranes, block entry of pathogens into the body.

- Invading microorganisms trigger the body's secondary defenses, which include phagocytosis, the complement cascade, the inflammatory response, and fever.

- The humoral immune response results in the production of antibodies that neutralize pathogens or trigger their destruction.

- The cell-mediated immune response results in the production of T cells that destroy infected body cells.

- Nutrition, hygiene, rest, exercise, stress reduction, and immunization protect the body against infection.

- Anything that weakens the body's defenses or increases the person's exposure to pathogens makes the person more susceptible to infection. Such factors include illness, injury, medical treatment, infancy or old age, frequent public contact, and various lifestyle factors.

- Medical asepsis requires that objects and surfaces in the healthcare environment be disinfected.

- Scrupulous hand washing markedly decreases the transmission of infection and is the most important aspect of medical asepsis.

- Standard precautions are used with all clients whenever there is a possibility of coming in contact with blood, body fluids (except sweat), excretions and secretions, mucous membranes, and any break in the skin.

- Transmission-based precautions are added to standard precautions when there is concern about transmission of infection via contact, droplets, or air currents.

- Isolation precautions are designed to prevent the spread of disease, not to isolate the person who has the disease.

- Surgical asepsis is an attempt to prevent the patient from coming in contact with *any* microorganisms.

- Sterile technique is required in many patient activities, such as administering an injection, starting an intravenous line, or performing a sterile dressing change.

- Exposure to blood, body secretions, or body tissues containing blood or secretions requires immediate action. Minimize the exposure by washing hands or flushing the area thoroughly. Contact the infection control or employee health nurse as soon after the exposure as possible, and complete an injury report.

- The task of the infection control nurse is to minimize the number of infections in the healthcare facility.

- A key factor in minimizing infectious outbreaks is recognizing unusual disease patterns.

Promoting Safety

Overview

Accidents or unintentional injuries (e.g., motor vehicle accidents, poisoning, and falls) are the fifth leading cause of death in the United States. A person's safety is influenced by developmental factors as well as lifestyle, cognitive awareness, and mobility status.

The main safety hazards in the home are poisoning, scalds and burns, fires, falls, firearm injuries, suffocation and drowning, and take-home toxins. Over half of all falls occur in the home; about 80% involve people over the age of 65 years. Smoking is the leading cause of home fire deaths.

Nursing interventions for promoting safety in the home focus on client teaching.

Hazardous agents in the community are a major contributor to illness, disability, and death worldwide. They include motor vehicle accidents, pathogens, improper sanitation, pollution (air, water, noise, and soil), and electrical storms.

Risks to safety in the healthcare agency include falls, equipment-related accidents, fires and electrical hazards, restraints, and mercury poisoning. Workplace hazards to nurses include back injuries, needlestick injuries, radiation injury, and violence. The Occupational Safety and Health Administration (OSHA) has enacted regulations to help prevent needlestick injuries.

Thinking Critically About Promoting Safety

The exercises in the following section allow you to practice the kind of thinking you will use as a full-spectrum nurse. Because these are critical-thinking activities, there is usually no single right answer. Discuss answers with your peers—discussion can stimulate critical thinking. If you have difficulty with any of the questions, consult with your instructor.

Caring for the Garcias

Refer to the database for Joseph Garcia on page 2. Use full-spectrum thinking to identify safety hazards for Mr. Garcia, his 3-year-old grandchild (Bettina Sanford, who lives with him), and his widowed mother, Katherine, who lives alone.

A. Without even using any patient data from the database (except ages), what theoretical knowledge do you have that will help you to identify risks that commonly occur in the developmental stages represented by these three clients?

Mr. Garcia

Mr. Garcia's 3-year-old grandchild, Bettina

Mr. Garcia's widowed mother, Katherine

B. From Mr. Garcia's database, what data can you put with your theoretical knowledge to identify the most likely safety risks for him? What are those risks?

C. From the risks and possible risks you have identified, for which one do you definitely need more data before deciding whether it increases his risk for accidents? That is, which piece of data is especially vague? What do you need to find out?

D. You know the theoretical (or possible) risks for Mr. Garcia's mother. What data do you need in order to determine her *actual* safety risks?

E. What, if any, data do you have that would help you to identify any *actual* safety risks for Mr. Garcia's grandchild? What, if any, are those risks?

F. What would you want to assess at the preschool to be sure that safety measures exist with respect to preventing falls?

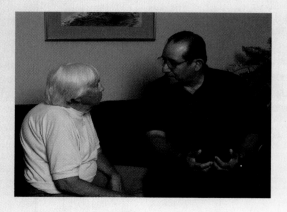

1 Recall from "Meet Your Patient" in Volume 1 the clients you encountered in the community setting. Teresa was caring for her 2-year-old son and her elderly grandmother. The grandmother has a fear of falling. In Volume 1 we addressed some of the issues related to "child-proofing" the home. You would like to suggest ways for Teresa to safe proof the home for her frail grandmother.

a Refer to the critical-thinking model and questions on the page facing the inside back cover of this text. What questions in the Inquiry section should you ask before making suggestions to Teresa?

b What specific information do you need about the grandmother? About the home?

c Once you have the necessary information, what suggestions could you make about safe proofing the home?

d Consider alternatives. What types of assistive devices might be helpful in preventing falls?

e Explore the alternatives. For example, are they practical? What do you need to know about this family to determine whether it is practical for them to obtain such devices?

f Think now about Teresa. Given the situation, what might create a safety risk for her?

thinking critically about promoting safety

2 Recall Alvin Lin (Meet Your Patients, in Volume 1), the 79-year-old man you were assigned to care for on your first day on the medical unit. The initial report you received was that he was alert and oriented, but you find that he is now confused and is becoming combative.

a What should be your first two priorities in this situation?

b What specific patient data do you need to determine what might have caused this change in behavior? How could you get that data?

c What steps could you take to ensure his safety?

d Would you consider calling the doctor to get an order for restraints?

e What alternatives to restraints might you consider?

3 A friend calls to tell you she thinks her 10-month-old daughter swallowed some of her sleeping pills. The child is very sleepy, and your friend is having difficulty arousing her. Your friend has ipecac in her medicine cabinet and wonders whether she should try to get her awake enough to take it.

a What is the first thing that you would recommend that the mother do?

b What is a major concern with inducing vomiting, given that you must assume from the mother that the child is very drowsy. What could go wrong if the child vomits?

c If the mother decides to take the daughter to the hospital instead of taking time to call the poison control center (PCC), what should you remind her to take with her?

4 An older couple both have health problems and are on several medications. The husband has assumed care for himself and his wife, Ethyl, because Ethyl has been exhibiting confusion at times. He says he sometimes becomes overwhelmed with everything he has to do, and he is not sure that he always gives the medicine at the right times.

a What information do you need to know to be able help with this situation? About the medications? About resources? How would you obtain the information?

b What suggestions can you make to help the husband organize the medications?

5 You are caring for a patient the first day after surgery following an abdominal hysterectomy. She asks you to help her to ambulate to a chair. You note that she has intravenous fluids infusing and is receiving narcotics via patient-controlled analgesia (PCA) pump. She states that she has not been out of bed since surgery and that she has just administered some medication and would like to get up while she has pain relief. You also notice that there is a Foley (indwelling urinary) catheter connected to a bedside drainage.

a What environmental factors could be safety hazards when this patient gets out of bed?

b What assessments and other interventions would help to ensure safe ambulation despite those obstacles?

6 For each of the following concepts, use critical thinking to describe how or why it is important to nursing, patient care, or promoting safety. Note that these are *not* to be merely definitions.

Environmental hazard

Pathogens

Poisoning

Scald injuries

Falls

Teaching firearm safety to children

Pollution

Radiation

Restraint

Ambularm

Heimlich maneuver

Refrigeration

Mosquito control

Rodent control

Reduce, reuse, recycle, respond

thinking critically about promoting safety

Back injuries

Needlestick injuries

Time, distance, and shielding

Gang culture

Morse Fall Scale

Practical Knowledge
knowing why

Nursing interventions to promote safety in the home focus mainly on patient teaching. In hospitals and long-term care facilities, however, you will take a more proactive role in preventing injury to patients. In addition to patient advocacy activities, you will need practical knowledge of measures other than restraints (e.g., bed and chair monitors) that can be used to prevent falls. You must also know how to apply and manage restraints safely.

PROCEDURES

PROCEDURE 21–1 Using a Bed Monitoring Device

 For steps to follow in *all* procedures, refer to the inside back cover of this book.

critical aspects
- Explain to the patient and family that the device alerts the staff when the patient tries to get out of the chair or bed.
- Apply or place the device; connect the control unit to the sensor pad.
- Connect the control unit to the nurse call system, if possible.
- Explain that the patient will need to call for assistance when she wants to get up.
- Disconnect or turn off the alarm prior to assisting the patient out of the bed or chair.
- Reactivate the alarm after assisting the patient back to the bed or chair.

Equipment
Bed or chair exit monitoring device. Check the alarm on the monitoring device to ensure that it is working properly.

Delegation
As the nurse, you must determine whether a monitoring device is needed. You must also select the appropriate device and provide ongoing evaluation of its effectiveness. You may delegate to a UAP the installation of the device, after verifying that the UAP has the necessary knowledge and skill

Assessments
- Assess the patient's risk for falls, including mobility status and level of awareness.
- Assess for the need for fall prevention measures.

➤

PROCEDURE 21–1   Using a Bed Monitoring Device *(continued)*

Procedural Steps

Step 1 Apply the device.

a. Place sensor pads for the bed or chair under the patient's buttocks.

The sensor will alarm when the patient attempts to get out of the bed or chair; it alarms when there is no weight on it for more than a few seconds. ▼

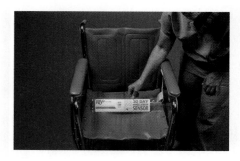

b. Alternatively, place leg sensors on the patient's thigh.

The alarm will sound when the leg assumes a near-vertical position. ▼

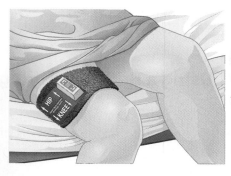

Step 2 Connect the control unit to the sensor pad.

a. Mount the control unit for the bed or chair sensor on the bed or chair.

b. Mount the control unit for a leg sensor directly on the leg sensor.

Step 3 Connect the control unit to the nurse call system, if possible.

Allows for a quicker response; however, not all call systems will accommodate this.

Step 4 Disconnect or turn off the alarm prior to assisting the patient out of the bed or chair.

Prevents false alarm.

Step 5 Reactivate the alarm after assisting the patient back to the bed or chair.

Helps prevent patient falls.

Evaluation

- Assess the sensitivity of the monitoring device, and adjust as needed to ensure that the alarm is activated if the patient tries to get out of the bed or chair.
- Continue to assess fall risk per agency policy and as indicated by the patient's physical and/or mental status.

Patient Teaching

- Explain to the patient and family that a bed or chair exit monitoring device alerts the staff when the patient tries to get out of the chair or bed.

Explaining that the purpose of the device is to help prevent falls using the least restrictive method possible will reassure the patient and family.

- Explain to the patient that she will need to call for assistance when she wants to get up.

Calling for assistance will prevent the alarm from sounding and help prevent the patient from falling.

PROCEDURE 21–1 **Using a Bed Monitoring Device** *(continued)*

Documentation

- Document the initial sensor placement, including type of sensor used and the location of placement.
- Place the patient on fall risk precautions according to agency policy.
- Document on fall risk assessment sheet, restraint flowsheet, and nurses' notes according to agency policy.

Example

8/22/06	1000	Bed sensor applied under buttocks due to confusion and repeated attempts to get out of bed. Family notified of pt. condition.
		S. Esrun, RN

PROCEDURE 21–2 **Using Restraints**

 For steps to follow in *all* procedures, refer to the inside back cover of this book.

critical aspects

- Follow agency policy and state laws for using restraints.
- Medicare standards allow for restraints only if the patient (1) is a danger to self or others, or (2) must be immobilized temporarily so that a procedure may be performed.
- Obtain a medical order for the restraint; in an emergency, apply restraints, and obtain a medical order within 24 hours. The order must be renewed every 24 hours. Guidelines are more restrictive when drugs are used for behavior management.
- Obtain patient and family consent when feasible; explain the need for the restraints.
- Pad bony prominences (e.g., wrists, ankles) as needed before applying the restraint.
- Tie and knot the restraints so that they can be released quickly in an emergency.
- Never tie restraints to a siderail.
- Adjust restraints to maintain good body alignment, comfort, and safety.
- Be sure that restraints do not impair blood circulation to any body area.
- At least every 2 hours:
  - Release restraints and provide skin care, passive and active range of motion, ambulation, toileting, hydration, and nutrition. Document.
  - Assess circulation, skin integrity, and need for continuing restraint. Document.
- Check the restraints every 30 minutes.

➤

PROCEDURE 21–2   **Using Restraints** (*continued*)

Equipment

- Restraint of the appropriate size: belt, vest, wrist or ankle, or mitt
- Soft gauze or cotton padding for bony prominences

Delegation

As the nurse, you must determine whether restraints are needed in each specific situation. You must also select the appropriate type of restraints, evaluate their effectiveness, and continue to assess for complications that may occur. You may delegate to UAP the application and periodic removal of ordered restraints, after verifying that the UAP has the knowledge and skill to do so.

Assessments

- Assess patient's risk for falls, including mobility status and level of awareness.
- Assess for need for restraints: (1) patient is a danger to self or others, or (2) patient must be temporarily restrained so that a procedure may be performed.
- Identify the appropriate restraint:
  - The least restrictive possible.
  - Does not interfere with care or exacerbate patient's medical condition.
  - Does not pose a safety risk to the patient.
  - Can be changed easily to keep it clean.

Procedural Steps

Step 1 Obtain a physician's order for restraint, including type of restraint, indications for use, site of restraint application, and duration.

Federal and state laws prohibit healthcare facilities from using restraints unless they are medically needed. If restraints are used, they must be based on a physician's order for a specified and limited time. You may apply restraint in an emergency, but patient should be medically evaluated and an order should be written within 24 hours. Guidelines are more restrictive when drugs are used for behavior management.

Step 2 Explain to the patient and family the need for restraints, and obtain patient and family consent when clinically feasible.

Patients have the right to refuse treatment. Consent may not be possible if there is an immediate threat to patient safety. However, as a rule the family must be notified of the use of restraints if the patient has cognitive impairment.

Step 3 Apply the appropriately sized restraint, using appropriate knotting techniques.

a. Use a quick-release knot, such as the half-bow, when tying restraints to the bed frame or wheelchair. Do not tie restraints to the siderails.

A quick-release knot is used to prevent patient injury and for ease of caring for the patient. Tie the knot on an immovable part of the bed to prevent injuring the patient if the siderails or head of bed are lowered. A half-bow knot will not tighten or slip when the patient moves about, but unties quickly when you pull on the loose end. ▼

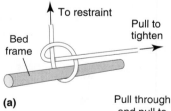

To restraint
Pull to tighten
Bed frame
(a)

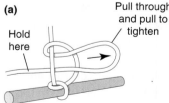

Pull through and pull to tighten
Hold here
(b)

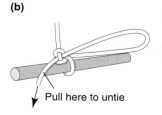

Pull here to untie
(c)

b. Belt restraint:
  1) Place belt restraint at the patient's waist, removing any wrinkles.
  2) Make sure that the belt is snug but does not constrict the patient's waist.
  3) Some belts have a key-locked buckle to prevent slipping.

A belt restraint is used mainly to prevent a patient from falling when getting up from a chair or wheelchair and may be used to remind a patient not to get out of bed unassisted. ▼

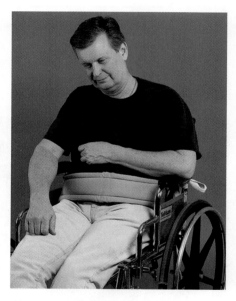

c. Vest or jacket restraint:
  1) Place the patient in the vest restraint. A zipper-style vest is preferred.

A vest restraint with a rear zipper is less likely to accidentally strangle the patient.

  2) Attach the vest straps to the bed or wheelchair.

PROCEDURE 21–2 **Using Restraints** *(continued)*

A vest restraint is used mainly to prevent a patient from falling out of a chair or wheelchair and may be used to prevent a patient from getting out of bed unassisted. ▼

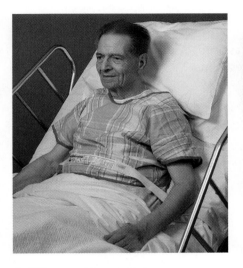

d. Wrist or ankle restraint:
1) Apply the padded portion of the wrist or ankle restraint around the patient's wrist or ankle.
2) Make the restraint snug enough to prevent the patient from being able to slip it off, but not tight enough to impair circulation. Generally, you should be able to slide two fingers under the restraint.
3) Attach the restraint strap to the bed frame. Do not attach to bed rails.

A wrist restraint is used mainly to prevent a patient from pulling at tubes, such as IV sites and nasogastric tubes. Wrist and ankle restraints are used with an extremely agitated patient. Ankle restraints are used in very limited situations. ▼

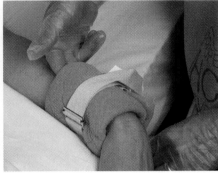

e. Mitt restraint:
1) Place patient's hand in mitt restraint, ensuring that fingers are slightly flexed in the mitt.
2) Attach restraint strap to the bed frame.

A mitt restraint is used mainly to prevent a patient from pulling at tubes, such as IV sites and nasogastric tubes. ▼

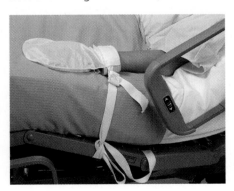

Step 4 Adjust the restraint to maintain good body alignment, comfort, and safety.

Step 5 Release restraints and provide skin care, passive and active range of motion, ambulation, toileting, hydration, and nutrition at least every 2 hours.

Prevents impaired circulation and injury. Medicare- and Medicaid-certified healthcare agencies must ensure that a patient's abilities do not decline unless the decline cannot be avoided because of the patient's medical condition. Patients often lose the ability to bathe, dress, walk, toilet, eat, and communicate when they are regularly restrained. If restraints are necessary, they must be used in a way that does not cause these losses.

Step 6 Assess the restraint every 30 minutes.

Ensures that it is still functioning as intended.

Step 7 Place the patient on fall risk precautions according to agency policy.

Helps prevent injury.

Evaluation
• Assess the initial restraint placement, circulation, and skin integrity. Observe for pallor, cyanosis, and coolness of extremities when extremities are restrained.
• Assess the need for continuing the use of the restraint every 2 hours, and remove it when it is no longer needed.

➤

PROCEDURE 21–2   **Using Restraints** *(continued)*

Patient Teaching

- Explain to the patient and family the need for the restraints.
- Explain that the restraints will be removed as soon as possible.

Home Care

- The same guidelines apply to clients in the home.
- Evaluate caregivers' knowledge and skill in using restraints, and provide teaching as needed (e.g., regarding padding bony prominences and the need to periodically release restraints).

Documentation

- Document the initial restraint placement, circulation, and skin integrity. Document reasons for placing the restraint (e.g., patient behaviors).
- Document on fall risk assessment sheet, restraint flowsheet, and nurses' notes according to agency policy.

Example

9/8/06   0800   Pt. oriented to self only. Attempting to remove IV lines and abd. dsg. Attempts to reorient unsuccessful. MD notified. Wrist restraints applied. Hands warm, sensation intact, capillary refill 2 seconds, skin intact. Will continue to monitor and attempt to reorient. – S. Max, RN

TECHNIQUES

The nursing interventions in this section focus on emergency procedures for choking. We describe the Heimlich maneuver for children and adults and a recommended procedure for infants under 12 months old.

TECHNIQUE 21–1	**Performing the Heimlich Maneuver on an Infant or Child**

The Heimlich maneuver is an emergency procedure for removing a foreign object lodged in the airway. It lifts the diaphragm and forces enough air from the lungs to create an artificial cough. The cough should move and expel the obstruction from the airway.

Caveats

- The American Heart Association does not recommend using the Heimlich maneuver on infants under 12 months of age.
- For maximum effectiveness and safety, these procedures should be learned by demonstration and supervised practice on a mannequin.
- Before doing the Heimlich maneuver, be certain that the airway is completely blocked. *If the child can talk or cry, do not do the maneuver*—have the child continue to try to cough up the foreign object on his own.
- The child may vomit after being treated with the Heimlich maneuver.

Infants Under 12 Months Old

- Perform this choking rescue procedure instead of the Heimlich maneuver.
- Sit, and rest your forearm on your thigh.
- Place the infant face down along your forearm, head lower than the trunk, supporting the head in your hand. Don't cover the infant's mouth.
- With the heel of your other hand, give four or five rapid blows to the infant's back between the shoulder blades.
- If the airway remains blocked, sandwich the infant between both your forearms, and turn him over so that he is lying face up, supported by the opposite arm (not the one you began with).
- Check the mouth for the object; look, but do not do blind finger-sweeps.

- With your free hand, use two finger on the center of the breastbone, and make four sharp upward chest thrusts.
- Look for the object in the baby's mouth. If you see it, remove it and give two rescue breaths.
- Continue alternating back blows and chest thrusts, observing for the foreign object, until the infant coughs up the object.
- Do not be too vigorous with back blows and chest thrusts; this can injure the infant's bones and internal organs.
- If you cannot dislodge the object call 911 and begin rescue breathing. Continue with back blows, chest thrusts, and rescue breathing until help arrives or the infant starts breathing.

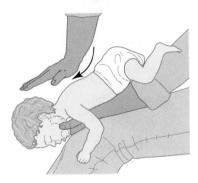

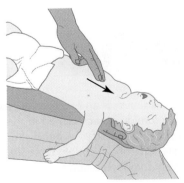

TECHNIQUE 21–1   Performing the Heimlich Maneuver on an Infant or Child (continued)

Children Over 12 Months Old

- If you suspect that a child has aspirated, encourage her to continue coughing as long as the cough remains forceful. If the cough becomes ineffective or the child is unable to make any sounds, then use the Heimlich maneuver in an attempt to dislodge the object.
- Tell the child you are going to help.
- Do not try to clear the airway.
- Call 911 if you are concerned about the child's breathing. ▼

- If the child is standing, the technique in children over 12 months old is the same as for adults, except that you use less force than for an adult to prevent damage to the child's ribs, breastbone, and internal organs.
- Deliver upward thrusts to the upper abdomen with your fisted hand, just below the rib cage. If the child becomes unresponsive, perform chest compressions similar to CPR.
- See Technique 21–2, following. ▼

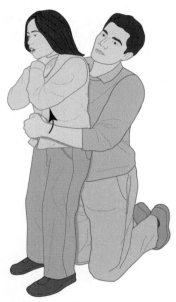

Child is conscious

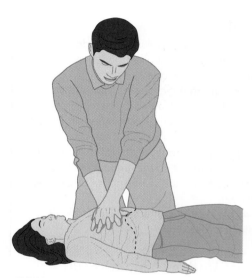

Child is unconscious

TECHNIQUE 21–2   Performing the Heimlich Maneuver on an Adult

The Heimlich maneuver is an emergency procedure for removing a foreign object lodged in the airway. It lifts the diaphragm and forces enough air from the lungs to create an artificial cough. The cough should move and expel the obstruction from the airway.

Caveats

- For maximum effectiveness and safety, these procedures should be learned by demonstration and supervised practice on a mannequin.

- Before doing the Heimlich maneuver, be certain that the airway is completely blocked. *If the person can talk or cry, do not do the maneuver*—have the person continue to try to cough up the foreign object on his own.
- The person may vomit after being treated with the Heimlich maneuver.

TECHNIQUE 21–2	**Performing the Heimlich Maneuver on an Adult** *(continued)*

Adults—Conscious

- Ask, "Are you choking?" Observe for the universal distress signal: clutching the neck between thumb and index finger.
- Indications that the airway is blocked:
  Person cannot speak or cough.
  Face turns blue.
  Person has weak, labored breathing that produces a high-pitched noise.
  Person becomes unconscious.
- If you determine that the airway is blocked, stand behind the victim (the victim may be sitting or standing).
- Place your arms under victim's armpits to encircle the chest.
- Make a fist with one hand; place the thumb toward the victim, below the ribcage and above the waist; place your other hand on top of the fist.
- Give a series of 6 to 10 quick, forceful, upward and inward thrusts to try to force the object back up the trachea.
- If the effort fails, keep repeating the series of 6 to 10 abdominal thrusts. As the victim loses consciousness,

the tracheal muscles relax slightly, so the object may be expelled on the second or third attempts.
- If the foreign object is removed and the victim is still not breathing, start CPR.

Adults—Unconscious

- If the person is (or becomes) unconscious, lay him on the floor.
- Shout for help. Call 911 and begin standard CPR, including chest compressions. See Procedure 35–12 in Chapter 35.
- Each time you open the airway in CPR, look for the object. If you see it, remove it. Do not perform blind finger sweeps.
- Do not perform abdominal thrusts.
- Continue CPR until the person breathes on his own or until help arrives.

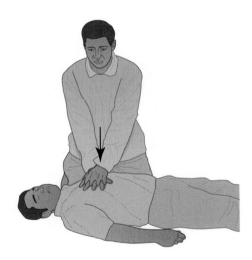

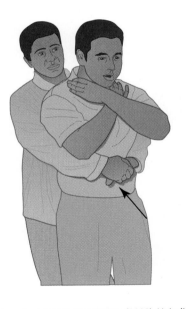

Sources: The American Heart Association. (2002). Heimlich maneuver: AHA recommendation. Retrieved January 11, 2004, from http://www.americanheart.org/presenter.jhtml?identifier=4605; National Institutes of Health (2004). Medical encyclopedia: Heimlich maneuver. Retrieved January 11, 2004, from http://www.nim.nih.gov/medlineplus/ency/article/000047.htm; CHC Thompson Corporation, Medical Library & Patient Education. (2004). Heimlich maneuver. Retrieved January 11, 2004, from www.chclibrary.org/micromed/00050520.html

TECHNIQUE 21–3   **Preventing Needlestick Injury**

- Avoid recapping a contaminated (used) needle; deposit it directly into an accessible sharps container. If you must recap, use a one-handed "scoop" method (see Procedure 23–9 in Chapter 23).
- When you must recap a sterile needle, use safety equipment or a modified "scoop" technique (see Procedure 23–9).
- Never carry syringes in your uniform pocket.
- Be sure that puncture-proof needle disposal containers are kept in every room.

If your agency does not use needleless systems or protective devices:

- Explain the OSHA Bloodborne Pathogens Standard (BPS) to your employer, including the need to provide needleless systems or protective devices for blood products and parenteral medication administration.
- Refer your employer to the OSHA web site at www.osha.gov/needlesticks/needlefaq.html

- OSHA requires worker involvement in evaluating, selecting, and implementing the use of safer needle products; volunteer to serve on that committee.
- Ask your agency for a copy of their exposure control plan, which is required by the BPS for monitoring compliance with the new law.
- Keep a record of needlestick injuries on your unit and of "near-misses" (e.g., overfilled sharps containers, sharps left on bed or overbed table).
- Submit written concerns to your employer.
- If your employer refuses to purchase safety devices, you may want to file an OSHA complaint (see www.osha.gov/as/opa/worker/complain.html). If you do, refer to Chapter 44, whistleblowing.

Source: Adapted from Wilburn, S. (2003). Health and safety: The needlestick law. *American Journal of Nursing, 103*(2), 104.

ASSESSMENT GUIDELINES AND TOOLS

Home Safety Checklist

Home Safety

____ Are smoke detectors installed in appropriate locations and operating properly?

____ Is water heater temperature set at a safe level to avoid scalds?

____ Do you keep extra fuses on hand?

____ Do small rugs have nonskid backing?

____ Do you have a proper step stool or ladder for in-home use?

____ Are there covers on electrical outlets where children play?

____ Are all firearms safely stored and locked according to current regulations?

____ Are emergency numbers posted at all telephones?

Entrances

____ Is there adequate lighting at entrances?

____ Are steps well maintained?

____ Are snow and ice immediately cleared from doorsteps?

____ Are shoes, boots, umbrellas, and so on, neatly stored inside?

____ Are other tripping hazards (toys, puddles from wet boots, and so on) cleaned away?

Stairways

____ Are stairways clear of all hazards, such as shoes and toys?

____ Are there full-length handrails in good repair?

____ Can stairways be well lighted?

____ Are treads, risers, and carpeting in good condition?

____ Are spills and wet surfaces cleaned up immediately?

Bathrooms

____ Do you use nonskid mats/surfaces in bathtubs to prevent falls?

____ Do you have a proper medicine cabinet?

____ Are expired medications disposed of properly?

____ Do you keep electrical appliances away from sinks, tubs, and other water receptacles?

____ Do you use a night-light to illuminate the way to the bathroom at night?

____ Is a ground fault circuit interrupter (GFCI) installed for bathroom circuits?

Kitchen

____ Do you clean the stove's exhaust hood and duct frequently?

____ Are cleaners, disinfectants, and other poisons secured out of reach of children and away from foods?

____ Do you always use a stepstool for climbing?

____ Are utensils and knives neatly stored?

____ Are handles of pots and pans always turned away from stove fronts?

____ Are cracked or chipped dishes and glassware disposed of immediately?

____ Are spills wiped up immediately?

____ Are cupboard contents kept orderly to prevent objects from falling?

____ Is a fully charged fire extinguisher readily available?

____ Are matches and lighters kept out of reach of children?

Living Rooms and Bedrooms

____ Is furniture arranged to avoid bumping the knees and shins?

____ Are electrical cords kept away from carpets?

____ Are fireplace screens used effectively?

____ Are throw rugs avoided to prevent tripping hazards?

____ Is furniture kept away from windows to prevent young children from falling out?

____ Are screens and windows secured to prevent young children from falling out?

____ Have plans been made for a fire escape route from bedrooms?

____ Are lamps located near beds to prevent tripping in the dark?

____ Are all chimneys checked for obstructions?

Exterior Building, Cellar, Barn, Garage, Grounds

____ Are walkways, aisles, and traffic areas clear of obstructions?

____ Is there adequate lighting in work areas and driveways?

____ Are stairs in good condition and equipped with handrails?

____ Are stairs kept clear of objects both on steps and landings?

Home Safety Checklist *(continued)*

_____ Are ladders in good condition and inspected regularly?

_____ Are all floors and driveways free of holes, cracks, and other defects?

_____ Are low ceilings and beams marked clearly with signs or fluorescent materials to prevent bumping into them?

_____ Are stored materials properly stacked to prevent them from falling?

_____ Are protrusions, such as nails, removed from walls, railings, and used lumber to prevent contact?

_____ Are spills wiped up immediately?

_____ Is there ample walking space between stored machines and materials?

_____ Are keys removed from stored machines?

_____ Do large doors open smoothly?

_____ Do you keep your tractor and/or other fuel-burning equipment in an outbuilding separate from the barn or other buildings?

_____ Do you avoid storing flammable liquids in garages, barns, or other structures?

_____ Do you keep the garage door down and locked at all times; test the automatic reverse mechanism monthly; and keep remote controls away from children?

_____ Do you always supervise children in the garage, where many hazards exist (e.g., motor oil, insecticides, power tools)?

_____ If you own a pool, is it covered when not in use and/or enclosed with a fence to prevent access without your knowledge. Is a flotation device or other rescue equipment within immediate reach? Are children always supervised when they are in or near a pool, pond, or other body of water?

Source: National Ag Safety Database (NASD). (2003). *Home safety 1, 2, and 3.* Retrieved November 13, 2003, from http://www.cdc.gov/nasd/docs/d001501-d001600/d001509/1.html

STANDARDIZED LANGUAGE

NANDA Diagnoses and NOC Outcomes for Safety Problems

NANDA Diagnostic Label	Associated NOC Outcomes (Examples)
Hyperthermia Hypothermia Ineffective Thermoregulation Risk for Imbalanced Body Temperature	Thermoregulation Thermoregulation: Newborn Vital Signs
Impaired Skin Integrity Risk for Impaired Skin Integrity Impaired Tissue Integrity	Tissue Integrity: Skin & Mucous Membranes Wound Healing: Primary Intention Wound Healing: Secondary Intention
Ineffective Airway Clearance (choking)	Aspiration Prevention Respiratory Status: Airway Patency Respiratory Status: Gas Exchange Respiratory Status: Ventilation
Ineffective Protection	Abuse Protection Endurance Immune Status Immunization Behavior Neurological Status: Consciousness
Latex Allergy Response Risk for Latex Allergy Response	Immune Hypersensitivity Response Tissue Integrity: Skin & Mucous Membranes
Risk for Aspiration Risk for Suffocation	Aspiration Prevention Respiratory Status: Ventilation Swallowing Status
Risk for Falls	Fall Prevention Behavior Falls Occurrence
Risk for Injury	Parenting: Psychosocial Safety Risk Control Safe Home Environment Personal Safety Behavior Physical Injury Severity
Risk for Poisoning Risk for Trauma	Safe Home Environment Personal Safety Behavior Physical Injury Severity Tissue Integrity: Skin & Mucous Membranes
Risk for Infection	Immune Status Infection Severity Risk Control: Sexually Transmitted Diseases (STD) Wound Healing: Primary Intention Wound Healing: Secondary Intention

NANDA Diagnoses and NOC Outcomes for Safety Problems *(continued)*

NANDA Diagnostic Label	Associated NOC Outcomes (Examples)
Risk for Perioperative Positioning Injury	Circulation Status Neurological Status: Spinal Sensory/Motor Function Respiratory Status: Ventilation Tissue Perfusion: Peripheral
Risk for Sudden Infant Death Syndrome	Risk Control Safe Home Environment

Sources: NANDA International. (2005). *Nursing diagnoses: Definitions and classification 2005–2006.* Philadelphia: Author; Moorhead, S., Johnson, M., & Maas, M. (Eds.). (2004). *Nursing outcomes classification (NOC)* (3rd ed.). St Louis: Mosby; Johnson, M., Bulechek, G., McCloskey Dochterman, J., Maas, M., & Moorhead, S. (2001). *Nursing diagnoses, outcomes, and interventions: NANDA, NOC, and NIC linkages.* St Louis: Mosby.

Examples of NIC Interventions Related to Safety

Examples of Interventions from the Safety Domain

Abuse Protection Support (Child, Domestic Partner, Elder, Religious)

Allergy Management

Area Restriction

Aspiration Precautions

Dementia Management

Elopement Precautions

Environmental Management: Safety

Fall Prevention

Fire-Setting Precautions

Infection Control

Latex Precautions

Physical Restraint

Radiation Therapy Management

Sports-Injury Prevention: Youth

Suicide Prevention

Surveillance: Safety

Vehicle Safety Promotion

Examples of Safety Interventions from Other Domains

Communicable Disease Management

Community Disaster Preparedness

Environmental Management: Community

Environmental Management: Worker Safety

Home Maintenance Assistance

Surveillance: Community

Source: Dochterman, J. M., & Bulechek, G. (Eds.). (2004). *Nursing interventions classification (NIC)* (4th ed.). St Louis: Mosby.

What Are the Main Points in this Chapter?

- Safety is a basic human need.
- Unintentional injuries are the fifth leading cause of death in the United States.
- Major causes of unintentional deaths in the United States are motor vehicle accidents, poisoning, and falls.
- The environment includes the physical and psychosocial factors that contribute to the life and well-being of each person. It may be identified as any setting where the nurse and client interact.
- A person's safety is influenced by developmental factors as well as individual factors, such as lifestyle, cognitive awareness, and mobility status.
- The main safety hazards in the home are poisoning, carbon monoxide poisoning, scalds and burns, fires, falls, firearm injuries, suffocation and drowning, and take-home toxins.
- Most fatal home fires occur while people are asleep, and most deaths result from smoke inhalation.
- Over half of all falls occur in the home; about 80% involve people over the age of 65 years.

- The Heimlich maneuver is performed to remove a foreign body from a choking victim.
- Nursing interventions for promoting safety in the home focus on client teaching.
- Community hazards include motor vehicle accidents, pathogens, improper sanitation, pollution (air, water, noise, and soil), and electrical storms.
- Safety hazards in the healthcare agency include falls, equipment-related accidents, fires and electrical hazards, restraints, and mercury poisoning.
- When possible, nurses should use alternative interventions instead of restraints.
- Workplace hazards to nurses include back injuries, needlestick injuries, radiation injury, and violence.
- The U.S. Occupational Safety and Health Administration (OSHA) has enacted regulations to help prevent needlestick injuries.
- All inpatients should be assessed for their risk for falls.

22 Facilitating Hygiene

Overview

Although many hygiene measures can be delegated to a UAP, as a nurse, you will retain full responsibility for each patient. One of your primary functions will be to teach patients about hygiene, with the goal of encouraging the patient's independence with the tasks.

Basic hygiene measures include care of the skin, perineum, genitals, feet, nails, mouth, hair, eyes, ears, and nose. Bathing removes perspiration and bacteria from the skin surface. Because skin function declines with age, older persons are more prone to skin infection, wound and rash formation, and delayed healing.

Numerous factors influence individual hygiene practices, including: personal preferences, cultural/religious/spiritual values and beliefs, economic status, living environment, developmental or knowledge level, and physical and emotional health. Demonstrate your caring by considering your patients' cultural, spiritual, and personal hygiene preferences and incorporating them into the care plan whenever possible.

Thinking Critically About Facilitating Hygiene

The exercises in the following section allow you to practice the kind of thinking you will use as a full-spectrum nurse. Because these are critical-thinking activities, there is usually no single right answer. Discuss answers with your peers—discussion can stimulate critical thinking. If you have difficulty with any of the questions, consult with your instructor.

Caring for the Garcias

Flordelisa Garcia works as a day-care teacher. She schedules a clinic visit to discuss a variety of concerns. For each of the concerns she mentions, answer the following four questions:

1. What theoretical knowledge do you need?
2. Where could you find it?
3. What, if any, additional patient information do you need?
4. How would you respond to Mrs. Garcia's concerns?

A. Flordelisa tells you that her skin is very dry and irritated.

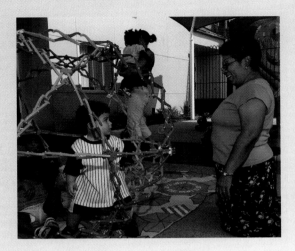

B. Flordelisa tells you that several of the children at the day-care center have recently been diagnosed with "head lice." She would like to know how to assess for pediculosis.

C. Flordelisa tells you that her 3-year-old granddaughter, Bettina, frequently refuses to bathe. She asks for advice on how to handle this.

1 You are caring for Mrs. Little, a 57-year-old woman who has been experiencing severe arthritic pain for the past 2 years. She rates her pain at an 8 or 9 on a 10-point pain-rating scale. During your assessment, you notice that Mrs. Little has a moderate body odor, long and untrimmed fingernails and toenails, oily hair, and unshaven legs and axillae. Mrs. Little readily admits that she has neglected her hygiene practices.

a What is the first hygiene-related nursing diagnosis (problem and etiology) that comes to your mind for Mrs. Little?

b What data do you have to support a diagnosis of Bathing/Hygiene Self-Care Deficit? What data do you have to support an etiology of "immobility secondary to pain"?

c With the information in the scenario, can you accurately rate her Self-Care Deficit on a scale of 1 to 4?

d Anything you could do to help relieve Mrs. Little's pain would facilitate her self-care abilities. However, to plan interventions in which you will assist with her hygiene care, what further patient data do you need?

e Suppose you assess Mrs. Little further and determine that she has arthritis in multiple joints, including her hands, shoulders, back, knees, and feet. You also determine that she will need a complete bath, either tub or shower, but that she can brush her own teeth if someone provides the necessary supplies. Could you delegate her A.M. hygiene care to an experienced UAP? If so, what instructions would you give the UAP?

2 Mr. Thomson is an 87-year-old African American man admitted 2 days ago after being found unconscious in his small apartment. Although Mr. Thomson denies being diabetic, his admission blood sugar was 653 mg/dL. His lower legs are swollen, red, and weeping a clear fluid. His toenails are long, thick, and yellow, and there is a small open sore on the great toe of his left foot. Mr. Thomson's skin is dry and scaly, his hair matted, and he has a strong odor of perspiration and urine. In addition, he is uncircumcised. He refuses help with hygiene, saying, "I've taken care of myself for 87 years, and I'll keep doing it. I take my bath once a week on Saturday evening. Now go away!"

a What theoretical knowledge will you need in order to know what to assess and how to provide his hygiene care?

b Self-knowledge is important in this case as well. What things in this situation would make caring for Mr. Thomson especially difficult for you? What things might interfere with your ability to give your best care?

3 Your instructor has assigned you to assist the following patients with their hygiene. You must assess the needs of each person, gather information on their bathing habits and preferences, plan nursing measures necessary to meet individual needs, and together with a UAP (unlicensed assistive personnel), provide care.

The first person on your assignment is Mrs. Williams, a 76-year-old Indian American woman who was admitted yesterday after suffering a stroke that paralyzed her right side. Since the stroke, she has been unable to speak clearly and becomes frustrated as she attempts to communicate her needs. Her daughter says Mrs. Williams is a proud, independent, and tidy woman who has been living alone since her husband's death last year. She has been driving her car, cleaning the house, doing her grocery shopping, and maintaining the yard and garden. She wears eyeglasses for reading and driving and has a hearing aid, although she rarely uses it.

The second person on your assignment is Mr. Gold, a 68-year-old man of Orthodox Jewish religion, admitted last week after he experienced a massive heart attack. Although his eyes are open, he is unresponsive to external stimuli. Because of Impaired Swallowing, Mr. Gold is unable to take food or fluid orally; his family has chosen to have a feeding tube placed to ensure adequate nutrition and hydration. His oral mucous membranes and lips are dry and crusty. He is incontinent of urine and stool. Mr. Gold's son, Ira, tells you that throughout his life Mr. Gold adhered to Orthodox Jewish law. The son requests that, in honor of his father, certain aspects of these laws be included in the care plan.

The following questions are about Mrs. Williams.

a To assess Mrs. Williams's self-care abilities, what important patient data do you still need?

b What problem has resulted from her stroke that will make it difficult for you to find out about Mrs. Williams's hygiene preferences and practices?

c From what you know of the patient situation, why do you think Mrs. Williams is becoming frustrated?

d How do you think you would react if this were to happen to you?

e How could you provide opportunities for Mrs. Williams to maintain her independence?

thinking critically about facilitating hygiene

The following questions are about Mr. Gold.

a What additional theoretical knowledge do you need to meet Mr. Gold's religious and cultural needs when providing hygiene care?

b Where could you obtain such information?

c If you decide to delegate Mr. Gold's bed bath to a UAP, how could you incorporate his religious and cultural needs into your delegation decisions?

5 For each of the following concepts, use critical thinking to describe how or why it is important to nursing, patient care, or facilitating hygiene. Note that these are *not* to be merely definitions.

Personal hygiene

Delegation of tasks

Cultural differences

Skin integrity

Life span variables

Self-Care Deficits

The nursing process

Patient teaching

Bathing

Oral care

Environment and comfort

Hair care

Nail care

thinking critically about facilitating hygiene

Practical Knowledge
knowing how

The following procedures and techniques provide the practical knowledge you will need to assist patients with personal cleanliness and grooming. As a nurse you are responsible for providing the necessary assistance and, at the same time, promoting as much self-care as possible. Self-care in ADLs promotes increased activity, independence, and self-esteem.

This "Practical Knowledge" section also contains a guideline for assessing hygiene needs, as well as standardized language tables for Self-Care Deficits and nursing diagnoses related to hygiene.

PROCEDURES

PROCEDURE 22–1 Bathing: Providing a Complete Bed Bath

 For steps to follow in *all* procedures, refer to the inside back cover of this book.

critical aspects
- Use warm, not hot, water.
- Prevent chilling or tiring the patient.
- Bathe the patient following the principles of "head to toe" and "clean to dirty."
- For extremities, wash and dry from distal to proximal.
- Change the water before cleansing the perineum and whenever the water becomes dirty or cool.

Equipment

- Basin for water
- Bath blanket
- Bath towels (2)
- Washcloths
- Soap; may use liquid rinse-free soap (e.g., Septisoft)
- Deodorant, lotion, and/or powder as needed
- Clean patient gown (gown with shoulder snaps or Velcro closures if the patient has an IV line)
- Clean bed linen
- Procedure gloves (for anal and perineal care)
- Bedpan or urinal
- Laundry bag

Delegation

You can delegate this procedure to the UAP if you conclude that the patient's condition and the UAP's skills allow. Perform the following assessments, and inform the UAP of the specific type of bath (e.g., basin, towel, bag bath) and the amount of help the patient needs. Inform the UAP of any special considerations, such as IV lines, drains, and so on. Ask the UAP to report the condition of the patient's skin, level of self-care, and ability to tolerate the procedure.

Assessments

- Assess the patient's mobility, activity tolerance, and type of bath needed.

A patient who has decreased activity tolerance or mobility (e.g., chest pain or shortness of breath with exertion or paralysis) may have limited ability to assist with the bath. Having the patient assist as much as possible increases mobility and sense of control and comfort.

PROCEDURE 22–1

Bathing: Providing a Complete Bed Bath

(continued)

• Check for positioning or activity restrictions (e.g., maintaining hip abduction following a total hip replacement).

Prevents injuring the patient during the procedure.

• Determine the number of people you need to safely bathe and reposition the patient.

Helps prevent injury to the patient or the nurse.

• Assess for personal and cultural issues that may be of concern to the patient regarding the bath.

Bathing may conflict with the patient's sense of privacy or modesty. Cultural norms and individual preferences must be considered.

• Assess for specific patient needs and preferences during a bath, such as special soaps or lotions and extra washcloths or towels.

The presence of skin conditions or breakdown may require special soaps and/or lotions. Incontinence or drainage may require additional washcloths, towels, and precautions. Meeting patient preferences helps prevent depersonalization.

Note: Assisting with or supervising the bath provides an excellent opportunity for you to assess the patient's level of consciousness, short- and long-term memory, ability to follow instructions, range of motion, skin condition, activity tolerance, and overall self-care ability.

Procedural Steps

Step 1 Provide for patient privacy and comfort.

• Close the door or privacy curtains, adjust room temperature, and assist patient with elimination as needed.
• Ask patient and family if they wish family members to assist with the bath.

Bathing practices differ among cultures, but are often private. The patient or family may wish to have a family member assist with the bath, or the patient may prefer that they leave the room. Assisting the patient with elimination before beginning the bath helps prevent interruptions during the procedure.

Step 2 Fill the basin with warm water (approximately 105°F or 41°C). Check the temperature with a thermometer or your hand. If possible, have the patient test the water temperature.

Hot water can injure the patient and removes protective skin oils. If the water is too cool, the patient may become chilled. Use water that is comfortable for the patient.

Step 3 Adjust the bed to working height, lower the siderail nearest you, and position the patient supine close to the side of bed you will be working on.

Prevents you from having to lean over the patient or reach across the siderail, possibly causing back strain or injury. ▼

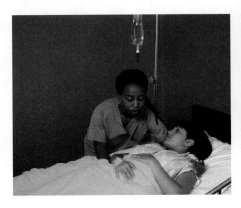

Step 4 Remove the bedspread, and spread the bath blanket over the top sheet; then have the patient hold the bath blanket in place while you remove the top sheet.

Protects modesty and prevents chilling. If no bath blanket is available, you can use the top sheet in its place. However, if the sheet becomes wet, it may chill the patient. ▼

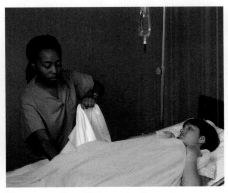

Note: Before proceeding, assist the patient with oral hygiene as needed. See Procedures 22–6 and 22–7.

Step 5 Remove the patient's gown, keeping the patient covered with the bath blanket. Keep the patient covered as much as possible during the bath, exposing just the part of the body you are bathing.

Maintains the patient's modesty and prevents chilling.

➤

PROCEDURE 22–1 Bathing: Providing a Complete Bed Bath
(continued)

Step 5 Variation Patient with an IV Line

If the patient has an IV line and is wearing a gown that does not have snap-open sleeves:

a. Remove the gown first from the arm without the IV.

b. Lower the IV container, and pass the gown over the tubing and the container, taking care to keep the container above the level of the patient's arm.

Keeps blood from backing up into the IV line. ▼

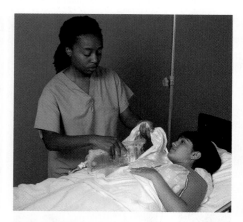

c. Rehang the container; check the flow rate.

Manipulating the IV equipment may change the flow rate; flow rate must be maintained as prescribed.

d. *Never* disconnect the IV tubing; this breaks the sterile system and provides a portal of entry for pathogens.

e. After the bath, replace the gown by threading the IV equipment from inside the arm of the gown and onto the affected arm. Then place the unaffected arm through the other arm of the gown.

Step 6 Don procedure gloves if exposure to body fluids is likely. Wash the patient's face, neck, and ears.

a. Fold the washcloth around the hand to make a mitt, tucking in loose corners.

Keeps loose ends from dragging across the skin. This is uncomfortable because loose ends cool quickly.

b. Wet the washcloth, wringing out excess water. You may wash the face without soap if the skin is dry or if the patient prefers.

Soap is a drying agent and may be inappropriate to use on the face.

c. Use a different corner of the washcloth (without soap) to gently wipe each eyelid outward from the inner canthus.

Soap is irritating to the eyes. A major principle is cleaning from "clean to dirty" to prevent contamination of a cleaner area. The inner canthus is considered the cleanest area. Prevents moving debris toward the nasolacrimal duct, which is located near the inner canthus. ▼

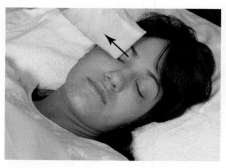

d. Wash the rest of the patient's face, neck, and ears.

Move sequentially through the bath to make it less tiring for the patient and more efficient for the nurse.

e. Rinse as needed, and pat face and neck dry.

Some soaps do not require rinsing. Pat the skin dry instead of rubbing to avoid irritation.

Step 7 Wash the patient's arms and chest.

a. Rinse and wring out the washcloth.

Rinse the washcloth frequently to ensure that it is clean and warm.

b. Fold the bath blanket off one arm at a time, and place a folded bath towel under the arm. Beginning with the patient's far arm, support the arm, and wash the arm from the hands upward using long strokes.

The folded towel keeps bottom sheet from getting wet and cold. Long strokes increase circulation in the extremity. Washing from hand upward toward the shoulder increases venous return from the periphery. Lifting the arm provides range of motion to preserve joint mobility. ▼

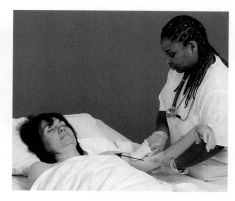

c. Continue to support the arm while washing the axilla.

Prevents potential injury to the joints. A sprain, subluxation, or dislocation of the joint can occur when an extremity is not properly supported, especially in older adults.

d. Rinse as needed, and pat the arms dry.

Rinsing preserves skin integrity by preventing the drying effect of the soap on the skin.

e. Apply deodorant and/or powder if desired.

Follow patient preferences whenever possible to increase feelings of comfort.

PROCEDURE 22–1

Bathing: Providing a Complete Bed Bath
(continued)

f. Repeat the preceding steps 7a–e for the arm nearest you.

g. Cover the patient's chest with a bath towel, and lower the bath blanket to the patient's waist.

Maintains patient comfort and modesty.

h. Wash the chest. For women, gently lift each breast to wash the skinfold if needed. Keep the chest covered between the wash and rinse.

Skinfolds can become reddened and irritated because of skin-to-skin irritation and dampness from perspiration. Skinfolds are also a source of odor. Cover to maintain privacy and warmth.

i. Rinse and pat the chest dry. Cover with a bath towel.

Rinsing preserves skin integrity by preventing the drying effect of soap on the skin.

Step 8 Wash the abdomen, legs, and feet.

a. Fold the bath blanket down to the perineal area, and cover the chest with a bath towel.

Maintains patient privacy and warmth.

b. Wash the abdomen, including the umbilical area; rinse and pat dry.

c. Cover the abdomen and chest with the bath blanket.

Prevents chilling.

d. Uncover one leg at a time, beginning with the leg farthest from you. Place the bath towel under leg.

Prevents chilling by keeping the sheet dry under the patient.

e. Place the basin of water on the towel. Supporting the ankle and heel with your hand, and the leg on your arm, help the patient bend his leg and place his foot in the basin of water to soak.

Support reduces strain on joints. Soaking allows for better cleansing of the foot, especially the toes and nails, and increases patient comfort.

f. Wash the leg from distal to proximal with long, gentle strokes. Rinse and pat the leg dry. Do not massage the calves of the legs.

Moving from distal to proximal may help to promote venous return. If a venous thrombus is present, massaging might dislodge the clot and cause an embolus. ▼

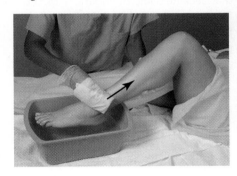

g. Thoroughly wash the foot and toes. Rinse and pat the foot dry; dry well between the toes. Apply lotion as needed.

Maintains healthy skin. Disease processes frequently decrease circulation to the feet and lower legs, increasing the likelihood that minor skin irritations may become more severe. Leaving damp areas between the toes can lead to skin breakdown.

h. Repeat the procedure on the other leg.

Step 9 Wash the back and buttocks.

a. Position the patient on his side with his back facing you, or in the prone position. Make sure the siderail on the far side of the bed, facing the patient, is still up.

Provides for clear visualization of back and access to the area.

b. Exposing only the back and buttocks, wash the back and then the buttocks. Rinse and pat dry, paying particular attention to gluteal folds. Observe for redness and skin breakdown in the sacral area.

Maintains the principle of "clean to dirty." The sacral area is a common site of pressure sores. ▼

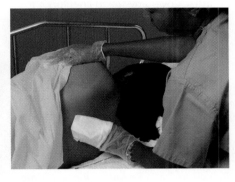

c. Unless contraindicated, give the patient a back rub, applying lotion to the back and buttocks (see Chapter 33, Procedure 33–1: Giving a Back Rub).

Stimulates circulation and maintains the health of the skin. Because the patient is in bed, he is at risk for skin irritation and breakdown from immobility and friction. A back rub may be contraindicated for patients with musculoskeletal injuries or cardiovascular disease.

d. Don procedure gloves if you have not already done so, and wash the rectal area, removing any fecal matter with tissues prior to washing with the washcloth. Wash from front to back. ▼

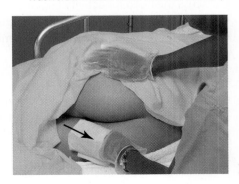

➤

PROCEDURE 22–1   Bathing: Providing a Complete Bed Bath
(continued)

Washing the rectal area at this time removes the need for the patient to turn to his side again and helps prevent soiling clean linen when changing the linen in an occupied bed. Fecal matter usually contains microorganisms.

e. Discard the soiled washcloth, and change the bathwater. Wash and wipe out the basin as needed before refilling it. Cover any soiled linen prior to repositioning the patient.

Prevents transferring microorganisms from anal to genital area—cleansing the gluteal and anal areas contaminates the washcloth, towel, and water. Maintains standard precautions during the bath and prevents soiling of clean linens during bed change.

Step 10 Wash the perineal area. See Procedure 22–4: Providing Perineal Care.

Step 11 After providing perineal care, reposition and cover the patient with the bath blanket. Remove soiled gloves. Help the patient put on a clean gown, and attend to other hygiene needs (e.g., hair grooming).

Prevents contaminating clean linen with soiled gloves. Ensures proper body position and warmth.

Step 12 Change the bed linen as needed, including soiled linen or linen that became damp during the bath. See Procedure 22–14: Making An Occupied Bed.

Ensures patient safety, comfort, and privacy.

Procedure Variations

Variation 1 If you are bathing the patient without assistance, or if you are too short to comfortably reach across the patient, you are at risk for back strain. Thus, you may want to bathe one side of the body—that is, the right arm, trunk, right leg—and then move to the other side of the bed to bathe the opposite side of the body (instead of the order given in steps 7 and 8, earlier.)

Variation 2 If you are bathing a patient in leg traction, you may decide to bathe the arms and trunk first. Then have the patient sit forward so that you can cleanse his back. Then have the patient lift up slightly so that you can wash his buttocks. Finally, wash the lower extremities.

Variation 3 Adapt the bathing order and procedure to individual patient needs.

Evaluation

- Assess how well the patient tolerated the procedure. Was there any discomfort, shortness of breath, and so on?
- Observe the patient's mobility, both range of motion and ease of movement.
- Note the condition of the patient's skin, including redness and other abnormal findings, especially in skinfolds.
- Ask the patient whether he feels comfortable.

Patient Teaching

- Discuss the need for activity (e.g., moving about in bed) and the hazards of immobility.
- Discuss usual skin care and how to increase the health of the skin.
- Demonstrate bathing procedure to family or other caregivers.

Home Care

- Evaluate home for safety considerations for bathing (not limited to bed bath):
  - Safety bars, stool for shower, nonskid pad for shower or tub
  - Availability of a safe water supply for bathing
  - Availability of bathing supplies
  - Patient's ability to help with bath

PROCEDURE 22–1   **Bathing: Providing a Complete Bed Bath**
(continued)

- Ask how the patient usually bathes (e.g., shower, at the sink). Follow patient's preference as much as possible.
- Ask what supplies the patient usually uses for the bath, and ask where they are stored. You will need to adapt the procedure depending on the available equipment and supplies.
- Suggest the use of large plastic trash bags or a shower curtain to protect the mattress during a bed bath.
- Instruct caregivers to wear gloves when handling linens that are soiled with blood or other body fluids. The linens should be washed in cold water, separately from other household laundry, and then washed again, using hot water, detergent and bleach.

Documentation

Chart the type of bath given, how much patient was able to help with the bath, how well the patient tolerated the procedure, the patient's mobility, and any abnormal findings. Hygiene care is charted on checklists and flowsheets in most agencies.

Example:

| 5/10/06 | 0800 | Complete bed bath given w/o c/o discomfort or SOB. 2 cm circular area of skin slightly reddened on coccyx—Skin Care Protocol initiated. Patient unable to assist with bath b/c "just too tired." Full ROM in all extremities. ————— S. Neal, RN |

PROCEDURE 22–2   Bathing: Providing a Towel Bath

For steps to follow in *all* procedures, refer to the inside back cover of this book.

Note: Because the towel bath is a variation of the bed bath, only the steps differing from a bed bath are listed.

critical aspects
- Refer to Procedure 22–1: Bathing: Providing a Complete Bed Bath.
- Check the temperature of the water.
- Begin at the feet and work toward the head (instead of "head to toe" as in Procedure 22–1).

Equipment
- Large plastic bag containing a bath blanket, bath towel, and two or three washcloths
- Dry bath blanket
- Dry bath towels
- Pitcher and approximately 2 qt (2000 mL) of warm water
- Liquid soap that does not require rinsing (e.g., Septisoft) or commercial solution of soap, moisturizer, and disinfectant
- Other supplies for a bed bath; see Procedure 22–1

Delegation
You can delegate this procedure to the UAP if you conclude that the patient's condition and the UAP's skills allow. Perform the following assessments, and inform the UAP of the amount of help the patient needs and any special considerations, such as IV lines, drains, and so on. Ask the UAP to report the condition of the patient's skin, level of self-care, and ability to tolerate the procedure.

Assessments
- Assess the patient's mobility and activity tolerance to determine whether she will be able to assist with the bath, if a bag bath is appropriate, and whether you will need another caregiver to assist.

A patient with decreased activity tolerance or mobility (e.g., because of chest pain or shortness of breath with exertion, or paralysis) may have a limited ability to assist with the bath, making a bag bath the most appropriate choice. For severely compromised patients, having two nurses administer the bath will make the procedure much quicker and less demanding on the patient.

- See Procedure 22–1: Bathing: Providing Complete Bed Bath, for further assessments.

Procedural Steps

Step 1 Prepare the bath bag.
a. Fill a large pitcher with warm water (approximately 105°F or 41°C).

The amount of water varies depending on the size of the bath blanket and bath towel. Use enough water to saturate them. Hot water can injure the patient and removes more of the skin's protective oils, but if the water is too cool, the patient may become chilled.

b. Add nonrinse soap or commercial solution to the water according to the manufacturer's instructions.

Adding the soap to the water prior to pouring into the bag prevents excessive sudsing.

c. Pour the solution into the bag, over the bath blanket and bath towel, to ensure even distribution.

Step 2 Spread the dry bath blanket over the patient.

Protects privacy and prevents chilling.

Step 3 Replace the dry blanket with the wet blanket:
a. Take the wet bath blanket or towel out of the bag, squeezing out excess water so that it does not drip.
b. Push the dry bath blanket down to the patient's waist, and place the wet bath blanket on the patient's chest.

c. Continue to unfold the wet bath blanket until it covers the patient, pushing the dry bath blanket out of the way as you do so.

The wet bath blanket will feel warm and relaxing when spread out over the patient. The dry bath blanket will be used to dry the patient, so you must keep it from becoming damp.

PROCEDURE 22–2 Bathing: Providing a Towel Bath *(continued)*

Step 4 Bathe the patient, beginning at the feet and working toward the head.

a. Keeping the patient covered, use the wet bath blanket to wash the legs, abdomen, and chest.

b. As you work, replace the wet bath blanket with the dry one.

Keeps the patient from chilling. ▼

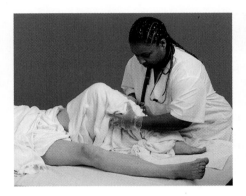

c. Use one of the wet washcloths to wash the patient's face, neck, and ears.

Notice that this varies from the order of most baths, which proceed from head to toe. However, this is the most efficient way to accomplish a towel bath. It does not really compromise the clean-to-dirty principle because the legs, abdomen, and chest are usually equally "clean," and you are washing those before the back, buttocks, and perineum. You will use separate, clean cloths to wash the face.

Step 5 Roll the client to one side, and use the wet bath towel to wash the back and then the buttocks.

Step 6 Wash the perineal area with a washcloth. See Procedure 22–4: Providing Perineal Care.

Step 7 Finish the bath as in Procedure 22–1: Bathing: Providing a Complete Bed Bath. Follow patient preferences whenever possible to increase feelings of comfort.

Step 8 Change linen as needed, including soiled linen or linen that became damp during the bath. You will almost certainly need to change the linen if you have not padded the bottom sheet well before the bath.

Ensures patient safety and comfort. Because the bath is finished rapidly, there is no real need to pad the bottom sheet if you know that you will have time to change the linens after the bath.

For Evaluation, Documentation, and Patient Teaching, see Procedure 22–1: Bathing: Providing a Complete Bed Bath.

PROCEDURE 22–3 Bathing: Providing a Packaged Bath

 For steps to follow in *all* procedures, refer to the inside back cover of this book.

critical aspects
- Refer to Procedure 22–1, Bathing: Providing a Complete Bed Bath.
- Check the temperature of the packaged bath after microwaving.

Equipment
- Packaged disposable washcloths (e.g., Comfort Bath)
- Lotion
- Deodorant and/or powder as needed
- Clean patient gown (gown with shoulder snaps or Velcro closures if the patient has an IV line)
- Clean linen
- Procedure gloves

➤

PROCEDURE 22–3   Bathing: Providing a Packaged Bath

(continued)

Delegation

You can delegate this procedure to the UAP if you conclude that the patient's condition and the UAP's skills allow. Perform the following assessments, and inform the UAP of the amount of help the patient needs and of any special considerations, such as IV lines, drains, and so on. Ask the UAP to report the condition of the patient's skin, level of self-care, and ability to tolerate the procedure.

Assessments

Assessments are the same as in Procedure 22–1, Bathing: Providing a Complete Bed Bath.

Procedural Steps

Step 1 Peel open the label on the commercial bath without completely removing it.

Allows for steam to escape as contents heat without spilling the contents. ▼

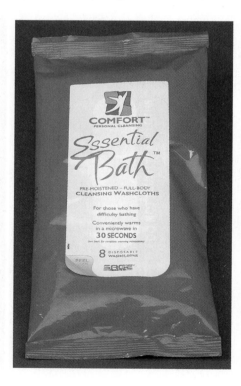

Step 2 Heat the package in the microwave for no longer than 1 minute. The temperature of contents should be approximately 105°F or 41°C. This is controversial. Some references suggest, for safety, using the commercial bag bath at room temperature.

Brings contents to a safe and comfortable temperature.

Step 3 Prepare the patient for the bath as described in Procedure 22–1: Bathing: Providing a Complete Bed Bath.

Step 4 Using one washcloth for each body area, wash the patient following the steps of Procedure 22–1.

Step 5 Discard each washcloth after use.

Ensures following the "clean to dirty" principle.

Step 6 Help patient don a clean gown.

For Evaluation, Documentation, and Patient Teaching, see Procedure 22–1: Bathing: Providing a Complete Bed Bath.

PROCEDURE 22–4   Providing Perineal Care

 For steps to follow in *all* procedures, refer to the inside back cover of this book.

critical aspects
- Provide privacy; keep the patient covered as much as possible.
- Use warm water.
- Perform perineal care following the principle of "clean to dirty" (front to back).

Equipment
- Procedure gloves
- Basin for water, or perineal wash bottle
- Waterproof pad
- Bedpan or portable sitz tub (optional)
- Bath towel
- Washcloth
- Toilet paper
- Cleansing solution or soap
- Perineal ointment or lotion if needed

Delegation
You can delegate perineal care to the UAP if you conclude that the patient's condition and the UAP's skills allow. Perform the following assessments, and inform the UAP of the amount of help the patient needs and any special considerations (e.g., presence of a urinary catheter, vaginal drainage). Ask the UAP to report the condition of the patient's perineum (skin, drainage), level of self-care, and ability to tolerate the procedure.

Assessments
- Assess the patient's mobility and activity tolerance.

Determine whether the patient will be able to assist with the perineal care. Doing as much self-care as possible increases the patient's sense of independence and maintains modesty.
- Check for positioning or activity restrictions, such as maintaining hip abduction following a total hip replacement.

Prevents injuring the patient during the procedure.
- Assess for psychosocial issues that may be of concern to the patient regarding perineal care.

You must consider cultural norms when providing perineal care to ensure that it is appropriate for that patient. For example, in some cultures a woman would find it completely unacceptable for a male nurse to perform her perineal care (pericare).
- Assess for any specific patient needs for perineal care.

For example, if there are lesions or skin breakdown, you may need to use special soaps and/or lotions. Incontinence or drainage requires assessment and follow-up to prevent Impaired Skin Integrity.
- Assess for the presence of a urinary drainage catheter, perineal surgery, or lesions.

You may need to adapt the procedure to clean around an indwelling urinary catheter or surgical incisions.

Procedural Steps

Step 1 Adjust room temperature, and assist with elimination as needed.

Assisting the patient with elimination prior to beginning perineal care helps prevent interruptions during the procedure and allows for thorough perineal care. Adjusting room temperature prevents chilling.

Step 2 Fill the basin or perineal wash bottle with warm water (the temperature should be approximately 105°F or 41°C).

Hot water can injure the skin, and cool water can cause chilling. Use water that is comfortable for the patient.

Step 3 Wash the perineal area.

a. Position the patient on her back (supine). Place waterproof pads under the patient if they are not already in place. You may wish to place the patient on a bedpan or portable sitz tub, especially if the perineum is grossly soiled.

➤

PROCEDURE 22–4   **Providing Perineal Care** *(continued)*

Placing the patient on a bedpan raises the hips to increase visualization and allows for more thorough cleansing. A bedpan also allows for using additional water when needed.

b. Wear procedure gloves (and other protective wear as needed) when providing perineal care. Wear a procedure gown and goggles if you are concerned about splashing (e.g., if the patient is confused and may be unable to follow instructions).

Follows Standard Precautions.

c. Drape the patient to protect privacy.
   Female patient:
   1) Drape the bath blanket so that one point faces the patient's head (drape it in the shape of a diamond).
   2) Take one of the side points of the diamond, and wrap it around the patient's leg. Anchor the end of the blanket under the patient's foot.
   3) Repeat on the other leg with other point of the diamond. ▼

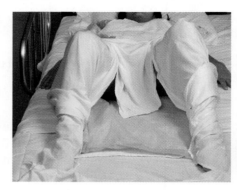

4) Fold the center lower point of the diamond up to expose the patient's perineum.

This draping technique covers the patient as much as possible, which helps maintain privacy and prevents chilling during the

procedure. The patient can also relax her legs against the bath blanket. ▼

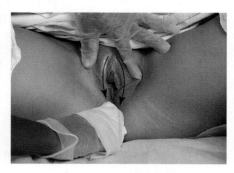

Male patient:
   1) Place the bath blanket over the patient's chest.
   2) Fold the bed linens down to expose only the patient's groin.

d. Remove any fecal material with toilet paper.

Prevents contamination of the perineum with feces, which can lead to bladder, vaginal, or incisional infections. If you are providing perineal care as part of giving a bed bath, you will have cleaned the anal area when the patient was in the lateral position.

e. Moisten the washcloth with the water in the basin, or spray the perineum with the perineal wash bottle.

Moistens the area or washcloth thoroughly to ensure adequate cleansing.

f. *Female patient:* Wash the perineum from front to back, using a clean portion of the washcloth for each stroke. Cleanse the labial folds and around the urinary catheter, if one is in place.

Prevents contaminating the urethra with fecal material. Any fecal particles that are left can cause skin breakdown and may

increase the risk of a urinary tract infection because of the presence of *E. coli* in the feces. ▼

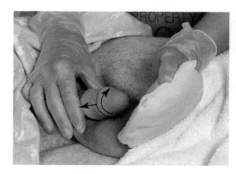

g. *Male patient:* Retract the foreskin, if present, and gently cleanse the head of the penis using a circular motion. Replace the foreskin, and finish washing the shaft of the penis, using firm strokes. Then wash the scrotum, using a clean portion of the washcloth with each stroke. Handle the scrotum with care, because the area is sensitive.

To adequately clean the head of the penis in an uncircumcised male, you must retract the foreskin. After cleaning, replace the foreskin to prevent constriction and edema of the penis. Firm strokes may help to prevent an erection. Using a clean portion of the washcloth for each wipe prevents fecal contamination of the urethra and perineum. ▼

h. In both males and females, cleanse the skinfolds of the groin area thoroughly, and pat dry. Examine the skin creases for redness or excoriation.

Detects and prevents excoriation in skinfold areas, where moisture accumulates.

PROCEDURE 22–4   Providing Perineal Care (continued)

Step 4 Rinse and pat dry.

Prevents skin injury secondary to maceration. If you are using perineal wash solution, rinsing is not required.

Step 5 If perineal care is *not* being done as part of the bath, also clean the anal area. Have patient turn to the side, and wash, rinse, and dry the buttocks and anal area as needed.

Fecal contamination of the perineum can lead to urinary tract infections and skin irritation. Therefore, the anal area is cleansed last.

Step 6 Apply skin protectants as needed. Powder only if patient requests it.

If urinary or fecal incontinence is present, skin barriers may be used to prevent urine, feces, or other drainage from contacting the skin. This helps prevent skin breakdown. For female patients, powder is a medium for bacterial growth.

Step 7 If the patient has an indwelling catheter and if agency policy requires special catheter care, you will usually provide the care at this point. Don clean gloves before providing catheter care, and follow the agency's procedure. For more information about catheter care, see Technique 27–7, Caring for a Patient with an Indwelling Catheter.

Step 8 Reposition and cover the patient with the bath blanket. Remove soiled gloves, discarding appropriately.

Prevents contaminating clean linen with soiled gloves.

Step 9 Change linen as needed, including soiled linen or linen that became damp during perineal care.

Ensures patient safety, comfort, and privacy.

Evaluation

- Assess the patient's responses to the procedure. Was there any discomfort?
- Observe for difficulty with movement or range of motion during the procedure.
- Note the condition of the skin, including redness and other abnormal findings.
- Ask the patient whether she feels comfortable now.

Patient Teaching

- Discuss adaptations to perineal care. For example, if the area is tender, (1) wash the area with warm water after going to the bathroom, instead of using toilet paper; or (2) use a skin protectant to the area.
- Review the importance of hand washing after elimination.
- If appropriate, teach the caregiver how to provide perineal care, including the major concept of cleaning front to back ("clean to dirty"). Stress the importance of wearing gloves and washing hands.
- Advise women not to douche because it disturbs the balance in normal vaginal flora and can irritate or injure mucosal cells.

- Explain that scented and deodorant feminine hygiene products are not necessary for cleanliness and may even be harmful. Plain soap and water are the most effective means of odor control.

Home Care

- Evaluate the ability of the patient or caregiver to provide perineal care.
- If needed, teach the caregiver how to provide perineal care, including the major concept of cleaning front to back ("clean to dirty").
- Determine the availability of supplies needed for perineal care.
- You will need to adapt the procedure depending on the available equipment and supplies. Major issues involved in perineal care in the home are the lack of clean water and/or linens. In some instances, you may need to use bottled water or boil water for the procedure. One option is to use prepackaged moistened towelettes to provide the care (e.g., Comfort Bath towelettes). These products may be heated in a water bath or microwave oven.

➤

PROCEDURE 22–4 **Providing Perineal Care** *(continued)*

Documentation

Usually this is part of routine hygiene care and is charted on a flowsheet. If you chart it, chart that perineal care was given, any patient responses to the procedure, and the condition of the perineal area.

Example:

8/16/06	1430	*Perineal care given. Patient had no c/o discomfort.*
		No redness or discharge noted. — N. Noyes, RN

PROCEDURE 22–5 **Providing Foot Care**

 For steps to follow in *all* procedures, refer to the inside back cover of this book.

critical aspects

- Inspect the feet thoroughly for skin integrity, circulation, and edema.
- Clean the feet with mild soap; clean the toenails; rinse; and dry well.
- Trim the nails straight across, unless contraindicated. Check institutional policy; many institutions do not allow nurses to trim nails.
- File the nails with an emery board.
- Lightly apply lotion, except between the toes.
- Ensure that footwear or bedding is not irritating to the feet.

Equipment

- Procedure gloves (if there are open lesions)
- Pillow (if procedure is done with the client in bed)
- Basin for water
- Liquid nonrinse soap
- Bath towel
- Waterproof pad
- Washcloth
- Orangewood stick
- Toenail clippers
- Nail file
- Lotion or prescribed ointment or cream

Delegation

You can delegate foot care to the UAP if you conclude that the patient's condition and the UAP's skills allow. For example, as a rule you should not delegate care if the patient has impaired peripheral circulation or foot ulcers. Perform the following assessments, and inform the UAP of the amount of help the patient needs and any special considerations (e.g., ability to sit in a chair). Ask the UAP to report the condition of the patient's skin and nails, level of self-care, and ability to tolerate the procedure.

PROCEDURE 22–5   **Providing Foot Care** *(continued)*

Assessments

- Assess bilateral dorsalis pedis pulses, skin color, and warmth. Compare right and left foot.

Palpate pulses at the same time bilaterally to determine whether one side is weaker than the other. Decreased circulation to the feet increases the risk for tissue injury and infection. A variety of diseases can cause poor circulation. For example, cardiac or renal disease may cause pedal edema, which impairs circulation to the skin, and diabetes causes vascular changes leading to poor circulation to the lower extremities.

- Thoroughly assess all areas of the feet for skin integrity, edema, condition of toenails, and any abnormalities. Check carefully between the toes.

Decreased circulation in the feet commonly causes such problems as thickened toenails, dry skin, and increased risk of infection. Changes in vision and mobility can increase the risk for injuries to the feet. Patients with diabetes also may have neuropathy, which prevents them from knowing when they have injured their foot. Identifying abnormalities enables you to provide interventions to help prevent potential problems. ▼

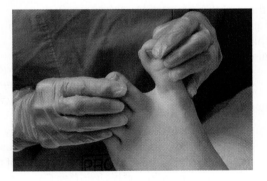

- Check institution policy to verify whether a nurse is allowed to trim nails. Obtain a physician's order for trimming the patient's nails, if necessary.

Patients who have diabetes or impaired circulation to the lower extremities require a physician's order for trimming their nails. Refer the patient to a podiatrist if the circulation is severely compromised or if edema would make the procedure difficult.

- Assess the patient's usual footwear.

Improperly fitting shoes, especially if they are too tight, are a common cause of foot problems.

- Assess the patient's self-care ability to provide foot care. Evaluate the need for a referral. Determine whether the patient has the necessary vision and mobility to be able provide his own foot care.
- Assess the patient's knowledge about foot care, including usual foot care practices.

Identify potential deficits in understanding of foot care needs that may require additional teaching or referral to a podiatrist, general practice physician, or advanced practice nurse. Many home remedies for foot problems can damage the tissue. For example, corn pads can increase pressure on the tissue, compromising circulation and causing local tissue ischemia. Cutting the sides of the toenails can lead to ingrown toenails.

Procedural Steps

Step 1 Wear procedure gloves and other protective wear as needed when providing foot care.

Follows Standard Precautions. The heel is a common place for skin breakdown, so use gloves if you are unable to see the area without lifting the foot. If the patient has significant drainage to the area, such as a draining wound, you may need to wear a protective gown.

Step 2 Have the patient sit in a chair with a waterproof pad or bath towel under the feet, if possible. If the patient is unable to sit in a chair, place him in semi-Fowler's position in bed; place a pillow under the knees.

It is easier to perform the procedure with the patient in a chair. The pillow supports the knee joints and prevents muscle fatigue.

Step 3 Fill the basin halfway with warm water (approximately 105 to 110°F or 40 to 43°C).

Hot water can injure the skin. Warm water promotes circulation. Filling the basin halfway prevents spilling when the patient places his foot in the water.

Step 4 Help the patient place one foot in the water, first checking with the patient that the temperature is comfortable.

- If the patient is in a chair, place the basin on the floor (on the waterproof pad).
- If the patient is in bed, place the basin near the foot of the bed on the waterproof pad; pad the basin with a towel.

➤

PROCEDURE 22–5   **Providing Foot Care** *(continued)*

The waterproof pad keeps the bed dry. Padding the basin prevents pressure on the back of the leg, which could cause discomfort and interfere with circulation.

Step 5 Allow the foot to soak for 5 to 20 minutes, depending on the patient's tolerance and the condition of his feet. Soaking is not recommended for patients with diabetes or peripheral vascular disease (PVD).

Soaking softens the skin and helps relax the patient. For patients who have diabetes or PVD, soaking is not recommended because it may remove natural oils, cause cracking of the skin, and may cause burns even if the water is at the recommended temperature.

Step 6 Clean the foot with mild or rinse-free soap.

Removes loose debris. Rinse-free soaps do not dry the skin. ▼

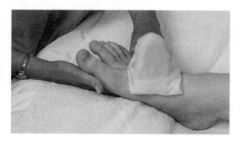

Step 7 Clean under the nails with the orangewood stick while the foot is still in the water.

Water softens the nails and makes cleaning easier.

Step 8 Rinse. Remove the foot from the water, and dry it gently and thoroughly.

Remaining moisture, especially between the toes, can cause maceration and promotes development of fungal infections.

Step 9 Change the water, if necessary.

Ensures proper temperature.

Step 10 Soak the opposite foot while performing steps 11 through 14 for the first (clean) foot.

Saves time.

Step 11 Gently push the cuticles back with the orange stick or towel.

Increases cuticle health. Do not damage the cuticle; doing so can increase the risk of infection.

Step 12 Trim the nails straight across with toenail clippers, if not contraindicated by patient's condition and if permitted by agency policy. Note whether the nail has cut into the skin of the toe being trimmed or the adjacent toes. If the nails are brittle or thick, allow the foot to soak for 10 to 20 minutes before trimming.

Trimming straight across prevents ingrown toenails. Early recognition and

treatment of problems will prevent further complications, such as infection. ▼

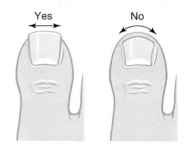

Step 13 File the nails with an emery board.

Smoothes the edges to prevent scratching the skin with the toenails.

Step 14 Apply cream or lotion or foot powder lightly to the feet and toes.

Cream hydrates the skin. Note, however, that excess cream can cause maceration. Foot powder absorbs moisture and functions as a nonirritating deodorant for patients whose feet perspire heavily.

Step 15 Repeat steps 11 through 14 with the second foot.

Step 16 Check the patient's footwear for rough edges that may injure feet. If patient has Impaired Bed Mobility, apply protective devices (e.g., lamb's wool) as needed. If the patient has an injury, lesions, or pain, you may need to use a bed cradle to keep the pressure of the bedding off his feet. (See Chapter 34 for measures to preserve skin integrity.)

Protects the feet from further injury from abrasion or pressure.

Evaluation

- Observe that feet are clean, smooth, and intact; nails are trimmed and smooth; skin is pink and warm.
- Be sure that foot problems are identified and interventions provided.
- Have patient demonstrate or describe correct foot care.

Patient Teaching

- Reinforce the following as necessary.
  1) Wash the feet daily with warm water and mild soap.
  2) Dry the feet well, especially between the toes.
  3) Inspect the feet daily (using a mirror to check the soles) for cracks, dry skin, cuts, redness, swelling, and change in temperature.

PROCEDURE 22–5   **Providing Foot Care** *(continued)*

4) Keep the toenails trimmed straight across.
5) Apply cream lightly to feet daily. Do not apply cream between the toes.
6) Report any abnormalities to the healthcare provider: numbness or tingling; decrease in sensation; skin redness, cracks, cuts, swelling; or decrease in skin temperature.

- Discuss the importance of properly fitting footwear and socks.
- Instruct the patient to avoid actions that would decrease circulation to the lower legs (e.g., wearing knee-high stockings, crossing the legs, smoking, sitting in chair without support to the feet).

Home Care

The procedure does not vary in the home. The nurse must:

- Work with the patient and care provider to determine the availability of supplies needed for foot care (clean water, and so on).
- Identify home care practices, and teach the patient and/or caregiver proper foot care techniques. Influencing older adults can be especially difficult if they have usual routines, such as walking barefoot, that put them at risk for injury. For patients with diabetes, the biggest risk to foot health is inadequate regulation of their blood glucose levels.

Documentation

In most agencies you will not document routine foot care (except, perhaps, on a checklist) unless there are problems. If you do document, chart that foot care was given, and chart assessment findings.

Example:

09/26/06	0900	Foot care given. 2 cm circular reddened area on right heel. Skin abrasion outer lateral aspect of 5th toe, left foot—bioocclusive dressing applied. ———————— A. Hopkins, RN

PROCEDURE 22–6   Brushing and Flossing the Teeth

For steps to follow in *all* procedures, refer to the inside back cover of this book.

critical aspects
- Assess the teeth, mucous membranes, and swallowing ability.
- Position the patient to prevent aspiration (sitting or side-lying position).
- Hold the brush at a 45-degree angle, and brush the patient's teeth (or assist).
- Floss and rinse.
- If the patient is at risk for choking, suction secretions as needed.

Equipment
- Toothbrush or sponge toothettes
- Toothpaste
- Dental floss (two pieces, each about 10 in. long)
- Floss holder (optional)
- Tonsil-tip suction connected to suction source (if aspiration is a concern)
- Emesis basin
- Towel
- Glass of water
- Mouthwash and/or lip moisturizer, if desired
- Procedure gloves; mask and goggles if splashing may occur

Delegation
You can delegate oral hygiene to the UAP if the patient's condition and the UAP's skills allow. Perform the following assessments, and inform the UAP of the specific type of oral care and the amount of help the patient needs. Ask the UAP to report the condition of the patient's mouth, level of self-care, and ability to tolerate the procedure.

Assessments
- Assess the patient's ability to assist with oral care.

Having the patient assist whenever possible promotes independence and supports a positive self-concept.
- Determine whether the patient has dentures, bridgework, or partial plates.

The presence of these devices determines how you will provide oral care.
- Assess the patient's general oral health, including the presence of the gag reflex and the condition of the teeth, gums, and mucous membranes. If a patient has dentures, examine the mouth with and without the dentures.

To prevent aspiration, you will need a suction set-up to provide oral care if the patient has a hypoactive or absent gag reflex. Any inflammation or lesions in the mouth increases the patient's risk of infection and may make eating difficult or painful, leading to malnutrition. Poorly fitting dentures can cause irritation of the gums.
- Assess the patient's usual oral care, including cultural practices.

Helps determine the type of oral care you will provide and identifies areas of patient teaching needed.

PROCEDURE 22–6   Brushing and Flossing the Teeth *(continued)*

Procedural Steps

Step 1 Position the patient to prevent aspiration: in high-Fowler's position or in a chair, if possible. Position the patient on the side if the head of bed cannot be elevated.

Prevents aspiration and makes the procedure easier.

Step 2 Set up suction, if needed. Attach suction tubing and tonsil-tip suction; check suction.

Suctioning equipment will be needed if the gag reflex is decreased or absent. Suctioning is done to prevent aspiration of secretions during the procedure.

Step 3 If the patient is able to perform self-care:

a. Arrange supplies within the patient's reach.

Promotes patient's ability to do self-care and therefore independence.

b. Assist the patient with brushing and flossing as needed.

Ensures that the teeth are thoroughly cleaned.

Step 4 For nurse-administered brushing and flossing:

a. Place the towel across the patient's chest.

Prevents getting the patient's gown or linen wet during the procedure.

b. Don procedure gloves and other protective garb as needed. Wear gown and goggles if splashing might occur, such as with a confused patient.

Follows Standard Precautions.

c. Moisten toothbrush, and apply a small amount of toothpaste. Use a soft toothbrush.

Excessive toothpaste does not increase the cleaning. Moistening the toothbrush increases patient comfort because patients frequently have dry mouths.

d. Place, hold, or have the patient hold the emesis basis under the chin.

e. Brush the teeth, holding the bristles at a 45-degree angle to the gum line.

1) Using short circular motions, gently brush the inner and outer surfaces of the teeth, from the gum line to crown of each tooth.

2) Brush the biting surface of the back teeth by holding the brush bristles straight up and down to the teeth and brushing back and forth.

This is the most effective technique for removing all food particles and plaque from the teeth and gums.

3) If the patient is frail, perform oral suctioning when fluid accumulates in the mouth.

Prevents choking and aspiration.

f. Gently brush the patient's tongue.

Removes coating and accumulated debris that can be a reservoir for bacteria. Brush gently to prevent gagging or vomiting. ▼

Brush teeth, holding bristles at a 45° angle to the gumline. Using short circular motions, gently brush the inner and outer surfaces of the teeth, including the gumline.

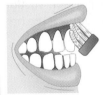

Clean front teeth.

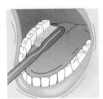

Clean both inner and outer surfaces of the teeth.

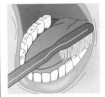

Brush the biting surfaces of the back teeth with the brush bristles straight up and down.

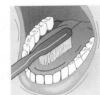

Brush the surface of the tongue.

g. Floss the teeth. Grasp dental floss in both hands, or use a floss holder. ▼

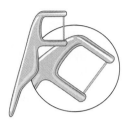

1) If you are not using a floss holder, wrap one end of the floss around the middle finger of each hand. ▼

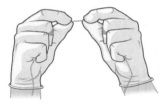

2) Stretch the floss between your thumbs and index fingers, and move the floss up and down against each tooth. ▼

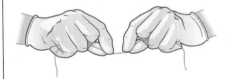

3) Floss between and around all teeth. ▼

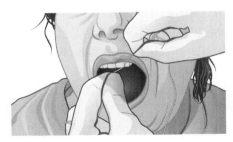

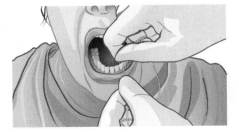

▶

PROCEDURE 22–6   Brushing and Flossing the Teeth *(continued)*

Moving the floss up and down instead of back and forth prevents damaging the gums.

h. Assist patient in rinsing mouth, suctioning as needed. Or, ask the patient to rinse vigorously and spit the water into the emesis basin.

Removes food particles from mouth. Suction if the patient has a decreased or absent gag reflex.

Step 5 Offer a mild or dilute mouthwash, and apply lip moisturizer, if desired.

Prevents irritation of the mucous membranes. Apply lip moisturizer for dry lips or patient preference.

Step 6 Reposition the patient as needed.

Evaluation

- Inspect the teeth, gums, and mucous membranes to verify that they are free of food particles.
- Inspect for abnormalities, such as bleeding, that may have been stimulated by the brushing or flossing.
- Observe for patient discomfort or gagging during procedure.

Patient Teaching

- Discuss the importance of daily oral care.
- Review any areas of brushing or flossing that the patient has not been performing adequately.
- Discuss any problems that need further follow-up, such as inflammation, bleeding, or dryness.

Home Care

The procedure does not vary in the home. The issues are that the nurse must:

- Work with the patient and care provider to determine supplies needed for the home.
- Determine whether suction is needed (e.g., if the patient is unconscious or has a decreased gag reflex). Explain to the patient and/or caregiver how to obtain a portable suction unit.
- Demonstrate how to position the patient and perform the procedure if the height of the bed is not adjustable or if both sides of the bed are not accessible.

Documentation

Document that oral care was given, the patient's response, any abnormal findings, and nursing interventions. Oral care is usually charted on a flowsheet.

Example:

| 12/27/06 0815 | *Oral care given. Mucous membranes intact, pink, and dry. No choking or complaints of discomfort. Patient encouraged to increase fluid intake. ——————— N. Botha, RN* |

PROCEDURE 22–7 Providing Denture Care

For steps to follow in *all* procedures, refer to the inside back cover of this book.

critical aspects
- Refer to Procedure 22–6: Brushing and Flossing the Teeth.
- Remove (and replace) the top denture before the lower denture.
- Tilt dentures slightly when removing and replacing.
- Handle dentures carefully, and place towel in sink to avoid breaking the dentures if you drop them.
- Use cool water and a stiff-bristled brush.

Equipment
- See Procedure 22–6: Brushing and Flossing the Teeth.
- Denture cup

Delegation
You can delegate denture care to the UAP if the patient's condition and the UAP's skills allow. Perform the following assessments, and inform the UAP of the specific care and the amount of help the patient needs. Ask the UAP to report the condition of the patient's mouth and dentures, level of self-care, and ability to tolerate the procedure.

Assessments
See Procedure 22–6: Brushing and Flossing the Teeth.

Procedural Steps

Step 1 Don gloves, and remove dentures (if the client cannot do so).

a. *Upper denture:* With a gauze pad, grasp the denture with your thumb and forefinger, and move it gently up and down. Tilt denture slightly to one side to remove it, without stretching the lips. Place the denture in the denture cup.

The gauze gives you a better grip. Breaking the seal on the top dentures can be difficult; movement breaks the suction. Always place dentures in a denture cup as soon as you remove them to prevent accidental breakage. ➤

b. *Lower denture:* Use your thumbs to push up gently on the denture at the gum line to release from lower jaw. Grasp the denture with your thumb and forefinger, and tilt it to remove it from the patient's mouth. Place the denture in the denture cup.

Generally, a gauze pad is not needed to grasp the lower dentures; however, you can use one if the dentures are difficult to grasp. Pushing up on the dentures breaks the seal. Rotating the dentures is necessary to remove the dentures from the patient's mouth. ▼

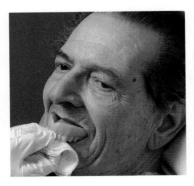

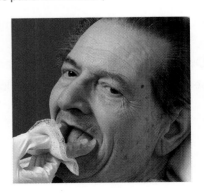

➤

PROCEDURE 22–7   **Providing Denture Care** (*continued*)

Step 2 Place the towel in the sink, and cleanse the dentures under cool running water.

Heat can damage some dentures. Towel helps prevent the dentures from breaking if they are accidentally dropped. Dentures are expensive.

a. Apply a small amount of toothpaste to a stiff-bristled toothbrush.

Assists in cleaning. Follow patient's preference in use of denture cleaner. Some patients prefer to soak their dentures in a cleanser overnight. If dentures have been soaking, rinse them well before placing them in the patient's mouth.

b. Brush all surfaces of each denture.

Loosens all food particles and any old denture adhesive.

c. Rinse thoroughly with cool water.

Removes loosened particles and the cleaning agent. Do not use hot water with dentures, because hot water can react to make the denture material sticky.

d. You can soak stained dentures in a commercial cleaner, following the manufacturer's instructions. Do not soak the denture overnight if the appliance has metal parts.

Can cause corrosion.

Step 3 Inspect dentures for rough, worn, or sharp edges.

These can irritate the tongue, gums, or mucous membranes of the mouth.

Step 4 Inspect the mouth under the dentures for redness, irritation, lesions, or infection.

If present, refer to a dentist to check the fit of the dentures or to make needed repairs.

Step 5 Apply denture adhesive as needed (ask the patient whether he uses denture adhesive).

Adhesives are needed to "seal" some dentures and prevent slipping and irritation of the gums.

Step 6 Moisten the top denture, if it is dry. Then insert the top denture, at a slight tilt, and press it up against the roof of the mouth.

Moisten the dentures if they are dry to ease the insertion. You can tell when you have securely seated the dentures by checking to feel for any slippage or to confirm that the dentures stay in place. Because the top denture is larger, it is removed first and inserted first for ease of insertion.

Step 7 Moisten the bottom denture, if it is dry. Then insert bottom denture, rotating it as you put it in the patient's mouth.

Because it is smaller, the bottom denture is inserted last. ▼

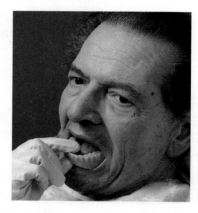

Step 8 Ask the patient whether the dentures are comfortable.

Ensures that the dentures are properly placed.

Step 9 If the client does not wish to wear the dentures, cover them with water in a denture container with a lid. Label the container with the patient's name and the agency identifying number.

Step 10 Offer mouthwash.

Evaluation
* See Procedure 22–6: Brushing and Flossing the Teeth.
* Check to see that dentures are comfortable and fit properly.

Documentation, Patient Teaching, and Home Care
See Procedure 22–6: Brushing and Flossing the Teeth.

PROCEDURE 22–8   Providing Oral Care for an Unconscious Patient

➤ For steps to follow in *all* procedures, refer to the inside back cover of this book.

critical aspects
- Assess the condition of the teeth (or dentures), gums, and mucous membranes.
- Assess for the gag reflex.
- Position the patient to prevent aspiration.
- Brush and floss the patient's teeth.
- Suction secretions as needed.

Equipment
- Toothbrush with soft bristles or sponge oral swabs
- Toothpaste
- Denture cup, if patient has dentures
- 4 × 4 gauze pad to remove dentures if present
- Tonsil-tip suction connected to suction source (you may use a product that combines the toothbrush or oral swab with the suction device)
- Tongue blade (padded) or bite-block
- Towel
- Waterproof linen protector
- Emesis basin
- Water-soluble lip moisturizer
- Procedure gloves and goggles

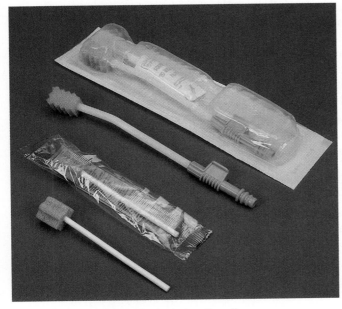

Source: Courtesy of Sage Products, Inc., Cary, IL.

Delegation
As a rule, you probably should not delegate oral hygiene for an unconscious patient to a UAP. However, in some situations it may be acceptable—for example, when the UAP has a great deal of experience caring for unconscious patients and when the UAP's ability to perform oral hygiene safely for them is documented. Perform the following assessments, and inform the UAP of any special considerations for care (e.g., if the patient must have the head of the bed elevated to facilitate breathing). Ask the UAP to report the condition of the patient's mouth and the patient's ability to tolerate the procedure (e.g., ask the UAP to take vital signs before and after the procedure, or to note the oxygen saturation if it is being monitored).

Assessments
- Determine whether the patient has dentures or partial plates.

The presence of these appliances determines how you will provide oral care. You may leave dentures out for an unconscious patient to decrease the risk of the dentures' being damaged or blocking the airway. However, when possible keep the dentures in place to prevent difficulty in getting an adequate denture fit later. Partial plates should be removed in an unconscious patient to prevent the plate from causing aspiration or damage to the mouth if it becomes loosened.

- Assess the patient's gag reflex.

If the patient has an intact gag reflex, the risk of aspiration is lower.

- Assess the patient's general oral health, including the condition of the teeth and gums, and hydration of the mucous membranes. If a patient has dentures, examine the mouth with and without the dentures.

➤

PROCEDURE 22–8

Providing Oral Care for an Unconscious Patient
(continued)

Unconscious patients tend to breathe through the mouth, so oral mucosa are often dry. Because the oral mucosa act as a barrier against microorganisms, any inflammation or lesions in the mouth increase the risk for infection. The lips, gums, and mucous membranes should be pink, moist, and intact. The teeth should be intact and clean. The condition of the mouth determines what you will use to provide oral care. Assess the fit of dentures and the condition of the skin under the dentures to determine whether the fit is proper and whether any irritation is present.

Procedural Steps

Step 1 Position the patient in a side-lying position, with head turned to the side and, if possible, with head of bed down.

Secretions will pool in the dependent side of the mouth. This position helps prevent aspiration and facilitates the removal of secretions by gravity.

Step 2 Set up suction. Attach suction tubing and tonsil-tip suction; check suction.

Suctioning helps ensure that the patient does not aspirate oral secretions during the mouth care procedure.

Step 3 Brush the patient's teeth.
a. Place the waterproof pad and then the towel under the patient's cheek and chin.

Prevents getting the linen wet during the procedure.

b. Place emesis basin under the patient's cheek.

Catches the secretions draining from the patient's mouth. ▼

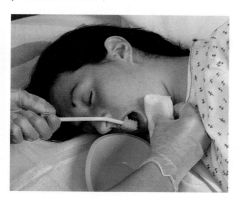

c. Don procedure gloves and eye goggles.

Follows Standard Precautions. Eye protection is needed when suctioning because of the risk of splashing.

d. Moisten the toothbrush, and apply a small amount of toothpaste.

Excessive toothpaste does not increase the cleaning. Brushing the teeth with a soft-bristled brush stimulates the mucosa, which increases the health of the gums.

e. Brush the teeth, holding the bristles at a 45-degree angle to the gum line, and using a padded tongue blade or bite-block to hold the patient's mouth open.
1) Using short circular motions, gently brush the inner and outer surfaces of the teeth, including the gum line.
2) Brush the biting surface of the back teeth by holding the brush bristles straight up and down to the teeth and brushing back and forth.
3) Brush the patient's tongue.

This is the most effective technique for removing plaque and debris from the teeth and gums. The tongue can be a reservoir for bacteria. A padded tongue blade or bite block is used to hold the mouth open so you can visualize and reach the different areas of the mouth without injuring the oral mucosa.

f. Draw about 10 mL of water or mouthwash (e.g., dilute hydrogen peroxide) into a syringe; eject it gently into the side of the mouth. Allow the fluid to drain out into the basin, or suction as needed.

Rinsing with water or dilute hydrogen peroxide removes any toothpaste residue, which may have a drying effect. Remove all fluid from the mouth to prevent aspiration into the lungs.

Step 4 Provide denture care, if necessary. See Procedure 22–7: Providing Denture Care.

Step 5 Clean the tissues in the oral cavity according to agency policy. Use foam swabs or a moistened gauze square wrapped around a tongue blade. Use a clean swab for each area of the mouth: cheeks, tongue, roof of the mouth, and so on.

Oral tissues may be dry and sticky from mouth breathing. Using separate swabs prevents transfer of microorganisms from one area to another.

Step 6 Remove the basin, dry the patient's face and mouth, and apply water-soluble lip moisturizer.

PROCEDURE 22–8

Providing Oral Care for an Unconscious Patient
(continued)

Use of petroleum-based lip moisturizers (e.g., mineral oil, petroleum jelly) is not recommended because of the possibility of aspiration, which might cause pneu-

monia. Never use petroleum-based jelly for patients on oxygen therapy; it can cause burns.

Step 7 Reposition the patient as needed. Maintains good body alignment.

Evaluation

- Inspect the teeth, gums, and mucous membranes for cleanliness.
- Observe oral mucosa and gums for hydration, inflammation, bleeding, or infection.
- Observe the patient's overall responses to the procedure (e.g., gagging, coughing, vital signs, skin color).

Patient Teaching

- Discuss with family members any problems that need further follow-up.
- Teach oral hygiene measures, as needed.

Home Care

The procedure does not vary in the home.

- Work with the patient and caregiver to determine supplies needed for the home.
- Determine whether suction is needed, and explain to caregivers how to obtain a portable suction unit.
- Demonstrate how to position the patient and perform the procedure if the height of the bed is not adjustable or if both sides of the bed are not accessible.

Documentation

Document that oral care was given, any abnormal findings, and nursing interventions.

Example:

| 09/16/06 | 0730 | Oral care given. Mucous membranes pink and moist. White coating on tongue—physician notified. Patient had no coughing during the procedure. Gag reflex is intact. Patient did not aspirate. Respiratory rate 18. — S. Hiam, RN |

| PROCEDURE 22–9 | **Shampooing the Hair for a Patient on Bedrest** |

 For steps to follow in *all* procedures, refer to the inside back cover of this book.

critical aspects

- Determine the type of procedure needed. Assess the patient's ability to help and the condition of the hair and scalp.
- Identify hair care products needed for the procedure.
- Protect the bed from getting wet.
- Wash the hair with warm water.
- Protect the patient's eyes and ears from soap and water.
- Towel-dry the hair.
- Take care not to burn the patient with the hair dryer, if one is used.

Equipment

- Shampoo
- Conditioner, optional
- Shampoo tray or commercial system, if available
- Washbasin or plastic pail
- Towels (2)
- Washcloth
- Bath blanket
- Waterproof pads or plastic trash bag
- Brush and comb
- Procedure gloves, if indicated by the presence of lesions or infestation

- Hair dryer
- Commercial system (e.g., EZ-Shower), if available

Delegation

You can delegate this procedure to the UAP if you conclude that the patient's condition and the UAP's skills allow. Perform the following assessments, and inform the UAP of the specific type of procedure needed (e.g., in bed, at sink, disposable shampoo equipment) and the amount of help the patient needs. Inform the UAP of any special considerations, such as positions the patient cannot assume or presence of scalp lesions. Ask the UAP to report the condition of the patient's scalp and hair, level of self-care, and ability to tolerate the procedure.

Assessments

- Assess for any contraindications to a shampoo.

For example, if the patient has scalp sutures, you may need special measures to keep them dry. Or, you might find that a patient has limited head or neck movement. A rinse-free shampoo would be more appropriate in these cases.

- Determine the patient's ability to assist with the procedure.

Promotes independence and provides active range of motion.

- Assess the condition of the patient's hair and scalp.

Dry and brittle hair may indicate hypothyroidism or malnutrition and may require special shampoos or conditioners. Note any dryness or irritation of the scalp.

- Determine the need for special hair care products, such as medicated shampoo.

Dandruff, lice, and dry hair are examples of conditions that require medicated shampoos or conditioners.

- Ask the patient how she normally cares for her hair.

Follow cultural practices, and identify personal preferences.

PROCEDURE 22–9   Shampooing the Hair for a Patient on Bedrest
(continued)

Procedural Steps

Step 1 If lesions or infestation are present, don procedure gloves.

Observes standard precautions.

Step 2 Unless contraindicated (e.g., by a neck condition), lower the head of the bed, take the pillow from under the patient's neck, and place it under her shoulders.

Hyperextends the neck and helps keep water from the eyes.

Step 3 Place the waterproof pad or plastic trash bag under patient's shoulders, and cover with towels.

Protects the bed from getting wet.

Step 4 Place the shampoo tray under patient's shoulders (or head, depending on how it is made). If you are using a hard plastic tray, liberally pad it with towels. An inflatable shampoo tray needs minimal padding.

Protects the patient from lying on a hard surface and prevents water from leaking out onto the bed.

Step 5 Ensure that the tray will drain into the washbasin or plastic pail.

Prevents water draining onto the bed or floor.

Step 6 Fold the top linens down to the patient's waist, and cover her upper body with a bath blanket.

Keeps the linen dry; keeps the patient warm.

Step 7 Work your fingers through the patient's hair, or comb the hair to remove tangles prior to washing.

Removing the tangles prior to washing helps prevent creating worse tangles while shampooing. Note that very tangled or matted hair may sometimes indicate a lice infestation.

Step 8 Wash the hair.
- Wet the hair using warm water, then apply shampoo and lather well, working from the scalp out and from the front to the back of the head.
- Gently lift the patient's head to rub the back of the head.

Cleaning the scalp is the most important part of a shampoo.

Step 9 Rinse thoroughly.

Shampoo is drying if left in the hair. ▼

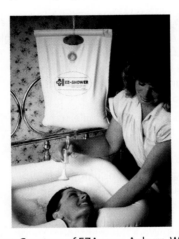

Source: Courtesy of EZAccess, Auburn, WA.

Step 10 If desired, apply conditioner to the hair. Conditioner should be used for patients with hair that tangles easily, such as dry, long, curly, or kinky hair. Rinse if needed. Leave-in conditioner can be used and is recommended for curly hair.

Step 11 Remove the tray, and blot-dry the hair with the towel. Do not use circular motions to dry the hair.

Circular motions will increase tangles.

Step 12 Comb or brush hair to remove tangles, starting at the ends and working toward the scalp.

Prevents excessive pulling on the patient's hair, which may cause breakage.

Step 13 If desired, dry hair with hair dryer at a medium temperature.

Use a medium temperature to prevent burning the patient.

Procedure Variation

Shampooing the Hair of African American Clients

Step 1 If the hair is in cornrows or braids, do not take out the braids to wash the hair. Apply a stocking cap if one is available.

Cornrow braids are left in place during routine hair care.

Step 2 Handle the patient's hair very gently, being careful not to pull on the hair.

Many African Americans have fragile hair that breaks easily. Because it is fragile, apply moisturizer, if needed, to untangle the hair.

Step 3 When shampooing, thread your fingers through the hair from the scalp out to the ends. Do not massage the hair in circular motions.

A circular motion increases tangling.

Step 4 Use a conditioner on the hair.

A leave-in conditioner is often recommended because the hair is often dry and fragile.

Step 5 Comb through the hair.
a. Do not use a brush or fine-toothed comb on the patient's hair. Use a wide-toothed comb or hair pick.
b. Part the hair into four sections, and, using a wide-toothed comb or hair pick, begin combing near the ends of the hair, working through each section.
c. Use additional moisturizer to help soften and ease combing.

Never pull on the hair, because it will break easily.

Step 6 Apply a natural oil to the hair, if desired.

Examples of natural oils are coconut, sweet almond, shea butter, and avocado. There are many commercial products using these oils. Mineral oil and Vaseline tend to clog pores and damage the hair,

➤

PROCEDURE 22–9 **Shampooing the Hair for a Patient on Bedrest**
(continued)

so use them only if the patient still prefers them after receiving this information.

Step 7 Let the hair air-dry if possible.

Prevents the hair from becoming frizzy. A high temperature, such as from a hair dryer, will also damage the hair.

Procedure Variation
Shampooing the Hair Using Rinse-Free Shampoo

Equipment

- Rinse-free shampoo (no water is needed)
- Conditioner, optional
- Bath towel
- Brush or hair pick
- Comb
- Procedure gloves (if scalp lesion or infestation present)

Procedural Steps

Step 1 If possible, elevate the head of the bed.

Makes it easier to maintain good body mechanics during the procedure.

Step 2 Place the bath towel under the patient's shoulders.

Prevents the linen getting wet from the shampoo.

Step 3 Don procedure gloves if lesions or infestations are present.

Step 4 Work your fingers through the hair, or comb the hair to remove tangles prior to washing.
- If the patient has her hair in small braids, do not take out the braids to wash the hair.

Black curly hair is fragile, so handle it gently.

Step 5 Apply rinse-free shampoo.
- Apply enough shampoo to thoroughly wet the hair. One application is usually sufficient to clean the hair.

Step 6 Work the shampoo through the hair, from scalp down to ends.

Helps prevent pulling on and damaging the hair.

Step 7 Dry the hair with a bath towel.

Removes the shampoo. Leaves the hair feeling clean and soft.

Procedure Variation
Shampooing the Hair Using Rinse-Free Shampoo Cap

A commercial rinse-free shampoo cap is a microwavable cap that contains a rinse-free shampoo and conditioner.

Step 1 Warm the shampoo cap using a water bath or microwave according to package instructions. Be careful to not overheat. Check temperature before placing on patient's head to prevent burns.

Different products are available. Be sure to follow the directions on the package.

Step 2 Place the cap on the patient's hair, and gently massage.

The cap contains a rinse-free shampoo and water.

Step 3 Remove the cap, and towel-dry the patient's hair.

Removes the shampoo and excess water.

PROCEDURE 22–9   Shampooing the Hair for a Patient on Bedrest
(continued)

Evaluation
- Observe that the hair is clean, dry, and free of tangles.
- Observe for patient discomfort or fatigue during the procedure.
- Ask the patient how the hair and scalp feel.

Patient Teaching
- Advise patients with coarse hair to wash it less frequently (every 3 to 7 days, depending on dryness). Leave-in conditioners are often recommended for dry, curly, or kinky hair.
- Discuss potential adaptations in washing hair. Products such as rinse-free shampoos or a shampoo tray can make shampooing easier to accomplish for a bedridden patient.

Home Care
- In the home care setting, determine how the patient usually washes her hair.
- If the patient is bedridden, work with the caregiver to develop a plan for washing the patient's hair that will be effective. For example, if a shampoo tray is not available, you can make one by using a plastic garbage bag and pillows or rolled towels.
- The newer rinse-free products or the inflatable shampoo tray may be good choices for the patient.
- If the patient cannot afford the adaptive equipment needed, refer the caregiver to the local resources, such as senior services.
- If the patient is ambulatory, recommend a shower stool. The stool needs to fit into the shower or bathtub securely, without wobbling, to prevent the patient from falling.
- If the patient has only a bathtub, an adaptor for the faucet can be used to attach a hand-held showerhead. Again, using a shower stool will make the procedure easier.

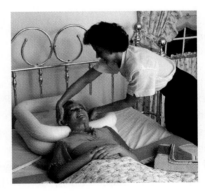

Source: Courtesy of EZAccess, Auburn, WA.

Documentation
Chart that hair was shampooed, the condition of the hair and scalp, and the patient's responses to the procedure.

Example:

| 09/16/06 | 2045 | Hair shampooed. Scalp without signs of irritation. Hair dry. Conditioner applied. No c/o discomfort. Pt states, "My hair feels wonderful now, and my head doesn't itch any more."————————— A. Nelson, RN |

PROCEDURE 22–10   Providing Beard and Mustache Care

➤ For steps to follow in *all* procedures, refer to the inside back cover of this book.

critical aspects
- Assess the skin for redness, dry areas, or lesions.
- Trim the beard and mustache to the desired length with a comb and scissors or beard trimmer.
- Shampoo the beard and mustache.
- Apply conditioner, if desired.
- Towel-dry the beard and mustache, and comb and style as desired.

Equipment
- Scissors or beard trimmer
- Wide-toothed comb
- Mild shampoo
- Conditioner for coarse and/or dry hair
- Bath towel
- Procedure gloves (if skin nicks occur, contact with blood may occur)

Delegation
You can delegate beard and mustache care to the UAP if the patient's condition and the UAP's skills allow. Perform the following assessments, and inform the UAP of the specific type of care needed (e.g., in bed, at sink, safety razor, electric razor), and the amount of help the patient needs. Inform the UAP of any special considerations, such as skin irritation or activity intolerance. Ask the UAP to report the condition of the patient's skin and beard, level of self-care, and ability to tolerate the procedure

Assessments
- Ask the patient or family about preferences for beard and mustache care.

Beards and mustaches may have personal and/or cultural meaning. Men in some cultures never cut or trim their beards. Some patients use a comb and scissors to do a small trim of their beard and/or mustache, whereas others use a beard trimmer for a closer trim.

- Assess the patient's skin and hair condition.

Determine whether the skin has any reddened or dry areas and whether skin treatments are needed.

Procedural Steps

Step 1 Trim the beard and mustache when they are dry.

The beard and mustache are often shorter when dry. If they are cut when wet, they may be shorter than desired after they dry.

Step 2 If you are using a comb and scissors:
a. Comb through the beard, and cut the hair on the outside of the comb. Be conservative; cutting too little is better than cutting too much.

Trimming too much off the beard can be very upsetting for the patient, whereas if you cut too little, you can always trim off more.

b. Trim from the front of the ear to the chin on one side, and repeat on the other.

Keeps the beard equal on both sides of the face.

Step 3 If you are using a beard trimmer:
a. Select the trimming guide to the correct length. Adjust the guide to a longer length rather than a shorter length so that you do not cut the beard too short.

b. Trim from the front of the ear to the chin on one side, and repeat on the other.

Step 4 Trimming the mustache:
a. Comb the mustache straight down.

Cuts the length equally so that the mustache is just above the upper lip. ▼

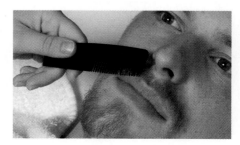

PROCEDURE 22–10   Providing Beard and Mustache Care *(continued)*

b. Using either scissors or a beard trimmer, start in the middle, and trim toward one side of the mouth and then toward the other. Do not trim the top of the mustache.

Trimming from the center out toward each side helps you cut both sides equally.

Step 5 Define the beard line by one of the following methods:

a. Using either the scissors or a beard trimmer, trim the line of the beard so that it is well defined.

Trim very little to ensure that you only define the beard and do not change the length. ▼

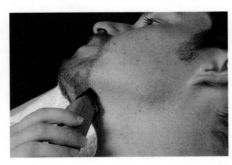

b. Shave the neck to define the beard line.

This is done particularly for short beards.

Step 6 Apply procedure gloves, if needed, and shampoo the beard and mustache using warm water and a mild shampoo.

The skin under beards and mustaches is tender, so treat it gently with a mild shampoo. Follow standard precautions, because it is possible to nick the skin and cause bleeding.

Step 7 Rinse well, and pat and wipe the beard and mustache dry with the towel.

Any shampoo left can irritate the skin, as can rubbing motions with the towel.

Step 8 Apply conditioner, if desired.

The hair in many beards and mustaches is coarse.

Step 9 Comb the beard and mustache with a wide-toothed comb or a brush.

Do not use a fine-toothed comb, because it will pull the hair.

Evaluation

- Make sure that the beard and mustache are trimmed to the desired length and are clean.
- Verify that skin problems are identified and treatment initiated.

Home Care

No adaptations are required in the home. Use supplies normally used by patient.

Documentation

Chart that beard and mustache were trimmed and shampooed; chart the condition of the skin.

PROCEDURE 22–11   Shaving a Patient

 For steps to follow in *all* procedures, refer to the inside back cover of this book.

critical aspects
- Wear procedure gloves.
- Assess the skin for redness or dry areas.
- To soften the beard and moisten the skin:
  - Apply a warm, damp towel to the face.
  - Apply shaving cream or soap.
- To prevent skin irritation:
  - Hold the skin taut, and shave the face and neck.
  - If using a safety razor, hold the blade at a 45-degree angle to the skin.
- Apply after-shave product, if desired.

Equipment
- Safety razor or electric razor
- Shaving cream or soap
- Shaving brush, if desired
- Warm water
- Face towel and bath towel
- After-shave lotion, if desired
- Procedure gloves (because blood contact can occur if skin is nicked)

Delegation
You can delegate shaving to the UAP if the patient's condition and the UAP's skills allow. Perform the following assessments, and inform the UAP of the specific type of care needed (e.g., safety or electric razor, in bed, or at the sink), and the amount of help the patient needs. Inform the UAP of any special considerations, such as skin irritation or activity intolerance. Ask the UAP to report the condition of the patient's skin, level of self-care, his ability to tolerate the procedure.

Assessments
- Determine how much assistance the patient needs.

Promote independence as much as possible.

- Assess the patient's skin and hair condition for redness, skin lesions, or moles.

Identify skin problems, and determine whether skin treatments are needed or the procedure must be modified. To prevent abrading the skin, do not shave any areas that have skin lesions or moles.

- Assess patient's usual shaving method, including use of electric razor or safety razor.

When possible, follow the patient's routine. The patient may or may not use shaving cream or shaving soap, shaving brush, and after-shave lotion.

- Check for any contraindications to shaving, such as an increased risk of infection or bleeding, neutropenia, thrombocytopenia, or the administration of anticoagulants, such as warfarin (Coumadin) or heparin.

Such patients must be shaved carefully using an electric razor, if at all. A razor scratch or cut causes a break in skin integrity, providing a portal of entry for pathogens. This could be serious for a patient whose defenses against infection are compromised. For a patient with a delayed clotting time, a cut could cause excessive blood loss.

- Assess the direction in which the hair is growing.

Shave in the same direction as the hair is growing to prevent skin irritation.

PROCEDURE 22–11   Shaving a Patient *(continued)*

Procedural Steps

Step 1 Don gloves.

Skin will bleed if it is nicked or scratched.

Step 2 Place a warm, damp face towel on the patient's face for 1 to 2 minutes.

Opens the pores and softens the beard to prevent pulling. Do not use hot water, because it will dehydrate the skin and can burn sensitive skin.

Step 3 Apply shaving lotion to the face with your fingers or a shaving brush. Lather well for 1 to 2 minutes.

Lathering well helps to further soften the beard. Do not use shaving creams that contain numbing agents, because they close the pores and stiffen the beard.

Step 4 Shave the patient.
a. Pull skin taut with your nondominant hand, and gently pull the razor across the skin. If you are using a safety razor, hold the blade at a 45-degree angle to the skin.

b. Shave the face and neck in the same direction of hair growth (the direction is not the same for all people). Using short strokes, start shaving at the sideburns, and work down to the chin on each side and then the neck.
c. Last, shave the chin and upper lip.

Usually the hair on the face will grow down toward the chin and on the neck up toward the chin. The hair is generally thickest on the chin and upper lip, so shaving them last allows more time for the shaving cream to soften the hair. ▼

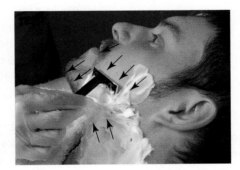

Step 5 Rinse the razor frequently while you are shaving.

Avoids clogging the blade.

Step 6 When you are finished shaving, rinse the patient's face with cool water, and gently pat it dry.

Cool water helps close the pores. Pat dry, do not rub, to prevent irritating the skin.

Step 7 Apply after-shave lotion, if desired.

After-shave lotions that contain alcohol are not recommended, because alcohol stings and dries out the skin. A moisturizer is recommended.

Evaluation

Inspect the patient's face for nicks or cuts.

Patient Teaching

Teach patients about changes that need to be made in their shaving technique as a result of changes in health status. For example, a patient who has begun taking anticoagulants may need to change from a blade to an electric razor because of an increased risk of bleeding.

Documentation

Chart that the patient was shaved and the condition of the skin. There will probably be a flowsheet or checklist for this information.

PROCEDURE 22–12   Removing and Caring for Contact Lenses

For steps to follow in *all* procedures, refer to the inside back cover of this book.

critical aspects
- Instill 1 to 2 drops of wetting solution.
- Gently remove the contact lenses; use your finger pads, not your fingernails.
- Clean and store contact lenses in sterile solution.
- Mark the containers "L" and "R" to identify the correct eye.

Equipment
- Contact lens wetting solution
- Contact lens case
- Contact lens soaking solution
- Contact lens remover (optional)
- Sterile saline (optional)
- Procedure gloves

Delegation

You can delegate this procedure if you conclude that the patient's condition and the UAP's skills permit. For example, if the patient is unconscious, you must determine whether contact lenses are present, and you should not delegate their removal.

Assessments
- Determine whether the patient is wearing contact lenses. As a part of the admission assessment, ask the patient whether he uses glasses or wears contact lenses. If the patient is unconscious, examine the eyes for the presence of contact lenses by shining a penlight across the eye. You should be able to see the edge of the lens. Some lenses are larger than others, so examine the surface of the cornea carefully.
- Determine the type of contact lenses in place. Hard lenses are smaller than soft lenses. Each type of contact lens has different care requirements. Hard lenses can be worn for only up to 18 hours. Rigid gas-permeable (RGP) lenses may be worn overnight or for 7 days, depending on the kind. Soft contacts are used for either short or longer periods.
- Ask the patient whether he is able to remove his contact lenses.

Promotes patient independence.

Procedural Steps

Note: It is difficult to remove a contact lens when wearing procedure gloves. For hard lenses, you can use a suction cup device if one is available. If you must use ungloved hands (e.g., in an emergency situation), it is extremely important to wash your hands thoroughly before and after the procedure. *Do not* use your fingernails.

Note: Lens cases are marked L and R to indicate left and right lenses. Clean, rinse, and place the lens you remove first into its designated cup before removing the second lens.

Step 1 Instill 1 to 2 drops of contact lens wetting solution to moisten the lenses.

Moistening the lens aids in removal.

Step 2 Variation: For a hard or gas-permeable contact lens:
a. If the lens is not centered over the cornea, place your finger on the patient's lower eyelid, and apply gentle pressure to move it into position.
b. Place your index finger at the outer corner of the eye, and gently pull sideways toward the ear; position your other hand below the eye to "catch" the lens. Ask the patient to blink. As the skin tightens, the contact will "pop" out.

As the palpebral fissure narrows, the lids catch on the edge of the lens and pop it out. ▼

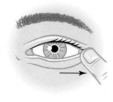 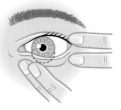

PROCEDURE 22–12 | **Removing and Caring for Contact Lenses**
(continued)

c. *Alternative 1:* Use a small suction cup contact lens remover. Gently press the suction cup end of the remover onto the contact lens, and lift straight up off the eye.

d. *Alternative 2:* Gently pull the top eyelid up and the lower lid down beyond the top and bottom edges of the lens. Then gently press the lower eyelid up against the bottom of the lens. When the lens is slightly tipped, move the eyelids together. This should cause the lens to slide out. ▼

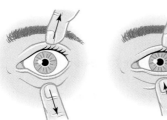

Step 3 Variation: For a soft contact lens:

a. Hold the eye open with your nondominant hand.

Allows you to visualize the contact lens.

b. Gently place the tip of your index finger on the contact lens, and slide it down off the pupil to the white area of the eye.

To prevent potential damage to the eye, do not pinch a lens directly over the pupil. ▼

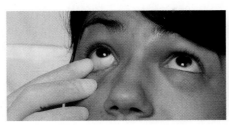

c. Using your thumb and index finger pads, gently pinch the lens, and lift it straight up off the eye.

A soft contact lens is very flexible and pinches easily. ▼

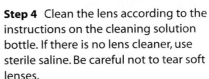

Step 4 Clean the lens according to the instructions on the cleaning solution bottle. If there is no lens cleaner, use sterile saline. Be careful not to tear soft lenses.

Step 5 Rinse the lenses with contact lens solution or sterile saline.

Removes any particles from the lenses.

Step 6 Place the lenses in a contact lens case containing soaking solution or sterile saline (see note above regarding lens cases).

Prevents bacterial growth on the contacts and keeps the lenses from drying out.

Evaluation

Examine the eyes for redness or irritation.

Patient Teaching

• Review with the patient and/or family the importance of keeping the contact lenses clean and moist.
• If hard contact lenses are used, they must be removed at bedtime to prevent hypoxia of the cornea.

Documentation

Chart that contacts were removed, what type of lenses they are, what solution they are stored in, and the condition of patient's eyes.

PROCEDURE 22–13   Making an Unoccupied Bed

> For steps to follow in *all* procedures, refer to the inside back cover of this book.

critical aspects
- Remove soiled linens without cross-contaminating other items in the room.
- Remake the bed with clean linens.
- Do not "shake" or "fan" linens.
- Work efficiently and safely.
- Ensure that there are no wrinkles in the bottom sheet or drawsheet.

Equipment
- Bottom and top sheets
- Drawsheet
- Pillowcase for each of the pillows
- Linen bag or hamper

Delegation
You can delegate this procedure to a UAP. You are responsible for supervising to ensure that the procedure is adequately performed.

Assessments
- Check to see whether the linen (including the mattress pad, blanket, and bed spread) needs to be changed.
- Determine what linens are needed.
- Assess whether the patient is able to be out of bed during the linen change.
- Assess for drainage or incontinence to determine whether personal protective equipment, such as procedure gloves and gown, is needed.

Procedural Steps

Step 1 Assist the patient to a chair. Provide a robe and/or blanket if needed.

Ensures that the patient is comfortable and will be warm enough during the bed change.

Step 2 Position the bed flat, raise to appropriate working height, and lower siderails.

Maintain good body mechanics during the procedure.

Step 3 Loosen all the bedding.

Step 4 If the blanket or bed spread is clean, fold it and place it on a clean area (e.g., on the back of a chair). Do *not* place on another patient's bed or furniture.

Reuse the blanket and/or bed spread if it is not soiled. Placing the item on a clean area prevents cross-contamination.

Step 5 Remove the bottom and top sheet, draw sheet, and pillowcases. Holding the items away from your body, place them in a laundry bag or hamper.

Never place linen on the floor, because cross-contamination can occur. Hold dirty linen away from your uniform to prevent contamination. ▼

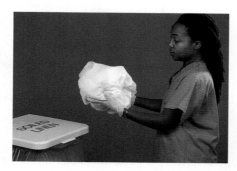

Step 6 From one side of bed:
a. Put the contour bottom sheet on one side of the bed, and smooth it out over half the mattress. If you are using a flat bottom sheet, position it so that approximately 10 inches hang over at the top and sides, and tuck in the sheet, mitering the corners (see Step 9).

Placing the linen on one side of the bed saves time. When using a flat bottom sheet, having extra sheet at the top helps keep it in place when the head of the bed is raised and lowered.

b. Place the drawsheet in the middle of the mattress, tuck the side in under the mattress, and smooth out over half of the mattress.

Ensures that all wrinkles are out of the bottom sheet and drawsheet. ▼

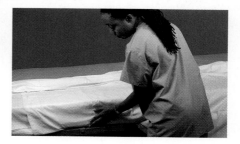

PROCEDURE 22–13 Making an Unoccupied Bed *(continued)*

Step 7 Go to the other side of the bed, straighten the linen, and finish tucking in the bottom sheet and drawsheet.
a. Make the drawsheet tight, and smooth any wrinkles in the bottom sheet and drawsheet.
b. If desired, place a waterproof pad on or under the drawsheet.

Pulling the drawsheet tight helps prevent wrinkles from developing under the patient when she moves around in bed. ▼

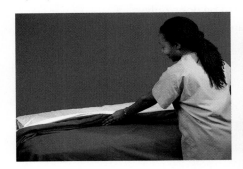

Step 8 Place the top sheet and bed spread along one side of the mattress.

Placing all linen on one side at a time saves steps. Center the top sheet and bed spread, so that when you straighten them from the other side of the bed, they fall equally over each side of the bed. ▼

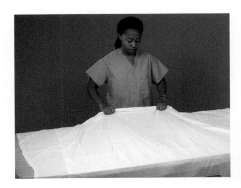

Step 9 At the foot of the bed, make a small pleat in the top sheet and bed spread.

Prevents the top covers from placing pressure on the patient's toes. ▼

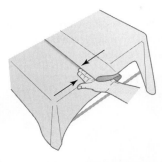

Step 10 Tuck in the top sheet and bed spread at the same time, mitering the corners.
a. Tuck in the sheet and bed spread at the bottom of the mattress. ▼

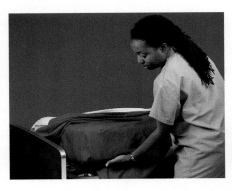

b. Bring the edge of sheet and the bedspread up to make a right angle. ▼

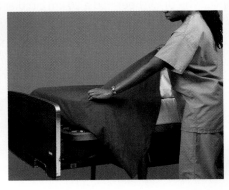

c. Tuck the lower edge of sheet and bed spread under the mattress.

Mitered corners help secure the linen at the foot of the bed. ▼

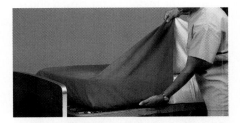

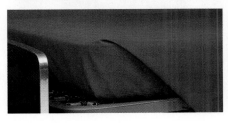

Step 11 Move to the other side of the bed, smooth top linens, and repeat step 10. At the head of the bed, fold the edge of sheet down over the bed spread.

Prevents the bed spread from rubbing against the patient's skin. ▼

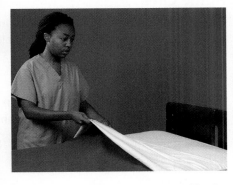

Step 12 Fanfold the top sheet and bed spread back to the foot of the bed.

Makes it easier for the patient to get into bed. ▼

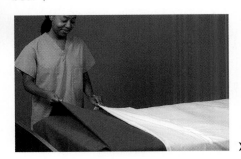

➤

PROCEDURE 22–13   **Making an Unoccupied Bed** (continued)

Step 13 Change pillowcases.
a. Turn the pillowcase wrong side out.
b. Grasp the middle of the closed end of the pillowcase.
c. Reaching through the pillowcase, grasp the end of the pillow. ▼

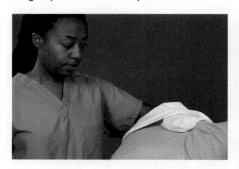

d. Continuing to grasp the end of the pillow, pull the pillowcase down over the pillow.

Do not hold the pillow under your arm or chin to put on pillowcase because contamination can occur. ▼

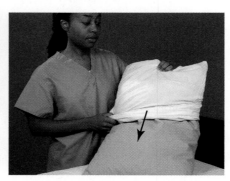

Step 14 Assist the client back to bed, return the bed to the low position, place the call signal within reach, and place the bedside table and overbed table so that they are accessible to the client.

Provides for client comfort and safety.

Evaluation

Evaluate the client's responses to activity (e.g., pulse and respirations)

Home Care

The only adaptations at home depend on the type of bed the patient has. If the height of the bed is not adjustable or the bed is not accessible from both sides, the procedure may be more difficult.

Documentation

Linen changes are generally recorded on a checklist. Additional charting would need to be done only if something abnormal occurred, for example, "The drawsheet had a 20 cm circular area of serosanguineous drainage."

PROCEDURE 22–14 **Making an Occupied Bed**

> For steps to follow in *all* procedures, refer to the inside back cover of this book.

critical aspects

- Maintain patient safety during the procedure.
- Position patient laterally near the far siderail, and roll soiled linens under him.
- Place clean linens on the side nearest you, and then tuck under the soiled linens.
- Roll the patient over the "hump," and position him on his other side, near you. Raise the near siderail.
- Move to other side of bed; pull soiled and clean linens through, and complete the linen change as in Procedure 22–13: Making an Unoccupied Bed.
- Place the bed in a low position, raise the siderails, and fasten the call light to the pillow.

Equipment

- Bottom and top sheets
- Drawsheet
- Pillowcase for each of the pillows
- Bath blanket (as needed)
- Linen bag or hamper
- Procedure gloves (if exposure to body fluids is possible)

Delegation

You can delegate this procedure if you conclude that the patient's condition and the UAP's skills permit. For example, if the client is very ill, in pain, or requires two people for turning and repositioning, you should assist with or perform the linen change yourself.

Assessments

- Determine the patient's ability to assist with the procedure and whether additional help is needed.
- Make other assessments listed in Procedure 22–13: Making an Unoccupied Bed.

Procedural Steps

Note: If linen change is done at the same time as the bed bath, some of these steps will vary.

Step 1 Position the bed flat if possible, and raise it to appropriate working height. Lower the siderail nearest you.

Maintain good body mechanics during the procedure. To prevent the patient from falling out of bed, lower the siderail *only* on the side where you are standing. Having the head of the bed flat makes it easier to smooth bottom sheet.

Step 2 Loosen all the bedding. Disconnect the call device, and remove the patient's personal items from the bed.

Prevents items from getting lost.

Step 3 Check that no tubes (e.g., IV, nasogastric) are entangled in the bed linens.

Prevents dislodging tubes accidentally.

Step 4 If the blanket or bed spread is clean, fold it and place it on a clean area. Cover the patient with a bath blanket, if available, or leave the top sheet over the patient.

Reuse the blanket and/or bedspread if it is not soiled. Covering the patient ensures that she will not become chilled and preserves modesty.

Step 5 Slide the patient to the side of bed farthest from you, and place her in a side-lying position, facing the siderail.

Place pillow under her head. If needed for support, place a pillow between the patient and the siderail. ▼

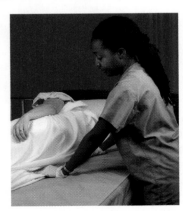

Placing the patient close to the side rail will allow you to place the clean linen over a larger area, making it easier to roll

PROCEDURE 22–14 **Making an Occupied Bed** (*continued*)

the patient back onto the clean linen. Patients who cannot maintain the side-lying position should have a pillow placed between their chests and the side-rail to prevent them from accidentally rolling into the siderail.

Step 6 Roll or tightly fanfold the soiled linens toward the patient's back. Tuck the roll slightly under the patient. Cover any moist areas with a waterproof pad.

Cover any moist areas to prevent contact with the clean linen or patient.

Step 7 Place the clean bottom sheet and drawsheet on the near side of the mattress, with the center vertical fold at the center of the bed. Fanfold the half of the clean linen that is to be used on the far side, folding it as close to the patient as possible and tucking it under the dirty linen. Tuck the lower edges of clean linen under the mattress. Smooth out all wrinkles.

Wrinkles under the patient can cause skin irritation. ▼

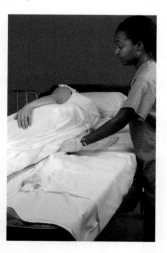

Step 8 Roll the patient over the clean and dirty linen. Explain to her that she will be rolling over a "lump," and then

gently pull the patient toward you so that she rolls onto the clean linen. ▼

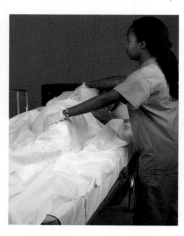

Step 9 Raise the siderail on the clean side of the bed.

Prevents the patient from falling.

Step 10 Move the pillows to the clean side. Position the patient comfortably on her side, near the siderail.

Always ensure patient comfort and safety before going to the other side of the bed.

Step 11 Go to the opposite side of bed, and lower the rail. Pull the soiled linen from under the clean linen, and place it in laundry bag or hamper.

Never place linen on the floor; cross-contamination can occur. ▼

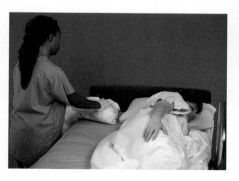

Step 12 Pull clean linens through, and tuck them in. Pull taut, starting with the middle section.

Ensures that no wrinkles will be under the patient. ▼

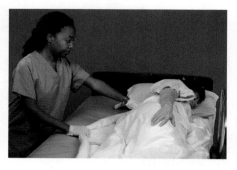

Step 13 Assist the patient to a supine position close to center of the mattress.

Makes it easier to place the top linen.

Step 14 Place the top sheet and bed spread along one side of the mattress, and continue making the bed as in Procedure 22–13, Steps 8 through 13, *except* remove the bath blanket from under the top linens before tucking them in. ▼

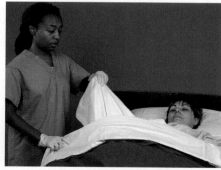

Step 15 Return the bed to the low position, raise the siderails, and attach the call light within patient's reach. Position the bedside table and overbed table within patient's reach.

For Evaluation, Documentation, and Patient Teaching, see Procedure 22–13: Making an Unoccupied Bed.

Home Care

The only adaptations at home depend on the type of bed the patient has. If the height of the bed is not adjustable or the bed is not accessible from both sides, the procedure may be more difficult.

TECHNIQUES

TECHNIQUE 22–1 Assisting with a Shower or Tub Bath

- Assess the patient's self-care abilities: sensorimotor, musculoskeletal, and cognitive function; activity tolerance; level of knowledge.
- Ensure that there is a nonskid surface or mat in the shower or tub.
- For patients who have impaired mobility or activity intolerance, use a shower chair in the shower or tub.
- Be sure that the shower or tub is clean and safe. Most hospitals and long-term care facilities have grab bars and handrails in the bathrooms, but these may need to be installed in the home.
- Ensure that the patient has the necessary supplies (e.g., soap, washcloth, towel, clean gown, and so forth).
- Assist the patient to the shower or bathroom as needed.
- To avoid burns, you will need to verify water temperature for clients with impaired cognition or decreased sensory perception. Water should be 110 to 115°F (43 to 46°C).
- Provide a call device for the patient to obtain help if needed; point out the emergency call device if there is one in the

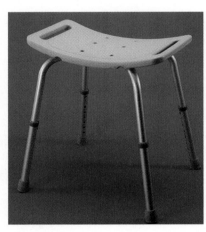

Shower chair

bathroom (usually it is a red button or cord on the wall).
- Hang a sign on the door to ensure privacy.
- Help wash and dry any areas that the patient cannot reach (e.g., feet, back).

Patient Teaching for Self-Care

- Encourage patients and families to install hand bars on the sides of the bathtub and on the wall next to the tub.
- Advise parents never to leave a child alone in the tub or shower and to have a way to unlock the bathroom door from outside the room.
- Advise older adults or those who are ill to avoid locking the door when they are in the bathroom, in case they require assistance.

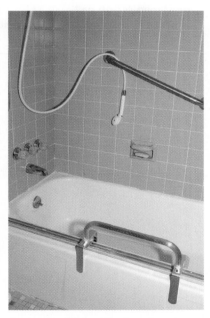

Bathtub with handrail and grab bars

TECHNIQUE 22–2 Caring for Artificial Eyes

To remove and clean an artificial eye, you will need procedure gloves, saline for cleaning, a labeled container filled with saline or tap water, and cotton balls. Follow these steps:

- Position the patient lying down so that if you accidentally drop the eye when removing it, it will fall onto the bed instead of the floor.
- To remove the artificial eye, raise the upper eyelid, and depress the lower lid with your dominant hand. Apply slight pressure below the eye to release the suction holding it in place. Alternatively, you can use a small bulb syringe, place it directly on the eye, and squeeze to create suction and lift the eye from the socket.
- Clean the eye with saline, and store it in a labeled container filled with saline or tap water.
- Wipe the edge of the patient's eye socket with a moistened cotton ball.
- Inspect the socket for redness, swelling, or drainage.

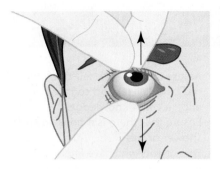

To remove a prosthetic eye, apply pressure.

- To reinsert the eye, remove the eye from the container, but do not dry it, because it will slide into place more easily when it is wet. Hold the eye between your thumb and the index finger of your dominant hand; with your nondominant hand, pull down on the lower lid while lifting the upper lid; and guide the eye into the socket.

TECHNIQUE 22–3 Caring for Hearing Aids

- To remove the hearing aid, turn it off. Rotate the earmold slightly forward (toward the nose), and gently pull it out.
- If the hearing aid is to remain out of the ear for a few days, remove the battery, label the hearing aid with the patient's name, and store it in a safe place (not exposed to heat or moisture). This helps prevent damage in case the battery corrodes.
- If the earmold is detachable, disconnect it, and soak it in soapy water. Rinse and dry well, and then reattach it. Do not use alcohol because it may damage the earmold. *Never immerse a hearing aid in water; only the earmold.*
- If the earmold is glued or fastened by a small metal ring, do not detach it. Wipe it with a damp cloth, and remove earwax and other debris with a pipe cleaner, cotton-tipped applicator, or toothpick.

- Check the device tubing for cracks and loose connections.
- Before reinserting the hearing aid, check that the battery is functioning. Hold the hearing aid in your hand, turn the power on, turn the volume high, and listen for a whistling sound, which indicates proper functioning. If you do not hear whistling, be sure that the battery has been put in correctly (i.e., that the negative (−) and positive (+) symbols on the battery match their location on the hearing aid). Replace the battery if necessary.
- Before reinserting earmold, clean the outer ear using the corner of a washcloth or a cotton-tipped applicator.
- Next, turn off the hearing aid, and set the volume control as low as possible to protect the ear from sudden, loud sound.

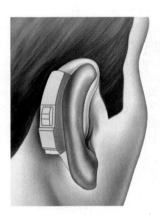 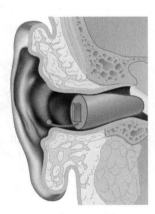 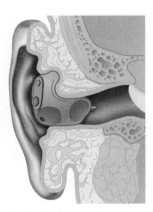

A, *A postaural hearing aid.*   B, *An in-the-canal hearing aid.*   C, *An in-the-ear hearing aid.*

ASSESSMENT GUIDELINES & TOOLS

Assessment Guidelines: Hygiene

The Environment

- Is the room temperature comfortable?
- Are the siderails up, when indicated? Is the bed in low position?
- Are bed wheels locked?
- Are bed linens clean and wrinkle free?
- Is the patient's call device within reach?
- Is the overbed table clean and uncluttered?
- Is the walking space uncluttered?
- Are there unpleasant odors?

Skin

Subjective Data

Patients may be sensitive about skin problems or poor hygiene practices, so direct your questions to the patient in a nonjudgmental, respectful manner. General questions to ask include the following:

- How often do you prefer to bathe?
- How do you usually care for your skin?
- What soaps, lotions, or other skin care products do you use?
- Do you have difficulty controlling body odor?
- Have you ever had an allergic skin reaction to food, medications, plants, skin care products, or other materials?
- What problems have you had with your skin in the past?
- What problems are you having with your skin now?

For each problem identified, ask:

- What symptoms are you having (e.g., any rash or itching)?
- Where is the problem located?
- How long have you had this problem?
- What have you done to provide relief from the symptoms?
- Do you use any prescription, over-the-counter (OTC), or herbal remedies to treat this problem?
- Have you seen a healthcare provider about this problem?
- Was a diagnosis made? If so, what was it?
- How has this problem affected your life?
- How can I best help you with your skin care?

Also ask about the presence of diseases or other factors that are known to cause skin problems; for example, decreased mobility, decreased circulation, incontinence, inadequate nutrition, or deficient knowledge.

Objective Data

- Inspect each area of the skin in an orderly, head-to-toe manner.
- Note the skin's overall cleanliness, condition, color, texture, turgor, hydration, and temperature.
- Observe for rashes, lumps, lesions, and cracking.
- Look for drainage from wounds or around tubes.
- Observe for four significant color changes:
  1. **Pallor** in a light-skinned person may appear as pale skin without underlying pink tones. However, in a dark-skinned person, you will need to observe for an ashen gray or yellow color.
  2. **Erythema** is redness of the skin. It is difficult to see in dark-skinned people, so you may discover it by palpating the skin for areas of increased warmth.
  3. **Jaundice,** a yellow discoloration of the skin, is most readily seen in the sclera of the eye.
  4. **Cyanosis,** a bluish coloring of the skin, is caused by decreased peripheral circulation or decreased oxygenation of the blood. In dark-skinned patients, you can most readily see cyanosis by examining the conjunctivae, tongue, buccal mucosa, and palms and soles for a dull, dark color.

Feet

Subjective Data

Ask the patient the following questions or obtain the data from his records:

- What is your normal foot care routine?
- What type of footwear do you usually wear? (Observe what the patient is wearing.)
- Have you had any foot problems; what treatments have you had for them?
- Do you examine your feet on a regular basis?
- Do you have diabetes mellitus or peripheral vascular disease?

Objective Data

Compare findings for both feet:

- Observe for cleanliness and skin integrity. Note open areas, drainage, or redness.
- Inspect for swelling, inflammation, or infection.
- Palpate for edema.

(continued)

- Check the skin between the toes for cracks or signs of a fungal infection.
- Notice the color and temperature of the feet; are they the same bilaterally? The color and temperature provide data about circulation and oxygenation. For example, cold, dusky feet may indicate impaired circulation or tissue perfusion secondary to a peripheral vascular disease.
- Check capillary refill. How many seconds does it take for the color to return after you apply pressure?
- Note the presence foot odors, if any.

Nails

Subjective Data

Ask about the patient's usual nail care practices, history of nail problems, and their treatments.

Objective Data

Inspect the nails for the following:

- Shape, contour, and cleanliness
- Presence of broken nails, hangnails, or cracked cuticles
- Hands: Do the fingernails appear neatly manicured, or does the patient bite the nails?
- Feet: Are the toenails trimmed appropriately, straight across?
- Presence of redness or swelling at the nail base or sides

Oral Cavity

Subjective Data

- Usual hygiene practices.
- History of periodontal disease or other oral problems.
- Financial or insurance problems that limit access to dental care.
- Nutritional status and dietary habits (e.g., intake of refined sugars).
- Medications, such as anticonvulsants or diuretics.
- Medical treatments, such as radiation therapy, oxygen therapy, and nasogastric tubes.
- Other factors known to cause oral problems (smoking, alcohol use, NPO status, dehydration, mouth breathing).
- Self-care deficits (e.g., cognitive impairment, activity intolerance, impaired mobility, depression, lack of knowledge, lack of motivation).

Objective Data

- Observe the lips, which should be pink and moist without lesions.
- Inspect the oral mucosa and gums, which should also be pink, moist, smooth, and free of lesions. Healthy gums should have a well-defined margin at each tooth. There should be no visible bleeding.
- Instruct the patient to stick out his tongue and to move it around. It should move freely. The tongue should be symmetrical and pink, with a slightly rough surface.
- Assess the teeth for the presence of any loose, missing, or decaying teeth.
- Examine the hard and soft palates for color, lesions, patches, or petechiae.
- Note any unusual mouth odors or halitosis.

Hair

Subjective Data

- Use of special products or medicated shampoos.
- History of hair problems or current conditions needing treatment (e.g., pediculosis).
- History or presence of disease or therapy that affects the hair (e.g., chemotherapy).
- Factors influencing the patient's ability to manage hair and scalp care (e.g., Impaired Mobility).
- Personal or cultural preferences for styling of the hair.

Objective Data

- Note the condition, cleanliness, texture, and oiliness of the hair.
- Inspect the scalp for dandruff, pediculosis (head lice), alopecia (hair loss), secretions or lesions.

Eyes

Subjective Data

- If the patient wears glasses, ask when he uses them (e.g., for reading, for driving); and ask how well he sees without them.
- If the patient wears contact lenses, determine:
  1. The type of lens (hard, soft, long-wearing, disposable).
  2. How often he wears them (daily, occasionally) and for how long at a time. Are they worn during sleep?
  3. History of, or present, problems with lens usage (e.g., cleaning, removal).
  4. Usual practices for cleaning and storage.
  5. History of, or current, problems with the eyes (e.g., redness, tearing, irritation, dryness or "scratchy feeling").

Objective Data

- Inspect the eyes for redness, lesions, swelling, crusting, excessive tearing or discharge.
- Check the color of the conjunctivae.

STANDARDIZED LANGUAGE

Selected Standardized Outcomes and Interventions for Self-Care Deficit Diagnoses

NANDA Diagnosis	NOC Outcomes	NIC Interventions
Bathing/Hygiene Self-Care Deficit	Self-Care: Activities of Daily Living (ADL) Self-Care: Bathing Self-Care: Hygiene	Bathing Ear Care Eye Care Oral Health Maintenance Foot Care Hair Care Nail Care Perineal Care Self-Care Assistance: Bathing/Hygiene Energy Management
Dressing/Grooming Self-Care Deficit	Self-Care: Activities of Daily Living (ADL) Self-Care: Dressing	Self-Care Assistance: Dressing/Grooming Energy Management Environmental Management Hair Care
Toileting Self-Care Deficit	Self-Care: Activities of Daily Living (ADL) Self-Care: Hygiene Self-Care: Toileting	Self-Care Assistance: Toileting Environmental Management Bathing Perineal Care Bowel Management Urinary Elimination Management

When using NOC outcomes to write goals, rank the patient's abilities by using the NOC scale for self-care indicators: (1) dependent, does not participate, (2) requires assistive person and device, (3) requires assistive person, (4) independent with assistive device, and (5) completely independent. For example:

> Chooses clothing (5)
> Buttons clothing (4)

NANDA International (2005). *Nursing diagnoses: Definitions & classification 2005–2006.* Philadelphia: Author; Johnson, M., Bulechek, G., Dochterman, J., Maas, M., & Moorhead, S. (2001). *Nursing diagnoses, outcomes, & interventions: NANDA, NOC, and NIC linkages.* St. Louis: Mosby; Moorhead, S., Johnson, M., & Maas, M. (Eds.). (2004) *Nursing outcomes classification (NOC)* (3rd ed.). St. Louis: Mosby; and Dochertman, J., & Bulechek, G. (2004). Nursing interventions classification (NIC). (4th ed.). St. Louis: Mosby.

Selected NOC Outcomes and NIC Interventions for Hygiene Problems

NANDA Diagnoses	NOC Outcomes	NIC Interventions
	Skin	
Impaired Skin Integrity Risk for Impaired Skin Integrity	Immobility Consequences: Physiological Tissue Integrity: Skin and Mucous Membranes Wound Healing: Primary Intention Wound Healing: Secondary Intention	*For Impaired Skin Integrity:* Bathing Cutaneous Stimulation Incision Site Care Perineal Care Pressure Management Pressure Ulcer Care Skin Surveillance Wound Care *For Risk for Impaired Skin Integrity,* *in addition to those above:* Bed Rest Care Circulatory Precautions Pressure Ulcer Prevention Positioning
	Feet	

Impaired Skin (or Tissue)
  Integrity
Risk for Impaired Skin
  Integrity (feet)
	Tissue Integrity: Skin and Mucous Membranes
	Wound Healing: Primary (and Secondary)
	  Intention
	The following may also apply:
	Knowledge: Health Behavior
	Health-Seeking Behavior
	Self-Care: Activities of Daily Living
		Foot Care
		Circulatory Care: Arterial Insuf-
		  ficiency
		Circulatory Care: Venous Insuf-
		  ficiency
		Infection Protection
		Self-Care Assistance
		Skin Surveillance
		Teaching: Individual
		  Wound Care

	Nails	
Risk for Impaired Tissue Integrity Risk for Infection	Tissue Integrity: Skin and Mucous Membranes Self-Care: Hygiene Knowledge: Health Behavior Health-Seeking Behavior	Nail Care Infection Protection Self-Care Assistance Teaching
	Mouth	
Risk for Infection Impaired Dentition Impaired Oral Mucous Membrane	Oral Hygiene Knowledge: Health Behavior Self-Care: Oral Hygiene	Oral Health Maintenance Teaching: Individual Self-Care Assistance

NANDA International (2005). *Nursing diagnoses: Definitions & classification 2005–2006.* Philadelphia: Author; Johnson, M., Bulechek, G., Dochterman, J., Maas, M., & Moorhead, S. (2001). *Nursing diagnoses, outcomes, & interventions: NANDA, NOC, and NIC linkages.* St. Louis: Mosby; Moorhead, S., Johnson, M., & Maas, M. (Eds.). (2004) *Nursing outcomes classification (NOC)* (3rd ed.). St. Louis: Mosby; and Dochertman, J., & Bulechek, G. (2004). Nursing interventions classification (NIC). (4th ed.). St. Louis: Mosby.

Selected NOC Outcomes and NIC Interventions for Hygiene Problems *(continued)*

NANDA Diagnoses	NOC Outcomes	NIC Interventions
Hair		
Impaired Skin Integrity Risk for Impaired Skin Integrity Situational Low Self-Esteem	Tissue Integrity: Skin and Mucous Membranes Self-Esteem	Hair Care Skin Surveillance Infection Protection
Eyes		
Disturbed Sensory Perception: Visual	Sensory Function: Vision	Medication Administration: Eye Eye Care Contact Lens Care Prosthesis Care
Ears		
Disturbed Sensory Perception: Auditory	Sensory Function: Hearing	Ear Care Medication Administration: Ear

NANDA International (2005). *Nursing diagnoses: Definitions & classification 2005–2006.* Philadelphia: Author; Johnson, M., Bulechek, G., Dochterman, J., Maas, M., & Moorhead, S. (2001). *Nursing diagnoses, outcomes, & interventions: NANDA, NOC, and NIC linkages.* St. Louis: Mosby; Moorhead, S., Johnson, M., & Maas, M. (Eds.). (2004) *Nursing outcomes classification (NOC)* (3rd ed.). St. Louis: Mosby; and Dochertman, J., & Bulechek, G. (2004). Nursing interventions classification (NIC). (4th ed.). St. Louis: Mosby.

What Are the Main Points in this Chapter?

- Personal hygiene contributes to physical and psychological well-being by promoting comfort, improving self-image, and decreasing infection and disease.

- Although a patient may need assistance with hygiene measures, the goal is to encourage as much independence with these tasks as possible.

- Numerous factors influence individual hygiene practices, including: personal preferences, cultural/religious/spiritual values and beliefs, economic status, living environment, developmental or knowledge level, and physical and emotional health.

- Maintain a respectful, nonjudgmental attitude about cultural and spiritual differences. Avoid the temptation to impose personal values about hygiene practices onto patients.

- Consider patients' personal hygiene preferences, and incorporate them into the care plan whenever possible. This reflects caring and promotes maximum participation and independence with ADLs.

- Although many hygiene measures can be delegated to UAP, the nurse retains full responsibility for each patient and must instruct the UAP about the patient's limitations and restrictions, amount of assistance necessary, use of any assistive devices, any specific safety precautions to be undertaken, and any other factors influencing the patient's hygiene practices.

- Teaching patients about hygiene is a primary function of the professional nurse.

- Intact skin is the body's first line of defense to keep pathogenic microorganisms from entering the body and causing infection.

- Bathing removes perspiration and bacteria from the skin surface. It promotes relaxation and comfort, improves circulation, reduces odor, and enhances well-being by increasing self-image. However, it can be stressful for some patients.

- Careful assessment of the feet allows for early detection of common foot problems, such as calluses, corns, tinea pedis, ingrown toenail, or foot odor.

- Because dirt and debris can collect under the nails and serve as a source of infection, nail care is an important part of hygiene, especially in patients with diabetes mellitus or peripheral neuropathy.

- To maintain healthy mucous membranes, teeth, and gums, and to prevent tooth loss and gum disease, regular dental checkups and daily mouth care, including brushing and flossing the teeth, are necessary.

- The condition of the hair is a measure of an individual's overall health. Shampooing and daily brushing of the hair massages the scalp, stimulates the circulation, and distributes the natural oils.

- The eyes normally require very little care; however, when necessary, they may be gently cleansed from the inner to the outer canthus.

- Unconscious or critically ill patients who no longer have a blink reflex may need eye care at least every 2 to 4 hours. Keeping the eyes lubricated protects them from corneal abrasions and drying.

- Some contact lenses can be worn for only about 12 hours at a time; others may be worn for up to 30 days. All types must be cleaned carefully and regularly.

- Hearing aids are expensive and should be properly handled and stored. They should not be immersed in water.

- Usually no special care is required for the nose. Excess secretions can be removed by gentle blowing with both nostrils open.

- Clean, wrinkle-free bed linens help to promote comfort and a sense of well-being.

- Room temperature, adequate ventilation, low noise level, and neat and clean surroundings all contribute to a comfortable patient environment.

23 Administering
Medications

Overview

Pharmacokinetics refers to the absorption, distribution, metabolism, and excretion of a drug, all of which are affected by route of administration, solubility of the drug, effects of pH, blood flow to the body area, total body surface area and other patient characteristics, and the form of the drug (e.g., tablet, elixir). In general, intravenous medications are absorbed most rapidly, followed by intramuscular, subcutaneous, buccal, and oral medications. *Metabolism* is the chemical inactivation of a drug into a form that the body can excrete; drug metabolism takes place mainly in the liver. The primary route of drug *excretion* is from the kidneys; other routes are the liver, gastrointestinal tract, lungs, and exocrine glands.

Nurses are legally responsible for the medications they administer, including knowledge of drug actions and side effects and the questioning of orders they believe to be incorrect. One study (*AJN* Reports, 2003) indicated that approximately 19% of medication doses administered by nurses are erroneous. Medication errors should be reported immediately after they are discovered, and an evaluation process to identify and address causative factors should be in place. To help prevent medication errors, observe the "three checks" (before and after pouring or drawing up a medication, and at the bedside) and "six rights" (right drug, right dose, right time, right route, and right patient, as well as right documentation immediately after giving the medication).

Parenteral medications require the use of sterile technique to prevent infection. Needleless systems reduce the likelihood of needlestick injury. Always dispose of needles in special "sharps" containers. If an unusual circumstance forces you to recap a used needle, use a one-handed technique.

The ventrogluteal site is the preferred intramuscular injection site for adults. Other sites are the vastus lateralis and the deltoid. Use the dorsogluteal and rectus femoris sites only if no other sites are available. Choose the gauge and length of the needle on the basis of the route of the injection (e.g., intramuscular, subcutaneous), the amount of subcutaneous and muscle tissue, and the type of medication being given.

Thinking Critically About Administering Medications

The exercises in the following section allow you to practice the kind of thinking you will use as a full-spectrum nurse. Because these are critical-thinking activities, there is usually no single right answer. Discuss answers with your peers—discussion can stimulate critical thinking. If you have difficulty with any of the questions, consult with your instructor.

Caring for the Garcias

Bettina Sanford, the 3-year-old granddaughter of Joe and Flordelisa Garcia, has been tired and observed to be sitting down a lot at preschool. Last week, she developed coughing, wheezing, shortness of breath, nasal congestion, and extreme fatigue. The pediatrician at the Family Medicine Center diagnosed asthma. He gave her an injectable steroid in the office, prescribed a 7-day tapering course of prednisone, Singulair 4 mg orally daily at bedtime, and periodic treatments with albuterol through a home nebulizer system.

Joe's mother, Katherine, became very upset when she saw the bottle of prednisone elixir. She was even more upset when she learned that Bettina received an injection of the medicine in the office. She advised Flordelisa not to give Bettina the medicine because, she said, it causes weak bones and stunts growth. Flordelisa has called the clinic asking for advice on how to handle this problem.

A. What theoretical knowledge do you need to answer these concerns?

B. What are some reliable sources where you might find this information?

C. What explanation could you offer to Flordelisa to explain the safety of the prednisone orders? You will need to use a variety of references to answer this question.

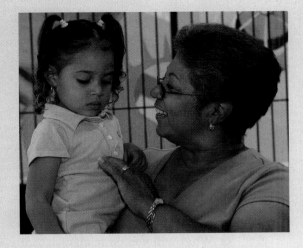

D. Flordelisa asks you to explain why Bettina received both a shot and pills. How would you respond?

E. Why is Bettina receiving Singulair orally and albuterol by nebulizer? Look up the medications, and use your knowledge of different routes of administration.

1   Your patient is ordered Humulin R insulin 30 units subQ. You have available in a multidose vial Humulin R insulin; the label reads "100 units per mL."

a What equipment and supplies do you need to give this medication? Be specific.

b What practical knowledge (psychomotor skills) will you need?

c With regard to the psychomotor skills, what are the two aspects that require the most careful attention? Explain your thinking.

d What will you do to ensure that you have the correct dosage?

e What specific technique steps will you take to decrease the risk for infection?

f Suppose that after drawing the insulin into the syringe, you see that instead of the 30 units ordered, you have only 20 units in the syringe. What will you do?

2   The physician orders heparin 4000 units subQ q12hr for Mr. Dale. You have on hand heparin 10,000 units/mL. How many milliliters should you draw up?

VOL 1 Recall the patients from Chapter 23, **Meet Your Patients,** in Volume 1. The next exercises refer to these patients.

- Margaret Marks is an 82-year-old woman who has a fractured hip and experiences periods of confusion throughout the day. She has returned home. She tries to be compliant with her medications but has limited income and many times is unable to purchase all of her medication.
- Cary Pearson is a 70-year-old man with feeding and swallowing difficulties. He uses a gastrostomy tube to receive his medications. He resides in an assisted living facility, where a personal aide assists him with his care and medications.
- Cyndi Early is a 32-year-old woman with diabetes who is scheduled for surgery at 10:00 A.M. today. Cyndi was admitted to the hospital for right upper quadrant abdominal pain associated with nausea and vomiting. She is scheduled today for a cholecystectomy (removal of the gallbladder).
- James Bigler is a 44-year-old man who has had a repair of a compound fracture of the right arm and is receiving intravenous fluids and medications, including narcotics and antibiotics.
- Rebecca Jones is an 84-year-old woman with compression fractures of the vertebrae resulting from a fall. She has returned to an assisted living facility. Rebecca has hearing and vision problems; she does not always see her medications clearly and frequently takes them according to color and tablet size rather than reading the label.

3 It is 0800, and you have begun organizing your medication pass for this shift by verifying the MAR entries against the physicians' orders. You notice that Mr. Bigler has been ordered Toradol 30 mg IM q6hr. His last dose was supposed to have been given at 0600, and there is no documentation that the medication was administered.

a What should you do?

b Should you assume the night shift nurse gave the medication but forgot to document that she had given it, and give the 0600 dose late? Why or why not?

c When should the next dose be given?

d If the night nurse did *not* give the medication as ordered, what type of medication error did she make? What are some of the things that could have caused this error?

e Assuming that the nurse *did* give the medication as ordered at 0600, what error did the night nurse make? Which of the "six rights" was violated?

4 You receive the laboratory results for Cary Pearson's potassium level and find it to be 3.1 mEq/L. You notify the physician and receive a verbal order to add 20 milliequivalents of KCl to the running IV of D_5 $\frac{1}{2}$ NS (5% dextrose in half-strength normal saline) to infuse at 125 mL per hour. (The running IV is in a new 1000 mL bag that is still almost full.)

a Write the order as you would write it on the order sheet.

b What information must you put on the additive label for this bag?

c Suppose the situation were slightly different. There is only 100 mL of IV fluid left in Mr. Pearson's IV bag when you call the physician. The physician says to you, "Add 10 mEq to the IV, and infuse it at 125 mL per hour." Would you ask for clarification of this order? Why or why not?

d Change the situation again. You have taken the order in this way: "Add 20 mEq of KCl to 1000 mL of D_5 $\frac{1}{2}$ NS and run at 125 mL per hour." You are preparing this medication and find that Mr. Pearson currently has 500 mL remaining in his IV. Should you add the KCl to this infusing IV or wait until you hang a new 1000 mL bag? If you do add it, how much KCl will you add? What is your rationale for your decision?

e You begin preparing the infusion with the 20 mEq of KCl to be added and find you have available only a vial containing KCl 40 mEq in a 10 mL vial. How many milliliters of KCl will you add to the bag of fluids?

5 Dr. Xi has ordered heparin 8000 units subQ q12hr for Mrs. Marks.

a You have vials of heparin containing 10,000 units per mL. How many mL of heparin will you administer?

b To prevent tissue trauma and hematoma, and to help ensure adequate absorption, what precautions should you take while administering heparin?

c What syringe and needle will you select for administration, and why?

6 You are checking Mrs. Early's chart and find that the physician has ordered a medication the patient lists as an allergy. What steps should you take?

7 A patient has been taking warfarin sodium (Coumadin) 3 mg daily for the past 3 years. She has tolerated the medication well, but recently she has noticed more bleeding tendencies, such as nosebleeds and hematuria (blood in the urine). You assess the patient and find that she has gross hematuria today and numerous bruises over her body. To answer the following questions, what theoretical knowledge do you need, and where can you find it? (Note: After you get the information you need, answer the following questions.)

a What could be causing these bleeding episodes?

b What laboratory test is indicated in this situation, and what do you expect the result to be?

c What actions should you take in this situation?

8 James Bigler ("Meet Your Patients") has had a postoperative repair of a compound fracture of the right arm and is receiving intravenous fluids and medications, including opioid analgesics and antibiotics. Coincidentally, he has for some time now had a herniated intervertebral disk, and he has begun to have severe muscle spasms. He was given his first dose of oral Flexeril (a muscle relaxer), 10 mg at midnight. At 8:00 A.M. he received another dose. At 9:00 A.M. he received an IV antibiotic, and, while awake, he has been self-administering his opioid analgesic by IV pump about every 4 hours in a low dose. Consider these facts:

- The most common side effect of Flexeril is drowsiness. It has a half-life of 24 to 72 hours.
- Common side effects of opioids are drowsiness, decreased respiratory rate and depth, decreased blood pressure, and constipation (if taken long term).
- Aside from allergies, the most common adverse effect of Mr. Bigler's antibiotic is diarrhea.

Mr. Bigler's Flexeril is to be given every 8 hours. When you enter his room to give it again at 4:00 P.M., you find that he is extremely sleepy. He will awaken when you shake him or speak to him, but he falls right back to sleep, and he is slurring his words. These are new symptoms for him.

a Is there anything obvious about his medical diagnosis that might be producing these symptoms. If so, what?

b Which of his medications could cause these symptoms, and why?

c What would you do? Would you give the 4:00 P.M. dose of Flexeril?

9 Mrs. Jones lives alone and until a few months ago was able to take care of herself. When her eyesight began to deteriorate, she experienced difficulty self-administering her medications.

a Discuss the assessment required to determine whether she is at risk for ineffective management of her medication regime.

b Mrs. Jones has an order for Ativan 1 mg orally. Is this order complete? If not, what is missing? What actions should you take?

c Mrs. Jones has an order for Lanoxin 1.25 mg orally each A.M. You have available Lanoxin 0.25 mg, and you calculate that the dose to be given would be 5 tablets. You check a drug guide and find that the usual dose is 0.125 mg to 0.25 mg orally daily. What actions should you take?

thinking critically about administering medications

10 Calculate dosages for the following medications that you will be administering during your medication pass today. Are there any orders you would question? If so, why?

a Keflex 500 mg IV q6hr. You have on hand Keflex 1 g in 1 mL of solution.

b Lasix 280 mg orally daily. You have 40 mg tablets of Lasix available.

c Demerol 10 mg intramuscularly, to a child. You have Demerol 25 mg/mL available in a prefilled syringe. In addition to calculating the dosage, describe the equipment you would use to administer the Demerol to a child.

d Morphine gr 1/4. You have morphine labeled 10 mg per mL. How many milliliters of morphine will you give?

11 Describe the procedure for giving meperidine (Demerol) 50 mg and hydroxyzine (Vistaril) 50 mg intramuscularly using the same syringe. The Demerol is in a prefilled 2.5 mL Carpuject cartridge containing 50 mg of Demerol in 1 mL of fluid. The Vistaril is in a single-dose vial containing 50 mg Vistaril in 1 mL of fluid.

12 You have an order to give injectable phenytoin (Dilantin) and furosemide (Lasix). You would like to give them in the same syringe. What theoretical and practical knowledge do you need to decide whether you can do this?

13 For each of the following patient problems, (1) state what you think might be the cause and (2) state one thing you might have done to prevent the problem.

a When you give Mrs. King an intramuscular injection in her ventrogluteal muscle, she complains of pain.

b Several weeks after receiving an intramuscular injection in the dorsogluteal site, Mr. Aguilar begins having pain in his left lower back and hip; the pain proceeds down his leg. He is beginning to limp when he walks.

c Several days after receiving a subcutaneous injection, Patti Deal's upper arm is red, hot, painful, and swollen. There is pus oozing from the injection site.

d Immediately after an intramuscular injection, a patient starts showing severe, unexpected symptoms.

14

For each of the following concepts, use critical thinking to describe how or why it is important to nursing, patient care, or administering medications. Note that these are *not* to be merely definitions.

Pharmacology

Drug classification systems (e.g., according to use or chemical traits)

The *United States Pharmacopoeia (USP)* and the *National Formulary* (US), the *British Pharmacopoeia*, and the *Canadian Formulary*

Drug excretion

Therapeutic levels

Side effects and adverse reactions

The apothecary system

Household measurements

Units and milliequivalents

Standing orders

"Six rights" of medication administration

Ventrogluteal site for intramuscular injection

Medication errors

Practical Knowledge
knowing how

The practical knowledge you will need to administer medications safely and effectively includes procedures and techniques for measuring dosages and administering medications by a variety of routes. This section also includes information about assessments focused on medications, as well as standardized outcomes and interventions related to medications.

PROCEDURES

Procedures in this section will assist you to prepare, measure, and administer various types of medications, to locate injection sites, and to handle needles safely. Use the following Medication Guidelines for all types and routes.

Medication Guidelines: Steps to Follow for All Medications (Regardless of Type or Route)

 For steps to follow in *all* procedures, refer to the inside back cover of this book.

Regardless of the type or route of the medication you are giving, you should always follow the steps below. For specific routes of administration, refer to the procedures in this chapter.

Equipment

- Medication administration record (MAR)
- Medication drawer or cart
- Keys to the cart as needed
- Procedure gloves, as needed
- Other supplies and equipment needed for the specific procedure (e.g., water, alcohol wipes)

Delegation

As an RN, you can usually delegate administration of medications (except for intravenous medications) to a licensed practical nurse (LPN/LVN). You cannot usually delegate this task to a UAP. You can instruct a UAP in the therapeutic effect and side effects of medications and to report any effects observed. Nurse practice acts governing medication administration vary from state to state, and policies vary further among healthcare agencies. Even if specially trained UAPs can administer some (e.g., oral) medications in your facility (e.g., as do "medication aides" in some long-term care settings in some states), as the RN you are always responsible for evaluating client responses, both therapeutic effects and side effects.

Assessment

- Assess your knowledge of the medication (e.g., drug action, purpose, recommended dosage, time of onset and peak action, common side effects, contraindications, drug interactions, and nursing implications).
- Determine whether the prescribed dosage is appropriate for the patient's age and weight.

Dosages are generally decreased for children and older patients because of both age and weight. Both groups have less efficient liver and renal function, increasing the life span of a drug. Many medications are ordered by body weight, especially for children.

- Check for any history of allergies to medications or food.

Some medications (e.g., penicillin and the cephalosporins) have cross-sensitivity; that is, a patient with a penicillin allergy is at high risk for also being allergic to cephalosporins. Medications can also have cross-sensitivity with certain foods.

- At least on the first administration, assess the patient's knowledge about the medications being given.

The patient will be more likely to take the medication correctly if she understands why she is taking the medication.

- Assess the patient's ability to cooperate during the procedure.

If the patient is unable to cooperate, you may need assistance to prevent the patient from moving during the injection or to help position the patient.

- Assess for any factors that would interfere with drug absorption (e.g., diarrhea, inadequate circulation, other medications).
- Before administering the medication, assess vital signs and check lab studies specific to the medication to determine whether the medication can be safely administered.
- Assess for patient findings that might affect absorption and/or metabolism of the medication, such as impaired liver function, edema, inflammation, or age-related changes.

Medications are metatabolized more slowly in a person with decreased liver function. Children and older adults are likely to metabolize and excrete medications more slowly, so they require lower dosages.

- Assess for any reasons that would preclude administering the medication, such as oral medications prescribed for a patient who is NPO for surgery or a test, who is vomiting, who has difficulty swallowing, or who is too sedated.

Medication Guidelines: Steps to Follow for All Medications (Regardless of Type or Route) *(continued)*

Procedural Steps

Step 1 Check the MAR for the patient's name and identification number, medication, dose, route, time, and drug allergies.

The six rights of medication administration are the right patient, right drug, right dose, right route, right time, and right documentation. Initially check the MAR to determine when medications are due. Frequently check for new orders during the shift, so that you do not miss medication changes.

Step 2 Compare the medication on the MAR against the physician's order.

Clarify any discrepancies before giving the medication.

Step 3 Follow agency policies for medication administration, including the time frame for medication administration. Most agencies allow medications to be given 30 minutes before or 30 minutes after the time indicated on the MAR. Do not prepour medications.

The time of administration is more important for some medications. For example, if an anti-infective agent is given early or late, a therapeutic blood level may not be maintained.

Step 4 Wash your hands.

Minimizes transmission of microorganisms.

Step 5 Access the patient's medication drawer, unlock the medication cart, or log onto the medication dispensing computer.

Depending on the agency, the patient's medications may be in a centralized cart or in a locked drawer in the patient's room. Follow agency policy for obtaining the medication.

Step 6 If administering a narcotic or barbiturate, obtain the narcotic cabinet key, and sign out the medication, including the patient's name, drug, dose, and other information per agency policy. Note the drug count when removing a narcotic.

Federal law governs administration of narcotics and barbiturates. All narcotics and barbiturates must be accounted for on every shift.

Step 7 Select the ordered medication, and compare medication with the MAR for the first five rights (patient, drug, dose, route, time); check for drug allergies. (First check.)

Ensure that the *correct drug* is being given to the *correct patient* at the *correct time* in the *correct dose* by the *correct route*. An inpatient should be wearing an identification band with the drug allergies identified; allergies should be clearly marked in the chart and on the MAR. Question the patient about allergies prior to giving a newly ordered medication.

Step 8 Calculate medication dosage.

Double-check any calculations. If you are unable to measure the dose exactly, contact the pharmacist.

Step 9 Check the expiration date (on the label or on the box) of all medications.

A medication that has expired is no longer guaranteed to contain the correct dose.

Step 10 After preparing the medications, do a second check to verify the correct medication, dose, route, and time. (Second check.)

Verifies the first five rights of medication administration.

Step 11 Lock the medication cart.

Never leave an unlocked medication cart unattended. Locking the cart guards against pilferage and protects children who might wander near it.

Step 12 Administer the medications.
a. Take the medication and MAR into the patient's room.

You must be able to do the final check in the patient's room and verify that you are administering the correct medication to the correct patient.

b. Identify the patient according to agency policy: checking the identification bracelet, having the patient state her name, comparing the patient to a posted picture of the patient.

Agencies may have different means of identifying patients, but you must identify all patients carefully prior to administering medications. ▼

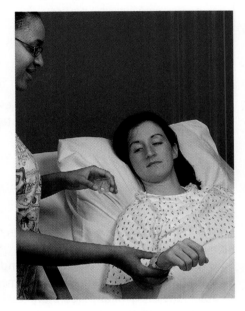

c. Do a third check of the medication for the right patient, right medication, right dose, right route, and right time.

Three checks for the first five rights are required for all medications to prevent medication errors. An error does not occur until the patient has taken a medication that is incorrect.

d. Perform any assessments needed, such as checking the pulse or blood pressure.

Some medications can be given only if physical findings are within certain parameters. For example, when you administer digoxin you must assess the apical pulse and administer the drug only if the pulse is above 60 beats per minute; and antihypertensive medications may need to be held if the blood pressure is lower than normal.

➤

Medication Guidelines: Steps to Follow for All Medications (Regardless of Type or Route) *(continued)*

e. Explain to the patient that you are there to administer the medication and answer any questions about the medication.

Increases the patient's understanding of and compliance with treatment. Also, the patient may identify potential errors in medication administration. If the client questions a medication, double-check the medication. For example, you are about to give the patient her pill, when she says, "It is the wrong color." Always believe the patient and determine why the tablet is different from what the patient is used to taking.

f. Administer the medication using appropriate technique (see the procedures for administering medications by the specified route).

g. Remain with the client until you are sure that she has taken the medication.

Never leave medication at the bedside. Someone else (e.g., another patient or a child) might take it, or the patient might discard it.

Evaluation

- Perform any assessments indicated to evaluate the therapeutic effects of medication, such as checking blood pressure after administering an antihypertensive medication or pain level after an analgesic.
- Be alert for any adverse reactions, side effects, or allergic reactions. If present, notify the appropriate care provider.

Patient Teaching

- Explain the purpose, common side effects, and drug interactions of the medications the patient is taking.
- Describe how the drug is prescribed and when the patient should take the medication.
- Discuss the importance of taking the medication as prescribed.
- Explain the need for any laboratory tests for monitoring the medication, such as tests to measure drug level in the blood, if appropriate.
- Teach the patient to observe for side effects that signal the need to contact the physician.
- Discuss ways to minimize the side effects of a medication, such as avoiding the sun when taking a medication that causes photosensitivity or rising slowly when taking a medication that causes orthostatic hypotension.
- Discuss potential cultural issues related to taking the medication. An example is the concept of hot and cold conditions and treatments in the Hispanic/Latino culture. If the medication is interpreted as "hot" when the appropriate treatment is "cold," the patient may not take the medication.
- Teach the patient to self-administer medications (e.g., ear drops), as appropriate.

Home Care

- Assess the client's ability to self-administer medications safely.
- Determine the client's financial ability to obtain medications.
- Instruct the client in safe storage of medications.
- Provide instruction for each medication.
- Determine whether the patient or caregiver has had past problems or present concerns about taking the medications as prescribed.
- If problems have occurred in the past or there are present concerns, discuss potential remedies, such as a preparing the patient's medications in a container with compartments for the times and days of the week, or setting up a schedule that will work for the patient.

Medication Guidelines: Steps to Follow for All Medications (Regardless of Type or Route) *(continued)*

Documentation

- Chart the medication, time, dose, and route given, preadministration assessments, and your signature.
- Do not document before giving the drug; do not document for anyone else; do not ask another nurse to document a drug you have given.
- Chart any therapeutic or adverse effects of the medication.
- Record the scheduled medications on the MAR. Record PRN medications in the nurse's notes, as well, including the reason the drug was given and the patient's response.
- If the client is unable or refuses to take the medication, document on the MAR that that medication was not administered, along with the reason, and inform the physician.
- For parenteral medications, chart the site of injection.

Sample documentation (for a PRN medication):

| 5/25/06 | 0930 | Tylenol #3, tabs ii, given by mouth for complaint of incision pain (rated 7 on a scale of 1 to 10). — S.Kline, RN |

| 5/25/06 | 1035 | Rates pain as 4 on a scale of 1 to 10 now. States, "I feel a little sleepy, but no other problems." Assisted to chair, splinting incision, but able to stand erect. — S.Kline, RN |

PROCEDURE 23–1 Administering Oral Medications

For steps to follow in *all* procedures, refer to the inside back cover of this book. Also refer to Medication Guidelines: Steps to Follow for All Medications (Regardless of Type or Route).

critical aspects

- Observe the "three checks" and "six rights": right drug, dose, time, route, patient, and documentation.
- *Tablets and capsules:* Pour the correct number into the medication cup.
- *Liquids:* Hold the plastic medication cup at eye level to measure the dose.
- Assist the patient to a high-Fowler's position, if possible.
- For enterically administered medications, check for correct placement of the nasogastric or gastric tube.
- Correctly administer the medication.
  Powder: Mix with liquid, and give it to the patient to drink.
  Lozenge: Instruct the patient not to chew or swallow it.
  Tablet or capsule: Place the tablet or medication cup in the patient's hand or mouth, and have the patient swallow with sips of liquid.
  Sublingual: Have the patient place the tablet under the tongue and hold it there until it is completely dissolved.
  Buccal: Have the patient place the tablet between the cheek and teeth and hold it there until it is completely dissolved.

Equipment

- Desired liquid for taking medications
- Disposable medication cup
- Drinking straw, if needed
- Procedure gloves, if you will need to place a tablet in the patient's mouth
- For enterically administered medications:
  – Water (for diluting and flushing the feeding tube)
  – 60 mL catheter tip syringe
  – Clean gloves
- Stethoscope (to check for placement prior to administering enteric medications through a tube; to check the apical pulse before administering some cardiac medications)

Delegation

As a rule, you can delegate this skill to an LPN/LVN, but not to a UAP, except under special policies and situations.

Assessment

- Assess the patient's condition to determine whether there are contraindications to oral medications or to the specific medication; for example, the patient's ability to swallow.

Impaired swallowing increases the patient's risk for aspiration.

- Check fluid needs and restrictions.

To decide how much fluid to give with the medications. Give additional fluid to a patient with dehydration, and give only sips for the patient with a fluid restriction. If the patient is NPO (nothing by mouth), check with the physician to determine whether the medication should be given by another route or can be given with small sips of water.

PROCEDURE 23–1   Administering Oral Medications *(continued)*

Procedural Steps

Step 1 Prepare the medication for administration.

Variation For Tablet or Capsule

a. If you are pouring from a multidose container, do not touch the medication. Pour the tablet into the cap of the bottle, then into the medication cup.

b. If the medication is unit-dose, do not open the package. Place the entire unit-dose package into the cup.

c. Pour all medications scheduled at the same time for the same patient into the same cup. However, you will need separate cups for any medications that require preadministration assessment (e.g., check the apical pulse rate prior to administering digoxin).

Because the medications are being given at the same time, they can be placed in the same cup. If a medication is held because of a preadministration assessment finding, it will be readily identified because it was poured into a separate cup.

d. You may break scored tablets with a knife or a pill cutter if necessary.

Only scored tablets may be broken, because breaking an unscored tablet would deliver an imprecise dose.

e. If a patient has difficulty swallowing, check to see whether the pill can be crushed. If so, use a mortar and pestle to grind it. If the pill is in a unit-dose package, grind the pill while it is still inside the package. Mix the ground pill with a small amount of soft food, such as applesauce or pudding.

Some medications, such as capsules, enteric-coated tablets, and sustained-release formulas cannot be crushed. Crushing such a medication may alter its effectiveness or result in an overdose due to rapid absorption.

Variation For Liquid Medications

f. Check to see whether you must shake the liquid before opening the container.

Some liquids, such as suspensions, will precipitate and need to be shaken well before they are administered.

g. Remove the bottle cap, and place it upside down on the cart or counter.

Prevents contaminating the inside of the cap.

h. Hold the bottle with the label in the palm of your hand.

Prevents the liquid from dripping down onto the label and obscuring it. ▼

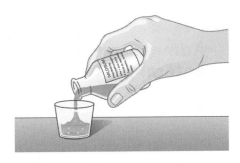

i. Hold or place the plastic medication cup at eye level, and pour the desired amount of medication (or place the cup on a level surface, pour the medication, then hold the cup at eye level to read the amount). Read the dose at the lowest part of the concave surface (meniscus).

Measuring liquids above or below eye level will cause you to make an error in the dose.

j. When you are finished pouring medication, slightly twist the bottle to prevent the medication from dripping down the lip of the bottle. If medication does drip down over the lip, wipe the lip with a tissue or paper towel.

Helps prevent contamination. Wipe only outside the lip of the bottle.

Step 2 Administer the medication.

a. Assist the patient to a high-Fowler's position, if possible. If the patient is unable to sit upright, raise the head of bed as much as possible, or assist the patient into a side-lying position.

Prevents choking and facilitates swallowing.

b. *Powder:* Mix with liquid at the bedside, and give the mixture to the patient to drink.

Some powders thicken very quickly, so they need to be mixed immediately before administration.

c. *Lozenge:* Instruct the patient not to chew or swallow it.

The medication is absorbed through the oral mucosa and is generally inactivated by the acidity in the stomach.

d. *Tablet or capsule:*
   1) If the patient is able to hold the medication in her hand, place the tablet or medication cup in her hand.

Encourages independence and is easier for the patient.

   2) Give the patient water or other liquid.

Moistens the mouth and helps the patient swallow the pill.

   3) If the patient is unable to hold the tablet, place the medication cup up to her lips, and tip the pill into her mouth.

Encourage the patient to do as much as possible. Getting the pill to the back of the mouth will assist in swallowing.

e. *Sublingual medications:* Have the patient place the tablet under the tongue and hold it there until it is completely dissolved.

➤

PROCEDURE 23–1   **Administering Oral Medications** *(continued)*

Sublingual medications are made to be rapidly absorbed through the oral mucosa. The area under the tongue is very vascular, so sublingual medications act very rapidly. Sublingual medications are inactivated by gastric acid if swallowed. ▼

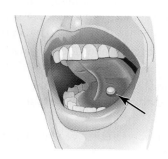

f. *Buccal medications:* Have the patient place the tablet between the cheek and teeth.

Buccal medications may act by being absorbed through the oral mucosa or by being dissolved and swallowed in the saliva. ▼

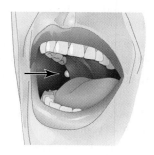

Step 3 Stay with the patient until all medications have been swallowed or dissolved.

Ensures that the patient took the medication.

PROCEDURE 23–1A   **Administering Medication Through an Enteral Tube**

➤ *Note:* Follow Steps 1a through 1j of Procedure 23–1: Administering Oral Medications. Also, follow precautions for administering enteral medications:

 VOL 1 Go to Chapter 23, **Enteral (Nasogastric and Gastrostomy) Medications,** in Volume 1.

Preparation

- If the patient is receiving a continuous tube feeding, disconnect it before giving the medications. Leave the tube clamped for a few minutes after administering the medication, according to agency protocol.

- If the enteral tube is connected to suction, you will usually discontinue the suction for 20 to 30 minutes after administration, and keep the tube clamped, to allow time for the drug to be absorbed.

Procedural Steps

Step 1 Verify that the medication can be crushed and given through an enteral tube.

Some tablets (e.g., time-release or enteric-coated tablets) should not be crushed because doing so changes their action.

Step 2 Crush the tablet and mix it with approximately 20 mL water or obtain a

liquid medication. If you are giving several medications, mix and administer each one separately.

If you are using a small-bore tube, such as a PEG tube, Keofeed NG feeding tube, or jejunostomy tube, always obtain the liquid form of the medication, because the small-bore tubes clog easily. Ensure that the medication is diluted enough to pass easily

through the tube. Instilling drugs one at a time allows you to identify each medication.

Step 3 Don nonsterile procedure gloves.

Maintains standard precautions.

Step 4 Place patient in a sitting (high-Fowler's) position, if possible.

PROCEDURE 23–1A

Administering Medication Through an Enteral Tube *(continued)*

Step 5 For nasogastric tubes, check tube placement (see Chapter 26, Technique 26–4).

Nasogastric tubes can become displaced or positioned in the lungs. If medications are given through a misplaced nasogastric tube, the patient may develop aspiration pneumonia.

Step 6 Check for residual volume (see Chapter 26, Procedure 26–3).

Step 7 Flush the tube. Based on the type of tube, use a piston tip or Luer-Lok syringe (usually a 30 to 60 mL syringe). Remove the bulb or plunger, attach the barrel to the tube, and pour in 20 to 30 mL of water.

Ensures patency of the tube.

Step 8 Instill the medication by depressing the syringe plunger or using the barrel of the syringe as a funnel and pouring in the medication. A smaller tube or thicker medication will require instilling the medication with a 30 to 60 mL syringe, but when larger tubes are used, the medication can be poured. ▼

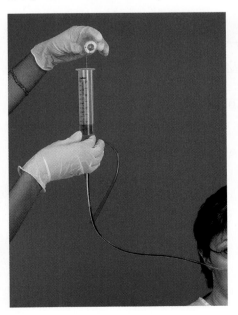

Step 9 Flush the medication through the tube by instilling an additional 20 to 30 mL of water.

Ensures that all the medication has been administered and prevents the tube from clogging.

Step 10 If there is more than one medication, give each separately, flushing after each.

Some medications are less effective when given in combination with others, or there may be an additive effect if they have similar actions.

Step 11 Have the patient maintain a sitting position for at least 30 minutes after you administer the medication.

Minimizes risk of aspiration.

Special Considerations: Older Adults (Oral)

- Check level of consciousness.
- Check for potential aspiration risk by checking the patient's swallow and gag reflexes.

Special Considerations: Children

- Because of the small size of the feeding tube, only use medications that come in a liquid preparation.

Prevents occlusion.

- Position an infant in a prone or side-lying position for 30 minutes to 1 hour following medication administration.

Special Considerations: Patients Who Have Difficulty Drinking from a Cup

If the patient has difficulty taking liquids from a cup, you can use a syringe without a needle to place the medication in his mouth. Place the patient in a side-lying or upright position to help prevent choking and aspiration. Place the syringe between the gum and cheek, and slowly push the plunger to administer the liquid.

Special Considerations: Patients on Fluid Restrictions

If the patient is on fluid restrictions, use the smallest amount of water needed to swallow or dissolve tablets and to flush enteral tubes.

Special Considerations: Patients Who Are Cognitively Impaired

Have the patient open his mouth to see whether he has swallowed the medication; look under the tongue.

➤

PROCEDURE 23–1 **Administering Oral Medications** *(continued)*

Evaluation

- Refer to **Medication Guidelines: Steps to Follow for All Medications (Regardless of Type or Route).**
- For medications administered through a feeding tube:
  - Note whether the patient gags or coughs.
  - Evaluate for gastric discomfort.
  - Assess that the nasogastric tube is patent before and after administering the medication.

Patient Teaching

- Refer to **Medication Guidelines: Steps to Follow for All Medications (Regardless of Type or Route).**
- Discuss drug safety measures with the patient, including use of child-proof caps, keeping the medication in its original container, discarding expired medications, and carefully reading the label and directions for each medication.
- Discuss the relationship between food and the medication, if needed. For example, is the medication to be taken with food or not? Does the medication interact with any foods?

Documentation

- Refer to **Medication Guidelines: Steps to Follow for All Medications (Regardless of Type or Route).**
- For enteral (feeding tube) medications: Document any difficulty with administering the medications through the feeding tube. Document patency, residual volume, and placement of tube.
- Be sure to document on the intake and output record the amount of liquid medication and the water used for flushing.

  Sample documentation:

09/26/06	1000	Medications given via Keofeed tube (see MAR). Tube placement verified before administration 20 mL residual.———————————— S. Smith, RN

PROCEDURE 23–2   Administering Ophthalmic Medications

For steps to follow in *all* procedures, refer to the inside back cover of this book. Also refer to the Medication Guidelines: Steps to Follow for All Medications (Regardless of Type or Route).

critical aspects
For Instillations
- Assist the patient to high-Fowler's position, with head slightly tilted back.
- If necessary, clean the edges of the eyelid from the inner to outer canthus.
- Apply the medication into the conjunctival sac.
- Do not apply the medication to the cornea.
- Do not let the dropper or tube touch the eye.
- For eye drops, press gently against the same side of the nose for 1 to 2 minutes to close the lacrimal ducts. For eye ointment, ask the patient to gently close the eyes for 2 to 3 minutes.

For Irrigations
- Assist the patient to low-Fowler's position.
- Check the pH in the conjunctival sac, if indicated.
- Use a Morgan lens or IV tubing to irrigate the eyes.
- For direct-flow irrigation, irrigate from the inner canthus to the outer canthus.
- Irrigate for 20 minutes or until the pH reaches the desired level.

Equipment
- Eye drops or ointment
- Tissue

For irrigation, add:
- Prescribed eye irrigation solution (e.g., 500 to 1000 mL of normal saline or lactated Ringer's solution are commonly used)
- IV tubing or eye irrigation insert, such as the Morgan lens (Follow manufacturer's directions for this specialized equipment.)
- Ocular anesthetic, according to protocol or physician orders
- pH paper
- Basin
- Towel

Delegation
As an RN, you can usually delegate administration of eye instillations to a licensed practical nurse. You usually cannot delegate this task to a UAP unless the UAP has special training for a specific, defined situation (e.g., "medication aides" in some long-term-care settings). See **Medication Guidelines: Steps to Follow for All Medications (Regardless of Type or Route),** at the beginning of the **Procedures** section.

Assessment
- Assess the patient's eyes for redness, discharge, or other signs of irritation.
- Determine whether the eyes need to be cleansed prior to administration of the medication.

Establishes a baseline to determine the effectiveness of the medication.

- Check the order for where to instill medication (*Note:* We do not advise using these abbreviations—they have been disallowed by the JCAHO—but you may still see them written in orders).
  OD = right eye
  OS = left eye
  OU = both eyes

For irrigations, also assess the following:
- Determine the cause of the eye problem—acid, alkaline, or other chemical burn or body fluid splash; or nonembedded foreign body.

Irrigations are generally done to remove chemical or physical irritants, but they may be done following surgery or to treat a severe infection. The type of problem determines the irrigation solution and volume used. Normal saline (NS) or lactated Ringer's is the solution generally recommended for high-volume eye irrigations because the pH of 6 to 7.5 is ➤

PROCEDURE 23–2 Administering Ophthalmic Medications
(continued)

closest to the normal tear pH of 7.1. Volumes of 500 to 1000 mL are generally used.

- Assess the patient's eyes for swelling, redness, drainage, or complaints of pain.

Establishes a baseline to determine need for and effectiveness of irrigation. Sclera should be smooth, white, and glistening.

- Determine the patient's level of discomfort and ability to cooperate with the procedure.
- Eye irritants can be extremely painful. The eye may need to be anesthetized prior to irrigation or a general systemic pain medication given. Notify the physician if the patient cannot hold still for the procedure, because he may need to be sedated.

Procedural Steps

Step 1 If possible, assist the patient to a high-Fowler's position, with head slightly tilted back.

Keeps eye drops in the eye and helps prevent eye drops from draining into lacrimal duct. Do not tilt the head back if the patient has a neck injury or other contraindication.

Step 2 Don procedure gloves.

Maintains standard precautions.

Step 3 If needed, cleanse the edges of eyelid from the inner to outer canthus.

Follows principle of "clean to dirty." Avoids transferring debris into the nasolacrimal duct.

Step 4 To administer eye drops:
a. Gently rest your dominant hand, with the eyedropper, on the patient's forehead.

Stabilizes hand in the event the patient moves—prevents accidental injury to the eye.

b. With your nondominant hand, pull the lower lid down to expose the conjunctival sac.

Allows visualization of the area where you will administer the medication.

c. Position the eyedropper about 13 to 19 mm ($\frac{1}{2}$ to $\frac{3}{4}$ inch) above the patient's eye. Ask the patient to look up, and drop the prescribed number of drops into the conjunctival sac. Do not let the dropper touch the eye.

Prevents accidental injury to the eye and avoids contamination of the dropper. Having the patient look up helps decrease the blink reflex. Instilling the eye drops directly onto the cornea could injure the cornea, so drops are instilled into the conjunctival sac. ▼

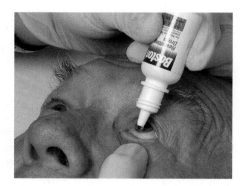

d. Ask patient to gently close and move the eyes.

Helps distribute the medication.

e. If the medication has systemic effects, press gently against the same side of the nose for 1 to 2 minutes to close the lacrimal ducts.

Prevents systemic absorption through the lacrimal duct. ▼

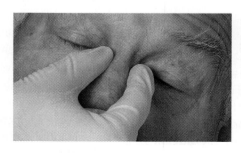

Step 5 To administer eye ointment:
a. Gently rest your dominant hand, with the eye ointment, on the patient's forehead.

Stabilizes your hand in the event the patient moves—prevents accidental injury to the eye.

b. With your nondominant hand, pull the lower lid down to expose the conjunctival sac.

Allows visualization of area where you will administer the medication.

c. Ask the patient to look up, and apply a thin strip of ointment—usually about 2 to 2.5 cm (1 inch)—in conjunctival sac, and twist your wrist to break off the strip of ointment. Do not let the tube touch the eye.

If the medication ribbon is not broken off, lifting the tube will pull the medication out of the conjunctival sac. ▼

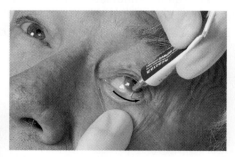

PROCEDURE 23–2 | Administering Ophthalmic Medications
(continued)

d. Ask the patient to gently close eyes for 2 to 3 minutes.

Distributes medication.

e. Explain to patient that his vision will be blurred for a short amount of time after administration of ointment.

The viscosity of the ointment can cause blurring.

PROCEDURE 23–2A | Irrigating the Eyes

Procedural Steps

Step 1 If possible, assist patient to a low-Fowler's position, with the head tilted toward the affected eye.

Helps drain the irrigating solution from the eye and prevents contamination of unaffected eye.

Step 2 Place the towel and basin under the patient's cheek to absorb the drainage.

Increases patient comfort.

Step 3 Check the pH by gently touching the pH paper to secretions in the conjunctival sac.

Determines the correct irrigating solution and whether the irritant is alkaline or acidic. The normal pH of tears is approximately 7.1.

Step 4 If on agency protocol or ordered by the physician, instill ocular anesthetic drops.

Increases patient comfort. The ocular anesthetic will be washed out by the irrigation fluid, so it needs to be reinstilled every 2 to 3 minutes, or it can be added to the irrigation solution.

Step 5 Connect the solution and tubing, and prime the tubing.

Prevents blowing air across the cornea, which would be uncomfortable.

Step 6 Irrigate the eye.
a. Hold the tubing about 2.5 cm (1 inch) from eye.

Keeps you from accidentally touching the eye.

b. Separate the eyelids with your thumb and index finger.

Allows you to irrigate the cornea.

c. Direct the flow of solution over the eye from the inner canthus to the outer canthus.

Follows the principle of "clean to dirty." ▼

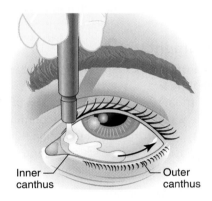

Inner canthus — Outer canthus

Step 7 Recheck pH, and continue to irrigate the eye as needed.

With alkaline or acidic chemical injuries, the pH of the eye needs to be returned to normal as soon as possible to prevent further eye injury.

Evaluation
- Examine the eyes for redness or drainage.
- Observe the patient's ability to follow instructions during procedure (e.g., close and move eyes), and note any reports of discomfort.
- Check for decrease in eye pain (for irrigations).

Patient Teaching
- Discuss with patient how to prevent contaminating eye drops or ointment.
- Instruct patient how to instill eye drops or ointment.

➤

PROCEDURE 23–2   Administering Ophthalmic Medications
(continued)

- If patient needs assistance with instilling drops, discuss use of an eyedrop guide.
- Discuss with the patient the signs and symptoms that need to be reported to the physician, including eye pain and increased redness or drainage.

For irrigations:

- Discuss with the patient the cause and prevention of eye injuries, including the use of protective goggles.
- Discuss with the patient the need for follow-up treatment. If patient will be instilling eye medications or applying eye patches, ensure that patient is able to use the correct technique.

Home Care

If a splash occurs to the eyes in the home, immediately flood the eyes with water:

- Hold the lids open and put the head under a faucet or pour water from a clean container.
- Roll the eyes as much as possible while running water across the eyes.
- Flood the eyes for at least 20 minutes.
- Get medical help immediately after rinsing the eyes.

Documentation

- For instillations: Chart assessment data before and after instillation. Record on the MAR, as for all medications.
- For irrigations: Chart the condition of the patient's eyes before the irrigation, including the patient's complaints of pain or burning. Document the eye pH, instillation of anesthetic drops, the type and amount of irrigation fluid used, the eye pH following irrigation, and the patient's response. You also need to chart other treatment, such as instillation of lubricating and/or antibiotic ointment and application of eye patches.

Sample documentation:

11/14/06	1530	Patient admitted for chemical splash to both eyes. Eyes reddened, lids swollen bilaterally, profuse tearing present. Patient complaining of severe pain in both eyes. pH = 8.4 bilaterally. 2000 mL lactated Ringer's administered free-flow. pH = 7.6 after irrigation. An additional 150 mL lactated Ringer's irrigation administered via eye irrigation insert at 50 mL/hr for 3 hours. pH = 7.1.————————— S. Suske, RN

| PROCEDURE 23–3 | **Administering Otic Medications** |

 For steps to follow in *all* procedures, refer to the inside back cover of this book. Also refer to Medication Guidelines: Steps to Follow for All Medications (Regardless of Type or Route).

critical aspects
- Warm the solution to be instilled.
- Assist the patient to a side-lying position, with the appropriate ear facing up.
- Straighten the ear canal. For an adult client, pull the pinna up and back; for a child 3 years or younger, down and back.
- Instill the ordered number of drops into the ear canal.
- Do not force the solution into the ear or occlude the ear canal with the dropper.
- Instruct the patient to remain on his side for 5 to 10 minutes.

Equipment
- Ear drops
- Dropper with flexible rubber tip
- Cotton-tipped applicators
- Cotton ball

Delegation
As an RN, you can usually delegate administration of otic medications to a licensed practical nurse. You usually cannot delegate this task to a UAP unless the UAP has special training for a specific, defined situation (e.g., "medication aides" in some long-term care settings in some states). See the **Medication Guidelines** at the beginning of the **Procedures** section.

Assessment
- Assess the external ear and canal for redness, drainage, and cerumen.

You may need to clean the external ear to remove obstructions so that the medication can be distributed throughout the ear canal. Use the otoscope to evaluate the tympanic membrane if the drainage is bloody or the patient complains of pain or decreased hearing acuity. If the tympanic membrane is ruptured, use sterile technique.

- Assess for any ear pain or hearing impairment.
- Establish a baseline that can be used to evaluate the effects of treatment.

Procedural Steps

Step 1 Hold the eardrop bottle in your hand to warm it, or place it in warm water (not hot).

Placing cool solutions in the ear can cause dizziness. Promotes comfort.

Step 2 Assist patient to a side-lying position, with the appropriate ear facing up.

Facilitates administering the drops and prevents drops escaping from the ear.

Step 3 Don procedure gloves.

Maintains standard precautions.

Step 4 Clean the external ear with a cotton-tipped applicator, if necessary.

Allows eardrops to reach all areas of the ear canal. Be careful not to push cerumen further into the ear canal.

Step 5 Fill the dropper with the correct amount of medication. ➤

PROCEDURE 23–3   **Administering Otic Medications** *(continued)*

Step 6 For infants and young children, ask another caregiver to immobilize the child while you administer the medication.

Helps to prevent injury should the child struggle during the procedure.

Step 7 Straighten the ear canal.
a. For a child less than 3 years old, pull the pinna down and back. ▼

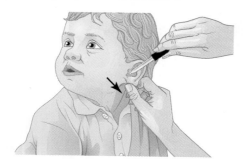

b. For older children and adults, pull the pinna up and back.

Straightens the ear canal for proper channeling of the medication. ▼

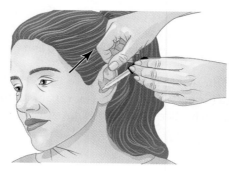

Step 8 Instill the ordered number of drops along the side of the ear canal, being careful not to touch the end of the dropper to any part of the ear.

Prevents contamination of the dropper.

Step 9 Massage or press on the tragus of the ear.

Facilitates flow of medication into the auditory canal.

Step 10 Instruct the patient to remain on his side for 5 to 10 minutes.

Assists in distributing the medication and prevents drops from escaping the ear canal.

Step 11 Place a cotton ball, or a piece of it, loosely at the opening of the auditory canal for 15 minutes.

Prevents drops from escaping the canal when the patient changes position.

Evaluation

- Refer to **Medication Guidelines: Steps to Follow for All Medications (Regardless of Type or Route).**
- Assess for discomfort or pain during the procedure and for relief afterward.
- Evaluate for wax buildup, redness, swelling, or drainage.

Documentation

- Refer to **Medication Guidelines: Steps to Follow for All Medications (Regardless of Type or Route).**
- Assess the amount, color, character, and odor of drainage, if indicated.
- Note any swelling or redness in the ear canal.
- Document pain or discomfort and any hearing loss.

Sample documentation:

7/21/06	0345	*Otic medication instilled (see MAR). No drainage observed and no redness or edema in ear canal. Patient states "no pain," but does have "ringing in my left ear."*
		— P. Stith, RNC

PROCEDURE 23–4 Administering Nasal Medications

For steps to follow in *all* procedures, refer to the inside back cover of this book. Also refer to Medication Guidelines: Steps to Follow for All Medications (Regardless of Type or Route).

critical aspects

- Determine head position: Consider the indication for the medication and the patient's ability to assume the position.
- Explain to the patient that the medication may cause some burning, tingling, or unusual taste.
- Position the patient appropriately.
- Have the patient blow his nose, occlude one nostril, and exhale.
- Administer the spray or drops while the patient is inhaling.
- Repeat for other nostril.
- If nose drops are used, ask the patient to stay in the same position for approximately 5 minutes.

Equipment

- Medication drops, spray, or aerosol
- Tissues

Delegation

As an RN, you can usually delegate administration of nasal instillations to a licensed practical nurse. You usually cannot delegate this task to a UAP.

Assessment

- Check for nasal obstruction and congestion.

Nasal obstruction or congestion could prevent the medication from reaching the nasal mucosa.

- Assess nasal discharge for color, consistency, and odor.

Establishes baseline data. The appearance of drainage is not always diagnostic of infection, especially for people with chronic sinus problems or polyps.

- Assess whether the patient is experiencing sinus pain.

Will determine proper administration technique if medication is to drain into sinuses.

- Assess nasal mucous membranes for redness, color, and moisture.

Establishes baseline and identifies signs of irritation.

Procedural Steps

Step 1 Explain to the patient the possibility that the medication may cause some burning, tingling, or unusual taste.

The taste of nasal medications can cause patients to become nauseated or vomit after administration. The medication is more likely to cause burning or tingling if the nasal mucosa is inflamed.

Step 2 Don procedure gloves.

Maintains standard precautions.

Step 3 Have the patient blow his nose.

Removes discharge so that the medication can come into contact with the mucous membranes.

➤

PROCEDURE 23–4   **Administering Nasal Medications** *(continued)*

Step 4 Position the patient.

a. "Head down and forward"—if the patient can assume these positions, have him lean forward or kneel on the bed with his head down. Administer the medication, and then have the patient tilt his head back to medicate the nasal passages.

   If the patient cannot assume one of these positions, have him tilt his head back to administer the drops or spray.

Radionuclide studies have demonstrated that using nasal drops or sprays with the patient sitting and leaning the head back causes poor distribution of the medications into the nasal complex and sinuses. ▼

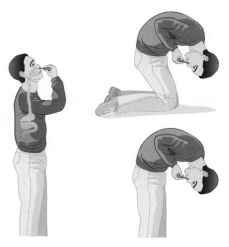

Wrong position   Correct positions

b. To medicate the ethmoid and sphenoid sinuses, assist the patient into a supine position, with his head over the edge of the bed. Support the patient's head. Alternatively, place a towel roll behind the patient's shoulders, and allow the head to drop back.

Prevents straining the neck muscles. ▼

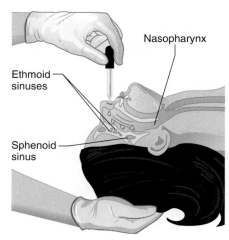

Ethmoid sinuses

Sphenoid sinus

Nasopharynx

c. To medicate the frontal and maxillary sinuses, tilt the head toward the affected side.

Uses gravity to distribute the medication to the frontal sinuses. ▼

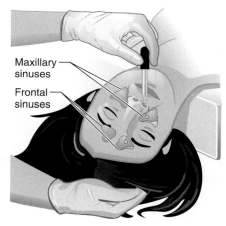

Maxillary sinuses

Frontal sinuses

Step 5 Have the patient close one nostril and exhale.

Provides for larger inhalation.

Step 6 Administer the spray or drops while the patient breathes through the mouth. If a dropper is used, do not touch the sides of the nostril.

Inhaling through the mouth prevents aspiration of the drops into the trachea and bronchi. Touching the dropper to the nostril will contaminate the dropper.

Step 7 Repeat for the other nostril.

Step 8 If nose drops are used, ask the patient to stay in the same position for 1 to 5 minutes (depending on manufacturer's guidelines).

Allows for better absorption by using gravity to disperse the medication throughout the nasal passages and sinuses.

Step 9 Instruct patient to not blow his nose for several minutes.

Prevents expelling of the medication.

PROCEDURE 23–4   **Administering Nasal Medications** *(continued)*

Evaluation

Assess for a reduction of symptoms 15 to 20 minutes after administration.

Patient Teaching

* Teach the procedure for administering nasal drops or sprays, including proper positioning.
* Discuss the correct use of the medication and the adverse effects of overusing nasal deconges-tants.
* Explain the implications of the color of nasal secretions.

Documentation

Chart according to **Medication Guidelines: Steps to Follow for All Medications (Regardless of Type or Route).** For example, record the administration of the medication on the MAR.

PROCEDURE 23–5   **Administering Vaginal Medications**

 For steps to follow in *all* procedures, refer to the inside back cover of this book. Also refer to Medication Guidelines: Steps to Follow for All Medications (Regardless of Type or Route).

critical aspects

For Instillation
* Position the patient in a dorsal recumbent or Sims' position.
* Inspect and cleanse the vaginal area before administering the medication.
* Use water-soluble lubricant.
* Insert the suppository or applicator along the posterior vaginal wall about 8 cm (3 inches).
* Instruct the client to maintain the position for 5 to 15 minutes after the medication is inserted.

For Irrigation (Douche)
* Warm the irrigation solution to approximately 105°F (40.6°C).
* Hang the irrigation solution approximately 30 to 60 cm (1 to 2 ft) above the level of the patient's vagina.
* Position the patient in a dorsal recumbent position on a waterproof pad and bedpan.
* Insert the nozzle approximately 7 to 8 cm (3 inches) into the vagina, and start the flow of irriga-tion solution.

➤

PROCEDURE 23–5   **Administering Vaginal Medications** (continued)

Equipment

- Medication: foam, jelly, cream, suppository, douche, or irrigating solution
- Applicator (if indicated)
- Washcloth and warm water for perineal care as needed
- Water-soluble lubricant
- Toilet tissue
- Perineal pad
- Bath blanket
- For irrigation: you will also need a waterproof pad, bedpan, vaginal irrigation set (may be disposable; consists of a solution container, nozzle, tubing, and clamp) and IV pole

Delegation

As an RN, you can usually delegate the administration of vaginal medications to a licensed practical nurse. You usually cannot delegate this task to a UAP. Nurse practice acts governing medication administration do vary from state to state, and policies vary further among healthcare agencies. However, as the RN you are always responsible for evaluating client responses, both therapeutic effects and side effects. You can instruct a UAP in the therapeutic effect and side effects of medications and to report any effects observed.

Assessment

- Assess for complaints of vaginal burning, pruritus, and pain.

Determines the patient's level of comfort and baseline data. Infections can cause vaginal burning, itching, and pain.

- Inspect the labia and vaginal orifice for redness and lesions.
- Check for vaginal drainage, including color, amount, consistency, and odor.

Helps determine the cause and establish baseline data.

Procedural Steps

Step 1 Have the patient void before you insert the vaginal medication.

The increased pressure associated with a full bladder could cause discomfort during the instillation of vaginal medications.

Step 2 Position the patient in a dorsal recumbent or Sims' position; drape the patient with a bath blanket so that only the perineum is exposed.

a. Dorsal recumbent position— supine with knees flexed and legs rotated outward.

b. Sims' position—semiprone on the left side with the right hip and knee flexed.

These two positions allow for visualization during administration and promote retention of the medication following administration. Draping respects patient's modesty.

Step 3 Prepare the medication. Remove wrapper from the suppository and place the suppository on the wrapper or in a medication cup; or fill the applicator according to the manufacturer's instructions. For irrigation, use a warm solution of approximately 105°F.

Some suppositories come with applicators. Using a warm irrigation solution promotes patient comfort and prevents injury to the vaginal tissue. ➤

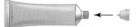

Invert cap and pierce end of medication tube

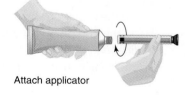

Attach applicator

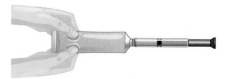

Squeeze medication into applicator

PROCEDURE 23–5   Administering Vaginal Medications *(continued)*

Step 4 Don procedure gloves.

Follow standard precautions to prevent contaminating your hands and spreading of microorganisms.

Step 5 Inspect and clean around vaginal orifice.

Prevents introduction of microorganisms into the vagina during medication administration.

Step 6 Administer the medication.

Variation A Suppository

a. Apply water-soluble lubricant to the rounded end of the suppository and to your gloved index finger on your dominant hand.

Eases insertion and prevents injury to the vaginal tissue.

b. Separate the labia with your non-dominant hand.

Allows visualization of the vaginal orifice.

c. Insert the suppository as far as possible along the posterior vaginal wall (about 8 cm, or 3 inches) or as far as it will go. If the suppository comes with an applicator, place the suppository in the end of the applicator, insert the applicator into the vagina, and press the plunger.

The posterior vaginal wall is about 2.5 cm (1 in.) longer than the anterior wall. ▼

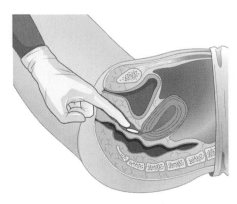

d. Have the patient remain in a supine position for 5 to 15 minutes. You may wish to elevate her hips on a pillow.

Promotes retention and absorption of the medication.

Variation B Applicator Insertion of Cream, Foam, or Jelly

e. Separate the labia with your non-dominant hand.

f. Insert the applicator approximately 8 cm (3 inches) into the vagina along the posterior vaginal wall.

g. Depress the plunger on the applicator, emptying the medication into the vagina.

h. Dispose of the applicator, or place it on a paper towel if the applicator is reusable. You will later wash it with soap and water.

Prevents spread of microorganisms.

i. Have patient remain in a supine position for 5 to 15 minutes.

Promotes retention and absorption of the medication.

Variation C Irrigation

j. Hang the irrigation solution approximately 30 to 60 cm (1 to 2 ft) above the level of the patient's vagina.

Creates enough pressure for continuous irrigation without increasing the pressure so high that it causes the patient discomfort and possibly damages the vaginal tissue. ▼

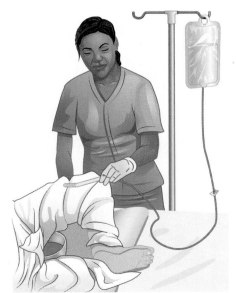

k. Assist patient into a dorsal recumbent position, and position a waterproof pad and bedpan under the patient.

The dorsal recumbent position is the easiest for performing a vaginal irrigation. Positioning the patient on the bedpan and using a waterproof pad protects the bedding.

l. If using a vaginal irrigation set with tubing, open the clamp to allow the solution to completely fill the tubing.

Prevents introducing air into the vagina, which can cause discomfort.

m. Lubricate the end of the irrigation nozzle.

n. Insert the nozzle approximately 8 cm (3 inches) into the vagina, directing it toward the sacrum.

o. Start the flow of the irrigation solution, and rotate the nozzle intermittently as solution flows.

Ensures even distribution of the solution throughout the vagina.

p. If the labia are reddened, run some of the solution over the labia.

Decreases the irritation of the tissue and promotes patient comfort.

q. After all irrigating solution has been used, remove the nozzle.

r. Assist the patient to a sitting position on the bedpan.

Promotes removal of all the irrigating solution.

Step 7 Cleanse the perineum with toilet tissue or with warm water and a washcloth. Dry the perineum.

Drainage could cause skin irritation.

Step 8 Apply a perineal pad if there is excessive drainage.

➤

PROCEDURE 23–5   **Administering Vaginal Medications** *(continued)*

Evaluation

- Assess for complaints of vaginal burning, pruritus, or pain.
- Assess for purulent vaginal discharge.

Patient Teaching

- Discuss with the patient personal hygiene and pericare.

Documentation

- For vaginal medications, chart according to **Medication Guidelines: Steps to Follow for All Medications (Regardless of Type or Route).**
- For vaginal irrigations, chart assessment findings, the type and amount of solution given, any discomfort the patient experienced during the procedure, and patient's report of decreased vaginal pain, itching, and/or burning following the procedure.

Sample documentation:

| 08/14/06   0645 | Moderate amount of yellow-green, thick, foul-smelling vaginal discharge. Irrigated vagina with 350 mL of medicated solution (see MAR), warmed. Patient stated no discomfort during procedure, but after procedure stated she is still having "a lot of" vaginal itching. Labia and vagina are deep red, but mucosa intact. Peri-pad applied. Taught front-to-back pericare.— C. Ivy, RN |

PROCEDURE 23–6 Inserting a Rectal Suppository

 For steps to follow in *all* procedures, refer to the inside back cover of this book. Also refer to Medication Guidelines: Steps to Follow for All Medications (Regardless of Type or Route).

critical aspects
- Before inserting the suppository, assess for contraindications, such as rectal surgery, rectal bleeding, or cardiac disease.
- Position the client in Sims' position (left lateral with the upper leg flexed).
- Lubricate the suppository.
- Never force the suppository during insertion.
- Insert the suppository past the internal sphincter about 10 cm (4 inches).
- Have the client stay on his side for 5 to 10 minutes and to retain (not expel) the suppository for about 30 minutes.

Equipment
- Suppository
- Water-soluble lubricant
- Toilet tissue

Delegation
As an RN, you can usually delegate administration of rectal medications to a licensed practical nurse. Although in some institutions you can delegate the administration of a glycerin suppository (non-medicated) to a UAP, you generally cannot delegate administration of rectal medications to a UAP.

Assessment
- Determine the presence of contraindications for rectal administration, such as recent rectal surgery, rectal bleeding, or cardiac disease.
- Assess the rectal area for hemorrhoids or irritation.

Procedural Steps

Step 1 Ask whether the patient needs to defecate prior to the suppository insertion.

Allows insertion of medication against the rectal wall and promotes retention of the medication.

Step 2 Don procedure gloves.

Prevents exposure to feces and spread of microorganisms; maintains standard precautions.

Step 3 Assist patient to Sims' position—lying on the left side with the right hip and knee flexed—keeping the patient covered as much as possible.

Allows visualization of the anus and promotes retention of the medication because the descending colon is on the left side. Sims' position also aids in relaxing the external anal sphincter. Keeping the patient covered prevents chilling and maintains privacy.

Step 4 For an uncooperative patient, such as a confused patient or young child, have someone help immobilize the patient while you insert the suppository.

Allows proper instillation of medication and prevents injury to the rectal mucosa.

Step 5 Remove the suppository wrapper. Using water-soluble lubricant, lubricate the smooth end of the suppository and the tip of glove on the index finger.

➤

PROCEDURE 23–6   Inserting a Rectal Suppository *(continued)*

Lubrication eases insertion and prevents friction damage to the rectal mucosa during insertion.

Step 6 Explain that there will be a cool feeling from the lubricant and a feeling of pressure during insertion.

The patient should not experience severe pain with the insertion of a suppository but will feel the coolness of the lubricant and pressure as the suppository is inserted past the rectal sphincter.

Step 7 Using your nondominant hand, separate the buttocks.

Allows visualization of the anus.

Step 8 Have the patient take deep breaths in and out through the mouth.

Relaxes the rectal sphincter. Pushing a suppository through a constricted sphincter produces pain.

Step 9 Administer the suppository.
a. Using the index finger of your dominant hand, gently insert the lubricated smooth end first, or follow the manufacturer's instructions.

Using the smooth end eases insertion. ▼

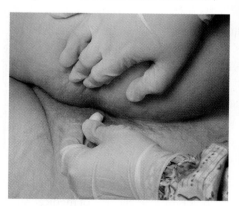

b. Never force the suppository during insertion.

Forcing the insertion of the suppository into a fecal mass would affect absorption or may cause rectal damage.

c. Push the suppository past the internal sphincter and along the rectal wall (about 10 cm or 4 inches in an adult). For a child, insert the suppository 5 cm (2 inches) or less (just past the internal sphincter).

The suppository must be in contact with the rectal wall for the medication to be absorbed. Inserting the suppository past the internal sphincter promotes retention. For a child, inserting the suppository too far could damage the rectal mucosa. ▼

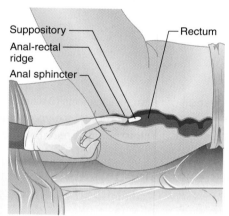

Step 10 Ask the patient to try to retain the suppository if he is able. If the client has difficulty retaining the suppository, hold the buttocks together for a short time.

Promotes retention.

Step 11 Wipe the anus with toilet tissue.

Maintains hygiene and comfort.

Step 12 Explain to the patient the need to remain in the side-lying position for 5 to 10 minutes.

Promotes retention and absorption of the medication. Explanation promotes compliance.

Step 13 Leave the call light and bedpan within reach if the suppository was a laxative.

In case the patient cannot retain the suppository for the recommended time.

PROCEDURE 23–6   **Inserting a Rectal Suppository** *(continued)*

Developmental Modifications

- For pediatric clients, it may be necessary to gently hold the buttocks for 5 to 10 minutes.
- Older adults may have difficulty retaining a suppository because of poor sphincter control.

Evaluation

- Assess for pain or burning during insertion of the medication.
- Determine that the patient retained the suppository for the desired length of time after insertion (reinsertion may be required).
- Assess for rectal pain, if indicated.

Patient Teaching

Explain that suppositories may take up to 30 minutes to be absorbed, depending on the medication.

Documentation

- Refer to **Medication Guidelines: Steps to Follow for All Medications (Regardless of Type or Route).**
- Chart the condition of anal tissue if abnormalities are present, any complaints of discomfort during administration, and the length of time that the suppository was retained.
- Chart responses to medication (e.g., symptom relief, side effects).

Sample documentation:

11/04/06	0900	Dulcolax suppository inserted (see MAR). No abnormalities of anus or perineum noted. Pt retained suppository for 5 minutes, then passed small amount of dark brown formed stool. No c/o pain, but states, "I still feel full and bloated."————S. Kneeley, RN

PROCEDURE 23–7 | Preparing and Drawing Up Medications

For steps to follow in *all* procedures, refer to the inside back cover of this book. Also refer to Medication Guidelines: Steps to Follow for All Medications (Regardless of Type or Route).

critical aspects
- Maintain sterile technique.
- Recap the needle or injection cannula using a needle recapping device or the one-handed method (see Procedure 23–9).
- Change the needle, if indicated.

Ampules
- Tap the ampule to remove medication trapped in the top of the ampule.
- Use an ampule opener to break the ampule neck. If one is not available, wrap gauze or an unopened alcohol wipe around the neck of the ampule, and snap the ampule away from you.
- Use a filter needle or filter straw to withdraw the medication.
- Withdraw all of the medication from the ampule by inverting or tipping the ampule.
- Dispose of the top and bottom of ampule and filter needle in a sharps container.

Vials
- Thoroughly clean the rubber top of the vial with an alcohol prep pad (for a multiple-dose vial only).
- Draw air into the syringe equal to the amount of medication to be withdrawn.
- When inserting the needle through the rubber top of the vial, avoid coring by inserting the needle at a 45 to 60° angle, bevel up, or by using a filter needle.
- Keeping the needle above the fluid line, inject air into the vial before withdrawing the medication.
- Remove bubbles, hold the vial at eye level, and check that the dose is correct before removing the needle.

Equipment
- Medication ampule or vial
- Alcohol prep pads (70% alcohol)
- 2 × 2 gauze pad or ampule snapper
- Filter needle or filter straw
- Needle and syringe the appropriate size for medication volume, viscosity, and site of administration
- Vial access device, or filter needle

Note: Vial access devices can be used only for single-use vials and vials that are specifically made for vial access devices, such as Life-Shield vials. The access pins leave too large a hole for multiuse vials. Also, when some vial access devices are removed from the vial, the injection pin remains in the vial, and only the access cannula is left, which is then used for intravenous injections.

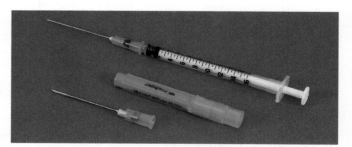

Top: Syringe with regular needle. Bottom: Filter needle.

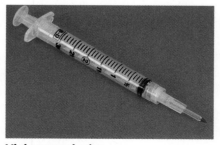

Vial access device

PROCEDURE 23–7   Preparing and Drawing Up Medications
(continued)

Delegation

As an RN, you can delegate administration of some parenteral medications to a licensed practical nurse. You usually cannot delegate this task to a UAP. Nurse practice acts governing medication administration vary from state to state, and policies vary further among healthcare agencies. Nevertheless, as the RN you are always responsible for supervising and evaluating delegated care. You can instruct a UAP in the therapeutic effect.

Assessment

Check the ampule or vial for intactness, cloudiness, particles, and color.

Ensures that the medication is not compromised. A change in color, cloudiness, particles, or cracks indicate that the medication is altered or contaminated and should not be used.

PROCEDURE 23–7A   Drawing Up Medications from Ampules

Procedural Steps

Step 1 With your index finger, gently flick or tap the top of the ampule to remove medication trapped in the top of the ampule. An alternate approach to remove trapped medication is to shake the ampule by quickly turning and snapping your wrist, like shaking down a mercury thermometer.

Medication left in the top of the ampule may lead to administering an inadequate dose. All the medication must be in the bottom of the ampule before you withdraw it.

Step 2 Wrap 2 × 2 gauze pad (or an unwrapped alcohol wipe) around the neck of the ampule, or slip on an ampule snapper. Using your dominant hand, snap the top off, breaking it away from you.

Prevents you from accidentally cutting your fingers or spraying glass fragments toward you. Do not use an opened alcohol wipe to break the ampule, because it is not thick enough to prevent injury. ➤

Step 3 Attach a filter needle or filter straw to the syringe. If the syringe has a needle in place, remove both the needle and the cap, and place them on a sterile surface (e.g., a newly unwrapped alcohol pad still in the open wrapper), and attach the filter needle.

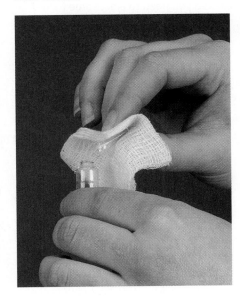

The use of a 5 μm filter needle minimizes the possibility of injecting small glass fragments into the patient. Ensures that the sterility of the injection needle is maintained.

Step 4 Withdraw the medication from the ampule by using one of the following techniques. Be careful not to touch the neck of the ampule with the needle while withdrawing medication.

Touching the neck of the ampule with the needle increases the risk of contamination.

a. Invert the ampule, place the needle tip in the liquid, and withdraw the prescribed amount of medication. Be careful not to insert needle through the medication into the air at the top of the inverted ampule.

PROCEDURE 23–7A   Drawing Up Medications from Ampules

(continued)

This method is particularly useful with large ampules. The medication's surface tension will prevent the liquid from leaking from the ampule while the ampule is inverted. However, if you insert the needle too far (into the air pocket above the medication), the medication will run out. ▼

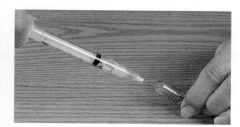

b. Alternatively, tip the ampule, place needle in the liquid, and withdraw all medication. Reposition the ampule so that needle tip remains in the liquid.

Allows for easier stabilization of the ampule while you withdraw the medication. ▼

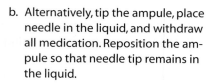

Step 5 Hold the syringe vertically, and draw 0.2 mL of air into the syringe (see Technique 23–4). Measure the exact medication dose, plus 0.2 mL of air (the syringe plunger should be at 0.2 mL more than the ordered dose). See Technique 23–4.

Step 6 Remove the filter needle, and reattach the "saved" needle for administering the injection.

Step 7 Next, eject the 0.2 mL of air, and read the dose. If after all of the air is ejected you need to eject some medication to make the dose correct, tip

the syringe horizontally to eject the medication.

Use a filter needle only to withdraw the medication. For injection, use a needle of the correct gauge and length. Pushing the medication out of the syringe with the filter needle in place could cause the filter to break and release the glass fragments. Pulling air into the syringe allows for an exact dose when the medication is injected; the air will clear the needle so that the patient receives all the medication that was drawn up in the syringe. *Note:* This is not the old "air lock" technique; you will eject the air before injecting the medication into the patient.

The syringe must be vertical to eject air; however, if you eject the medication while holding the syringe vertically, the drug will run down the needle and then track through the patient's tissue during the injection.

Step 8 Alternatively, for a medication that is irritating to tissues, you can leave the 0.2 mL of air in the syringe for injection. But be sure to account for the air when you read the dose markings on the syringe.

Step 9 Dispose of the top and bottom of the ampule and the filter needle in a sharps container.

Prevents accidental injury.

PROCEDURE 23–7B   Preparing and Drawing Up Medications from Vials

Procedural Steps

Step 1 Mix the solution in the vial, if necessary, by gently rolling the vial between your hands.

Aqueous suspensions will settle to the bottom of the vial, so they need to be mixed. Rolling the vial between your hands will mix the medication without

forming air bubbles. Shaking the vial will trap air in the medication.

Step 2 Place the vial on a flat work surface, and thoroughly clean the rubber top of the vial, with an alcohol prep pad. This step can usually be omitted for single-dose vials.

Removes dust, grease, and microorganisms.

Step 3 Uncap the needle without touching the needle tip or shaft. If you are using a vial access device, attach the device to the syringe, and remove the cap.

Maintains sterility of the needle. Vial access devices can be used only with single-use vials, unless the vial is designed for use with access pins, such as a Life-Shield vial.

PROCEDURE 23–7B

Preparing and Drawing Up Medications from Vials *(continued)*

Step 4 Place the needle cap on a clean surface, or hold the cap open-side out between two fingers of your nondominant hand.

Prevents getting the needle cap dirty, which might contaminate the needle during recapping.

Step 5 Draw air into the syringe equal to the amount of medication to be withdrawn.

Makes withdrawing the medication easier. For small unit-dose vials, you may not have to instill air prior to withdrawing the medication, but you will need to maintain backward pressure on the plunger until the needle is completely withdrawn. If you release the plunger, the negative pressure in the vial will pull the medication back in.

Step 6 Maintaining sterile technique, insert the needle or vial access cannula into the vial without coring.

a. Place the tip of the needle or vial access cannula in the middle of the rubber top of the vial, with the bevel up at a 45 to 60° angle. ▼

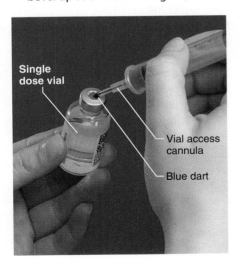

Single dose vial
Vial access cannula
Blue dart

b. While pushing the needle or vial cannula device into the rubber top, gradually bring the needle upright to a 90° angle.

Coring occurs when a small piece of the rubber top is trapped inside the needle when the needle is inserted. Coring is more likely to occur with large-gauge needles and vial access devices. ▼

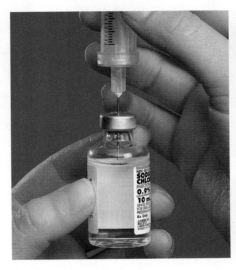

Step 7 With the bevel of the needle above the fluid line, inject the air in the syringe into the air in the vial.

Injecting air into the vial creates positive pressure, making the medication easier to withdraw. Injecting the air into the medication will create air bubbles, which interfere with dosage measurement. ▼

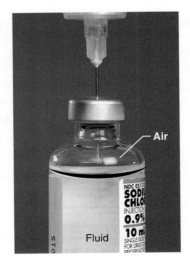

Air
Fluid

Air to air.

Step 8 Invert the vial, keep the needle or vial access device in the medication, and slowly withdraw the medication.

The vial needs to be inverted so that all the medication can be withdrawn. Keeping the needle in the medication and slowly drawing the medication will help prevent you from drawing excess air into the syringe. ▼

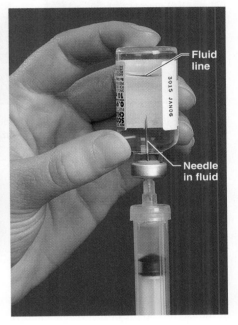

Fluid line
Needle in fluid

➤

PROCEDURE 23–7B   **Preparing and Drawing Up Medications from Vials** (*continued*)

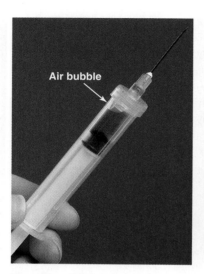

Incorrect—If syringe is not vertical, air is trapped near the hub.

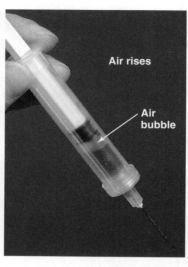

Incorrect—If needle is down, air is trapped at the plunger.

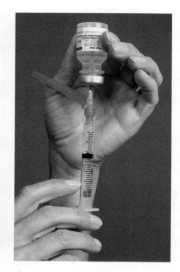

Correct—Syringe is vertical.

Step 9 Keeping the needle or vial access device in the vial, expel air bubbles from the syringe back into the vial. ▲

a. Carefully stabilize the vial and syringe, and firmly tap the syringe below the air bubbles.

The volume of air in the hub of the needle and inside the needle, dead space, will be drawn back into the syringe. Air bubbles alter the dose of medication being administered, so they must be expelled. A pen can be used to tap the syringe if extra force is needed.

b. When the air bubbles are at the hub of the syringe, make sure the syringe is vertical (straight up and down), and push the air back into the vial.

Remember that air rises, so if the syringe is tilted, air will be trapped in it.

c. Withdraw additional medication, if necessary, to obtain the correct dose.

When the needle is connecting the vial and syringe, a sterile unit is formed. With-

drawing and reinstilling medication into the vial can be done as many times as needed to expel the air bubbles from the syringe and obtain the correct medication dose.

Step 10 When the dose is correct, withdraw the needle or vial access device from the vial at a 90° angle.

Prevents accidental contamination or bending of the needle.

Step 11 Hold the syringe upright at eye level to recheck the medication dose.

Reading the syringe at an angle can result in inaccurate measurement.

Step 12 Recap the needle or injection cannula using a needle recapping device or the one-handed method (see Procedure 23–9).

Although recapping a sterile needle does not present a threat of bloodborne pathogen exposure, using a mechanical

recapping device or the one-handed method helps develop safe habits.

Step 13 If you are administering an irritating medication or if you used a vial access device or filter needle to draw up medication, change the needle before you inject the medication. Before changing the needle, draw back on the syringe plunger to remove all medication from dead space in the old needle (or vial access device), remove the old needle, and reattach a new one (see Technique 23–6). Hold the syringe vertically and expel the air; if it is necessary to expel some medication, hold the syringe horizontally to do so.

The difficulty with changing the needles is that you may slightly alter the dose. If you are planning to change the needles, draw slightly more than the ordered dose. After changing the needle, remeasure the dose. Holding the syringe horizontally prevents medication from running down the needle and tracking into the patient's skin.

Evaluation

No patient responses, because this procedure does not involve the patient.

Documentation

No documentation.

PROCEDURE 23–8	**Mixing Medications in One Syringe**

For steps to follow in *all* procedures, refer to the inside back cover of this book. Also refer to Medication Guidelines: Steps to Follow for All Medications (Regardless of Type or Route).

critical aspects

- Make sure the medications are compatible.
- Maintain the sterility of the needles and medication.
- Avoid contaminating a multidose vial with a second medication.
- Carefully expel air bubbles.
- When you withdraw the second medication, the medications are mixed as you pull back the plunger; therefore, you must withdraw the exact amount. If there is any excess, you must discard the contents of the syringe and start over.
- When opening ampules, protect yourself from injury.
- Use a filter needle or straw to withdraw medication from ampules; change to a needle of the proper length and gauge for administering the medication.
- When drawing up from a single-dose vial and ampule, draw up from the vial first.
- Do not use prefilled cartridges for intramuscular injections unless they have a safety device; transfer the medication to a syringe with a safety device before administering.
- Always recap a sterile needle using a needle capping device or the one-handed scoop method (see Procedure 23–9).

Equipment

- Medication vials, ampules, and/or prefilled syringe
- Alcohol prep pad (70% alcohol)
- Syringe of the appropriate size for medication volume
- Needle of the appropriate size or vial access device
- Filter needle or straw, and gauze pad or ampule snapper, if you are using ampules

Delegation

As an RN, you can usually delegate administration of parenteral medications to a licensed practical nurse (LPN). You usually cannot delegate this task to a UAP.

Assessment

- Check the compatibility of the medications.

Some medications are either chemically or physically incompatible and cannot be mixed. Other medications may be compatible for only 20 to 30 minutes, so they must be given promptly after they are mixed. Although physically incompatible medications can frequently be identified by a change in appearance, such as precipitation, no such indication exists for chemically incompatible medications.

- Determine the total volume of medications and whether the total volume is appropriate for the administration site.

Although the reason for mixing medications is to limit the number of injections a patient receives, the total volume of the injections must not be greater than what is appropriate for the site, such as 1 mL for deltoid or 3 to 4 mL for the vastus lateralis or ventrogluteal.

➤

PROCEDURE 23–8

Mixing Medications in One Syringe *(continued)*

Procedural Steps

Procedure Variation A

Using Two Vials

First review Procedures 23–7 and 23–9.

Step 1 Clean the tops of both vials with an alcohol prep pad (note: some experts omit this step for single-dose vials).

Not all pharmaceutical companies guarantee the sterility of the rubber top on vials, even when they are first opened. However, be aware that once your fingers touch the alcohol pad, it is no longer sterile, either; so, you are not sterilizing, but rather are cleaning the vial tops, removing any tiny particles that might be on them.

Step 2 Draw up the same amount of air into the syringe as the total medication doses for both vials (e.g., if the order is for 0.5 mL for vial A and 1 mL for vial B, then draw up 1.5 mL of air). ▼

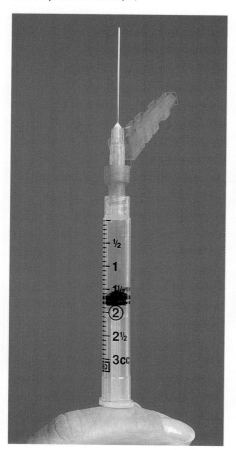

Step 3 Keeping the tip of the needle (or vial access device) above the medication, inject an amount of air equal to the volume of drug to be withdrawn from the first vial (e.g., 0.5 mL for vial A in step 2); then inject the rest of the air into the second vial. Take care to prevent coring (see Procedure 23–7B, step 6). ▼

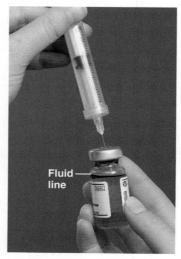

Vial A

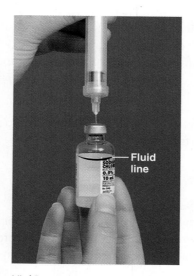

Vial B

Makes withdrawing the medication easier by creating positive pressure. For small unit-dose vials, it may be possible to withdraw the medication without instilling air, but you will need to maintain a slight backward pressure on the plunger until the needle is completely withdrawn. If you release the plunger, the negative pressure in the vial will pull the medication back in. Therefore, it is always safer to instill air.

Note: If one vial is a multidose vial, inject air into the single-dose vial first, and change the needle before injecting air into the multidose vial. You must withdraw medication from the multiple-dose vial before withdrawing from the single-dose vial.

This is an extra precaution to prevent contamination of the multidose vial with medication from the single-dose vial. However, the needle tip should stay above the medication at all times in step 3 anyway.

Note: If you are mixing two types of insulin, put air into the regular insulin last (see Technique 23–5 for mixing two types of insulin).

Step 4 Without removing the needle (or access device) from the second vial (B), invert the vial and withdraw the ordered amount of medication. Expel any air bubbles, and measure the dose. Remove the needle from the vial, then pull back on the plunger enough to pull all medication out of the needle (or access device) into the syringe (see Technique 23–4). Read the dose at eye level. Tip the syringe horizontally if you need to eject any medication.

This allows you to withdraw all the medication. Keeping the needle in the medication and slowly withdrawing the

PROCEDURE 23–8   **Mixing Medications in One Syringe** *(continued)*

medication will help prevent withdrawing excess air into the syringe and prevent bubbles. ▼

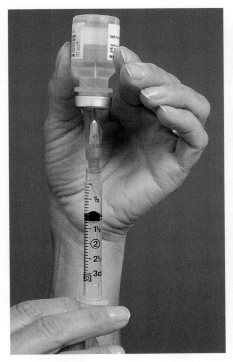

Vial B (Step 4)

Step 5 Insert the needle into the first vial, invert, and withdraw the exact ordered amount of medication. Be very careful not to withdraw excess medication; keep your index finger or thumb on the flange of the syringe to prevent it being forced back by pressure. If this occurs, you must discard the medication in the syringe and start over. (Using the example in step 2, you should have 1.5 mL of the mixed medications in the syringe.)

Because the medications are mixed, withdrawing extra from the second vial makes the entire mixture incorrect. If you eject excess medication from the syringe, you do not know how much of either medication you have ejected; so, even if you have the correct amount of fluid (e.g., 1.5 mL in our example), you would not know how much of that is medication A and how much of it is medication B.

There is no need to change the needle before step 5 because even if one vial is a multidose vial, you would have withdrawn the medication from it first (in step 4). It will not matter if you track medication into the single-dose vial. ▼

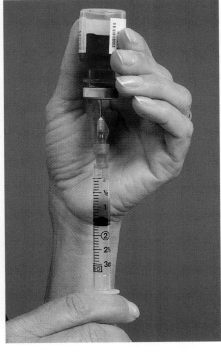

Vial A (Step 5)

Step 6 Remove the needle from the vial, and then recap the needle, using a needle capping device or the one-handed scoop method (see Procedure 23–9).

Although recapping a sterile needle does not present a threat of bloodborne pathogen exposure, using a mechanical recapping device or the one-handed method helps develop safe habits. As a rule, we do not recommend using the one-handed scoop for *sterile* needles; however, this needle will be discarded anyway, so if it is accidentally contaminated with a one-handed scoop, it will not be a major error.

Step 7 Put a new sterile needle on the syringe for the injection. Hold the needle vertically to expel all air and recheck the dosage (the total for both medications). If you have used a filter needle or vial access device, refer to Technique 23–4.

By the time you are finished withdrawing both medications, you will have put the needle through a rubber vial top at least three times. This dulls the needle. A sharp needle causes less trauma to the patient on injection. A new needle also prevents tracking of the medication through the skin and subcutaneous tissues.

Procedure Variation B
Using One Ampule and Vial
Review Procedures 23–7A and B and 23–9.

Step 8 Begin with the vial. Cleanse the stopper of a multiple-dose vial. Draw up the same volume of air as the dose of medication ordered for the vial. Inject air into the vial, and withdraw the medication. See Procedure 23–7B.

Because you do not need to add air to ampules before drawing up the medication, you should draw from the vial first. Additionally, if it is a multidose vial, you would contaminate it with the medicine if you withdrew from the ampule first (unless you change the needle, and that is an unnecessary expense).

Injecting air into the vial makes withdrawing the medication easier. For small unit-dose vials, it may be possible to withdraw the medication without instilling air, but you will need to maintain a slight backward pressure on the plunger until the needle is completely withdrawn. If you release the plunger, the negative pressure in the vial will pull the medication back in. Therefore, it is safer always to instill air.

Step 9 Remove the injection needle, and place it on an opened, sterile alcohol pad.

Keeps the needle sterile; you will reuse it.

Step 10 Attach the filter needle or straw to the syringe. Flick or tap the top of the ampule (or snap your wrist) to remove medication from the neck of the ampule.

The use of a 5 μm filter needle minimizes the possibility of withdrawing small glass fragments.

➤

PROCEDURE 23–8 Mixing Medications in One Syringe *(continued)*

Step 11 Open the ampule by wrapping the neck with a gauze pad or an unopened alcohol wipe or use an ampule snapper. Snap open away from you.

Prevents you from accidentally cutting your fingers or spraying glass fragments toward your face. Do not use an opened alcohol wipe to break the ampule, because it is not thick enough to prevent injury.

Step 12 Withdraw the exact ordered amount of medication from the ampule into the syringe. See Procedure 23–7A. Be very careful in drawing up the second medication; if the total amount of the two medications is incorrect, you must discard the syringe contents and start over.

See Step 5.

Step 13 Draw about 0.2 mL of air into the syringe to clear the filter needle (see Technique 23–4). Using a one-handed technique, recap and remove the filter needle or straw and discard it in a sharps container. Replace the filter needle with an administration needle.

(1) Prevents accidental needlestick injury. (2) You cannot measure the dose accurately with a filter needle. You should not eject medication through the filter needle because of risk of breaking the filter. See Steps 5 and 7 and Technique 23–4.

Step 14 Confirm that the dose is correct.

Ensures that the total volume in the syringe equals the ordered amount of both medications plus 0.2 mL of air. ▼

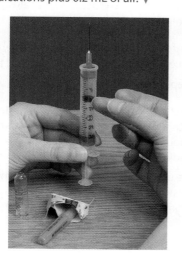

Step 15 Discard the syringe and needle into a sharps container.

Prevents needle-stick injury.

Procedure Variation C:

Using a Prefilled Cartridge and Single-Dose Vial—For Intravenous Administration

Note: It is best to *not* use this technique with multidose vials because there is a risk of contaminating the multidose vial with the cartridge medication.

Step 16 Cleanse the vial thoroughly with an alcohol prep pad.

See Step 1.

Step 17 Assemble the prefilled cartridge and holder (see Technique 23–2).

Step 18 Remove the needle cap from the prefilled cartridge, expel the air, and measure the correct dose of medication.

You must confirm that the dose of the first medication is correct before you mix it with the second medication.

Step 19 Holding the cartridge with the needle up, withdraw an amount of air equal to the volume of medication you need from the vial.

Step 20 While continuing to hold the syringe with needle straight up (vertically), insert the needle into the inverted vial, and inject the air into the vial. Maintain pressure on the plunger so that air and/or medication does not flow back into the syringe.

Makes medication easier to withdraw. ➤

Step 21 While maintaining pressure on the plunger, allow the pressure in the vial to push the medication into the syringe. Withdraw the ordered amount of vial medication, being careful not to withdraw any excess.

See Step 5.

Step 22 The pressure will generally push a little less than you need, so withdraw the correct amount.

Withdrawing any excess will result in an altered dose, so you would need to discard the syringe and start over.

Step 23 Recap the needle (use a one-handed method), and if possible, remove the needle from the prefilled syringe and replace with an injection cannula for intravenous administration.

The cannula prevents needlestick injury. Unless there is a needle safety device for the prefilled syringe, it is not recommended for IM injections.

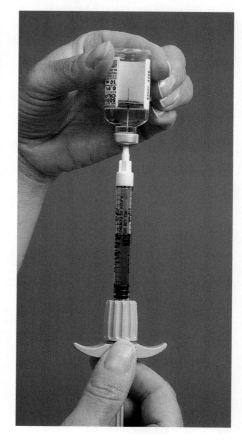

PROCEDURE 23-9	**Recapping Needles Using One-Handed Technique**

 For steps to follow in *all* procedures, refer to the inside back cover of this book. Also refer to Medication Guidelines: Steps to Follow for All Medications (Regardless of Type or Route).

critical aspects

Recapping Contaminated Needles
- Recap a contaminated needle only if doing so is unavoidable.
- Do not place your nondominant hand near the needle cap when recapping the needle or engaging the safety mechanism.
- If you are using a safety needle, engage the safety mechanism to cover the needle.
- If available, place the needle cap in a mechanical recapping device.
- If recapping devices are not available and you must recap the needle for your own and/or the patient's safety, use the one-handed scoop technique.

Recapping Sterile Needles
- Be sure to keep the needle and cap sterile.
- Do not place your nondominant hand near the needle cap when recapping the needle or engaging the safety mechanism.
- Use one of the following methods:
  - Place the needle cap in a medication cup, and recap the needle.
  - Place the cap on a clean surface so that the end of the needle cap protrudes over the edge of the counter or shelf, and scoop with the needle.
  - Use a hard syringe cover: Insert the needle cap into the cover, and then insert the needle.
  - Place the needle cap on a sterile surface, such as on open alcohol prep pad, and use the one-handed scoop technique.

Equipment
- Mechanical recapping device, if available
- Needle cover
- Other supplies depending on the method used.

Delegation

Delegation is not usually an issue because recapping needles is done in conjunction with administering parenteral medications, which you will usually not delegate. If you do delegate

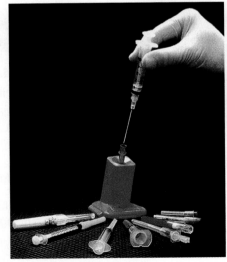

Needle recapping devices.

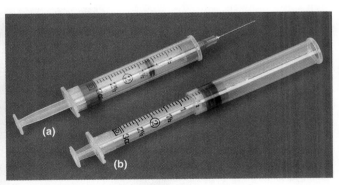

A: Before injection; B: After injection.

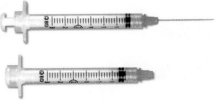

Top: Before injection; Bottom: Needle retracted after injection.

administration of parenteral medications to a licensed practical nurse (LPN), you must supervise and evaluate recapping to ensure that the nurse uses proper technique.

Preparation

• Assess the need to recap the needle.

Recap a contaminated needle only if doing so is absolutely unavoidable, according to OSHA standards. As a rule, place a contaminated syringe and needle directly into a puncture-proof sharps container, without capping, bending, or breaking the needle.

• Identify whether the needle is sterile or dirty.

Although a one-handed technique is used to recap both sterile and dirty needles, different considerations exist. When you use the one-handed method for recapping a sterile needle, it is easy to contaminate the needle without realizing it; so, you should modify the technique to help prevent that. The danger in recapping a dirty needle is that you will stick yourself with it, exposing yourself to pathogens.

• Determine the availability of mechanical recapping device.

Always use a mechanical recapping device, if one is available.

Procedural Steps

Procedure Variation A
Recapping Contaminated Needles

Step 1 If you are using a safety needle, engage the safety mechanism to cover the needle. (See Equipment.)

OSHA regulations require the use of safety syringes to prevent needlestick injuries. You must engage the safety mechanism before placing the needle and syringe into the sharps container.

Step 2 Alternatively, place the needle cap in mechanical recapping device, if one is available. (See Equipment.)

Step 3 If a mechanical recapping device is not available, use the one-handed scoop method to recap the needle.
a. Place the needle cover on a flat surface. ▼

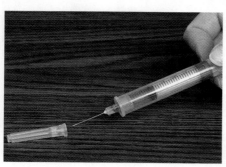

b. Then, holding syringe in your dominant hand, scoop the needle cap onto the needle. Tip the syringe vertically to slip the cap over the needle. Do not hold onto the needle cap with your nondominant hand while scooping.

A mechanical recapping device protects against accidental needlesticks. If it is unavailable, the one-handed method of recapping will prevent accidental injuries when your own or the patient's safety is a concern. ▼

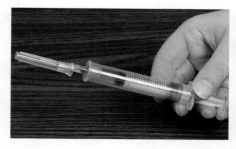

c. Secure the needle cap by grasping it near the hub.

Prevents an accidental stick if the needle goes through the needle cap. Needles are sharp enough to go through the needle cap if inserted at an angle. ▼

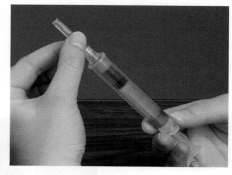

Procedure Variation B
Recapping Sterile Needles

Use one of the following techniques to ensure that you do not contaminate a sterile needle.

If you contaminate the needle, microorganisms will be introduced with the injection.

Step 4 Place the needle cap in a mechanical recapping device, if one is available.

The device is specially developed to provide safe recapping.

PROCEDURE 23–9

Recapping Needles Using One-Handed Technique *(continued)*

Step 5 Alternatively, place the cap into a medication cup with the open end facing up. You can then insert the sterile needle into the cap, keeping your free hand well away from the cup.

This step performs the same function as a mechanical recapping device. ▼

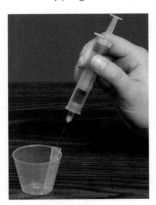

Step 6 Alternatively, place the cap on a clean surface so that the end of the needle cap protrudes over the edge of the counter or shelf, and scoop with the needle; keep your free hand well away from the needle and cap as you are recapping.

Prevents you from inadvertently hitting an unsterile surface with the needle. ▼

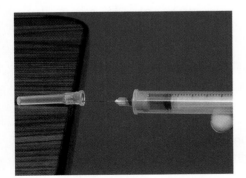

Step 7 Alternatively, if the syringe is packaged in a hard plastic tubular container, stand the container on its large end, invert the needle cap, and place it in the top of the hard container. Insert the needle downward into the cap. ▼

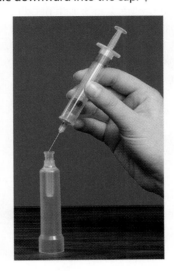

Step 8 Alternatively, place the needle cap on a sterile surface, such as on open alcohol prep pad, and use the one-handed scoop technique.

Provides a sterile barrier. If the needle does contact the sterile surface, it will remain sterile. ▼

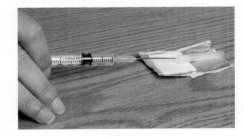

PROCEDURE 23–10 | Administering Intradermal Medications

 For steps to follow in *all* procedures, refer to the inside back cover of this book. Also refer to Medication Guidelines: Steps to Follow for All Medications (Regardless of Type or Route).

critical aspects
- Maintain sterile technique and standard precautions.
- Use a 1 mL syringe and a 25- to 28-gauge, $\frac{1}{4}$ to $\frac{5}{8}$ inch needle.
- Be aware that an intradermal dose is small, usually about 0.01 to 0.1 mL.
- Administer the injection on the ventral surface of the forearm, upper back, or upper chest.
- Hold the syringe parallel to the skin at a 5 to 15° angle, with the bevel up.
- Stretch the skin taut to insert the needle.
- Do not aspirate.
- Inject slowly, and create a wheal or bleb.
- Do not massage the site.

Equipment
- 1 mL syringe (tuberculin) with intradermal needle (25- to 28-gauge, $\frac{1}{4}$ to $\frac{5}{8}$ inch with short bevel)
- Alcohol prep pads
- 2 × 2 gauze pad
- Pen (ink or felt)

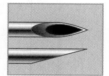
Regular bevel

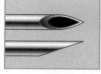
Intermediate bevel

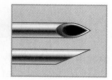
Short bevel

Delegation
As an RN, you can usually delegate administration of parenteral medications to a licensed practical nurse. You usually cannot delegate this task to a UAP.

Assessment
- Assess for previous reaction to skin testing.

Some skin tests, such as the tuberculin test, should not be repeated after positive test results.
- Assess for all types of allergies.

Because intradermal injections are also used for allergy testing, a client could have an anaphylactic reaction.
- Assess the skin at intradermal sites for bruising, swelling, tenderness, and other abnormalities.
- Do not give intradermal skin tests if skin abnormalities are present. Also avoid giving them in areas where reading the results may be difficult, such as areas of heavy hair growth.

Special Considerations
- Because intradermal injections are often given for allergy testing, the client is at risk for injury related to allergen sensitivity.
- Have appropriate antidotes (usually epinephrine hydrochloride, a bronchodilator, and an antihistamine) readily available before the start of the procedure.
- Know the location of resuscitation equipment (artificial airway, Ambu bag and code cart); allergic reactions can be fatal.

PROCEDURE 23–10

Administering Intradermal Medications
(continued)

Procedural Steps

Step 1 Draw up the medication from the vial. The usual dose is 0.01 to 0.1 mL. See Procedure 23–7B.

Intradermal sites can accommodate only small volumes of medication.

Step 2 Select the site for injection. Usual sites are the ventral surface of the forearm and upper back. The upper chest may also be used.

 Go to Chapter 23, **Figure 23–23,** in Volume 1.

Use areas where subcutaneous fat is less likely to interfere with administration and absorption. The forearm is the standard initial starting point because it has the least amount of subcutaneous tissue. The forearm and upper back usually have little hair, permitting easier visualization to interpret results accurately.

Step 3 Assist the patient to a comfortable position. If you are using the forearm, have the patient extend and supinate his arm on a flat surface. If you are using the upper back, have the patient lie prone or lean forward over a table or the back of a chair.

Stabilizes the injection site. The procedure will be more comfortable if the patient is able to relax his muscles. Tension, in general, increases pain perception.

Step 4 Cleanse the injection site with the alcohol prep pad by circling from the center of the site outward. Allow the site to dry before administering the injection.

Cleanse to remove microorganisms; follow the principle of "clean to dirty." Alcohol can interfere with the test results if a small amount is introduced during the injection; also, if the alcohol has not evaporated, it may cause the skin to sting during the injection.

Step 5 Don procedure gloves.

Procedure gloves are not required by OSHA for intradermal injections, but they are recommended by the CDC to prevent accidental exposure to bloodborne pathogens. You may prefer to don gloves before step 4; however, you can also do so while waiting for the alcohol to dry.

Step 6 Hold the syringe between the thumb and index finger of your dominant hand parallel to the client's skin; remove the needle cap.

Because of the low angle of administration, the syringe flange must be parallel to the skin surface. You must hold the syringe between your thumb and index finger to be able to administer the solution at the correct angle.

Step 7 Hold the client's skin taut by using one of the following methods, with your nondominant hand:
a. If using the forearm, you may be able to place your hand under the client's arm and pull the skin tight with your thumb and fingers.
b. Stretch the client's skin between your thumb and index finger.
c. Pull the client's skin toward the wrist or down with one finger.

Eases needle insertion. Holding the skin tight can be difficult because of the low angle of administration.

Step 8 While holding the client's skin taut with your nondominant hand, hold the syringe in your dominant hand with the needle bevel up (according to the CDC) and parallel to the client's skin at a 5 to 15° angle. Slowly insert the needle. Note that there is some controversy about whether it is better to have the bevel down or bevel up. You should read available resources and decide which seems better to you.

The low angle of insertion is necessary to place the needle tip in the intradermal layer instead of the subcutaneous tissue.

Having the bevel up is thought to decrease the chance of injecting the medication deeper into the subcutaneous tissue. ▼

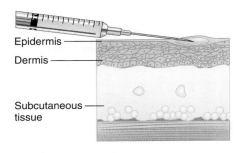

Epidermis
Dermis
Subcutaneous tissue

Step 9 Advance the needle approximately 3 mm ($\frac{1}{8}$ inch) so that the entire bevel is covered. The bevel should be visible just under the skin.

If the entire bevel is not inserted, the solution will leak out of the tissue. If you can see the bevel under the surface of the skin, you can be sure that the bevel is not in the subcutaneous tissue.

Step 10 Do not aspirate. Hold the syringe stable with your nondominant hand, and release the tightened skin.

Decreases pressure on the injection site.

Step 11 Slowly inject the solution. You should feel firm resistance. A pale wheal, about 6 to 10 mm ($\frac{1}{4}$ inch) in diameter, will appear over the needle bevel.

The dermis does not have room to absorb the solution, so a wheal forms, stretching the skin. Slow administration gives you time to terminate the injection should a systemic reaction occur. If a bleb (wheal) forms, you have administered the drug

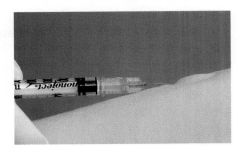

➤

PROCEDURE 23–10   Administering Intradermal Medications
(continued)

properly. The size of the bleb depends on the amount of medication you injected. ▼

Step 12   Remove the needle, engage the safety needle device, and dispose of the needle in a biohazard puncture-proof container. If there is no safety device, place the uncapped syringe and needle directly in biohazard puncture-proof container.

Prevents needlestick injuries.

Step 13   Gently blot any blood with a dry gauze pad. Do not rub the skin or cover it with an adhesive bandage.

Rubbing may cause the drug to leak out and alter absorption. An adhesive bandage can cause irritation and interfere with the skin test.

Step 14   With a pen, draw a 1-inch circle around the bleb/wheal.

Aids in later identification of the site for reassessment.

Evaluation

- Reassess the client 5 and 15 minutes after administration, because reactions (e.g., allergic reactions) may subsequently occur.
- Read the site within 48 to 72 hours of injection, depending on the test.
- Observe that a wheal (about 6 to 8 mm in diameter) forms at the site and that it gradually disappears.
- Observe for minimal bruising that may develop at the site of injection.

Patient Teaching

- Explain when the patient needs to have the intradermal injection read to determine whether the result is positive or negative.

Most intradermal skin tests must be read in 48 to 72 hours for accurate results.

- Explain that mild itching, swelling, or irritation may occur at the injection site and are normal.

If the patient has antigens to the injected solution, a histamine response occurs, causing itching, swelling, or irritation. This response generally subsides within a week.

- Discuss the significance of a positive or negative skin test result.

Explain that some signs of irritation may occur that do not mean a positive test result.

- Instruct the patient not to scratch, apply lotions or creams, cover the site with a bandage, or scrub the site.

Causes irritation and interferes with the test; may produce false-positive results.

Documentation

- See the information in **Medication Guidelines: Steps to Follow for All Medications (Regardless of Type or Route).**
- Some medications require documentation of lot numbers (check agency policy).
- Chart when the test is to be read.

Sample documentation:

| 6/23/06 | 0830 | Intermediate Strength PPD administered intradermally in left forearm (see MAR). Read 6/25/06 or 6/26/06.—M. Canna, RN |

PROCEDURE 23–11   Administering Subcutaneous Medications

For steps to follow in *all* procedures, refer to the inside back cover of this book. Also refer to Medication Guidelines: Steps to Follow for All Medications (Regardless of Type or Route).

critical aspects
- Maintain sterile technique and standard precautions.
- Use a 1 mL syringe and a 25- to 27-gauge needle that is less than 1 inch long (usually $\frac{3}{8}$ to $\frac{5}{8}$ inch).
- A subcutaneous dose must be no more than 1 mL.
- Injection sites: Use the outer aspect of the upper arms, abdomen, anterior aspects of the thighs, or the upper buttocks just below the waist.
- Pinch the skin to inject (as a general rule).
- For an average-weight or thin client, inject at a 45° angle; for an obese client, inject at a 90° angle.
- Aspiration is optional, but do not aspirate when injecting heparin or insulin.
- Do not massage the site.

Equipment
- Syringe and needle appropriate for volume and site
- Alcohol prep pad
- Gauze pad (optional)

Delegation
As an RN, you can usually delegate administration of parenteral medications to a licensed practical nurse. You usually cannot delegate this task to a UAP.

Assessment
- Check the site for previous injection.

Alternating among the arms, thighs, abdomen, and back changes the absorption rate of the medication. Absorption is fastest from the abdomen, then the arms, and lastly the thighs and back. It is recommended that you rotate sites within the same extremity or location, approximately 1 inch from the previous injection. Rotating the site helps prevent the development of lipodystrophy.

- Do focused assessments for the specific medication being administered.
  - *Insulin*—check capillary blood sugar level, and determine when the patient will be having her next meal; check for signs of hypoglycemia or hyperglycemia.

Insulin must be balanced with food intake to prevent the patient from developing insulin shock. Different insulins have specific rates of absorption, peak action, and duration. Some insulins such as Humalog and regular insulin, are rapid acting. Before you administer rapid-acting insulin, the capillary blood sugar must be within the normal range or above, and the patient must be ready to eat. With Humalog, the patient's food tray should be in front of him before you administer the insulin.

  - *Heparin*—check activated partial thromboplastin time (aPTT) and for signs of bleeding, such as bleeding from gums, intravenous injection sites, and so on.

Heparin is an anticoagulant, so the major side effect is bleeding. Besides overt bleeding, also check for occult blood loss through the urine and stool. The aPTT will not be monitored as frequently with the low-molecular-weight heparins (LMWHs), because bleeding is less likely to occur.

➤

PROCEDURE 23–11

Administering Subcutaneous Medications
(continued)

Procedural Steps

Step 1 Select an appropriate syringe and needle.

a. For insulin administration, you must use an insulin syringe.

Although both insulin and tuberculin (TB) syringes come in 1 mL size, they are not interchangeable. Insulin syringes are calibrated in units; they have a permanent needle and a very small amount of dead space.

b. For volumes less than 1 mL, use a tuberculin (TB) syringe with a 25- to 27-gauge, $\frac{3}{8}$ to $\frac{5}{8}$ inch needle.

Because of the small increments on the TB syringe, small doses can be more accurately measured. ▼

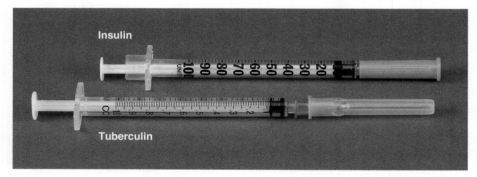

Insulin

Tuberculin

c. For administering a volume of 1 mL, you may use a 3 mL syringe with a 25- to 27-gauge, $\frac{3}{8}$ to $\frac{5}{8}$ inch needle.

Although you can measure 1 mL with a tuberculin (TB) syringe, it will be difficult to handle the syringe because the plunger will be pulled back as far as it can go. It is easy to pull it inadvertently out of the end of the syringe. Some medications are supplied in prefilled syringes. Examples are enoxaparin sodium (Lovenox) and the other low-molecular-weight heparins (LMWHs). These are usually supplied in unit-dose prefilled glass syringes.

Step 2 Draw up the medication. See Procedure 23–7.

Step 3 Select an injection site with adequate subcutaneous tissue.

 Go to Chapter 23, **Figure 23–24,** in Volume 1.

Helps you avoid accidentally injecting into the muscle.

a. The usual sites are the outer aspect of the upper arms, abdomen, anterior aspects of the thighs, and upper buttocks just below the waist.

These areas usually have good circulation and are easily accessible.

b. The abdomen is the only subcutaneous site used for administering heparin or low-molecular-weight heparins (LMWHs).

The subcutaneous tissue 2 inches away from the umbilicus poses less risk of bleeding when an anticoagulant is administered.

c. Check the site for inflammation, bruising, lumps, or other abnormalities.

Avoid areas with skin abnormalities, which may alter the absorption rates or increase patient discomfort during the injection.

Step 4 Position the patient so that the injection site is accessible and the patient is able to relax the appropriate area.

Makes performing the injection easier and helps decrease patient discomfort.

Step 5 Cleanse the injection site with an alcohol prep pad by circling from the center of the site outward. Allow the site to dry before administering the injection.

Cleanse to remove microorganisms; follow the principle of "clean to dirty." If the alcohol has not evaporated, it may cause the skin to sting during the injection.

Step 6 Don procedure gloves.

Procedure gloves are required to prevent exposure to bloodborne pathogens. You may prefer to don gloves before Step 5; however, you can also do so while waiting for the alcohol to dry.

Step 7 Remove the needle cap.

The needle cap is more difficult to remove when using a one-handed technique.

Step 8 With your nondominant hand, pinch the skin at the injection site, and determine the angle at which to inject the needle. If the "pinch" (adipose tissue) is greater than 2 inches, use a 90° angle. If the client is of average size or the "pinch" (adipose tissue) is less than 1 inch, use a 45° angle. If the client is obese and the adipose tissue pinches 2 inches or more, you should use a longer needle and spread the skin taut instead of pinching.

Grasping and lifting the skin prevents you from accidentally injecting into the muscle. Adjusting the angle of the injection allows you to deliver the medication into the subcutaneous tissue. *Note:* You can vary any or all of these techniques to be sure you are injecting into the subcutaneous tissue: needle length, "pinch or spread" technique, and injection angle. ▼

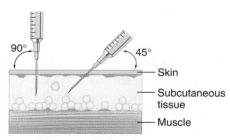

90°   45°
Skin
Subcutaneous tissue
Muscle

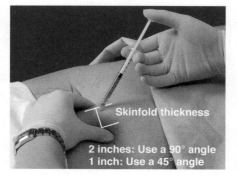

Skinfold thickness

2 inches: Use a 90° angle
1 inch: Use a 45° angle

PROCEDURE 23–11   Administering Subcutaneous Medications
(continued)

Step 9 Holding the syringe between thumb and index finger of your dominant hand like a pencil or dart, insert the needle at the appropriate angle into the skinfold.

Quickly inserting the needle through the skin minimizes discomfort.

Step 10 Stabilize the syringe with the fingers of your nondominant hand.

Prevents the needle from moving around in the tissue and thereby causing discomfort and possible tissue injury.

Step 11 Using the thumb or index finger of your dominant hand, press the plunger

slowly to inject the medication. Alternatively, after inserting the needle, you can continue to hold the barrel with your dominant hand and use your nondominant hand to depress the plunger.

Slow administration allows the medication to disperse and decreases discomfort. Subcutaneous injections do not need to be aspirated beforehand, because accidental entry into a blood vessel is very rare.

Step 12 Remove the needle smoothly along the line of insertion.

Prevents pulling against the skin and tissue and thus minimizes discomfort.

Step 13 Gently wipe the site with gauze if needed, engage the needle safety device, and dispose of the needle in biohazard container. If there is no safety device, place the uncapped syringe and needle directly into biohazard puncture-proof container.

Prevents needlestick injuries.

Step 14 Gently blot any blood with a gauze pad. Do not massage the site.

Massaging or rubbing the site will alter the rate of absorption of the medication.

Evaluation

- Observe for minimal bruising that may develop at the site of injection.
- Reassess patient for anticipated response and adverse reaction to medication.
  - For insulin, observe for signs that patient's blood sugar level has returned to normal and for signs of hypoglycemia.
  - For heparin, observe that patient has no signs of bleeding.
  - For other medications, observe for side effects.

Patient Teaching

- Discuss possible lifestyle adaptations that the client may need to undertake while receiving the medication, such as diet and exercise recommendations for managing diabetes mellitus.

Home Care

- Discuss with the patient or caregiver the options for insulin administration to determine the most appropriate choice for the person administering the injections.

Many options are available, including specially designed syringes that are easier to handle and read, pen injectors, and prefilled syringes.

- Teach the patient or caregiver that syringes and needles can be safely reused in the home. Teach them to discard the needle when it becomes dull, bent, or contaminated.

You will need to decide whether reusing syringes is appropriate for the patient. Contraindications include inadequate hygiene, immunocompromise, and difficulty handling equipment to prevent contamination of the needle. The very small insulin needles (30-gauge) bend very easily and are not recommended for reuse. For guidelines on reusing syringes and needles at home,

VOL 1 | Go to Chapter 23, the box **Home Care: Reusing Needles and Syringes,** in Volume 1.

PROCEDURE 23–11   **Administering Subcutaneous Medications**
(continued)

- Discuss safety concerns regarding subcutaneous medication administration in the home, such as how to dispose of biohazardous wastes correctly and where to obtain a puncture-proof bio-hazard container.

The patient or caregiver may use a large plastic bottle or a coffee can. Local regulations regarding disposal must be followed.

- Discuss with the patient the need to rotate sites. For insulin, explain to the patient that alternating among arms, thighs, and abdomen causes different absorption rates. The recommendation is to give the injections due at the same time of the day in the same body location about 1 inch from the previous injection site.

Repeatedly giving the medication in the same site can cause abnormalities in the tissue and alter absorption rates.

- If the patient is receiving heparin or LMWHs, discuss the need to avoid nonsteroidal anti-inflammatory medications, such as acetylsalicylic acid (aspirin) and ibuprofen (Motrin, Advil).

These drugs increase the risk of bleeding, so the patient should avoid them.

- For patients receiving heparin or LMWHs, discuss home safety and the need to avoid falls.

Patient is at risk for bleeding and needs to follow safety guidelines to prevent injury.

Documentation

- Chart according to **Medication Guidelines: Steps to Follow for All Medications (Regardless of Type or Route).**
- Some agencies have a specific coded form for documenting subcutaneous injections, which allow exact site documentation on an outline of the body.
- In the nurse's notes, document any related patient assessment findings, such as capillary blood sugar, signs of hypoglycemia or hyperglycemia, bruising, and so on. Document in the nurse's notes as well as MAR any medication that was given PRN.

Sample documentation:

6/24/06	8:00 AM	Blood glucose 210 g/dL. 10 Units of NPH insulin administered SubQ in upper left arm. See MAR. ———— G. Smith, RN

PROCEDURE 23–12   Locating Intramuscular Injection Sites

For steps to follow in *all* procedures, refer to the inside back cover of this book. Also refer to Medication Guidelines: Steps to Follow for All Medications (Regardless of Type or Route).

critical aspects

- Always palpate the landmarks and the muscle mass to ensure correct placement.
- *Deltoid:* The injection site is an inverted triangle. The base is two to three fingerbreadths below the acromion process, and the tip is even with the top of the axilla.
- *Vastus lateralis:* Midlateral thigh: On adults, one handbreadth below the head of the trochanter and one handbreadth above the knee. The site is the middle third of this area. This is the preferred site for infants under 7 months.
- *Ventrogluteal:* On adults, a triangle formed between your fingers when you place your palm on the head of the trochanter, index finger on the anterior superior iliac spine, and middle finger on the iliac crest. This is the preferred site for adults and children over 7 months (some authorities say over 12 months).
- *Dorsogluteal:* Locate the site by drawing an imaginary line between the head of the trochanter and the posterior superior iliac spine. At the middle of the line, go up approximately 1 inch. Use this site only if no others are accessible.
- *Rectus femoris:* Middle third of the anterior thigh. Use this site only if no others are accessible.

Assessment

Note: Always palpate the landmarks and the muscle mass to ensure correct placement.

Because patients come in different sizes, the site locations will vary slightly. Always palpate the muscle mass to ensure proper placement.

Delegation

As an RN, you can usually delegate administration of parenteral medications (including locating injection sites) to a licensed practical nurse. You usually cannot delegate this task to a UAP. If you delegate the skill, you are responsible for evaluating the LPN's ability to locate injection sites correctly.

Procedural Steps

Procedure Variation A

Ventrogluteal site:

1. Have the patient assume a side-lying position, if possible.

   Makes the site easier to locate.

2. Locate the greater trochanter, anterior superior iliac spine, and the iliac crest.

3. Place the palm of your hand on the greater trochanter, your index finger on the anterior superior iliac spine, and your middle finger pointing toward the iliac crest. (Use your right hand on the patient's left hip; use your left hand on the patient's right hip.) ➤

4. The middle of the triangle between your middle and index fingers is the injection site.

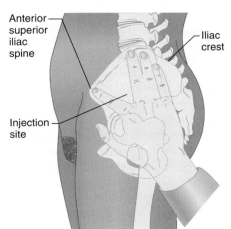

Anterior superior iliac spine

Iliac crest

Injection site

This is a safe site for IM administration because it is not in close proximity to any major blood vessels or nerves. It is safe for patients of all ages and the preferred site for adults and children over 7 to 12 months old (there is some disagreement over the age; always palpate to assess adequacy of muscle mass, regardless of age). ▾

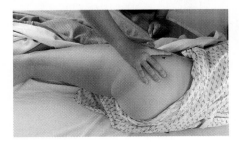

➤

PROCEDURE 23–12 Locating Intramuscular Injection Sites
(continued)

 Go to Chapter 23, **Figure 23–26,** in Volume 1.

Procedure Variation B
Dorsogluteal site:

1. Do not use this site unless all others are inaccessible and another medication route is not feasible.

The proximity of the sciatic nerve creates a risk for injury to the patient.

2. Have the patient lie prone.

If the patient is not prone, you may incorrectly locate the site, especially if the gluteal area is not firm.

3. Locate the greater trochanter and the posterior superior iliac spine. ▼

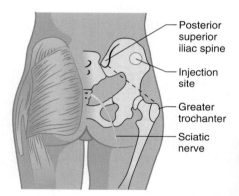

Posterior superior iliac spine

Injection site

Greater trochanter

Sciatic nerve

4. Draw an imaginary line between the greater trochanter and the posterior superior iliac spine. ▼

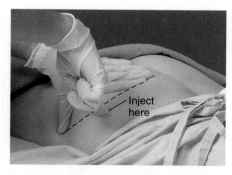

Inject here

5. In the middle of the line, go up approximately 1 inch to locate the site.

Never use this site in children, because the muscle is not well developed enough and because it is close to the sciatic nerve. Use it for adults only as a last resort. Using the upper outer portion of the muscle helps ensure a safe injection site. Do not use the upper outer quadrant of the buttock as a landmark, because you may locate the site too low and may compromise the sciatic nerve. That method (the "four quadrants" method) was taught in the past but should no longer be used.

Procedure Variation C
Deltoid site:

1. Completely expose the patient's upper arm. Remove the garment; do not roll up the sleeve.

Incomplete exposure of site and landmarks creates a risk of injecting into other than muscle tissue. This is a small site, and it is easy to make an error in location.

2. Locate the lower edge of the acromion process, and go two fingerbreadths down. ▼

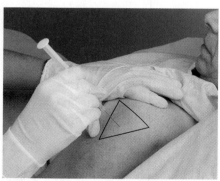

3. Draw an imaginary line out from the axillary crease.
4. The deltoid site is the resulting inverted triangle.
5. An alternative approach is to place four fingerbreadths across the deltoid muscle, with your top finger on the acromion process. The injection goes three fingerbreadths below the process.

Locates the muscle body while avoiding the radial nerve and deep brachial artery. One of the recommended sites for many immunizations. Because it is a fairly small muscle, only 0.5 to 1 mL of medication can be administered.

 Go to Chapter 23, **Figure 23–27,** in Volume 1.

Procedure Variation D
Vastus lateralis site:

1. Have the patient lying supine or sitting.
2. Locate the greater trochanter and the lateral femoral condyle.
3. Place your hands on the thigh, with one hand against the greater trochanter, and the other edge of hand against the lateral femoral condyle.
4. Visualize a rectangle between your hands across the anterolateral thigh. The index fingers of your hands form the smaller ends of the rectangle. The long sides of the rectangle are formed by (1) drawing an imaginary line down the center of the anterior thigh and (2) drawing another line along the side of the leg, halfway between the bed and the front of the thigh. This box marks the middle third of the anterolateral thigh, which is the injection site. ▼

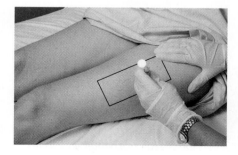

PROCEDURE 23–12   **Locating Intramuscular Injection Sites**
(continued)

Locates the body of the muscle. Because it is not near any major blood vessels or nerves, the vastus lateralis site is safe for patients of all ages and recommended site for children less than 7 months old. ▼

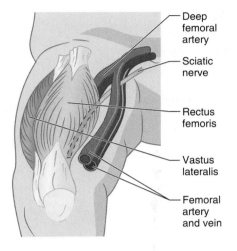

- Deep femoral artery
- Sciatic nerve
- Rectus femoris
- Vastus lateralis
- Femoral artery and vein

VOL 1   Go to Chapter 23, **Figure 23–28,** in Volume 1.

Procedure Variation E

Rectus femoris site:

Use this site only if no other sites are accessible and no other medication routes are feasible.

a. Divide the top of the thigh from the groin to the knee into thirds, and identify the middle third.

b. Visualize a rectangle in the middle of the anterior surface of the thigh. This is the location of the injection site. ➤

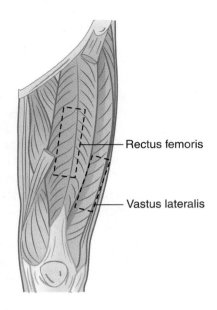

- Rectus femoris
- Vastus lateralis

PROCEDURE 23–13   Administering Intramuscular Injections

> For steps to follow in *all* procedures, refer to the inside back cover of this book. Also refer to Medication Guidelines: Steps to Follow for All Medications (Regardless of Type or Route).

critical aspects

- Maintain sterile technique and standard precautions.
- Use a 1 to 3 mL syringe and a 21- to 25-gauge, 1 to 1½ inch needle.
- The usual dose per injection is no more than 3 mL.
- Select an appropriate injection site, and identify the site using anatomical landmarks:
  - Ventrogluteal site is preferred for IM injections
  - Deltoid site is acceptable for IM doses of 1 mL or less (check agency policy)
- Aspirate the needle before injecting. If blood appears, remove the needle, discard it, and start over.
- Inject at a 90° angle.
- Z-track technique is recommended. Mnemonic:

Deliver	**D**isplace
All	**A**spirate
Injections	**I**nject (wait 10 seconds)
With	**W**ithdraw
Responsibility	**R**elease

Equipment

- Syringe and needle appropriate for volume and site
- Alcohol prep pad
- Gauze pad or Band-Aid
- Biohazard container

Delegation

As an RN, you can usually delegate administration of parenteral medications to a licensed practical nurse. You cannot delegate this task to a UAP.

Assessment

- Identify the site of the previous injection.

Alternating the sites for injections helps prevent tissue damage and increases patient comfort.

- Assess the chosen site for adequate muscle mass, bruises, edema, tenderness, redness, or other abnormalities.

Muscle mass must be large enough to absorb the amount of medication prescribed. Abnormalities at the site will increase patient discomfort and alter the absorption rate of the medication.

- Assess for factors that might affect absorption of the medication, such as decreased intramuscular blood flow, as found in shock or muscle atrophy.

Decreased peripheral circulation or muscle atrophy will decrease the absorption of the medication.

PROCEDURE 23–13

Administering Intramuscular Injections
(continued)

Procedural Steps

Step 1 Select the appropriate syringe and needle.

a. The usual syringe size is 1 to 3 mL, depending on volume of medication to be given.

For doses less than 1 mL, you can use a tuberculin syringe with an intramuscular needle.

b. The usual needle size is 21- to 23-gauge, $1\frac{1}{2}$ inch in length.

For IM administration, the needle gauge must be appropriate for the viscosity of the medication, and the needle must be long enough to deliver the medication into the muscle.

c. Some medications are supplied in prefilled syringes, which are used for administration.

An example is ketorolac tromethamine (Toradol), which is supplied in both a vial and a prefilled syringe.

Step 2 Draw up the medication. See Procedures 23–7A and 23–7B.

Step 3 Select the site for injection. If the client is to receive more than one injection, rotate sites.

Volumes of 1 to 3 mL may be given, depending on the muscle size (for adults, 0.5 to 1 mL in the deltoid and up to 3 mL in the vastus lateralis and ventrogluteal sites). Rotating sites reduces discomfort and tissue trauma.

Step 4 Position the patient so that the injection site is accessible and the patient is able to relax the appropriate muscles.

Makes performing the injection easier and helps decrease patient discomfort.

a. Deltoid site: Position the patient with the arm relaxed at the side or resting on a firm surface, and completely expose the upper arm.

b. Ventrogluteal site: Position the patient on the opposite side, with the upper hip and knee slightly flexed.

This position may cause the trochanter to become more prominent, making it easier to locate the site.

c. Vastus lateralis: Position the patient supine or sitting.

d. Rectus femoris: Position patient supine. Because this site often causes more discomfort than others, use it only if all other sites are inaccessible and no other route is feasible.

e. Dorsogluteal: Position the patient prone, with the toes pointing inward. Do not attempt to locate this site with the patient side-lying or standing. Because the sciatic nerve and major blood vessels are located near this site, use it only if all other sites are inaccessible and no other route is feasible.

Position the patient so that (1) you can fully visualize and safely access the site and (2) the muscle is relaxed to decrease patient discomfort while you administer the injection.

Step 5 Using appropriate landmarks, identify the injection site. See Procedure 23–12.

Step 6 Cleanse the injection site with an alcohol prep pad (or other antiseptic swab) by circling from the center of the site outward. Place the alcohol wipe on the patient's skin *outside the injection site,* with a corner pointing to the site. Allow the site to dry before administering the injection.

Cleanse to remove microorganisms; follow the principle of "clean to dirty." Leaving the alcohol prep pad on the skin with a corner pointing to the injection site helps identify the location for the injection. If the alcohol has not evaporated, it may cause the skin to sting during injection.

Step 7 Don procedure gloves.

Procedure gloves are required by OSHA to prevent exposure to bloodborne pathogens. You may prefer to don gloves before Step 6; however, you can also do it while waiting for the alcohol to dry.

Step 8 Remove the needle cap.

Note: Steps 9 through 16 are the traditional method; we recommend Steps 17 through 24 (Z-track method) for all IM injections.

Step 9 With your nondominant hand, hold the patient's skin taut by spreading the skin between your thumb and index finger.

Facilitates quick insertion of needle through the skin and minimizes pain.

Step 10 Holding the syringe between thumb and fingers of your dominant hand like a pencil or dart, insert the needle at a 90° angle to the skin surface. Insert fully.

Quickly inserting the needle through the skin minimizes discomfort. A 90° angle is needed for the needle to penetrate through the subcutaneous and adipose tissue to the muscle.

Step 11 Stabilize the syringe with the fingers of your nondominant hand.

Prevents the needle from moving around in the tissue and thereby causing discomfort and possible tissue injury.

Step 12 Aspirate the needle by pulling back on the plunger and waiting for 5 to 10 seconds. If you obtain a blood return, remove the needle, discard it, and prepare the medication again.

Aspirating blood indicates that the needle is in a blood vessel. Continuing would result in administering the medication intravenously instead of intramuscularly. If the needle is in a small vessel, it may take a few seconds for the blood to appear in the syringe. Some authors have questioned whether aspiration is necessary; however, they say only that there is no research to support aspirating. Beyea and Nicoll (1995) assert that there are data to support a research-based protocol for aspirating. There seems to be no reason for *not* aspirating.

➤

PROCEDURE 23–13

Administering Intramuscular Injections
(continued)

Step 13 Using the thumb or index finger of your dominant hand, press the plunger slowly to inject the medication (5 to 10 seconds per milliliter).

Slow administration allows the medication to disperse and decreases discomfort.

Step 14 Remove the needle smoothly along the line of insertion.

Prevents pulling against the skin and tissue and thereby minimizes discomfort.

Step 15 Engage the safety needle device, and dispose of it in a biohazard container. If there is no safety device, place the uncapped syringe and needle directly into a biohazard puncture-proof container.

Prevents needlestick injuries.

Step 16 Gently massage the site with a gauze pad, and apply a Band-Aid as needed.

Massaging or rubbing will increase medication dispersal and absorption.

Procedure Variation
Z-Track Administration

Follow Steps 1 through 8 for intramuscular injections.

Step 17 With the side of your nondominant hand, displace the skin away from the injection site, about 2.5 to 3.5 cm (1 to 1.5 inches).

This stretches the skin over the muscle, so that when it is released after the injection, the medication is sealed in the muscle. ▼

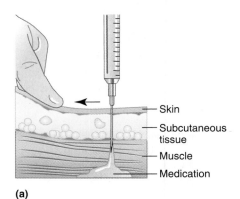

(a)

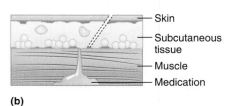

(b)

Step 18 Holding the syringe between thumb and fingers of your dominant hand like a pencil or dart, insert the needle at a 90° angle to the skin surface.

Quickly inserting the needle through the skin minimizes discomfort. A 90° angle is needed for the needle to penetrate through the subcutaneous and adipose tissue to the muscle.

Step 19 Stabilize the syringe with fingers of your nondominant hand. Do not release the skin to stabilize the syringe.

Prevents the needle from moving around in the tissue, thereby causing discomfort and possible tissue injury. You must keep the skin retracted to create a seal after the medication is injected and the skin released.

Step 20 Aspirate the needle by pulling back slightly on the plunger for 5 to 10 seconds. If you obtain a blood return, remove the needle, discard it, and prepare the medication again.

Aspirating blood indicates that the needle has penetrated a vein. Continuing could result in administering the medication intravenously instead of intramuscularly. ▼

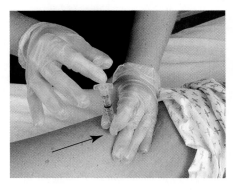

Step 21 Using the thumb or index finger of your dominant hand, press the plunger slowly to inject the medication (5 to 10 seconds per milliliter).

Slow administration allows the medication to disperse and decreases discomfort.

Step 22 Wait for 10 seconds, then remove the needle smoothly along the line of insertion; then immediately release the skin.

Prevents pulling against the skin and tissue to minimize discomfort. Leaves a zig-zag needle track that traps the medication in the muscle, preventing it from leaking up into the subcutaneous tissue.

Step 23 Engage the safety needle device, and dispose of it in a biohazard container. If there is no safety device, place the uncapped syringe and needle directly in a biohazard puncture-proof container.

Prevents needlestick injuries.

Step 24 Do not massage the site.

Massaging and rubbing can force medication into the subcutaneous tissues.

PROCEDURE 23–13   **Administering Intramuscular Injections**
(continued)

Developmental Modifications: Infants and Children

- *Sites.* Because an infant's muscles are not fully developed, site selection for injections is limited.
  1) Do not use the ventrogluteal site for children under the age of 7 months.
  2) The vastus lateralis site is the recommended site for IM injections after age 7 to 12 months.
- *Preparation.* If time permits, apply EMLA cream topically over the injection site 1 to 2.5 hours prior to injection to minimize pain. If time does not permit, choose one of the other techniques to minimize pain:
  1) Distract the child with conversation, or give him something to do, such as squeeze a hand.
  2) Spray vapocoolant on the site prior to injection.
  3) Apply a cold compress or wrapped ice cube over the site or to the contralateral site.
- *Syringe selection.* Usually no more than 1 mL in a single injection; 0.5 mL in small infant.

The small muscles are unable to tolerate a larger amount.

- *Needle size.* 22- to 25-gauge, with a needle length of $\frac{5}{8}$ to 1 inch.

The smaller the needle, the less discomfort.

- *Administration.* Restrain the child as needed to ensure that the medication is administered safely. Parents can help by holding the child during the injection.

Children are unpredictable and may not cooperate during the injection procedure.

- In infants and small children, grasp the muscle with your thumb and index finger; in obese children, spread the skin and then grasp the muscle.

This localizes and stabilizes the site for injection (Wong & Hockenberry-Eaton, 2001).

Developmental Modifications: Older Adults

Administration. Because older adults may have less muscle mass, you may need to modify your injection technique. If there is little muscle mass, use a shorter needle; spread the skin and then grasp the muscle to localize and stabilize the site for injection.

Evaluation

- Observe for minimal bruising that may develop at the site of injection.
- Observe for local reactions at site (e.g., pain, swelling, redness).

Patient Teaching

- Refer to **Medication Guidelines: Steps to Follow for All Medications (Regardless of Type or Route).**

Home Care

- Discuss safety concerns with administering medication intramuscularly in the home, such as correct disposal of biohazardous wastes and where they can obtain a puncture-proof biohazard container.

The caregiver or patient can use a large plastic bottle. The local regulations must be followed for disposal.

- Discuss with the patient the need to rotate sites.

Repeatedly giving the medication in the same site can cause abnormalities in the tissue and alter absorption rates.

➤

PROCEDURE 23–13   **Administering Intramuscular Injections**
(continued)

Documentation
- Refer to **Medication Guidelines: Steps to Follow for All Medications (Regardless of Type or Route).**
- Document related assessment findings, such as pain level or presence of nausea.
- Unless the medication is PRN, you will typically document it only on the MAR.

Sample documentation for PRN medication:

> 6/24/06   1445   *Toradol 20 mg given intramuscularly in LVG*
> *area for incision pain (rated 7 on a 1–10 scale).*
> *See MAR.* —————————— *B. Kuhl, RN*

PROCEDURE 23–14   **Adding Medications to Intravenous Fluids**

 For steps to follow in *all* procedures, refer to the inside back cover of this book. Refer also to Medication Guidelines: Steps to Follow for All Medications (Regardless of Type or Route).

critical aspects
- Check the compatibility of the intravenous solution and medication.
- Assess the patency of the intravenous site.
- Maintain the sterility of intravenous fluids and medication admixture.
- Affix the medication label to the bag, with the name and dose of medication, date and time administered, and your name or initials.

Equipment
- Prescribed intravenous solution
- Syringe for measuring medication
- Needleless access device or needle (if a device is not available)
- Antimicrobial swab
- Label with medication, dose, date, time, and your initials

PROCEDURE 23–14

Adding Medications to Intravenous Fluids

(continued)

Delegation

As an RN, you should usually not delegate adding medications to intravenous fluids to licensed practical or vocational nurses because of the high potential for harm. Nurse practice acts governing IV medication administration vary from state to state, and policies can further vary among healthcare agencies regarding which additives may be added by LPNs/LVNs. Even if you delegate the skill, as the RN you are always responsible for evaluating the patient's responses, both therapeutic effects and adverse effects.

Assessment

- Assess the patency of the intravenous site.
- Assess the appearance of the IV site.
- Check the medication insert or PDR for appropriate time or rate for infusion and for preparation.

PROCEDURE 23–14A

Adding Medication to a New IV Bag or Bottle

Procedural Steps

Step 1 Determine whether the ordered medication(s) are compatible with the intravenous solution and with each other.

Not all medications or other additives can be mixed with the glucose or saline normally found in the primary IV bag. Multiple additives increase the possibility of incompatibility.

Step 2 Calculate the amount of medication to be instilled into the intravenous solution, and the rate of administration.

Ensures that the correct amount of medication is instilled in the fluid.

Step 3 Remove any protective covers, and inspect the bag or bottle for leaks, tears, or cracks. Inspect the fluid for clarity, color, and presence of any particulate matter. Check the expiration date.

Prevents infusing contaminated or outdated solutions.

Step 4 Using the appropriate technique, draw up the ordered medication (see Procedures 23–7A and 23–7B, as needed). Alternatively, insert a vial access device into the medication vial.

Medications can come in vials, ampules, or bags.

Step 5 Cleanse the injection port on the bag with an antimicrobial swab.

Decreases transmission of microorganisms and maintains the sterility of the solution.

Step 6 Remove the cap from the syringe, insert the needle or the needleless vial access device into the injection port, and inject the medication into the bag, maintaining aseptic technique.

Maintains sterility of the intravenous solution. ▼

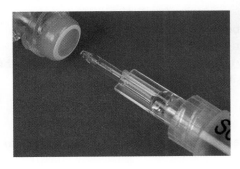

Step 7 Mix the intravenous solution and medication by gently turning the bag from end to end.

Ensures even distribution of the medication or additive into the solution.

Step 8 Place a label on the bag so that it can be read when the bag is hung; be sure the label does not cover the solution label or volume marks.

Provides information for others regarding additives to IV solutions. Allows easy visualization when bag is hanging. ▼

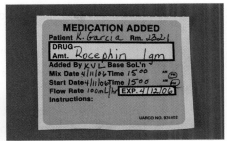

Step 9 Dispose of used equipment, syringe, or needleless access device appropriately.

Maintains standard precautions.

PROCEDURE 23–14B   Adding Medication to a Running IV

Step 1 Determine the compatibility of the medication being added to the existing solution.

Not all medications and solutions are compatible.

Step 2 Note the volume in the existing IV bag and the amount needed for dilution of medication.

Adequate solution is needed to dilute the medication.

Step 3 Clamp the running IV line.

Prevents medication from directly infusing into the client.

Step 4 Cleanse the IV additive port with the antimicrobial swab.

Decreases transmission of microorganisms and maintains the sterility of the solution.

Step 5 Remove the cap from the syringe, insert the needle or the needleless vial access device into the injection port, and inject the medication into the bag, maintaining aseptic technique.

Maintains the sterility of the intravenous solution. ▼

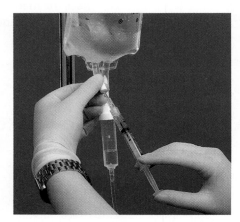

Step 6 Mix the intravenous solution and medication by gently turning the bag from end to end. Keep the bag above the level of the patient's IV insertion site.

Ensures even distribution of the medication or additive into the solution. The height of the bag keeps blood from backing up in the IV tubing.

Step 7 Place the label on the bag so that it can be read when the bag is hung; be sure the label does not cover the solution label or volume marks.

Provides information for others regarding additives to IV solutions.

Step 8 Unclamp the IV line, and run the IV at the prescribed rate.

Ensures that the medication is being administered at the correct dosage and rate.

Step 9 Dispose of used equipment, syringe, or needleless access device appropriately.

Maintains standard precautions.

Evaluation

- Check the IV line at least once every hour to ensure that the ordered or calculated rate is maintained.
- Assess the patient for complaints of pain at the infusion site.

Patient Teaching

- Discuss reasons why the medication is being given intravenously.
- Explain whether it is a continuous or intermittent infusion.
- Explain the need to report immediately any reactions to the medication, such as breathing problems, rashes, or pain at the IV insertion site.

Documentation

- Document information according to **Medication Guidelines: Steps to Follow for All Procedures (Regardless of Type or Route).**
- If you added medication to an existing IV setup, document related patient assessment findings, such as appearance of IV site and complaints of pain or discomfort during administration. Findings are usually documented on an IV flow record rather than in the nurse's notes. Chart a nursing note only if there is a problem (e.g., if the IV has infiltrated).

PROCEDURE 23–15   Administering IV Push Medications

 For steps to follow in *all* procedures, refer to the inside back cover of this book. Also refer to Medication Guidelines: Steps to Follow for All Medications (Regardless of Type or Route).

critical aspects

- Determine the type and amount of dilution needed for the medication.
- Determine the amount of time needed to administer medication.
- Ensure the patency of the line prior to administration.
- Flush the line before and after administering the medication.
- Maintain sterility.

Equipment

- Syringe appropriate for medication volume
- If you are administering through an intermittent device:
  - Two 5 to 10 mL syringes, or one 10 mL syringe with 2 to 10 mL of normal saline for flushing flush the line

Although either is acceptable, separate syringes pose less risk of contamination.

  - Depending on site and facility policy, one 5 to 10 mL syringe containing 2 to 5 mL of heparin flush (or saline) solution

Agency procedures differ: Some use saline to flush; others use heparin.

- Alcohol prep pad, or povidone-iodine (Betadine) and gauze pad
- Procedure gloves

Delegation

As an RN, you may, in some situations, be able to delegate administration of parenteral medications to a licensed practical nurse. However, this is not a widespread practice.

Assessment

- Check the compatibility of the medication with the existing intravenous (IV) solution, if it is infusing.

Medications can be physically or chemically incompatible with the IV solution. Physical incompatibility will often be obvious because precipitation may occur. Chemical incompatibility is not obvious and may result in the medication's having a weaker or a stronger effect than anticipated.

- Assess the patency of the IV line.

If the line is occluded, you will not be able to instill the medication.

- Check the site for redness, swelling, tenderness, and other signs of infiltration or phlebitis.

Some medications are very irritating and may be toxic to the tissue. If the IV line is infiltrated, the medication may leak into the tissue and cause injury. IV medications can also irritate the veins and cause phlebitis. Do not infuse a medication into a compromised site.

➤

PROCEDURE 23–15   Administering IV Push Medications *(continued)*

Procedural Steps

Step 1 Determine how fast the medication may be administered and whether the medication needs to be diluted for administration.

IV push medications are frequently injected over 1 minute. Some medications must be administered over a longer time period, and some medications require diluting prior to administration. Giving an IV push medication too fast and/or undiluted can result in speed shock or other adverse reactions.

Step 2 Prepare the medication from a vial or ampule. Dilute as needed.

Refer to Procedure 23–7A and Procedure 27–7B. Some medications must be diluted to prevent adverse reactions during administration.

PROCEDURE 23–15A   Administering IV Push Through a Running Primary IV Line

Step 1 Follow Steps 1 and 2 above.

Step 2 Don procedure gloves. Thoroughly cleanse the injection port closest to the patient with the alcohol prep pad or the povidone-iodine solution (Betadine).

Follow agency policy. Some facilities require nurses to use povidone-iodine or cleanse the port with alcohol for 1 minute when accessing venous access devices. Using the port closest to the patient minimizes the distance the medication must travel and gets it into the patient's circulation faster. You must use an injection port, which is self-sealing. If you puncture the plastic IV tubing, it will leak.

Step 3 Insert the medication syringe cannula into the injection port. If a needleless system is not available, insert the syringe needle into the port.

Using a needleless system prevents needlestick injuries.

Step 4 Pinch or clamp the IV tubing between the IV bag and the port.

Prevents the medication from being injected back toward the IV bag. ▼

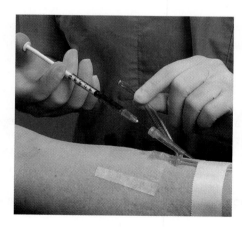

Step 5 Gently aspirate by pulling back on the plunger to check for a blood return.

A blood return is an indication that the IV catheter is in the vein. An IV site may still be patent if no blood is returned, and an infiltrated IV line may have a blood return. Use the blood return as one indication of patency (Phillips, 2001).

Step 6 If blood is returned, administer a small increment of the medication while observing for reactions to the medication.

a. If blood is not returned, further assess the patency of the IV line by administering a small amount of the saline flush and monitoring for ease of administration, swelling at the IV site, or patient complaint of discomfort at the site.

b. Another technique to determine patency is to lower the IV bag below the level of the IV site—a blood return should occur. Do not give IV push medication until you can verify the patency of the IV site.

c. If the IV catheter is a small gauge, a blood return may not always be aspirated.

(1) Prevents you from administering the drug too rapidly and allows you to observe adverse reactions to the medication before all the medication has been injected. Administering IV push medications carries the highest potential risk to the patient, because immediate, life-threatening reactions can occur. (2) Injecting an IV medication into an IV site that is not patent administers the medication into the local tissue at the IV site. Some medications will cause tissue irritation and even necrosis if infused into the subcutaneous tissue. In addition, the patient would not receive the immediate therapeutic benefit from the drug. If the patency of the IV site is questionable, restart the IV at another site.

PROCEDURE 23–15A

Administering IV Push Through a Running Primary IV Line *(continued)*

Step 7 Administer another increment of the medication (you may pinch the tubing while injecting medication and release it when not injecting; this is optional).

Step 8 Repeat Steps 6 and 7 until the medication has been administered over the correct amount of time.

Ensures slow administration and allows quick intervention in case of an adverse reaction. Medications require different administration times. Follow agency guidelines, physician orders, and pharmaceutical information regarding whether the medication needs to be diluted and the rate of administration.

PROCEDURE 23–15B

Administering IV Push Through an Intermittent Device (IV Lock) When No Extension Tubing Is Attached to the Venous Access Device

Step 1 Select the appropriate size of syringe for flush solution.

Smaller syringes exert more pressure against the wall of the IV catheter than do larger syringes. With 5 lb of force, a 3 mL syringe generates 56 PSI of pressure, whereas a 10 mL syringe delivers 19.75 PSI. Check with the IV catheter company for specific recommendations, and follow agency policy. ▼

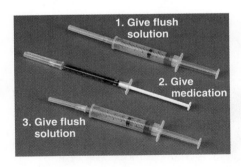

1. Give flush solution
2. Give medication
3. Give flush solution

Step 2 Don procedure gloves. Thoroughly cleanse the injection port closest to the patient with an alcohol prep pad or the povidone-iodine solution (Betadine).

Follow agency policy. Some facilities require nurses to use povidone-iodine or cleanse the port with alcohol for 1 minute when accessing venous access devices. Using the port closest to the patient minimizes the amount of medication in the IV line.

Step 3 Insert the saline flush syringe cannula into the injection port.

Allows you to check for patency before injecting the medication.

Step 4 Gently aspirate by pulling back on the plunger to check for a blood return.

A blood return is an indication that the IV catheter is in the vein. An IV site may still be patent if no blood is returned, and an infiltrated IV may have a blood return. Use the blood return as one indication of patency (Phillips, 2001).

Step 5 If blood is returned, administer a flush solution using a forward pushing motion on the syringe, with a push-stop-push technique.

If blood is not returned, further assess the patency of the IV line by administering a small amount of the IV flush and monitoring for ease of administration, swelling at the IV site, or patient complaint of discomfort at the site.

(1) Using a push-stop-push technique causes turbulence in the intravenous device, which helps remove any blood cells or fibrin buildup. (2) Injecting an IV medication into an IV site that is not patent administers the medication into the local tissue at the IV site. Some medications will cause tissue irritation and even necrosis if infused into the subcutaneous tissue. If the patency of the IV site is questionable, restart the IV at another site.

Step 6 Continuing to hold the injection port, remove the flush syringe, cleanse the port with the alcohol prep pad or povidone-iodine, and attach the medication syringe.

Cleanse the port again to prevent injection of microorganisms into the bloodstream.

Step 7 Administer the medication in small increments over the correct time interval.

➤

PROCEDURE 23–15B

Administering IV Push Through an Intermittent Device (IV Lock) When No Extension Tubing Is Attached to the Venous Access Device *(continued)*

For example, if 1 mL of the medication is to be given over 1 minute, inject approximately 0.25 mL every 15 seconds. ▼

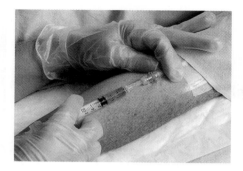

Step 8 Continuing to hold the injection port, remove medication syringe, cleanse port with alcohol prep pad or povidone-iodine, and attach the flush syringe.

Prevents contamination of the port.

Step 9 Administer the flush solution.

Ensures that all the medication has been administered and prevents occlusion of the IV catheter.

Step 10 Use positive-pressure technique when removing the syringe: Continue to

administer the flush solution while withdrawing the syringe cannula from the injection port. Follow equipment guidelines, because some injection ports maintain positive pressure by removing the syringe and then closing the clamp. Others instruct the nurse to clamp the tubing and then remove the syringe.

Prevent any blood backflow into the IV catheter, which might cause an occlusion.

PROCEDURE 23–15C

Administering IV Push Through an Intermittent Device with IV Extension Tubing

Step 1 Determine the amount of volume of any extension tubing attached to the access port.

The volume of extension sets can be greater than the IV push medication being given. If not accounted for, all the medication may be injected into the patient's bloodstream at once when the second flush solution is given.

Step 2 Don procedure gloves. Cleanse the injection port with an antiseptic wipe. Administer the saline flush. Then again cleanse the port, and inject a volume of medication equal to the volume of the extension set, at the same rate as the flush solution.

This clears the line of saline solution and fills it with medication; it also flushes the IV catheter with saline as the medication pushes the saline through the catheter. Flush solutions are administered briskly when a 5 mL syringe is used for peripheral lines and a 10 mL syringe for central lines. When you use a smaller syringe, the rate needs to be slower to prevent excess pressure damaging the IV cannula. ➤

Step 3 Using the push-stop-push method, administer the remainder of the medication in small increments over the correct time interval for the specific medication.

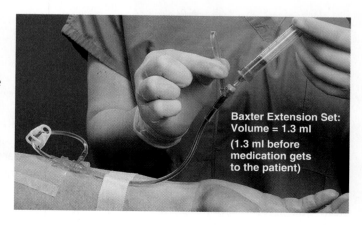

Baxter Extension Set: Volume = 1.3 ml

(1.3 ml before medication gets to the patient)

PROCEDURE 23–15C

Administering IV Push Through an Intermittent Device with IV Extension Tubing *(continued)*

When the medication begins to enter the patient's bloodstream, administering it in small increments prevents adverse reactions.

Step 4 Continuing to hold the injection port, remove the medication syringe, cleanse the injection port, and attach the flush syringe.

Step 5 Administer the flush solution at the same rate as the medication in Step 3. Then administer the remainder of the flush solution. For example, if the extension tubing has a volume of 1.3 mL, give the first 1.3 mL of the flush solution at the same rate as the medication.

(1) At this step, the extension tubing contains all the medication. Administering the flush solution all at once pushes the medication too fast (it will enter the vein all at once). (2) Once you have cleared the medication from the line and all the medication is already in the vein, then the rate no longer matters as far as the medication is concerned.

Evaluation

- Assess the patient for complaints of pain or discomfort at the site.

Patient Teaching

- Discuss the reason why the medication is being administered intravenously.
- Explain the need to report immediately any reaction to the medication.

Home Care

Discuss with the patient and/or caregiver how to care for the IV site, including flushing. Many IV push medications need to be administered by a nurse. However, cost-cutting efforts have led to short hospital stays, and some clients are now being taught to give their own IV antibiotics at home (Skokal, 2000).

- Explain how to identify problems with the IV site, such as infiltration and phlebitis.
- Determine whether the patient has adequate facilities for storing the medication, such as refrigeration if needed.
- Discuss safety issues, such as keeping medications and needles and syringes secure and away from children and pets.

Documentation

Besides charting according to **Medication Guidelines: Steps to Follow for All Medications (Regardless of Type or Route),** document related patient assessment findings, such as the appearance of the IV site and patient complaints of pain or discomfort during IV administration. You will usually document on an IV flow record and/or MAR rather than in the nurse's notes. Chart a nursing note only if there is a problem (e.g., if the patient experiences pain when you administer the medication).

PROCEDURE 23–16 | Administering Medications by Intermittent Infusion

> For steps to follow in *all* procedures, refer to the inside back cover of this book. Also refer to Medication Guidelines: Steps to Follow for All Medications (Regardless of Type or Route).
> For step-by-step instructions in using intermittent infusion devices (pumps), see Procedure 36–3.

critical aspects

- Ensure the compatibility of the IV solution and medication, both the solution in the primary IV systems and the diluent in the secondary system.
- Assess the IV site and the patency of the line.
- Calculate the amount of medication to add to the solution.
- Use the correct amount and type of diluent solution.
- Use the correct rate of administration.
- Determine the correct primary line port in which to infuse the medication.
- Affix the correct label to the secondary bag, with start date and hour, discard date and hour, and your initials.

Equipment

- Correct size syringe for measuring medication
- Needle or needleless access cannula
- Volume-control IV set (e.g., Buretrol, Volutrol, Soluset) or small bag of diluted medication with piggyback or secondary tubing
- Primary IV solution and tubing (unless one is already infusing)
- Antimicrobial swabs
- Labels for the IV tubing and medication administration system

Delegation

Nurse practice acts governing intravenous medication administration vary from state to state, and policies can further vary among healthcare agencies, regarding which medications or methods of administration the LPN/LVN may perform. You should not delegate this procedure to a UAP.

Assessment

- Check the compatibility of the medication with the intravenous (IV) solution.

Medications can be physically or chemically incompatible with the IV solution. Physical incompatibility will be obvious if precipitation occurs. Chemical incompatibility is not obvious and may result in the medication's having a weaker or a stronger effect than anticipated.

- Assess the patency of the IV line.

If the line is occluded, or if the fluid has infiltrated, the medication will not infuse.

- Check the site for redness, swelling, tenderness, and other signs of infiltration or phlebitis.

Some medications are irritating to the tissue. If the IV fluid has infiltrated, medication would leak into the tissue and cause injury. IV medications can also irritate the veins and cause phlebitis. Do not infuse a medication into a compromised site.

- Determine the amount of IV solution needed to administer the specific medication.

Most medications specify (on the order or on the label) specific dilution to prevent potential harm to the patient.

- Determine the time period over which the solution needs to be infused.

Infusing a medication too slowly may result in an inadequate blood level to achieve therapeutic levels, and infusing a medication too rapidly can cause harm.

- Perform assessments that will provide a basis for evaluating the drug's effectiveness, such as checking blood pressure after administering an antihypertensive agent.

Procedural Steps

If you have not already done so, affix a label to the secondary bag indicating the name and amount of medication, date and time given, and your name or initials.

PROCEDURE 23–16A   Using a Volume-Control Administration Set

Procedural Steps

Step 1 Prepare the volume-control set tubing.

a. Close both the upper and lower clamps on the tubing.

Prevents air bubbles from forming in the tubing.

b. Open the clamp of the air vent on the volume-control chamber.

Allows air to escape, which lets the IV solution enter the chamber.

c. Maintaining sterile procedure, attach administration spike of the volume-control set to the primary IV bag. See Procedure 36–1.

d. Fill the volume-control chamber with the desired amount of IV solution by opening the clamp between the IV bag and the volume-control chamber. When the correct amount of solution is in the chamber, close the clamp.

Provides solution for priming the tubing and diluting the IV medication.

e. Prime the rest of the tubing by opening the clamp below the chamber and running the IV fluid until all the air has been expelled.

Ensures that IV line is free of air.

f. Recheck the volume, and, if needed, add additional fluid to desired amount.

Priming the tubing alters the volume in the chamber. You must fill to the desired amount.

Step 2 Cleanse the port with an antimicrobial swab.

Maintains sterility of the system.

Step 3 Connect the end of the volume-control IV line to the patient's IV site. Attach it directly to the IV catheter, to the extension tubing, or to the injection port closest to patient.

Step 4 Cleanse the injection port on the volume-control chamber, attach the medication syringe (preferably with a blunt, needleless device), and inject the medication into the solution in the chamber.

Maintains sterility of the system.

Step 5 Gently rotate the chamber to mix the medication in the IV solution.

Ensures even distribution in the IV solution.

Step 6 Open the lower clamp, and start the infusion at the correct flow rate.

Administers the medication over the correct amount of time and prevents a toxic reaction to the medication.

Step 7 Label the volume-control chamber with the date, time, medication and doses added, and your initials, according to agency policy.

Allows continual monitoring of administration of the medication.

Step 8 When the medication has finished infusing, add a small amount of the primary fluid to the chamber, and flush the tubing. Use two times the volume in the dead space of the tubing as the flush volume; check the tubing package for the amount (Ford, Drott, & Cieplinski-Robertson, 2003).

This flushes the medication all the way through the tubing so that all medication is given to the patient; the medication or fluid does not stagnate in the tubing. ▼

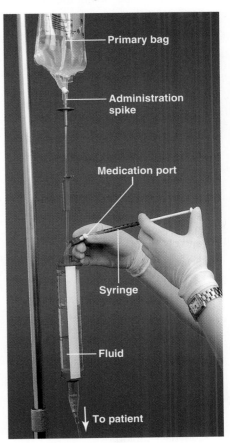

Primary bag

Administration spike

Medication port

Syringe

Fluid

To patient

PROCEDURE 23–16B   **Using a Piggyback Set**

Procedural Steps

Step 1 Draw up the medication, and inject it into the piggyback solution (see Procedure 23–14). This step is not necessary if the medication comes premixed from the pharmacy, which is frequently the case.

Ensures medication is diluted properly.

Step 2 Be sure you have the correct tubing. Attach the piggyback tubing to the medication bag. Do not touch the spike.

Tubing connects the piggyback to the primary line. Prevents contamination of tubing and solution. Piggyback tubing is short. Secondary tubing is long.

Step 3 Squeeze the drip chamber, filling it one-third to one-half full.

Prevents excess air coming into the line when you are priming the tubing.

Step 4 Open the clamp and prime the tubing, holding the end of the tubing lower than the bag of fluid. Do not let more than one drop of fluid escape from the end of the tubing. Close the clamp.

Variation "Backflushing" the Piggyback Line

a. As an alternative, you can clamp the piggyback tubing, cleanse the primary "Y" port, and attach the piggyback setup with needleless system.

b. Open the clamp on the piggyback tubing, and lower the bag below the primary to prime the piggyback line.

c. Once the line is primed, clamp the piggyback tubing.

Removes air from the tubing and maintains sterility of the system. Medications are diluted in small amounts of fluid (usually 50 to 100 mL), so you should take care not to waste any medication. The backflush method ensures that you will not lose any of the medication.

Step 5 Label the bag with the date, the medication, the dosage, and your initials. Label the tubing with the time, the date, and your initials.

Allows continual monitoring of administration of the medication. Tubing used for intermittent infusions can be used for 48 to 72 hours, depending on facility policy; labeling allows the nurse to know when it must be changed.

Step 6 Hang the piggyback container on the IV pole. Lower the primary IV container to hang below the level of the piggyback IV.

Gravity causes the higher bag (the piggyback IV setup) to flow *instead of* the primary IV setup. When the piggyback IV solution has infused, the primary IV line will resume infusing.

Step 7 Open the clamp of the piggyback line, and regulate the drip rate with the roller clamp on the primary line. Regulate to the prescribed infusion rate for the medication.

Because the piggyback is the only bag running, the primary roller clamp regulates the speed of the piggyback bag. Piggyback tubing does not have a roller clamp on it. ➤

Step 8 At the end of the infusion, clamp the piggyback tubing, and move the primary tubing back to its original height. Use the rollerclamp to reset the primary bag to its correct infusion rate.

This ensures that the primary fluids flow at their ordered rate rather than flowing at the rate the piggyback medication was flowing—which would probably be either faster or slower than the prescribed primary fluid rate.

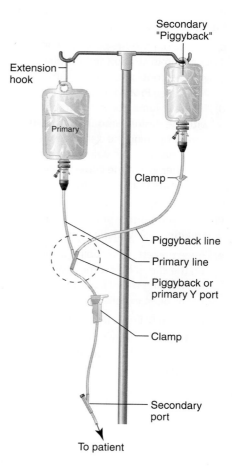

Secondary "Piggyback"

Extension hook

Primary

Clamp

Piggyback line

Primary line

Piggyback or primary Y port

Clamp

Secondary port

To patient

PROCEDURE 23–16C   **Using a Tandem (Secondary) Set**

Procedural Steps

Step 1 Draw up the medication, and inject it into the tandem (secondary) solution (see Procedure 23–14). This step is not necessary if the medication comes premixed from the pharmacy, which is frequently the case.

Ensures that the medication is diluted properly.

Step 2 Be sure you have the correct tubing (the secondary tubing is long; the piggyback tubing is short). Attach the secondary tubing to the secondary (medication) bag. Do not touch the spike.

Tubing connects the secondary to the primary line. Prevents contamination of tubing and solution.

Step 3 Squeeze the drip chamber, filling it one-third to one-half full.

Prevents excess air in line when priming tubing.

Step 4 Open the clamp and prime the tubing, holding the end of the tubing lower than the bag of fluid. Do not let more than one drop of fluid escape from the end of the tubing. Close the clamp.

Variation: "Backflushing" the Tandem Line

a. As an alternative, you can clamp the tandem tubing, cleanse the secondary port (the one nearest the patient), and attach the tandem tubing with the needleless system.

b. Open the clamp on the secondary tubing, and lower the bag below the primary line to prime the secondary line.

c. Once the line is primed, clamp the secondary tubing.

Removes air from the tubing and maintains sterility of the system. Medications are diluted in small amounts of fluid (usually 50 to 100 mL), so you should take care not to waste any medication. The backflush method ensures that you will not lose any of the medication while clearing the line of air.

Step 5 Label the bag with the date, the medication, the dosage and your initials. Label the tubing with the time, the date, and your initials.

Allows continual monitoring of administration of the medication. Tubing used for intermittent infusions can be used for 48 to 72 hours, depending on facility policy; labeling allows the nurse to know when it must be changed.

Step 6 Hang the secondary bag at the same height as primary bag.

Step 7 Cleanse the lower (secondary) port of the primary line with an antimicrobial swab, and connect the secondary tubing to this port with needleless system. (If you back-flushed in Step 4, the tubing will already be connected.)

Prevents contamination. Prevents risk of needlestick injury. ➤

Step 8 If you are using a tandem (secondary) set, both the secondary and primary sets run simultaneously. Unclamp the secondary tubing, and regulate the secondary rate at its prescribed infusion rate—the secondary line has its own roller clamp. You also need to re-verify the primary set flow rate.

Ensures that the medication is administered at a rate that will provide desired therapeutic effects and reduce possibility of adverse reactions. Infusing the secondary set may change the rate of infusion of the primary set.

Step 9 At the end of the infusion, clamp the secondary tubing. The primary bag should continue to flow at its prescribed rate.

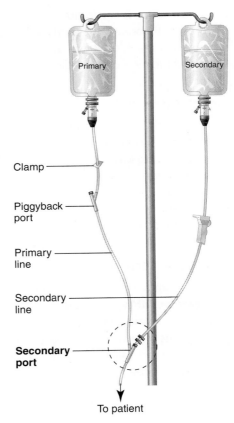

Primary   Secondary

Clamp

Piggyback port

Primary line

Secondary line

Secondary port

To patient

➤

| PROCEDURE 23–16 | **Administering Medications by Intermittent Infusion** *(continued)* |

Evaluation

- Assess for patient complaints of pain or discomfort at the site.
- Intermittent infusions are generally infused over 15 to 60 minutes; therefore, you need to assess the patient as soon as the medication begins infusing and every 15 to 20 minutes until it is absorbed.

Patient Teaching

- Discuss the reason why the medication is being administered intravenously.
- Explain the need to report immediately any reaction to the medication.

Special Situation

If the medication is *not* compatible with the primary infusion:
- Stop and disconnect the primary infusion.
- Hang a compatible flush solution in its place.
- Connect the secondary (medication) tubing to the flush solution tubing, and hang the secondary bag.

Home Care

- Discuss with the patient and/or caregiver how to care for the IV site. Only a nurse should add medications to the IV.
- Explain how to identify problems with the IV site, such as infiltration and phlebitis.
- Assess whether the patient has adequate facilities for storing the medication, such as refrigeration if needed.
- Discuss safety issues, such as keeping medications and needles and syringes secure and away from children and pets.

Documentation

- Chart information according to **Medication Guidelines: Steps to Follow for All Medications (Regardless of Type or Route).**
- Document related patient assessment findings, such as the appearance of the IV site and patient complaints of pain or discomfort during the administration.
- Usually you will merely document on the MAR and/or an IV flowsheet. Write a nurse's note only if there is any problem.

TECHNIQUES

This section suggests techniques for reconstituting, mixing, measuring, and administering various medications, including insulin and heparin.

TECHNIQUE 23–1   Applying Medications to the Skin

Cleanse the skin with soap and water and pat dry before applying to enhance absorption.

Lotions, Creams, and Ointments

- Warm the medication in your gloved hands. This will be more comfortable for the patient and make the preparation easier to apply.
- Use gloves or an applicator to apply and spread the medication evenly, following the direction of hair growth and coating the area.
- When using topical medications to treat skin and wound infections or skin disease, rub them into the skin until they are no longer visible.
- Use a sterile cotton swab, tongue blade, or gloved finger to apply corticosteroid creams and other topical medications so that you will not absorb them systemically.

Topical Aerosol Sprays

- Shake the container to mix the contents.
- Hold the container at the distance specified on the label (usually 6 to 12 inches), and spray over the prescribed area.
- You will need to hold most containers upright when spraying.
- If you are spraying near the patient's head, cover his face with a towel to prevent him from inhaling the spray.

Powders

- Be careful that the patient does not inhale the powder.
- Apply the powder to clean, dry skin.

- Spread apart skinfolds, and apply a very thin layer.
- Do not use powders merely to mask unpleasant odors. Powder is not a substitute for cleanliness.

Transdermal Medications

- Wash your hands, and don protective gloves.
- Remove the previous patch, folding the medicated side to the inside. Cleanse the skin of traces of remaining medication.
- Dispose of the old patch carefully, keeping it away from children and pets.
- Remove the patch from its protective covering, and then remove the clear, protective covering without touching the adhesive or the inside surface that contains the medication.
- Apply the patch to a clean, dry, hairless, intact skin area, pressing it down for about 10 seconds with your palm.
- Rotate application sites. Common sites are the trunk, lower abdomen, lower back, and buttocks.
- Avoid areas where lesions are present, because they decrease absorption.
- Teach the client to *not* use a heating pad over the area. This increases the rate of absorption.
- Write the date, the time, and your initials on the new patch.
- Wash your hands again.
- Observe for local side effects, such as skin irritation, itching, and allergic contact dermatitis.
- Nitroglycerine (NTG) comes in an ointment form that you must apply to NTG paper. Wear gloves. The paper is marked in increments, and the ointment is applied in a continuous motion along those marks to measure the required dose. Fold the paper in half to distribute the ointment evenly on the patch.

TECHNIQUE 23–2　Using Prefilled Unit-Dose Systems

Currently the use of prefilled systems is limited to some office practices and self-administration. They are no longer widely used in healthcare facilities, because the manipulation required to remove the cartridge from the holder creates a needlestick risk for nurses. However, because you may encounter these systems in your clinical rotations, we include the technique.

- Check each medication cartridge and dose carefully, because all of the cartridges look alike.
- No medication preparation is necessary.
- Slide the cartridge into the holder.
- Swing the plunger into place and lock at the needle end.
- Attach (screw on) the plunger, if necessary. (The system may come with plunger attached.)

- If the needle gauge or length is not correct for the patient, you can transfer the medication into a regular syringe. Maintaining sterile technique:
  1. Pull back on the plunger of the regular syringe (have a capped sterile needle ready).
  2. Insert the cartridge needle through the open tip of the regular syringe.
  3. Eject the medication into the regular syringe.
  4. Replace the capped needle onto the regular syringe.
- Expel air and excess medication.
- Don gloves
- Administer the medication
- Dispose of the empty cartridge. The Carpuject (or other) holder is available for reuse.

Note: It is not necessary to glove when drawing up medication, even though these photos show gloved hands.

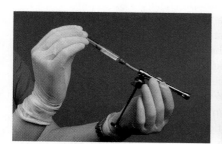

Slide the cartridge into the holder.

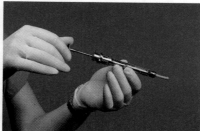

Seat the cartridge, and lock it at the needle end.

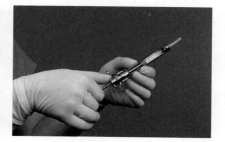

Screw in the plunger if necessary.

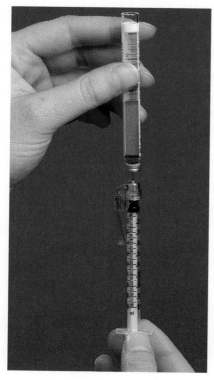

Note: The tops can be removed from some prefilled cartridges, allowing the cartridge to be used as a vial. This allows you to draw the medications into a different syringe. Do not inject air into a cartridge, because the excess pressure may eject the movable bottom.

TECHNIQUE 23–3 Reconstituting Medications

1. Remove the caps of both the medication and diluent vials.
2. If a vial was previously opened, clean the top with alcohol wipe or other antiseptic to clean the cap of dust and reduce the number of microorganisms.
3. If agency policy allows, attach a filter needle to the syringe to prevent withdrawing glass and rubber particles, which have been found in medications withdrawn from vials and ampules.
4. Draw up the diluent into the syringe:
   a. Draw air into the syringe in a volume equal to the amount of diluent you will be withdrawing.
   b. Insert the needle (or vial access cannula) carefully through the center of the rubber cap, and, keeping the bevel of the needle (or cannula) above the diluent, inject the air. The air prevents negative pressure inside the vial when you withdraw the diluent, allowing you to withdraw the diluent easily. Keeping bevel above diluent helps prevent bubbles.
   c. Withdraw the diluent in the specified amount. ▼

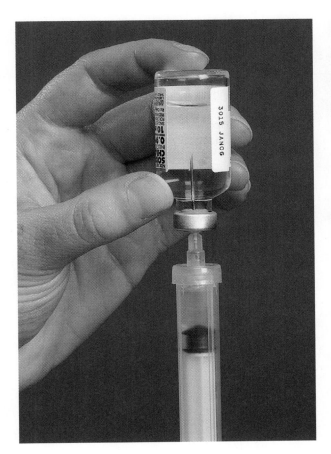

5. Insert the needle or vial access cannula carefully through the center of the rubber cap, and inject the diluent into the medication vial. ▼

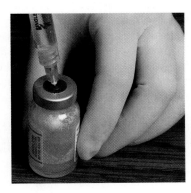

6. Mix the medication, taking care not to create bubbles. If medication does not mix easily, remove the needle or cannula from the vial, and place syringe and needle on sterile field (e.g., the wrapper the syringe came in) while you mix more. Alternatively, recap the sterile needle (see Procedure 23–10). ▼

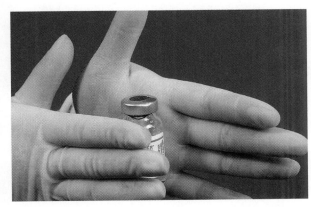

Steps 5 and 6

7. Reinsert needle or cannula (if it was removed), and withdraw the reconstituted medication into the syringe.
8. Remove the filter needle or the vial access cannula, and replace it with a sterile needle before measuring the medication. This ensures that the dose is correct and minimizes discomfort. It also prevents tracking of medication through the tissues; filter needles are usually larger than you will need for an injection.
9. Hold syringe vertically, and carefully eject all air from the syringe, but do not eject the medication.
10. If necessary, eject unneeded medication from the syringe to reach the prescribed dose.

Note: You do not need procedure gloves for this technique.

For a Non-Filter Needle

Note: These are *not* the old "air lock" techniques.

You should always use a filter needle to withdraw medications, if one is available, but you must use a needle of the correct gauge and length for the injection. You must eject air to measure the medication; however, pushing medication out of the syringe with the filter needle in place could cause the filter to break and release glass (and other) fragments. Pulling air into the syringe allows for exact dosage when the medication is injected; when ejected, the air will clear the needle so that the patient receives all the medication that is in the syringe.

1. Withdraw the correct amount of medication with the first needle. Eject air (keeping the syringe vertical) and medication (keeping the syringe horizontal) as needed to obtain correct dose.
2. Change to the needle you are going to use for injection.
3. Pull back on the plunger, and draw in 0.2 mL of air.
4. Measure the medication. Your plunger should be 0.2 mL more than the ordered dose.
5. When you inject the patient, she will receive the correct dose; the air will drive the medication from the needle into the patient's tissues. This is important when giving irritating medications such as iron.

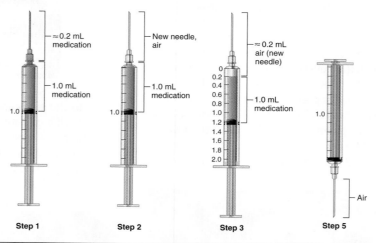

For a Filter Needle

1. Withdraw the exact amount of medication.
2. Pull back on the plunger to withdraw all the medication from the needle (or filter needle or vial access device) into the syringe. Depending on the size of the access device, this may be as much as 0.2 mL. It will now appear that you have more than the ordered dose in the syringe.
3. Change to the needle you are going to use for injection.

4. Hold the syringe vertically, and eject air until you see a drop of medication at the tip of the needle ("drop to the top").
5. Measure the medication. It should be at the correct syringe marking. If it is not, then tip the syringe horizontally, and eject the medication until the dose is correct.
6. When you inject the patient, she will receive the correct dose even though some medication will remain in the needle.
7. If you are giving an irritating medication (e.g., iron) draw 0.2 mL of air into the syringe before giving the injection.

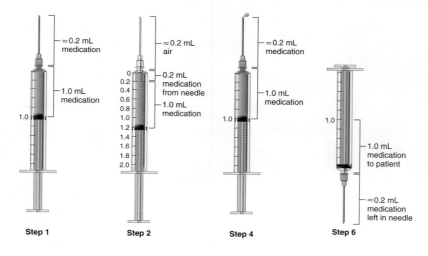

TECHNIQUE 23–5   Mixing Two Kinds of Insulin in One Syringe

Various combinations of rapid-acting, intermediate-acting, and long-acting insulin may be prescribed. Some can be mixed; some cannot. Insulins are classified as either rapid acting, short acting (regular), intermediate acting, long acting, or premixed.

- Many people use rapid- or short-acting insulin with an intermediate- or long-acting insulin.
- Always check to be certain the two insulins are compatible. As a general rule: (a) Insulin glargine cannot be mixed with other forms of insulin and (b) NPH (neutral protamine Hagedorn) insulin can be mixed with rapid- and short-acting insulins.
- Read labels carefully. The old "clear and cloudy" rule no longer differentiates types of insulin. Regular insulin is clear, but so are the long-acting insulins, glargine, and detemir.
- When mixing, draw up the regular insulin first, to avoid transferring modified insulin (e.g., NPH), into the unmodified (regular) vial.

Follow these steps when drawing up insulin from two vials into one syringe. The procedure assumes you are mixing regular (unmodified) insulin with a modified (e.g., NPH) insulin.

1. Maintain sterile technique throughout.
2. Prior to preparation, rotate the insulin vials between the palms of your hands for at least 1 minute, and invert them to ensure an adequate concentration. Do not shake the vials because this can create bubbles, which take up space and make it difficult to measure the dose precisely.
3. Clean vial stoppers with alcohol or other antiseptic (they are usually multiple-dose vials).
4. Using an insulin syringe and needle, inject an amount of air equal to the amount of insulin to be withdrawn from the vial of modified insulin vial. Do not allow the needle tip to touch the insulin.
5. Using the same syringe, inject the appropriate amount of air into the vial of regular insulin (clear vial).
6. Do not withdraw the needle; withdraw the correct dose of regular insulin.

7. Remove the syringe from the regular insulin. Eject air, and remove all air bubbles to measure the correct dose.
8. Calculate the total amount on the syringe that the combined types of insulin should measure.
9. Return to the (first) vial of modified insulin, and draw the correct dose into the syringe. For example, if you have 5 units of regular insulin in the syringe and you need 10 units of NPH, the plunger should be at the 15-unit mark when you have drawn up the NPH.
10. Recall that you have already added air to this vial in a previous step. Draw up the medication slowly, being very careful not to create bubbles and to withdraw only the amount needed. You cannot return any excess to the vial because it is now a mixture of two medications.
11. Administer the insulin mixture within 5 minutes after preparation. Even NPH insulin will bind with regular insulin and delay the onset of its action.

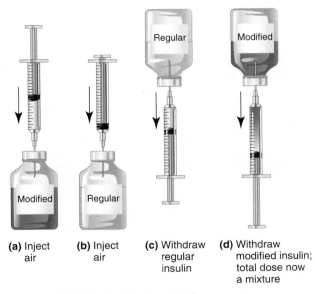

(a) Inject air   **(b)** Inject air   **(c)** Withdraw regular insulin   **(d)** Withdraw modified insulin; total dose now a mixture

Mixing two kinds of insulin in one syringe.

TECHNIQUE 23–6   Administering Heparin Subcutaneously

Because of the anticoagulant properties of heparin, you will need to adapt your technique for subcutaneous injections in the following ways:

- Give the injection subcutaneously deep on the abdomen, at least 2 inches away from the umbilicus.
- Use a $\frac{3}{8}$ in, 25- or 26-gauge needle.
- After drawing up the correct dose, add 0.2 mL of air to the syringe to ensure that all of the heparin is injected into the subcutaneous tissue and is not tracked into the superficial tissue.
- With your nondominant hand, pinch or spread the skin and insert the needle at a 90° angle, using your dominant hand. If the patient has very little subcutaneous tissue, use a slightly longer needle and insert it at a 45° angle.
- Do not aspirate before injecting, because doing so can traumatize tissue and cause bruising.
- Do not massage the site after injecting, because doing so can cause bleeding and bruising. It may also cause the heparin to be absorbed more rapidly than desired.
- Rotate injection sites on the abdomen; keep a record of the sites used. Most agencies have a chart of the body on which to record the sites used.

MEASURING AND CALCULATING DOSAGE

Medications are not always available in the exact dosage the patient needs. Therefore, you must be proficient in calculating drug dosages to be sure your patients receive the correct amount of medication.

Drugs in solid form (e.g., pills, powders) are measured by weight (e.g., milligrams, grains). Drugs used for irrigation, infusion, and injection are liquids (usually solutions), measured by volume, generally milliliters. When measuring and calculating, you can think of solutions as a quantity of "solid" drug dissolved in a quantity of "liquid" diluent. The diluent merely carries the medication. When you see a vial marked "50 mg/mL," for example, you will know this means that in each milliliter of diluent there are 50 mg (in weight) of the solid, active, medication. Your task is to determine how many milliliters of liquid you need to give the patient the number of milligrams of active drug ordered.

A solution can be either a solid dissolved in a fluid or a given volume of one liquid dissolved in a given volume of another liquid. Solution concentrations may be expressed as a proportion. A 1/100 solution is a solution of 1 gram of solid dissolved in 100 mL of fluid, or 1 mL of fluid mixed with 100 mL of another fluid.

Medication Measurement Systems

Medications are usually ordered and measured using the metric system; however, there are still a few medications that use the apothecary and household systems, so you need to learn how to work with all three systems.

Metric System

The metric system is the preferred system. The basic metric units of measurement are the **meter** (the unit for linear measurement), the **liter** (for capacity or volume), and the **gram** (for weight). A meter is a little longer than a yard, a liter a little larger than a quart, and a gram a little more than the weight of a steel paper clip. The metric system promotes accuracy by allowing for calculation of small drug dosages. A disadvantage of this system in the United States is its limited use among people outside of health care. The following are the metric units you will use in preparing medications.

Weights

1 mg (milligram)	=	1000 mcg or (micrograms)
1 gm (gram)	=	1000 mg (milligrams)
1 kg (kilogram)	=	1000 g or gm (grams)

Volume

1000 mL (milliliters)	=	1 L (Liter)
1000 (cubic centimeters)	=	1 L (Liter)

The following are examples of medication orders using the metric system:

Milk of Magnesia 30 mL orally daily at bedtime

Ancef 1 gm IV q8hr

Apothecary System

The British apothecary system of measurement has been in use in the United States since Colonial times.

Only a few medications (e.g., aspirin) are measured using this system because it is less convenient and less precise. Apothecary measurements are usually written using Roman numerals, but you may also see them in Arabic numerals. For example, *5 grains* might be written as *gr V* or *5 gr.* The system uses fractions (e.g., gr 1/4) instead of decimals (e.g., 0.25 gr). The following are the units you will use in preparing medications:

Volume
1 minim (m) = 1 drop (gtt)
1 fluid dram (dr) = 60 minims
1 fluid ounce (oz) = 8 fluid drams

Weight
1 dram (dr) = 60 grains (gr)

The following are Roman numerals you will use most often:

M	= 1000	x	= 10
D	= 500	v	= 5
C	= 100	i	= 1
L	= 50	ii	= 2

The following are examples of medication orders using the apothecary system:

Tylenol gr (grains) X orally q4hr PRN for fever >101° F

Chloromycetin otic 2 gtts in each ear 3 × daily

Household Measurements

Because most people are familiar with the household system, it is easier to teach a patient about home medications using this system. However, nurses use it only occasionally because dosages measured in this system are usually only approximate. The following are household units of measurement:

Volume
1 tablespoon (tbsp or T)	=	3 teaspoons (tsp)
6 tsp or 2 T	=	1 ounce (oz)
6 oz or 12 T	=	1 cup (c)
16 T or 8 oz	=	1 glass
2 C	=	1 pint (pt)
2 pt	=	1 quart (qt)
4 qt	=	1 gallon (gal)

Weight
16 oz	=	1 pound (lb)

Length
12 inches (in.)	=	1 foot (ft)
3 feet (ft)	=	1 yard (yd)

The following is an example of a medication order using the household system:

Amoxicillin 250 mg per 5 mL. Give 1 tsp po tid

Special Measurements: Units and mEq

Insulin, a drug used by diabetics to assist in the control of blood sugar, is measured in **units,** with 100 international units (U100) being the standard strength preparation. In this strength, 1 mL of the fluid medication contains 100 units of insulin. Heparin, an anticoagulant, and penicillin are also ordered in units. Be aware that not all units are the same. For example, 1 mL of heparin does *not* contain 100 units of heparin. You must always read the container label to know the number of units per milliliter. The following are medication orders using units:

NPH insulin 14 units SubQ q a.m.

Heparin 4000 units SubQ 2 × per day

Milliequivalents (mEq) indicate the strength of the ion concentration in a drug. A milliequivalent is the number of grams of a solid contained in one milliliter of a solution. Electrolytes, such as potassium chloride (KCl), are measured in mEq. The following are medication orders using mEq:

KCl 20 mEq orally 2 × daily

D_5W 1000 mL with KCl 40 mEq q8hr

Note that units and mEq *cannot* be directly converted to the apothecary, metric, or household systems.

Calculating Dosages

You should be able to calculate accurately using several different methods and formulas. Inaccurate calculations result in incorrect dosages and could harm the patient. One easy formula to remember is the following:

$$\frac{\text{Dose on hand}}{\text{Quantity (or volume) on hand}} = \frac{\text{Desired dose}}{\text{Quantity (or volume) desired}} \quad \text{or} \quad \frac{DH}{QH} = \frac{DD}{X}$$

Remember:
You must pay attention to *both* the milligrams (weight of the drug) marked on the medication container *and* the milliliters (amount of liquid in which the medication is dissolved). For example, suppose you have a prefilled syringe containing 50 mg of Demerol in 1 mL volume, but you wish to administer only 25 mg to the patient. How much of the liquid (how many mL) would you give?

$$\frac{DH}{QH} = \frac{DD}{X} \quad \text{or} \quad \frac{50 \text{ mg}}{1 \text{ mL}} = \frac{25 \text{ mg}}{X}$$

Therefore (recalling your algebra),

$$50X = 25 \text{ mL},$$
so X = 25 divided by 50,
so X = 0.5 mL

Here is an alternative formula you can use for calculating dosages:

$$\frac{\text{Dose desired (DD)}}{\text{Dose on hand (DH)}} \times \frac{\text{quantity}}{\text{on hand (QH)}} = \frac{\text{desired}}{\text{quantity}}$$

CriticalThinking 23–1 (Vol. 2)

Mr. Pearson ("Meet Your Patients") has been ordered nifedipine (Procardia XL) 60 mg orally daily. You have available Procardia XL (extended-release nifedipine) 30 mg tablets. Calculate the number of tablets you will need for one dose. How many tablets per day?

Conversions Within One System

When the physician's drug order is written in the same system as the preparation you have on hand, you can easily make conversions by using the equivalents identified in the preceding sections. For example, in the metric system, if you want to convert grams to milligrams, you simply multiply by 1000 (because 1 g = 1000 mg). So, if you have 2.5 grams,

$$2.5 \text{ gm} \times 1000 = 2500 \text{ mg}$$

To change milligrams to grams, *divide* by 1000—move the decimal three places to the left. For example, if you wanted to know, in grams, the equivalent of 250 mg:

You know that 1000 mg = 1 g
By dividing: 250 mg ÷ 1000 mg = 0.25 g
Or by moving the decimal point three places to the left: 250.0 mg = .250 g

Use exactly the same procedures to convert liters (L) and milliliters (mL). For example, if you wanted to know how many milliliters are the equivalent of 0.25 L:

You know that 1 L = 1000 mL
By multiplying: 0.25 L × 1000 = 250 mL
By moving the decimal point three places to the right, 0.250 L = 250 mL (Notice that you must add a zero to *have* three places to the right.)

Within the apothecary system or the household system, use the equivalents and follow a similar process of multiplying and dividing (of course, you cannot just move the decimal in these systems). For example, suppose you have a dr ii (2 dram) tablet and you need to know how many grains you have (apothecary system). You know that 2 dram = 60 gr, so multiply:

$$2 \text{ dr} \times 60 \text{ gr} = 120 \text{ gr}$$

In the household system, suppose you have 4 tbsp of a liquid and you need to know what part of a cup that represents. You know that 1 cup = 16 tablespoons, so substitute the equivalent and divide:

$$16 \text{ tbsp} = 1 \text{ cup}$$

So,

$$4 \text{ tbsp} = 16 \div 4 = 1/4 \text{ cup}$$

KnowledgeCheck 23–1 (Vol. 2)

Lanoxin 0.25 mg orally daily is ordered for a patient with congestive heart failure. The label on the package you have reads " Lanoxin 0.125 mg." How many tablets will you give? Use the "dose on hand (DOH)" formula just explained.

 Go to Chapter 23, **Knowledge Check Response Sheet and Answers,** on the Electronic Study Guide.

Conversions Between Systems

You will sometimes need to make conversions from one measurement system to another. For example, you may need to convert pounds to kilograms because many medications are ordered as milligrams per kilograms (e.g., "Give 2 mg per kg of body weight"). The table on the next page identifies the most frequently used equivalents to help you convert among the three measurement systems.

The following are the basic methods for converting between systems.

- **Metric and Apothecary—Weights**

  Grams and grains

  (Memorize: 1 g = 15 gr)

  To convert grams to grains—*multiply* the grams by 15

  To convert grains to grams—*divide* the grains by 15

  Grains and milligrams

  (Memorize: 1 gr = 60 mg)

  To convert grams to milligrams—*multiply* the grains by 60

  To convert milligrams to grains—*divide* the milligrams by 60

- **Metric and Apothecary and Household— Liquid Volume**

  Liters and ounces

  (Memorize: 1 L = 32 oz)

  To convert liters and quarts to ounces—*multiply* the liters by 32

  To convert ounces to liters and quarts—*divide* the ounces by 32

  Ounces and milliliters

  (Memorize: 1 oz = 30 mL)

  To convert ounces to milliliters—*multiply* the ounces by 30

To convert milliliters to ounces—*divide* the milliliters by 30

Milliliters and drops

(Memorize: 1 mL = 15 drops or 15 minims)

To convert milliliters to minims or drops—*multiply* milliliters by 15

To convert minims and drops to milliliters—*divide* the minims or drops by 15

KnowledgeCheck 23–2 (Vol. 2)

Work the following conversions:
* How many drops in 4 mL?
* How many mL in 2 oz?
* Convert 16 oz to liters.
* You have 3 g. How many grains is this?
* You have 10 mg. How many grains is this?

 Go to Chapter 23, **Knowledge Check Response Sheet and Answers,** on the Electronic Study Guide.

Developmental Variations: Pediatric Dosages

You must be very careful when calculating medication dosages for children and infants. Most drug references list normal pediatric ranges, which can serve as additional verification.

Orders for pediatric dosages are usually either calculated by the prescriber or stated in terms of "milligrams per kilogram of body weight." For example, you might have an order for "Erythromycin 30 mg/kg of body weight." From the equivalents table, you know that 1 kg equals 2.2 lb. If the child weighs 44 lb, then to convert to kilograms you divide 44 by 2.2; the child thus weighs 20 kg. So, 30 mg/kg would be 30 mg × 20, or 600 mg (the dosage for a 20 kg child).

You should only rarely need to calculate a child's dosage on the basis of an adult dose, because medication orders should specify the exact dosage for the individual child. However, you can use either of the following two methods to double-check the safety of pediatric orders.

BSA Formula for Children

Pediatric dosages are most accurately calculated according to the child's *body weight* or *body surface area (BSA)*. Although it is not used much any more, a chart called a nomogram uses the child's height and weight to estimate body surface area. To see a nomogram,

 Go to Chapter 23, **Tables, Boxes, Figures: ESG Figure 23–2,** on the Electronic Study Guide.

Approximate Equivalents: Metric, Apothecary, and Household

Metric	Apothecary	Household
Volume		
1 mL	15–16 minims (m)	15–16 drops (gtt)
4–5 mL	1 fl dram	1 tsp
15–16 mL	4 fl dr	1 tbsp
30 mL	1 oz or 8 dr	2 tbsp or 6 tsp
180 mL	6 oz	1 cup
240 ml	8 fluid ounces	1 glass
0.5 L (480 mL)	1 pint	1 pint
1 L (960 mL)	1 quart	1 quart
4 L (3840 mL)	1 gallon	1 gallon
Weight		
1 kilogram	2.2 lb	
30 grams	1 oz	
15 grams	4 drams	
1 g (1000 mg)	15–16 gr	
0.5 g (500 mg)	$7\frac{1}{2}$ gr	
0.3 g (300 mg)	5 gr	
0.1 g (100 mg)	$1\frac{1}{2}$ gr	
0.06 g (60–65 mg)	1 gr	
0.03 g (30–32 mg)	$\frac{1}{2}$ gr	
0.01 g (10 mg)	$\frac{1}{6}$ gr	
0.6 mg	$\frac{1}{100}$ gr	
0.3 mg	$\frac{1}{200}$ gr	

To find a child's BSA using the nomogram, you must know the child's height and weight. If the height is 30 inches and the weight is 20 lb, the BSA will be 0.42 m² (square meters). To calculate a proper dosage for a child based on a usual adult dose, use the following formula:

$$\frac{\text{BSA (child)}}{\text{BSA (adult)}} \times \text{adult dose} = \text{child dose}$$

The average BSA for adults is 1.73 m² (you need to memorize that). So for this child, if a *usual adult dose* for erythromycin is 250 to 500 mg, then

$$\frac{0.42}{1.73} \times 250 \text{ mg} = 0.243 \times 250 \text{ mg} = 60.69 \text{ mg (62 mg)}$$

To obtain the safe range for the child, enter the *maximum adult dose* (500 mg) into the same formula, obtaining 121 mg. So, the safe range for this child is 62 to 121 mg of erythromycin.

For a web-based pediatric dose calculator,

Go to **Manuel's Web** web site at http://www.manuelsweb.com/nrs_calculators.htm

Clark's Rule for Children

For children aged 2 years and younger, *Clark's rule* is sometimes used. Using this formula, you must assume that an average adult weighs 150 lb (68 kg).

$$\text{Adult dose} \times \frac{\text{child's weight in lb}}{150} = \text{child's dose}$$

According to Clark's rule, if the maximum adult dose of erythromycin is 500 mg, then the maximum dose for an infant weighing 15 lb is

$$500 \times 0.1 = 50 \text{ mg.}$$

The Electronic Study Guide contains several practice problems.

 Go to Chapter 23, **Practice Dosage Problems,** on the Electronic Study Guide.

If you cannot work the practice problems easily, you should obtain a dosage calculation book and practice the various formulas until you are proficient with conversion.

MEDICATION-RELATED ABBREVIATIONS

Because abbreviations can be easily misread, it is better to write words in full, especially when you are working with medications. However, you may still see other people using the medications in this box, so you should be familiar with them. Be sure you are familiar with the list of abbreviations approved for use in your particular agency.

Abbreviation	Explanation	Example of Administration Time
ac	before meals	0700, 1100, 1700 hours
ad lib	as desired	
AM	morning	
aq	water	
bid	twice a day	0900, 2100 hours
c̄	with	
cc*	cubic centimeters	
Cap	capsule	
Comp	compound	
DC or D/C*	discontinue, discharge	
Dil	dissolve, dilute	
dr	dram	
elix	elixir	
fl oz	fluid ounce	
gr	grain	
g, gm, or GM	gram	
gtt	drop	
h, hr	hour	
hs*	at bedtime (hour of sleep)	
ID	intradermal	
IM	intramuscular	

(continued)

Abbreviation	Explanation	Example of Administration Time
IV	intravenous	
IVPB	intravenous piggyback	
Kg or kg	kilogram	
KVO	keep vein open	
Ⓛ	left	
L or l	liter	
M	minim	
M or m	mix	
Mcg or μg*	microgram	
mEq	milliequivalent	
M\mg or mgm	milligram	
mL or ml	milliliter	
No.	number	
Non rep	do not repeat	
∅	none	
OD*	right eye	
OS*	left eye	
OU*	both eyes	
OTC	over-the-counter	
Oz	ounce	
pc	after meals	0900, 1300, 1900 hours
PM	evening	
po or PO	by mouth	
PRN	as needed	
pt	patient	
q	every	
qam	every morning	1000 hours
QD or qd*	every day	
qh, qr (q1h, q1hr)	every hour	
q2h, q2hr	every 2 hours	0800, 1000, 1200 hours, and so on
q3h, q3hr	every 3 hours	0900, 1200, 1500 hours, and so on
q4h, q4hr	every 4 hours	1000, 1400, 1800 hours, and so on
q6h, q6hr	every 6 hours	0600, 1200, 1800 hours, and so on
qid	four times a day	1000, 1400, 1800, 2200
qod*	every other day	0900 on odd dates
qs	sufficient quantity	
®	right	
rept	may be repeated	
Rx	take	
s̄	without	
sc or SC or SQ*	subcutaneous	
Sig or S	label	
SL	sublingual	
sos	if it is needed, one dose only	
S̄s or s̄s̄	one half	
Stat or STAT	at once	
sup or supp	suppository	
susp	suspension	
tab	tablet	
Tbsp	tablespoon	
tid	three times a day	1000, 1400, 1800 hours
TO	telephone order	
tr or tinct	tincture	

➤

Medication-Related Abbreviations *(continued)*

Abbreviation	Explanation	Example of Administration Time
T\tsp	teaspoon	
U*	unit	
VO or vo	verbal order	
i, ii	one, two	
x	times	
>	greater than	
<	less than	
=	equal to	
↑	increasing, increase	
↓	decreasing, decrease	

*Indicates an abbreviation that has been disallowed by the Joint Committee on Accreditation of Healthcare Organizations (JCAHO).

STANDARDIZED LANGUAGE

Standardized Diagnoses, Outcomes, and Interventions Related to Medication Administration

Nursing Diagnosis	NOC Outcomes*	NIC Interventions
Deficient Knowledge r/t lack of motivation to learn and/or decreased energy available for learning	Knowledge: Medication Knowledge: Treatment Regimen	Teaching: Individual Teaching: Prescribed Medication Teaching: Psychomotor Skill
Noncompliance with medication schedule r/t (e.g., lack of confidence in its effectiveness, forgetfulness, denial of illness, cost of medications, visual impairment)	Adherence Behavior Compliance Behavior Motivation Treatment Behavior: Illness or Injury	Culture Brokerage Discharge Planning Health System Guidance Patient Contracting Self-Modification Assistance Teaching: Prescribed Medication Telephone Consultation Values Clarification
Ineffective Management of Therapeutic Regimen r/t polypharmacy, deficient knowledge, confusion, sensory deficits, self-treatment	Adherence Behavior Compliance Behavior Knowledge: Treatment Regimen Participation in Health Care Decisions Treatment Behavior: Illness or Injury	Behavior Modification Decision-Making Support Health System Guidance Mutual Goal Setting Patient Contracting Self-Modification Assistance Self-Responsibility Facilitation Teaching: Procedure/Treatment
Risk for Poisoning r/t polypharmacy, confusion, impaired memory	Knowledge: Medication Medication Response Risk Control: Drug Use Risk Detection Self-Care: Non-Parenteral Medication Self-Care: Parenteral Medication	Environmental Management Safety Health Education Medication Management Surveillance: Safety

(continued)

Nursing Diagnosis	NOC Outcomes*	NIC Interventions
Anxiety r/t learning to self-administer insulin (or other parenteral drugs)	Anxiety Self-Control Coping Impulse Self-Control	Anxiety Reduction Teaching: Prescribed Medication
Risk for Aspiration r/t decreased level of consciousness, impaired swallowing	Aspiration Prevention Respiratory Status: Airway Patency Self-Care: Non-Parenteral Medication Swallowing Status	Airway Management Aspiration Precautions Positioning Respiratory Monitoring Surveillance Swallowing Therapy Vomiting Management
Risk for Injury r/t adverse and/or toxic effects of medications	Risk Control	Health Education Risk Identification
Constipation r/t narcotic usage	Bowel Elimination Hydration	Constipation/Impaction Management Medication Management Nutrition Management
Impaired Comfort: pruritus r/t allergic reaction to medication	Comfort Level	Pruritus Management
Bowel Incontinence (or Diarrhea) r/t side effect of antibiotic therapy	Bowel Continence Bowel Elimination	Bowel Incontinence Care Bowel Management Diarrhea Management Perineal Care

*For 5-point scales to use in describing desired outcomes or goals, see Chapter 5, **Noc Measurement Scales.**

Sources: Johnson, M., Bulechek, G., Dochterman, J., Maas, M., & Moorhead, S. (2001). *Nursing diagnoses, outcomes, & interventions: NANDA, NOC, and NIC linkages.* St Louis: Mosby; Moorhead, S., Johnson, M., & Mass, M. (Eds.). (2004). *Nursing outcomes classification (NOC)* (3rd ed.). St Louis: Mosby; Dochterman, J., & Bulechek, G. (Eds.). (2004). *Nursing interventions classification (NIC)* (4th ed.). St Louis: Mosby; and NANDA International (2004). *Nursing diagnoses: Definitions and classification 2003–2004,* Philadelphia: Author. Used with permission.

What Are the Main Points in This Chapter?

- Drugs are classified according to their use, body systems, and chemical or pharmacological traits. Learning the classifications helps you to remember the characteristics of individual drugs.

- The form (preparation) of a drug affects its speed of onset, intensity of action, and route of administration.

- In the United States, the Food and Drug Administration (FDA) regulates the manufacturing, sale, and effectiveness of all medications. Various state and federal agencies and legislation also regulate the administration of medications.

- Controlled substances must be stored, handled, disposed of, and administered according to regulations established by the U.S. Drug Enforcement Agency (DEA).

- In general, intravenous medications are absorbed most rapidly, followed by intramuscular, subcutaneous, buccal, and oral medications.

- Metabolism is the chemical inactivation of a drug into a form that the body can excrete; drug metabolism takes place mainly in the liver.

- The primary route of drug excretion is from the kidneys; other routes are the liver, gastrointestinal tract, lungs, and exocrine glands.

- The therapeutic level of a drug is the concentration in the blood serum that produces the desired effect without toxicity.

- Medication effects can be primary (therapeutic and intended) or secondary (nontherapeutic and unintended). Secondary effects include side effects, adverse reactions, toxic reactions, allergic reactions, and idiosyncratic reactions.

- The metric system is preferred for medications; however, for a few medications, the apothecary and household systems are still used.

- You are legally responsible for the medications you administer. You must question orders you believe to be incorrect.

- To help prevent medication errors, observe the "three checks" (before and after pouring or drawing up a medication, and at the bedside) and "six rights" (right drug, right dose, right time, right route, and right patient, as well as right documentation immediately after giving the medication).

- The oral route is the one most commonly used; it is convenient and safe.

- Buccal and sublingual medications are held in the mouth so that they will be absorbed through the mucous membrane.

- For patients who cannot swallow or who have feeding tubes, you can give oral medications through enteric (e.g., nasogastric and gastrostomy) tubes; the medications are given one at a time; the tube must be flushed before and after each medication.

- Topical medications may have local and systemic effects; transdermal patches are applied for their systemic effect.

- Nebulization is the production of a fine spray, fog, powder, or mist from a liquid drug.

- Parenteral medications require the use of sterile technique to prevent infection.

- Needle length and gauge are chosen based on the type of medication and the route of administration.

- Needleless systems reduce the likelihood of needle-stick injury.

- Always dispose of needles in special "sharps" containers. If you must recap a needle, use a one-handed technique.

- The ventrogluteal site is the preferred intramuscular injection site for adults. Other sites are the vastus lateralis and the deltoid. Use the dorsogluteal and rectus femoris sites only if no other sites are available.

- Experts agree that the anterolateral thigh (vastus lateralis) is preferred for infants under 7 months of age. For older infants, there is some controversy about when to begin using the ventrogluteal site. Some say it is the preferred site after 7 months of age; others continue to recommend the anterolateral thigh throughout childhood. The deltoid can be used for older children if you are certain that the muscle mass is adequate.

- Medications may be given intravenously by adding the medication to a large-volume (primary infusion), by the IV push technique, or by intermittent (piggyback and tandem setup) infusion.

- You should report medication errors immediately after they are committed, and an evaluation process for causative factors should be in place.

Teaching Clients

Overview

Teaching, both formal and informal, is an essential component of professional nursing. Along with cooperation between the learner and the teacher, effective teaching involves: motivating the learner, demonstrating tasks and skills, requiring learner participation, and providing written materials for reference.

Learning is a change in behavior, knowledge, skills, or attitudes that occurs as a result of exposure to environmental stimuli (Bastable, 2003). Bloom (1956) identified three domains of learning: cognitive, psychomotor, and affective.

Some common barriers to teaching include failure to see teaching as a priority and lack of time, preparation, space, privacy, and third-party reimbursement for teaching. Barriers to learning include illness, physical discomfort, anxiety, low literacy, environmental distraction, overwhelming amount of behavioral change needed, lack of positive reinforcement, and feelings of discouragement.

When a client requires extensive teaching, you will want to create a separate teaching plan, which is similar to a nursing care plan. Be sure to document specifically what teaching you provided as well as your evaluation of the learning that occurred.

Thinking Critically About Teaching Clients

The exercises in the following section allow you to practice the kind of thinking you will use as a full-spectrum nurse. Because these are critical-thinking activities, there is usually no single right answer. Discuss answers with your peers—discussion can stimulate critical thinking. If you have difficulty with any of the questions, consult with your instructor.

Caring for the Garcias

Joe Garcia has been diagnosed with hypertension, type II diabetes mellitus, obesity, osteoarthritis, and tobacco abuse. Based on the information you know about Joe and his family, consider the following questions.

A. What kinds of information does Joe probably need?

B. What would be the best approach to teach Joe about his healthcare conditions?

C. You have been asked to teach Joe about weight loss. What theoretical knowledge must you have, and where can you obtain it?

D. What patient information do you need to know prior to planning your teaching?

E. Joe tells you that he is overwhelmed with all of his recent diagnoses. He does not believe he can begin a weight loss program or attend any teaching sessions. How might you handle this concern?

F. Joe has been prescribed the following medicines:

Lisinopril 20 mg PO daily
Hydrochlorothiazide 25 mg PO daily
Metformin 500 mg PO BID

Devise one or more teaching sessions focused on these medications. You will need to use your pharmacology reference books to devise this plan. As you plan your teaching, recall that Joe is overwhelmed by his recent diagnoses.

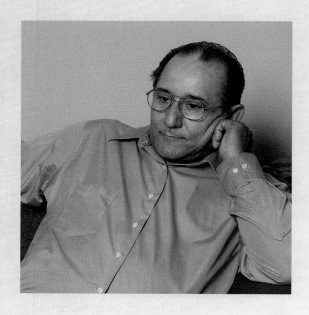

1 For the following *NOC* standardized outcomes (Moorhead, Johnson, & Maas, 2004), try to figure out which NANDA diagnoses might be linked to each outcome. Consult the NANDA handbook as necessary.

Knowledge: Breastfeeding

Knowledge: Child Physical Safety

Knowledge: Diabetes Management

Knowledge: Diet

Knowledge: Disease Process

Knowledge: Energy Conservation

Knowledge: Health Behavior

Knowledge: Illness Care

Knowledge: Infant Care

Knowledge: Infection Control

2 Recall that Heather ("Meet Your Patient" in Volume 1) is a 20-year-old mother of a 3-year-old toddler. They have come to a family practice clinic for a well-child checkup. You notice that the child speaks in one- or two-word phrases. Heather seems impatient with her and continually tells her to "stop using that baby talk." Your nursing instructor tells you that you need to assess for teaching needs and provide anticipatory guidance to the mother regarding safety, nutrition, and normal toddler growth and development.

a Heather says, "Gosh, I don't know what I'm doing wrong. All her little friends are bigger and talking more. She was even small when she was born, so I suppose it's my fault." How do you assess Heather's learning needs without reinforcing her perception that "it's my fault"?

b Your assessment shows that although the child is below the 5th percentile for height and weight, she has grown appropriately since her last clinic visit. What teaching could you provide that might help address her mother's learning needs related to childhood growth and development?

c In addition to information on growth and development, your anticipatory guidance should include safety measures and nutrition for a 3-year-old. How can you evaluate whether your teaching has been effective and further promote Heather's retention of all of this new information?

3 As a student, you have learned about discharge planning. Your instructor tells you that you need to begin teaching for discharge as soon as the client is admitted. You hear the nurses grumbling that they just don't have time for any teaching. So where do you begin? You will need to use the teaching process for your assigned client.

Your client is a 9-year-old girl who is being admitted to the outpatient procedures unit for testing because of chronic recurrent urinary tract infections. She receives daily an antibiotic, Ritalin for her diagnosed attention deficit disorder, and an asthma inhaler for sports activities. She is accompanied by her mother and father, a younger sister, and her big, pink teddy bear. She is scheduled for x-ray studies and blood work. Depending on the results of her tests, she may require surgery or dilatation of her ureters. The parents appear very anxious and tell you that their daughter is "a little slow and needs a lot of repetition." You have an hour to prepare her for the procedures and testing.

a Assessment

1) What information do you already have that will be significant for your teaching plan?

2) What other information will you need to gather?

b Diagnosis

1) What possible diagnoses are involved in this situation? Consider a diagnosis for your client and another one for at least one of her family members.

c Planning

1) What information will you present first?

2) What teaching techniques would you use for this situation?

3) Who would you include in the teaching?

4) Where would you complete the teaching?

d Goals and interventions

1) Write an appropriate goal for your client (the child). Remember to make the goal client centered, timed, and realistic. You have only an hour to complete this teaching.

2) What content and methods would you include in your teaching plan?

3) How can you incorporate the teddy bear in your teaching?

e Evaluation

1) How would you determine whether your teaching was effective?

2) What further teaching do you need to continue to prepare your client for discharge?

4 For each of the following situations, determine which teaching techniques would be most effective.

a A group of adolescents with diabetes need to plan for their prom. The prom lasts until 6:00 A.M. and will interfere with their usual schedule for insulin administration. You need to help them decide how to manage this problem. They are all busy with after-school activities and attend three different schools.

b An 80-year-old man has experienced a cerebrovascular accident (CVA) with right-sided weakness. He will need mobility training and assessment of his home situation for safety hazards. Currently he lives alone.

c A new mother must learn how to feed her infant, who has a cleft palate. She is in considerable pain after an emergency cesarean section and unexpected blood loss.

5 You are assigned to a client with a diagnosis that you are unfamiliar with. You are expected to prepare a teaching session for this client and family as well as for your classmates. How should you prepare for this assignment?

6 Give an example of teaching content you might need to present to a 58-year-old patient who has been diagnosed with hypertension. What chapters in this text (Volume 1) might be useful if you need theoretical knowledge about hypertension to answer this question? Where would you look to verify where this information is located?

thinking critically about teaching clients

thinking critically about teaching clients

7 Do you think it is appropriate for a nurse to offer personal experiences in the teaching process? Explain your thinking.

8 A client refuses to make eye contact during a teaching session. This makes it difficult for you to determine whether she is actually paying attention to what you are saying. How can you assess whether she is focused on the teaching session?

9 For each of the following concepts, use critical thinking to describe how or why it is important to nursing, patient care, or teaching clients. Note that these are *not* to be merely definitions.

Role of teaching in professional nursing

Principles of teaching and learning

Factors that affect the learning process

Factors that affect the teaching process

Timing

Choice of techniques

Relevance

Learning styles

Amount of information to be presented

Practical Knowledge
knowing how

ASSESSMENT GUIDELINES AND TOOLS

Learning Assessment Guidelines

Pre-assessment

Before assessing the learner, think about the following:

- *Time constraints.* How much information do you need to present? How much time do you have to do it?

- *Available resources.* What equipment and supplies do you have to work with? Do you have audiovisual equipment? A chalkboard? A copy machine? Books?

Assessing the Learner

You can assess the learner in several ways: through informal conversations, structured interviews, focus groups, questionnaires, tests, observations, and information obtained from the client's chart. You will pick up many cues in your initial comprehensive assessment of the client. A teaching/learning assessment should include the following:

- *Intended audience.* Who are you teaching? What is the person's age, occupation, developmental level, and cultural affiliation? Will you be teaching a person or a group?

- *Learning needs.* The client's need for information is based on actual or anticipated healthcare or developmental needs. What is the client's medical (or other) problem? What behavioral changes are needed? What self-care knowledge and skills does the client need?

- *Client's knowledge level.* Determine what the client already knows so that you can reinforce correct information, correct misinformation, and adapt the teaching plan to the client's learning needs. Ask questions such as: "What do you think caused your health problem? What are your concerns about it? How has the problem affected your usual activities? What are your concerns about treatment (tests, surgery, and so on)?"

- *Health beliefs and practices.* Teaching will not be effective unless it falls into the range of beliefs and practices that are acceptable to the client. People are unlikely to incorporate changes that do not fit into their value system. Ask the client to give a general description of her health. Ask: "What do you usually do to stay healthy? What problems do you think you are at risk for? What lifestyle changes would you be willing to make in order to improve your health?"

- *Physical readiness.* The client must have adequate concentration, manual dexterity skills, and minimal pain to be able to listen and learn.

- *Emotional readiness.* Find out if the client is experiencing anxiety or emotional distress that will interfere with the learning process. Also ask the client whether she would like a family member or friend to be present during the learning.

- *Ability to learn.* What are the learner's cognitive and psychomotor developmental level and ability? How does the client learn best (e.g., by memorization or recall, or by problem solving or applying information)? How well does the client recall previously presented material?

- *Literacy level.* Can the person read and write? Adults who have a low literacy level may exhibit a variety of behaviors. These include reacting to learning situations by withdrawal, avoidance, or repeated noncompliance. They may claim that they were too tired, were too busy, or just didn't feel like reading. They may also ask you to read to them with the excuse that their eyes are tired, they are not interested, or they have no energy. They may hold the reading material upside down or act excessively nervous in fear of getting "caught." They may not be able to follow directions, or they may fail to ask questions or ask for clarification.

- *Neurosensory factors.* What is the client's ability to feel, see, hear, and grasp? Does the client have a medical condition that causes neurosensory compromise?

- *Learning styles.* Ask the person: "How do you prefer to learn new things? For example, do you prefer to read about them, talk about them, watch a video, be shown how to do it, listen to the teacher, or use a computer? Do you like to read? Where do you get information about your health—from books, magazines, your family, your physician? Do you like learning alone or with other people?"

STANDARDIZED LANGUAGE

NOC Outcomes for Health Knowledge

Health Knowledge outcomes are those that describe a client's understanding in applying information to promote, maintain, and restore health. They are as follows:

Knowledge: Body Mechanics

Knowledge: Breastfeeding

Knowledge: Cardiac Disease Management

Knowledge: Child Physical Safety

Knowledge: Conception Prevention

Knowledge: Diabetes Management

Knowledge: Diet

Knowledge: Disease Process

Knowledge: Energy Conservation

Knowledge: Fall Prevention

Knowledge: Fertility Promotion

Knowledge: Health Promotion

Knowledge: Health Resources

Knowledge: Illness Care

Knowledge: Infant Care

Knowledge: Infection Control

Knowledge: Labor and Delivery

Knowledge: Medication

Knowledge: Ostomy Care

Knowledge: Parenting

Knowledge: Personal Safety

Knowledge: Postpartum Maternal Health

Knowledge: Preconception Maternal Health

Knowledge: Pregnancy

Knowledge: Prescribed Activity

Knowledge: Sexual Functioning

Knowledge: Substance Use Control

Knowledge: Treatment Procedure(s)

Knowledge: Treatment Regimen

Source: Moorhead, S., Johnson, M., & Maas, M. (Eds.). (2004). *Nursing outcomes classification (NOC)* (3rd ed.). St Louis: Mosby, p. 115.

NIC Interventions for Patient Education

The following are interventions to assist another to build on his own strengths, to adapt to a change in function, or to achieve a higher level of function.

Chemotherapy Management

Family Planning: Contraception

Health Education

Learning Facilitation

Learning Readiness Enhancement

Parent Education: Adolescent

Parent Education: Childrearing Family

Parent Education: Infant

Preparatory Sensory Information

Teaching: Disease Process

Teaching: Foot Care

Teaching: Group

Teaching: Individual

Teaching: Infant Nutrition

Teaching: Infant Safety

Teaching: Infant Stimulation

Teaching: Preoperative

Teaching: Prescribed Activity/Exercise

Teaching: Prescribed Diet

Teaching: Prescribed Medication

Teaching: Procedure/Treatment

Teaching: Psychomotor Skill

Teaching: Safe Sex

Teaching: Sexuality

Teaching: Toddler Nutrition

Teaching: Toddler Safety

Teaching: Toilet Training

Source: Dochterman, J., & Bulechek, G. (2004). *Nursing interventions classification (NIC)* (4th ed.). St Louis: Mosby, p. 121.

What Are the Main Points in This Chapter?

- Teaching is an essential component of professional nursing.
- Nurses do formal and informal teaching for individuals and groups.
- To be effective, teaching requires cooperation between the learner and the teacher.
- Learning is a change in behavior, knowledge, skills, or attitudes that occurs as a result of exposure to environmental stimuli.
- Bloom and Krathwohl (1956) identified three domains of learning: cognitive, psychomotor, and affective.
- Teaching includes motivating the learner.
- Readiness means that the learner is both motivated and able to learn at a specific time.
- Other factors that affect learning include emotions, timing, active involvement, feedback, repetition, environment, amount and complexity of the content, communication, developmental stage, culture, and literacy.
- Common barriers to teaching include failure to see teaching as a priority and lack of time, preparation, space, privacy, and third-party reimbursement for teaching.

- Barriers to learning include illness, physical discomfort, anxiety, low literacy, environmental distraction, overwhelming amount of behavioral change needed, lack of positive reinforcement, and feelings of discouragement.
- The teaching process is similar to the nursing process.
- The nursing diagnosis Deficient Knowledge may be the primary problem or the etiology of other problems; this diagnosis is often used incorrectly.
- A teaching plan is similar to a nursing care plan, except that (1) the interventions are actually teaching strategies and (2) the plan includes the content of the teaching, the sequencing of the content, and the materials to be used.
- Demonstration and return demonstration are the most effective strategies for teaching psychomotor skills.
- A certain amount of forgetting is normal. You can aid learner retention by using strategies that require learner participation and by providing printed materials to use at a later time.
- It is important to document specifically what teaching you did as well as your evaluation of the learning that occurred.

Knowledge Map

Teaching and Learning

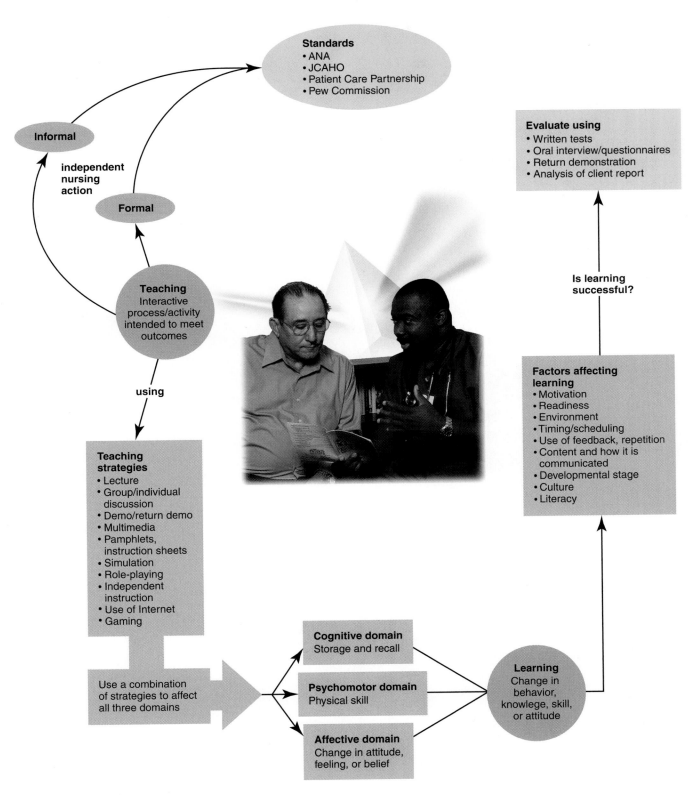

Standards
- ANA
- JCAHO
- Patient Care Partnership
- Pew Commission

Informal

independent nursing action

Formal

Teaching
Interactive process/activity intended to meet outcomes

using

Teaching strategies
- Lecture
- Group/individual discussion
- Demo/return demo
- Multimedia
- Pamphlets, instruction sheets
- Simulation
- Role-playing
- Independent instruction
- Use of Internet
- Gaming

Use a combination of strategies to affect all three domains

Cognitive domain
Storage and recall

Psychomotor domain
Physical skill

Affective domain
Change in attitude, feeling, or belief

Learning
Change in behavior, knowlege, skill, or attitude

Factors affecting learning
- Motivation
- Readiness
- Environment
- Timing/scheduling
- Use of feedback, repetition
- Content and how it is communicated
- Developmental stage
- Culture
- Literacy

Is learning successful?

Evaluate using
- Written tests
- Oral interview/questionnaires
- Return demonstration
- Analysis of client report

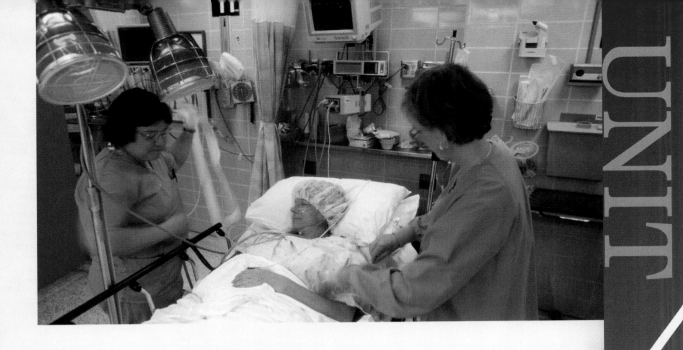

How Nurses
Support Physiological Functioning

25 STRESS & ADAPTATION

26 NUTRITION

27 URINARY ELIMINATION

28 BOWEL ELIMINATION

29 SENSORY PERCEPTION

30 PAIN MANAGEMENT

31 ACTIVITY/EXERCISE

32 SEXUAL HEALTH

33 SLEEP/REST

34 SKIN INTEGRITY & WOUND HEALING

35 OXYGENATION

36 FLUID/ELECTROLYTES & ACID/BASE BALANCE

37 PERIOPERATIVE NURSING

25 Stress

& Adaptation

CHAPTER

Overview

Stress is a disturbance in normal homeostasis caused by internal or external stimuli—physical, mental, spiritual, developmental, situational, psychosocial, or psychological—that are called stressors.

Adaptive coping techniques are healthful choices that reduce the negative effects of stress. A client's perception of the stressor, overall health status, and support system influence how well the client will adapt. Unsuccessful adaptation can lead to organic disease (e.g., stomach ulcers), somatoform disorders (e.g., hypochondriasis), and psychological disorders (e.g., mental illness). Prolonged stress can result in crisis and burnout.

Interventions tailored to the individual should include (1) health promotion; (2) anxiety, fear, and anger management;
(3) stress management; (4) techniques to alter perception, such as positive self-talk; (5) identifying and using support systems; (6) spiritual support; (7) crisis intervention; and (8) referrals.

Thinking Critically About Stress and Adaptation

The exercises in the following section allow you to practice the kind of thinking you will use as a full-spectrum nurse. Because these are critical-thinking activities, there is usually no single right answer. Discuss answers with your peers—discussion can stimulate critical thinking. If you have difficulty with any of the questions, consult with your instructor.

Caring for the Garcias

After having a comprehensive physical exam at the family health center, Flordelisa Garcia has been scheduled to have a mammogram and screening laboratory work. When she arrives at the clinic for her mammogram, she tells you she is very nervous. "I have a good friend who just found out she has breast cancer. She's very depressed now. Do I really have to do this test?"

A. What kind of stress is Flordelisa experiencing?

B. Three days later, the radiologist contacts Flordelisa requesting that she return to the family health center for additional films of the upper outer quadrant of the right breast. "There are some calcifications I want to check out," explains the radiologist.

- What factors might affect Flordelisa's adaptation to this stress?

- Evaluate what you know about Flordelisa's perception of her stress, her overall health status, her support system, and her coping methods.

- What more do you need to know about these topics to fully answer this question?

C. Later, Flordelisa calls the office frantically explaining that she is very upset about this recent event. She says, "Not knowing is killing me. I'm so nervous I can't stand it. I can't sleep. I can't eat." She asks how she can handle the stress until she comes in for the additional tests next week. What strategies would you recommend to help Flordelisa deal with the stress?

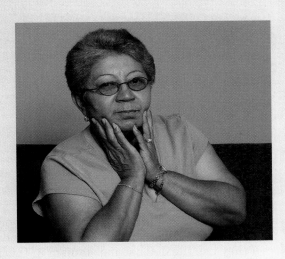

1 (From "Meet Your Patient" in Volume 1.) Gloria and her husband, John, live in a residential community from which John commutes to work in a nearby city. Gloria runs an accounting business from their home. They have two teenage boys, who are active in sports, church activities, Boy Scouts, and the school band. The boys need transportation to activities. Gloria and John teach Sunday school and are Boy Scout leaders. Gloria's mother needs knee replacement surgery and so cannot take care of Gloria's father, who has beginning Alzheimer's disease. In addition to her own home responsibilities, Gloria must go to her parents to prepare meals and to provide care for her parents during the day. Gloria's sister comes at 8:00 P.M. to sleep in the parent's home during the night.

a What resources may be available to help Gloria?

b What stress-reducing techniques can you suggest to help Gloria?

c What may reduce John's stress?

d On a scale of 1 to 10, (1 being low and 10 being high), what number will you give to Gloria's stress level?

2 Look again at Gloria and John's situation. Using the following defense mechanisms, create a possible scenario for each. That is, what might Gloria (or John) say and/or do if they use the defense mechanism in this situation? Review Table 25–2 in Volume 1 as needed.

a *Avoidance*—unconsciously staying away from events or situations that might open feelings of aggression or anxiety.

b *Conversion*—emotional conflict is changed into physical symptoms that have no physical basis.

c *Denial*—transforming reality by refusing to acknowledge thoughts, feeling, desires, or impulses. This is unconscious; the person is *not* consciously lying.

d *Displacement*—"kicking the dog." Transferring emotions, ideas, or wishes from one original object or situation to a substitute inappropriate person or object that is perceived to be less powerful or threatening.

e *Reaction formation*—similar to compensation, except the person develops the exact opposite trait. The person is aware of her feelings but acts in ways opposite to what she is really feeling.

3 Mary is a nursing student. She works part time to maintain health insurance coverage for herself and her children and to earn tuition money for school. She has to do her studying after the children are in bed, so she gets little sleep herself. Her grades are low and do not reflect Mary's true knowledge level. Nursing faculty suggest that Mary seek counseling for exam anxiety and test-taking strategies. Mary realizes she may fail out of nursing school without this counseling, but she does not know how she will fit weekly sessions into her already full schedule.

a List Mary's stressors.

b Self-Knowledge

- What life experiences do you have that may help you to understand Mary's situation?

- How could these same life experiences, on the other hand, interfere with your empathy for and understanding of Mary?

- How much of Mary's story can you identify with as being part of your own experience now?

c Which type of intervention do you think would be most helpful to Mary: (1) helping her to change her perception of her stressors, or (2) the health promotion activities discussed in Volume 1? Explain your reasoning.

d Before deciding specifically how to help Mary, what data do you still need?

e Based on the information you have, what do you think Mary's two most important goals are?

f If you discover that Mary's most important goals are to (1) provide for her children and (2) succeed in nursing school, how might you use this information to help her?

4 (Self-knowledge) In Volume 1, you listed your stressors. Let's assess further.

a What are your two (or three) *most* important goals? List them in order of importance.

b What supports do you have that can help you to achieve each of these goals?

5 (Self-knowledge and theoretical knowledge) Use the "Script for Visualization" to lead a partner through a visualization exercise; then reverse roles, and have your partner lead you through it. To see the script,

Go to Chapter 25, **Tables, Boxes, Figures: ESG Box 25–2,** on the Electronic Study Guide.

a Before beginning, what were your thoughts and feelings about the exercise?

b After doing the visualization exercise, how did you feel? Did you feel more relaxed?

c How do you think your attitudes and perceptions prior to the exercise affected how you felt *after* the exercise?

thinking critically about stress & adaptation

6 For each of the following concepts, use critical thinking to describe how or why it is important to nursing, patient care, or stress and adaptation. Note that these are *not* to be merely definitions.

Stress

Developmental stressors

Coping strategies

Ego defense mechanisms

Inflammatory response

Somatoform disorders

Relaxation techniques for stress reduction

Practical Knowledge
knowing how

TECHNIQUES

TECHNIQUE 25–1	Dealing with Angry Patients

Anger Management

- Be aware of how you are responding to angry clients. Are you relieving your own stress, or are you relieving the client's stress? If you respond angrily to relieve your own stress, you may provoke further anger in the client and even escalate the situation to the point of violence.
- Keep reminding yourself not to take anger personally; remind family members of this as well.
- Recognize the client's right to be angry. Do not discount feelings by saying something like, "Please don't be so angry," or "You shouldn't talk like that."
- Encourage the client and family to express feelings verbally and appropriately.
- Listen instead of defending. If the client yells, "Everything about this place stinks," don't respond with something like, "This hospital is highly rated by JCAHO," or, "We really are all trying to do the best we can for you." Instead, say something to encourage the person to express his feelings or give you more information: "You seem really angry; what's going on?" or "Maybe I can help. Tell me a little more about what stinks."
- Do not take responsibility for the client's anger. It is not your fault, so don't apologize (unless you really *do* have something to apologize for). In the preceding example, for instance, it is not your fault that "the place stinks" or that the patient feels that way. So do *not* say, "I'm sorry we haven't been meeting your expectations."
- Remain calm; this reassures the client.
- Help the client identify what is causing the anger and try to meet those needs.
- Be alert to your own and to the client's safety needs. If the person seems violent, do not allow him to get between you and the door. Be sure you know how to call for help from staff or security personnel if you think you or someone else is in danger.
- Refer to the NIC intervention, Anger Control Assistance (Dochterman & Bulechek, 2004, p. 166), for other suggestions.

TECHNIQUE 25–2   Crisis Intervention Guidelines

For nurses who are at an entry level of practice, the goals of crisis intervention include the following (Brammer, 1998; Neeb, 2001):

1. Assess the situation.
    What is the nature of the patient's condition and the severity of the crisis?

2. Ensure safety.
    • Call for help if you or the patient is in physical danger.
    • Do not leave the patient unless you think you are in imminent danger.
    • First ensure your own safety; then provide for the patient's safety.

3. Defuse the situation.
    • Keep in mind that a person in crisis may not be in control of his actions.
    • Try to calm the person verbally.
    • Attempt physical restraint only as a last resort and only when there is enough help to do it safely for both the staff and the patient.

4. Decrease the person's anxiety.
    • Reassure the person that he is in a safe place and that you are concerned and want to help.
    • Explain gently but firmly that you need his help and cooperation.
    • Help the person to vent feelings of fear, guilt, and anger.
    • Use physical contact very cautiously. The person in turmoil may interpret touch as aggression or a sexual approach.

5. Determine the problem.
    • Find out what the patient believes to be the cause of the crisis.
    • Remain calm, and do not pressure the patient to give reasons. Any tension on your part will create further panic in the patient.

6. Decide on the type of help needed.
    • You may be able to calm the person enough for him to understand what just happened, or you may not. Evaluate your ability to calm the patient based on your assessment of his coping skills and resources.
    • Put in place the help needed to restore the person to a minimal level of functioning. This may require long-term treatment. In that case, make the referrals.

7. Return the person to precrisis level of functioning. This may involve crisis counseling and/or home crisis visits.
    • The goal of **crisis counseling** is to provide immediate relief, solve the most urgent problems, and give long-term counseling if needed. Crisis centers often rely on telephone counseling ("hotlines").
    • If telephone counseling is not adequate, or if observations of the home environment are needed, home visits may be necessary.

ASSESSMENT GUIDELINES AND TOOLS

The Holmes-Rahe Social Readjustment Scale

This is a way to check your stress level, measured in "life change units." Of course it is not possible to score the exact "amount" of stress. However, this will give you a general idea of your stress level and should provide some insight about the sources of your stress. The following are based on the number of life change units over a 1- to 2-year period:

Over 300 points (major amount of change): 80% chance of major illness
200–299 (Moderate amount of change): 50% chance of major illness
150–199 (Mild amount of change): 33% chance of major illness
0–149 (Insignificant amount of change): Minimal chance of major illness

Of course, your personality and your ability to cope also determine the likelihood of your becoming ill.

Life Event	Life Change Units	Life Event	Life Change Units
Death of spouse	100	Trouble with in-laws	29
Divorce	73	Outstanding personal achievement	28
Marital separation	65	Spouse begins or stops work	26
Imprisonment	63	Begin or end school	26
Death of a close family member	63	Change in living conditions	25
Personal injury or illness	53	Revision of personal habits	24
Marriage	50	Trouble with boss	23
Dismissal from work	47	Change in work hours or conditions	20
Marital reconciliation	45	Change in residence	20
Retirement	45	Change in schools	20
Change in health of family member	44	Change in recreation	19
Pregnancy	40	Change in church activities	19
Sexual difficulties	39	Change in social activities	18
Gain of new family member	39	Minor mortgage or loan	17
Business readjustment	39	Change in sleeping habits	16
Change in financial state	38	Change in number of family reunions	15
Change in number of arguments with spouse	35	Change in eating habits	15
Major mortgage	32	Vacation	13
Foreclosure of mortgage or loan	30	Christmas	12
Change in responsibilities at work	29	Minor violation of the law	11
Son or daughter leaving home	29		

Source: Reprinted from Holmes, T., & Rahe, R. (1967) Social readjustment rating scale. *Journal of Psychosomatic Research, 11*(2), 213–218, with permission from Elsevier.

Assessing for Stress: Questions to Ask

1. **Assess stressors and risk factors.** Have the client complete a stress inventory, such as the preceding Holmes-Rahe Social Readjustment Scale. Then ask the client the following questions:

   - What is causing the most stress in your life?
   - On a scale of 1 to 10 (where 1 is "not much" and 10 is "extreme"), rate the stress you are experiencing in each of these areas: work or school, finances, community responsibilities, your health, health of a family member, family relationships, family responsibilities, relationships with friends.
   - How long have you been dealing with the stressful situation(s)?
   - Can you track the accumulation of stress in your life?
   - How long have you been under this stress?
   - Note the client's developmental stage, and determine whether he is functioning as expected for this stage. Review the expanded version of Chapter 9 to help you identify developmental milestones. To help you assess for stressors that can be predicted to occur in each stage, you might ask questions such as:

     What challenges do you face as a result of your life and your age?

     Have you had recent life changes?

     Do you anticipate any life changes?

 Go to **Chapter 9** on the Electronic Study Guide.

 Go to Chapter 25, **Box 25–1: Stressors Throughout the Life Span,** in Volume 1.

2. **Assess coping methods and adaptation.**

   - What coping strategies have you used previously? What was successful, and what was not successful?
   - Tell me about previous experiences you have had with stressful situations in your life.
   - What do you usually do to handle stressful situations? (If the client needs prompting, you can ask, "Do you cry, get angry, avoid people, talk to family or friends, do physical exercise, pray? Some people laugh or joke, others meditate, others try to control everything, others just work hard and look for a solution. What is your usual response?")
   - How well do these methods usually work for you?

   - What have you been doing to cope with the *present* situation?
   - How well is that working?
   - During the interview, you should also observe for the use of psychological defense mechanisms.

 Go to Chapter 25, **Table 25–1: Psychological Defense Mechanisms,** in Volume 1.

   - If the patient has not exhibited any defense mechanisms, you could ask about the common ones. For example, "Do you ever cope with a situation by denying that it exists or just by trying to put it out of your mind?"
   - Also ask the client about physiological changes and diseases caused by ongoing stress. Check the client's records for a history of somatoform disorders. Ask the client:

     What physical illnesses do you have? How long have you had them?

     What, if any, physical changes have you noticed?

     Do you have other physical conditions, for example, hypertension, cardiac disease, diabetes, arthritis, joint pains, cancer?

     For data that might indicate maladaption to stress,

 Go to Chapter 25, **Stress-Induced Organic Responses,** in Volume 1.

3. **Assess physiological responses to stress.** The following are examples of questions you should ask:

   - What do you do to stay healthy?
   - Tell me about your health habits.
   - How often do you have a checkup?
   - What are your health concerns?

4. **Assess emotional and behavioral responses to stress.**

Emotional Responses

- Anger
- Anxiety
- Depression
- Fear

(continued)

- Feelings of inadequacy
- Low self-esteem
- Irritability
- Lack of motivation
- Lethargy

Behavioral Responses

- Crying, emotional outbursts
- Dependence
- Poor job performance
- Substance use and abuse
- Sleeplessness (or sleeping too much)
- Change in eating habits (e.g., loss of appetite, overeating)
- Decrease in quality of job performance
- Preoccupation (i.e., daydreaming)
- Illnesses
- Increased absenteeism from work or school
- Increased number of accidents
- Avoiding social situations or relationships
- Rebellion, acting out

Examples of Assessment Questions

- Do you smoke?
- How much alcohol do you drink every day?
- What do you eat? What is your typical eating pattern?
- How much fluid do you drink daily?
- How many hours do you sleep at night? Do you feel rested when you wake up?
- What prescribed medications, vitamins, over-the-counter medications, or herbs do you take?
- What regular physical activity or exercise do you engage in?
- How much time do you spend at work versus at leisure and play?
- How do you relax?

- How do you express anger?
- Do you try to be perfect?
- Would you describe yourself as having the stress-filled lifestyle of a type A personality?
- How often do you find yourself feeling hopeless? Sad?

5. Assess cognitive responses to stress.
Observe for the following responses when you assess other functional areas:

- Difficulty concentrating
- Poor judgment
- Decrease in accuracy (e.g., in counting money)
- Forgetfulness
- Decreased problem-solving ability
- Decreased attention to detail
- Difficulty learning
- Narrowing of focus
- Preoccupation, daydreaming

6. Assess support systems.
Ask the following questions:

- Tell me about your home. Describe your living environment. (Make a home visit if possible, or contact the case manager or social worker to arrange a home evaluation.)
- Who are the persons that provide the most support for you? In what ways do they support you?
- What support is available from family, friends, significant others, community agencies, and clergy that you may not have required until now?
- Do you have or do you seek spiritual support?
- How has your stress affected the family?
- What are the your financial resources? What are your financial obligations?

STANDARDIZED LANGUAGE

Standardized Outcomes and Interventions for Stress-Related Nursing Diagnoses

Examples of NOC Outcomes

Anxiety Level	Family Resiliency
Caregiver Stressors	Nutritional Status
Coping	Psychosocial Adjustment: Life Change
Decision-Making	Rest
Family Coping	Sleep

NIC Interventions Listed Under "Stress" in the NIC Index

Anxiety Reduction	Counseling
Art Therapy	Dementia Management
Caregiver Support	Emotional Support
Case Management	Relocation Stress Reduction
Cognitive Restructuring	Resiliency Promotion
Coping Enhancement	Sleep Enhancement

Sources: Moorhead, S., Johnson, M., & Maas, M. (Eds.). (2004). *Nursing outcomes classification (NOC)* (3rd ed.). St Louis: Mosby; Dochterman, J. M., & Bulechek, G. M. (Eds.). (2004). *Nursing interventions classification (NIC)* (4th ed.). St Louis: Mosby.

What Are the Main Points in This Chapter?

- Stress is a disturbance in normal homeostasis caused by internal or external stimuli called stressors.

- Stressors can be physical, mental, spiritual, developmental, situational, psychosocial, or psychological in origin.

- Adaptive coping techniques are those that offer healthy choices to the person and reduce the negative effects of stress.

- Approaches to coping include altering the stressor, adapting to the stressor, and avoiding the stressor.

- Whether the outcome of stress is positive (adaptation) or negative (disease) depends on the balance between the strength and duration of the stressors and the effectiveness of the person's coping methods.

- The three stages of Selye's general adaptation syndrome (GAS) are alarm, resistance, and exhaustion. Each stage in the GAS produces different physical or psychological responses.

- In the alarm stage of the GAS, responses are primarily produced by adrenal hormones, epinephrine, mineralocorticoids, and the sympathetic nervous system.

- The exhaustion stage can lead to stress-induced illness, burnout, or death.

- The two most common responses of the local adaptation syndrome (LAS) are the reflex pain response and the inflammatory response.

- Examples of psychological responses are anxiety, fear, anger, and ego defense mechanisms.

- Ego defense mechanisms are unconscious mental mechanisms that help to decrease the inner tension associated with stressors; when overused, they are maladaptive.

- Unsuccessful adaptation can lead to crisis, organic disease (e.g., stomach ulcers), somatoform disorders (e.g., hypochondriasis), and psychological disorders (e.g., mental illness).

- Crisis exists when (1) an event in a person's life drastically changes his or her routine and is perceived as a threat to self, and (2) the person's usual coping methods are ineffective, resulting in high anxiety and reduced ability to function.

- Burnout occurs when nurses or other professionals cannot cope effectively with the demands of the workplace.

- You should assess for data about the patient's stressors, risk factors, coping and adaptation, support systems, and psychosocial and physiological responses to stress.

- Interventions for stress must be individualized to the patient. They include (1) health promotion activities for preventing and improving the ability to cope with stressors; (2) managing anxiety, fear, and anger; (3) stress management techniques that focus on discharging tension or producing relaxation; (4) techniques to alter perception (i.e., cognitive restructuring and positive self-talk); (5) identifying and using support systems; (6) providing spiritual support, (7) crisis intervention, and (8) making referrals.

Knowledge Map

Stress and Adaptation

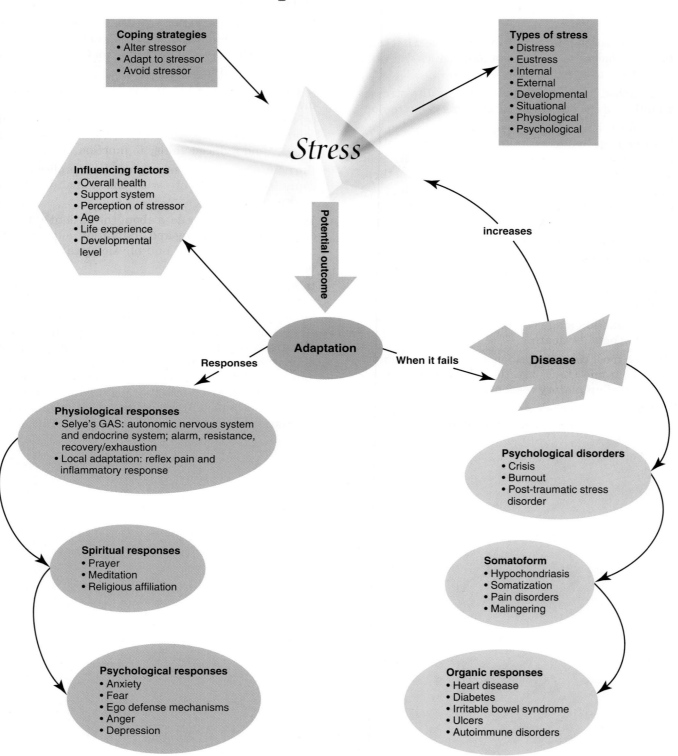

Coping strategies
- Alter stressor
- Adapt to stressor
- Avoid stressor

Types of stress
- Distress
- Eustress
- Internal
- External
- Developmental
- Situational
- Physiological
- Psychological

Stress

Influencing factors
- Overall health
- Support system
- Perception of stressor
- Age
- Life experience
- Developmental level

Potential outcome

increases

Adaptation

Responses

When it fails

Disease

Physiological responses
- Selye's GAS: autonomic nervous system and endocrine system; alarm, resistance, recovery/exhaustion
- Local adaptation: reflex pain and inflammatory response

Psychological disorders
- Crisis
- Burnout
- Post-traumatic stress disorder

Spiritual responses
- Prayer
- Meditation
- Religious affiliation

Somatoform
- Hypochondriasis
- Somatization
- Pain disorders
- Malingering

Psychological responses
- Anxiety
- Fear
- Ego defense mechanisms
- Anger
- Depression

Organic responses
- Heart disease
- Diabetes
- Irritable bowel syndrome
- Ulcers
- Autoimmune disorders

Nutrition

Overview

To function, the cells and tissues of the body depend on building blocks called nutrients. Energy nutrients are carbohydrates, proteins, and fats. Other important nutrients are water and the micronutrients: fat-soluble vitamins, water-soluble vitamins, and minerals.

The body changes and uses nutrients in a process called metabolism. During metabolism, a series of reactions causes the release of energy to maintain a balance between supply and demand.

You can determine an individual's nutritional balance by assessing nutritional history, physical findings, anthropometric measurements, and biochemical values. The body mass index (BMI), skinfold measurements, and circumferences are estimates of body composition. The most accurate method for obtaining data about a client's actual food intake is the food record.

Interventions for underweight/undernutrition include measures to improve the patient's appetite and providing enteral and parenteral nutrition. The preferred bedside technique for checking enteral tube placement is to aspirate stomach contents and measure the pH (normally 1 to 4 for stomach contents). Potential complications associated with enteral feedings include aspiration, infection, diarrhea, and electrolyte imbalance. You must follow meticulous sterile technique when administering parenteral nutrition because the solution is delivered into a large central vein; if infection occurs, sepsis is almost immediate.

Nurses can help support nutrition for patients who have Self-Care Deficits or Impaired Swallowing by assisting patients with meals and providing swallowing therapy.

Thinking Critically About Nutrition

The exercises in the following section allow you to practice the kind of thinking you will use as a full-spectrum nurse. Because these are critical-thinking activities, there is usually no single right answer. Discuss answers with your peers—discussion can stimulate critical thinking. If you have difficulty with any of the questions, consult with your instructor.

Caring for the Garcias

Joseph Garcia has been diagnosed with hypertension, type II diabetes mellitus, obesity, osteoarthritis, and tobacco abuse. Jordan Miller has advised an 1800 kcal diabetic diet with no added salt and a brisk daily 30-minute walk. Joe discusses these challenges with his daughter, Carmen.

A. Why might Jordan have selected this diet plan? Discuss the rationale for each component (i.e., 1800 kcal, diabetic diet, no added salt).

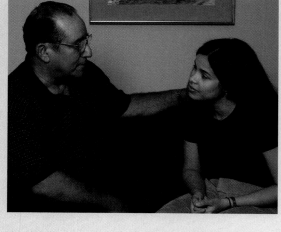

B. Mr. Garcia's diet is complex. He tells you he is overwhelmed by the many changes asked of him. How might Jordan streamline his instructions about Mr. Garcia's diet?

D. Identify teaching tools that might help Joe understand his diet.

C. Joe asks what is the best way for him to monitor his weight loss progress at home and how Jordan Miller will monitor his progress. How would you respond?

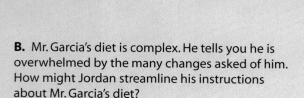

1   Recall the employees interviewed in the "Meet Your Patient" scenario. In addition, you now have two more patients. Their information is provided below.

- Isaac Schwartz, a 50-year-old accountant, works long hours. He describes a sedentary lifestyle, no tobacco use, infrequent alcohol use, no medical problems, and a nutritional history of skipping meals and daily consumption of restaurant food. You measure his height and weight as 69 inches tall and 245 lb.

- Sujing Lee, a 29-year-old project manager, regularly works 65 hours per week. Sujing is 30 weeks pregnant. She does not smoke or drink and has never been hospitalized or had surgery. She has gained a total of 25 pounds so far this pregnancy. Her diet consists mainly of traditional Chinese food. She eats three meals a day and always brings lunch from home. Lately she has felt "tired all the time." At the screening, she weighs 126 lb and measures 63 inches tall.
- Wakenda Pierre is a 38-year-old administrative assistant. She exercises at the gym 4 to 5 days per week, smokes an occasional cigarette, has two to three drinks every night before dinner, struggles with keeping her blood pressure under control, and eats fast food for breakfast and lunch every day. She is 72 inches tall and weighs 165 lb.
- Luceno Jarin is a 65-year-old business executive. He tells you he was diagnosed with type II diabetes mellitus 5 years ago. He is struggling to follow his prescribed diet. He drinks alcohol sporadically and briskly walks 30 minutes every day of the week. He is 67 inches tall and weighs 205 pounds.

a Determine each client's BMI. Based on these results, what conclusions can you make about their weight status?

b What are the likely causes of each person's weight status?

c What additional workup would be recommended for each individual?

d What indications would lead you to believe that each client has adopted a healthier lifestyle?

2   The following are three clients admitted to the medical-surgical unit of your local hospital. On their admission, the primary nurse collected the following information.

	Client 1	Client 2	Client 3
Weight	175 lb	100 lb	250 lb
Height	70 inches	59 inches	65 inches
Gender/Age	Male/40 years old	Female/18 years old	Male/65 years old
Usual Daily Caloric Intake	2500 kcal	1000 kcal	2500 kcal
Usual Activity Level	Moderate	High	Light
Serum Albumin	Normal	Low	Normal
Serum Glucose	Normal	Low	High

a   Identify which client(s) is/are at risk for nutritional imbalance.

b   Which client is at risk for developing malnutrition?

c   What additional information would support this conclusion?

d   What nursing interventions would you initiate at this time?

3 After 3 days, you examine how well each of these clients is doing using the same parameters as admission day.

	Client 1	Client 2	Client 3
Weight	170 lb	103 lb	250 lb
Current Daily Caloric Intake	2500 kcal	1500 kcal	1500 kcal
Intake (mL)	2000	2000	1000
Output (mL)	1800	1900	500
Current Activity Level	Up as tolerated	Up as tolerated	Bed rest
Serum Albumin	Normal	Low	Normal
Serum Glucose	Normal	Low	High

a In comparison with the admission data, there are some changes. Which client's health status is a priority now, and why?

b What is the most likely cause(s) of this concern?

c Which nursing interventions should be initiated for this client while hospitalized? Focus on nutritional needs.

d Identify appropriate education that should begin during hospitalization for this client.

4   For each of the following concepts, use critical thinking to describe how or why it is important to nursing, patient care, or nutrition. Note that these are *not* to be merely definitions.

Energy balance

Basal metabolic rate

Body mass index

Nutrients

Weight management

Nutritional history

Body weight standards

Enteral feedings

Total parenteral nutrition

Special diets

Practical Knowledge
knowing how

To support patient nutrition, you will need to master techniques for assessing nutritional status, feeding patients, administering supplemental feedings, and working with nasogastric and nasoenteric tubes.

PROCEDURES

PROCEDURE 26–1	Checking Fingerstick (Capillary) Blood Glucose Levels

 For steps to follow in *all* procedures, refer to the inside back cover of this book.

critical aspects
- Have the patient wash hands with warm soap and water. Some agencies may still require that you cleanse the patient's finger with an alcohol prep pad.
- Check the reagent test strips for expiration date.
- Engage the sterile lancet, hold it perpendicular to the skin, and puncture the skin.
- Wipe off the first drop of blood; then allow contact between the drop of blood and the test patch.
- Place the correct reagent strip into the blood glucose meter.
- After the indicated amount of time, read the blood glucose level indicated on the digital display. (Most meters include instructions from the manufacturer. Follow the instructions.)

Equipment
- Blood glucose meter
- Reagent strip
- Sterile lancet (and injector, if available)
- Alcohol (or other antiseptic) pad, if required
- 2 × 2 gauze pad
- Procedure gloves
- Cotton ball

Delegation
You can delegate this procedure to an LPN or UAP who has been adequately trained in performing the skill if the patient's condition allows. Assess the patient first; if the patient's condition is unstable, do not delegate the procedure.

Assessment
- Assess the patient's comprehension of the procedure.

Understanding allays anxiety and promotes cooperation.

- Assess potential puncture sites for bruising, inflammation, open lesions, poor circulation, or edema.

Avoid sites containing bruising, inflammation, open lesions, or edema because of risk for infection and inaccurate results.

- Check for factors such as anticoagulant therapy, bleeding disorders, or low platelet count.

These place the patient at risk for bleeding after skin puncture.

- Assess the patient's ability to perform fingerstick blood glucose monitoring independently if the patient typically performs testing at home.

A change in the patient's condition may not allow the patient to perform testing. Certain conditions, such as arthritis and limited vision, may limit dexterity. ➤

PROCEDURE 26–1

Checking Fingerstick (Capillary) Blood Glucose Levels *(continued)*

Procedural Steps

Step 1 Verify the medical order for frequency and timing of testing.

A physician's order is necessary for testing. Timing and frequency of testing are crucial for accurate insulin dosing.

Step 2 Have the patient wash his or her hands with soap and warm water, if able.

Reduces the risk for infection and dilates capillaries at the puncture site.

Step 3 Assist the patient into a semi-Fowler's position.

Provides accessibility to puncture site.

Step 4 Turn on the blood glucose meter. Calibrate it according to manufacturer instructions.

Readies the meter for testing.

Step 5 Check the expiration date on the container of reagent strips. If the strips are outdated, replace them.

Outdated strips may alter test results.

Step 6 Remove the reagent strip from container, then tightly seal the container. Check that the strip is the correct type for the monitor.

Protects reagent strips from exposure to the air and light. Different brands of monitors require use of different kinds of reagent strips.

Step 7 Don procedure gloves.

Protects against exposure to blood.

Step 8 Select a puncture site on the lateral aspect of a finger in the adult or child; select the heel or great toe for an infant.

The lateral aspect of the finger contains fewer nerve endings than the central fingertip.

Step 9 Promote blood flow to the site.
a. Position the finger in a dependent position, and massage toward the tip of the finger.

Promotes blood flow to the site via gravity and pressure, ensuring an adequate specimen. May prevent the need for repuncture.

b. As an alternative for infants, older adults, and people who have poor circulation, place a warm cloth on the site for about 10 minutes before obtaining the blood sample.

Capillaries in infants are very small; older adults may have poor peripheral circulation. The warmth may dilate the capillaries, helping you obtain an adequate amount of blood.

Step 10 Clean the site with an alcohol (or other antiseptic) pad, according to facility policy, and dry it thoroughly with a gauze pad.

Protects the patient from infection by removing some surface microorganisms. Dry thoroughly because alcohol can affect the meter reading. Using alcohol is controversial (it may interfere with the reagent on the strip), so follow agency policy, and consult practice guidelines frequently.

Step 11 Engage the sterile lancet, and remove the cover. Place the back of the client's hand on the table, or otherwise secure the finger so it does not move when pricked. Position the sterile lancet firmly against the skin, perpendicular to the chosen puncture site. Push the

release switch, allowing the needle to pierce the skin. If there is no injector, use a darting motion to prick the site with the lancet.

Proper positioning ensures that the lancet pierces to the correct depth. This prevents patient injury and allows for adequate blood sampling. ▼

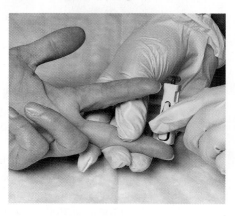

Step 12 Lightly squeeze the patient's finger above the puncture site until a droplet of blood has collected.

Ensures adequate blood sample for testing without causing injury to puncture site.

Step 13 Wipe away the first drop and squeeze again to form another droplet.

The first drop of blood contains more serous fluid and can alter test results.

Step 14 Place the reagent strip test patch close to the drop of blood. Allow contact between the drop of blood and the test patch until blood covers the entire patch. Do not "smear" the blood over the reagent strip.

PROCEDURE 26–1   **Checking Fingerstick (Capillary) Blood Glucose Levels** *(continued)*

Ensures adequate blood sample for testing. ▼

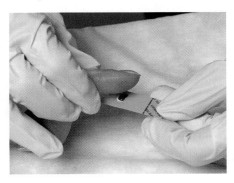

Step 15 Allow the blood sample to remain in contact with the reagent strip for the amount of time specified by the manufacturer.

The blood sample must be in contact with the reagent strip for the specified amount of time to ensure accurate test results.

Step 16 Using a gauze pad, gently apply pressure to the puncture site.

Stops bleeding at the puncture site.

Step 17 Place the reagent strip into the blood glucose meter. (Some manufacturers require you to first wipe the reagent strip with a cotton ball so that no blood remains on the test patch. Follow the manufacturer's instructions).

Step 18 After the meter signals, read the blood glucose level indicated on the digital display. ▼

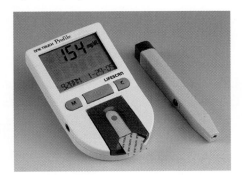

Step 19 Turn off the meter, and dispose of the reagent strip, cotton ball, gauze pad, alcohol pad, and lancet in the proper containers.

Proper disposal prevents the spread of infection via bloodborne pathogens.

Step 20 Remove the procedure gloves, and dispose of them in the proper container.

Promotes infection control.

Evaluation

- Assess the puncture site for bleeding.
- Evaluate the patient's understanding of the procedure and the test results.
- Promptly notify the physician of abnormal test results, or administer sliding scale insulin based on test results, if prescribed.

Patient Teaching

- Explain the procedure, test results, and treatment to the patient.

Involves patient in the plan of care and promotes compliance with the therapeutic regimen.

- If the patient will be performing fingerstick blood glucose testing at home, teach the patient how to perform the procedure. Have the patient perform a return demonstration.
- Discuss the importance of maintaining glycemic control.

➤

| PROCEDURE 26–1 | **Checking Fingerstick (Capillary) Blood Glucose Levels** *(continued)* |

Home Care

- Advise the patient about purchasing home glucose monitoring equipment.
- Explain how to dispose of lancets in a labeled, puncture-proof container, such as an empty bleach container.
- Instruct caregivers to wear gloves when obtaining a blood sample for glucose monitoring.
- At home, patients do not need to cleanse their finger with an alcohol wipe before puncturing it. However, they should wash their hands with soap and water.

Documentation

- Record the fingerstick blood glucose result in the progress notes or special flowsheet, including the date and time the test was performed.
- Note whether the physician was notified and record any treatment given.
- Document patient teaching.

Sample narrative note:

10/13/06	0730	*Fingerstick blood glucose level 210 mg/dL.*
		Dr. Gonzales notified. 4 U of regular insulin
		Sub Q ordered and administered in back of
		upper arm. ———————————— L. Smith, RN

PROCEDURE 26–2 Inserting Nasogastric and Nasoenteric Tubes

 For steps to follow in *all* procedures, refer to the inside back cover of this book.

critical aspects

- Place the patient in a sitting or high-Fowler's position.
- Measure the length of the nasogastric tube by measuring from the tip of the nose to the earlobe and from the earlobe to the xiphoid process. For nasoenteric tubes, add 8 to 10 cm (3 to 4 in.) to this measurement.
- Lubricate the tube with water-soluble lubricant.
- Have the patient hyperextend the neck.
- Insert the tube gently through the nostril.
- When the patient begins to gag, instruct him to tilt the head forward, drink water, and swallow.
- Withdraw the tube immediately if respiratory distress occurs during insertion.
- Confirm tube placement by testing the pH of aspirate, by auscultation, and/or by x-ray film.
- Tape the tube in place.

Equipment

- Nasogastric tube (12 Fr, 14 Fr, 16 Fr, or 18 Fr) or nasoenteric tube (8 Fr, 10 Fr, or 12 Fr)
- Stylet or guidewire (for small-bore tubes), according to agency policy (most critical care units allow nurses to use a stylet or guidewire, but it is not a widespread practice on other units)
- Procedure gloves
- Linen-saver pad or towel
- Water-soluble lubricant
- 50–60 mL catheter-tip syringe or bulb syringe
- Hypoallergenic tape (about 2.5 cm or 1 in.) or tube fixation device
- Skin adhesive
- Stethoscope
- Emesis basis
- Basin with warm water (for plastic tube) or ice (for rubber tube)
- Glass of water with a straw
- Penlight
- Tongue blade
- pH test strip
- Tissues
- Safety pin
- Gauze square or small plastic bag
- Rubber band
- Suction equipment (if tube is being connected to suction)

Delegation

This procedure usually should not be delegated because it requires knowledge of anatomy and physiology and the ability to adapt the procedure based on client responses. You can, however, delegate associated oral hygiene needs.

Assessment

- Assess the patient's need for nasogastric (NG) or nasoenteric (NE) intubation, such as surgery involving the GI tract, impaired swallowing, or decreased level of consciousness.

NG or NE intubation decreases the risk for aspiration in these patients.

- Assess each naris for patency, deviated septum, and skin breakdown.

A septal defect or facial fracture may cause obstruction, placing the patient at risk for nasal membrane trauma if insertion is attempted through the affected naris.

- Check medical history for anticoagulant therapy, coagulopathy, nasal trauma, nasal surgery, epistaxis, or deviated septum.

Patient history may place the patient at risk for injury during NG or NE insertion.

- Assess for gag reflex.

Absence of gag reflex places the patient at risk for aspiration.

➤

PROCEDURE 26–2

Inserting Nasogastric and Nasoenteric Tubes *(continued)*

Procedural Steps

Step 1 *Plastic tube:* Place in basin of warm water for 10 minutes.

Rubber tube: Place in basin of ice for 10 minutes.

Small-bore tube: Insert stylet or guide-wire and secure into position, according to agency policy. (Small-bore tubes may come with the guidewire in them. Leave the wire in place until the tube is positioned and its placement has been checked on x-ray film. Once the guide-wire is removed, do not reinsert it.)

Warm water softens a plastic tube, and ice stiffens the rubber tube to make them easier to insert. Guidewire facilitates passage of small-bore tube but can cause trauma if not secured in proper position.

Step 2 Assist the patient into a high-Fowler's position.

This position facilitates tube insertion and prevents aspiration should the patient vomit during tube insertion. Gravity facilitates passage of the tube.

Step 3 Measure the tube for placement.

a. *Nasogastric tube:* Measure the length of tube to be inserted by measuring from the tip of the nose to the earlobe, and from the earlobe to the xiphoid process. Mark the length with tape or indelible ink.

Determines the distance the tube must be inserted to reach the stomach. ▼

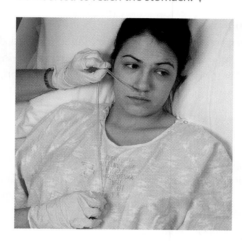

b. *Nasoenteric tube:* Add 8 to 10 cm (3 to 4 in.) to NG tube measurement, and mark the tube with tape.

Step 4 Drape a linen saver pad over the patient's chest, and hand her an emesis basin.

Protects the patient's gown from becoming soiled during tube insertion.

Step 5 Cut a 10 cm (4 in.) piece of hypo-allergenic tape.

Secures NG tube after insertion.

Step 6 Don procedure gloves if you have not already done so.

Reduces the spread of microorganisms.

Step 7 Lubricate the distal 10 cm (4 in.) of the tube with a water-soluble lubricant.

Facilitates passage of the tube and prevents injury to the nasal mucosa. Water-soluble lubricant will dissolve if it accidentally gets into the lungs, whereas oil-based lubricants do not dissolve in the respiratory tract and would cause complications if they enter the lungs.

Step 8 If the patient is awake, alert, and able to swallow, hand her a glass of water with a straw.

Instructing the client to swallow water during insertion eases passage.

PROCEDURE 26–2 Inserting Nasogastric and Nasoenteric Tubes *(continued)*

Step 9 Gently insert the tip of the tube into the nostril. Have the patient hyperextend her neck and advance the tube slowly aiming downward and toward the ear. You'll feel some resistance when the tube reaches the nasopharynx; use gentle pressure, but do not force the tube to advance. The patient's eyes may tear; if so, provide tissues.

Gentle insertion prevents trauma to the nasal mucosa. Hyperextending the neck straightens the curve where the nasal passage meets the pharynx (*nasopharyngeal junction*). Tearing is normal. Forcing against resistance can traumatize the mucosa.

Step 10 After the tube passes through the nasopharynx, have the patient flex her head toward the chest.

This maneuver closes the trachea and opens the esophagus. ▼

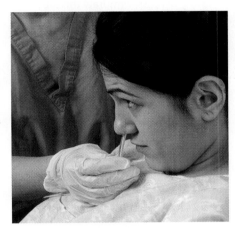

Step 11 Rotate the tube 180°.

Redirects the tube so that it will not reenter the patient's mouth.

Step 12 Direct the patient to sip and swallow the water as you slowly advance the tube. Advance the tube 5 to 10 cm (2 to 4 in.) with each swallow until the tube is advanced the desired distance.

Moving the tube with each swallow uses normal peristaltic movement to advance the tube into the stomach. Swallowing closes the epiglottis so that the tube cannot advance into the trachea.

Variation Difficulty Advancing the Tube

a. If the patient gags, stop advancing the tube. Have the patient take deep breaths and drink a few sips of water.

Helps suppress the gag reflex.

b. If gagging continues, use a tongue blade and penlight to check the tube position in the back of the throat.

The tube may be coiled in the back of the throat.

➤

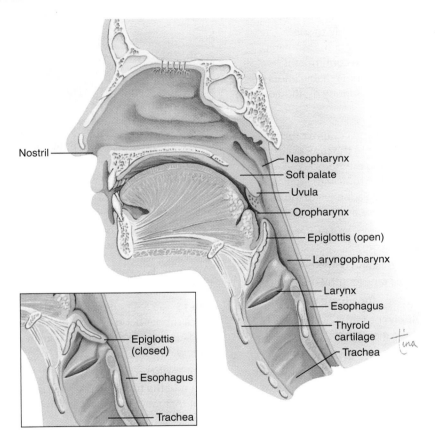

Nostril

Nasopharynx
Soft palate
Uvula
Oropharynx
Epiglottis (open)
Laryngopharynx
Larynx
Esophagus
Thyroid cartilage
Trachea

Epiglottis (closed)
Esophagus
Trachea

PROCEDURE 26–2   **Inserting Nasogastric and Nasoenteric Tubes** (*continued*)

c. If the tube is coiled in the back of the throat, the patient coughs excessively during insertion, the tube does not advance with each swallow, or the patient develops respiratory distress, withdraw the tube and allow the patient to rest before reinserting.

The tube may be in the patient's trachea.

Variation To Advance the NE Tube into the Duodenum

d. After the tube is in the stomach, position the patient on the right side.

Allows gravity to assist NE tube passage through the pyloric sphincter.

e. Advance the tube 5 to 7.5 cm (2 to 3 in.) hourly, over several hours (up to 24 hours) until radiographic study confirms placement.

Radiographic study must confirm duodenal placement.

Step 13 Once the tube is in, temporarily secure it with one piece of tape so that it does not move while you are confirming placement. Then verify tube placement (see Technique 26–5). Radiographic verification is the most reliable method. You can verify placement at the bedside by using the following methods.

If you do not secure the tube, at least temporarily, it may move out of position—especially if you are waiting for placement to be confirmed by x-ray film.

a. Aspirate stomach contents and measure aspirate pH.

Stomach contents normally measure a pH of 1 to 4; however, if the patient is receiving medications to control stomach acidity, the pH may be as high as 6. Intestinal contents usually have a pH of 6 or greater.

b. Inject air into the nasogastric tube. Use this only to confirm other methods; do not use as the primary method of verification because it is not reliable.

If the tube is in the stomach, injecting 5 to 30 mL of air with a bulb syringe or catheter-tip syringe produces a gurgling sound audible by listening with a stethoscope over the stomach.

c. If the patient is able to speak, the tube is probably in the stomach. Use this only to confirm other methods; it is not reliable enough to use as the primary method of verification.

Step 14 After you confirm proper placement, secure the tube using one of the following methods.
a. Securing the tube with tape:
   1) Apply skin adhesive to the patient's nose, and allow it to dry.

Helps tape adhere and protects skin from breakdown.

   2) Tear one end of the hypoallergenic tape lengthwise 5 cm (2 in.).

Prepares tape for adherence to tube.

   3) Apply the intact end of tape to the patient's nose.

Helps secure tube at insertion site.

   4) Wrap the 5 cm (2 in.) strips around the tube where it exits the nose.

Secures tube in the proper position.

b. Alternatively you can use 2.5 cm (1 in.) tape. Apply one end to the patient's nose (see photo) and wrap the other

end around the tube and secure on the opposite side of the nose. ▼

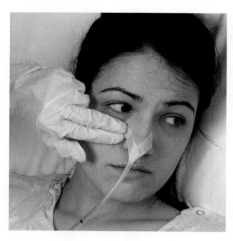

c. Securing the tube with a tube fixation device:
   1) Place the wide end of the pad over the bridge of the nose.

Helps secure the fixation device.

   2) Position the connector around the NG or NE tube where it exits the nose.

Secures the tube to the fixation device.

Step 15 Tie a slipknot around the tube with a rubber band. Secure the rubber band (or tape) to the patient's gown with a safety pin.

Reduces discomfort produced by the weight of the tube and prevents movement that may cause dislocation of the tube.

Step 16 Plug or clamp the nasogastric or nasoenteric tube, or attach it to suction tubing if suction is ordered.

Procedure Variation
Patients Who Are Confused, Combative, or Comatose

1. If the patient is comatose, place the patient into a semi-Fowler's position. Have a coworker help position the patient's head for insertion.
2. If the patient is confused and combative, ask a co-worker to assist you with insertion.

PROCEDURE 26–2   **Inserting Nasogastric and Nasoenteric Tubes** *(continued)*

Evaluation

- Assess how well the patient tolerated the procedure; did the patient have any discomfort, coughing, or gagging?
- Note the color, consistency, and pH of NG or NE aspirate.
- Ask the patient whether he or she feels comfortable.

Patient Teaching

- Discuss the need for frequent mouth care while the tube is in place.
- Explain the importance of immediately reporting tension on the tube or displacement of the tape or fixation device.

Home Care

- Assess the patient or caregiver's ability to maintain an NG or NE tube at home.
- Assess the home environment to determine the patient's risk for infection.
- Instruct the patient or caregiver about aspirating stomach contents and measuring pH.
- Teach the patient or caregiver how to verify tube placement.
- Explain to the patient or caregiver how to properly secure the NG or NE tube.
- Reinforce the need for frequent mouth care.

Documentation

Chart the date and time of insertion, size of the NG or NE tube and insertion site, tolerance of the procedure, any abnormal findings, and methods for verifying NG or NE tube placement. NG or NE tube insertion is documented in the progress notes and flow sheets in most agencies.

Sample of a narrative note:

| 9/5/06 | 1400 | 14 Fr NG tube was inserted in the L naris w/o difficulty. Patient offered no c/o discomfort. No coughing and only minimal gagging noted. Tube placement verified. Aspirated stomach contents were greenish brown with a pH of 2. Placement was also verified by injecting air into the NG tube; gurgling noted over the stomach during auscultation. — S. Brown, RN |

PROCEDURE 26–3

Administering Feedings Through Gastric and Enteric Tubes

 For steps to follow in *all* procedures, refer to the inside back cover of this book.

critical aspects

- Check the medical order for the type of formula, rate, route, and frequency of feeding.
- Verify tube placement before administering the feeding.
- Elevate the head of the bed at least 30 degrees while administering the feedings and for an hour after administration.
- Check residual volume before feeding.
  - *For continuous feeding:* Check gastric residual volume every 4 to 6 hours. If residual is 10% greater than the formula flow rate for 1 hour (or alternatively, a total of 150 ml), hold the feeding for 1 hour and recheck. Notify the physician if residual is still not within normal limits.
  - *For gastrostomy and percutaneous endoscopic gastrostomy (PEG) tubes:* (1) Check residual volume every 4 hours. (2) Residual volumes are not checked for jejunostomy tubes.
- Flush tubing with 30 mL of water every 4 hours and before and after medication administration.
- Change the tube feeding administration set every 24 hours.

Equipment

- Prescribed feeding formula at room temperature
- Tube feeding administration set
- 60 mL Luer-Lok or catheter-tip syringe (2 are needed for syringe feeding)
- Connector to connect administration set to the feeding tube
- Stethoscope
- Enteral feeding infusion pump (if being used)
- IV pole
- Linen-saver pad
- Graduated container
- pH strip
- *For gastrostomy and jejunostomy tubes:* a small, precut, gauze dressing

Delegation

You can delegate the procedure to the UAP or LPN if the patient's condition is stable and the UAP's skills allow. You must verify peristalsis, tube placement, and feeding tube patency before the feeding is started. Remind the UAP to position the patient upright and to report patient discomfort and any difficulty with the infusion.

Assessment

- Assess fluid status by checking breath sounds, mucous membranes, skin turgor, edema, and intake and output.

Identifies imbalanced fluid volume.

- Obtain baseline weight and laboratory studies.

Helps monitor effectiveness of enteral nutrition in restoring nutritional status.

- Auscultate for bowel sounds before each feeding or every 4 to 8 hours for continuous feedings. Also check for distention, nausea, vomiting, and diarrhea.

These symptoms may indicate intolerance of tube feedings.

- Assess frequency of bowel movements.

Diarrhea may indicate intolerance of the formula, excessive feeding, or gastrointestinal disease.

- Check patient history for food allergies.

Helps prevent allergic reaction to ingredients in the feeding formula.

- *For gastrostomy and jejunostomy tubes:* Also assess exit site every shift. Report drainage to the physician.

Leaking of gastric or intestinal contents may cause skin breakdown.

PROCEDURE 26–3

Administering Feedings Through Gastric and Enteric Tubes *(continued)*

Procedural Steps

Step 1 Check the medical order for the type of feeding, rate of infusion, and frequency of feeding.

A physician's order is required for enteral feedings. Rate and frequency of feeding are crucial for providing adequate nutrition.

Step 2 Check the expiration date of the tube feeding formula.

Expired formula should be discarded.

Step 3 Warm the formula to room temperature.

Because the formula goes directly into the stomach and is not warmed by the mouth and esophagus, cold formula may cause abdominal cramping and increase the risk for diarrhea.

Variation Continuous Feeding

Keep continuous-feeding formulas cool, but not cold.

Heat can coagulate some feedings (e.g., those containing egg). Cold feedings may cause vasoconstriction and cramps.

Step 4 Shake the feeding formula well.

Ensures feeding formula is well mixed.

Step 5 Prepare the equipment for administration.

Readies feeding for administration

Variation Open System with Feeding Bag

a. Fill a disposable tube feeding bag with a 4- to 6-hour supply of feeding formula and prime the tubing.

Prevents bacterial growth and prevents air from entering the GI tract.

b. Label the feeding bag with the date, time, formula type, and rate.

Identifies the formula and helps avoid administering formula past the expiration date.

c. Hang the disposable tube-feeding bag on an IV pole.

Prepares feeding formula for administration.

Variation Open System with Syringe

d. Prepare the syringe by removing the plunger.

Prepares syringe barrel to receive feeding formula.

Variation Closed System with Prefilled Bottle with Drip Chamber

e. Attach the administration set to the prefilled bottle of feeding formula, and prime the tubing.

Prevents air from entering the GI tract.

f. Hang the prefilled bottle on an IV pole. A prefilled container can safely hang for 24 to 36 hours.

Closed systems decrease the risk of contamination.

Step 6 Elevate the patient's head of the bed at least 30°.

Helps prevent aspiration and promotes digestion.

Step 7 Place a linen-saver pad under the connection end of the feeding tube.

Prevents soilage of the patient's bed linens and gown.

Step 8 For the first feeding verify tube placement using these three methods. (See Technique 26–5):

a. Aspirating stomach contents.

Gastric contents are normally greenish brown; intestinal contents are yellow-green because of the influence of bile.

b. Aspirating stomach content and measuring aspirate pH.

Stomach contents normally measure a pH of 1 to 4; however, if the patient is receiving medications to control stomach acidity, the pH may be as high as 6. Intestinal contents (jejunostomy tubes) usually have a pH of 6 or greater.

c. Injecting air into the nasogastric tube. Do not use this method for gastrostomy or jejunostomy tubes.

If the tube is in the stomach, injecting 5 to 30 mL of air with a bulb syringe or catheter-tip syringe produces a gurgling sound audible by listening with a stetho-

scope over the stomach. For gastrostomy and jejunostomy tubes, the tube has been placed through the upper abdominal wall so the tube cannot be inadvertently introduced into the airway. Injecting air into the tube unnecessarily introduces air into the GI tract.

Step 9 For subsequent feedings aspirate and measure gastric residual volume.

Helps assess gastric emptying.

a. Connect the syringe to the proximal end of the feeding tube, draw back on syringe to aspirate contents.

Allows aspiration of gastric contents.

b. Measure the volume of aspirated contents using a syringe (if volume is more than 60 mL, use graduated container).

Helps assess gastric emptying and verifies tube placement.

c. Reinstill aspirate unless the volume is more than the formula flow rate for 1 hour (or alternatively, a total of 150 mL).

Reinstilling aspirate prevents fluid and electrolyte imbalance. If the aspirate volume is more than the formula flow rate for 1 hour or 150 mL, hold the feeding for 1 hour and recheck the residual. Notify the physician if the residual is still elevated. High residual volumes indicate delayed gastric emptying.

Variation Jejunostomy Tube

Do not measure residual volume.

Residual volumes evaluate gastric emptying. The jejunum isn't normally a reservoir; therefore, no residual volume is present in the jejunum.

Step 10 Flush the feeding tube with 30 mL of tap water.

Maintains tube patency.

➤

PROCEDURE 26–3

Administering Feedings Through Gastric and Enteric Tubes *(continued)*

Step 11 Begin the feeding.

Provides prompt nutritional supplementation.

Variation Infusion Pump

a. Thread the administration tubing through the infusion pump according to the manufacturer's instructions. Pinch off the end of the feeding tube.

Prevents air from entering the feeding tube. ▼

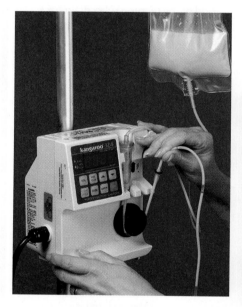

b. Attach the connector, if needed, to the proximal end of the feeding tube. Connect the distal end of the administration tubing to the connector. Alternatively, if no connector is needed, attach the distal end of the administration tubing to the proximal end of the feeding tube.

Prepares the tubing for administration.

c. Turn on the infusion pump. Set the infusion pump with the correct infusion rate and volume to be infused.

Delivers continuous tube feeding at the prescribed rate and volume.

Variation Open System Syringe

d. Pinch off the end of the feeding tube.

Prevents air from entering the feeding tube.

e. Attach the syringe to the proximal end of the feeding tube.

Prepares the syringe for feeding administration.

f. Fill the syringe with the prescribed amount of formula. Release the feeding tube, and elevate the syringe. Do not elevate the syringe more than 18 inches above the insertion site.

Gravity allows the formula to flow through the feeding tube. Rate of flow is determined by the height of the syringe. ▼

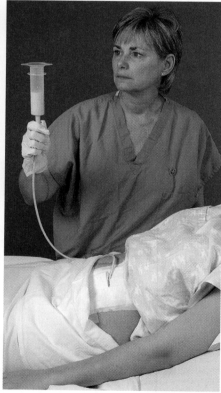

g. Allow the feeding to flow slowly.

Prevents sudden stomach distention, which can lead to diarrhea, cramping, nausea, and vomiting.

h. When the syringe is nearly empty, refill the syringe until the prescribed amount of feeding has been administered.

Variation Closed System with Prefilled Bottle with Drip Chamber

i. Pinch off the end of the feeding tube.

Prevents air from entering the feeding tube.

j. Attach the connector, if needed, to the proximal end of the feeding tube. Connect the distal end of the administration tubing to the connector. Alternatively, if no connector is needed, attach the distal end of the administration tubing to the proximal end of the feeding tube.

Prepares tubing for administration.

k. Open the roller clamp on the administration tubing and regulate the flow rate manually or with the pump.

Ensures administration at the prescribed rate. ▼

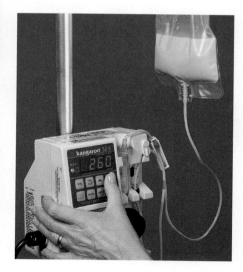

PROCEDURE 26–3

Administering Feedings Through Gastric and Enteric Tubes *(continued)*

Step 12 When the feeding is infused, pinch off the proximal end of the feeding tube.

Prevents air from entering the feeding tube.

Variation Infusion Pump

If an infusion pump was used, turn off the pump before pinching off the proximal end of the feeding tube.

Step 13 Disconnect the syringe or administration tubing from the feeding tube. Flush the feeding tube with 30 mL of tap water.

Helps maintain feeding tube patency.

a. If administering a continuous feeding, flush the tube with the prescribed amount of water (typically 50 to 100 mL) every 4 to 6 hours.

Provides the patient with free water to maintain fluid and electrolyte balance.

Step 14 Cap the proximal end of the feeding tube.

Prevents spillage of gastric contents and stops air from entering the stomach.

Step 15 Change tube feeding bag, administration set, and syringes every 24 hours.

Prevents bacterial growth.

Step 16 Keep the patient's head of bed elevated at least 30° for 1 hour after administering the tube feeding.

Reduces the risk for aspiration.

Procedure Variation

Gastrostomy or Jejunostomy Tubes

Clean the insertion site daily with soap and water. You may apply a small, precut gauze dressing to the site.

Helps prevent infection.

Procedure Variation

Cuffed Tracheostomy Tube

If the patient has a cuffed tracheostomy tube, inflate the cuff before administering the feeding, and keep the cuff inflated at for least 15 minutes afterward.

Helps prevents aspiration.

Evaluation

- Evaluate the patient's tolerance to the tube feeding; did the patient have any abdominal discomfort, nausea, vomiting, or diarrhea?
- Auscultate bowel sounds every 4 hours.
- Check gastric residual volume every 4 hours.
- Monitor intake and output every 8 hours.
- Weigh patient at least 3 times per week.
- Assess the exit site for signs of skin breakdown.
- Check laboratory values to evaluate nutritional status.

Patient Teaching

- Demonstrate the procedure to the patient and caregiver if the patient will be continuing tube feedings at home.
- Explain the importance of flushing the feeding tube with tap water every 4 hours while the patient is awake to maintain tube patency and fluid and electrolyte balance.
- Discuss the importance of remaining upright for at least 1 hour after the feeding.

PROCEDURE 26–3   Administering Feedings Through Gastric and Enteric Tubes (continued)

Home Care

- Explain to the patient and caregiver how to measure the prescribed amount of tube feeding formula and water for flushes by using household measuring equipment.
- Explain the importance of washing reusable equipment thoroughly with soap and water to prevent the spread of infection.
- Discuss how and where to purchase and store the formula.

Documentation

- Chart the type of tube feeding, rate and volume of infusion, amount of gastric residual volume (if any), and tolerance of procedure.
- Tube feeding intake is typically documented on the intake and output portion of the flowsheet in most agencies.

Sample of a narrative note (nasogastric and nasoenteric tubes):

12/10/06	0500	Jevity infusing at 70 mL/hour via feeding tube x 20 hours per day. Placement verified by aspirating stomach contents. 30 mL residual noted. HOB maintained at 45°. Abd. round, soft, nontender. (+) bowel sounds auscultated. Patient denies nausea or abdominal cramping. No diarrhea or vomiting noted. Weight this A.M. 63 kg. Instructed patient to notify staff of any nausea, vomiting, diarrhea, or abdominal discomfort. ——— R. Stephens, RN

Sample note (gastrostomy and jejunostomy tubes):

12/10/06	0500	Glucerna infusing via PEG tube at 60 mL/hour. 100 mL water flushes given every 4 hours, as ordered. Residuals minimal, pH of aspirate 5. Patient had 1 small semiformed stool. No complaints of nausea, vomiting, or abdominal cramping. See lab results. Skin warm and dry, mucous membranes moist, breath sounds clear. Patient tolerating tube feeding without difficulty. ——— R. Stephens, RN

PROCEDURE 26–4 Removing a Nasogastric or Nasoenteric Tube

 For steps to follow in *all* procedures, refer to the inside back cover of this book.

critical aspects
- Assist the patient to a sitting or high-Fowler's position.
- Clear the tube of secretions by injecting 10 mL of air through the main lumen.
- Have the patient hold his breath, and gently, but quickly, withdraw the tube.
- Discard the equipment.

Equipment
- Linen-saver pad
- 60-mL Luer-Lok or catheter-tip syringe
- Procedure gloves
- Stethoscope
- Disposable plastic bag

Delegation
This procedure should not be delegated to the LPN or UAP.

Assessment
- Auscultate the abdomen for the presence of bowel sounds.

Bowel sounds verify peristalsis, which indicates bowel function is present.

- Assess the patient's ability to consume an oral diet.

Confirms readiness for discontinuing the nasogastric (NG) or nasoenteric (NE) tube.

Procedural Steps

Step 1 Assist the patient to a sitting or high-Fowler's position.

Proper body alignment facilitates tube removal.

Step 2 Place plastic bag on bed or within reach.

Step 3 Drape a linen-saver pad across the patient's chest, and don procedure gloves.

Protects the gown and linens from soilage. Maintains universal precautions.

Step 4 Attach the syringe to the proximal end of the NG or NE tube and flush tube with 10 mL of air.

Clears the tube of gastric secretions that could cause irritation during tube removal.

Step 5 Unpin the tube from the patient's gown, and then untape the tube from the patient's nose.

Readies the tube for removal.

Step 6 Pinch the proximal end of the tube in your hand.

Step 7 Ask the patient to hold his or her breath.

Closes the epiglottis to prevent aspiration.

Step 8 Quickly and gently withdraw the tube and place it in the plastic bag or on the linen-saver pad.

Prevents tissue trauma.

Step 9 Hand the patient a tissue.

Patients often ask to blow the nose after this procedure.

Step 10 Provide mouth care.

Promotes patient comfort and prevents infection.

Step 11 Remove and dispose of gloves and used supplies in nearest receptacle according to facility policy.

Proper disposal prevents the spread of infection.

➤

PROCEDURE 26–4   Removing a Nasogastric or Nasoenteric Tube *(continued)*

Evaluation

- Assess the insertion site for signs of skin breakdown.
- Assess the patient for signs of GI dysfunction, such as food intolerance, nausea, vomiting, and abdominal distention.
- Monitor intake and output every 8 hours.
- Weigh patient regularly.
- Check laboratory values to evaluate nutritional status.

Patient Teaching

- Instruct the patient or caregiver how to remove the nasogastric or nasoenteric tube.
- Explain the importance of reporting nausea, vomiting, food intolerance, or abdominal distention to the physician.

Home Care

- Have the patient or caregiver place a towel over the patient's chest to prevent soiling with removal.
- Instruct the patient and caregiver to place the tube in a plastic zippered storage bag before discarding it in the trash can.

Documentation

- Chart the date and time of removal as well as the patient's tolerance of the procedure.
- Note any complications following NG or NE tube removal, such as food intolerance, nausea, vomiting, and abdominal distention.

Sample documentation:

11/29/06	0800	NG tube removed. No coughing or gagging. Left naris slightly red, but skin intact. Patient drank 100 mL water. ———— S. Carpenter, RN

11/29/06	1130	Taking clear liquids since 0800 with no nausea, vomiting, or stomach distention. Bowel sounds faint, but audible. ———— S. Carpenter, RN

TECHNIQUES

TECHNIQUE 26–1   Measuring Triceps Skinfold

- Locate the midpoint on posterior of the dominant upper arm.
- With the client's arm hanging loosely at the side, palpate the measurement site at the midpoint to become familiar with distinguishing muscle from adipose soft tissue.
- From 1 cm above the midpoint, grasp a vertical pinch of skin and only the subcutaneous fat layer between the thumb and index finger. Gently pull the skinfold away from the underlying muscle.
- Place the skinfold caliper at the midpoint, and slowly release the jaw of the caliper while maintaining a grasp of the skinfold (see the figure).

- Take three readings in quick succession, and average the results to the nearest 0.1 mm. Take each reading as soon as the jaws of the caliper come into contact with the skin and the reading has stabilized.

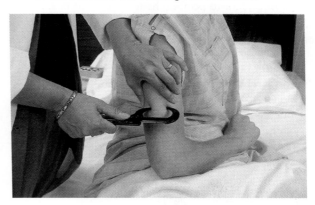

TECHNIQUE 26–2   Measuring Circumferences to Evaluate Body Composition

Measuring Mid-Upper Arm Circumference

- Keeping the client's dominant arm parallel to the body, bend the elbow 90°.
- Using a tape measure, measure the distance between the acromion (the bony protrusion of the back of the upper shoulder) and the olecranon process (tip of the elbow).
- Mark the midpoint between these two landmarks.
- Ask the client to relax the arm, so that it hangs loose and parallel to the body.
- Position the tape around the upper arm at the marked midpoint. Make sure the tape is snug but not so tight as to indent or pinch the skin.
- Record the circumference to the nearest 0.1 cm.

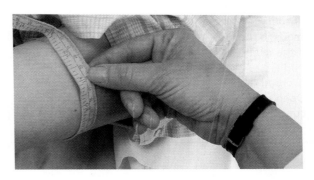

Calculating Waist-to-Hip Ratio (WHR)

- Use a tape measure to measure the circumference of the waist (at the umbilicus with stomach muscles relaxed).
- Use a tape measure to measure the circumference of the hips at their widest point.
- Calculate the waist-to-hip ratio using the following formula:

  waist circumference in inches ÷ hip circumference in inches

  Example: Robert's waist measurement is 32 inches, and his hip measurement is 34 inches. His WHR is 32 ÷ 34 = 0.94

TECHNIQUE 26–3 — Interventions for Patients with Impaired Swallowing

Nutritional support for patients with Impaired Swallowing includes the following activities from the NIC intervention Swallowing Therapy (Dochterman & Bulechek, 2004, pp. 697–698):

- Provide/use assistive devices, as appropriate.
- Avoid use of drinking straws.
- Assist patient to position head in forward flexion in preparation for swallowing (chin tuck).
- Assist patient to place food at back of mouth and on unaffected side.
- Monitor patient's tongue movements while eating.
- Check mouth for pocketing of food after eating.
- Monitor body hydration (e.g., intake, output, skin turgor, mucous membranes).

In addition, you must also take Aspiration Precautions (Dochterman & Bulechek, 2004, p. 175):

- Monitor level of consciousness, cough reflex, gag reflex, and swallowing ability.
- Position upright 90° or as far as possible.
- Keep suction setup available.
- Feed in small amounts.
- Avoid liquids or use thickening agent.
- Cut food into small pieces.
- Keep head of bed elevated for 30 to 45 minutes after feeding.

TECHNIQUE 26–4 — Assisting Patients with Meals

- Provide an opportunity for toileting, oral hygiene, and hand washing prior to meals.
- If the patient's condition allows, encourage him to get out of bed for meals.
- Encourage residents in long-term care settings to eat meals in the dining room instead of in the bedroom.
- If the patient must eat in bed, place the head of the bed at the highest tolerable level, and adjust the overbed table to be in easy reach.
- Open food containers, and arrange and prepare (e.g., cut, mash) food to the client's preferences.

- If the client is visually impaired, identify the locations of the meal on the tray based on a clock face (e.g., "The coffee is at 1 o'clock above the plate on the right").
- Feed the patient if she is unable to feed herself. Be sure to provide adequate time for her to chew and swallow. If possible, ask her what food she would like next.
- Record the amount of food and fluid the patient consumed.
- Help the client to wash hands or use the rest room after the meal.

TECHNIQUE 26–5   Checking Feeding Tube Placement

Aspirating Stomach Contents

- Don procedure gloves. This is a clean, not sterile, technique.
- Just before feeding, draw up 10 to 30 mL of air in a 30- to 60-mL syringe, insert the syringe in the distal end of the feeding tube, and inject air to flush out formula, medications, and other substances. This also helps keep a small-bore tube from collapsing when you aspirate.
- With the same syringe, aspirate the air and 20 to 30 mL of stomach or intestinal contents. Gastric contents are normally greenish brown and liquid. Intestinal contents are usually yellow-green because of the influence of bile.
    a. If you did not aspirate any fluid, inject another 20 mL of air and use a smaller syringe to aspirate again. Using a small (<10 mL syringe) for very small tubes also decreases the likelihood of collapse because it creates less negative pressure.
    b. If you still do not aspirate, repeat the procedure with this variation: Insert air with the large syringe; insert the small syringe into the end the tubing, and leave it for 15 minutes to allow fluid to accumulate before aspirating.
    c. If you are still unsuccessful, reposition the patient. This may move the tube into a place where fluid has pooled.

Measuring the pH of the Aspirate

This is currently the most effective way to check tube placement at the bedside.

- Follow the preceding procedure for aspirating stomach contents.
- Measure the pH of the aspirated fluid by using nitrazine paper. See the accompanying figure.
- Because of the action of hydrochloric acid in the stomach, gastric contents measure a pH of 1 to 4. However, if the client is receiving medications to control stomach acidity (e.g., antacids, H_2 blockers, or proton pump inhibitors), the pH may be as high as 6. Intestinal contents usually have a pH of 6 or

greater. The pH of respiratory secretions is 7 or more; however respiratory secretions may occasionally have a pH as low as 6.

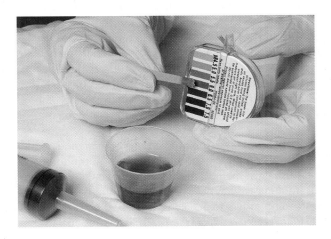

Injecting Air into the Tube to Confirm Other Methods

Use this method only to confirm other methods. It has been shown to be unreliable (Metheney, 1998).

- Draw 5 to 30 mL of air into a syringe; place the tip of the syringe in the end of the feeding tube.
- Place a stethoscope over the stomach.
- Listen with stethoscope as you inject the air through the tube.

Air injected into the stomach produces a gurgling or whooshing sound in the left upper quadrant. If the tube has been inadvertently placed in the lungs, you will hear no gurgling.

Because none of these methods is foolproof, it is wise to use a combination. Auscultate as you are injecting air prior to aspiration; aspirate fluid; and check the pH. In addition, as confirmation, if the patient can talk, the tube is probably in the stomach. However, Rombeau and Rolandelli (1997) found that some clients can speak even when the tube is in the lung.

TECHNIQUE 26–6   Monitoring Patients Receiving Enteral Nutrition

For patients receiving enteral nutrition, monitor the following:

- *Position of the feeding tube.* Periodically check the placement of the tube to ensure that it is correct. As a rule, check on each shift or at each intermittent feeding.
- *Tube insertion site.* An NG or NE tube is secured by tape to the nose. Regularly check the skin, gently cleanse the area, and retape the tube as needed. Report tissue breakdown, epistaxis (nosebleed), or sinusitis; they may signal a need for insertion of a PEG. Inspect a PEG insertion site for erythema or drainage, which are signs of infection.
- *Weight.* To assess the adequacy of the feeding, regularly weigh patients receiving enteral nutrition. There is usually a medical order for frequency of weighing. Frequent weight checks allow adjustment of the feeding orders to achieve the desired goal.
- *Tube feeding residual volume.* To assess residual volume, aspirate the feeding tube to determine the amount of feeding remaining in the stomach. If you are able to aspirate a quantity equal to or greater than the formula flow rate for 1 hour (or alternatively, a total of 150 mL), the patient may be receiving too much fluid or may have delayed gastric emptying. However, you should not automatically stop the feeding; if you obtain a single elevated residual volume,

recheck it in 1 hour (American Gastrointestinal Association, 1995). See Technique 26–5.

- *Frequency of bowel movements.* Bowel movements should occur regularly. Constipation is usually due to inadequate water or fiber. Some commercial feedings contain fiber. To alleviate constipation, you may add free water and perhaps fiber to the formula. Diarrhea may indicate intolerance of the formula, excessive feeding, or gastrointestinal disease.
- *Bowel sounds.* Check before each feeding, or every 4 to 8 hours for continuous feedings. Peristalsis must be present.
- *Abdominal distention.* Measure abdominal girth daily, at the umbilicus.
- *Serum electrolyte levels.* Monitor regularly.
- *Urine for sugar and acetone.* This is sometimes done as a bedside screen for hyperglycemia. However, treatment is based on blood sugar levels.
- *Skin turgor, hematocrit, and urine specific gravity.* If the patient is not receiving enough water, dehydration may occur.
- *Serum blood urea nitrogen (BUN) and sodium levels.* This is especially important for high-protein formulas. Insufficient fluid intake combined with high protein intake may overload the kidneys so that nitrogenous wastes are not excreted adequately.

TECHNIQUE 26–7   Monitoring Patients Who Are Receiving Total Parenteral Nutrition

For patients receiving TPN, you will need to monitor the following:

- *Tube insertion site.* Check the insertion site frequently. Any signs of erythema or drainage may indicate infection. Because the catheter is inserted into a central vessel, infection at the site can lead rapidly to sepsis.
- *Weight.* To assess the adequacy of the IV nutrition, regularly weigh the patient (according to medical order or agency policy). Frequent weight checks

allow adjustment of the formula to achieve the desired goal.

- *Glucose.* Because of the high proportion of glucose in the formulas, monitor blood glucose every 6 hours.
- *Diuresis and dehydration.* These can occur if hypertonic dextrose is infused too rapidly.
- *Lab values.* Patients receiving TPN require regular lab studies (electrolytes, blood sugar, albumin, BUN, and creatinine) for formula adjustment. The frequency of the studies depends on the patient's condition.

ASSESSMENT GUIDELINES AND TOOLS

Nutritional History

Item	Components
Demographic data	Name, date, age, sex, date of birth, address, occupation, workplace, insurance
Chief complaint	Client's subjective statement of health problem, including onset and duration
Present illness and current health	Detailed data about chief complaint as it relates to nutrition status Recent diet changes and reasons Recent weight loss or gain and over what period of time Usual body weight: 20% above or below desirable weight? Change in appetite Unusual stress/trauma (surgery, job, family) Medications, prescriptions Alcohol, nicotine, caffeine consumption
Health history	Previous illnesses, trauma, major dental problems, or issues that could interfere with ability to shop, prepare food, chew, or swallow Allergies (i.e., environmental, foods, drugs) Eating disorders Chronic disease or surgery that affects gastrointestinal tract Substance abuse Nutritional programs
Family health history	Genetic/familial disorders that could affect nutritional status: cardiovascular or gastrointestinal disorders, Crohn's disease, diabetes, cancer, sickle cell anemia, allergies, celiac disease, other food intolerances, obesity
Dietary history	Current food intake pattern using one of the following methods: 24-hour–7-day recall, as appropriate; food frequency food record, and comparison to dietary guidelines and RDAs Special dietary considerations, restrictions Fad diets Vitamin and mineral supplements Commercial dietary supplements Nonconventional dietary supplements Food preferences, dislikes Dietary influences from ethnic, cultural, or religious practices Counseling needs (based on food knowledge)
Medication history	Recent use of steroids, immunosuppressants, chemotherapy, anticonvulsants, or oral contraceptives
Socioeconomic factors	Adequate food storage, refrigeration, food prep Payments: Supplemental Security Income (SSI), food stamps, WIC Who shops, prepares, and cooks food?
Personal factors	Stress/coping mechanisms, self-concept, social supports Daily activity level and exercise regimen

Assessing for Nutritional Problems

Clients who are found to be at risk for nutritional problems should be further evaluated using one of the three following methods.

I. Subjective Global Assessment

Using the subjective global assessment (SGA) method, an experienced clinician examines subjective and objective parts of a medical history and physical examination to evaluate a client's nutritional status. There are six components pertinent to nutritional status:

1. *Weight history*—over previous 6 months
2. *Dietary history*—including a comparison of usual, recommended, and current intake
3. *Gastrointestinal symptoms history*—for example, anorexia, nausea, vomiting, and diarrhea
4. *Energy level*—including activity level and functional status
5. *Existing disease*—evaluation of the metabolic demands of any disease states along with acute stressors that may alter those demands
6. *Physical examination data*—regarding loss of fat stores, muscle wasting, and the presence of edema and ascites

As a clinician, you would analyze these components to rate the client's nutritional status as normal, mild, moderate, or severe. Effectiveness of this method depends largely on the experience of the clinician (Barone, Milosavljevic, & Gazibarich, 2003).

II. Nutrition Screening Initiative

Recognizing the importance of nutrition in our aging population, the American Academy of Family Physicians, the American Dietetic Association, and the National Council on Aging developed the Nutrition Screening Initiative (NSI) (1995). The NSI addresses nutritional concerns associated with chronic diseases that older adults frequently experience. The NSI requires collection and evaluation of data in four areas: clinical, dietary, body composition, and biochemical. In addition, it identifies indicators of impaired nutritional status (following). To obtain copies of patient education materials and screening tools,

 Go to the **American Academy of Family Physicians** web site at **www.aafp.org/nsi.xml**

Indications of Impaired Nutritional Status

Major Indicators	Minor Indicators	Symptoms	Physical Signs	Lab Values
• Significant weight loss over time • Significant high or low weight for height • Significant change in functional status • Significant and inappropriate food intake • Significant reduction in midarm circumference • Significant decrease in skinfold • Osteoporosis or osteomalacia • Folate or vitamin B deficiency	• Concurrent syndromes • Alcoholism • Cognitive impairment • Chronic renal insufficiency • Multiple concurrent medications • Malabsorption syndromes	• Anorexia, nausea, or dysphagia • Early satiety • Changed bowel habits • Fatigue or apathy • Memory loss	• Poor oral or dental status • Dehydration • Poorly healing wounds • Loss of subcutaneous fat or muscle mass • Fluid retention	• Reduced levels of serum albumin, transferrin, or pre-albumin • Folate deficiency • Iron deficiency • Zinc deficiency • Reduced levels of ascorbic acid

Assessing for Nutritional Problems *(continued)*

III. Mini Nutritional Assessment

The Mini Nutritional Assessment (MNA) is a quick and easy method of identifying individuals with nutritional risk or with malnutrition. (See the accompanying figure). This tool was developed primarily for use with older clients. It con-

sists of two parts. The first part screens for nutritional risk. The second part is completed only if the individual is identified to be at risk. The final score, which tallies the scores of both parts, is the Malnutrition Indicator Score. Indications of malnutrition require multidisciplinary follow-up.

NESTLÉ NUTRITION SERVICES

Mini Nutritional Assessment
MNA®

Last name: _____ First name: _____ Sex: _____ Date: _____

Age: _____ Weight, kg: _____ Height, cm: _____ I.D. Number: _____

Complete the screen by filling in the boxes with the appropriate numbers.
Add the numbers for the screen. If score is 11 or less, continue with the assessment to gain a Malnutrition Indicator Score.

Screening

A Has food intake declined over the past 3 months due to loss of appetite, digestive problems, chewing or swallowing difficulties?
0 = severe loss of appetite
1 = moderate loss of appetite
2 = no loss of appetite

B Weight loss during the last 3 months
0 = weight loss greater than 3 kg (6.6 lbs)
1 = does not know
2 = weight loss between 1 and 3 kg (2.2 and 6.6 lbs)
3 = no weight loss

C Mobility
0 = bed or chair bound
1 = able to get out of bed/chair but does not go out
2 = goes out

D Has suffered psychological stress or acute disease in the past 3 months
0 = yes   2 = no

E Neuropsychological problems
0 = severe dementia or depression
1 = mild dementia
2 = no psychological problems

F Body Mass Index (BMI) (weight in kg) / (height in m)²
0 = BMI less than 19
1 = BMI 19 to less than 21
2 = BMI 21 to less than 23
3 = BMI 23 or greater

Screening score (subtotal max. 14 points)
12 points or greater   Normal – not at risk – no need to complete assessment
11 points or below   Possible malnutrition – continue assessment

Assessment

G Lives independently (not in a nursing home or hospital)
0 = no   1 = yes

H Takes more than 3 prescription drugs per day
0 = yes   1 = no

I Pressure sores or skin ulcers
0 = yes   1 = no

J How many full meals does the patient eat daily?
0 = 1 meal
1 = 2 meals
2 = 3 meals

K Selected consumption markers for protein intake
• At least one serving of dairy products (milk, cheese, yogurt) per day?   yes ☐   no ☐
• Two or more servings of legumes or eggs per week?   yes ☐   no ☐
• Meat, fish or poultry every day?   yes ☐   no ☐
0.0 = if 0 or 1 yes
0.5 = if 2 yes
1.0 = if 3 yes

L Consumes two or more servings of fruits or vegetables per day?
0 = no   1 = yes

M How much fluid (water, juice, coffee, tea, milk…) is consumed per day?
0.0 = less than 3 cups
0.5 = 3 to 5 cups
1.0 = more than 5 cups

N Mode of feeding
0 = unable to eat without assistance
1 = self-fed with some difficulty
2 = self-fed without any problem

O Self view of nutritional status
0 = views self as being malnourished
1 = is uncertain of nutritional state
2 = views self as having no nutritional problem

P In comparison with other people of the same age, how does the patient consider his/her health status?
0.0 = not as good
0.5 = does not know
1.0 = as good
2.0 = better

Q Mid-arm circumference (MAC) in cm
0.0 = MAC less than 21
0.5 = MAC 21 to 22
1.0 = MAC 22 or greater

R Calf circumference (CC) in cm
0 = CC less than 31   1 = CC 31 or greater

Assessment (max. 16 points)

Screening score

Total Assessment (max. 30 points)

Malnutrition Indicator Score
17 to 23.5 points   at risk of malnutrition
Less than 17 points   malnourished

Ref.: Guigoz Y, Vellas B and Garry P.J. 1994. Mini Nutritional Assessment: A practical assessment tool for grading the nutritional state of elderly patients. *Facts and Research in Gerontology.* Supplement #2:15-59.
Rubenstein LZ, Harker J, Guigoz Y and Vellas B. Comprehensive Geriatric Assessment (CGA) and the MNA: An Overview of CGA, Nutritional Assessment, and Development of a Shortened Version of the MNA. In: "Mini Nutritional Assessment (MNA): Research and Practice in the Elderly". Vellas B, Garry PJ and Guigoz Y, editors. Nestlé Nutrition Workshop Series. Clinical & Performance Programme, vol. 1. Karger, Bale, in press.

© Nestlé, 1994, Revision 1998. N67200 12/99 10M

Nutrition-Focused Physical Examination

Correlate the following physical examination findings with the dietary history, screening methods, anthropometric measurements, and laboratory results.

I. The General Survey

Assess vital signs, height, weight, and overall impressions.

- *Overall appearance.* Does the client look ill? Does he appear adequately nourished? You will want to investigate any hunches as you move through the physical exam.
- *Temperature.* An increase in temperature raises the client's metabolic rate and need for fluid, is a sign of infection, and may decrease the client's appetite.
- *Blood pressure (BP) and heart rate* are affected by fluid status. An elevated BP may be related to fluid volume excess; a low BP may be a sign of dehydration. Heart rate usually increases when fluid volume is low.
- *Height and weight.* Calculate the body mass index (BMI) on the basis of these measures. The normal BMI for adults ranges from 18.5 to 24.9.

BMI = weight in kilograms ÷ (height in meters)^2

Classification of Body Mass Index Values

Classification	BMI (kg/m^2)	Risk of Comorbidities
Underweight	< 18.5	Low
Normal weight	18.5–24.9	Average
Pre-obese	25.0–29.9	Mildly increased
Class I obesity	30.0–34.9	Moderate
Class II obesity	35.0–39.9	Severe
Class III obesity	≥ 40.0	Very severe

II. Integumentary System

- *Skin turgor* is an indicator of fluid status. Poor skin turgor may result from dehydration. Swelling may result from overhydration.
- *Skin integrity* reflects overall nutritional status. Poor wound healing may suggest inadequate intake of protein, vitamin C, or zinc. Patients with uncontrolled diabetes often experience slow-healing wounds, especially in the feet and legs.
- *Areas of warmth or erythema.* These are signs of inflammation or infection.
- *Other nutrition-related skin changes* include red, swollen skin lesions (due to niacin deficiency); excessive bleeding seen as petechiae or ecchymoses (due to vitamin K or C deficiency); and xerosis (dry skin).
- *Abnormal nail findings* include spoon-shaped, brittle nails (due to iron deficiency); dull nails with transverse ridge (due to protein deficiency); pale, poor blanching, or mottled nails (due to vitamin A or C deficiency); bruising or bleeding beneath nails (due to protein or caloric deficiency); and splinter hemorrhages (due to vitamin C deficiency).
- *Hair* will grow slowly, thin, or break easily if protein is deficient.

III. The Head and Neck

The condition of the mouth, teeth, and gums has a major effect on a client's choice of food, ability to chew, and ability to swallow.

- *Facial paralysis or drooping* of one side of the face may be a result of stroke, injury, or nerve irritation, which also affects the ability to chew and swallow (dysphagia).
- *Enlarged thyroid gland.* Look for swelling of the thyroid, which may be related to hypothyroid or hyperthyroid states. Both disorders affect metabolic rate and energy requirements.

Nutrition-Focused Physical Examination *(continued)*

- *Eyes.* Nutritional deficits may cause the eyes to be red and dry and the conjunctiva pale.
- *Lips and tongue.* The lips may be chapped, red, or swollen. The tongue may be bright red, purple, or swollen or may have longitudinal furrows.
- *Teeth and gums.* Look for cavities, mottled or missing teeth, and for spongy, bleeding, or receding gums.

IV. Cardiovascular System

You will have gained initial information about the cardiovascular system by taking the vital signs. As you follow up and listen to the heart and check pulses, you should explore any abnormal vital signs.

- *Bounding pulses* are associated with fluid overload, fever, and hypertension.
- *Weak, thready pulse* may indicate dehydration, shock, or hypotension.
- *Edema in the extremities* may be a sign of fluid overload, inadequate protein stores, or electrolyte imbalance.

V. Abdominal Exam

- A *scaphoid or concave abdomen* indicates loss of subcutaneous fat, possibly caused by malnutrition.
- A *round or protuberant abdomen* points to obesity due to excess caloric and/or high fat intake.
- A *generalized enlarged abdomen* may signify **ascites** (fluid in the abdominal cavity) due to liver malfunction. Ascites results from three mechanisms: abnormal movement of protein and water into the abdomen; sodium and fluid retention; and decreased albumin production in the liver.
- *Hyperactive bowel sounds* are heard with gastrointestinal infection, laxative use, and malabsorption disorders.
- *Hypoactive bowel sounds* suggest sluggish motility through the GI tract.

VI. Musculoskeletal System

- *Thin extremities with excess skinfolds* indicate muscle atrophy and fat loss related to malnutrition, especially protein and calories. This may also occur as a result of prolonged bed rest and inadequate food intake. Skinfold measurement is also useful in assessing muscle and fat stores.
- Look for any obvious *swelling, deformities, or limitation in range of motion of the joints.*
- *Kyphosis* of the spine may indicate osteoporosis and possible insufficient calcium intake.

- *Joint pain* on palpation or with movement is a sign of arthritis or gout. Arthritis may affect ability to shop for groceries, prepare food to eat, and use utensils for eating and drinking. Gout is often induced by diets high in **purines** (food substances that break down into uric acid), obesity, and excess alcohol intake.

VII. Neurological System

The neurological examination will give you insight into the client's ability to perform independent tasks.

- Look for *altered level of consciousness or signs of behavioral disturbances and dementia* through general conversation and appropriateness of answers to specific questions.
- Assess *coordination and reflexes.*
- Assess for *cognitive deficits or severe psychiatric disorders:* A client with cognitive deficits or severe psychiatric disorders may have difficulty preparing food or judging appropriate nutrient choices.
- Assess for *motor or sensory deficits.* Clients with motor or sensory deficits may be unable to purchase, prepare, or eat a variety of foods.
- *Confusion, weakness, diminished reflexes, paresthesia, and sensory loss* may be cues to vitamin B deficiencies.
- *Tetany or severe and generalized muscle spasm* may indicate calcium or magnesium deficits.

VIII. What Are the Signs of Severe Malnutrition?

Malnutrition is a condition of impaired development or function caused by a long-term deficiency, excess, or imbalance in energy and/or nutrient intake.

- Symptoms of undernutrition due to insufficient food include reduced physical activity, weight loss, and reduced height.
- Children, older adults, and people with chronic illnesses such as cancer, HIV infection, and chronic obstructive pulmonary disease (COPD) are most likely to experience malnutrition.
- To assess for malnutrition in children, compare weight, height, and head circumference to the standards (norms) for the child's age.
- Other indicators in children include the presence of iron deficiency anemia.
- In adolescents, look for a delay of stages of sexual maturation (Matarese & Gottschlich, 1998).

STANDARDIZED LANGUAGE

NOC Outcomes and NIC Interventions Related to Nutrition

NOC Outcomes

The following outcomes are directly linked to nutritional diagnoses:

- Nutritional Status
- Nutritional Status: Food and Fluid Intake
- Nutritional Status: Nutrient Intake
- Weight Control

NIC Interventions

The following interventions are directly linked to nutrition problems:
- Nutrition Management
- Nutrition Therapy
- Nutritional Counseling
- Nutritional Monitoring

The following interventions are also found in the class Nutrition Support. They address specific etiologies of nutrition problems.

- Diet Staging
- Eating Disorders Management
- Enteral Tube Feeding
- Feeding
- Gastrointestinal Intubation
- Self-Care Assistance: Feeding
- Swallowing Therapy
- Teaching: Prescribed Diet
- Total Parenteral Nutrition (TPN) Administration
- Tube Care: Gastrointestinal
- Weight Gain Assistance
- Weight Management
- Weight Reduction Assistance

Sources: Moorhead, S., Johnson, M., & Maas, M. (Eds.). (2004). *Nursing outcomes classification* (*NOC*) (3rd ed.). St Louis: Mosby; Dochterman, J. M., & Bulechek, G. M. (Eds.). (2004). *Nursing interventions classification* (*NIC*) (4th ed.). St Louis: Mosby.

NOC Outcomes and NIC Interventions for Overweight/Obesity and Underweight/Malnutrition

For Overweight/Obesity

Nursing Diagnoses	Imbalanced Nutrition: More Than Body Requirements Risk for Imbalanced Nutrition: More Than Body Requirements
NOC Outcomes	Weight Control Nutritional Status: Food and Fluid Intake Nutritional Status: Nutrient Intake
NIC Interventions	Weight Management—to balance caloric intake and energy expenditure Nutritional Counseling—to provide information based on identified knowledge deficits regarding nutrition Nutrition Management—to balance metabolic needs with nutrient intake Weight Reduction Assistance—to balance caloric intake and energy expenditure

For Underweight/Malnutrition

Nursing Diagnoses	Imbalanced Nutrition: Less Than Body Requirements Risk for Imbalanced Nutrition: Less Than Body Requirements Adult Failure to Thrive
NOC Outcomes	Weight Control Nutritional Status: Food and Fluid Intake Nutritional Status: Nutrient Intake
NIC Interventions	• Nutrition Management—to balance metabolic needs with nutrient intake • Eating Disorder Management—if anorexia nervosa or bulimia nervosa is present • Nutritional Counseling—to provide information based on identified knowledge deficits regarding nutrition • Nutritional Monitoring—to evaluate the effectiveness of the counseling and nutritional therapy • Nutritional Therapy—for the treatment of nutritional imbalance • Swallowing Therapy—to treat dysphagia or difficulty swallowing • Weight Gain Assistance—used when the focus is to help the client gain weight • Weight Management—used to maintain a balance in caloric intake and energy expenditure • Enteral Tube Feeding, Gastrointestinal Intubation, Total Parenteral Nutrition (TPN) Administration, and Tube Care: Gastrointestinal—are used when the patient cannot tolerate oral feedings

Sources: Moorhead, S., Johnson, M., & Maas, M. (Eds.). (2004). *Nursing outcomes classification (NOC)* (3rd ed.). St Louis: Mosby; Dochterman, J. M., & Bulechek, G. M. (Eds.) (2004). *Nursing interventions classification (NIC)* (4th ed.). St Louis: Mosby.

What Are the Main Points in This Chapter?

- Energy nutrients are carbohydrates, proteins, and fats. Other important nutrients are water and the micronutrients: fat-soluble vitamins, water-soluble vitamins, and minerals.

- Water is an essential nutrient.

- Carbohydrates include simple sugars called monosaccharides and disaccharides, and complex carbohydrates called polysaccharides.

- Glucose, a monosaccharide, is the primary form of energy for the brain, as well as for the body during moderate-to-intense physical activity.

- Proteins are made up of amino acids and are required for cell and tissue growth, maintenance, and repair.

- Lipids, including fats and oils, are classified as triglycerides or sterols. They are essential components of cells, fuel the body at rest and during light activity, aid in absorption of fat-soluble vitamins, and promote a sense of satiety when eaten.

- Saturated fats and trans fats are less healthful lipid choices than mono- and polyunsaturated fats.

- Nutrients must be consumed at least at a minimal level in order to meet the body's physiological needs. This level is called Dietary Reference Intake (DRI).

- Reliable guidelines for designing a nutritious diet include the DRIs, the Dietary Guidelines for Americans 2005, Food Guide Pyramids, and the Nutrition Facts panel found on packaged foods in the United States.

- The basal metabolic rate (BMR) is a measure of the energy required by resting tissue to maintain basic function.

- Factors influencing a client's nutritional status include developmental stage, education, lifestyle choices, vegetarianism, dieting for weight loss, culture, religion, disease processes, functional limitations, and economic factors.

- Many people must follow a modified diet to assist in managing their illness. In addition, all inpatients must have a diet ordered by their primary care provider.

- When examining an individual's nutritional balance, it is important to thoroughly assess nutritional history, physical findings, anthropometric measurements, and biochemical values.

- A food record is the most accurate method of obtaining data about a client's actual food intake.

- The body mass index (BMI), skinfold measurements, and circumferences are estimates of body composition.

- Laboratory or biochemical indicators of nutritional status include blood glucose and serum protein levels or indices such as albumin, urea, and hemoglobin.

- Vitamin and mineral supplementation may be appropriate for some people, but they do not replace the need for a balanced diet.

- Government programs provide some assistance for clients who cannot afford to buy food.

- Nutritional requirements of older adults are similar to those for adults, with a slight reduction in the need for calories. Nutritional problems are also similar, but the incidence is higher among older adults.

- Nurses can help support nutrition for patients who have Self-Care Deficits or Impaired Swallowing by assisting patients with meals and providing swallowing therapy.

- Nutritional imbalance can range from either inadequate or excessive amounts of a single nutrient to overall caloric intake.

- Interventions for underweight/undernutrition include measures to improve the patient's appetite and providing enteral and parenteral nutrition.

- The most accurate way to check enteral tube placement is by radiographic verification; but this is too expensive for ongoing bedside use.

- The preferred bedside techniques for checking enteral tube placement are to aspirate stomach contents and measure the pH (normally 1 to 4 for stomach contents).

- Potential complications associated with enteral feedings include aspiration, infection, diarrhea, and electrolyte imbalance.

- You must follow meticulous sterile technique when administering parenteral nutrition because the solution is delivered into a large central vein; if infection occurs, sepsis is almost immediate.

Urinary Elimination

Overview

The urinary system consists of two kidneys, two ureters, the urinary bladder, and the urethra. The kidneys filter nitrogen and other metabolic wastes, toxins, excess ions, and water from the bloodstream and excrete them as urine. Voiding and control of urination require normal functioning of the bladder and the urethra, as well as an intact brain, spinal cord, and nerves supplying the bladder and urethra.

As an adult ages, the number of functional nephrons gradually decreases, along with the ability to dilute and concentrate urine. An adequately hydrated adult produces clear yellow urine. Concentrated urine is darker in color, but dilute urine can appear colorless. Substances that contain caffeine act as diuretics and increase urine production. Decreased urine production can be caused by a diet high in salt. Medications with anticholinergic effects inhibit the free flow of urine and may also contribute to urinary retention.

A routine urinalysis is one of the most commonly ordered laboratory tests. It is used as an overall screening test as well as an aid to diagnose renal, hepatic, and other diseases. Urinary retention, an inability to empty the bladder, may be caused by obstruction, nerve problems, infection, surgery, medications, or anxiety. To allow drainage of urine, a pliable tube is introduced into the bladder in a procedure called urinary catheterization. Nurses can independently perform the primary interventions to manage urinary incontinence (UI), a lack of voluntary control over urination. Pelvic floor muscle exercises (PFME) are a mainstay of UI treatment for women. PFME strengthen perineal muscles and help to prevent and treat stress, urge, and mixed UI. Kegel exercises are the most commonly used.

Thinking Critically About Urinary Elimination

The exercises in the following section allow you to practice the kind of thinking you will use as a full-spectrum nurse. Because these are critical-thinking activities, there is usually no single right answer. Discuss answers with your peers—discussion can stimulate critical thinking. If you have difficulty with any of the questions, consult with your instructor.

Caring for the Garcias

At a recent visit to the Family Health Center, Joe and Flordelisa Garcia confide that Joe's mother, Katherine, has had several "accidents." She has denied the problem but Flordelisa tells you that she helped her mother-in-law with laundry recently and many of the clothes smell of urine. They ask you how to approach Katherine about this problem.

A. How would you respond?

B. What suggestions, if any, could you make to the Garcias about treatment for Katherine?

C. Flordelisa tells you that she has been told that surgery is the best form of treatment. She asks you whether this is true. How would you answer her question?

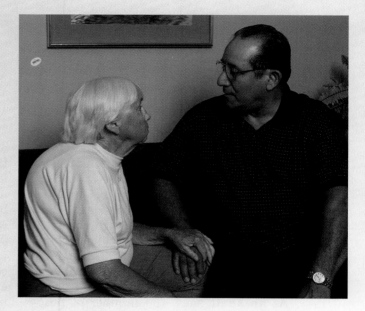

1 You receive report from a UAP that a patient with no history of urinary elimination problems has had 150 mL of oral liquids in 6 hours and has voided 100 mL of clear, dark amber urine. His vital signs at the start of the shift were as follows: blood pressure, 108/76 mm Hg; pulse, 72 bpm; respirations, 18; temperature, 98.6°F. The most recent check revealed blood pressure, 112/80 mm Hg; pulse, 88 bpm; respirations, 22; and temperature, 100.4°F.

a What conclusion might you draw about what has caused these symptoms?

b What actions should you take?

2 As you make rounds, you discover a collection bag for an indwelling catheter placed on the bed above the level of the patient's bladder.

a What should you do first? What assessments should you make?

b What teaching would be important in this situation?

3 Unlicensed assistive personnel complain that Mr. Jones, a patient with dementia, keeps urinating in his trash can and in the hallway.

a What special measures could be taken to assist Mr. Jones in finding the bathroom?

b What data could be helpful in developing a plan for Mr. Jones?

4 For each of the following concepts, use critical thinking to describe how or why it is important to nursing, patient care, or urinary elimination. Note that these are *not* to be merely definitions.

Blood pressure

The kidney tubules

Developmental stage

Privacy

Hydration

Specific gravity

Urinary incontinence

Practical Knowledge
knowing how

This section provides procedures and techniques you will need to support your patients' urinary function. You will also find assessment guidelines, information about diagnostic tests of urinary function, and standardized nursing language tables.

PROCEDURES

PROCEDURE 27–1 | Collecting a Clean-Catch Urine Specimen

 For steps to follow in *all* procedures, refer to the inside back cover of this book.

critical aspects

- Don clean procedure gloves.
- Wash the perineum or the end of the penis first with soap and water, then with antiseptic solution. (For women, wash from front to back; for men, use a circular motion from the urethra outward.)
- Have the patient begin voiding. After the stream begins, collect a 30 to 60 mL specimen.
- Maintain sterility: Do not touch the inside of the container or the container lid.
- Place the lid on the container, label the container, and transport it to the lab in a timely manner.

Equipment

- Prepackaged collection kit
- If no kit is available:
  - Sterile specimen container
  - Antiseptic solution
  - Sterile cotton balls or 2 × 2 gauze pads
- Washcloth or towel
- Mild soap and water
- 2 pairs of clean procedure gloves
- Patient identification labels
- Bedpan or bedside commode for an immobile patient

Delegation

This procedure may be delegated to unlicensed assistive personnel (UAP), but you must be sure that the UAP knows how to perform the procedure correctly, including proper cleansing and maintaining sterility of the container. You must complete the following assessments and instruct the UAP to report any abnormalities seen in the urine (e.g., blood, foul odor, mucus). In addition, the UAP should report any complaints of dysuria by the patient and bring the specimen to you for inspection.

Assessment

- Cognitive status

To determine whether the patient can be instructed to complete this procedure on her own and/or whether she can follow directions.

- Mobility status

To determine where the specimen will be collected (e.g., bed, commode, bedpan)

- Urinary status

Patients with impaired ability to control urinary flow may not be able to collect a specimen in this manner.

➤

PROCEDURE 27–1

Collecting a Clean-Catch Urine Specimen
(continued)

Procedural Steps

Step 1 If the patient is immobile or needs assistance, assist the patient to the toilet, to a bedside commode, or onto the bedpan.

See Procedure 28-2 for placing a patient on the bedpan.

Step 2 Open the prepackaged kit (if available), and remove the contents.

Step 3 Wash your hands and don clean procedure gloves.

Prevents the transmission of bacteria.

Step 4 Cleanse, or instruct the patient to cleanse, around the urinary meatus.

Prevents the contamination of the specimen with surface bacteria.

Variation For Women

a. Have the patient spread her legs. Wash the perineal area with warm water and mild soap.

Cleanses the area of bacteria so that any bacteria found in the specimen can be assumed to have come from the bladder and urethra rather than the perineal skin.

b. Open the antiseptic towelette provided in the prepackaged kit. If there is no kit, pour the antiseptic solution over the cotton balls. With one hand, spread the labia; with the other, cleanse the perineal area in a front-to-back direction, making sure to cleanse over the urinary meatus. Clean the perineal area at least twice. Use each towelette or cotton ball only once.

Following the "clean-to-dirty" principle decreases the likelihood of contamination of the specimen with feces. Antiseptic helps reduce the number of bacteria. ▼

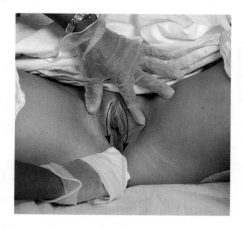

Variation For Men

c. If the penis is uncircumcised, retract the foreskin back from the end of the penis.

Allows better access for cleansing the area around the meatus.

d. Use the towelette provided in the prepackaged kit or pour antiseptic solution over cotton balls. With one hand, grasp the penis gently. With the other hand, cleanse the meatus in a circular motion from the meatus outward, and cleanse for a few inches down the shaft of the penis. Cleanse around the meatus at least twice, using each towelette or cotton ball only once.

Helps prevent contaminating the specimen with bacteria.

Note: Some lab manuals recommend rinsing the antiseptic solution from the meatus to prevent contamination of the specimen with antiseptic.

Step 5 Remove gloves. Wash your hands, and don the second pair of clean procedure gloves.

Prevents transmission of bacteria when opening sterile specimen container.

Step 6 For the patient using a bedpan, raise the head of the bed to a semi-Fowler's position.

Facilitates correct direction of urine flow down into the specimen container you are holding. Additionally, this is the anatomical position for voiding.

Step 7 Open the sterile specimen container, being careful not to touch the inside of the lid or container.

Prevents the contamination of the specimen.

Step 8 Holding the container near the meatus, instruct the patient to begin voiding. Some resources suggest holding the female labia apart during this step (or teaching self-care patients to do so). For the male patient who is unable to assist, it will be necessary to hold the penis.

Clears the distal urethra of bacteria, keeping skin bacteria from contaminating the urine specimen.

Step 9 Allow a small stream of urine to pass, and then place the specimen container into the stream, collecting approximately 30 to 60 mL. Do not let the end of the male patient's penis touch the inside of the container; do not touch the female perineum with the container.

Prevents specimen contamination.

Step 10 Remove the container from the stream, and allow the patient to finish emptying his bladder. *Note:* If the penis is uncircumcised, replace the foreskin over the glans when the procedure is finished.

Step 11 Carefully replace the container lid, touching only the outside of the cap and container. Clean the outside of the container of urine, if necessary.

Maintains sterility of specimen; prevents cross-contamination of others with urine.

PROCEDURE 27–1

Collecting a Clean-Catch Urine Specimen
(continued)

Step 12 Label the container with the correct patient information (in many institutions, labels are preprinted or bar-coded). Place the container in a facility-specific carrier (usually a plastic bag) for transport to the lab.

Step 13 Remove your gloves and wash your hands. If the specimen has been obtained from a patient on a bedpan, leave your gloves on until you have removed, emptied, and stored the bed-pan properly.

Prevents bacteria transmission.

Step 14 Assist the patient back to bed, or remove the bedpan, if applicable. (See Procedure 28-2 for removing a bedpan.)

Step 15 Transport the specimen to the lab in a timely manner.

Delayed testing can cause inaccurate test results (e.g., casts in the urine will break up if urine is allowed to sit for an extended period of time).

Evaluation
- Note any unusual characteristics of the urine (e.g., color, odor).
- Note any difficulties with urination (e.g., pain, dribbling, difficulty beginning).

Patient Teaching
Teach cognitively intact ambulatory patients to complete the steps of this procedure independently.

Home Care
- Teach the patient the steps of the procedure, focusing on how to maintain sterility of the specimen.
- Tell the patient to refrigerate the specimen until it can be transported to the lab. Instruct the patient to place the specimen in a plastic bag, separate it from food items, and label it appropriately.
- Teach the patient that prepackaged antiseptic wipes cannot be flushed down the toilet.
- Instruct the menstruating woman that perineal cleansing is especially important. The woman may use a tampon to prevent leakage during specimen collection. Instruct her to notify the lab that she is menstruating.

Documentation
- Document in the records, per agency protocol, the time and date that the specimen was collected.

Some facilities have a running sheet of procedures that are crossed off when they are completed. Other facilities have nurses chart specimen collection in the nurse's notes.

- Document the characteristics of the urine: color, odor, and so on.
- Document any difficulty with voiding.
- If the patient's intake and output are being recorded, remember to document the specimen amount on the I&O flowsheet.

PROCEDURE 27–2   Inserting a Urinary Catheter

➤ For steps to follow in *all* procedures, refer to the inside back cover of this book.

critical aspects

- Take an extra pair of sterile gloves and an extra sterile catheter into the room.
- Be sure that you have good lighting, especially if the patient is a woman. Take a procedure lamp to the bedside if necessary.
- Work on the right side of the bed if you are right-handed; the left side, if you are left-handed.
- Drape the patient for privacy.
- Perform perineal care before the procedure; wash your hands; open the kit.
- Don sterile gloves and maintain sterile technique while manipulating kit supplies and performing the procedure.
- Once you have touched the patient with your nondominant hand, do not remove that hand from the patient.
- Lubricate the catheter tip before insertion.
- Insert the catheter 5 to 7.5 cm (2 to 3 in.) for women, 17 to 22.5 cm (7 to 9 in.) for men, until urine flows.
- Drain the bladder; collect needed samples; measure urine; and connect the drainage bag as needed.

Equipment

- Washcloth and towel
- Soap and water
- 1 pair of clean procedure gloves
- Catheter insertion kit containing:
  – Sterile gloves
  – Urinary catheter
  – Antiseptic cleansing agent
  – Forceps
  – Cotton balls

  – Sterile waterproof drapes (one fenestrated)
  – Sterile lubricant
  – Urine receptacle
  – Specimen container
- Extra pair of sterile gloves and extra sterile catheter

Prevents the need to leave the bedside to obtain additional supplies should the gloves or catheter become contaminated.

- Bath blanket
- Procedure lamp or flashlight
- 2% lidocaine (Xylocaine) gel (according to agency policy and patient need)

Delegation

In some institutions, unlicensed assitive personnel (UAPs) undergo special training to learn this skill. In such instances, you may delegate this task to the UAP. However, you must complete the following assessments and instruct the UAP when to stop the procedure and what abnormal findings to report. Otherwise, you should not delegate catheter insertion to a UAP.

Straight catheter kit

PROCEDURE 27–2   Inserting a Urinary Catheter *(continued)*

Assessment

- Assess the patient's cognitive level.

To determine whether the patient will be able to follow instructions.

- Assess for the presence of conditions that may impair the patient's ability to assume the necessary position.

To determine whether you will need assistance to help the patient maintain the correct position for catheter insertion.

- Assess the presence and degree of bladder distention.

To establish a baseline assessment.

- Determine time of last voiding or last catheterization.

To gain information you need to interpret the significance of the amount of urine obtained in this catheterization.

- Assess the general body size of the patient and size of the urinary meatus.

You may need to choose a different size catheter.

- Determine whether the patient has an allergy to iodine (if that is the antiseptic solution in the kit).

If the patient is allergic to iodine, you will need to use an alternative antibacterial agent other than povodine-iodine (Betadine).

- Determine whether the patient has an allergy to latex.

Many catheters are made of latex.

- Note signs and symptoms of bladder infection (e.g., elevated temperature, urinary frequency, dysuria).
- Note conditions (e.g., enlarged prostate in men) that may make it difficult to pass the catheter.
- Assess the need for extra lighting.

It is sometimes difficult to visualize a woman's urinary meatus. Supplemental, direct lighting helps.

PROCEDURE 27–2A   Inserting a Straight Urinary Catheter

Procedural Steps

Note: Allow adequate time for this procedure: Experienced nurses need at least 15 minutes. You will need more time if problems arise—and even more time if you are a novice.

Note: If lighting is poor and you cannot see the urinary meatus, ask an assistant to hold an extra light source, such as a flashlight.

Step 1 Place the patient supine, in a position to allow you to see and access the urinary meatus.

The urinary meatus is sometimes difficult to visualize on women because it may resemble skinfolds or other anatomical landmarks in the area.

a. *For women:* Flex the patient's knees, and place her feet flat on the bed (dorsal recumbent position). Instruct the patient to relax her thighs and allow them to rotate externally. *Note:* If the patient is confused, unable to follow directions, or unable to hold her legs in the correct position, obtain help.

You may need help both for patient comfort and for protecting your sterile field.

b. *For women who are unable to maintain dorsal recumbent position:* Use Sims' position (side-lying with the upper leg flexed at the hip). Cover the rectal area.

Prevents contamination from that area to the urethra and provides privacy.

c. *For men:* Position the patient in the supine position, with legs straight and slightly apart.

Allows easy access to the urinary meatus.

Step 2 If you are right-handed, stand and work at the patient's right side; if you are left-handed, stand and work on the patient's left side.

➤

PROCEDURE 27–2A   Inserting a Straight Urinary Catheter *(continued)*

Step 3 Drape the patient. (See Procedure 22-4 for draping.)

These methods preserve modesty and a feeling of security, while ensuring that you can expose the urinary meatus easily.

a. *For women:* Fold the blanket in a diamond shape, wrapping the corners around the patient's legs and folding the upper corner down over the perineum. ▼

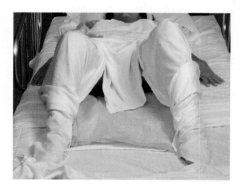

b. *For men:* Cover the patient's upper body with a blanket; fold bedsheets down to expose the penis.

Step 4 Don clean procedure gloves. Lift the corner of the privacy drape to expose the perineum; wash the perineal area with soap and water; dry. At the same time, visualize and locate the urinary meatus (for women).

Cleanses the area of skin bacteria, preventing transmission of microorganisms into the bladder. Locating the meatus during this step, especially if the patient is a woman, will help prevent delays at subsequent steps when it is important to maintain sterile technique.

Step 5 *For men:* If you are using 2% lidocaine (Xylocaine) gel, use a syringe (no needle) to insert it into the urethra now.

You will need to wait at least 5 minutes for the gel to take effect before inserting the catheter.

Step 6 Remove and discard gloves. Wash your hands.

Step 7 Organize the work area:
a. Arrange the bedside table or overbed table within your reach.
b. Open the sterile catheter kit according to directions, and place it on the bedside table.
c. Position a plastic bag or other trash receptacle so that you will not have to reach across the sterile field (between the patient's legs) to dispose of soiled cotton balls and so forth. For example, you may have a trash can on the floor beside the bed, or a trash bag on the bed near, but not between, the patient's feet.

Carrying contaminated objects above a sterile field can contaminate the field. The outer wrapping of the catheter kit may be used for collecting discarded waste.

d. Position the procedure light, or have an assistant hold a flashlight.

Step 8 Apply sterile drape(s) and underpad.

These drapes provide sterile work surfaces and help prevent contaminating your gloves and sterile supplies.

Variation Waterproof Drape Packed as Top Item in the Kit

a. Place the sterile underpad:
   1) *For women:* Remove the underpad from the kit carefully before donning sterile gloves. Do not touch other kit items. Allow the drape to fall open as you remove it from the kit. Place the drape flat on the bed, and tuck the top edge under the buttocks, taking care to touch only the corners of the drape.
   2) *For men:* Drop the sterile underpad across the thighs.
b. Don sterile gloves: Remove the sterile glove package, and don sterile gloves (see Procedure 20-5). *Note:* Once you have donned the sterile gloves, you may touch

items inside the catheter kit, arranging the supplies as needed.
c. Place the fenestrated drape: This has a hole in the center. Pick up the drape, allowing it to unfold as you remove it, without touching any other objects from the kit. For women, place the drape over the perineum with the hole over the labia. For men, place the fenestrated drape with the center hole over the penis. You will pull the penis up and through the opening when cleansing the meatus.

Variation Sterile Gloves Packed as Top Item in the Kit

d. Don sterile gloves: Remove the sterile glove package and don sterile gloves (see Procedure 20-5). *Note:* Once you have donned the sterile gloves, you may touch any item inside the catheter kit, arranging the supplies as needed.
e. Place the sterile underpad: Grasp the edges of the sterile drape. Fold the entire edge down (2.5 to 5 cm) (1 to 2 in.) and toward you, making a "cuff" to protect your gloves. Take care not to touch unsterile objects with your gloves or the drape.
   1) *For women:* Carefully slide the drape under the patient's buttocks without contaminating your gloves. Ask the patient to raise her hips slightly if she can. ▼

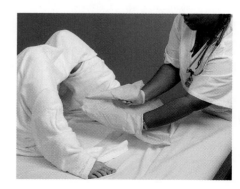

   2) *For men:* Drop the sterile underpad across thighs.

PROCEDURE 27–2A   Inserting a Straight Urinary Catheter *(continued)*

f. Place the fenestrated drape: Pick up the drape, allowing it to unfold as you remove it, without touching any other objects. Protect sterility as you did with the underpad (preceding step).

  1) *For women:* Place the fenestrated drape over the perineum so that the hole is over the labia. ▼

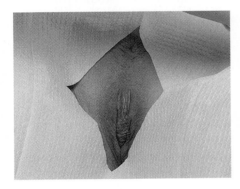

  2) *For men:* Place the fenestrated drape so that the center hole is over the penis. You will pull the penis up and through the opening when cleansing the meatus.

Step 9 Organize kit supplies on the sterile field, and prepare the supplies in the kit.

a. Open the antiseptic packet. Pour the solution over the cotton balls. *Note:* Some kits contain a packet of sterile antiseptic swabs. Open the end of the packet where you feel the "stick," leaving the swabs covered by the remainder of the packet.

b. Lay the forceps near the cotton balls.

c. Open the specimen container, if you are to collect a specimen.

d. Remove any unneeded supplies, such as a urine specimen container, from the urine collection basin.

e. Open the packet of sterile lubricant.

f. Remove the plastic covering (if there is one) from the catheter.

g. Squeeze sterile lubricant into the kit tray; lubricate the catheter by rolling it slowly in the lubricant.

  1) *For women:* Lubricate the first 2.5 to 5 cm (1 to 2 in.) of the catheter.

  2) *For men:* Do not lubricate the catheter if you have already inserted a lubricant (Xylocaine gel) directly into the urethra.

Allows for ease of insertion of the catheter. Prevents trauma to the mucosa.

Step 10 Cleanse the urinary meatus.

a. *For women:*

  1) Place your nondominant hand above the labia, and with your thumb and forefinger spread the patient's labia, pulling up (or anteriorly) at the same time, to expose the urinary meatus. Hold this position throughout the procedure—firm pressure is necessary. *If the labia slip back over the urinary meatus, it is considered contaminated, and you will need to repeat the cleansing procedure.*

When a woman is supine, gravity may cause tissues above the meatus to fall

downward and obscure the meatus from sight. Once placed on the patient's perineal area, your hand is considered contaminated, and you should not move it.

  2) With your dominant hand, pick up a wet cotton ball with the forceps and cleanse the perineal area, taking care not to contaminate your sterile glove. Use one stroke for each area, wiping from front (clitoris) to back (anus). Using a new cotton ball for each area, proceed in this order: Wipe the far labium majus, the near labium majus, inside far labium, inside near labium, and directly down the center over the urinary meatus. If the kit has only three cotton balls, cleanse only the inside far labium minora, inside near labium, and down the center directly over the meatus.

b. *For men:*

  1) With your nondominant hand, reach through the opening in the fenestrated drape and grasp the penis, taking care not to contaminate the surrounding drape. If the penis is uncircumcised, retract the foreskin to fully expose the meatus. *If the foreskin accidentally falls over meatus and does not remain retracted or if you drop the penis during cleansing, you must repeat the cleansing procedure.*

Allows for full cleansing of the area.

➤

PROCEDURE 27–2A   Inserting a Straight Urinary Catheter *(continued)*

(2) Continuing to hold the penis with your nondominant hand, hold the forceps in your dominant hand and pick up a cotton ball. Starting at the meatus, cleanse the glans in a series of circular motions and partially down the shaft of the penis. Repeat with at least one more cotton ball.

Following the "clean-to-dirty" principle prevents recontamination of the cleansed area. ▼

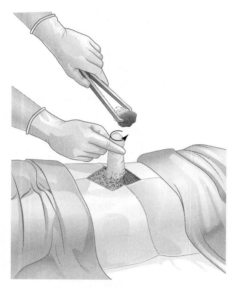

Step 11 Discard the used cotton balls as you use them, taking care not to move them across the open and sterile kit.

Prevents contamination of the sterile field.

Step 12 Prepare the urine receptacle. Place the plastic urine receptacle close enough to the urinary meatus so that the end of the catheter rests inside the container as urine drains.

a. *For women:* Place 10 cm (4 in.) from the meatus (women).

b. *For men:* Place the container between the patient's thighs.

The end of the catheter will need to reach into the container to catch the draining urine.

Step 13 Insert the catheter.

a. *For women:*

1) Ask the woman to bear down as though she is trying to void; slowly insert the end of the catheter into the meatus. Have the patient take slow, deep breaths until the initial discomfort has passed.

Helps relax the external sphincter and makes insertion easier and more comfortable.

2) Continue inserting the catheter gently until urine flows, for a distance of 5 to 7.5 cm (2 to 3 in.). After you see urine, insert the catheter another 2.5 to 5 cm (1 to 2 in.). You may feel slight resistance as the catheter goes through the sphincters. Twist the catheter slightly or apply gentle pressure, but do not force the catheter.

Deep breathing helps to relax the sphincters. Forcing may damage mucosa. Insert the catheter more deeply after urine flow to be sure the catheter is well into the bladder so that the bladder can empty completely.

3) If the catheter touches the labia or unsterile linens, or if you inadvertently place it in the vagina, it is contaminated; you must insert a new, sterile catheter. Leave the contaminated catheter in the vagina while you are inserting the new one into the meatus.

Helps you to avoid making the same mistake again.

b. *For men:*

1) Using your nondominant hand, hold the penis gently but firmly at a 90° angle to the body, exerting gentle traction.

Holding the penis at 90° and supporting the shaft with the fingers straightens the urethra, easing insertion of the catheter.

2) If you have not inserted lidocaine gel into the urethra, make sure the kit contains a prefilled syringe of lubricant rather than a packet of lubricant. Gently insert the tip of the prefilled syringe into the urethra and instill the lubricant. If the kit contains only a single packet of lubricant and if no other kits are available, then lubricate 12.5 to 17.5 cm (5 to 7 in.) of the catheter. This is not the technique of choice, however.

Allows for ease of insertion of the catheter and minimizes injury to urethral mucosa.

3) Ask patient to bear down as though trying to void; slowly insert the end of the catheter into the meatus. Have the patient take slow, deep breaths until the initial discomfort has passed.

Helps relax the external sphincter and makes insertion easier and more comfortable. ▼

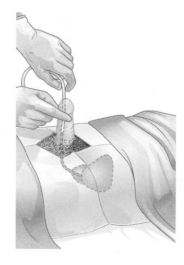

PROCEDURE 27–2A   Inserting a Straight Urinary Catheter *(continued)*

4) Continue inserting the catheter to about 17.5 to 22.5 cm (7 to 9 in.) or until urine flows. If you feel resistance, withdraw the catheter. Do not force against resistance. When urine appears, advance catheter 2.5 to 5 cm (1 to 2 in.) more.

You will commonly feel resistance at the prostatic sphincter. Hold the catheter firmly against the sphincter until the sphincter relaxes, and then advance it; but do not force it.

5) Lower the penis to allow the bladder to drain.

Step 14 Manage the catheter and or/urine collection device.
a. Continue to hold the catheter securely with your nondominant hand while the urine drains from the bladder.

Prevents catheter from being expelled by bladder or urethral contractions.

b. If you are to collect a urine specimen, use your dominant hand to take the specimen container and put it into the flow of urine until you obtain the correct amount of urine. Cap the container, maintaining sterile technique. See Procedure 27-1.

Prevents contamination of the specimen.

c. When the flow of urine has ceased and the bladder has been emptied, pinch the catheter and slowly withdraw it from the meatus. Discard the catheter.

Research (Nyman, Schwenk, & Silverstein, 1997) indicates that there is no longer a concern about the occurrence of hypotension or hematuria following the rapid removal of large volumes of urine. However, check your facility policy (some say not to remove more than 800 to 1000 mL). Pinching prevents urine from dribbling out of the end of the catheter.

d. Remove the urine-filled receptacle, and set it aside to be emptied when the procedure is finished.

Prevents spillage of the urine onto the bed.

Step 15 Cleanse the patient's perineal area as needed; dry. Replace the foreskin if it was retracted.

Removes residual antiseptic solution from the area, an especially important step if you used povidone-iodine (Betadine). Betadine left on intact healthy skin can cause irritation.

Prevents paraphimosis (constriction of foreskin behind the glans penis, which interferes with circulation to the glans).

Step 16 Remove your gloves and wash your hands.

Prevents transmission of bacteria.

Step 17 Return the patient to a position of comfort.

PROCEDURE 27–2B   Inserting an Indwelling Urinary Catheter

Equipment

An indwelling catheter is designed to remain in the urinary bladder. Therefore, in addition to the supplies contained in a straight-catheter kit, an indwelling catheter kit will include the following:

• A double-lumen or triple-lumen catheter with a balloon tip for inflation instead of a single-lumen rubber catheter.
• A syringe prefilled with sterile water (to inflate the catheter balloon)
• Urine collection bag with drainage tubing attached; sometimes the tubing is also attached to the catheter
• Tube holder, tape, or leg strap (to secure the catheter)
• Safety pin and elastic band (if needed to secure the tubing to the bed; you can usually use the clamp on the drainage tubing)

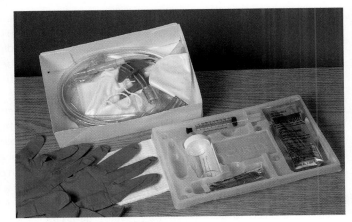

Indwelling catheter kit

➤

PROCEDURE 27–2B

Inserting an Indwelling Urinary Catheter
(continued)

Procedural Steps

Note: Allow adequate time for this procedure: Experienced nurses need at least 15 minutes. You will need more time if problems arise—and even more time if you are a novice.

Note: If lighting is poor and you cannot see the urinary meatus, ask an assistant to hold an extra light source, such as a flashlight.

Step 1 Place the patient supine, in a position to allow you to see and access the urinary meatus.

The urinary meatus is sometimes difficult to visualize on women because it may resemble skinfolds or other anatomical landmarks in the area.

a. *For women:* Flex the patient's knees, and place her feet flat on the bed (dorsal recumbent position). Instruct the patient to relax her thighs and allow them to rotate externally. *Note:* If the patient is confused, unable to follow directions, or unable to hold her legs in the correct position, obtain help.

You may need help both for patient comfort and for protecting your sterile field.

b. *For women who are unable to maintain a dorsal recumbent position:* Use Sims' position (side-lying with the upper leg flexed at the hip). Cover the rectal area.

Prevents contamination from that area to the urethra.

c. *For men:* Position the patient in the supine position, with legs straight and slightly apart.

Allows easy access to the urinary meatus.

Step 2 If you are right-handed, stand and work at the patient's right side; if you are left-handed, stand and work on the patient's left side.

Step 3 Drape the patient. (See Procedure 22-4 for draping.)

These methods preserve modesty and a feeling of security, while ensuring that you can expose the urinary meatus easily.

a. *For women:* Fold the blanket in a diamond shape, wrapping the corners around the patient's legs and folding the upper corner down over the perineum.

b. *For men:* Cover the patient's upper body with a blanket; fold the bedsheets down to expose the penis.

Step 4 Don clean procedure gloves. Lift the corner of the privacy drape to expose the perineum; wash the perineal area with soap and water; dry. At the same time, visualize and locate the urinary meatus (for women).

Cleanses the area of skin bacteria preventing transmission of microorganisms into the bladder. Locating the meatus during this step, especially for women, will help prevent delays at subsequent steps when it is important to maintain sterile technique.

Step 5 *For men:* If you are using 2% Xylocaine gel, use a syringe (no needle) to insert it into the urethra now.

You will need to wait at least 5 minutes for the gel to take effect before inserting the catheter.

Step 6 Remove and discard gloves. Wash your hands.

Step 7 Organize the work area:
a. Arrange the bedside table or overbed table within your reach.
b. Open the sterile catheter kit according to the directions, and place it on the bedside table.
c. Position a plastic bag or other trash receptacle so that you will not have to reach across the sterile field (between the patient's legs) to dispose of soiled cotton balls and so forth. For example, you may have a trash can on the floor beside the bed, or a trash bag on the bed near, but not between, the patient's feet.

Carrying contaminated objects above a sterile field can contaminate the field. The outer wrapping of the catheter kit may be used for collecting discarded waste.

d. Position the procedure light, or have an assistant hold a flashlight.

Step 8 Apply sterile drape(s) and underpad.

These drapes provide sterile work surfaces and help prevent contaminating your gloves and sterile supplies.

Variation Waterproof Drape Packed as Top Item in the Kit

a. Place the sterile underpad:
   1) *For women:* Remove the underpad from the kit carefully before donning sterile gloves. Do not touch other kit items. Allow the drape to fall open as you remove it from the kit. Place the drape flat on the bed and tuck the top edge under the buttocks, taking care to touch only the corners of the drape.
   2) *For men:* Drop the sterile underpad across thighs.
b. Don sterile gloves: Remove the sterile glove package and don sterile gloves (see Procedure 20-5). *Note:* Once you have donned the sterile gloves, you may touch any items inside the catheter kit, arranging the supplies as needed.
c. Place the fenestrated drape: This has a hole in the center. Pick up the drape, allowing it to unfold as you remove it, without touching any other objects. For women, place over the perineum with the hole over the labia. For men, place fenestrated drape with the center hole over the penis. You will pull the penis up and through the opening when cleansing the meatus.

PROCEDURE 27–2B Inserting an Indwelling Urinary Catheter
(continued)

Variation Sterile Gloves Packed as Top Item in the Kit

d. Don sterile gloves: Remove the sterile glove package and don sterile gloves (see Procedure 20-5). *Note:* Once you have donned the sterile gloves, you may touch any item inside the catheter kit, arranging the supplies as needed.

e. Place the sterile underpad: Grasp the edges of the sterile pad. Fold the entire edge down 2.5 to 5 cm (1 to 2 in.) and toward you, making a "cuff" to protect your gloves. Take care not to touch unsterile objects with your gloves or the drape.
   1) *For women:* Carefully slide the drape under the patient's buttocks without contaminating your gloves. Ask the patient to raise her hips slightly if she can.
   2) *For men:* Drop the sterile underpad across the thighs.

f. Place the fenestrated drape: Pick up the drape, allowing it to unfold as you remove it, without touching any other objects. Protect sterility as you did with the underpad (preceding step).
   1) *For women:* Place the fenestrated drape over the perineum so that the hole is over the labia.
   2) *For men:* Place the fenestrated drape so that the center hole is over the penis. You will pull the penis up and through the opening when cleansing the meatus.

Step 9 Organize the kit supplies on the sterile field, and prepare the supplies in the kit.

a. Open the antiseptic packet. Pour the solution over the cotton balls. *Note:* Some kits contain a packet of sterile antiseptic swabs. Open the end of the packet where you can feel the "stick," leaving the swabs covered by the remainder of the packet.

b. Lay the forceps near the cotton balls.

c. Open specimen container, if you are to collect a specimen.

d. Remove any unneeded supplies, such as a urine specimen container, from the urine collection basin.

e. Open the packet of sterile lubricant.
   1) *For women:* Squeeze sterile lubricant into the kit tray; lubricate the catheter by rolling it slowly in the lubricant. Lubricate the first 2.5 to 5 cm (1 to 2 in.) of the catheter.
   2) *For men:* Do not lubricate the catheter if you have already inserted a lubricant (Xylocaine gel) directly into the urethra.

f. Attach the saline-filled syringe to the side port of the catheter, and inflate the balloon. Once you have inspected it, deflate the balloon and return the catheter to the kit. Leave the syringe connected to the port.

Ensures before you insert the balloon that it does not leak. The inflated balloon keeps the catheter in the bladder. Leave the syringe attached because your nondominant hand will not be free to help attach it at a later step.

g. Touching only the box or sterile side of the wrapping, place the sterile catheter kit down onto the sterile field between the patient's legs (women) or beside or on top of the thighs (men). You may, as an alternative, set up the sterile field between the legs for a male patient.

Allows you to reach supplies during catheter insertion.

e. If the bedside bag is preconnected to the catheter itself, leave the bag on or near the sterile field until after the catheter is inserted.

The bag must hang lower than the level of the bladder so that urine can drain by gravity.

Step 10 Cleanse the urinary meatus. Discard the used cotton balls as you use them, taking care not to move them across the open and sterile kit.

Prevents contamination of the sterile field.

a. *For women:*
   1) Place your nondominant hand above the labia, and with your thumb and forefinger spread the patient's labia, pulling up (or anteriorly) at the same time, to expose the urinary meatus. Hold this position throughout the procedure—firm pressure is necessary. *If the labia slip back over the urinary meatus, it is considered contaminated and you will need to repeat the cleansing procedure.*

When a woman is supine, gravity may cause tissues above the meatus to fall downward and obscure the meatus from sight. Once placed on the patient's perineal area, your hand is considered contaminated and you should not move it.

➤

PROCEDURE 27–2B   Inserting an Indwelling Urinary Catheter
(continued)

2) With your dominant hand, pick up a swab or use forceps to pick up a wet cotton ball and cleanse the perineal area, taking care not to contaminate your sterile glove. Use one stroke for each area, wiping from front (clitoris) to back (anus). Using a new cotton ball for each area, proceed in this order: Wipe the far labium majora, the near labium majora, inside far labium, inside near labium, and directly down the center over the urinary meatus. If the kit has only 3 cotton balls, cleanse only the inside far labium minora, inside near labium, and down the center directly over the meatus. ▼

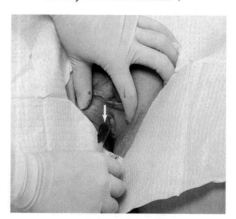

b. *For men:*
1) With your nondominant hand, reach through the opening in the fenestrated drape and grasp the penis, taking care not to contaminate the surrounding drape. If the penis is uncircumcised, retract the foreskin to fully expose the meatus. *If the foreskin accidentally falls over the meatus or if you drop the penis during cleansing, you must repeat the cleansing procedure.*

Allows for full cleansing of the area.

2) Continuing to hold the penis with your nondominant hand, hold the forceps in your dominant hand and pick up a cotton ball. Starting at the meatus, cleanse the glans in a series of circular motions from the inside to the outside and partially down the shaft of the penis. Repeat with at least one more cotton ball.

Following the "clean-to-dirty" principle prevents recontamination of the cleansed area.

Step 11   With your dominant hand, hold the catheter approximately 7.5 cm (3 in.) from the proximal end, keeping the rest of the catheter coiled in the palm of your hand or make sure the distal end of the catheter is connected to the drainage bag.

Keeps from soiling the bed.

Step 12   Insert the catheter.
a. *For women:*
1) Ask the woman to bear down as though she is trying to void; slowly insert the end of the catheter into the meatus. Have the patient take slow, deep breaths until the initial discomfort has passed.

Helps relax the external sphincter and makes insertion easier and more comfortable. ▼

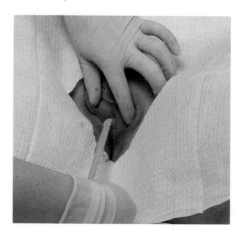

2) Continue inserting the catheter gently until urine flows. The distance is about 5 to 7.5 cm (2 to 3 in.) in a woman. After you see urine, insert the catheter another 2.5 to 5 cm (1 to 2 in.). You may feel slight resistance as the catheter goes through the sphincters. Twist the catheter slightly or apply gentle pressure, but do not force the catheter.

Forcing the catheter may damage mucosa. Insert the catheter more deeply after urine flows to be sure the catheter is well into the bladder so that complete emptying can occur.

3) If the catheter touches the labia or unsterile linens, or if you inadvertently place it in the vagina, it is contaminated and you must insert a new, sterile catheter. Leave the contaminated catheter in the vagina while you are inserting the new one into the meatus.

Helps you to avoid making the same mistake again.

b. *For men:*
1) Using your nondominant hand, hold the penis gently but firmly at a 90° angle to the body, exerting gentle traction.

PROCEDURE 27–2B

Inserting an Indwelling Urinary Catheter
(continued)

Holding the penis at 90° and supporting the shaft with the fingers straightens the urethra, easing insertion of the catheter.

2) Before beginning the procedure, make sure that the catheter kit contains a prefilled syringe or lubricant rather than a packet of lubricant. Gently insert the tip of the prefilled syringe into the urethra and instill the lubricant (unless you have already inserted Xylocaine gel). If the kit contains only a single packet of lubricant and if no other kits are available, then lubricate 5 to 7 inches (12.5 to 17.7 cm) of the catheter. This is not the technique of choice, however.

Allows for ease of insertion of the catheter and minimizes injury to urethral mucosa.

3) Ask the patient to bear down as though trying to void; slowly insert the end of the catheter into the meatus. Have the patient take slow deep breaths until the initial discomfort has passed.

Helps relax the external sphincter and makes insertion easier and more comfortable.

4) Continue inserting the catheter to the bifurcation. If you feel resistance, withdraw the catheter. Do not force against resistance. When urine appears, advance catheter 2.5 to 5 cm (1 to 2 in.) more.

You will commonly feel resistance at the prostatic sphincter. Hold the catheter firmly against the sphincter until the sphincter relaxes. Then advance it, but do not force it.

5) Lower the penis. When bladder is drained, replace the foreskin.

Prevents paraphimosis (constriction of foreskin behind the glans penis, interfering with circulation to the glans).

Step 13 Manage the catheter or urine collection device.
a. Continue to hold the catheter securely with the your nondominant hand until the urine begins to flow. After urine flows, stabilize the catheter's position in the urethra, and use your other hand to pick up the saline-filled syringe; inflate the catheter balloon.

Prevents the catheter from being expelled by the bladder or urethral contractions. The inflated balloon prevents the catheter from slipping out of the bladder. ▼

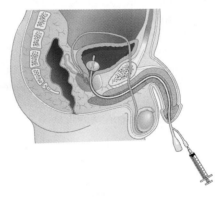

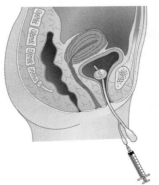

b. If the patient complains of pain on inflation of the balloon, allow the water to drain out of the balloon, and reposition the catheter by advancing it 1 inch (2.5 cm).

Pain usually indicates that the balloon was in the urethra instead of in the bladder.

c. Connect the drainage bag to the end of the catheter if it is not already preconnected. Hang the drainage bag on the side of the bed, below the level of the bladder.

Promotes adequate urinary drainage, preventing urinary stasis.

d. Using tape or a catheter strap, secure the catheter to the thigh. For men, you can secure the tape either to the thigh or the abdomen.

Prevents urethral irritation related to tugging or pulling of the catheter.

Step 14 Cleanse the patient's perineal area as needed; dry.

Removes residual antiseptic solution from the area, an especially important step if you used Betadine. Betadine left on intact healthy skin can cause irritation.

Step 15 Remove your gloves and wash your hands.

Prevents transmission of bacteria.

Step 16 Return the patient to a position of comfort.

►

PROCEDURE 27–2   **Inserting a Urinary Catheter** *(continued)*

Evaluation

- Note any difficulty with catheter insertion.

Can indicate structural problems, especially in the older male patient with an enlarged prostate gland.

- Note the characteristics of the urine obtained (e.g., amount, color, odor, presence of sediment or mucus).
- Continue to assess that drainage is not obstructed and that the drainage bag is below the level of the bladder.
- Assess for absence of bladder distention.

Indicates whether the bladder has been emptied. *Note:* Some facilities have a bladder-scanning device that will allow you to determine whether residual urine remains.

Home Care

You will need to teach self-catheterization to patients with compromised ability to spontaneously empty their bladders. In the home setting this is a clean procedure rather than a sterile one. It is referred to as clean intermittent self-catheterization, or CISC.

- In teaching the steps of the procedure, consider the patient's physical ability to manipulate the catheter and reach the urethra (e.g., range of motion, fine motor skills, degree of sensation).
- Home self-catheterization is a clean, rather than sterile, procedure. Teach the patient how to wash her hands before beginning. Also teach her to wash the reusable catheter in soap and water, rinse it, and store it in a clean dry place.
- The female patient must learn how to locate her urethra using a mirror.
- Teach the patient to report the signs and symptoms of urinary tract infection: burning, frequency, urgency, dull abdominal ache, fever, or malaise. Older adults may experience confusion before the other signs and symptoms occur.
- Teach the patient to drink 3000 mL of fluid per day unless contraindicated.

Variation Indwelling Catheter

In addition to the preceding, you will need to teach clients:
- When to change the catheter

Wilde (2002) suggests that patients who are at higher risk for catheter blockage may need to change catheters more frequently than the usual 4-week period.

- How to prevent catheter blockage (e.g., increase fluid intake, use bladder irrigation)

Fluids increase the urine volume, helping to reduce the deposit of sediment or other particles in the tubing.

- To empty the drainage bag frequently and to keep the bag below the level of the bladder
- How to prevent urinary tract infections (e.g., use new silver/hydrogel-coated catheters, use clean technique when inserting catheter, prevent blockage of urine outflow, avoid carbonated beverages)
- To take a shower rather than a bath, to decrease the risk for UTI
- How to prevent discomfort at the urethra
- Use of a leg bag
- To eat foods that help acidify the urine: meat, eggs, cheese, prunes, cranberries, and whole grains

PROCEDURE 27–2   Inserting a Urinary Catheter *(continued)*

Documentation

- Document the time and date of the procedure.
- Document the size of catheter used.
- Record the amount of urine obtained on the I&O portion of the graphics sheet. Record the color of urine, odor, presence of mucus, blood, and so on, in the nurse's notes.
- Record the patient's subjective statements.
- Document if you collected a specimen, and note the time it was sent to the lab.
- *For an indwelling catheter:* In addition, some facilities require that you record the amount of saline used to inflate the balloon.

Sample documentation:

5/3/07	10:00	Patient's lower abdomen mildly distended. Pt states, "I haven't urinated in 11 hours." #14F Foley catheter inserted. Spontaneous flow of clear yellow urine seen. Catheter to bedside drainage bag. Patient instructed how to carry bag when ambulating. —— S. Riley, RN

5/3/07	10:30	Patient states, "I feel so much more comfortable." S. Riley, RN

PROCEDURE 27–3 Intermittent Bladder or Catheter Irrigation

For steps to follow in *all* procedures, refer to the inside back cover of this book.

critical aspects

- Establish a sterile field under the specimen removal port or the irrigation port on a three-way catheter.
- Because of the risk of infection, never disconnect the drainage tubing from the catheter.
- Use sterile irrigation solution, warmed to room temperature.
- Instill the irrigation solution slowly.
- Repeat the process as necessary.

Equipment

For intermittent irrigation through a three-way catheter:
- Bag of sterile irrigation solution
- Connecting tubing (to connect the bag to the irrigation port)
- IV pole
- Antiseptic swabs
- Bath blanket

For intermittent irrigation via the specimen port using a syringe:
- Sterile container
- Sterile 60 mL syringe with large-gauge needle (16 to 18 Fr.)
- 2 pairs of clean procedure gloves

Delegation

Irrigation of an indwelling catheter requires nursing assessment and clinical decision making. Because of the high potential for urinary tract infection, you should not delegate this procedure to the UAP.

Assessment

- Note the characteristics of the urine (e.g., amount, color, odor, presence of clots or mucus)
- Assess for the presence and degree of bladder distention.
- Note patient complaints of discomfort.
- Assess the patient's cognitive status.

To determine patient's ability to remain still during the irrigation and the likelihood that the sterile field will be disrupted.

- Check the chart for the amount and type of sterile solution to use.
- Assess the type of catheter in place (e.g., two-way, three-way).

Procedural Steps

Note: This is the procedure for the closed methods of irrigation. The "open" method is no longer recommended. Because of the risk for infection, you would never disconnect the drainage tubing from the catheter.

Variation A

Intermittent Irrigation for the Patient with a Three-Way (Triple-Lumen) Indwelling Catheter

Step 1 Prepare the irrigation solution and connecting tubing as directed in Procedure 27-4 (steps 1 thru 5). Once the solution is connected to the irrigation port, complete the following steps.

Step 2 Prior to beginning the flow of irrigation solution, empty any urine that may be in the bedside drainage bag, and document the amount on the I&O record.

Provides a baseline for correct calculation of true urine output during irrigation.

PROCEDURE 27–3 Intermittent Bladder or Catheter Irrigation
(continued)

Step 3 Determine whether the irrigant is to remain in the bladder for any length of time. If the irrigant is to remain in the bladder for a certain time period, clamp the drainage tubing for that time.

Clamping the drainage tubing prevents immediate outflow.

Step 4 Slowly open the roller clamp on the irrigation tubing.

Slow instillation prevents patient discomfort.

Step 5 Instill or irrigate with the prescribed amount of irrigant.

Step 6 When the correct amount of irrigant has been used and/or the goals of the irrigation have been met, close the roller clamp on the irrigation tubing, leaving the tubing connected to the catheter for use during the next irrigation.

You can assess whether the goals of irrigation have been met by inspecting the color of the urine and assessing for presence of clots, mucus, or blood.

Variation B

Intermittent Irrigation for the Patient with a Two-Way Indwelling Catheter

Step 1 Don clean procedure gloves. Empty any urine currently found in the bedside drainage bag.

Prevents the transmission of bacteria. Emptying the bag will ensure accurate output results.

Step 2 Wash your hands and then reapply gloves.

Prevents the transmission of microorganisms.

Step 3 Drape the patient so that only the specimen removal port on the drainage tubing is exposed. Place a sterile waterproof drape beneath the exposed port.

Ensures patient privacy and prevents soiling of the bed linens.

Step 4 Open the sterile irrigation supplies. Pour approximately 100 mL of the irrigating solution into the sterile container, using aseptic technique.

Prevents the contamination of the irrigation solution with microorganisms.

Step 5 Swab the specimen removal port with antiseptic swab.

Cleanses the area of bacteria, preventing their transmission into the bladder.

Step 6 Draw up irrigation solution into the syringe. Insert the needle into the specimen port. Point the needle toward the bladder. (For catheter irrigation, use a total of 30 to 40 mL; for bladder irrigation the amount is usually 100 to 200 mL). *Note:* Hold the specimen port with your fingers. Do not lay the tubing or port in the palm of your hand when attempting to access the port.

Decreases the risk of sticking yourself with the needle of the irrigation syringe.

Step 7 Clamp the drainage tubing distal to the specimen port.

Prevents irrigant from going down and into the drainage bag instead of into the catheter and/or bladder.

Step 8 Inject the solution. Hold the specimen port slightly above the level of the bladder. If you meet resistance, have the patient turn slightly, and attempt a second time. If resistance continues, stop the procedure and notify the physician.

Holding the port above the level of the bladder enhances gravitational flow of irrigant into the bladder. ▼

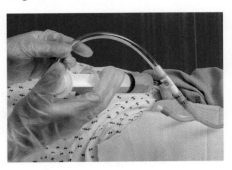

Step 9 When the irrigant has been injected, withdraw the needle. Refill the syringe if necessary. Do NOT recap the needle. If you need to repeat the irrigation, rest the needle end of the syringe in the irrigation solution container.

Decreases the likelihood of a needlestick injury and transmission of microorganisms.

Step 10 Unclamp the drainage tubing, and allow the irrigant and urine to flow into the bedside drainage bag by gravity. (If the solution is to remain in the bladder for a prescribed time, leave the tubing clamped for that time period.)

Step 11 Repeat the procedure as necessary until the prescribed amount has been instilled or until the goal of the irrigation is met (e.g., removal of clots and mucus, free flow of urine).

Step 12 Remove gloves, wash your hands, and return the patient to a position of comfort.

Prevents the transmission of microorganisms.

➤

PROCEDURE 27–3 Intermittent Bladder or Catheter Irrigation
(continued)

Evaluation

- Note the flow rate of irrigant and/or inability to instill irrigant into the catheter.
- Note the characteristics of urine output (e.g., presence of output, color, amount, clots, mucus).
- Note patient complaints of discomfort (e.g., pain, spasms).
- Assess for development of bladder distention accompanied by lack of urine outflow.

Home Care

- A patient who will be irrigating her catheter at home should be aware that the closed method offers the least risk for introducing bacteria into the bladder.
- For the syringe method, the patient will need access to syringes and needles and a process to dispose of them properly.
- Teach the patient and/or caregiver strict aseptic technique.
- Teach the signs and symptoms of urinary retention and urinary tract infection.

Documentation

- Document the time of procedure, the type of irrigant, and the total amount used.
- Document the color of urine and the presence of clots, mucus, sediment, and so on.
- Record evidence of catheter patency (e.g., flow of urine, absence of distention)

Sample documentation:

| 5/4/07 | 11:30 | Urine cloudy with many mucus shreds noted. Catheter irrigated with 60 mL of sterile normal saline. ———————— S. Riley, RN |

| 5/4/07 | 11:45 | Urine now more clear; fewer shreds. — S. Riley, RN |

PROCEDURE 27–4 Continuous Bladder Irrigation

 For steps to follow in *all* procedures, refer to the inside back cover of this book.

critical aspects

- Drape the patient, exposing the irrigation port of the indwelling catheter.
- Using aseptic technique, insert the connecting tubing into the irrigation solution container.
- Prime the tubing, removing all the air.
- Don clean procedure gloves.
- Pinch the irrigation port of the catheter; remove any plug, and connect the irrigation tubing to the port.
- Regulate the flow of the irrigant appropriately.
- Monitor for urine output.

Equipment

- Three-way (or triple-lumen) indwelling catheter in place
- Sterile irrigation solution at room temperature
- Connecting tubing
- Antiseptic swabs
- IV pole
- Bath blanket
- Measuring container
- Pair of clean procedure gloves

Delegation

You must use nursing judgment and clinical decision making when beginning continuous bladder irrigation. The flow rate is based on your knowledge of the purpose for the irrigation and the desired outcome. You should not delegate this procedure to the UAP.

Assessment

- Assess the characteristics of the urine prior to beginning the irrigation (e.g., color, presence of clots or mucus)

You should perform this assessment whether the patient already has an indwelling catheter or she is still voiding on her own.

- Assess for the presence of bladder distention.
- Assess urine output for the last 24 hours.
- Assess fall risk status and cognitive status.

The irrigation system adds extra tubing to the patient's environment, which may increase the likelihood of falls.

Procedural Steps

Step 1 If one is not already present, insert a three-way (triple-lumen) indwelling catheter. (See Procedure 27-2B.)

Provides an access for the irrigation solution.

Step 2 Prepare the irrigation fluid and tubing:
a. Roll the clamp on the connecting tubing to the "closed" position.

Prevents air from filling the tubing.

b. Spike the tubing into the appropriate portal on the irrigation solution container, using aseptic technique.

Prevents the introduction of microorganisms into the solution.

c. Invert the container, and hang it on the IV pole.

Allows the solution to flow by gravity.

d. Remove the protective cap from the distal end of the connecting tubing. Hold the end of the tubing over a sink or other receptacle. Open the roll clamp slowly, and allow the so-

lution to fill the tubing completely. Recap the tubing.

Flushes air from tubing, preventing bladder distention.

Step 3 Don clean procedure gloves.

Prevents the spread of microorganisms.

Step 4 Drape the patient so that only the connection port on the indwelling catheter is visible.

Provides patient privacy and prevents exposure of the genital area.

➤

PROCEDURE 27–4 Continuous Bladder Irrigation *(continued)*

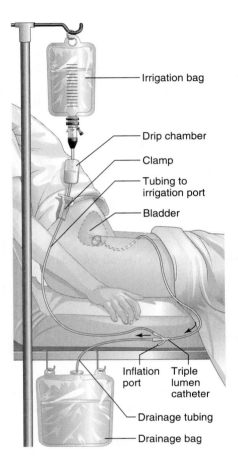

Irrigation bag

Drip chamber

Clamp

Tubing to irrigation port

Bladder

Inflation port | Triple lumen catheter

Drainage tubing

Drainage bag

Set-up for continuous bladder irrigation.

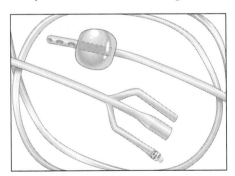

Triple lumen catheter.

Step 5 Place a sterile barrier drape under the irrigation port. Remove any plug from the port, pinching the tubing to prevent leakage of urine. Using aseptic technique, connect the end of the irrigation infusion tubing to the side port of the catheter.

Prevents the introduction of microorganisms into the bladder.

Step 6 Prior to beginning the flow of irrigation solution, empty any urine that may be in the bedside drainage bag, and document the amount on the I&O record.

Provides a baseline for correct calculation of true urine output during irrigation.

Step 7 Remove your gloves wash your hands.

Prevents the transmission of microorganisms.

Step 8 Cover the patient, and return him to a position of comfort.

Step 9 Open the roll clamp on the tubing, and regulate the flow of the irrigation solution to meet the desired outcome for the irrigation. (For example, the goal of continuous bladder irrigation for patients who have had a transurethral resection of the prostate is to keep the urine light pink to clear.)

Step 10 Monitor the flow rate for 1 to 2 minutes to ensure accuracy.

Prevents rapid introduction of solution into the bladder, which would cause patient discomfort.

PROCEDURE 27–4   **Continuous Bladder Irrigation** *(continued)*

Evaluation

At regular intervals, evaluate the:
- Flow rate of the irrigant.
- Characteristics of urine output (e.g., presence of output, color, amount, clots, mucus).
- Patient complaints of discomfort (e.g., pain, spasms).
- Development of bladder distention accompanied by lack of urine outflow.

Home Care

For patients who will have continuous bladder irrigation at home, you will need to teach the family the necessary steps.

Documentation

- Document the type and amount of irrigant.
- Note the time the irrigation was begun in the nurse's notes.
- Document the color of urine and the presence of clots or mucus.
- Record evidence of catheter patency (e.g., flow of urine, absence of distention).

Sample documentation:

10/31/06	0200	2000 mL bag of sterile normal saline irrigant hung. Urine dark pink with few dark red clots. Patient complains of some bladder spasms. ———————————— S. Riley, RN

10/31/06	0700	Urine now light pink, with rare clot. Patient offers no complaints of spasms. ———— S. Riley, RN

PROCEDURE 27–5 | Applying an External (Condom) Catheter

> For steps to follow in *all* procedures, refer to the inside back cover of this book.

critical aspects

- Application of a condom (external) catheter is a clean procedure.
- The penis should be clean and dry prior to catheter application.
- When applying the condom, stabilize the penis with your nondominant hand.
- Leave a gap of 2.5 to 5 cm (1 to 2 in.) between the condom and the tip of the penis to prevent skin irritation.
- Use only the tape supplied in the application kit to secure the catheter.
  For condom catheters that contain adhesive material on the inside of the condom, grasp the penis and gently compress the condom onto the shaft.
- Be certain that the tubing from the end of the catheter to the bedside drainage (or leg) bag is free from kinks.

Equipment

- Condom catheter
  - May have internal adhesive on the inside of the condom
  - May come with strip of special adhesive tape
- 2 pairs of clean procedure gloves
- Washcloth and towel
- Basin of soap and water
- Bath blanket
- Urine collection bag (e.g., bedside drainage bag or leg bag)
- Tape measure
- Skin prep (if allowed per your agency policy)
- Scissors

Delegation

You may delegate the application of a condom catheter to the UAP once you have completed the following assessments. Instruct the UAP to report any alterations in the skin integrity along the shaft of the penis.

Assessment

- Assess pattern of voiding (e.g., degree and time of incontinence).

To determine when the condom catheter will be applied and the length of time it will be worn.

- Assess the skin along the shaft of the penis, the glans, and the meatus (for swelling or excoriation).

The condom catheter cannot be used on excoriated, irritated skin or over areas of impaired skin integrity.

- Note the size of the penis.

There is an increased risk of nonadherence and leakage of urine in a patient with a retracted penis.

- Assess for the presence of neuropathy.

Patients with neuropathies that affect sensation in the penis may not feel skin irritation from the condom catheter and will need to be assessed more frequently.

Procedural Steps

Step 1 Prepare the leg bag or bedside drainage bag for attachment to the condom catheter by removing it from the packaging and placing the end of the connecting tubing near the perineal area.

Step 2 Place the patient in the supine position. For patients whose respiratory efforts may be impaired, raise the head of the bed to 30°.

Step 3 Fold down the bedcovers to expose the male genitalia, and drape the patient using the bath blanket.

Reduces patient embarrassment.

Step 4 Wash your hands and don clean procedure gloves.

Prevents the transmission of bacteria.

PROCEDURE 27–5   Applying an External (Condom) Catheter
(continued)

Step 5 Gently cleanse the penis with soap and water. Rinse and dry it thoroughly. If the patient is uncircumcised, retract the foreskin, cleanse the glans, and replace the foreskin.

Prevents infection and ensures a clean, dry surface that will enhance adherence of the condom catheter.

Note: McConnell (2001) suggests that excess hair along the shaft of the penis be carefully clipped off with the scissors to ensure better adherence of the condom catheter.

Step 6 Wash your hands and change procedure gloves.

Step 7 Measure the circumference of the penis. Be sure that you have a condom catheter of the appropriate size.

A catheter that is too small will impair circulation. A catheter that is too large will allow leakage of urine.

Step 8 Apply skin prep (if used by your agency), and allow it to dry. *Note:* Some external condom catheters require the placement of the special adhesive strip onto the penis prior to the application of the condom. Read the manufacture's directions.

Increases adherence.

Step 9 Hold the penis in your nondominant hand. With your dominant hand, place the condom catheter at the end of the penis, and slowly unroll it up and along the shaft. Leave 2.5 to 5 cm (1 to 2 in.) between the end of the penis and the drainage tube on the catheter.

Prevents irritation of the glans due to rubbing and allows for expansion of the penis if an erection were to occur. ▼

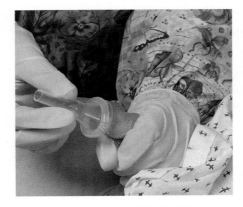

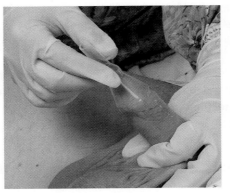

Step 10 Secure the condom catheter in place on the penis.
a. Ensure that the condom is not twisted.

Twisting can obstruct urine flow.

b. For condom catheters with internal adhesive, gently grasp the penis and compress so that the entire shaft comes in contact with the condom.

c. For condom catheters with external adhesive strips, wrap the strip around the outside of the condom in a spiral direction, taking care not to overlap the ends.

Prevents constriction of blood flow to the penis.

d. Do not use regular bandage or surgical dressing tape to hold an external condom catheter in place.

Regular surgical dressing does not expand and could lead to decreased blood flow to the penis.

Step 11 Assess the proximal end of the condom catheter. If there is a large portion of the condom still rolled above the adhesive strip, you may need to clip the roll (McConnell, 2001).

Clipping the roll prevents constriction of blood flow.

Step 12 Attach the tube end of the condom catheter to a drainage system (e.g., a leg bag). Make sure there are no kinks in the tubing.

Kinks impede the flow of urine. Urine that does not drain away from the meatus can cause irritation and skin breakdown and possibly cause the condom catheter to fall off.

Step 13 Secure the drainage tubing to the patient's thigh using tape or a commercial leg strap (follow facility protocol).

Controls movement of the tubing and accidental pulling on the condom catheter. ▼

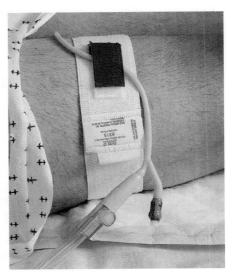

Step 14 Cover the patient. Remove your gloves, and wash your hands.

Step 15 Change the condom daily or more often if needed.

➤

PROCEDURE 27–5   **Applying an External (Condom) Catheter**
(continued)

Evaluation

Within 30 minutes of condom application, assess for:
- Urine flow (should not be obstructed)
- Swelling or discoloration of the penis

Swelling or discoloration might indicate that the condom is too tight.

Make ongoing evalutions of:
- The penis for circulatory changes
- The position and patency of the drainage tubing
- Characteristics of the urine (e.g., color, odor, bleeding)
- Patient comfort
- Leakage of urine

Home Care

Teach the patient to:
- Change the external condom catheter every 24 hours.
- Recognize the signs and symptoms of skin irritation and excoriation.
- Notify the care provider and discontinue use of the condom catheter if skin irritation or swelling occurs.
- Empty the urine collection device. The collection bag should be emptied before it becomes completely full to prevent the weight of the urine from pulling the condom catheter off.
- Not use any type of household tape to secure the condom catheter.

Documentation

- Document the date and time of application of the external condom catheter in the nurse's notes.
- Note any unusual findings in your assessment of the skin on the penis.

Sample documentation:

> 04/16/06   0900   External condom cath applied. Skin intact on penis and perineal area. ————— S. Riley, RN

> 04/16/06   0925   Scant clear, yellow urine in drainage tubing and bag. No leaks. Condom and tubing without kinks. No edema or discoloration of the penis. Patient states it "feels strange, but isn't uncomfortable." ————— S. Riley, RN

TECHNIQUES

TECHNIQUE 27–1 Measuring Voided Urine and Obtaining a Specimen

Measuring Urine Output from a Bedpan or Urinal

- Have the client void directly into the bedpan or urinal.
- While wearing clean gloves, pour the urine into a graduated cylinder or calibrated measuring device.
- Place the measuring device on a flat surface (e.g., shelf, table), and read the amount at eye level.
- Observe the urine for color, clarity, and odor.
- Discard the urine in the toilet. If a specimen is required, transfer at least 30 mL of urine to the designated container.
- Record the time and amount on the I&O record.
- Clean the measuring container.

Obtaining a Urine Specimen for Testing

After collecting the specimen, do not discard the urine in the toilet. Instead, do the following:
- Pour the urine into a specimen container that is labeled with the patient's name, the date, and the time of collection.
- Follow agency policy on additional packaging. (Many facilities require packaging the container in a specimen handling bag.)
- Transport the specimen to the lab as soon as possible. If there is a delay in getting the specimen to the lab, most facilities recommend refrigeration.

TECHNIQUE 27–2 Measuring Urine from an Indwelling Catheter

- While wearing clean gloves, place the drainage spout for the collection bag inside a calibrated measuring device.
- Unclamp the drainage spout, and direct the flow of urine into the measuring device. Avoid touching the spout to the inside of the container.
- Reclamp the spout when the collection bag is empty.
- Wipe the drainage spout with an alcohol pad, and replace the spout into the slot on the collection bag.
- Record the time and amount on the I&O record; record your observations of urine color, clarity, and odor.
- Discard the urine in the toilet.

Note:
- Measure urine output from the indwelling catheter at the end of each shift unless otherwise ordered.
- Clients who require close monitoring of I&O will have a special collection bag with a measuring chamber. Often this is used to assess hourly urine output.
- Do not use a measuring device for more than one patient.

TECHNIQUE 27–3   Obtaining a Sterile Urine Specimen from a Catheter

Supplies

- Clean gloves
- Antiseptic swab
- Sterile specimen container
- Sterile syringe with a sterile 21- to 25-gauge needle (a 5 to 10 mL syringe is usually sufficient)

Steps

- Empty the drainage tube of urine.
- Clamp the drainage tube below the level of the specimen port for 15 to 30 minutes to allow a fresh sample to collect. If the client's urine is flowing briskly, you may not need to clamp the catheter.
- Don clean gloves, and swab the specimen port with an antiseptic swab.
- Insert the needle into the specimen port, and aspirate to withdraw the amount of urine you need.
- Once you have the sample, transfer the specimen into a sterile specimen container.
- Discard the needle and syringe into the sharps container.
- Tightly cap the specimen container.
- Remove the clamp from the catheter.

- Label and package the specimen according to agency policy.
- Transport the specimen to the lab. If immediate transport is not possible, refrigerate the sample.

Note: Never disconnect the catheter from the drainage tube to obtain a sample. Interrupting the system creates a portal of entry for pathogens, thereby increasing the risk of contamination.

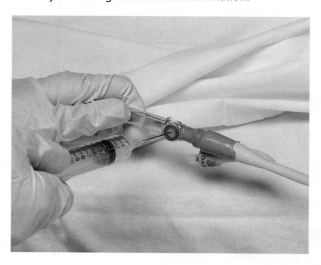

TECHNIQUE 27–4   Collecting a 24-Hour Urine Specimen

- Check with the laboratory to determine whether the specimen needs to be kept in a basin of ice during the 24-hour collection.
- Use a large collection container, and collect all urine voided in the 24-hour period. Occasionally you will be asked to collect each voiding in a separate container.
- To begin collection, have the client void, and record the time. Discard this first voiding.

- Collect all urine voided during the next 24 hours (e.g., if the first voiding was at 9:00 A.M. on Monday, collect all urine voided until 9:00 A.M. on Tuesday).
- Inform the client and all staff about the collection.
- Post signs in prominent locations, such as the client's bathroom or entry door, to remind staff of the ongoing collection.

It is essential to collect *all* urine voided during the 24-hour period.

TECHNIQUE 27–5 Dipstick Testing of Urine

- Read the kit label to be certain that you are using the correct reagent and that the kit has not passed the expiration date.
- Follow the manufacturer's directions carefully regarding the amount of urine needed.
- Select a test strip, and recap the bottle. Exposure to moisture or light can damage the remaining test strips.
- Wear clean procedure gloves when collecting and testing the urine.
- Dip the test strip into the urine, and begin timing. Follow the manufacturer's directions regarding the time needed for the reagent to develop.
- At the specified time, compare the results to the color chart. You will need good lighting to evaluate the results.

You may delegate bedside urine testing to a UAP if you know that he has the knowledge and skill to perform the procedure. Ask the UAP to report the test results to you and to save the urine sample in case you should need to repeat the test.

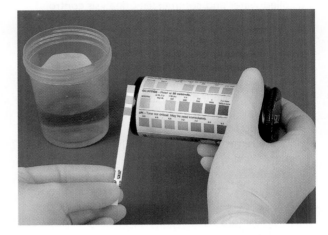

TECHNIQUE 27–6 Measuring Specific Gravity of Urine

- *Equipment:* Refractometer, procedure gloves, distilled water, dropper, small urine sample.
- Confirm the refractometer calibration by testing with distilled water and commercial urinalysis controls (follow manufacturer's instructions).
- Use fresh urine; if you cannot perform the test within 1 hour, refrigerate the specimen.
- Clean the surface of the cover and prism with a dampened lens paper; dry with lens paper. Close the cover.
- Wearing procedure gloves, use the dropper to place 1 or 2 drops of urine on the prism surface (at the notched bottom of the cover).
- Hold the refractometer horizontally, and turn toward a bright light.
- Rotate the eyepiece until the scale is in focus.
- Read the scale at the point where the dividing line between bright and dark fields crosses the scale. The scale reads from 1.000 to 1.035 in increments of 0.001.
- Record the results.
- When you are finished, dry the refractometer, and add a drop of distilled water to cleanse the prism. Dry the prism with lens paper.

Source: Point of care (posted December 2000). Procedures: Specific gravity procedure, refractometer. Retrieved May 20, 2004, from http://www.pointofcare.net/procedures/SpecificGravityProcedure.htm. Website hosted by Medical Automation Systems, Charlottesville, VA.

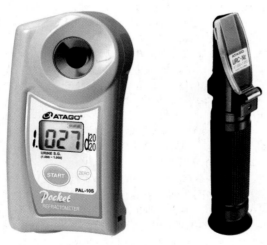

A refractometer indicates urine concentration by measuring the extent to which a beam of light is refracted ("bent") when it is passed through the urine. (Photo courtesy of Atogo USA, Inc., Bellevue, WA)

Variation: Testing Specific Gravity With a Hydrometer (Urinometer)

Note: This method is less desirable because it is slightly less precise, requires 20 to 30 mL of urine, and poses the risk of spilling urine. However, it is easy to do and cost-effective, so you may still find it used in practice.

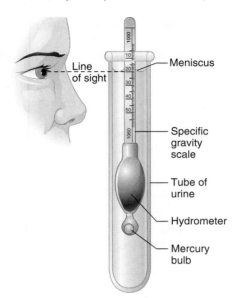

A hydrometer measures specific gravity using the principle that the higher the concentration of solid substances in a liquid, the higher a body will float. Read the hydrometer at eye level.

- *Equipment:* a test tube or cylinder and a calibrated hydrometer (urinometer).
- Wear procedure gloves.
- Obtain freshly voided urine sample, at least 20 mL.
- Pour at least 20 mL of the urine into the cylinder.
- Carefully place the hydrometer in the urine, with the weighted bulb at the bottom. Use caution when handling the glass hydrometer to avoid breaking it.
- Spin the urinometer gently to keep it from sticking to the sides of the tube.
- Hold the urinometer at eye level, and read the number at the bottom of the meniscus at the surface of the urine.
- Discard the urine.
- Clean the equipment with soap and water.
- Document the test results.
- Some older hydrometers may have mercury in the base. They should be replaced with newer ones that have steel weights in the base.

Interpreting the Test

Recall that the normal range for urine specific gravity is 1.002 to 1.028. The depth to which the hydrometer sinks indicates the specific gravity. The hydrometer floats better in concentrated urine, so the reading will be high. In dilute urine, it will sink more, so the reading will be lower.

TECHNIQUE 27–7 Caring for a Patient with an Indwelling Catheter

An indwelling catheter is connected to a drainage tube and collection bag, which constitute a closed system.

Nursing Goals

1. Prevent urinary tract infection.
2. Maintain free flow of urine.
3. Prevent transmission of pathogens to others.
4. Promote normal urinary elimination.
5. Maintain perineal skin integrity.

Goal 1: Prevent Urinary Tract Infection

- Do not disconnect the tubing or open the drainage system at any point. For example, do not disconnect the system to obtain specimens or measure the urine. A closed system minimizes the chance for pathogens to enter the system and infect the urinary tract.
- Regularly check connections between the catheter and drainage tubing and the drainage tube and collection bag. Any breaks in the system cause leaks and serve as entry points for pathogens.
- If the system inadvertently becomes disconnected at any connection, wipe the ends of both tubes with antiseptic before reconnecting them.
- If the catheter becomes soiled from drainage or feces, cleanse the catheter with mild soap and water by cleaning from the meatus outward. Rinse the catheter well, and pat it dry. This removes the medium for growth of microorganisms.
- Empty the collection bag at least every 8 hours and more frequently if urine output is high. This prevents stagnation of urine.
- When emptying the collection bag, avoid touching the spout to any surfaces. If the spout is accidentally contaminated, cleanse it with an antiseptic (e.g., alcohol or Betadine).
- Always make sure the collection bag is placed below the level of the bladder. Never place the bag on the bed. This prevents backflow of stale urine into the bladder.
- Assist the patient to take a shower regularly if his condition permits.
- Encourage foods that increase urine acidity (e.g., cranberry juice, prunes, plums, tomatoes, meat, cheese, citrus fruits, and eggs). This discourages bacterial growth.
- Teach the patient to report signs of UTI (e.g., burning at the meatus); observe for cloudy, strong-smelling urine, chills, or fever.

- Change the indwelling catheter only when necessary. Some agencies have a policy specifying that catheters be changed at specified intervals (e.g., weekly). However, this is not advisable because the more often a catheter is changed, the more likely an infection will develop. The catheter needs to be changed when any of the following occurs:

    Sediment collects in the tubing or the catheter.

    The urine does not drain well.

    The sandy particles that build up inside the drainage tubing cannot be freed by rolling the tubing between your hands.

Goal 2: Maintain Free Flow of Urine

Maintaining free flow of urine prevents backflow of urine into the bladder, which can cause bladder distention and injury. Stasis of urine also provides a medium for growth of microorganisms.

- Make sure the tubing and bag remain below the level of the bladder to prevent backflow. Urine drains by gravity in this system.
- If the collecting bag must be higher than the bladder at any time, you must clamp the catheter to prevent backflow of stagnant urine into the bladder.
- Frequently inspect the tubing to ensure that urine flows freely in the tubing. Any kinks, coils, or compression of the catheter or tubing may impede flow and cause backup into the bladder.
- If urine is not flowing, check to be sure the patient is not lying on the tubing.
- Do not allow the collection bag to lie on the floor. This decreases the effect of gravity. It also increases the likelihood of contamination.

Goal 3: Prevent Transmission of Infection

When providing catheter care, observe universal precautions:

- Wear gloves when handling the catheter or drainage system to prevent possible exposure to body fluids.
- Always wash your hands before and after providing care to any client, including one with an indwelling catheter.

Goal 4: Promote Normal Urine Production

Adequate urine production flushes pathogens out of the bladder, provides natural irrigation of the tubing, and prevents stasis of urine.

➤

Caring for a Patient with an Indwelling Catheter *(continued)*

- Unless contraindicated by other health problems, encourage oral intake of at least 8 to 10 glasses (approximately 3000 mL) of fluid per day. For patients who are unable to take oral liquid, provide an equivalent amount of parenteral or enteral fluids.
- Monitor the patient's intake and output at least every 8 hours. More frequent monitoring may be required if the patient is experiencing fluid and electrolyte problems. Although the urine collection bag has volume markings, they are only approximate.
- For accurate determination of output, you must empty the urine into an accurately calibrated container.
- Observe the urine output for color and characteristics. Report evidence of blood, sediment, or infection to the primary care provider.
- Encourage the patient to be active and out of bed as much as possible.

Goal 5: Maintain Skin and Mucosal Integrity

Perineal skin and mucosa can be irritated by feces and by movement or encrustation of the catheter.

- Although the inflated balloon helps maintain the catheter in the bladder, you will need to secure the tubing to the leg to prevent traction on the bladder. Secure the tubing by taping it to the thigh or applying a Velcro band to the thigh through which the tubing is secured. For men, if the catheter will remain in place for an extended period, you should secure the tubing to the abdomen to prevent damage to the penile-scrotal juncture. Failure to secure the tubing may cause significant injury to the bladder neck and urethra.
- Routine hygiene care normally provides adequate cleanliness. Cleanse the area around the meatus with mild soap and water daily, after each bowel movement, and more often if there is drainage or excessive sweating. Be sure to carefully rinse the area well and pat dry to avoid irritating the skin.
- Avoid using powders or lotions in the perineal area.
- Monitor the urethral meatus and upper drainage tube. Encrustation, as evidenced by sandy particles at the meatus, is irritating to the mucosa and signals a need to change the catheter.

TECHNIQUE 27–8 Removing an Indwelling Catheter

Equipment

- Syringe (to deflate the catheter balloon; 5 to 30 mL, depending on balloon size)
- Towel or drape
- Hygiene supplies (washcloth, warm water, a second towel)

Steps to Remove the Catheter

- Wash hands before and after removing the catheter.
- Wear clean gloves during the removal.
- Explain that this procedure is nearly always pain-free.
- Have the patient assume a supine position.
- Place the catheter receptacle near the patient (e.g., on the bed).
- Place a towel or waterproof drape between the patient's legs and up by the urethral meatus.
- Obtain a sterile specimen (see Technique 27-3), if needed. Some agencies require a culture and sensitivity test of the urine when an indwelling catheter is removed.
- Remove the tape securing the catheter to the patient.
- Deflate the balloon completely by inserting a syringe into the balloon valve and aspirating the fluid. Verify that the total fluid volume has been removed by checking the balloon size written on the valve port. If you cannot aspirate all the fluid, do not pull on the catheter, because you may injure the urethra. Report to the charge nurse or the primary care provider before continuing the procedure.
- Have the patient relax and take a few deep breaths as you slowly withdraw the catheter from the urethra.
- Wrap the catheter in the towel or drape.
- Use warm water and a washcloth to cleanse the perineal area. A mild soap may also be used. Be sure to rinse well if you use soap.
- Measure the urine and then empty it in the toilet; discard the catheter, drainage tube, and collection bag in the biohazard waste.
- Explain to the patient that you need to monitor the first few voidings after catheter removal to ensure that he does not have difficulty reestablishing bladder control and to observe for signs of infection. If the patient toilets independently, ask him to notify you when he voids and to save the urine. Place a receptacle in the toilet or commode.
- Encourage the patient to increase fluid intake if not contraindicated by other health conditions.
- Record the date and time of the procedure; the amount, color, and clarity of the urine; and your patient teaching.
- Monitor the next few voidings. Note the time of the first voiding and the amount voided. Observe the urine for color, odor, and presence of blood. Compare voidings over the next 8 to 10 hours to the patient's intake, and monitor for bladder distention.

TECHNIQUE 27–9 Managing Urinary Incontinence

Most urinary incontinence (UI) is managed with skin care and behavioral interventions, but medications and other collaborative treatments are sometimes used.

Perineal Skin Care

- Provide dry clothing and bedding as soon as possible after incontinence occurs.
- Wash the perineum with soap and warm water after each episode to remove urine from the skin. Rinse and dry well.
- Use body lotion to moisturize the skin.
- Use petroleum-based ointment to provide a protective barrier.
- Antifungal creams (e.g., nystatin [Mycostatin]) may be prescribed for fungus growth.

Normal urine is acidic. When it remains in contact with the skin, it becomes alkaline, causing encrustations to collect on the skin. The skin then becomes macerated and excoriated.

Lifestyle Modification

Make the following recommendations to clients:
- Increase daily oral fluids (to 8 to 10 glasses, or 3000 mL) to encourage flushing of the bladder.
- Limit daily caffeine intake to less than 100 mg.
- Try limiting the intake of alcohol, artificial sweeteners, spicy foods, and citrus fruits, which are thought to irritate the bladder.
- Lose weight (for persons with a BMI>30). Studies have shown this to be more effective for women than for men.
- Stop smoking. Smoking has been linked to stress UI and urge UI among women, and to urge UI in men.
- Take prescribed diuretics early in the morning.
- Avoid constipation. Fecal impaction and chronic constipation, especially in older adults, is associated with increased risk of UI. (See Chapter 28 for interventions to promote normal bowel elimination.)
- Be aware that high-impact exercise (e.g., running, jumping rope) is associated with increased stress UI.

Bladder Training

The goal of bladder training is to enable the patient to hold increasingly greater volumes of urine in the bladder and to increase the interval between voidings. This involves patient teaching, scheduled voiding, and self-monitoring using a voiding diary.
- Teach the mechanisms of urination.

- Teach distraction and relaxation strategies to help inhibit the urge to void. For example:
  - Instruct the patient to perform serial subtractions or become involved in an activity that requires concentration (e.g., a crossword puzzle) when she feels the urge to void.
  - Alternatively the patient might perform several rapid pelvic floor muscle contractions to quiet the sensations from the bladder.
  - Other techniques include deep breathing and guided imagery.
- **Scheduled voiding** is a form of bladder training involving timed voiding and habit retraining. The client must be mentally and physically capable of self-toileting.
  - Assist the patient to the toilet, commode, or bedpan on a timed schedule. Initially this may be every 2 hours or even more often.
  - As a pattern develops and the person gains greater control, the length of time between voiding may be increased.
  - Scheduled voiding is usually combined with other techniques, including lifestyle adjustments and pelvic muscle exercises.
- Have the patient keep a daily record of her adherence to the schedule and of the number of incontinence episodes.
- If the patient can adhere to the schedule without frequent changes due to urgency, the voiding interval can be increased by 15 to 30 minutes each week.

Kegel Exercises

Pelvic floor muscle exercises (PFME) strengthen perineal muscles and help to prevent and treat stress, urge, and mixed UI. Kegel exercises are the most commonly used.

Teach patients the following routine to strengthen pelvic floor muscles:
- Imagine that you are urinating and wish to stop the flow; also tighten your rectum as though you are trying to keep from passing gas. The muscles you contract to interrupt flow are the pelvic floor muscles. (*Note:* Caution the patient against doing Kegel exercises while actually urinating because this may cause backflow of urine.)
- You should feel your rectum tighten. Women may also feel the vagina tighten. However, your abdomen should not tighten—check by placing your hand lightly on your abdomen. Also, do not contract the thigh and gluteal muscles.

TECHNIQUE 27–9   Managing Urinary Incontinence *(continued)*

- Hold each contraction for 5 to 10 seconds and then rest for 5 to 10 seconds. Some people may be able to hold for only 3 seconds at first. Count, "one-and-two-and-three . . ." Keep contraction and relaxation times equal. That is, if you hold a contraction for 5 seconds, rest 5 seconds before the next contraction.
- A recommended daily exercise routine is to perform 40 to 60 PFME divided into two to four sets of 15 exercises each time. Do one set sitting, one standing, and one lying down. Do not do all 40 to 60 exercises at one time; spread them out through the day.
- One way to remember to perform your exercises it to associate them with an activity. For example, do a Kegel at every stoplight or stop sign when you are in the car. Or, do a Kegel every time you go to the bathroom—but not while you are urinating.
- **Vaginal weight training** is another form of PFME. The woman inserts a small cone-shaped weight in the vagina for two 15-minute periods per day. The woman must contract the pelvic floor muscles to keep the weight in her vagina. Some women prefer this form of PFME because it helps them identify the correct muscles for contraction. However, this method has not been shown to produce better outcomes than Kegel exercises.

Anti-incontinence Devices

Anti-incontinence devices (e.g., a pessary) are designed to reduce the incidence of UI or provide a pathway for urine flow. When anti-incontinence devices are used, it is important to observe for vaginal or urinary tract infection, blood in the urine, and vaginal erosion.

Supportive Interventions

Supportive interventions focus on helping the patient reach the toilet and perform toileting self-care.
- Provide a bedside commode, raised toilet seat, bedpan, urinal, or other aids to make it easier to urinate independently.
- Advise and assist the patient with gait and strength training to improve the person's ability to reach the toilet in time.
- When continence cannot be achieved, provide absorbent products with waterproof coverings. Meticulous skin care must be given when these are used. Under no circumstances should you refer to these as "diapers." To do so is disrespectful of the patient's dignity.

Home Care Guidelines

- Routinely ask clients and families about incontinence. Patients and families often do not raise the issue.
- Phrase the question indirectly. Patients are likely to answer no if you ask directly, "Are you incontinent?" For example, ask; "Do you wear a pad to keep your clothes dry?" "Do you ever wet your clothing?" "Do you sometimes not make it to the toilet in time?"
- Ask where the toilet is and whether the patient can get there easily. For example, must he go upstairs?
- In a two-story house with a toilet on only one floor, place a commode on the other floor in the room where the patient spends most of his time. With a written prescription, Medicare may reimburse this expense.
- For some patients, a commode should be placed by the bedside on a large, absorbent, washable mat (to absorb any urine that leaks).
- Teach behavioral techniques for incontinence management.
- Because most home caregivers are middle-aged or older women, they may have continence problems of their own. Teach them pelvic floor muscle exercises and the best techniques for lifting and turning the patient in bed.

Source: Lewis, L. (2003). Managing incontinence at home. *American Journal of Nursing, 3* (suppl.), 41.

TECHNIQUE 27–10   Caring for Patients with Urinary Diversions

The overall goal is for the patient to become comfortable with his changed body and to assume self-care.

- Perform a thorough assessment. A healthy stoma ranges in color from deep pink to brick red, regardless of skin color, and is shiny and moist at all times. A pale, dusky, or black stoma often indicates inadequate blood supply; immediately document and report such findings to the surgeon.
- Assess the skin surrounding the stoma for signs of irritation, such as redness, tenderness, and skin breakdown. When the normally acid urine remains in contact with the skin, it becomes alkaline. Encrustations collect on the skin, and the skin becomes macerated and excoriated. Skin breakdown may lead to infection, pain, and leakage.
- A moisture-proof skin barrier is usually placed around the stoma to protect surrounding skin.
- Be available to discuss the patient's reaction to the stoma.

- Show acceptance when working with the patient and the stoma.
- Pay close attention to the skin surrounding the stoma.
- Be certain that the collection device fits snugly against the skin to prevent leakage.
- Monitor the amount and type of drainage from the stoma.
- Empty the device frequently during the day; connect it to a larger collection bag during the night when the patient is sleeping.
- Provide ample time to explain stoma care and use of ostomy appliances. For most patients this is a lifelong task; therefore patient teaching is essential.
- Barrier creams may be prescribed for irritated skin; if fungal infection develops, nystatin may be prescribed.

ASSESSMENT GUIDELINES AND TOOLS

Urinary Elimination History Questions

Usual Urination Pattern

- How often do you urinate?
- Do you get up in the middle of the night to urinate?
- Do you have difficulty getting to the bathroom in time to urinate?
- Do you ever leak urine when you cough, laugh, or exercise?
- Do you ever leak urine on the way to the bathroom?
- Do you need to use pads or tissue in your underwear to catch urine?
- Do you have any difficulty starting to void?

Appearance of Urine

- How would you describe your urine?
- Have you noticed unusual odor with urination?

Changes in Urination Habits or Urine Appearance

- Have you experienced any changes in your voiding pattern recently?
- Have you experienced any changes in the appearance or odor of your urine?

History of Urination Problems

- What has been your experience with urination problems?
- Have you experienced any problems with urinary tract infections or kidney and bladder problems?

- Have you ever lost control of your urination?
- Have you ever had urinary tract surgery or diagnostic procedures?

Use of Urination Aids

- What aids, if any, do you use to help you urinate?
- What is your usual fluid intake over the course of a day?
- What medications are you taking? Have they had any affect on your urination pattern?

Lifestyle Questions

- Where is your bathroom located? Can you get to it easily?
- Can you manage your clothing when you go to the bathroom?
- How much fluid do you drink each day?
- How much caffeine do you drink?
- Do you smoke?
- Are you bothered with constipation?
- Do you do high-impact exercise (e.g., jogging)?

Presence of Urinary Diversions

- Have you ever had surgery of your urinary tract?
- If so, what and when?

For Infants and Young Children

- Has the child been toilet-trained?
- What elimination routines have been established?

Guidelines for Physical Assessment for Urinary Elimination

Physical assessment for urinary elimination includes examination of the kidneys, bladder, urethra, and skin surrounding the genitals, as appropriate. For a complete discussion of physical examination of the genitourinary system, See Chapter 19, Procedures 19-17 and 19-18, in this volume.

The Kidneys

Technique: The **costovertebral (CV) angle** is formed by the junction of the 12th rib and the spine on both sides of the back. Place one palm flat on the CV angle and lightly strike it with the closed fist of the other hand (see the accompanying figure).

Rationale: You cannot usually palpate the kidneys. Instead, examine them by assessing for costovertebral angle tenderness (CVAT). If kidney inflammation is present, percussion of this angle produces pain.

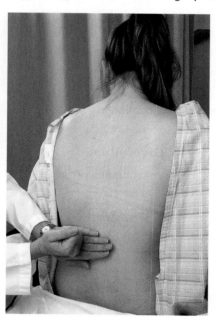

The Bladder

Inspect, palpate, and percuss the lower abdomen. Correlate your findings with data about the client's fluid intake and voiding.

Technique: Inspect the lower abdomen.

Rationale: An empty bladder, or one with limited urine, is small and sits below the symphysis pubis. In contrast, a distended bladder rises above the symphysis pubis. If it is very distended, you may be able to see a rounded swelling above the symphysis pubis.

Technique: Lightly palpate the lower abdomen to define the bladder margin. Observe the patient's response to palpation, noting signs of tenderness or discomfort.

Rationale: An empty bladder, or one with limited urine, will not be palpable.

Technique: Percuss the area.

Rationale: A distended bladder produces a dull sound as opposed to the normal tympanic sound of intestinal air.

The Urethra

Technique: Inspect the urethral orifice. Look for erythema, discharge, swelling, or odor.

Rationale: These are all signs of infection, trauma, or inflammation.

The Perineal Area

Guideline: Frequently inspect skin color, condition, texture, turgor, and presence of urine or stool.

Rationale: Clients who have urine leakage or a urinary catheter are at risk for perineal skin problems. Ammonia in the urine may result in skin excoriation, skin breakdown, and subsequent infection. If both urine and stool are present on the skin, the likelihood of skin breakdown increases.

DIAGNOSTIC TESTING

Urinalysis

Characteristic	Expected Findings	Variations
Color	A freshly voided sample is pale yellow to deep amber.	Urine becomes lighter in color and may even be clear if fluid intake is high or urine output is excessive. Urine becomes dark in color as it becomes more concentrated with decreased fluid intake or excessive fluid loss. Color is also affected by diet and medications.
pH	4.6–8.0, with an average of 6.0	Indicates kidneys' ability to help maintain balanced hydrogen ion concentration in the blood. pH increases (more alkaline) if the client eats dairy products or citrus fruits or has a vegetarian diet. pH decreases (more acidic) if the client eats a high-protein diet or consumes cranberry juice.
Specific gravity	1.002–1.028	Reflects ability of kidneys to concentrate urine. Specific gravity rises with limited fluid intake or dehydration. It may also rise with kidney disease. Specific gravity decreases as fluid intake increases.
Clarity	A freshly voided sample should be translucent. If the urine sits for a period of time, it will become cloudy.	Cloudiness in a freshly voided sample indicates the presence of other constituents in the urine. These may include bacteria, RBCs, WBCs, sperm, prostatic fluid, or vaginal discharge.
Odor	Fresh urine is aromatic.	Certain foods, such as garlic, onions, and asparagus, may give urine a distinctive odor. Bacteria will give urine an ammonia-like odor. A sweet syrup odor may indicate a congenital metabolic disorder.
Protein	< 20 mg/dL	Proteinuria is the most common indicator of renal disease. Protein is increased in diabetic nephropthy, glomerulonephritis, nephrosis, and toxemia of pregnancy. May be increased in benign proteinuria secondary to stress or physical exercise.
Glucose	Negative	Increased with elevated blood sugars and diabetes.
Ketones	Negative	Presence indicates impaired carbohydrate metabolism. Increased with diabetes, fever, fasting, high-protein diets, starvation, vomiting, postanesthesia period.
Hemoglobin	Negative on dipstick. If RBCs are assessed via microscopic exam: < 5/hpf	Increased with infection of the urinary tract, disease of the bladder, glomerulonephritis, pyelonephritis, trauma, nephrolithiasis, hemolytic reactions, or trauma. May be present in samples from women who are currently menstruating.
Bilirubin	Negative	Increased with liver disease.
Urobilionogen	Up to 1 mg/dL	Increased in cirrhosis, heart failure, liver disease, infectious mononucleosis, malaria, and pernicious anemia.
Nitrite	Negative	Used to test for bacteriuria. Increased in the presence of nitrite-forming bacteria.
Leukocyte esterase	Negative If WBCs are assessed via microscopic exam: < 5/hpf	Increased in bacterial infection, calculus formation, fungal or parasitic infection, glomerulonephritis, interstitial nephritis, or tumor.

➤

Urinalysis *(continued)*

Characteristic	Expected Findings	Variations
Renal cells	None seen	Renal cells come from the lining of the collecting ducts. Their presence indicates damage to the tubular network.
Transitional cells	None seen	Transitional cells line the renal pelvis, ureter, bladder, and proximal urethra. Their presence is seen with infection, trauma, and malignancy.
Squamous cells	Rare	Typically insignificant: squamous cells line the vagina and distal portion of the urethra.
Casts	Rare hyaline; otherwise negative	Large numbers of hyaline casts seen in renal disease, hypertension, with diuretic use, and fever. Granular casts seen in renal disease, viral infection, or lead intoxication.
Crystals	Absent in freshly voided sample	Presence may indicate an old sample, stone formation in the urinary tract, gout, high dietary intake of oxalates, liver disease, or side effect of chemotherapy.
Bacteria, yeast, parasites	None seen	Seen in infection of the urinary tract.

Source: Adapted from Schnell, Z., Van Leeuwen, A., & Kranpitz, T. (2003). *Davis's comprehensive handbook of laboratory and diagnostic tests with nursing implications.* Philadelphia: F. A. Davis company.

Blood Studies: BUN and Creatinine

Normal Ranges

Blood Urea Nitrogen (BUN)	8–20 mg/dL
Creatinine	0.5–1.1 mg/dL

Levels may be increased in:
- Renal failure
- Impaired renal perfusion
- Kidney infection or inflammation
- Kidney obstruction
- Dehydration
- Excessive protein intake
- Use of total parenteral nutrition (TPN)

Levels may be decreased in:
- Inadequate protein intake
- Malabsorption syndromes
- Liver disease

Source: Adapted from Schnell, Z., Van Leeuwen, A., & Kranpitz, T. (2003). *Davis's comprehensive handbook of laboratory and diagnostic tests with nursing implications.* Philadelphia: F. A. Davis Company.

diagnostic testing

Studies of the Urinary System

Direct Visualization Studies

Cystoscopy—Direct visualization of the urethra, bladder, and ureteral orifices by insertion of a scope. May be used to obtain biopsies and treat pathology of visualized areas.

Preparation
- Instruct the patient the procedure is performed under anesthesia.
- Ensure that a signed consent form is on the chart.
- Restrict food and fluids for 8 hours if the patient is receiving general anesthesia. For local anesthesia, allow clear liquids only for 8 hours prior to the procedure.

Post-Procedure Care
- Monitor vital signs and I&O.
- Observe the characteristics of urine after the procedure.
- Encourage increased fluid intake.
- Report suprapubic or flank pain, chills, or difficulty urinating.

Cystometry—Urodynamic testing of bladder function; measures bladder pressure and volume.

Preparation
- Ensure that a signed consent form is on the chart.
- Explain that patient cooperation with positioning and activity is crucial during the test.
- There are no food or fluid restrictions prior to the test.

Post-Procedure Care
- Monitor vital signs and I&O.
- Encourage increased fluid intake.
- Report suprapubic or flank pain, chills, or difficulty urinating.

Indirect Visualization Studies

Intravenous pyelogram (IVP)— Uses radiopaque contrast medium to visualize the kidneys, ureters, bladder, and renal pelvis. Evaluates renal function by analyzing flow of contrast over time.

Retrograde pyelogram—Uses radiopaque contrast medium to visualize the renal collecting system. Contrast media is injected via a ureteral catheter inserted through a cystoscope.

Preparation
- Obtain history of allergies. This test is contraindicated for patients with allergies to shellfish or iodinated dye.
- Ensure that baseline BUN and Creatinine results are available. This test is contraindicated for patients who are in renal failure.

- Ensure that a signed consent form is on the chart.
- NPO 8 hours before the procedure.
- Some patients may require a laxative the evening before the surgery to clear the GI tract and improve visualization.

Post-Procedure Care
- Encourage increased fluid intake.
- Monitor vital signs and I&O.
- Observe for reactions to the contrast media: rash, nausea, hives.
- For a retrograde pyelogram, ureteral catheters may be in place. They will require separate monitoring of I&O for each side.

Ultrasound—Uses sound waves to produce an image of the organs

Preparation
- Ensure that a signed consent form is on the chart.
- Fluid restrictions may be applied based on the organ to be scanned.

Post-Procedure Care
- No special care is required.

Computerized tomography—Using contrast media, examines body sections from different angles using a narrow x-ray beam to produce a three-dimensional picture of the area of the body being scanned.

Preparation
- Obtain history of allergies. This test is contraindicated for patients with allergies to shellfish or iodinated dye.
- Ensure that a signed consent form is on the chart.
- NPO 8 hours before the procedure.
- Remove all metal objects from the patient's body (e.g., eyeglasses, rings, safety pins).
- *Post-Procedure Care*
- Monitor vital signs and I&O.
- Observe for reactions to the contrast media: rash, nausea, hives.

Renal biopsy—Removal of a piece of kidney tissue for microscopic evaluation.

Preparation
- Ensure that baseline coagulation studies and hemoglobin results are available.
- Ensure that a signed consent form is on the chart.
- NPO 8 hours before the procedure.
- Instruct the patient that sedation and/or pain medication may be given.

Post-Procedure Care
- Monitor vital signs and I&O.
- Have patient rest in bed on affected side for at least 30 minutes with a pillow or sandbag under the site to prevent bleeding.
- The patient should be on bedrest for 24 hours.
- Monitor biopsy site for bleeding.
- Monitor urine for presence of blood.

Source: Schnell, Z., Van Leeuwen, A., & Kranpitz, T. (2003). *Davis's comprehensive handbook of laboratory and diagnostic tests with nursing implications.* Philadelphia: F. A. Davis Company.

STANDARDIZED LANGUAGE

NIC Interventions for Urinary Problems

Interventions When Altered Urination is the Problem

Biofeedback

Bladder Irrigation

Environmental Management

Fluid Management

Fluid Monitoring

Medication Administration

Medication Management

Pelvic Muscle Exercise

Perineal Care

Pessary Management

Prompted Voiding

Self-Care Assistance: Toileting

Specimen Management

Teaching: Individual

Tube-Care: Urinary

Urinary Bladder Training

Urinary Catheterization

Urinary Catheterization: Intermittent

Urinary Continence Care

Urinary Elimination Management

Urinary Habit Training

Urinary Incontinence Care

Urinary Incontinence Care: Enuresis

Urinary Retention Care

Weight Management

Interventions when Altered Urination is the Etiology of Other Problems

Fluid Management

Infection Protection

Ostomy Care

Perineal Care

Self-Esteem Enhancement

Skin Care: Topical Treatments

Skin Surveillance

Source: Dochterman, J. M., & Bulechek, G. M. (Eds.). (2004). *Nursing interventions classification (NIC)* (4th ed.). St Louis: Mosby.

What Are the Main Points in This Chapter?

- The urinary system consists of two kidneys, two ureters, the urinary bladder, and the urethra.
- The kidneys filter nitrogen and other metabolic wastes, toxins, excess ions, and water from the bloodstream and excrete them as urine.
- The bladder has a normal average storage capacity of 500 mL (1 pint), but it may distend, when needed, to a capacity twice that amount.
- Voiding occurs when contraction of the detrusor muscle pushes stored urine through the relaxed internal urethral sphincter into the urethra.
- The kidneys produce urine at a rate of approximately 60 mL per hour, or 1500 mL per day. Most people urinate about five to six times per day.
- Voiding and control of urination require normal functioning of the bladder and the urethra, as well as an intact brain, spinal cord, and nerves supplying the bladder and urethra.
- As an adult ages, the number of functional nephrons gradually decreases, along with the ability to dilute and concentrate urine. The potential volume of the bladder also decreases as the bladder wall loses elasticity; thus, older adults need to urinate more frequently.
- Substances that contain caffeine act as diuretics and increase urine production.
- A diet high in salt causes water retention and decreases urine production.
- Medications with anticholinergic effects inhibit the free flow of urine and may contribute to urinary retention.
- An adequately hydrated adult produces clear yellow urine. Concentrated urine is darker in color, but dilute urine can appear colorless.
- A clean-catch urine specimen is preferred for many diagnostic tests. To collect this specimen, the client must cleanse the genitalia before voiding and collect the sample in midstream.
- Sterile urine specimens may be obtained by inserting a catheter into the bladder or withdrawing a sample from an indwelling catheter.
- A 24-hour urine collection requires collection of all urine voided in the time period. The first-voided urine is discarded before timing begins.
- A routine urinalysis is one of the most commonly ordered laboratory tests. It is used as an overall screening test as well as an aid to diagnose renal, hepatic, and other diseases.
- Normal urine is free of bacteria, viruses, and fungi. Urinary tract infections are often caused by the introduction of *Escherichia coli (E. coli),* which normally live in the colon, into the urethra and bladder.
- Urinary retention is an inability to empty the bladder. It may be due to obstruction, nerve problems, infection, surgery, medications, or anxiety.
- Urinary catheterization is the introduction of pliable tube (catheter) into the bladder to allow drainage of urine.
- Urinary incontinence (UI) is a lack of voluntary control over urination. Nurses can independently perform the primary interventions to manage UI.
- A urinary diversion, or urostomy, is a surgically created opening for elimination of urine.
- A patient with a urinary diversion requires physical and psychological care. The goal is to have the patient become comfortable with his changed body and assume self-care.

28 CHAPTER Bowel Elimination

Overview

Bowel elimination is a normal process by which waste products (feces) are eliminated from the body. Feces is a mixture of insoluble fiber and other undigestible material, bacteria, and water. During defecation, the internal and external anal sphincters relax, the rectum contracts, and peristalsis increases in the sigmoid colon, propelling feces through the anus.

The frequency of BMs varies. The bowel pattern set in childhood normally continues into adulthood. Adequate fiber, fluid, and exercise are required to maintain this pattern; stress, anesthesia, medications, pregnancy, and pathological conditions can alter the pattern.

Diarrhea is the passage of frequent, watery stools. Assess for fluid losses in patients with diarrhea by monitoring intake and output, body weight, and vital signs. Be sure to provide hygiene measures to protect the skin.

Constipation is a decrease in the frequency of BMs and the passage of dry, hard stool that requires more effort to pass. Bulking agents rather than laxatives are the preferred medications for treating constipation. Fecal impaction is detected by digital examination of the rectum. To treat a fecal impaction, enemas or digital removal of stool is required. A bowel training program can be used to promote a healthy pattern of bowel elimination.

A bowel diversion is a surgically created opening for elimination of digestive waste products. The effluent of an ostomy ranges from liquid to solid, depending on the part of the bowel that is being diverted. A healthy stoma ranges in color from deep pink to brick red and is shiny and moist at all times. A client with a bowel diversion must adapt to an altered body image and learn to care for his stoma.

Thinking Critically About Bowel Elimination

The exercises in the following section allow you to practice the kind of thinking you will use as a full-spectrum nurse. Because these are critical-thinking activities, there is usually no single right answer. Discuss answers with your peers—discussion can stimulate critical thinking. If you have difficulty with any of the questions, consult with your instructor.

Caring for the Garcias

Flordelisa Garcia arrives at the family health center for a scheduled appointment, accompanied by her granddaughter, Bettina. Recently, Flordelisa has been constipated and has had several episodes of bleeding with BMs. She has read that a change in bowel habits is a sign of colon cancer and is very worried about that. She brought her granddaughter along because she is also having bowel problems. Bettina's bowel habits are erratic. At times she has a soft BM daily. However, she has also had bouts of constipation and diarrhea. Flordelisa would like advice on her granddaughter's elimination status. As a critical thinker, you will begin by obtaining accurate, credible information.

A. What history questions would be appropriate to ask Flordelisa regarding her bowel concerns? What data do you need? How can you get it? Are the data accurate? What information is important; what is not? Write some specific questions, just as you would ask them in an interview.

B. What physical assessments would you conduct for Flordelisa to add to, and possibly to validate, your subjective data?

C. Now you must consider the context. What factors must you consider when gathering a history on Bettina?

D. The family nurse practitioner (FNP) examines Flordelisa and determines that she has external hemorrhoids that have been bleeding because of recent straining at stool. The FNP orders rectal suppositories to decrease the swelling of the hemorrhoids and asks you to teach Flordelisa about necessary lifestyle changes. What additional information will you need to gather to provide this teaching? Recall that you have already gathered a significant amount of information from the history questions. Again, think about context: Whatever the content of your teaching, Flordelisa will be using that information to care for herself and her granddaughter in her home.

E. The FNP examines Bettina and tells you that the examination is normal. Use your theoretical knowledge of bowel elimination and Bettina's developmental stage to think of possible reasons for her erratic bowel pattern.

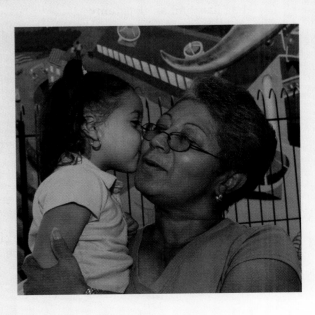

1

Your neighbor is aware that you are a nursing student and calls you for advice. She has a 12-year-old daughter with diarrhea. "Everything runs through her," states the mother. There are also two other children in the house, ages 6 years and 18 months. Both have had watery stools this morning. Your neighbor explains that her husband has an ileostomy and has been hospitalized since yesterday. Your neighbor has no symptoms but is very worried. She asks, "Do we all need to go to the hospital?"

a Consider alternatives. What are the most likely explanations for the diarrhea?

b Based on your theoretical knowledge, how would you explain why her husband was hospitalized, while the rest of the family remains at home with the same symptoms?

c After reassuring her, what advice should you offer your neighbor about self-care for her and the children's elimination problem?

2

Consider the following patients:

- A 54-year-old man diagnosed with colon cancer who now has a new sigmoid colostomy
- A 21-year-old female with Crohn's disease (an inflammatory bowel disorder) who has just had an ileostomy
- A 36-year-old trauma victim who has a new double-barreled transverse colostomy

a How are these patients similar?

b In regard to their surgery, what nursing care priorities do these clients share?

c How do the major concerns for these clients differ? (Consider the context. How are their surgical and self-care situations different?)

3 For each of the following concepts, use critical thinking to describe how or why it is important to nursing, patient care, or bowel elimination. Note that these are *not* to be merely definitions.

Digestion (in the mouth, esophagus, stomach, and small intestine)

Large intestine (colon)

Rectum and anus

Fluid intake

Location of a bowel diversion

Bowel sounds

Providing privacy

Diarrhea

Practical Knowledge
knowing how

To help you promote normal bowel elimination and support patients who have bowel elimination problems, this section provides practical knowledge of procedures and techniques for identifying problems and providing interventions. You will also find in this section assessment guidelines for assisting patients who are having diagnostic studies of the gastrointestinal system and a list of NOC outcomes and NIC interventions associated with bowel elimination.

PROCEDURES

The procedures in this chapter will help you provide care to patients who have problems with bowel elimination.

| PROCEDURE 28–1 | **Testing Stool for Occult Blood** |

 For steps to follow in *all* procedures, refer to the inside back cover of this book.

critical aspects
- Use a clean, dry collection container.
- Take care that the sample is not contaminated by urine or menstrual blood.
- Be careful not to contaminate the outside of the collection container with feces.
- Test two small stool samples from separate areas of the large sample.
- Spread each sample thinly, one at a time, onto the "windows" of the Hemoccult slide.
- Place the correct number and size of drops of developer solution into the "windows" of the opposite side on the Hemoccult slide.
- Record a positive result if the slide windows turn blue.

Equipment
- Clean gloves
- Tongue blade or other wooden applicator
- Clean, dry collection container to place in the commode, or a clean, dry bedpan
- Facility-specific Hemoccult slide or test paper
- Developing solution

Delegation
You can delegate the collection and testing of a stool sample for occult blood to the unlicensed assistive personnel (UAP) if the UAP has the necessary skills and the patient's condition is stable. Inform the UAP of any special considerations (e.g., the need to assist the patient with ambulation or the need for a bedpan). Instruct the UAP to inform you if there is visible blood in the stool and to show you the Hemoccult slide for evaluation of results when the test is complete.

Assessment
- Assess the mobility status of the patient.

Determines the patient's ability to participate in stool collection, the need for a bedpan or commode, and so forth.

- Assess the patient's dietary history for the past 24 to 48 hours.

Some foods, such as red meat, chicken, or raw vegetables, may lead to a false-positive reading. Vitamin C in excess of 250 mg per day can produce a false-negative result.

- Assess medication history.

Some medications, such as salicylates, NSAIDs, iron, anticoagulants, and colchicine, may cause a false-positive reading.

- Assess for the presence of hemorrhoids.

Fresh blood from bleeding hemorrhoids in the stool sample may cause a positive reading. The test is intended to check for blood higher up in the intestines, which is not visibly obvious when passed through the stool.

PROCEDURE 28–1 Testing Stool for Occult Blood *(continued)*

- If the patient is female, ask whether she is menstruating.
Menstrual blood may cause a false-positive reading.
- Check the expiration date on the developing solution for the Hemoccult test slide.

- Assess the patient's or family's understanding of the need for the stool test.
Provides a baseline for health teaching.

Procedural Steps

Step 1 Determine whether the test will be done by the nurse at the point of service or by lab personnel.

Because of the regulatory and billing practices in some settings, this test may be completed by lab personnel.

Step 2 Have the patient void before collecting the stool specimen.

Helps prevent contaminating the stool with urine.

Step 3 Don procedure gloves and place a clean, dry container for the stool specimen into the toilet or bedside commode in such a manner that the urine falls into the toilet and the fecal specimen falls into the container. Obtain a clean, dry bedpan for a patient who is immobile.

Using a sample of stool that comes in contact with either urine or water may produce an inaccurate test result.

Step 4 Instruct the patient to defecate into the container, or place the patient on the bedpan. Do not contaminate the specimen with toilet tissue.

Step 5 Wash your hands, and don clean procedure gloves.

Prevents the spread of intestinal bacteria.

Step 6 Once the specimen has been obtained, gather the necessary testing supplies. Be sure you understand the directions for the testing kit you are using.

This procedure gives instructions for using the Hemoccult slide method.

Step 7 Explain the purpose of the test. Explain to the patient that serial specimens may be needed.

Testing serial specimens decreases the chances of a false-negative finding.

Step 8 Open the specimen side of the Hemoccult slide. With a wooden tongue blade or other applicator, collect a small sample of stool and spread it thinly onto one "window" of the Hemoccult slide.

Step 9 With a different applicator or the opposite end of the tongue blade, collect a second small sample of stool from a different location in the large sample. Spread the second sample thinly onto the second "window" of the slide.

Reduces the possibility of a false-negative result. ▼

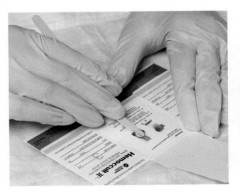

Step 10 Wrap the tongue blade in tissue and paper towel; place it in waste receptacle. Do not flush it.

Prevents transfer of microorganisms. Flushing would likely clog the plumbing.

Step 11 Close the Hemoccult slide.

Prevents the transfer of microorganisms from the specimen smears on the slide.

Step 12 If the test is to be done by laboratory personnel, label the specimen properly, and place it into the proper receptacle for transportation to the lab.

Step 13 If you are to perform the test, turn the slide over, and open the opposite side of the Hemoccult slide. Place one or two drops of developing solution onto each "window."

Follow the directions on the package regarding the number of drops of the developing solution to use to ensure an accurate reading. ▼

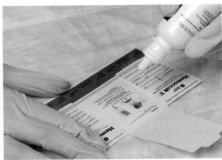

➤

PROCEDURE 28–1   **Testing Stool for Occult Blood** *(continued)*

Evaluation

- Observe the color of the paper inside the Hemoccult slide windows for 30 to 60 seconds.
- If the paper turns blue, consider the test for occult blood to be positive.

Patient Teaching

- Inform the patient of the reasons for performing the test.
- Explain the possible implications of a positive occult blood test, if one is obtained.

Home Care

- Determine the client's level of cognition and manual dexterity to assess his ability to follow instructions and physically perform the test.
- Explain necessary dietary and medication restrictions, as discussed in the "Assessment" section of this procedure.
- Instruct the client to collect the stool specimen in a clean, dry container. If an appropriate container is not available, the client may flush the toilet immediately prior to obtaining the sample. If commercial toilet bowl cleaners are in use, remove them from the tank, and flush twice.
- Protect the slide from heat, light, and household chemicals.
- Home collection slides come in a kit, connected together as a set of three. Instruct the patient not to tear them apart.
- Emphasize to the patient that each sample should be from separate bowel movements on separate days.
- After all three specimens have been collected over the course of at least 3 days, store the slide in a paper envelope to air-dry.
- The client must place the slides in the special mailing pouch that comes with the slides, if they are to be mailed back to the lab. The slides should be returned to the care provider or lab no later than 14 days after the first sample was collected.
- For additional instructions,

 Go to the **Hemoccult web site at www.hemoccultfobt.com**

Documentation

- Document the date and time of the specimen collection, both in the patient record and on the specimen container or Hemoccult kit.
- Note the appearance of the stool (e.g., color, odor) and the presence of blood, mucus, or other abnormal constituents.
- Note any rectal bleeding or discomfort during and after defecation.

PROCEDURE 28–1   Testing Stool for Occult Blood *(continued)*

- Document the test results on the appropriate agency form.
- Notify the appropriate care provider of the results.

Sample documentation

06/14/07	0915	*Specimen taken from 2 separate sections of*
		yellowish brown, liquid stool containing mucus.
		No rectal bleeding or discomfort with defecation.
		Specimen sent to lab; test results pending.
		— *S. Hoeszle, RN*

PROCEDURE 28–2   Placing and Removing a Bedpan

 For steps to follow in *all* procedures, refer to the inside back cover of this book.

critical aspects

- Determine whether the patient will need to use a regular bedpan or a fracture pan.
- Don clean procedure gloves.
- Help the patient to achieve a position on the bedpan that will be most helpful in facilitating urinary or bowel elimination. Place the patient in semi-Fowler's position whenever possible. Modify the position based on the patient's condition.
- Provide clean washcloths and towels for the patient to perform personal hygiene when elimination is complete. Assist if patient cannot perform these tasks independently.

Equipment

- Bedpan
- Two pairs of clean gloves
- Toilet tissue
- Two washcloths, towel, and basin
- Waterproof pad
- Bedpan cover

Delegation

You may delegate the placement and removal of a bedpan to the UAP after ensuring that the UAP has the necessary skills and that the patient's condition is stable. Complete the following assessments, and inform the UAP of any special considerations (e.g., medical or surgical conditions that will necessitate the use of a fracture pan, extra care with turning or required positioning based on medical condition).

Assessment

- Assess the patient's level of consciousness, ability to follow directions, and mobility status.

Helps determine whether one or two persons are needed to complete the procedure.

- Determine the patient's level of comfort—note the presence of rectal or abdominal pain or the presence of hemorrhoids or perianal irritation.

Pain can cause difficulty with positioning and bearing down during defecation. Any unexplained pain should be evaluated by the primary care provider.

➤

PROCEDURE 28–2   **Placing and Removing a Bedpan** *(continued)*

- Assess the physical size of the patient and whether the patient is allowed to sit up or lie flat when using a bedpan.

Determines the type of bedpan to use and whether you need additional personnel to assist.

- Identify factors that will necessitate the use of a fracture pan.

Examples include fracture of the pelvis; total hip replacement; lower back surgery; presence of casts, splints, or braces on lower limbs; or obese patient who cannot be placed on a regular bedpan.

- Auscultate bowel sounds, and palpate for distention if necessary.

The colon when full with fecal matter is a rounded, firm mass. A smooth, round mass above the symphysis pubis is a distended bladder.

- Review the patient's chart to determine the need to obtain a stool specimen.

Allows you to obtain a specimen container before placing the patient on the bedpan.

Procedural Steps

Placing a Bedpan

Step 1 Obtain the necessary supplies, and proceed to the patient's room. Leave clean washcloths, towel, and basin with warm water at the bedside for use during bedpan removal.

The patient may wish to wash her hands after using the bedpan.

Step 2 If the bedpan is metal, place it under warm, running water for a few seconds. Then dry it, making sure bedpan is not too hot.

A metal bedpan is very cold. Running it under warm water allows the patient to be more comfortable and helps relax the anal sphincter.

Step 3 Raise the siderail on the opposite side from where you are working.

Prevents patient from falling out of bed and gives the patient something to hold onto while moving around in bed.

Step 4 Raise the bed to a comfortable height.

Encourages the use of good body mechanics and prevents muscle strain for the nurse.

Step 5 Prepare the patient by folding down the covers to a point that will allow for placement of the bedpan.

Step 6 Don clean procedure gloves.

Prevents the spread of bacteria via contact with urine or feces.

Step 7   Variation A For the Patient Able to Move/Turn Independently in Bed

a. Observe for the presence of dressings, drains, intravenous fluids, and traction.

These appliances may hinder the patient from assisting with the procedure and may necessitate the use of more assistance.

b. With the patient in a supine position, lower the head of the bed.

c. Ask the patient to lift her hips. The patient may need to raise her knees to a flexed position, place her feet flat on the bed and push up. You can also assist the patient to raise her hips by sliding a hand under the small of her back.

d. As an alternative, place the patient in semi-Fowler's position. Ask the patient to raise her hips by pushing up on raised siderails or by using an overhead trapeze.

e. Place the bedpan under the patient's buttocks so that the wide, rounded end is toward the back. Do not push the pan under the patient's buttocks. When using a fracture pan, place the wide, rounded end toward the front.

Step 8   Variation B For the Patient Unable to Move/Turn Independently

a. Ask for help from another health-care worker if the patient's condition warrants.

b. With the patient in the supine position, lower the head of the bed.

c. Assist the patient to the side-lying position. Use a turn sheet, if necessary.

d. Place the bedpan up against the patient's buttocks so that the wide, rounded end is toward the head. When using a fracture pan, place the wide, rounded end toward the feet. ▼

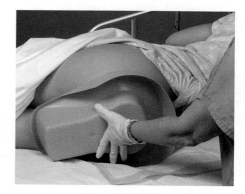

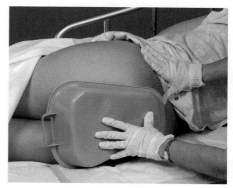

PROCEDURE 28–2 Placing and Removing a Bedpan *(continued)*

e. Holding the bedpan in place, slowly roll the patient back and onto the bedpan.

Step 9 Replace the covers; raise the head of the bed to a position of comfort for the patient. Place a rolled towel, blanket, or small pillow under the sacrum (lumbar curve of the back). Place the call light and toilet tissue within the patient's reach. Make certain that the bed is back at its lowest position and that the upper siderails are raised.

Provides privacy, comfort, and safety.

Step 10 Remove your gloves and wash your hands.

Prevents the transmission of intestinal bacteria.

Removing a Bedpan

Step 11 Don clean procedure gloves. Wet the washcloths with warm water and place them near the work area.

Step 12 If the patient is immobile, lower the head of the patient's bed. Pull down the covers only as far as needed to remove the bedpan.

Lowering the head of the bed is necessary only if the patient is immobile.

Step 13 Offer the patient toilet paper.

Assist patients who are unable to complete this task independently.

Step 14 Ask the patient to raise her hips. Stabilize and remove the bedpan. If the patient is unable to raise her hips, stabilize the bedpan and assist her to the side-lying position.

Stabilizing the bedpan prevents spillage of urine.

Step 15 Cleanse the buttocks with a warm, wet washcloth. Dry with a towel.

Provides for patient comfort and hygiene and decreases the risk of skin irritation and breakdown.

Step 16 Replace covers, and position the patient for comfort. Offer the patient the second washcloth moistened with warm water to cleanse her hands.

Allows patient to perform personal hygiene and decreases transmission of bacteria.

Step 17 Empty the bedpan into the patient's toilet. Measure the output if measuring I&O is part of the treatment plan. Clean the bedpan following facility-specific guidelines.

If there is no toilet in the patient's room, use a bedpan cover and carry the bedpan to the nearest toilet or soiled utility room for emptying.

Step 18 Remove the soiled gloves and wash your hands.

Prevents transmission of infectious microorganisms.

Evaluation
- Assess the amount and characteristics of any urine and/or stool.
- Observe the skin on the perineum and buttocks for redness and breakdown.

Home Care
Teach the patient's family the steps of this procedure.

Documentation
- Document the amount of urine voided if intake and output are being recorded.
- Document a bowel movement on the graphics record.
- Note the presence of any unusual characteristics of either stool or urine. If there are none, it is enough to document the passage of stool or urine in the graphic records.

PROCEDURE 28–3   Administering an Enema

For steps to follow in *all* procedures, refer to the inside back cover of this book.

critical aspects

- Determine the patient's ability to retain the enema solution.
- If the patient is immobile, have a bedpan or bedside commode available.
- Warm the solution.
- Lubricate the tip of the enema tubing generously.
- Insert the tubing only about 7 to 10 cm (3 to 4 in.) into the rectum.
- Hold the container at the correct height above the level of the hips.
- Instill the solution at a slow rate.
- Encourage the patient to take slow, deep breaths and hold the solution for 3 to 15 minutes, depending on the type of enema.
- Assess the patient for cramping or inability to retain the solution.
- Document the results.

Equipment

- Enema administration container, correct enema solution, or prepackaged enema—depends on the type of enema ordered
  - Enema kit: This may be a grouping of supplies that includes a small plastic bucket or a 1 L plastic bag with attached tubing, disposable toweling, lubricant, and castile soap
  - Prepackaged enema solution: If a prepackaged enema (e.g., Fleets) is ordered, you may need to obtain the preparation from the pharmacy or central supply department
- Washcloths, towels, and/or toilet tissue
- Bath blanket
- Waterproof pad
- Bedpan with cover or bedside commode, if needed
- Water-soluble lubricant
- Clean procedure gloves
- IV pole

Delegation

You may delegate this procedure to the UAP. Complete the following assessments, and instruct the UAP about conditions under which the procedure should be stopped (e.g., severe abdominal pain occurs, bleeding is seen, or the patient is unable to retain the solution). Instruct the UAP to report the results of the enema and show you any stool that appears to be abnormal (e.g., containing blood or pus).

Assessment

- Assess for history of bowel disorders (e.g., diverticulitis, ulcerative colitis, recent bowel surgery, abdominal pain, abdominal distention, hemorrhoids).

Some disorders put the patient at risk for complications, such as mucosal irritation or perforation. Abdominal pain along with hypoactive bowel sounds and distention could indicate a bowel obstruction.

- Inspect the abdomen for the presence of distention.

Establishes baseline for effectiveness of the enema.

- Review the patient's chart for the presence of increased intracranial pressure, glaucoma, or recent rectal or prostate surgery.

These conditions contraindicate this procedure.

- Note the patient's last bowel movement, recent bowel movement pattern, and bowel sounds.

Establishes baseline for bowel function.

- Assess the patient's cognitive level and mobility status.

Determines the patient's ability to follow instructions and the need for placing him on a bedpan.

- Assess the patient's degree of rectal sphincter control.

Will determine whether you need to administer the enema with the patient on the bedpan. Determines the amount of solution to instill.

- Assess for the presence of a fecal impaction.

May necessitate the use of a different type of enema than that prescribed.

PROCEDURE 28–3A Administering a Cleansing Enema

Procedural Steps

Step 1 Open the enema supplies or kit. Attach the tubing to the enema bucket, if you are using a bucket.

The 1L enema bag comes with preconnected tubing.

Step 2 Close the clamp on the tubing, and fill the container with 500 to1000 mL of warm solution. The water temperature should be 105 to 110° F (lukewarm). Check the temperature with a bath thermometer. Never warm the enema solution in a microwave oven.

a. For infants: Use 50 to 150 mL of solution.

b. For toddlers: Use 250 to 350 mL of solution.

c. For school-age children, use 300 to 500 mL of solution.

Cold solution causes intestinal cramping. Very hot solution can damage the intestinal mucosa. Use the correct amount of solution to decrease the necessity of repeating the procedure.

Step 3 Add castile soap (or the soap solution used by your facility) to the fluid at this time if a soapsuds enema has been ordered.

Soap causes mucosal irritation, which stimulates peristalsis and defecation.

Step 4 Hang the container on the IV pole. Holding the end of the tubing over a sink or waste can, open the clamp and slowly allow the tubing to prime (fill) with solution. Reclamp the tubing when the tubing is filled.

Expresses air from the tubing. Air introduced into the bowel may cause intestinal distention and discomfort.

Step 5 Have the patient turn, or assist the patient to turn, to a left side-lying position with the right knee flexed. You may elevate the head of the bed very slightly if the patient has shortness of breath associated with respiratory conditions.

Do not assist the patient to the toilet for enema administration, because the curved rectal tubing can scrape the rectal wall.

Allows the enema solution to fill the rectum and intestine following the natural flow of gravity. Avoid the semi-Fowler's position, because it increases the likelihood that gravity will cause the solution to leak out. If the patient has a poor sphincter control, position the patient on the bedpan in comfortable dorsal recumbent position, because he will not be able to retain all of the enema solution.

Step 6 Drape the patient with the bath blanket, exposing only the buttocks and rectum. See Procedure 22-4 to review the procedure for draping.

Allows for patient privacy.

Step 7 Don clean procedure gloves.

Prevents the transmission of intestinal bacteria.

Step 8 Place the waterproof pad under the patient's buttocks or hips.

Prevents soiling of bed linens.

Step 9 Depending on the patient's mobility status:

a. Place the bedpan flat on the bed, directly beneath the rectum, up against the patient's buttocks.

b. Place the bedside commode near the bed.

Step 10 Lubricate the tip of the enema tubing generously.

Allows for ease of insertion and decreases patient discomfort.

Step 11 If necessary, lift the buttock to expose the anus. Slowly and gently insert the tip of the tubing approximately 7 to 10 cm (3 to 4 in.) into the rectum. Have the patient take slow, deep breaths as you complete this step. If the tube does not pass with ease, do not force it. Allow a small amount of fluid to infuse and then retry, inserting the tube slowly.

Helps the patient to relax and decreases reflex tightening of the anal sphincter. ▼

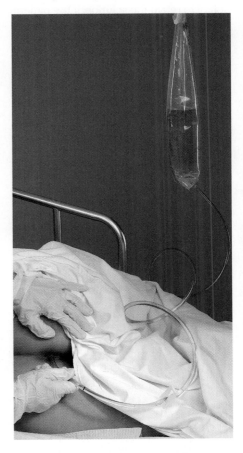

Step 12 Remove the container from the IV pole, and hold it at the level of the patient's hips. Begin instilling the solution.

Lowering the container slows the force of the instillation, decreasing pressure, cramping, discomfort, and reflex expulsion of the solution.

Step 13 Slowly raise the level of the container, so that it is 30 to 45 cm (12 to 18 in.) above the level of the hips. Adjust the pole and rehang the container. Continue a slow, steady instillation of the enema solution.

The height of the container determines the speed of the flow. A slow, steady rate of infusion decreases cramping and increases the patient's ability to retain the solution.

➤

PROCEDURE 28–3A   **Administering a Cleansing Enema** *(continued)*

Step 14 Continuously monitor the patient for pain or discomfort. Assess his ability to retain the solution. If the patient has difficulty with retention, lower the level of the container, stop the flow for 15 to 30 seconds, and then resume the procedure. If the patient feels pain or you meet with resistance at any time during the procedure, stop and consult with the primary care provider.

Allows patient to rest and adjust to sensation of rectal fullness, increasing the patient's ability to retain the solution. Prevents injury.

Step 15 When the correct amount of solution has been instilled, clamp the tubing, and slowly remove the tubing from the rectum. If there is stool on the tubing, wrap the end of the tubing in a washcloth or toilet tissue until it can be rinsed or disposed of.

Prevents transmission of bacteria.

Step 16 Clean the patient's rectal area, re-cover the patient, and instruct him to hold the enema solution for approximately 5 to 15 minutes. Place the call light within reach.

Retention of the enema solution will distend the bowel and increase the stimulus to defecate.

Step 17 Dispose of the enema supplies or, if they are reusable, clean and store them in an appropriate location in the patient's room.

Maintains pleasant environment and helps prevent transfer of pathogens.

Step 18 Remove your gloves and wash your hands.

Prevents transmission of intestinal bacteria.

Step 19 Depending on the patient's mobility status, assist him onto the bedpan, to the bedside commode, or to the toilet when he feels compelled to defecate. Wash your hands and use clean procedure gloves as necessary.

Step 20 After the patient has defecated, inspect the stool for color, consistency, and quantity.

Step 21 Assist the patient in cleansing his rectal area and buttocks as needed. Dispose of the fecal material and cleanse the bedpan according to agency policy.

PROCEDURE 28–3B   **Administering a Prepackaged Enema**

Procedural Steps

Step 1 Open the prepackaged enema. Remove the plastic cap from the container. The tip of the prepackaged enema container comes prelubricated. However, you may need to add extra lubricant.

Extra lubricant decreases discomfort and eases insertion of the tube into the rectum.

Step 2 Follow Steps 5 through 11 of Procedure 28-3A.

Step 3 Tilt the container slightly and slowly roll and squeeze the container until all of the solution is instilled.

Ensures that the container empties completely and that an adequate amount of solution is instilled. ▼

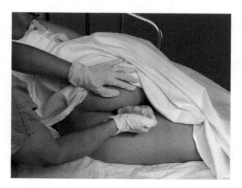

Step 4 Withdraw the container tip from the rectum. Wipe the area with a washcloth or toilet tissue.

Prevents transmission of bacteria.

Step 5 Recover the patient, and instruct him to hold the enema solution for approximately 5 to 10 minutes. Place the call light within reach.

Retention of the enema solution will distend the bowel and increase the stimulus to defecate.

Step 6 Dispose of the empty container.

Maintains pleasant environment.

Step 7 Follow steps 18 through 20 of Procedure 28-3A.

PROCEDURE 28–3 **Administering an Enema** *(continued)*

Evaluation

- Observe the amount, color, and consistency of the stool.
- Evaluate the patient's tolerance of the procedure (e.g., amount of cramping, discomfort).
- Determine whether the physician's orders require subsequent enema administration.
- Some bowel exams require repeated enemas or enemas administered until the returns are "clear." For the latter, it will be necessary for you to examine the return and determine whether stool particles are still present. "Clear" does not mean absence of color, but rather absence of stool particles and transparency of the liquid.

Patient Teaching

- Teach the patient that dependence on enemas to achieve a regular bowel elimination pattern can disrupt the normal process that stimulates defecation.
- Teach dietary and lifestyle changes that promote regular elimination (e.g., increased fluid intake, diet high in fiber, increased exercise).

Home Care

- Show the patient the box in which a prepackaged enema comes, and instruct him that he may purchase this type of enema at a local grocery or drugstore.
- Assess the patient's ability to administer his own enema. If you determine that he will be unable to accomplish the task, encourage him to seek assistance and instruct the caregiver in the task.
- Teach the patient or caregiver proper hand washing. Encourage them to purchase clean procedure gloves.

The layperson may not be aware of the serious infections that can be caused by gram-negative intestinal bacteria.

- If the patient will be attempting to self-administer a cleansing enema, help him determine how and where to hang the container so that it is at the proper height.
- If a soapsuds enema is to be administered in the home setting, teach the patient which household soaps may be substituted for castile soap.

Some soaps used in the home for cleaning purposes may be too harsh and irritating to the intestinal mucosa.

Documentation

- Document the type of enema given and, if applicable, the amount of the solution instilled on the nurse's notes.
- For prepackaged enemas, some facilities require documentation (of the time given and the nurse's initials) on the medication administration record (MAR).
- Document the patient's tolerance of the procedure.

➤

PROCEDURE 28–3   **Administering an Enema** *(continued)*

- Document the characteristics and amount of the stool.
- If the order is to administer enemas until the returns are clear, document the color of the return solution and the amount of stool seen.

Sample documentation

06/04/07   0825   *Fleets enema administered (see MAR). Patient had no cramping; retained enema for 5 minutes. Passed moderate amount of solid, formed, brown stool with no mucus, but with a streak of bright red blood on the surface.*

                                                      — R. Kline, RN

PROCEDURE 28–4   **Removing Stool Digitally**

 For steps to follow for *all* procedures, refer to the inside back cover of this book.

critical aspects

- Trim and file your fingernails if they are long. Nails should not extend over the end of the fingertips.
- Obtain baseline vital signs, and determine whether the patient has a history of cardiac problems or other contraindications.
- Determine whether the procedure will be accompanied by suppository insertion or enema administration (e.g., will an oil-retention enema be given first?)
- Use only one or two fingers, and remove stool in small pieces.
- Allow the patient periods of rest, and monitor for signs of vagal nerve stimulation.
- Teach the patient lifestyle changes necessary to prevent stool retention.

Equipment

- Two pairs of clean procedure gloves
- Water-soluble lubricant (containing lidocaine, if agency policy permits)
- Bedpan and cover
- Washcloth, soap, and towel or toilet tissue (or moistened towlettes)
- Basin of warm water
- Bath blanket
- Waterproof pad

Delegation

This procedure should not be delegated to the UAP. Ongoing assessment of the patient by the professional nurse is required when stool is manually removed from the rectum. The nurse must monitor the patient for complications, such as bleeding and vagal nerve stimulation. Nursing judgment is necessary in determining the need to halt the procedure.

PROCEDURE 28–4   **Removing Stool Digitally** *(continued)*

Assessment

- Assess the patient's baseline vital signs and history of heart disease.

Digital removal of stool can stimulate the vagus nerve, causing bradycardia. Patients who have a history of heart disease or dysrhythmia have a greater risk. Be sure to monitor patient's pulse before and during procedure.

- Assess the patient's cognitive level and mobility status.

Determines the patient's ability to follow directions and turn in bed.

- Assess the patient's white blood cell (WBC) count.

If the patient has a compromised immune status, evidenced by a low WBC count, you should discuss this procedure with the primary care provider to evaluate the risks and benefits of the procedure.

- Determine the time of the patient's last bowel movement.

Infrequent defecation increases the chance that hard stool may form in the rectum.

- Assess the patient for history of fecal impaction.

Can be a recurrent problem for bedridden, disabled, or institutionalized patients.

- Assess stool consistency.

Patients who are immobilized may become incontinent of watery stool. They may be able to pass small sections of hard stool or small quantities of watery stool. The latter, which may be intermittent or continuous, is a symptom of high colon impaction.

- Assess the patient's ability to defecate: Does the patient have the desire but is unable to have a BM?

Large amounts of stool can cause distention in the rectum.

- Determine whether the patient experiences pain on defecation.

Pain can exacerbate the problem because the patient tends to suppress defecation.

- Assess the patient's pattern of bowel movements, diet, exercise, mobility status, and medications (e.g., iron supplements or narcotic analgesics).

You should determine whether any of these factors contribute to the problem and then add this information to the nursing care plan to help prevent recurrence.

- Assess bowel sounds and any abdominal distention.

There can be peristalsis without gastrointestinal patency, which creates distention. Abdominal distention can add to constipation.

Procedural Steps

Note: Some practitioners may order an oil-retention enema prior to the procedure. Also, many advise that you follow digital removal of stool with either an oil-retention and/or tap water enemas.

An oil-retention enema, given prior to the procedure, softens and moistens the stool, making removal easier. Enema(s) given after the procedure ensure the evacuation of stool that may not be reached by digital removal.

Step 1 Determine whether lubricant containing lidocaine is to be used, and obtain the correct lubricant.

May decrease rectal discomfort for the patient.

Step 2 Drape the patient with the bath blanket. Go to Procedure 22-4 to review the procedure for draping. Assist him to turn on his left side, with his right knee flexed toward his head. Place the waterproof pad halfway beneath his left hip.

Provides privacy and exposes the anus for visualization. The pad protects the bed from being soiled.

Step 3 Don clean procedure gloves. Some sources recommend double-gloving.

Prevents the transmission of intestinal bacteria.

Step 4 Expose the buttocks. Place a clean, dry bedpan on the waterproof pad next to the buttocks in line with the rectum.

The bedpan serves as a receptacle for stool that is removed.

Step 5 Wet a washcloth, or have toilet tissue or moist towelettes ready to cleanse the rectal area when you complete the procedure.

Step 6 Generously lubricate either the gloved forefinger and/or middle finger on your dominant hand.

Prevents discomfort, pain, and mucosal injury.

➤

PROCEDURE 28–4 **Removing Stool Digitally** (*continued*)

Step 7 Slowly slide one lubricated finger into the rectum. Observe for perianal irritation.

Patient may need skin care to reduce pain during additional bowel evacuation. ▼

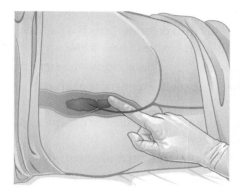

Step 8 Gently rotate your finger around the mass and/or into the mass.

Assists in determining the amount and texture of the fecal bulk.

Step 9 Begin to break the stool into smaller pieces. At this point, you may insert a second finger and gently "slice" apart the stool, using a scissoring motion. Remove pieces of stool via the rectum as they become separated, and place them in the bedpan. ▼

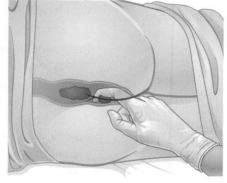

Step 10 As you proceed, instruct the patient to take slow, deep breaths.

Helps the patient to relax his anal sphincter.

Step 11 Continue to manipulate and remove pieces of stool, allowing the patient to rest at intervals. Reapply lubricant (containing lidocaine, if permitted) each time you reinsert your fingers.

Allows for assessment of and attention to the patient's comfort level and tolerance for the procedure.

Step 12 Assess the patient's heart rate at regular intervals.

Stimulation of the vagus nerve may cause bradycardia and poses a risk for dysrhythmias in susceptible patients. Stop the procedure if the patient's heart rate falls or the rhythm changes from your initial assessment.

Caution: Some resources (including the website Medline Plus, an online medical encyclopedia) suggest that this procedure should be done in small steps (no more than 4 finger insertions in one session), giving a series of suppositories in between stool removal episodes.

Prevents patient fatigue and pain. Reduces the risk of injury to the rectal tissue and vagal stimulation.

Step 13 When removal of stool is complete, cover the bedpan and set it aside. Use washcloth and/or toilet tissue to cleanse the rectal area.

Provides personal hygiene and decreases pathogen transmission.

Step 14 Assist the patient to return to a position of comfort. Note the color, amount, and consistency of the stool, and dispose of it properly.

Step 15 Remove your gloves and wash your hands.

Prevents transmission of intestinal pathogens.

Evaluation

- Determine whether evacuation of the retained stool was complete. Perform a rectal exam to assess for presence of stool.
- Reassess vital signs, and compare the results to the initial assessment. Continue to monitor for 1 hour for bradycardia.

Determines whether there is any vagal stimulation.

- Assess bowel sounds.

Determines whether there is any peristaltic activity.

- Palpate abdomen for nontenderness and softness.
- Ask the patient whether he feels relief from rectal pressure or abdominal discomfort.

PROCEDURE 28–4   **Removing Stool Digitally** *(continued)*

Patient Teaching

Retained stool is most often the result of poor dietary habits, lack of fluid intake, lack of exercise, inattentiveness to the urge to defecate, and laxative abuse. Focus patient teaching on lifestyle changes that will facilitate a regular bowel elimination pattern (e.g., high-fiber foods, drinking at least eight glasses of water per day).

Home Care

Home care related to this procedure focuses on preventing constipation that would require the digital removal of stool. You should teach clients about high-fiber foods, adequate water intake, and the importance of exercise. Digital removal of stool may be necessary for some clients as part of a bowel program (e.g., patients who are paraplegic or quadriplegic). You can teach this procedure to the care provider in the home.

Documentation

- Document the bowel movement on the graphics record.
- Document the procedure and the patient's tolerance for the procedure in the nurse's notes.
- Document the patient's pulse rate on the vital signs record.
- Document any unusual characteristics of the stool (e.g., black or green color, blood, or mucus)

Sample documentation

7/11/06	6:15 P.M.	Impacted stool removed digitally. No perianal irritation noted. Removed moderate amount (approximately 6 oz [170g]) dry, hard, gray-colored stool. Pulse 78 before removal; 84 after. Encouraging 8 oz fluids every hour. ———— C. Bryan, RNC

| PROCEDURE 28–5 | **Changing an Ostomy Appliance** |

> For steps to follow in *all* procedures, refer to the inside back cover of this book.

critical aspects

- Change the pouch every 3 to 5 days. Frequency will also depend on the type of stoma, the equipment used (e.g., one- or two-piece pouch), the effluent, the patient's preference, and the climate (i.e., change more frequently during the summer).
- Empty the old pouch prior to removing it, if possible.
- Remove the wafer or pouch slowly and gently, pulling down from the top with one hand while holding counter-tension with the other.
- Assess the stoma and the peristomal skin area for abnormalities (e.g., discoloration, swelling, redness, irritation, excoriation, bleeding).
- Use a measuring guide to determine the size of the stoma.
- Trace the size of the opening onto the back of the wafer, and cut the wafer opening about 2 to 3 mm ($\frac{1}{16}$ to $\frac{1}{8}$ inch) larger.
- Apply the new wafer with gentle pressure.
- *Note:* Some pouches come with the wafer attached, some without. These instructions assume that the wafer is attached.

Equipment

- Ostomy pouch
  - One-piece pouch with the wafer attached, or a two-piece system with a separate wafer and pouch
  - Clamp for pouches with an opening at the bottom (a new clamp is not used each time; usually one clamp is packaged with each box of pouches).

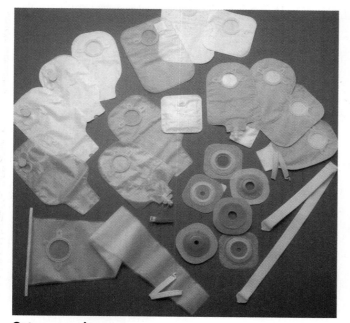

Ostomy equipment.

- Skin care items per agency protocol or those recommended by the enterostomal therapist (e.g., skin prep, skin barrier, adhesive remover, adhesive paste)
- Stoma measuring guide (or precut template)
- Scissors
- Pen or pencil
- Two pairs of clean procedure gloves
- Washcloth, towel, basin with warm water
- Toilet tissue
- 4 × 4 gauze pad
- Bedpan or container for effluent
- Plastic bag (for disposal of used pouch)
- Waterproof pad
- Ostomy deodorant
- Hypoallergenic paper tape (optional) or ostomy belt
- Bath blanket

Delegation

During the immediate postoperative period, the professional nurse must assess the newly created stoma and peristomal skin area and use clinical judgment when changing a pouch. You may delegate to a UAP if it is a preexisting, stable stoma and if you are sure the UAP is qualified to perform the task. If you do delegate this task, instruct the UAP to report any changes or unusual findings (e.g. changes in stoma color, swelling, peristomal redness, excoriation,

PROCEDURE 28–5   **Changing an Ostomy Appliance** *(continued)*

deviations from expected amount) and color and consistency of drainage from the stoma.

Assessment

- Assess the type of stoma (e.g., ileostomy, colostomy, urostomy), number of stomas, and location on the abdomen (for example, is the stoma near structures that will impact care?).

Determines the type of pouch or system to use.

- Assess stoma color, shape, size, and/or length of protrusion or retraction; stoma construction (end, loop, double barrel); and direction of stoma lumen.

Alterations in stoma color may indicate poor circulation and possible necrosis and should be reported to the physician. Protruding or retracted stomas will need special adjustments in wafer measurement and placement.

- Assess peristomal skin for redness, rash, irritation, or excoriation. Observe existing skin barrier and pouch for leakage and length of time in place. You may have to remove the pouch to observe the stoma fully, depending on the type of pouch (i.e., if the pouch is opaque).

Skin excoriation may indicate an ineffective seal between the wafer and the skin and leakage of effluent.

- Determine the changing schedule for the pouch.

Pouches are usually changed every 3 to 5 days, preferably before leakage occurs. Frequency also depends on the type of stoma, the equipment used (e.g., one- or two-piece pouch), the effluent, the patient's preference, and the climate (i.e., pouches are changed more frequently during the summer). Avoid changing entire system to decrease skin irritation. In a one-piece or two-piece pouching system, change the skin barrier only every 3 to 7 days, never daily.

- Measure the stoma with each pouching system.

Determines the correct size of equipment needed. Follow the manufacturer's directions and measuring guide for the size of ostomy pouch and the patient's stoma size.

- Observe abdominal shape and incision, if present.

Abdominal shape determines the proper placement of the pouch. Because of stomal and abdominal characteristics, some patients may need convexity in their ostomy pouching system to avoid leakage.

- Assess the patient's willingness to look at the stoma, touch the appliance, and discuss or participate in the task.

May indicate a readiness or desire to learn.

- Assess the patient's condition. Consider vision, dexterity or mobility, and cognitive ability.

Helps determine best type of appliance to use. Poor vision may indicate the need to use magnification mirrors and yellow-tinted sunglasses to help reduce glare and improve contrast. Immobility or spinal cord injuries may necessitate using equipment that has a longer pouch that the patient can easily empty independently when sitting. Impaired dexterity or vision may warrant the use of a one-piece system or precut pouch and skin barrier, whereas a two-piece system may be preferable for patients who need to keep the skin barrier in place for several days and change just the pouch. Patients who are blind can also be taught to change their own equipment.

- Auscultate for bowel sounds.

Determines the presence of peristalsis.

- Observe for effluent from the stoma, and document your findings.

Change the skin barrier pouch at times of lower effluent output. Avoid changing after meals, when the gastrocolic reflux increases chance of fecal effluent output.

- Check for pouch leakage.

Leakage may indicate the need for a different type of pouch system or sealant.

- Assess whether a new clamp will be needed or the one on the pouch can be used again.

➤

PROCEDURE 28–5 Changing an Ostomy Appliance *(continued)*

Procedural Steps

Step 1 Wash your hands and don clean procedure gloves.

Prevents transmission of pathogens.

Step 2 Fold down the bed covers to expose the ostomy site. Place a clean towel across the patient's abdomen under the existing pouch.

Helps prevent spillage of effluent onto the patient.

Step 3 Position the patient so that no skinfolds occur along the line of the stoma.

Ensures an adequate seal between the wafer and the skin, preventing leakage.

Step 4 Place towel or linen-saver pad underneath the pouch. If it is drainable, empty the existing ostomy pouch into the bedpan.

Pouches should be drained when they are one-third to one-half full because the weight of the contents may dislodge the skin seal; ostomy drainage is irritating to the skin. The pouch also collects flatus, which needs to be expelled because it can disrupt the skin seal.

a. To calculate the amount of output in milliliters for an ostomy with a liquid effluent (e.g., ileostomy or urostomy), use a graduated measuring container.

b. For pouches that you open by unrolling them at the bottom, you must remove a clamp to empty the pouch. Save this clamp for reuse.

Note: Some pouches cannot be drained.

Step 5 With one hand, gently remove the old wafer from the skin, beginning at the top and proceeding in a downward direction. At the same time, use your other hand to hold tension on the skin in the opposite direction of the pull. If you encounter resistance and the wafer is difficult to remove, you may use adhesive remover or rubbing alcohol if your facility protocol allows.

Prevents skin irritation or tearing and patient discomfort. ▼

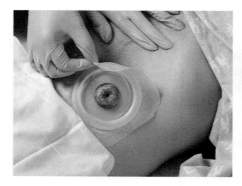

Step 6 Place the old pouch and wafer in the plastic bag for disposal. If you were unable to drain the pouch, dispose of it according to agency protocol.

Prevents transmission of infections caused by fecal bacteria.

Step 7 Inspect the stoma and peristomal skin area (see "Assessment," preceding).

Step 8 Cleanse the stoma and surrounding skin using warm water and mild soap. Allow the area to dry.

Removes old adhesive and any effluent that has leaked. Helps prevent skin irritation and/or breakdown.

Note: When you wash the stoma, slight bleeding may occur. This is normal. Report excessive bleeding to the physician.

Step 9 Remove your gloves, wash your hands, and don clean gloves.

Decreases the spread of intestinal bacteria.

Step 10 Measure the size of the stoma. You can accomplish this in several ways.
• Place a standard stoma measuring guide over the stoma.
• Reuse a previously cut template.
• Measure the stoma from side to side (approximating the circumference).

The stoma may need to be remeasured frequently during the initial postoperative period. The size of the stoma may change as edema subsides. ▼

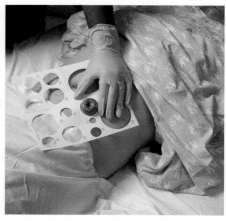

Step 11 Place a clean 4 × 4 gauze pad over the stoma.

Gauze will absorb any leaking effluent, keeping the skin clean and dry during application of the new pouch.

Step 12 Trace the size of the opening obtained in step 9 onto the paper on the back of the new wafer. Cut the opening. The opening in the wafer should be approximately 1/16 to 1/8 (1.5–3 mm) inch larger than the circumference of the stoma.

Allows for skin movement with activity and prevents impaired circulation to the stoma.

Step 13 Peel the paper off the wafer. Some resources suggest first holding the wafer between the palms of your hand to warm the adhesive ring.

Enhances the integrity of the seal by making the ring more "sticky" so that it will bond better with the skin.

Note: Some ostomy wafers come with an outer ring of tape attached. Do not remove the backing on this tape until the wafer is securely positioned (step 16).

PROCEDURE 28–5   Changing an Ostomy Appliance *(continued)*

Step 14 At this time, you may apply ostomy skin care products per your clinical judgment, hospital protocol, or following the recommendations of the enterostomal therapist (e.g., wipe around stoma with skin prep, apply skin barrier powder or paste, or apply extra adhesive paste).

These products prevent or treat excoriated skin and/or ensure a tight seal between the wafer and the skin.

Step 15 Remove the gauze. Center the wafer opening around the stoma, and gently press it down.

a. If you are using a one-piece pouch, make sure the bag is pointed toward the patient's feet.

b. If you are using a two-piece system, place the wafer on first. When the seal is complete, attach the bag following manufacturer's instructions. ▼

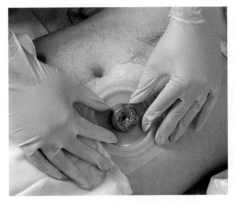

c. For an open-ended pouch, fold the end of the pouch over the clamp,

and close the clamp, listening for a "click" to ensure that it is secure.

Note: McConnell (2002) and information from the University of Pittsburgh Medical Center suggest that the patient place her hand over the newly applied wafer. Heat from the hand warms the adhesive ring, making it adhere better. Some sources also suggest taping down the edges of the wafer.

Step 16 Return the patient to a comfortable position. Dispose of the used ostomy pouch following your facility's policy for biohazardous waste.

Step 17 Remove your gloves and wash your hands.

Prevents transmission of bacteria.

Evaluation

- Note the characteristics of stoma: color, size, presence of edema, and shape.
- Note the presence of blisters, redness, or excoriation on peristomal skin.
- Note the amount and characteristics of effluent: color, odor, consistency.
- Note whether the patient expressed a desire to participate in the task.
- Note whether the patient demonstrated nonverbal cues that she is ready to learn about the task (e.g., looking at the stoma, picking up the equipment).

Patient Teaching

Patient teaching is aimed at preparing the patient to complete this skill at home. She will need to be instructed in how to complete all the steps of the procedure.

Home Care

- The patient may need to stand in front of a mirror or sit to change her ostomy appliance if she is unable to view the stoma easily.
- Teach the patient that slight bleeding is normal when the stoma is washed.
- A patient with a colostomy can complete the removal of her pouch and cleansing of the peristomal skin in the shower.
- Soaps and lotions containing oils should not be used. They decrease the adhesiveness of the wafer.

➤

PROCEDURE 28–5 **Changing an Ostomy Appliance** *(continued)*

- The appliance and wafer cannot be flushed down the toilet.
- Teach the patient to report changes in the color or size of the stoma and/or the presence of peri- stomal irritation or skin breakdown to the physician.
- Provide information about community support groups, such as Ostomates.
- Provide contact information for ostomy supply vendors.

Documentation

- Document your assessment of the stoma and peristomal skin area.
- Document the type of appliance used.
- Document the use of any special ostomy skin care products.
- Document the amount of liquid effluent on the I&O portion of the graphics record.
- Document patient teaching.

Sample documentation

| 3/16/07   4:30 P.M. | Ostomy pouch changed. 300 mL effluent obtained. (See I&O record.) Reapplied Hollister 2-piece appliance. Stoma deep pink; peristomal skin slightly red for about 1/2 inch around stoma. Patient observed procedure, but not ready yet for teaching. —S. King, RN |

PROCEDURE 28–6 Irrigating a Colostomy

For steps to follow in *all* procedures, refer to the inside back cover of this book.

critical aspects
- Determine the patient's normal bowel pattern before surgery.
- Use 500 to1000 mL, preferably 1000 mL, of warm tap water, priming the tubing prior to irrigation.
- Position the patient in front of or on the toilet or bedside commode. If the patient is immobile, place her in left side-lying (Sims') position, and use a bedpan.
- Remove the existing colostomy appliance. Examine the stoma and periostomal skin.
- Place the irrigation sleeve over the stoma.
- Lubricate the cone at the end of the irrigation tubing. Through the top of the irrigation sleeve, gently insert the cone into the stoma.
- Open the clamp, and begin the irrigation.
- When the irrigation is complete, clamp the top of the sleeve. Allow approximately 30 minutes for evacuation.
- Remove the sleeve, and rinse, dry, and store it. Apply a new colostomy appliance.

Equipment
- Irrigation equipment
  – One-piece system with a fluid container connected to tubing with cone or two-piece system with a container separate from tubing with cone
  – Irrigation sleeve; a sleeve without adhesive backing requires a belt to hold it in place
  – Clamp for a sleeve with an opening at the top
- IV pole
- Chair
- Water-soluble lubricant
- Toilet tissue
- Washcloth, towel
- Waterproof pad

- Two pairs of clean procedure gloves
- Bedpan or bedside commode (for the patient with Impaired Mobility)
- New ostomy appliance and skin barrier or stoma cap cover
- Ostomy deodorant (optional)
- Plastic bag for the disposal of the used pouch
- Skin barriers
- Toilet facilities that include a flushable toilet and a hook or some other device to hold the irrigation container

Delegation
The initial irrigation of a newly created colostomy requires nursing judgment and clinical decision making. Initially, this procedure should not be delegated to the UAP, although in some situations it may be delegated to an LPN, depending on agency policy.

Assessment
- Evaluate the occurrence of defecation, nature of stool, placement of stoma, abdominal distention, and nutritional pattern.

Findings may indicate the need to irrigate to stimulate elimination function; consistency of stool varies along the length of the GI tract.

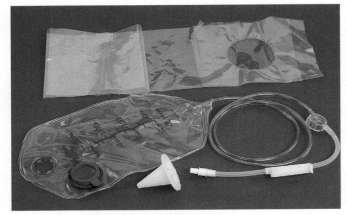

Colostomy irrigation equipment.

PROCEDURE 28–6   Irrigating a Colostomy *(continued)*

- Assess the type of ostomy.

An ileostomy drains liquid containing high concentrations of sodium, chloride, potassium, magnesium, and bicarbonate. Ileostomies should never be irrigated, except in cases of food blockage near the stomal outlet. Only a qualified person, such as an enterosotmal therapy nurse, may perform a gentle lavage. For lavage, normal saline is preferred because excessive lavage could lead to a serious fluid and electrolyte imbalance.

- Assess the patient's usual bowel pattern.

The purpose for irrigating a colostomy is to promote a regular pattern for bowel elimination.

- Assess for the presence of abdominal distention.

Distention may indicate excess gas or inflammation and should be reported to the primary care provider.

- Assess hydration status.

The colon may absorb some of the irrigation fluid if the patient is sufficiently dehydrated.

- Assess cognitive level and mobility status.

Determines the necessity for a bedpan or bedside commode. Also determines whether patient teaching will be effective.

- Assess the patient's ability to maintain a sitting position.
- Assess the characteristics of the stoma (see Procedure 28-5).

Procedural Steps

Step 1 Place the IV pole near the location of the procedure (e.g., in the bathroom, next to the bedside commode, or next to the bed).

Allows you to work efficiently.

Step 2 If possible, assist the patient to the bathroom or commode. Ask the patient if she prefers to sit directly on the toilet or on a chair in front of it.

Patients with impaired mobility can sit directly on or in front of the bedside commode, or they may remain in bed in the side-lying position.

Step 3 Prepare the irrigation container.
a. For two-piece systems, connect the tubing to the container.
b. Clamp the tubing. Fill the container with 500 to 1000 mL of warm tap water.

Water that is too cold will cause cramping, nausea, and discomfort. Water that is too hot will damage the intestinal mucosa.

c. Prime the tubing. Unclamp the tubing to allow it to fill.

Removes air from the tubing, preventing gas pains.

Note: Some ostomy resources suggest that using 1000 mL of water will promote a more effective irrigation of the entire colon and decrease the necessity to irrigate more than once a day.

Step 4 Hang the solution container on the IV pole. Adjust the IV pole so that it reaches the height of the patient's shoulder (approximately 45 cm, or 18 inches, above the stoma).

The height of the container regulates the force of the flow.

Step 5 Wash your hands and don clean procedure gloves.

Prevents the transmission of pathogens.

Step 6 Remove the existing colostomy appliance (if the patient is wearing one) following the steps in Procedure 28-5. Inspect the stoma and surrounding skin area.

Use of ostomy skin care preparations may be needed when you replace the pouch.

Step 7 Dispose of the used colostomy appliance properly. Empty the contents into the bedpan or toilet, and discard the pouch in a moisture-proof (e.g., plastic) bag.

Prevents transmission of intestinal bacteria.

Step 8 Apply the colostomy irrigation sleeve, following the manufacturer's directions.
a. Apply sleeves with adhesive backing according to the steps described in Procedure 28-5.
b. For sleeves without an adhesive backing, place the belt around the patient's waist, and attach the ends to the pouch flange on either side.
c. For patients sitting in front of the toilet or bedside commode, place a waterproof pad under the sleeve over the patient's thighs.

Prevents leakage and spilling of irrigation fluid and effluent.

Note: For patients sitting directly on a toilet or bedside commode, the end of the sleeve should hang down past the patient's pubic area, but not down into the water. For a patient in bed, the end of the sleeve should go into the bedpan.

Step 9 Generously lubricate the cone at the end of the irrigation tubing with water-soluble lubricant.

Prevents irritation and damage to the stoma and intestinal lumen.

PROCEDURE 28–6 Irrigating a Colostomy *(continued)*

Step 10 Open the top of the irrigation sleeve; insert the cone gently into the colostomy stoma, and hold it solidly in place.

Gentle insertion prevents damage to the mucosa. ▼

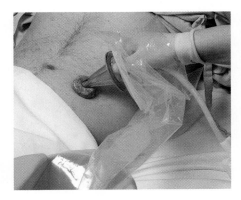

Step 11 Open the clamp on the tubing, and slowly begin the flow of water. The fluid should flow for about 10 to 15 minutes or as the patient can tolerate.

Proceeding slowly will allow the patient to adjust to the distention of the bowel.

Step 12 If the patient complains of discomfort, stop the flow for 15 to 30 seconds, and have the patient take deep breaths.

Allow the patient to rest and adjust to the pressure of solution.

Step 13 When the correct amount of solution has instilled, clamp the tubing, and remove the cone from the stoma.

Step 14 Wrap the end of the cone in tissue or paper towel until you can clean or dispose of it properly.

Prevents transmission of intestinal bacteria.

Step 15 Close the top of the irrigation sleeve with a clamp.

Prevents spillage of irrigation fluid and feces.

Step 16 Have the patient remain sitting until most of the irrigation fluid and bowel contents have evacuated. Alternatively, you can clamp the end of the sleeve and have the patient ambulate to stimulate compete evacuation of stool.

This should take approximately 30 minutes on average.

Step 17 When evacuation is complete, open the top clamp, and rinse and remove the irrigation sleeve. Set it aside.

The irrigation sleeve is reusable, but it should be rinsed promptly to make thorough cleansing easier in the following steps.

Step 18 Cleanse the stoma and peristomal skin area with a warm washcloth. Apply a new colostomy appliance, if the patient is wearing one, following the steps in Procedure 28-5. Otherwise, cover the stoma with a small gauze bandage.

Step 19 Clean the irrigation sleeve with mild soap and water. Allow it to dry. Place the irrigation supplies in the proper place (e.g., in a plastic container or plastic bag).

The irrigation sleeve is reusable, but it must be cleaned well to avoid odors and transmission of pathogens.

Step 20 Remove your gloves and wash your hands.

Prevents nosocomial infections.

Step 21 Assist the patient back to a position of comfort.

Evaluation

- Note the characteristics of the stool: color, amount, consistency.
- Note any signs of bleeding from stoma or bowel.
- Note the presence or absence of abdominal distention.
- Note the patient's tolerance of procedure (e.g., cramps, fatigue).
- Note the ability of the patient to participate in the irrigation.

Patient Teaching

- Teach the patient the purpose for the procedure.
- Explain that using sufficient fluid will decrease the likelihood of multiple irrigations during the day.
- Teach the steps of the irrigation procedure to prepare the patient to complete the task at home.
- Explain that it takes approximately 6 to 8 weeks for the bowel to become regulated with irrigations.

➤

PROCEDURE 28–6 **Irrigating a Colostomy** *(continued)*

Home Care

- Help the patient determine where this procedure will be completed in the home setting.
- Make sure the patient has resources for purchasing the supplies for the irrigation. Provide contact information.
- Help the patient locate a place to hang the irrigation container. There may be a hook on the bathroom wall, for instance.
- If the irrigating solution does not flow well, the patient should:
  - Check the tubing for kinks.
  - Change the position of the cone.
  - Put the container at a slightly higher level.
- Explain and demonstrate how to care for the irrigation supplies (e.g., how to rinse and clean the sleeve and/or belt, if used).

Documentation

- Document your assessment of the stoma and peristomal area.
- Document the amount of irrigation solution used.
- Document the date and time that you performed the irrigation.
- Document the characteristics of the stool returned in the irrigation fluid.
- Document patient teaching.

Sample documentation

06/14/07	8:30 A.M.	Ostomy irrigated with 750 mL warm tap water. Small amount of loosely formed, flaky stool returned in the fluid, with some undigested food apparent. No blood; very small amount of mucus. Stoma pink, peristomal area without redness. Explained procedure steps to patient as it was performed. Patient stated he will do some of the steps tomorrow. — C. Hiam, RNC

TECHNIQUES

TECHNIQUE 28–1 Testing for Pinworms

Pinworms (an intestinal parasite) live in the cecum and migrate to the anal area to deposit eggs during the night; they go back into the rectum during the day. Pinworm infestation is frequently seen in children. The test may need to be repeated on several consecutive days.

- While the child is sleeping, spread the buttocks, and examine the anus to see whether any pinworms are visible to the naked eye.

- Test in the morning, as soon as the person awakens and before he gets out of bed to use the bathroom or bathe. Press clear (not frosted) cellophane tape against the anal opening. Remove it immediately and place it on a slide. Eggs will be visible.
- Alternatively, or in addition, insert a cotton-tipped swab gently into the rectum for not more than 2.5 cm (1 in.). Smear the specimen on a slide to inspect for parasites and eggs.

TECHNIQUE 28–2 Administering an Oil-Retention Enema

An oil-retention enema may be used in a variety of circumstances. It may be administered to help a client pass hard stool; it also may be administered prior to digital removal of stool; or it may be given at least 1 hour prior to a cleansing enema.

Also see Procedure 28-3.
- Obtain a commercial oil-retention enema kit; these kits include a small rectal tube. If a commercial kit is not available, use a small tube (to minimize cramping and promote retention) and about 90 to 120 mL of the prescribed solution.

- Warm the oil to body temperature by running warm tap water over the container. Test a drop on your arm. (If the oil is too cold, it will cause cramping and expulsion of the oil. If it is too warm, it may injure the patient.)
- Instill the oil into the rectum (to soften stool and lubricate the rectum for easier passage of stool).
- Instruct the patient to retain the oil for at least 30 minutes.

TECHNIQUE 28–3 Administering a Return-Flow Enema

A return-flow enema, known as a *Harris flush,* may be ordered to help a patient expel flatus and relieve abdominal distention.
- You will need a rectal tube and solution container (e.g., bag or pail).
- Prepare 100 to 200 mL (for adults) of tap water or saline.
- Instill all the solution into the patient's rectum.

- Lower the tube and container below the level of the rectum, and allow the solution to flow back into the container.
- Repeat this process several times, or until the distention is relieved.
- If the solution becomes thick with fecal matter, discard it and begin again with new solution.

TECHNIQUE 28–4 Inserting a Rectal Tube

A rectal tube may be used to facilitate the passage of gas for clients experiencing intestinal distention.

- Use a 22 to 34 French rectal tube for adults. Choose the size according to the size of the client. For children or petite adults, a smaller size tube may be required.
- Position the patient on his left side.
- Wear clean gloves.
- Thoroughly lubricate the tip of the rectal tube, and insert the tube 10 to 12.5 cm (4 to 5 in.) into the rectum.
- Attach a collecting device to the end of the rectal tube. You may use a waterproof pad, or a graduated cylinder partially filled with water. An advantage of using water in the container is that gas generates bubbles, and you will be able to assess the effectiveness of the rectal tube based on the amount of bubbling in the container.
- Alternatively, you may attach the tube to a urine collection bag. You will need to provide a vent system by nicking the top of the collection bag to allow the flatus to exit the bag.
- Leave the rectal tube in place for 15 to 20 minutes. If distention persists, you may reinsert the tube every 2 to 3 hours.
- Assist the patient to move about in bed to promote gas expulsion. A knee-chest position is ideal because gas is lighter than fluid or solid; the position, therefore, promotes passage of flatus. Unfortunately, many patients cannot tolerate this position.

ASSESSMENT GUIDELINES AND TOOLS

Focused Assessment: Bowel Elimination

Nursing History

Ask questions such as the following

1. Normal bowel pattern
   - How often do you have a bowel movement (BM)?
   - What time of day do you usually have a BM?
   - Do you follow any routines to help you have a BM?

2. Appearance of stool
   - How would you describe your stool?
   - What color is your stool?
   - How would you describe the texture of your stool—hard, soft, or watery?
   - What shape is the stool?
   - Have you noticed unusual odor with your stool?

3. Changes in bowel habits or stool appearance
   - Have you had any changes in your bowel pattern recently?
   - Have you noticed any changes in the appearance, texture, or odor of your stool?

4. History of elimination problems
   - What has been your experience with bowel elimination problems?
   - Have you had any problems with constipation, diarrhea, or severe bloating or gas?
   - Have you ever lost control of your bowels?
   - Have you ever had bowel surgery or diagnostic procedures of the digestive tract?

5. Use of bowel elimination aids, including diet, exercise, medications, and remedies
   - What aids, if any, do you use to help you have a BM?
   - What foods help you maintain your bowel pattern?
   - What foods do you avoid? What affect do these foods have on you?
   - What is your usual fluid intake over the course of a day?
   - What is your usual exercise pattern?
   - What medications are you taking? Have they had any effect on your bowel elimination pattern?
   - What is your current stress level? What effect does stress have on your bowel elimination pattern?

6. For clients with a bowel diversion, you will also gather data on the client's usual care of the stoma, use of appliances, and adjustment to the ostomy.

Physical Assessment

Examine the abdomen, rectum, and anus.

- Recall that in abdominal assessment, the order of the exam is inspection, auscultation, percussion, and palpation.
- Observe the size, shape, and contour of the abdomen, and listen to bowel sounds.
- Percuss and palpate the abdomen for tenderness, presence of air or solid, and presence of masses.
- Inspect the anus for signs of hemorrhoids.
- Depending upon the policies of your institution as well as your skill with assessment, you might also palpate the anus and rectum for the presence of stool or masses.
- When listening to bowel sounds, note the presence and timing of the sounds and the presence of any bruits.

Normal bowel sounds are high-pitched, with approximately 5 to 35 gurgles every minute.

Hyperactive bowel sounds are very high-pitched and more frequent than normal. They may occur with small bowel obstruction and inflammatory disorders.

Hypoactive bowel sounds are low-pitched, infrequent, and quiet. A decrease in bowel sounds indicates decreased peristalsis.

- If after listening for 3 to 5 minutes you hear no bowel sounds, you can describe them as *absent*.

For a complete discussion of physical examination of the abdomen, rectum, and anus, see Procedures 19-14 and 19-19.

DIAGNOSTIC TESTING

Direct Visualization Studies of the Gastrointestinal Tract

- Because all of these studies are invasive procedures, you should ensure that the patient has signed an informed consent.
- All of the tests require some degree of advance preparation, such as fasting. Check agency policy, because preparation may vary from what is described in this box.
- Preparing the patient includes telling him what he will experience and feel during the test.
- When the patient is sedated (e.g., with Versed or Valium), a crash cart must be in the room during the procedure, and the patient monitored with pulse oximetry.
- All of the tests require teaching for aftercare.
- For all tests, explain that rectal bleeding is normal for a few days if polyps were removed or a biopsy was taken.

Esophagogastroduodenoscopy (EGD)

Provides direct visualization of the upper GI system. A *fiberoptic endoscope*, a long flexible tube with a light and lens, is introduced through the mouth and advanced for visualization of the esophagus, stomach, and duodenum. The physician may also perform tissue biopsies or coagulate bleeding sites through the endoscope.

Preparation
- Instruct the patient to fast for 6 to 12 hours before the test.
- Remove dentures and eyewear prior to the test.
- Because the tube is introduced through the mouth, patients often require sedation to limit gagging.

During the Test
The patient will be sedated, but awake. A local anesthetic will be sprayed into his mouth and throat to lessen the gag reflex.

Post-test Care
- Check vital signs and gag reflex (per agency protocol).
- Keep the patient NPO until the gag reflex returns; then instruct him to eat lightly for 12 to 24 hours.
- Instruct the patient to resume normal activity, medications, and diet in 24 hours.
- Observe, and teach patient to observe, for Potential Complication: esophageal or bowel perforation—cyanosis, substernal or abdominal pain, vomiting blood, continuing difficulty swallowing, or black, tarry stools.
- Explain to the patient that he will have a sore throat and hoarseness for a few days. Suggest gargling with saltwater and using throat lozenges.
- Caution the patient to notify the physician immediately if he experiences severe pain, fever, difficulty breathing, or expectoration of blood.
- Inform the patient that belching, bloating, or flatulence is a result of introducing air into the intestine and will be temporary.

Sigmoidoscopy

Allows visualization of the anal canal, rectum, and sigmoid colon. A rigid metal scope or a flexible fiberoptic scope may be used for this exam. The patient is usually not sedated. During the examination, the physician may perform a biopsy, remove polyps (small growths), or coagulate sources of bleeding in the area. A sigmoidoscopy is recommended as a screen for colon cancer at the age of 50. Subsequent screening depends on the findings of the sigmoidoscopy as well as patient and family history.

Preparation
- A light meal before the test is allowed.
- Administer two Fleet (or other commercially prepared, small-volume) enemas before the test.
- Have the patient void before the procedure.

During the Test
The patient may feel the urge to defecate; encourage slow, deep breathing through the mouth to help alleviate the feeling.

Post-test Care
- Observe for Potential Complication: bowel perforation (see discussion of EGD).
- The patient may resume normal activity.
- Explain that air was introduced into the intestines to distend them for better visibility and that, as a result, the patient may experience gas pains or flatulence for a few hours.

Fiberoptic Colonoscopy

Provides direct visualization of the rectum, colon, large intestine, and distal small bowel. A flexible scope is inserted through the anus and advanced to the cecum. Colonoscopy is useful in detecting lower GI disease. Many patients and healthcare providers choose a colonoscopy for cancer screening instead of a sigmoidoscopy, because colonoscopy provides greater visualization of the colon. This is the preferred test for clients with suspected problems above the level of the sigmoid colon.

Preparation
- Instruct the patient to consume a clear liquid diet for 24 to 48 hours before test.

- Instruct the patient to take strong cathartic and Dulcolax tablets the day before the test and an enema on day of the test, until returns are clear. *Or*
- Instruct the patient to drink a gallon of a strong cathartic (e.g., GoLytely) in 1 hour or less. It is important that returns be clear.
- The patient will be sedated before the test.

Post-test Care
- Monitor vital signs (per agency protocol).
- Observe for Potential Complication: bowel perforation (see discussion of EGD).

- Explain that air was introduced into the intestines to distend them for better visibility and that, as a result, the patient may experience gas pains or flatulence for a few hours.
- Instruct the patient to resume a normal diet when he has recovered from sedation.

Source: Schnell, Z. B., Leeuwen, A. M., & Kranpitz, T. R. (2003). *Davis's comprehensive handbook of laboratory and diagnostic tests with nursing implications.* Philadelphia: F. A. Davis Company.

Indirect Visualization Studies of the Gastrointestinal Tract

Abdominal Flat Plate

An anterior to posterior x-ray view of the abdomen used to detect gallstones, fecal impaction, and distended bowel. This test requires no preparation and no special post-test care.

Barium Enema (BE)

Radiological examination of the rectum, colon, and distal small bowel. A rectal tube is inserted into the rectum or an existing ostomy. Barium (a contrast medium) is instilled. The patient must retain the barium through several position changes while radiographs are obtained. The test is especially useful for visualizing polyps, diverticula, and tumors. In addition, it may be used to reduce certain obstructions. As a rule, patients are not sedated.

Preparation
- The test is invasive, so a signed informed consent is necessary.
- Instruct the patient to consume a low-residue diet for several days prior to the procedure.
- Instruct the patient to consume only clear liquids the evening before the procedure.
- Make sure the patient is NPO for 8 hours before the test.
- Administer a laxative, suppository, or cleansing enema the day before the test and cleansing enemas on the morning of the procedure (check agency policy). Enema administration is discussed in this chapter. For complete instructions for inserting a suppository, see Chapter 23, Procedure 23-6.

Post-test Care
- Instruct the client to resume food, fluids, and medications withheld before the procedure.

- Instruct the client to take a mild laxative and increase fluid intake (four glasses) to aid in elimination of barium (unless contraindicated).
- Explain that stools will be white or light-colored for 2 to 3 days; if patient is unable to eliminate barium, she should call the physician.

Ultrasonography (Ultrasound)

Detects tissue abnormalities such as masses, cysts, edema, or stones. An ultrasound probe, called a transducer, is moved over the skin surface of the abdomen. The probe emits a sound wave that abdominal tissue and organs reflect back based on their density. The sound waves may be transformed into images visible on a computer screen.

Computed Tomography (CT) Scan

Examines body sections from different angles using a narrow x-ray beam. It produces a three-dimensional picture of the area of the body being scanned. This test is useful in diagnosis of many abdominal disorders. A CT scan may be enhanced by injection of contrast dye that allows for improved visualization of circulatory function. Sometimes the patient is asked to drink about 450 mL of a dilute barium solution 1 hour before the CT scan to distinguish GI from other abdominal organs.

Preparation
If contrast dye is to be used:
- Determine that the patient is not allergic to contrast medium, iodine, or shellfish.
- Check blood urea nitrogen and creatinine levels to assure adequate kidney function.
- Patients taking metformin (Glucophage) should discontinue it on the day of the test and withhold it for 48 hours after to prevent lactic acidosis.
- Restrict food and fluids for 6 to 8 hrs if contrast medium is to be given.

During the Test
Explain that patient may feel nausea, warmth, a metallic taste, or a transient headache after injection of contrast medium. Instruct the patient to take slow, deep breaths if this occurs.

Post-test Care
- Patient may resume normal diet, activity, and medication; renal function should be assessed before metformin (Glucophage) is restarted.
- Instruct the patient to increase fluid intake to help eliminate contrast medium.
- Diarrhea may occur after ingestion of oral contrast medium. Observe for delayed allergic reactions (e.g., hives, headache, nausea, vomiting) if contrast medium was used.

Magnetic Resonance Imaging (MRI)

Produces cross-sectional images of the body. MRI utilizes a strong magnetic field in conjunction with radiofrequency waves. This type of diagnostic test does not use ionizing radiation, so it is free of the hazards of x-rays. MRIs are very sensitive and may be used to detect edema, hemorrhage, blood flow, infarcts, tumors, and infections in organ structures. When used, the contrast medium is noniodinated, administered intravenously to enhance contrast between normal and abnormal tissues.

Preparation
- Determine the presence of metal in the body, such as shrapnel or flecks of ferrous metal in the eye.
- Instruct the patient to remove all external metallic objects before entering the scanning room (e.g., jewelry, body piercing rings, eyeglasses, hairpins, credit cards).
- Food and fluids are not restricted.
- Have the patient void before the procedure.

Post-test Care
- The patient can resume normal activity, medication, and diet.
- If a contrast medium is used, observe for delayed allergic reactions.

Source: Schnell, Z. B., Leeuwen, A. M., & Kranpitz, T. R. (2003). *Davis's comprehensive handbook of laboratory and diagnostic tests with nursing implications.* Philadelphia: F. A. Davis Company.

STANDARDIZED LANGUAGE

Selected Standardized Outcomes and Interventions for Bowel Elimination Diagnoses

Nursing Diagnosis	NOC Outcomes and Scale*	NOC Outcome Indicators	NIC Interventions and Activities
Bowel Incontinence	Bowel Continence (m, t)	Recognizes urge to defecate Maintains control of stool passage Responds to urge in timely manner	*Bowel Incontinence Care* Determine … cause of fecal incontinence Keep bed and clothing clean Place on incontinent pads as needed
	Bowel Elimination (a, n)	Control of bowel movements Diarrhea Mucus in stool Elimination pattern	*Bowel Management* Teach patient/family members to record color, volume, frequency, and consistency of stools *Bowel Training* Initiate an uninterrupted, consistent time for defecation Teach patient/family the principles of bowel training
Constipation	Bowel Eliminaton (a, n)	Stool color Stool soft and formed Ease of stool passage Comfort of stool passage Passage of stool without aids	*Bowel Management* Monitor BMs, including frequency, consistency, shape, volume, and color, as appropriate Instruct patient on foods high in fiber, as appropriate Insert rectal suppository, as needed
	Hydration (a, n)	Skin turgor Moist mucous membranes Adequate fluid intake Dark urine	*Constipation/Impaction Management* Monitor for … impaction Explain etiology of problem and rationale for actions to patient
	Symptom Control (m)	Uses relief measures Reports symptoms controlled	Institute a toileting schedule as appropriate Teach patient/family on the relationship of diet, exercise, and fluid intake to constipation/impaction *Fluid Management* Monitor hydration status (e.g., moist mucous membranes …) Monitor food/fluid ingested … Promote oral intake (e.g., … offer fluids between meals)
Constipation, Perceived	Health Beliefs (l)	Perceived importance of taking action Perceived threat from inaction Perceived benefits of action	*Teaching: Individual* Determine patient's learning needs Determine … ability to learn specific information (i.e., developmental level, pain, fatigue, emotional state …) Reinforce behavior as appropriate
	Bowel Elimination (a, n)	Abuse of aids not present Passes stool without aids Elimination pattern in expected range	*Values Clarification* Encourage patient to list values that guide behavior in various settings and types of situations Help patient define alternatives and their advantages and disadvantages Encourage consideration of the issues and consequences of behavior
Diarrhea	Bowel Elimination (a, n)	Elimination pattern Fat in stool Blood in stool Mucus in stool Diarrhea	*Bowel Management* Monitor BMs, including frequency, consistency, shape, volume, and color, as appropriate

➤

Selected Standardized Outcomes and Interventions for Bowel Elimination Diagnoses *(continued)*

Nursing Diagnosis	NOC Outcomes and Scale*	NOC Outcome Indicators	NIC Interventions and Activities
	Electrolyte and Acid-Base Balance (a)	Apical heart rate and rhythm Respiratory rate, rhythm Serum Na, K, Ca (etc.) Mental alertness Muscle strength 24-hr intake and output balance	*Diarrhea Management* Evaluate medication profile for gastrointestinal side effects Encourage frequent, small feedings, adding bulk gradually Suggest trial elimination of foods containing lactose Instruct patient to notify staff of each episode of diarrhea Monitor skin in perianal area for irritation and ulceration Measure diarrhea/bowel output
	Fluid Balance (a, n)	Skin turgor Moist mucous membranes	
	Symptom Severity (n)	Symptom intensity Impaired life enjoyment	*Fluid/Electrolyte Management* Monitor for abnormal serum electrolyte levels, as available Consult physician if signs and symptoms of fluid and/or electrolyte imbalance persist or worsen

Sources: Moorhead, S., Johnson, M., & Maas, M. (Eds.). (2004). *Nursing outcomes classification (NOC)* (3rd ed.). St Louis: Mosby; Dochterman, J. M., & Bulechek, G. M. (Eds.). (2004). *Nursing interventions classification (NIC)* (4th ed.). St Louis: Mosby; NANDA International. (2003). *NANDA nursing diagnoses: Definitions and classification 2005–2006*. Philadelphia: Author.

*For a list of NOC measurement scales, see Chapter 5, Volume 2.

What Are the Main Points in This Chapter?

- Bowel elimination is a normal process by which waste products are eliminated from the body.
- Feces is a mixture of insoluble fiber and other undigestible material, bacteria, and water.
- During defecation, the internal and external anal sphincters relax, the rectum contracts, and peristalsis increases in the sigmoid colon, propelling feces through the anus.
- The frequency of BMs varies. As long as stools are passed without excessive urgency, with minimal effort and no straining, and without the use of laxatives, bowel function may be regarded as normal.
- The bowel pattern set in childhood normally continues into adulthood. Adequate fiber, fluid, and exercise are required to maintain this pattern.
- Factors affecting bowel function include stress, anesthesia, medications, pregnancy, and pathological conditions.
- A bowel diversion is a surgically created opening for elimination of digestive waste products.
- The effluent of an ostomy ranges from liquid to solid, depending on the part of the bowel that is being diverted.
- Constipation is a decrease in frequency of BMs and the passage of dry, hard stool that requires more effort to pass.
- Diarrhea is the passage of frequent, watery stools.
- To promote regular defecation, provide privacy for the patient and allow time to use the toilet.

- Monitor patients with diarrhea for intake and output, body weight, and vital signs to assess for fluid losses; provide hygiene measures to protect the skin.
- Bulking agents are the preferred medications for treating constipation.
- Habitual use of laxatives, except bulking agents, may cause reliance on medication for bowel elimination.
- Fecal impaction is detected by digital examination of the rectum. To treat a fecal impaction, enemas or digital removal of stool is required.
- An enema is the introduction of solution into the rectum to soften feces, distend the colon, and stimulate peristalsis and evacuation of feces.
- Flatulence can be managed by avoiding foods that trigger this response and maintaining regular bowel movements.
- Bowel incontinence may be managed by providing assistance to the bathroom at regular intervals and at times BMs are most likely to occur, and by beginning a bowel training program.
- A healthy stoma ranges in color from deep pink to brick red and is shiny and moist at all times.
- A moisture-proof skin barrier is usually placed around a stoma to protect surrounding skin.
- A client with a bowel diversion must adapt to the stoma for elimination and learn to care for the stoma.

29

Sensory Perception

Overview

We experience the world through vision, hearing, smell, taste, touch, and the sense of our body in space. These senses help us to interpret and interact with our environment.

A sensory experience involves four components: stimulus, reception, perception, and an arousal mechanism. Reception is the process of receiving stimuli from nerve endings in the skin and body. Perception is the ability to interpret the impulses transmitted from the receptors (stimuli) and give them meaning. Humans respond to sensations when they are alert and receptive to stimulation. Developmental issues, culture, health status, medications, stress level, and individual preferences, however, can affect sensory perception.

Sensory deprivation, a lack of meaningful stimuli, can be due to environmental conditions or to interference with the reception or perception of stimuli. Impaired vision and hearing are the sensory deficits most commonly encountered in nursing practice.

Sensory overload, by contrast, develops when either environmental or internal stimuli—or a combination of both—becomes too much for a person to process. It can also occur in clients with neurological or psychiatric disorders.

Assessment of sensory perceptual function focuses on factors affecting sensory perception, mental status, recent changes in sensory stimulation, use of sensory aids, the client's environment, and the support network.

Nursing strategies to address impaired sensory perception include activities that:

- Promote sensory function.
- Prevent and treat sensory overload and deprivation.
- Assist clients with sensory deficits.
- Promote communication with clients with altered mental status.

Thinking Critically About Sensory Perception

The exercises in the following section allow you to practice the kind of thinking you will use as a full-spectrum nurse. Because these are critical-thinking activities, there is usually no single right answer. Discuss answers with your peers—discussion can stimulate critical thinking. If you have difficulty with any of the questions, consult with your instructor.

Caring for the Garcias

Katherine Garcia, Joe Garcia's mother, has been experiencing blurred vision. At a recent ophthalmology appointment, she was told she has bilateral cataracts that will require surgical removal. She reports to the clinic today, accompanied by her son, Joe. Katherine tells you, "I don't know what happened. I was pulling into a parking space at the grocery store, and the next thing you know, I hear this loud boom. I don't know how I did it, but I hit the car next to me. I just didn't see it."

Joe is very concerned and questions whether his mother should be allowed to drive. Katherine is visibly upset. "I don't want to hurt anyone, but I don't want to lose all my freedom." Joe insisted on this appointment to discuss his concerns.

A. What data will you need to gather from Katherine and Joe?

B. What assessments will you need to perform?

C. How will cataract surgery most likely affect Katherine? You will need to learn about the surgery and recovery to answer this question. Use a textbook, or, for a list of helpful web sites you can access,

 Go to Chapter 29, **Resources for Caregivers and Healthcare Professionals,** on the Electronic Study Guide.

D. What information would you offer to Katherine and Joe?

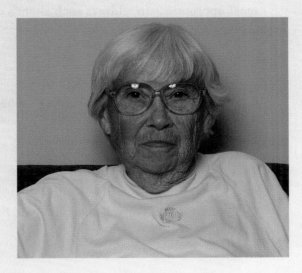

1

Review the following client scenarios.

- Client A is 84 years old. She is a retired school teacher who loves to read, work in her garden, and volunteer at the local children's hospital. She has developed macular degeneration and is progressively losing her sight.
- Client B is 55 years old. He is a former guitar player in a heavy-metal band. He now works in music production. He has significant hearing loss related to chronic exposure to loud music. Most recently he has developed tinnitus, which has exacerbated his hearing loss.
- Client C is 31 years old. He is a chef at a local four-star restaurant. He suffered a head injury in a motor vehicle accident and has lost his sense of smell.
- Client D is 26 years old. She is a licensed architect working for a firm in the downtown area. She has been taking birth control pills for 5 years. Recently she has been under a lot of stress. She began drinking lots of coffee, smoking cigarettes, and working long hours. She was admitted to the hospital with right-sided weakness and slurred speech. She is being evaluated for a cerebrovascular accident.
- Client E is 15 years old. He has cerebral palsy. As a result, he has a "scissor walk" and dysarthric speech. He has recently had a series of falls due to increasing problems with balance.

a For each client, write a nursing diagnosis to reflect their sensory perception problem. Write one other nursing diagnosis that might result from the sensory perception problem. Explain your thinking.

b Each of the clients is experiencing a sensory deficit. What interventions would be most appropriate to address each client's concerns?

c Which client(s) is/are most likely to have difficulty adapting to the sensory deficit? How would you determine how each client is adapting?

d Which client, if any, is most likely to be experiencing sensory overload?

2 Examine the clinical unit that you are visiting for your current clinical rotation. What unit factors contribute to the development of sensory overload?

3 What factors in the clinical unit contribute to the development of sensory deprivation?

4 For each of the following concepts, use critical thinking to describe how or why it is important to nursing, patient care, or sensory perception. Note that these are *not* to be merely definitions.

Sensory stimulation

Sensory overload

Sensory deprivation

Sensory deficits

Sensory aids

Practical Knowledge
knowing how

To provide support for patients with sensorineural alterations, you will need practical knowledge about assessing and diagnosing sensorineural functions. Other nursing interventions involve caring for patients who have vision and hearing deficits. This section includes a procedure for otic irrigations, which may be used to correct hearing loss resulting from a cerumen-blocked ear canal. Some procedures to support sensory function, such as instilling medications and irrigating the eye, are presented in the procedures in Chapter 23 of this volume. For other interventions,

 Go to **Chapter 23: Administering Medications,** and **Chapter 29: Sensory Perception,** in Volume 1.

In this section you will also find techniques for communicating with patients who have visual or hearing deficits, assessment guidelines, and a standardized language table.

PROCEDURES

| PROCEDURE 29–1 | **Performing Otic Irrigation** |

 For steps to follow in *all* procedures, refer to inside back cover of this book.

critical aspects
- Warm the irrigating solution to body temperature.
- Assist the patient into a sitting or lying position, with the head tilted away from the affected ear.
- Straighten the ear canal by pulling up and back on the pinna. For a young child, pull down and back to straighten the canal.
- Instruct the patient to notify you if he experiences any pain or dizziness during the irrigation.
- Place the tip of the nozzle (or syringe) into the entrance of the ear canal, and direct the stream of irrigating solution gently along the top of the ear canal toward the back of the client's head.
- Continue irrigating until the canal is clean.

Equipment
- An ear irrigation system, such as the Welch Allyn ear wash system, Asepto syringe, or rubber bulb syringe
- Irrigating solution (usually water, but may be an antiseptic solution)
- Bath towel and moisture-resistant towel
- Emesis basin
- Otoscope
- Cotton balls
- Procedure gloves

Delegation
You must assess the client before performing this procedure and evaluate client responses during and after the procedure. The procedure requires knowledge of anatomy and physiology, use of an otoscope, and, sometimes, use of sterile technique. Therefore, you should not delegate otic irrigation to unlicensed assistive personnel (UAP).

Assessment
- Determine whether there are contraindications for ear irrigation.

Contraindications include ruptured tympanic membrane, the presence of a middle ear infection, or acute inflammation of the ear canal.

- Assess the external ear for drainage.

PROCEDURE 29–1   **Performing Otic Irrigation** *(continued)*

Do not irrigate the ears if drainage is present. Drainage from the ear may be a sign of rupture of the tympanic membrane.

• Assess the external ear for cerumen.

Impacted cerumen is the most common reason for performing an ear irrigation.

• Assess the external ear canal for redness, swelling, or foreign objects.

Establishes baseline. If a foreign object is present, attempt to remove it prior to irrigation.

• Assess for pain or hearing loss.

Establishes baseline. Cerumen blockage in the ear canal may result in a conductive hearing loss.

Procedural Steps

Step 1 Warm irrigating solution to body temperature (37°C [98.6°F]), and fill the reservoir of the irrigator.

Placing cool solutions in the ear can cause dizziness.

Step 2 Assist the client into a sitting or lying position, with the head tilted away from the affected ear.

Facilitates administering the solution and allows fluid to flow from the auditory canal.

Step 3 Drape the client with a plastic drape, and place a towel on the client's shoulder on the side being irrigated. Have the client hold an emesis basin under the ear to collect the irrigating fluid as it drains out of the ear.

Note: An emesis basin is not necessary if a comprehensive ear wash system is used.

Step 4 If you are using an ear wash system, flush the system to remove air. If you are using an Asepto or rubber bulb syringe, fill the syringe with about 50 mL of the irrigating solution, and expel any remaining air. ▼

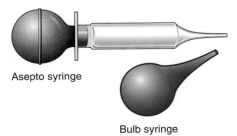

Asepto syringe

Bulb syringe

Step 5 Straighten the ear canal.

Developmental Modification For infants and young children, you will need another caregiver to immobilize the child.
a. For a child less than 3 years old, pull the pinna down and back.
b. For older children and adults, pull the pinna upward and outward.

Straightens the ear canal so that the solution can flow through the length of the canal.

Step 6 Instruct the client to notify you if he experiences any pain or dizziness during the irrigation. Explain to the client that he may feel warmth, fullness, or pressure when the fluid reaches the tympanic membrane.

Pain or dizziness may indicate a contraindication to the procedure.

Step 7 Place the tip of the nozzle (or syringe) about 1 cm (1/2 in.) above the entrance of the ear canal, and direct the stream of irrigating solution gently along the top of the ear canal toward the back of the client's head. Instill the solution slowly. Do not occlude the ear canal with the nozzle; allow the solution to flow out as it is instilled. Repeat this procedure for

5 minutes or until you can see cerumen in the return solution. ▼

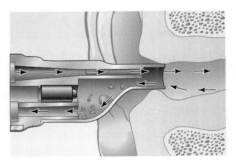

Ear irrigation system

Directing the flow directly onto the tympanic membrane could injure the membrane. Strong pressure can cause discomfort and may even damage the tympanic membrane.

Step 8 Inspect the ear with an otoscope to evaluate cerumen removal. See Procedure 19–7 for a review of otoscopic examination.

Allows visualization of the canal.

Step 9 Continue irrigating until the canal is cleaned. Do not block the ear canal with the syringe or irrigation tip.

The irrigating solution will soften the cerumen, easing removal. Blocking the canal prevents the outward flow of the solution.

Step 10 Place a cotton ball loosely in the ear canal, and have the client lie on the side of the affected ear.

The cotton ball will absorb excess fluid that drains by gravity.

➤

PROCEDURE 29–1   **Performing Otic Irrigation** *(continued)*

Evaluation

- Observe the quantity and quality of ear cerumen you removed.
- Observe the appearance of the ear canal.
- Assess for complaints of pain or dizziness.
- Assess for improvement in hearing acuity.
- Re-assess for drainage on the cotton ball.

Patient Teaching

- Avoid use of cotton swabs. They simply push cerumen deeper into the ear.
- Clean ears daily with washcloth, soap, and water.
- If earwax is a problem, over-the-counter preparations can be used to prevent wax buildup.

Home Care

Provide caregiver with instructions on ear care as stated above.

Documentation

- Document the ear solution used, the quantity, character, and odor of cerumen or drainage.
- Chart the condition of the ear canal and tympanic membrane after the irrigation.

Sample documentation

| 10/18/06 | 1400 | Pt c/o decreased hearing acuity in both ears. External ear canals occluded with dried cerumen. Irrigated with warm water. Large amount of dry brown cerumen removed with irrigation. External canals and tympanic membrane intact to otoscopic inspection after irrigation. —————— N. Ephrain, RN |

TECHNIQUES

| TECHNIQUE 29–1 | **Communicating with Visually Impaired Clients** |

- Introduce yourself when you enter the room.
- Call the client by her name so that she can be certain you are addressing her.
- When you enter a room with a client who is visually impaired, describe the room, room layout, and activities that are occurring.
- Orient the client to new surroundings, for example, "The couch is directly ahead 3 feet. There is a table next to it."
- Provide an uncluttered environment, and do not rearrange furniture.
- If the client has limited vision, be sure to position yourself in the client's field of vision.
- Speak to the visually impaired person before you touch him so that he is prepared for your touch.
- Do not raise your voice unless the client has a hearing impairment.
- Let the client know when you are leaving the room.
- Use the words "see" and "look" as you would with a sighted person.
- Avoid expressions such as "over there," or "right here." Guide the client to the location or place her hand on the object.
- Place the call bell, phone, and frequently used items within easy reach.
- Consider books on tape or Braille for the client's enjoyment.

| TECHNIQUE 29–2 | **Communicating with Hearing-Impaired Clients** |

- Make sure you have the hearing-impaired person's attention and are clearly visible to her before you start speaking. You may have to touch her lightly to attract attention.
- Face the person directly while speaking, and keep your hands away from your mouth.
- Many clients use lip reading to help them interpret your speech. Do not talk while chewing or eating.
- Help the listener by providing visual clues. Use gestures for clarification.
- Speak as clearly as possible in a natural way and at a moderate pace. Don't shout. Shouting often results in distortion of speech.
- Don't drop your voice at the end of a sentence.
- For better speech understanding, eliminate as much background noise as possible.
- Articulate your words clearly.
- If the person does not hear or understand something you've said, rephrase your statements. Do not repeat your words.
- Observe the client's verbal responses, facial expressions, and body language for clues to understanding. An inappropriate response indicates misunderstanding.
- If you are giving specific information, such as a time or place, be sure the person repeats it back to you. Many numbers and words sound alike (e.g., "fifteen" and "fifty").

ASSESSMENT GUIDELINES AND TOOLS

As a nurse, you should always consider your client's sensory perceptual status. Sensory deficits and excess or inadequate stimulation have a significant influence on quality of life and may be especially troublesome for institutionalized clients.

Nursing History: Sensory Perceptual Status

Usual Sensory Function

Ask questions such as the following:

- How would you rate your vision?
- How would you evaluate your ability to see objects up close or at a distance?
- Do you have any difficulty hearing conversations or listening to the radio or television?
- Have you experienced any difficulty locating sounds?
- Do you experience ringing or buzzing in your ears?
- Do you enjoy the taste of food?
- Do you notice any difficulty with your ability to smell?
- Are you experiencing any pain or discomfort?
- Do you have any areas of numbness or tingling on your body?
- Do you have any difficulty with sensing hot or cold?
- Describe your level of coordination.
- What medications are you taking? Have they had any effect on your vision, hearing, sense of taste, smell, touch, or balance?
- What is your current stress level?
- What is your usual activity level?
- What is your preferred activity level?

Risk Factors for Impaired Sensory Function

Assess:

- Developmental level (e.g., older adults)
- Health status (usual and current state of health, current health concerns, history of hospitalizations and surgeries)
- Medications (i.e., look up side effects to determine what, if any, effect the medications have on sensory function)
- Stress (current and usual stress level, major sources of stressors, usual coping mechanisms)
- Lifestyle (normal activity, noise, interaction levels, hobbies, and usual lifestyle)

Changes in Sensory Function

Ask questions such as the following:

- Have you experienced any changes in your vision or hearing?

- Have you had to turn up the sound of the television or radio recently?
- Have you had any changes in your appetite or interest in food?
- Have you noticed any changes in the taste of food?
- Do things smell the same as usual?
- Have you lost or gained weight recently?
- Have you had any recent falls? If so, describe the circumstances.
- Have family or friends commented on any changes in your vision, hearing, or function?
- Have you had any recent changes in activity level?

History of Sensory Problems

Ask the client:

- Have you experienced any problems with blurred vision, double vision, sensitivity to light, blind spots, objects moving in front of your eyes, or eye pain?
- Have you ever felt unable to follow a conversation because of difficulty hearing?
- Have you ever had problems with your ability to taste or smell?
- Have you ever had areas of numbness or tingling?
- Has anyone in your family ever been diagnosed with a stroke or circulation problem?
- Have you ever had episodes of confusion or disorientation?

Use of Sensory Aids, Including Diet, Exercise, Medications, and Remedies

- Does the client wear glasses or contact lenses at any time? If so, determine the following:
  - When was the client's last eye exam?
  - Are the glasses clean and in good repair? Are the glasses within easy reach?
  - Are contact lenses in good condition? Is the client able to care for them?
- Does the client wear a hearing aid? If so, determine the following:
  - Can the client hear adequately with the hearing aid in place?
  - Are the batteries working?

(continued)

- Is the hearing aid clean?
- How much help does the client need to place the aid in his ear?

- Does the client use a cane or walker? If so:
  - Has the cane or walker been properly fitted to the client?
  - How often does the client use the device when walking?
  - What factors determine when the device will be used?

Assess Mental Status

- Assess behavior, appearance, response to stimuli, speech, memory, and judgment. See Technique 19–7.

- Assess level of orientation: Have the client tell you his name, the date, and his current location. If he can answer these questions correctly, describe him as "awake, alert, and oriented to person, place, and time (AA&Ox3).

 Go to Chapter 19, **Table 19-5: Glasgow Coma Scale,** in Volume 1.

Assess Support Network for Clients with Sensory Deficit

- Are there support persons to help the client by assuming chores he can no longer perform?

- Are there people who provide comfort to ease the client's distress about sensory losses?

- Who can provide sensory stimulation?

- Who can help reorient and calm the client?

Bedside Assessment of Sensory Function

Sense	Assessment Process
Vision	Use the Snellen chart, or have the client read a newspaper. Observe for squinting.
Hearing	Perform the whisper test. Inspect the ear canals for hardened cerumen. Observe client conversations. Are there frequent requests for repeating information or misunderstandings? How loud is the client's radio or television?
Smell	Ask the client to close his eyes and identify common smells (e.g., coffee, vanilla, cloves, tobacco).
Taste	Ask the client to close his eyes and identify common tastes (e.g., salt, lemon, and sugar). Give water between tastes.
Tactile	With his eyes closed, touch the client with a wisp of cotton. Have him identify when you have touched him. Repeat this process with a sharp object, such as a needle. With his eyes closed, ask the client to identify where you are touching his body.
Kinesthesia	Have the client perform the Romberg test. See Procedure 19–7 on page 265. Have the client perform alternating rapid motions, such as tapping heels or clapping. Observe the client's gait and movement.

STANDARDIZED LANGUAGE

Selected NOC Outcomes and NIC Interventions for Sensory Perceptual Nursing Diagnoses

NANDA Diagnoses	NOC Outcomes	NIC Interventions
Disturbed Sensory Perception (specify): Visual	Sensory Function: Vision Vision Compensation Behavior	Communication Enhancement: Visual Deficit Environmental Management Fall Prevention
Auditory	Communication: Receptive Sensory Function: Hearing Hearing Compensation Behavior	Communication Enhancement: Hearing Deficit Ear Care
Kinesthetic	Sensory Function: Proprioception Balance Body Positioning: Self-Initiated Coordinated Movement	Body Mechanics Promotion Exercise Therapy: Balance Environmental Management
Gustatory and Olfactory	Sensory Function: Taste & Smell Appetite Nutritional Status: Food & Fluid Intake	Nausea Management Nutrition Management Feeding Environmental Management
Tactile	Sensory Function: Cutaneous	Teaching: Foot Care Lower Extremity Monitoring Peripheral Sensation Management
Acute Confusion	Cognitive Orientation Information Processing Neurological Status: Consciousness	Delirium Management Delusion Management Environmental Management
Chronic Confusion	Cognitive Orientation Concentration Information Processing Neurological Status: Consciousness	Dementia Management Dementia Management: Bathing Mood Management Cognitive Stimulation Environmental Management
Impaired Environmental Interpretation Syndrome	Cognitive Orientation Concentration Fall Prevention Behavior Memory Neurological Status: Consciousness	Dementia Management Dementia Management: Bathing Reality Therapy
Impaired Memory	Cognition Memory Neurological Status	Memory Training Neurologic Monitoring Surveillance: Safety
Risk for Peripheral Vascular Dysfunction	Body Positioning: Self-Initiated Neurological Status: Cranial Sensory/Motor Function Neurological Status: Spinal Sensory/Motor Function	Exercise Therapy: Joint Mobility Lower Extremity Monitoring Neurologic Monitoring Peripheral Sensation Management
Unilateral Neglect	Adaptation to Physical Disability Body Positioning: Self-Initiated Coordinated Movement	Unilateral Neglect Management Environmental Management: Safety Positioning Touch

NANDA International. (2005). *Nursing diagnoses: Definitions and classification 2005–2006.* Philadelphia: Author; Johnson, M., Bulechek, G., Dochterman, J., Maas, M., & Moorhead, S. (2001). *Nursing diagnoses, outcomes, and interventions: NANDA, NOC, and NIC linkages.* St Louis: Mosby; Moorhead, S., Johnson, M., & Maas, M. (Eds.). (2004). *Nursing outcomes classification (NOC)* (3rd ed.). St Louis: Mosby; and Dochterman, J. M., & Bulechek, G. M. (Eds.). (2004). *Nursing interventions classification (NIC).* (4th ed.) St Louis: Mosby.

What Are the Main Points in This Chapter?

- The purpose of sensation is to allow the body to respond to changing situations and maintain homeostasis.

- A sensory experience involves four components: stimulus, reception, perception, and an arousal mechanism.

- Reception is the process of receiving stimuli from nerve endings in the skin and body.

- Perception is the ability to interpret the impulses transmitted from the receptors and give meaning to the stimuli.

- Humans respond to sensations when they are alert and receptive to stimulation. The response to a stimulus is based on intensity, contrast, adaptation, previous experience, illness, or injury.

- Sensory deprivation is caused by a deficiency of meaningful stimuli.

- Sensory deprivation can be due to environmental conditions or to interference with the reception or perception of stimuli.

- Sensory overload develops when either environmental or internal stimuli—or a combination of both—exceed a level that the client's sensory system can effectively process. It can also occur in clients with neurological or psychiatric disorders who are unable to adapt to continuing, nonmeaningful stimuli.

- Impaired vision and hearing are the sensory deficits most commonly encountered in nursing practice.

- The client with impaired vision, hearing, tactile sensation, olfactory sensation, or kinesthesia is at risk for injury.

- Visual and hearing changes may diminish the ability to communicate and may hamper social interaction.

- Developmental issues, culture, health status, medications, stress level, and individual preferences affect sensory perception.

- To assess sensory perceptual function, assess factors affecting sensory perception, mental status, recent changes in sensory stimulation, use of sensory aids, the client's environment, and the support network.

- Nursing strategies to address impaired sensory perception include activities to promote sensory function, prevent and treat sensory overload and deprivation, assist clients with sensory deficits, and communicate with clients with altered mental status.

30 CHAPTER Pain Management

Overview

Pain should be considered the fifth vital sign and be assessed continuously. It can be classified by its origin, cause, duration, and quality. Pain exists whenever your patient says it does. Emotional factors, developmental variations, past pain experiences, sociocultural factors, inability to communicate, and cognitive impairment influence a person's perception of pain. Serious physiological as well as psychological problems can result from unrelieved pain.

Because it warns of potential or actual tissue damage, pain is protective. It begins when mechanical, thermal, or chemical stimuli activate nociceptors, which initiate the transmission of pain impulses to the spinal cord. Pain can be modulated by the endogenous analgesic system or by pain relief measures.

Nonpharmacological pain relief measures include cutaneous stimulation, immobilization, and cognitive-behavioral intervention. Pharmacological measures include nonopioid analgesics, opioid analgesics, and adjuvant analgesics. Opioid addiction among individuals being treated for pain is rare. A pain management program includes discovering the patient's goals, educating the patient and family, and developing a nursing plan of care. Be sure to assess continually the effectiveness of pain management strategies.

Thinking Critically About Pain Management

The exercises in the following section allow you to practice the kind of thinking you will use as a full-spectrum nurse. Because these are critical-thinking activities, there is usually no single right answer. Discuss answers with your peers—discussion can stimulate critical thinking. If you have difficulty with any of the questions, consult with your instructor.

Caring for the Garcias

Review the introduction to the Garcias at the front of this volume. Joseph Garcia has bilateral knee pain secondary to osteoarthritis. To develop a pain management plan, what patient data do you need to know?

A. How will you get the data you need? What sources should you use?

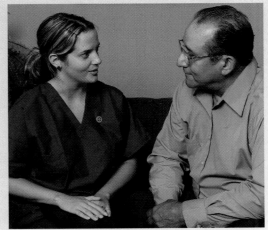

B. What types of nursing knowledge (theoretical, practical, ethical, or self-knowledge) are needed to develop a pain management plan?

1 Mrs. J is a 29-year-old woman with terminal metastatic breast cancer. She knows she is dying. She has a devoted husband and two children ages 2 and 4. Her husband has been taking care of her at home, but she is currently hospitalized for intractable pain. She does not want to be heavily sedated because she wants to spend as much time with her family as she can. She has no pain management plan.

   a What is it about the patient's situation that may intensify her pain?

   b Would you suggest using alternative therapies? Why or why not?

2 Mr. L is a 39-year-old construction worker who fell from a roof at a construction site 8 months ago and is still having back pain from the accident. His pain medication is an oral opioid prescribed every 4 hours on a PRN basis. He is still out of work and has great difficulty walking, so that he spends most of the day in a recliner watching TV and drinking beer. Mr. L also sleeps most nights in the recliner. He states that the alcohol is the only thing that helps his pain. How would you alter his pain management plan to get better relief? What is your rationale for these changes?

3 How might you encourage a facility to enact a pain assessment strategy of pain as the fifth vital sign if this is not their current policy?

4 If you were delegating vital signs to a UAP, what instructions would you give?

5 For each of the following concepts, use critical thinking to describe how or why it is important to nursing, patient care, or pain management. Note that these are *not* to be merely definitions.

Nociceptive pain

Neuropathic pain

Unrelieved pain

Fear of addiction

Nonpharmacological pain management

Nonopioid pain medications

Opioid pain medications

Adjuvant therapies

Pain as the fifth vital sign

Pain scales

Pain flowsheets

thinking critically about pain management

Practical Knowledge

knowing how

When caring for patients with pain, you will need to be skilled in medication administration, including use of PCA pumps and caring for patients who have an epidural catheter.

PROCEDURES

PROCEDURE 30–1	Connecting a Patient-Controlled Analgesia Pump

 For steps to follow in *all* procedures, refer to the inside back cover of this book.

critical aspects

- Determine the patient's baseline vital signs, cognitive status, and pain level.
- Determine (calculate as needed): the initial bolus (loading) dose, the basal rate, the demand dose, the lockout interval between each dose, and the 1-hour or 4-hour lockout dose limit.
- Prime the connecting tubing.
- Insert into the pump the device containing the medication.
- Lock the pump, and turn it on.
- Set the pump for the loading dose (if ordered), basal rate, demand dose, lockout interval, and the 1-hour or 4-hour lockout dose limit.
- Connect the tubing into the patient's maintenance IV line.
- Start infusing the medication (loading, then basal, dose).
- Put the button that controls dosing within reach of the patient.

Equipment

- PCA pump
- Manufacturer's instructions for the pump
- Cartridge, syringe, or other type of sealed unit containing the medication
- Connecting tubing (to connect the PCA device to the patient's IV line)
- Maintenance IV supplies (if patient does not already have an IV line)
- IV pole
- Antiseptic swab
- Flowsheet
- 1 pair of clean procedure gloves (if venipuncture is necessary)

Delegation

Patient controlled analgesia is a system by which a narcotic medication is delivered intravenously to the patient. This procedure is outside the scope of practice of a UAP and should never be delegated. Furthermore, the UAP should not administer a dose for the client, even if he asks her to do so. You can inform the UAP of expected side effects and ask her to report her observations to you.

Assessment

- Assess physical conditions that can affect respirations.

Respiratory diseases, such as chronic obstructive pulmonary disease (COPD) and asthma, and conditions such as head injury and sleep apnea may put the patient at increased risk for respiratory depression that can occur with opioid use.

- Assess for the presence of hepatic and renal disease processes.

May negatively affect the clearance and elimination of opioid narcotics from the body.

- Assess baseline respiratory rate, pulse, and blood pressure.

PROCEDURE 30–1

Connecting a Patient-Controlled Analgesia Pump *(continued)*

A negative response to narcotic administration can be measured by a change in vital signs (e.g., hypotension, respiratory rate below 12).

- Check the patient's age and weight.

As with the use of any form of opioid narcotic, age is a factor when you are considering the dose. Older patients and very young children are at increased risk for respiratory suppression.

- Determine the baseline pain level and pain level that is acceptable to the patient.

Pain level is most commonly measured using a numerical scale ranging from 0 to 10.

- Assess level of consciousness and cognitive level.

Determines whether the patient will be able to understand and/or follow directions for self-dosing.

- Assess the patient's manual dexterity.

Patients with poor or impaired fine-motor control may not be able to operate the self-dosing mechanism.

- Identify medications currently in use.

The risk of respiratory suppression increases when a patient-controlled analgesia pump is used in conjunction with other CNS depressants, such as Valium.

- Determine the presence of and/or involvement of the family. Identify any family anxiety over the patient's degree of pain.

The self-administration feature of the PCA pump is intended for patient use only. Hagle, Lehr, Brubakken, and Shippee (2004), the Institute for Safe Medication Practice, *Health, Medicine Week,* and others have found that "PCA by proxy" (someone other than the patient pushing the dosing button, such as families or nurses) is a major factor contributing to adverse patient outcomes.

Procedural Steps

Step 1 Don clean procedure gloves, and initiate IV therapy if the patient does not currently have an IV solution infusing. Refer to Procedure 36–1 as needed.

Step 2 Obtain the medication to be used. You may need to remove air from the vial by pushing the injector into the vial. Connect the PCA tubing to the vial (or cartridge).

Some vials may not be completely filled with medication. Ejecting the air makes it faster to prime the connecting tubing.

Step 3 Determine (calculate if necessary) the:
a. One-time "bolus" dose (also called the *loading dose,* which you administer after setting up the pump)
b. Basal rate (the amount of medication to be delivered automatically by the pump, slowly over each hour)
c. "On-demand" dose (the amount of drug to be delivered with each push of the button
d. The "lock-out" interval (the number of minutes allowed between each

administration of an on-demand dose (e.g., q8 minutes or q10 minutes). If the patient pushes the button more frequently, the PCA pump will lock out administration of a dose until the preset time between doses has been met.
e. The 1-hour or 4-hour lock-out dosage limit; this is a maximum dose allowed in that time frame. (For example, if the patient has a 4 mg on-demand dose with a 10 minute lockout interval, the patient can receive a maximum of six 4 mg doses per hour for a total of 24 mg per hour and a maximum dose of 96 mg in 4 hours.

Note: PCA orders are usually written in milligrams; however, pump settings may be in milliliters. In such cases, you must verify the concentration (milligrams per milliliter) to set the pump correctly.

Step 4 Prime the tubing; then clamp the tubing above the connector.

Prevents air from entering the pump and causing malfunction; prevents accidental bolus of medication to patient.

Step 5 Insert the container into the pump, and lock the pump. Follow the manufacturer's instruction manual (e.g., some pumps can be set only if the door is closed and locked).

Depending on the pump, it may be a syringe, a cartridge or other sealed container that can be "locked" into the pump. Locking the pump prevents unauthorized access to the narcotic and dosing features.

Step 6 Turn the pump on, and set the parameters according to the orders and your calculations. You may wish to verify your calculations with another registered nurse. The settings may include:
a. A one-time "bolus" dose, which you will administer after you finish setting up the pump
b. A basal dose
c. An "on-demand" dose
d. The "lockout" interval
e. The 1-hour or 4-hour limits as previously calculated

Step 7 Swab the port on the IV tubing closest to the patient, and connect the PCA pump tubing.

➤

PROCEDURE 30–1   Connecting a Patient-Controlled Analgesia Pump *(continued)*

Removes gross contamination and discourages pathogen growth.

Step 8 Open the clamp and administer the "bolus," or loading, dose if ordered. Remain present with the patient as the dose is delivered. To administer a loading dose, set the pump lockout time to 0 minutes. Set the volume to be delivered as the bolus volume you calculated (e.g., if 10 mg = 0.2 mL, set the volume to 0.2 mL); press the button that controls the loading dose.

A loading dose is usually larger than the basal and on-demand dosage because pain is likely to be more severe before the pump is initiated. Remaining with the patient allows you to observe for adverse effects.

Step 9 Close the pump door, and lock the machine with the key.

Step 10 Check for flashing lights or alarms that may indicate the need to correct settings.

Step 11 If you clamped the tubing after Step 9, be sure to release tubing clamps; press the start button to begin the basal infusion.

Step 12 Put the control button for on-demand doses within the patient's reach. ➤

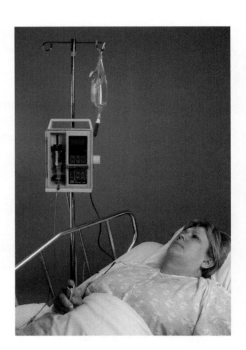

Evaluation

- Monitor the patient's pain level, sedation level, and respiratory rate every hour for the first 24 hours after initiating PCA.

Evaluates the effectiveness of the prescribed dosages and identifies need for dosage change. Promotes the early detection of respiratory depression, oversedation, or inadequate pain control.

- Perform routine assessment of medication use (e.g., number and frequency of doses) and pump settings as per facility protocol.
- Check the IV site for redness, infiltration, or phlebitis.
- Check the IV tubing (e.g., for kinks) to be sure the medication is infusing.

Patient Teaching

- Reinforce any patient (and if applicable, family) teaching about the safe and correct use of the PCA pump.

Decreases the likelihood of adverse outcomes.

- Teach the patient and family signs and symptoms of allergic reaction to report.
- Teach the patient how to rate the pain level.
- Teach families the rationale for not giving "doses by proxy."

PROCEDURE 30–1 **Connecting a Patient-Controlled Analgesia Pump** *(continued)*

Documentation

Documentation of PCA initiation is often completed on a specialized flowsheet. Items charted include:
- Time the pump was begun
- Patient's baseline pain level and evaluation of subsequent pain level performed at intervals determined by facility policy
- Baseline respiratory rate, pulse, and blood pressure; routine evaluation of subsequent vital signs performed at intervals determined by facility policy
- Sedation level

Continuous monitoring of vital signs, level of consciousness, and pain status, as well as the number and frequency of doses, are usually also recorded on a special flowsheet. Document unusual occurrences (e.g., oversedation, IV infiltration) in the nurses' notes.

TECHNIQUES

TECHNIQUE 30–1 **Nursing Care of the Patient with an Epidural Catheter**

- Intraspinal analgesia is contraindicated in patients who have spinal defects, have local or systemic infections, have increased intracranial pressure, or are on anticoagulant therapy.
- Monitor for respiratory depression (every 1 hour for the first 24 hours, then every 4 hours if the patient is stable).
- Mark all epidural lines *clearly,* for patient safety. This line must not be confused with an IV line.
- Ensure that the tape on the tubing connected to patient is secure. Signs of catheter migration are nausea, a decrease in blood pressure, and a loss of motor function without a recognizable cause.
- Prevent infection. Watch the site for leaking or drainage. Use strict aseptic technique when changing tubing.
- Assess for urine retention. Keep careful intake and output (I&O) records.

- Observe for signs of headache in the patient as a result of dural puncture. Treatment consists of bed rest, analgesics, and liberal hydration. Caffeine is also helpful and may be administered IV. If unresolved after 72 hours, patient might receive an epidural blood patch.
- To discontinue the catheter, first loosen the tape securing the catheter. While wearing clean gloves, apply slow, steady pressure to withdraw the catheter. Inspect the catheter on removal. You must be able to see the tip of the catheter. If not, a portion of the catheter may still be lodged in the patient's epidural space. Notify the anesthesia team immediately of this finding.
- Cleanse the insertion site, and cover with a dry sterile dressing.

ASSESSMENT GUIDELINES AND TOOLS

Taking a Pain History

Taking a pain history is the most effective way to perform an assessment. Each agency has a different assessment form for this history, but the questions typically will include the following:

- Do you have pain now?
- When did the pain begin?
- Where is the pain located?
- How do you rate your pain? (Use a pain scale.)
- How would you describe your pain? Sharp? Dull? Achy? Burning?
- How often do you have pain? Is it constant or intermittent?
- Is there a rhythm or pattern to your pain?
- What makes the pain better?

- What makes it worse?
- How does the pain (if ongoing) affect your day-to-day life?
- Have you experienced this type of pain in the past?
- Do you have any other associated symptoms (such as nausea and vomiting) when you are experiencing pain?
- Have you used any medications to treat the pain? If so, were they effective?
- What, if any, alternative treatments have you used for pain?
- What past experiences or cultural factors, if any, influence the pain?

Observing for Nonverbal Indicators of Pain

Physiological (Involuntary) Responses

Sympathetic Responses (Acute Pain)

- Increased systolic blood pressure
- Increased heart rate and force of contraction
- Increased respiratory rate
- Dilated blood vessels to the brain, increased alertness
- Dilated pupils
- Rapid speech

Parasympathetic Responses (Deep or Prolonged Pain)

- Decreased systolic blood pressure, possible syncope
- Decreased pulse rate
- Changeable breathing patterns
- Withdrawal
- Constricted pupils
- Slow, monotonous speech

Behavioral Responses (Voluntary)

- Withdrawing from painful stimuli
- Moaning
- Facial grimacing
- Crying
- Agitation
- Guarding the painful area

Psychological (Affective) Responses

- Anxiety
- Depression
- Anger
- Fear
- Exhaustion
- Hopelessness
- Irritability

Using Pain Scales

The most commonly used pain scales are the visual analog scale (VAS), the numerical rating scale (NRS), the simple descriptor scale (SDS), and the Wong-Baker FACES rating scale.

The Visual Analog Scale

The Visual Analog Scale (VAS) is a 10 cm horizontal line in which "No pain" is written on the left side and "Worst pain imaginable" is written on the right. Patients point to a loca-

tion on the line that reflects their current pain. Although this rating system is simple and quick, some patients have problems with the abstract nature of the scale.

No
pain

Worst pain
imaginable

A visual analog scale for rating pain.

(continued)

The Numerical Rating Scale

The Numerical Rating Scale (NRS) is a line numbered from 0 to 10. Zero indicates no pain at all, whereas 10 indicates the worst possible pain. Patients choose a number from 0 to 10 to denote their level of pain. To use this scale, the patient must be able to count to 10. A scale of 0 to 5 may be more helpful for cognitively impaired patients.

The Simple Descriptor Scale

The Simple Descriptor Scale (SDS) is a list of adjectives that describe different levels of pain intensity. The simplest version of this scale uses the words *mild, moderate,* and *severe.* An SDS with many words is not recommended; it is time-consuming to describe and may not be understood by many patients.

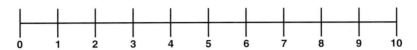

A numerical pain-rating scale.

The Wong-Baker FACES Pain Rating Scale

The FACES scale uses simple illustrations of faces to depict various levels of pain. It requires no numerical or reading skill. Initially developed for use with children over age 3, the scale has proven to be extremely useful for adults with communication and cognitive impairments as well.

Wong-Baker FACES Pain Rating Scale

0	1	2	3	4	5
No hurt	Hurts little bit	Hurts little more	Hurts even more	Hurts whole lot	Hurts worst

Explain to the person that each face is for a person who feels happy because he has no pain (hurt) or sad because he has some or a lot of pain. Face 0 is very happy because he doesn't hurt at all. Face 2 hurts a little more. Face 3 hurts even more. Face 4 hurts a whole lot. Face 5 hurts as much as you can imagine, although you do not have to be crying to feel this bad. Ask the person to chose the face that best describes how he is feeling. Rating scale is recommended for persons age 3 and older.

Wong's *essentials of pediatric nursing* (6th ed.). St Louis: Mosby, 1301. Copyright by Mosby, Inc. Reprinted with permission.

Revised Faces Pain Scales

We commonly ask patients to rate their pain on a scale of 0 to 10. However, the Wong-Baker FACES scale uses a 0 to 5 scale. To see a revised faces scale adapted to a 10-point scoring system, see Spragud, Piira, & Baeyer (2003), Children's self-report of pain intensity, *American Journal of Nursing, 103*(12), 62–64; or

Go to the **Pediatric Pain Sourcebook web site** at **www.painsourcebook.ca**

To see FACES scales using photos of children of various ethnicities,

Go to the **OUCHER! web site** at **www.oucher.org**

Sedation Rating Scale

1 = Awake and alert

2 = Slightly drowsy, easily aroused

3 = Frequently drowsy, arousable by voice

4 = Arousable by shaking

5 = Somnolent, not arousable

If the score on the sedation scale is 4, or higher, stimulate the patient and notify the physician. Before administering another dose, consider lowering the opioid dose, and investigate other potential causes of sedation.

If the respiratory rate is less than 8 to 10 per minute, respirations are shallow, or the patient is unresponsive to stimulation, attempt to stimulate the patient, notify the physician, and consider administering naloxone.

From *Pocket guide to pain management.* 2004. Distributed by Tufts-New England Medical Center Pain Clinic. Used with permission.

Client Pain Relief Diary

For pain relief I am using:

Medications _____

Alternative therapy (relaxation, distraction, etc.) _____

I will call my physician if _____ (filled in by nurse before discharge)

My goals are a pain rating of _____

Date	Time	Number of pills	Pain scale	Goal met?	Activity
			0 1 2 3 4 5 6 7 8 9 10	Yes No	

STANDARDIZED LANGUAGE

NOC Outcomes and NIC Interventions for Pain Diagnoses

NANDA Diagnosis	NOC Outcomes	NIC Interventions
Acute Pain	Comfort Level Pain Control Pain: Disruptive Effects Pain Level	Analgesic Administration Conscious Sedation Medication Management Pain Management Patient-Controlled Analgesia (PCA) Assistance
Chronic Pain	Comfort Level Pain Control Pain: Disruptive Effects Pain Level Depression Control Depression Level Pain: Psychological Response	Behavior Modification Cognitive Restructuring Coping Enhancement Mood Management Pain Management Patient Contracting

Sources: Dochterman, J. M., & Bulechek, G. M. (Eds.). (2004). *Nursing interventions classification (NIC)* (4th ed.). St Louis: Mosby; Johnson, M., Bulechek, G., Dochterman, J., Mass, M., & Moorhead, S. (2001). *Nursing diagnoses, outcomes,* and *interventions: NANDA, NOC, and NIC linkages.* St Louis: Mosby; Moorhead, S., Johnson, M., & Maas, M. (Eds.). (2004). *Nursing outcomes classification (NOC)* (3rd ed.). St Louis: Mosby.

What Are the Main Points in This Chapter?

- Pain is whatever the person says it is and exists whenever the person says it does.
- Pain has a protective function, warning us of potential or actual tissue damage and prompting us to take action.
- Pain can be classified by its origin, cause, duration, and quality.
- Pain begins when mechanical, thermal, or chemical stimuli activate nociceptors, which send pain impulses to the spinal cord.
- Fast-pain impulses are carried on large-diameter A-delta fibers, whereas slow-pain impulses are carried on thinner C fibers.
- Perception of pain occurs in the frontal cortex of the brain.
- Pain can be modulated by the endogenous analgesic system or by the gate-control mechanism.
- Some of the factors that influence pain are emotional factors, lifespan variations, past pain experiences, sociocultural factors, inability to communicate, and cognitive impairment.
- Serious physiological as well as psychological problems can result from unrelieved pain.

- Nonpharmacological pain relief measures include cutaneous stimulation, immobilization, and cognitive-behavioral intervention.
- Pharmacological measures include nonopioid analgesics, opioid analgesics, and adjuvant analgesics.
- Opioid addiction among individuals being treated for pain is extremely rare.
- Chemical and surgical pain relief measures are available.
- Pain should be considered the fifth vital sign and be assessed when the patient is admitted to a health-care facility, with each vital signs check, before and after an intervention, and when the patient complains of pain.
- Planning for the patient's pain management program includes discovering the patient's own goals, educating the patient and family, and developing a nursing plan of care.
- It is important to assess continually the effectiveness of pain management strategies.

31 Activity & Exercise

CHAPTER

Overview

The skeletal system, consisting of the bones, cartilage, ligaments, and tendons, forms the framework of the body and protects the internal organs. Movement depends on the interaction between the bones and the muscles, ligaments, tendons, and cartilage. Movement also requires balance. For your body to be balanced, your line of gravity must pass through your center of gravity, and your center of gravity must be close to your base of support. In the human body, the center of gravity is below the umbilicus at the top of the pelvis. The feet provide the base of support. Principles of body mechanics are the rules that allow you to move your body without causing injury.

The surgeon general of the United States recommends 30 minutes or more of moderate-intensity physical activity on all, or most, days of the week. A well-rounded exercise program focuses on flexibility, resistance training, and aerobic conditioning. Lack of exercise contributes to disease risk, especially cardiovascular disease, diabetes, and obesity. Severe illness associated with prolonged immobilization causes physiological changes in almost every body system.

When caring for immobilized or frail patients, provide a change of position at least every 2 hours to prevent skin breakdown, muscle discomfort, damage to superficial nerves and blood vessels, or contractures. Encourage range-of-motion exercises for a patient confined to bed so that she can maintain joint mobility and limit the complications of immobility. If the patient is unable to perform these exercises independently, you should move the joints in a process known as passive range of motion. Patients who have been confined to bed for more than a week or who have sustained major injury require conditioning before they are able to resume walking. Canes, braces, walkers, and crutches are available to assist a patient to walk. These aids promote stability and independence.

Thinking Critically About Activity and Exercise

The exercises in the following section allow you to practice the kind of thinking you will use as a full-spectrum nurse. Because these are critical-thinking activities, there is usually no single right answer. Discuss answers with your peers—discussion can stimulate critical thinking. If you have difficulty with any of the questions, consult with your instructor.

Caring for the Garcias

As you may recall, Joe Garcia has been advised to diet and exercise as part of the treatment plan for hypertension, type II diabetes mellitus, obesity, and osteoarthritis. Jordan Miller's exam has revealed no other cardiovascular problems.

A. Design an exercise program for Joe. Describe the program in detail. Recall that Joe has been relatively sedentary.

B. Compare the type of program you would recommend for Joe with the type of program appropriate for his granddaughter, Bettina.

C. What type of exercise program would be most appropriate for Katherine Garcia, Joe's mother? What additional information do you need to know to answer this question?

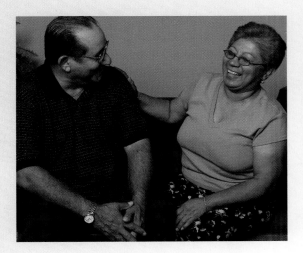

1 In Volume 1 you were introduced to Helen Jillian, a 72-year-old woman with hypertension, high cholesterol levels, and chest pain. She is 61 inches tall and weighs 290 pounds. Ms Jillian is admitted to the hospital for another episode of chest pain. You are assigned to care for her. Her physician has ordered her to be out of bed in the chair at least twice daily and to ambulate every day. How will you safely move this patient from bed to chair and assist her with ambulation? Work through that decision by answering the following questions.

a What aspects of this situation require the most careful attention (what are the risks; what could go wrong)?

b What steps can you take to prevent those difficulties?

2   Ms Jillian is refusing to get out of bed. "I'm sick," she tells you. "If you make me get out of bed, I'll probably have chest pain." How would you respond to this statement?

3   Vince Fulk is an 85-year-old man who sustained a massive cerebrovascular accident. He is unresponsive and immobile. What activity or mobility interventions should you incorporate into his plan of care? What is your rationale for these interventions?

4   For each of the following concepts, use critical thinking to describe how or why it is important to nursing, patient care, or activity and exercise. Note that these are *not* to be merely definitions.

Body mechanics

Exercise

Immobility

Activity tolerance

Assistive devices

Practical Knowledge
knowing how

In the next sections you will learn about procedures and techniques for positioning, moving, turning, transferring, and ambulating patients safely. Although the American Nurses Association (2005) recommends that you use assistive equipment for all patient lifting and transferring, you may encounter situations in which equipment is not available or you do not have time to get it. In such situations, using good body mechanics may help you decrease the risk of injury to you and the patient.

PROCEDURES

| PROCEDURE 31–1 | Moving and Turning Patients in Bed |

 For steps to follow in *all* procedures, refer to the inside back cover of this book.

critical aspects

31–1A: For Moving a Patient Up in Bed
- Use a friction-reducing device to move the patient if the patient can assist with movement. Use a full body sling if the patient cannot assist.
- Remove the pillow. Have the patient flex her neck, fold her arms across her chest, and place her feet flat on bed.
- Position a nurse on either side of the patient.
- Use a wide base of support.
- Have the patient, on the count of 3, push off with his heels as you shift your weight forward.

31–1B: For Turning a Patient in Bed
- Use a friction-reducing device and draw sheet to move the patient. Position at least one nurse on each side of the bed.
- Place the patient's near leg and arm (e.g., the left arm and leg when turning to the right) across his body, and abduct and externally rotate the far shoulder.
- Each nurse places one arm at the level of the patient's shoulders and the other at the level of the patient's hips. Each nurse shifts her weight as both simultaneously roll the patient in the intended direction.

31–1C: For Logrolling a Patient
- Move the patient as a unit to the opposite side of the bed; raise the siderail on that side.
- Move to the side of the bed that the patient will be turning toward; lower the siderail.
- Each staff member evenly distributes his arms across the patient's length. One nurse is responsible for moving the head and neck as a unit.
- Shift your weight backward as you roll the patient toward you.

➤

PROCEDURE 31–1   Moving and Turning Patients in Bed *(continued)*

Equipment

- Nonlatex gloves, if you may be exposed to body fluids
- Friction-reducing device, such as a transfer roller sheet or scoot sheet
- Pull or lift (draw) sheet
- Pillows, as needed

Delegation

You may ask unlicensed assistive personnel (UAP) to assist with moving a patient up in bed, turning a patient, or log-rolling a patient after ensuring that the UAP has the necessary skills and that the patient's condition is stable. Complete the assessment, and inform the UAP of any special considerations when moving the patient.

Assessment

- Assess the patient's level of consciousness, ability to follow directions, and ability to assist with the move.

Helps determine numbers of persons and equipment you need.

- Assess for any restrictions in movement or position by asking the patient and checking the physician's orders.

Helps determine how to proceed with the move.

- Assess the patient's level of comfort.

If the patient is uncomfortable, you may need to administer an analgesic prior to moving.

- Assess the physical size of the patient and the assistive devices available.

Helps determine how much assistance you need with the move.

- Observe for the presence of equipment such as IV set-ups, pumps, or casts.

PROCEDURE 31–1A   Moving a Patient Up in Bed

Procedural Steps

Note: This procedure employs the use of a transfer roller sheet. This device is inexpensive and readily available. Scoot sheets further reduce the risk of back and musculoskeletal injury; however, their availability varies.

Step 1 Lock the bed wheels. Lower the head of the bed, and place the patient in supine position. Position one nurse on each side of the bed. Lower the siderails. Raise the height of the bed to waist level.

Allows you to move the patient while maintaining good body mechanics and working with gravity.

Step 2 Remove the pillow from under the patient's head. Place it at the head of the bed.

Prevents patient from hitting his head on the head board.

Step 3 Instruct the patient to fold his arms across his chest. If an overhead trapeze is in place, ask the patient to hold the trapeze with both hands. Have the patient bend his knees with feet flat on the bed.

Position facilitates patient's assistance with move. ▼

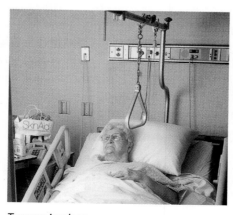

Trapeze in place.

Step 4 Instruct the patient to flex his neck.

Prevents hyperextension of the neck with movement.

Step 5 Ensure that a friction-reducing device, such as a transfer roller sheet, is in place under the draw sheet. If it is not in place, turn the patient from side to side to place the device under the draw sheet. You can improvise this device by placing a clean, unused plastic bag or plastic film under the draw sheet.

Facilitates movement by reducing friction. If a plastic bag is used, remove it after the patient is moved because it will allow moisture to pool under the patient.

Step 6 With a nurse positioned on either side of the patient, grasp and roll the draw sheet close to the patient.

PROCEDURE 31–1A   **Moving a Patient Up in Bed** *(continued)*

Step 7 Instruct the patient, on the count of 3, to lift his trunk and push off with his heels toward the head of the bed.

Coordinates and facilitates move.

Step 8 Position your feet with a wide base of support. Point your feet toward the direction of the move. Flex your knees and hips.

Allows you to maintain proper body mechanics while performing the move. ▼

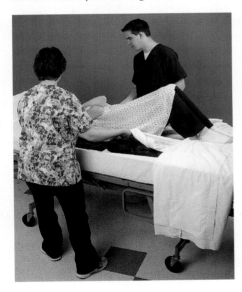

Step 9 Place your weight on your foot nearest to the foot of the bed. Count to 3, and shift your weight forward.

Shifting your weight allows you to use your momentum to move the patient.

Step 10 Repeat until the patient is positioned near the head of the bed.

Step 11 Straighten the draw sheet, and tuck it in tightly at the sides of the bed.

Prevents wrinkling, discomfort, and skin irritation.

Step 12 Place a pillow under the patient's head, and assist him to a comfortable position.

Provides comfort and good body alignment.

Step 13 Place the bed in low position, and raise the siderail.

Helps prevent falls.

Step 14 Place the call light in a position where the patient can easily reach it.

Allows patient to call for help, if needed.

Procedure Variation

Moving a Patient Up in Bed Who Is Obese or Unable to Assist

Step 15 Lock the bed wheels. Lower the head of the bed, and place the patient in supine position. Position at least one nurse on each side of the bed. Lower the siderails. Raise the height of the bed to waist level.

Step 16 Using the draw sheet, turn the patient to one side of the bed. Position the midline of the full body sling at the patient's back. Tightly roll the remaining half of the sling, and tuck the fabric under the draw sheet.

Positions the sling under the patient. ▼

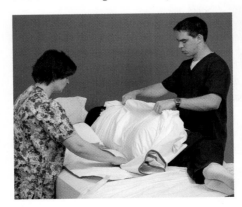

Step 17 Using the draw sheet, turn the patient to the opposite side of the bed. Unroll the full body sling, and reposition the patient supine.

Step 18 Attach the sling to the overbed lifting device or mechanical lift.

Allows the sling to be used as a lifting device.

Step 19 Engage the lift to raise the patient off the bed. Advance the lift toward the head of the bed until the patient is at the desired level. ▼

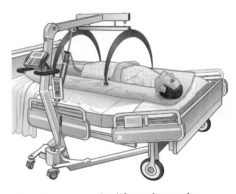

Step 20 Lower the lift, and turn the patient to the desired position. You may leave the sling in place for future movement, or you may remove it by turning the patient from side to side.

Note: If a full body sling is not available, use a friction-reducing device, such as a transfer roller sheet, and at least three staff members.

➤

PROCEDURE 31–1B

Turning a Patient in Bed

Procedural Steps

Note: This procedure employs the use of a transfer roller sheet. This device is inexpensive and readily available.

Step 1   Lock the bed wheels. Lower the head of the bed, and place the patient in supine position. Position one nurse on each side of the bed. Lower the siderails. Raise the height of the bed to waist level.

Allows you to move the patient while maintaining good body mechanics and working with gravity.

Step 2   Roll the patient side to side and place a friction-reducing device under the draw sheet. You can improvise this device by placing a clean, unused plastic bag or plastic film under the draw sheet. Move the patient to the side of the bed you are turning him away from by rolling up the draw sheet close to the patient's body and pulling it. Align the patient's legs and head with the trunk.

This allows you to position the patient in the center of the bed after turning. If a plastic film is used, remove it after you turn the patient. ▼

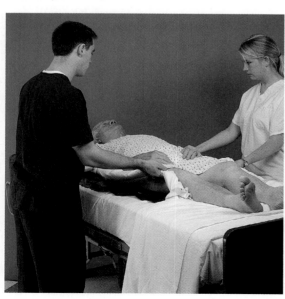

Step 3   Place the patient's near leg and foot across the far leg (e. g., when turning the patient to his right, place his left leg over his right leg).

This position facilitates the turn.

Step 4   Place the patient's near arm (e. g., left when turning right) across his chest. Abduct and externally rotate the other arm and shoulder.

Positioning the near arm in this way facilitates turning. Abducting and rotating the other arm prevents it from being caught under the patient during the turn.

Step 5   Each nurse positions her feet with a wide base of support, with one foot forward of the other. Bend from the hips, and place one hand on the draw sheet at the level of the patient's hip and the other at the level of the shoulder.

Allows you to maintain good body mechanics while performing the move.

Step 6   Instruct the patient that the turn will occur on the count of 3.

Coordinates and facilitates patient cooperation with the move.

Step 7   On the count of 3, flex your knees and hips and shift your weight. The nurse positioned on the side toward which the patient will turn shifts his weight to the back foot. The nurse on the opposite side shifts her weight forward.

Provides the best leverage to turn the patient. ▼

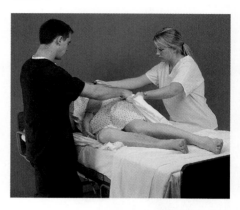

Step 8   Position the dependent shoulder forward.

Ensures that patient is not putting excess pressure on the inferior shoulder.

Step 9   Place pillows to maintain the patient in the lateral position.

Go to Chapter 31, **Table 31–4: Positioning a Bed-Bound Patient,** in Volume 1.

Provides support and maintains proper alignment.

Step 10   Place the bed in low position, and raise the siderail.

Helps ensure patient safety.

Step 11   Place the call light in a position where the patient can easily reach it.

Allows patient to call for help, if needed.

PROCEDURE 31–1C   **Logrolling a Patient**

Procedural Steps

Step 1 Lock the bed. Lower the siderail on the side where you are standing, but keep the opposite rail in the up position. Raise the height of the bed to waist level.

Allows you to move the patient while maintaining good body mechanics and working with gravity.

Step 2 Position one staff member at the patient's head and shoulders; she is responsible for moving the head and neck as a unit. Position the other person at the patient's hips. If you need three staff members, position one at the shoulders, one at the waist, and the third at thigh level. Instruct the patient to fold his arms across his chest.

One staff member must maintain the patient's head and neck in alignment. The other members assist with moving the rest of the body in alignment. ▼

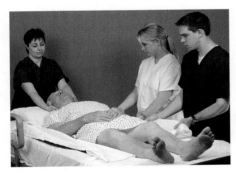

Step 3 Place a pillow between the patient's knees.

Prevents internal rotation of the hip and spine with movement. Maintains straight alignment of spine.

Step 4 Each nurse should position her feet with a wide base of support with one foot slightly more forward than the other.

Facilitates proper body mechanics and minimizes risk of injury to staff members.

Step 5 You should already have a draw sheet with an underlying friction-reducing device, such as a transfer roller sheet, to move the patient away from the side of the bed to which he will be turned. (You can improvise this device by placing a clean, unused plastic bag or plastic film under the draw sheet). One nurse should always support the head and shoulders. The move must be smooth so that the patient's head and hips are kept in alignment. Position the patient's head with a pillow.

Maintains straight alignment of the spine.

Step 6 Raise the siderail, and move to opposite side of the bed.

Ensures patient safety.

Step 7 Lower the siderail, and face the patient. All nurses should position their feet with a wide base of support, with one foot forward of the other. Place your weight on the forward foot. Bend from the hips, and position your hands evenly along the length of the draw sheet.

Provides the best leverage to turn the patient while maintaining spine alignment.

Step 8 All nurses flex their knees and hips and shift their weight to the back foot on the count of 3. Be sure to support the head as the patient is rolled.

Allows you to maintain straight alignment and body mechanics while performing the move. ▼

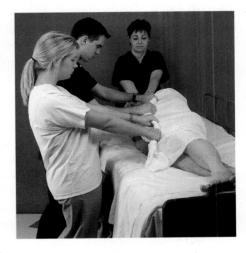

Step 9 Place pillows to maintain the patient in the lateral position.

 Go to Chapter 31, **Table 31-4: Positioning a Bed-Bound Patient,** in Volume 1.

Provides support and maintains proper alignment.

Step 10 Place the bed in low position, and raise the siderail.

Ensures patient safety.

Step 11 Place the call light in a position where the patient can easily reach it.

Allows patient to call for help, if needed.

Evaluation

- Assess the patient's comfort level after the position change.
- Assess body position and alignment after position change.
- Assess skin for pressure areas.

PROCEDURE 31–1   Moving and Turning Patients in Bed *(continued)*

Patient Teaching

- Explain to the patient the importance of maintaining spine alignment.
- Explain to the patient the importance of frequent position changes.
- Instruct the patient to ask the nurse when she needs to be turned sooner than scheduled.
- Teach the patient how he can assist with moving and turning.

Home Care

- Instruct the family member or caregiver in the proper technique for moving, turning, or logrolling the patient.
- Discuss the shearing effects on the skin from sliding down in bed (see Chapter 34).
- Provide instruction on importance of changing position and maintaining proper body alignment.

Documentation

Repositioning and turning patients are considered routine aspects of care and are not usually charted every time they are done. However, document in the nurse's notes any problems with positioning the patient or any areas of skin breakdown. You might also chart turning as an intervention when charting to a specific problem. For example, if the patient has Impaired Skin Integrity, you might describe the skin and chart, "Position changed hourly." Some facilities have flowsheets on which you indicate by a checkmark each time a patient is repositioned.

PROCEDURE 31–2   Transferring Patients

 For steps to follow in *all* procedures, refer to inside back cover of this book.

critical aspects

31–2A: For Transferring a Patient from Bed to Stretcher

- Move the patient to the side of the bed where the stretcher will be placed.
- Position the stretcher next to the bed, and lock it in place.
- Using the draw sheet, turn the client away from the stretcher.
- Place the transfer board against the patient's back halfway between the bed and stretcher. Position a friction-reducing device over the transfer board. Turn the patient to his back and onto the transfer board with the draw sheet.
- Use the draw sheet to slide the patient across the transfer board onto the stretcher.

PROCEDURE 31–2	**Transferring Patients** (continued)

31–2B: For Dangling a Patient at the Side of the Bed
- Place the patient in a supine position, and raise the head of the bed to 90°.
- Apply a gait transfer belt, and place the bed in the low position.
- Stand facing the patient with a wide base of support. Place your foot closest to the head of the bed forward of the other foot.
- Position your hands on each side of the gait transfer belt.
- Rock onto your back foot as you move the patient into a sitting position, and pivot to bring the patient's legs over the side of the bed.
- Stay with the patient as he dangles.

31–2C: For Transferring a Patient from Bed to Chair
- Have the patient wear nonskid slippers.
- Place the bed in low position, and lock the wheels.
- Assist the patient to dangle at the side of the bed (see Procedure 31–2B).
- Brace your feet and knees against the patient. Bend your hips and knees, and hold onto the transfer belt.
- If two nurses are available to assist with the transfer, one nurse should be on each side of the patient.
- Instruct the patient to place her arms around you between your shoulders and waist. Ask the patient to stand as you move to an upright position by straightening your legs and hips.
- Instruct the patient to pivot and turn with you toward the chair.
- Have the patient flex her hips and knees as she lowers herself to the chair. Guide her motion while maintaining a firm hold on her.

Equipment
- Nonlatex gloves, if you may be exposed to body fluids
- Transfer roller sheet
- Transfer board
- Pull or lift (draw) sheet (for transfers)
- Gait transfer belt (for dangling and transferring from bed to chair)

Delegation
You may ask a UAP to dangle, transfer a patient from bed to stretcher, or transfer a patient from bed to chair after ensuring that the UAP has the necessary skills and that the patient's condition is stable. Complete the assessment, and inform the UAP of any special considerations when dangling or transferring the client.

Assessment
- Assess the patient's level of consciousness, ability to follow directions, and ability to assist with the move.

Helps determine whether one or more persons are needed for the move.

- Assess for any restrictions in movement or position by asking the patient and checking the physician's orders.

Helps you determine how to proceed with the move.

- Assess the patient's level of comfort.

If the patient is uncomfortable, you may need to administer an analgesic prior to moving.

➤

PROCEDURE 31–2   **Transferring Patients** *(continued)*

- Assess the physical size of the patient and your own strength and ability to move the patient.

Helps determine whether you need assistance with the move.

- Observe for the presence of equipment such as IV setups, pumps, or casts.
- Assess possible side effects of medications (e.g., dizziness and sedation).

Evaluates the patient's ability to cooperate with the transfer.

- Assess vital signs, and check for postural hypotension.

If the patient is at risk for postural hypotension, you may need to allow additional time for the patient to change position and plan for adequate help.

- Before transferring a patient to a chair, assess the patient's tolerance of dangling.

Informs you about activity tolerance and readiness to get out of bed.

PROCEDURE 31–2A   **Transferring a Patient from Bed to Stretcher**

Procedural Steps

Step 1 Lock the bed. Position the bed so that it is flat (if the patient can tolerate being supine) and at the height of the stretcher.

Ensures client safety during the transfer. Helps prevent injury to staff, because the patient is easier to move if the bed is flat.

Step 2 Lower the siderails, and position at least one nurse on each side of the bed. Move the patient to the side of the bed where the stretcher will be placed by rolling up the draw sheet close to the patient's body and pulling it. Align the patient's legs and head with her trunk.

Positions patient to enable nurses to move her to the stretcher.

Step 3 Position the stretcher next to the bed. Lock the stretcher.

Locking the wheels keeps the stretcher from moving during the transfer; prevents falls.

PROCEDURE 31–2A

Transferring a Patient from Bed to Stretcher
(continued)

Step 4 Place the transfer board.

a. Place a friction-reducing device, such as a transfer roller sheet, over the transfer board. (You can improvise this device by placing a clean, unused plastic bag or plastic film under the draw sheet.)

b. The nurse on the side opposite the stretcher uses the draw sheet to turn the patient away from the stretcher, while the other nurse places the transfer board against the patient's back halfway between bed and stretcher. Turn the patient to her back and onto the transfer board.

Safely positions the transfer board under the patient, without friction. ▼

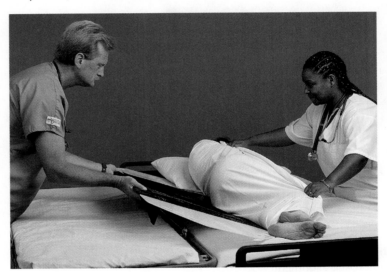

➤

PROCEDURE 31–2A

Transferring a Patient from Bed to Stretcher
(continued)

Step 5 Have the patient raise her head. Use the draw sheet to slide her across the transfer board onto the stretcher.

Using a transfer board and transfer roller sheet facilitates the move to stretcher; prevents friction on patient's skin. ▼

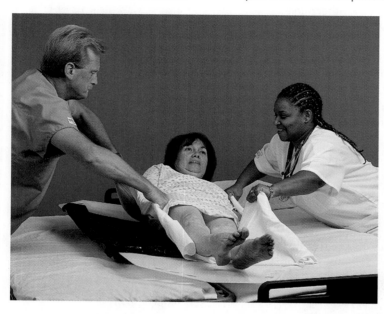

Step 6 Use the draw sheet to turn the patient away from the bed, and remove the board and roller sheet.

Step 7 Reposition the patient on the stretcher for comfort and alignment.

Provides support and maintains proper alignment.

Step 8 Provide a blanket if needed.

Step 9 Fasten safety belts, and raise the siderails on the stretcher.

Prevents falls.

Procedure Variation
Transferring a Client from Bed to Stretcher with a Slipsheet

Note: A slipsheet may be used instead of a transfer board. A slipsheet is a large, low-friction fabric that facilitates transfer.

Step 10 Lock the bed. Position the bed so that it is flat (if the patient can tolerate being supine) and at the height of the stretcher.

Ensures client safety during the transfer. Helps prevent injury to staff, because the patient is easier to move if the bed is flat.

Step 11 With the draw sheet, turn the patient to the side opposite where the stretcher will be placed. Position the midline of the slip sheet under the patient. Roll the remaining half tightly, and tuck it under the patient.

Step 12 Turn the patient to the opposite side, and pull the slip sheet from under the patient.

Step 13 Place the patient supine, and lower the siderail on the side where the stretcher will be placed.

Step 14 Move the stretcher next to the bed and lock the wheels on the stretcher.

Step 15 Position at least two nurses on the far side of the stretcher. Using the slip sheet, pull the patient onto the stretcher. ▼

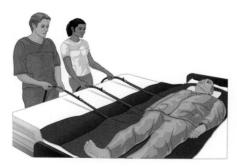

PROCEDURE 31–2B   Dangling a Patient at the Side of the Bed

Procedural Steps

Step 1 Lock the bed wheels. Place the patient in a supine position, and raise the head of the bed to 90°. Keep the siderail elevated on the side opposite where you are standing.

Locking the wheels prevents the bed from moving as you move the patient. Raising the head of the bed prepares the patient to be dangled and requires less effort from you to help the patient sit erect.

Step 2 Apply a gait transfer belt to the patient at waist level. Place the bed in the low position.

Ensures patient safety.

Step 3 Stand facing the patient with a wide base of support. Place your foot closest to the head of the bed forward of the other foot. Lean forward, bending at the hips, with your knees flexed.

Allows you to maintain proper body mechanics and prevents injury.

Step 4 Position your hands on each side of the gait transfer belt.

Prepares the patient for the move to the dangling position. ▼

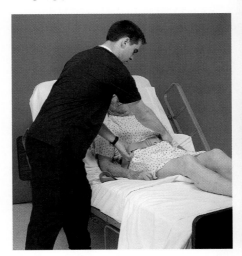

Step 5 Rock onto your back foot as you pull the patient toward you with the gait transfer belt, thereby moving the patient into a sitting position at the side of the bed.

Uses your body weight as leverage to reposition the patient, preventing injury to your back. ▼

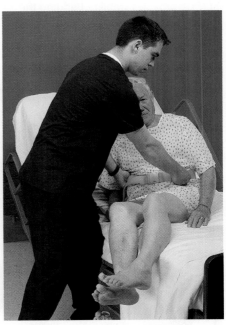

Step 6 Stay with the patient as he dangles.

Ensures patient safety.

PROCEDURE 31–2C   Transferring a Patient from Bed to Chair

Procedural Steps

Step 1 Position the chair next to the bed. If possible, lock the chair.

Prevents chair from moving during transfer. Ensures client safety.

Step 2 Put nonskid slippers on the patient.

Prevents patient from slipping during transfer.

Step 3 Apply the transfer belt.

Facilitates transfer of patient to chair and helps prevent back injury to the nurse.

Step 4 Place the bed in low position, and lock the bed.

Prevents the bed from moving during the transfer.

Step 5 Assist the patient to dangle at the side of the bed (see Procedure 31–2B).

➤

PROCEDURE 31–2C

Transferring a Patient from Bed to Chair
(continued)

Step 6 Face the patient. Brace your feet and knees against the patient. Pay particular attention to any known weakness. Bend your hips and knees, and, keeping your back straight, hold onto the transfer belt. If two nurses are available to assist with the transfer, one nurse should be on each side of the patient.

Bracing provides stability. Bending the hips and knees allows you to use the major muscle groups and limit the risk of injury. Lifting the patient at waist level prevents injury to the arm or shoulder. ▼

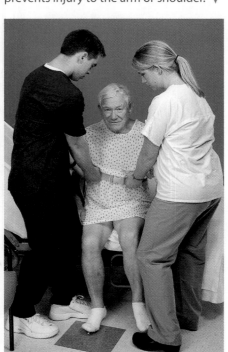

Step 7 Instruct the patient to place his arms around you between the shoulders and waist (the location depends on your height and the height of the patient). Ask the patient to stand as you move to an upright position by straightening your legs and hips.

Having the patient hold you on your trunk prevents injury to your neck. Straightening your thighs and hips uses your large muscle groups and prevents injury to your back.

Step 8 Allow the patient to steady himself for a moment.

Allows the patient an opportunity to rest before further movement. Allows you to evaluate her tolerance to activity before progressing.

Step 9 Instruct the patient to pivot and turn with you toward the chair.

Positions the patient to sit in the chair.

Step 10 Assist the patient to position himself in front of the chair, and to place his hands on the arms of the chair. Have the patient flex his hips and knees as he lowers himself to the chair. Guide his motion while maintaining a firm hold of the patient and keeping your back straight.

Maintains good body mechanics and balance and ensures client safety. ▼

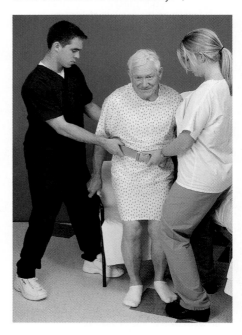

Step 11 Assist the patient to a comfortable position in the chair.

Step 12 Provide a blanket if needed.

Step 13 Place the call light in reach of the patient.

Note: If the patient is obese or unable to assist, use a full body sling that allows the patient to assume a seated position, if one is available. You may also use a powered standing assist lift, if one is available.

PROCEDURE 31-2 **Transferring Patients** *(continued)*

Evaluation

- Assess the patient's comfort level after the position change.
- Assess proper body position and alignment after position change.
- Assess vital signs for postural hypotension after dangling or transferring to a chair.

Patient Teaching

- Explain to the patient the importance of frequent position changes.
- Explain the importance of movement and getting out of bed to avoid problems of immobility.

Home Care

- Instruct the family member or caregiver in the proper technique for assisting the patient to dangle at the bedside or transfer to a chair.
- Provide instruction in the importance of changing position and maintaining proper body alignment.

Documentation

Patients are usually moved to a stretcher for transport to a test or procedure. The movement is a routine aspect of care and is not documented. When dangling or transferring a patient to a chair, document in the nurse's notes how much assistance was required, any problems with positioning the patient, and how long the patient was out of bed.

Sample documentation

| 10/4/06 | 1100 | Pt assisted to dangle at the side of the bed for 5 minutes. Pt experienced some initial feelings of vertigo with BP 108/60, P 110, RR 28. After 5 minutes BP 126/72, P 90, RR 24. Pt assisted back to bed. ———— S. Jones, RN |

| 11/11/06 | 0630 | Pt dangled at side of bed and assisted to chair with minimal assistance. Able to sit up for 90 minutes with no pallor and no change in vital signs. ———— B. Bowen, RN |

| PROCEDURE 31–3 | **Assisting with Ambulation** |

For steps to follow in *all* procedures, refer to inside back cover of this book.

critical aspects

- Have the patient wear nonskid slippers.
- Place the bed in low position, and lock the wheels.
- Assist the patient to dangle at the side of the bed (see Procedure 31–2B).
- If using two nurses, each should stand facing the patient on opposite sides of the patient.
- Brace your feet and knees against the patient. Bend your hips and knees, and hold onto the transfer belt. Pay attention to any known weakness.
- Instruct the patient to place her arms around you between your shoulders and waist (the location depends on the height of the patient and the nurses). Ask the patient to stand as you move to an upright position by straightening your legs and hips.
- Allow the patient to steady herself for a moment.
- One nurse: Stand at the patient's side, placing both hands on the transfer belt. If the patient has weakness on one side, position yourself on the weaker side.
- Two nurses: Each nurse stands at the patient's sides, grasping hold of the transfer belt.
- Slowly guide the patient forward. Observe for signs of fatigue or dizziness.
- If the patient must transport an IV pole, allow the patient to hold onto the pole on the side where you are standing. Assist the patient to advance the pole as you ambulate together.

Equipment

- Nonlatex gloves, if you may be exposed to body fluids
- Transfer belt

Delegation

You may ask a UAP to assist with ambulation after ensuring that the UAP has the necessary skills and that the patient's condition is stable. Complete the assessment, and inform the UAP of any special considerations when assisting a client with ambulation.

Assessment

- Assess the patient's level of consciousness, ability to follow directions, and ability to assist with the move.

Assesses ability of the patient to ambulate with your help.

- Assess for any restrictions in movement or position by asking the patient and checking the physician's orders.

Helps you determine how to proceed with the move.

- Assess the patient's level of comfort.

If the patient is uncomfortable, you may need to administer an analgesic prior to moving.

- Assess the physical size of the patient and your own strength and ability to move the patient.

Helps determine whether you can help the patient by yourself.

- Observe for the presence of equipment, such as IV set-ups, pumps, or casts.
- Assess possible side effects of medications (e.g., dizziness and sedation).

Evaluates the patient's ability to cooperate with the transfer.

- Assess vital signs, and check for postural hypotension.

If the patient is at risk for postural hypotension, you may need to allow additional time for the patient to change position and to plan for adequate help.

- Assess the patient's tolerance of dangling.

Informs you about activity tolerance and readiness to get out of bed.

PROCEDURE 31–3A   Assisting with Ambulation (One Nurse)

Procedural Steps

Step 1 Put nonskid slippers on the patient.

Prevents the patient from slipping during transfer.

Step 2 Apply the transfer belt.

Allows you to support the patient during ambulation.

Step 3 Place the bed in a low position, and lock the bed.

Prevents the bed from moving during transfer. Makes it easier for patient's feet to reach the floor.

Step 4 Assist the patient to dangle at the side of the bed (see Procedure 31–2B).

Step 5 Face the patient. Brace your feet and knees against the patient. Pay particular attention to any known weakness. Bend your hips and knees, and hold onto the transfer belt.

Bracing provides stability. Bending the hips and knees allows you to use the major muscle groups and limit injury. Lifting at the patient's waist level prevents injury to his arm or shoulder.

Step 6 Instruct the patient to place his arms around you between the shoulders and waist (the location depends on your height and the height of the patient). Ask the patient to stand as you move to an upright position by straightening your legs and hips.

Having the patient hold you on your trunk prevents injury to your neck. Straightening your thighs and hips uses your large muscle groups and promotes good body mechanics.

Step 7 Allow the patient to steady himself for a moment.

Allows the patient an opportunity to rest before further movement and to regain equilibrium before walking.

Step 8 Stand at the patient's side, placing both hands on the transfer belt. If the patient has weakness on one side, position yourself on the weaker side.

Helps patient maintain an erect posture. ▼

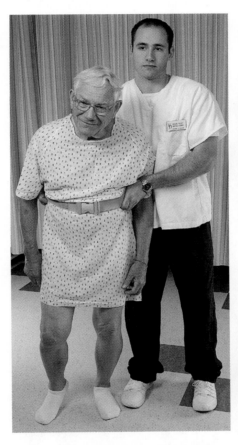

Step 9 Slowly guide the patient forward. Observe for signs of fatigue or dizziness.

Ensures client safety.

Step 10 If the patient must transport an IV pole, allow the patient to hold on to the pole on the side where you are standing. Assist the patient to advance the pole as you ambulate. Be sure the patient does not rely on the pole for support.

Provides a grip for the patient and positions the IV pole near you so that you can assist the patient to move the pole. ▼

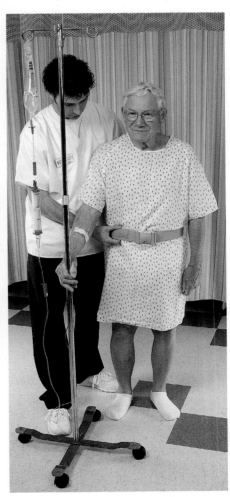

PROCEDURE 31–3B   Assisting with Ambulation (Two Nurses)

Procedural Steps

Step 1 Put nonskid slippers on the patient.

Prevents the patient from slipping during transfer.

Step 2 Apply the transfer belt.

Allows you to support client during ambulation.

Step 3 Place the bed in low position, and lock the bed.

Prevents the bed from moving during transfer and prevents the patient from falling.

Step 4 Assist the patient to dangle at the side of the bed (see Procedure 31–2B).

Step 5 Each nurse should stand facing the patient on opposite sides of the patient. Brace your feet and knees against the patient, paying particular attention to any known weakness. Bend from the hips and knees and hold onto the transfer belt.

Bracing provides stability. Bending the hips and knees allows you to use the major muscle groups and limit injury. Lifting at the patient's waist level prevents injury to his arm or shoulder.

Step 6 Instruct the patient to place his arms around each of you between the shoulders and waist (the location depends on your height and the height of the patient). Ask the patient to stand as each of you move to an upright position by straightening your legs and hips.

Step 7 Allow the patient to steady himself for a moment.

Allows the patient an opportunity to rest before further movement, to regain equilibrium.

Step 8 Each nurse stands at the patient's sides, grasping hold of the transfer belt. If no belt is available, the nurses grasp each other's arms at the patient's waist.

Helps patient maintain an erect posture. ▼

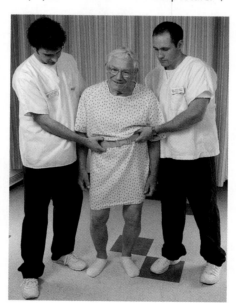

Step 9 Slowly guide the patient forward. Observe for signs of fatigue or dizziness.

Ensures client safety.

Step 10 If the patient must transport an IV pole, one nurse advances the IV pole along the side of the patient by holding the pole with the outside hand. Remind the patient not to use the IV pole for support.

Positions the IV pole out of the path of the patient.

Evaluation

- Assess patient comfort with ambulation.
- Assess posture and base of support.
- Assess vital signs for postural hypotension.

PROCEDURE 31–3   **Assisting with Ambulation** *(continued)*

Patient Teaching

- Instruct patient to inform you if he feels dizzy or weak.
- Explain the importance of ambulation.

Home Care

- Instruct family member or caregiver of proper technique for assisting client with ambulation.
- Provide instruction on importance of ambulation.

Documentation

Document in the nurse's notes how much assistance was required, any problems with ambulation, and the distance walked.

Sample documentation

| 11/11/06 | 0630 | *Pt assisted to ambulate to doorway in room. Required minimal assistance from one nurse. Placed in chair for 30 minutes and then assisted back to bed. Required maximum assist from two nurses to return to bed.* ———*B. Bowen, RN* |

TECHNIQUES

TECHNIQUE 31–1	Applying Principles of Body Mechanics

Principles of body mechanics are the rules that enable you to move your body without causing injury. As a nurse, you will be moving and lifting patients. Use the following guidelines to decrease the risk of back and other injuries. Teach them to your patients as well. Remember that the ANA states you should use mechanical equipment for lifting and transferring when possible and not rely on body mechanics alone to prevent injury.

- *Stand in good alignment* (erect posture).
- *Use a wide base of support* (feet spread apart).
- *Minimize bending and twisting.* These movements increase the stress on the back. Instead, face the object or person, and bend at the hips or squat.
- *Squat to lift heavy objects from the floor.* (Squatting lowers your center of gravity.) Push against the strong hip and thigh muscles to raise yourself to a standing position. Avoid bending at the waist.
- *Keep objects close to your body when you lift, move, or carry them.* The closer an object is to the center of gravity, the greater the stability and the less strain on the back.
- *Use both hands and arms* when you lift, move, or carry heavy objects.
- *Raise the height of the bed and bedside table to waist level* when you are working with a patient.

- *When possible, keep your elbows bent* when you carry an object.
- *Use the muscles in your legs as the power for lifting.* Bend your knees, keep your back straight, and lift smoothly. Repeat the same movements for setting the object down.
- *Do not stand on tiptoes to reach an object.* If you must use a ladder or stepstool to reach an object, make sure it is stable and adequate to position your body close to the object.
- *Push, slide, or pull heavy objects* whenever possible rather than lift them.
- *Make sure you have a good grip* on the patient or object you are moving before attempting to move it.
- *Work with smooth and even movements.* Avoid sudden or jerky motions.
- *Get help to move a heavy object or patient.* Assess the object or patient you are going to lift. **If you have any doubt that you can do it by yourself, get help from a co-worker.**
- *Use assistive devices at all times* to limit the risk of back and musculoskeletal injury.
- *Familiarize yourself with new assistive devices* as they become available.

TECHNIQUE 31-2 Making a Trochanter Roll

1. Fold a towel or bath blanket lengthwise.
2. Roll the towel or bath blanket tightly.
3. Invert the roll. Turning the patient to one side, place the bath blanket or towel under the patient's hip and thigh. Repeat on other side if needed.
4. Roll the sheet or towel under until it is snug against the patient's hip and thigh. The patient's weight should keep the roll from unrolling and help to prevent external rotation of the hips.
5. Alternately, you can place the patient on a sheet that has been folded so that the top edge is at the top of the hips, and the lower edge is about one-third the way down the thighs. Then place the rolled towels under the sheet and roll the sheet under tightly.

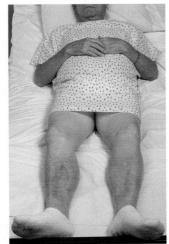

External rotation occurs without a trochanter roll.

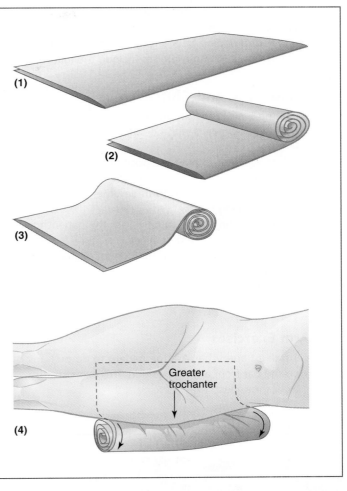

(1)

(2)

(3)

(4)

Greater trochanter

TECHNIQUE 31-3 Performing Passive Range-of-Motion Exercises

Passive range of motion (PROM) is the movement of the joints through their full range of motion by another person. Nurses frequently perform PROM to maintain function.

- Explain to the patient the purpose of PROM. You may also wish to teach family members and caregivers about the importance of ROM exercises and enlist their help in exercising the patient when they visit.
- Observe the patient as you perform PROM. You may need to perform the exercises in several short segments if the patient tires easily.
- Support the patient's limb above and below the joint that is to be exercised.
- Move the joint in a slow, smooth, rhythmic manner. Avoid fast movements; they may cause muscle spasm.

- Never force a joint. Some patients may have limited ROM. Move each joint until there is resistance, not pain.
- Perform PROM at least twice daily. Move each joint through ROM three to five times with each session. Consider incorporating PROM into care activities, for example, while bathing or turning the patient.
- Return the joint to a neutral position when exercise is complete.
- Encourage active exercise whenever possible.

For a guide to move each joint through the range of motion it is able to attain,

 VOL 1 Go to Chapter 31, **Table 31–3: Range of Motion at the Joints,** in Volume 1.

Assisting with Physical Conditioning Exercises to Prepare for Walking

Patients who have been confined to bed for more than a week or who have sustained major injury require conditioning before they are able to resume walking. Conditioning exercises include the following.

Quadriceps and Gluteal Drills

- Ask the patient to tighten her thigh muscles by pushing downward with her knees and flexing her feet.
- Ask the patient to hold the position for a count of 5 and then relax.
- Repeat this process two to three times per hour during the waking hours.
- To exercise the gluteal muscles, ask the patient to pinch her buttocks together.
- Repeat this exercise when the patient exercises the quadriceps muscles.
- Instruct the patient not to hold her breath as she exercises.

Arm Exercises

- Install a trapeze bar. Ask the patient to do pull-ups on the bar from a lying position. This exercises the biceps muscles.

- To exercise the triceps muscles, ask the patient to lift his upper body off the mattress by firmly pressing down with the palms.
- The patient can also do push-ups from a seated position at the side of the bed or from a stationary chair or wheelchair.

Dangling

- Dangling is a seated position at the side of the bed, feet resting on the floor.
- Provide a footstool if the patient's feet do not reach the floor.
- Observe for light-headedness or orthostatic hypotension.
- Do not progress to ambulation until the patient is comfortable and stable in the dangling position.

Daily Activities

- Encourage your patient to be active in bed.
- Encourage the patient to get out of bed and into a chair prior to attempting to walk.
- Encourage the patient to perform ADLs as much as possible.
- ADLs exercise many of the muscle groups used in ambulation.

TECHNIQUE 31–5 **Sizing Walking Aids**

Sizing Canes

- Have the patient stand erect, and place the cane tip 20 cm (4 inches) to the side of the foot.
- The top of the cane should reach to the top of the hip joint so that the patient can hold the cane with her elbow flexed 30°.

Sizing Walkers

- Have the patient stand erect, holding onto the walker.
- The walker should extend from the floor to the hip joint so that the patient can comfortably hold the walker with 30° flexion of the elbow.

Sizing Crutches

To measure a patient for an axillary crutch, follow these guidelines:

- Have the patient lie down wearing the shoes she will use when walking.
- Measure the distance between the heel and the anterior fold of the axilla, then add 2.5 cm (1 inch).
- Select a crutch that adjusts to this height.
- Have the patient stand, and position the crutch tip 10 to 15 cm (4 to 6 inches) to the side of the heel. Adjust the axillary crutch pad three fingerbreadths below the axilla.
- Adjust the handgrips so that the patient can comfortably grasp the bar while the elbow is slightly flexed.

| TECHNIQUE 31–6 | **Teaching Patients to Use Canes, Walkers, and Crutches** |

Canes

Instruct patients to do the following:
- Hold the cane on the stronger side.
- Distribute weight evenly between the feet and cane.
- Advance the cane and weaker leg simultaneously, then swing the stronger leg through.
- Avoid leaning over onto the cane.

Walkers

Instruct the patient to:
- Stand between the back legs of the walker. Be sure not to stand too far behind the walker.
- Pick up the walker, and advance it as you step ahead. Do not advance it so far as to lose balance.
- If one leg is weaker, move it forward with the walker.
- Pick up, rather than slide, the walker (unless it has wheels).

Crutches

- When first instructing the patient in crutch use, have him stand near a wall with a chair behind him. Help the patient to stand and grip the crutches. Ask the patient to sway from side to side on the crutches to become accustomed to weight bearing by the arms.
- *Tripod position* is the basic crutch gait standing position. Place crutches 15 cm (6 inches) in front of the feet, with the crutch point 15 cm from the patient's center. In this position, a triangle is formed by the crutches and the body.
- Five crutch gaits exist (see accompanying chart): 2-point gait, 3-point gait, 4-point gait, swing-to gait, and swing-through gait.
- To teach the patient how to go up and down stairs, instruct him to lead with the unaffected leg when going up the stairs and to lead with the affected leg coming down the stairs.
- Navigating stairs with crutches can be quite dangerous. When possible, have the patient practice this technique before discharge. When having a patient practice, the nurse should always be below the patient on the stairs to prevent falling.

TECHNIQUE 31–6 | Teaching Patients to Use Canes, Walkers, and Crutches (continued)

2-Point gait	3-Point gait	4-Point gait	Swing to	Swing through
• Partial weight bearing, both feet; faster, but less support than a 4-point gait	• Non-weight bearing; faster than a 4-point gait; can use with walker	• Partial weight bearing, both feet; patient must shift weight constantly	• Weight bearing, both feet; can use with walker	• Weight bearing; requires the most coordination and balance
4. Advance right foot and left crutch	4. Advance right foot	4. Advance right foot	4. Lift both feet; swing them forward, landing feet next to the crutches	4. Lift both feet; swing them forward, landing feet in front of the crutches
3. Advance left foot and right crutch	3. Advance left foot and both crutches	3. Advance left crutch	3. Advance both crutches	3. Advance both crutches
2. Advance right foot and left crutch	2. Advance right foot	2. Advance left foot	2. Lift both feet; swing them forward, landing feet next to the crutches	2. Lift both feet; swing them forward, landing feet in front of the crutches
1. Advance left foot and right crutch	1. Advance left foot and both crutches	1. Advance right crutch	1. Advance both crutches	1. Advance both crutches
Tripod position	Tripod position	Tripod position	Tripod position	Tripod position

ASSESSMENT GUIDELINES AND TOOLS

Suggested History Questions for Assessing Activity and Exercise

Usual Activity

- Describe your typical daily activity level.

If the patient has very restricted activity, proceed with the following questions:

- Are you able to care for yourself in regard to hygiene, dressing, toileting, and getting out of bed?
- [If the patient has ADL limitations:] Who helps you with these daily activities?

If the patient does not indicate restricted activity, proceed with the following questions:

- What is your usual form of exercise?
- How often do you exercise?
- How long are your exercise sessions?
- How long have you been engaged in this type of activity?
- What types of exercise or sports have you participated in in the past?
- Describe your activity level over the last 10 years.
- Are you exercising more or less than in the past?
- What factors have changed your activity level?

Fitness Goals

- What aspects of exercise do you enjoy? What aspects of exercise do you dislike?
- What do you think are the benefits of exercise?
- How do you schedule your exercise?
- What motivates you to exercise?
- What are your current fitness goals?

Mobility Concerns

- Do you have any pain or discomfort with activity?
- Do you avoid any activities because of pain, discomfort, shortness of breath, or chest pain?

If yes to either question, describe the following:

- Type of problem
- Onset of concern

- Frequency of problem
- Activities that trigger and relieve
- Severity and type of symptoms
- Effect of problem on day-to-day activities
- Treatments used to alleviate and how they worked

Underlying Health Concerns

- Do you have any healthcare problem that affects your ability to engage in activity or exercise?
- If so, describe the problem and the effect.
- What medications do you take?
- Have you ever been told you have a bone problem? If so, what was the nature of the problem?
- Have you ever experienced a fracture, strain, or sprain? If so, where was the problem? When did it occur? How did it occur?
- Have you ever had weakness of the muscles or problems coordinating movement?
- Do you have any cardiac or respiratory problems that affect your ability to perform activities?
- Have you ever experienced anxiety or depression that affected your ability to participate in activities?

Lifestyle

- What kind of work do you do?
- Describe your typical work activities.
- How many hours per week do you work?
- What other commitments do you have (school, family, obligations)?

External Factors

- Are there any restrictions in your home that limit your ability to be active?
- Do you feel you need an assistive device?
- Are you comfortable exercising outside your home or in your neighborhood?

Focused Physical Assessments for Activity and Exercise

Body Alignment

- With the patient standing, observe from the anterior, posterior, and lateral views. Check for the following:
  - Shoulders and hips are level.
  - Toes are pointed forward.
  - The spine is straight, with no abnormal curvatures noted.
  - The posture is not slumped.
- Ask the patient to sit down; observe as he does so.
  - Does he have difficulty lowering his torso?
  - Can he control the movement?
  - Is he able to get into this position with ease?
  - When he sits, does he slump?
- If the patient cannot stand or sit, assess his alignment in bed. Look for ability to move in bed, as well as the posture the patient maintains.

Joint Function

- Assessing joint function includes inspection and palpation of the joints and assessment of range of motion.
- Begin your assessment at the neck and systematically work your way through each of the joints.
- At each joint observe for swelling, erythema, symmetry, or obvious deformity.
- Compare the size of the muscles above and below the joint and on each side of the body.
- Palpate the joint for temperature and crepitus. Warmth over a joint indicates inflammation or infection. Be sure to compare body temperature over several joints and right to left. **Crepitus** is a grating sensation when the joint is moved. It can often be heard as well as felt. Crepitus is associated with degenerative joint disease or arthritic changes in the joint.
- As you palpate the joint, move it through its range of motion. For a description of the anticipated range of motion for the joints,

 Go to Chapter 31, **Table 31–3: Range of Motion of the Joints,** in Volume 1.

Muscle Strength

- Assess muscle strength by having the patient push and then pull against your hands.
- Start at the neck, and test the strength of all major joints' range of motion.

Gait

- Gait is divided into two phases: stance and swing.

- *Stance*—In the stance phase, the heel of one foot strikes the ground while the opposite foot pushes off and leaves the ground.
- *Swing*—In the swing phase, the leg from behind moves in front of the body. When the right leg is in stance mode, the left leg is in swing mode.

- You must observe the patient walking. Normal gait includes the following features:
  - Head is erect, gaze forward.
  - Heel strikes the ground before the toe.
  - Opposite arm moves forward at the same time.
  - Feet are dorsiflexed in the swing phase.
  - Gait is coordinated and rhythmic.
  - Weight is evenly distributed with minimal swing from side to side.
  - Movement starts and stops with ease.
  - Movement is at a moderate pace.

- If the patient uses an assistive device, such as a cane, crutch, or walker, pay attention to how he uses it. Ask the patient to ambulate a short distance with and without the device to determine if the device is actually providing stability.

Activity Tolerance

- Assess and record vital signs before having the patient engage in 3 minutes of activity.
- Select an activity appropriate for the patient. For example, if the patient uses a walker, ask the patient to walk down the hallway. For a patient without obvious health limitations, consider asking her to run in place for 3 minutes.
- Observe the patient throughout the exercise. If she shows any signs of distress, stop the exercise, immediately take a set of vital signs, and repeat the vital signs every minute until they have returned to baseline.
- If the patient can exercise continuously for 3 minutes, assess the patient at the end of the 3-minute period and at 1-minute intervals. Note the change in heart rate, blood pressure, and respiratory rate.
- This type of approach is not appropriate for patients who easily become short of breath, develop chest pain, or are very unsteady on their feet. Instead, for example, limit your assessment to determining the amount of assistance the patient needs to turn in bed or get out of bed.
- As you observe the patient, compare muscle mass on the right and left sides. If you notice an obvious discrepancy in size, measure the circumference of the limbs and compare.

Muscle Mass and Strength

- To assess strength, ask the patient to push against your hand with the hands and feet. Once again, compare differences between sides.

(continued)

- The following are terms used to describe problems with muscle mass, strength, or mobility.

  - *Atrophy* is a decrease in the size of muscle tissue due to lack of use or loss of innervation.
  - *Clonus* is spasmodic contractions of opposing muscles resulting in tremorous movement.
  - *Flaccidity* is a decrease or absence of muscle tone.
  - *Hemiplegia* is paralysis of one side of the body.
  - *Hypertrophy* is an increase in the size or bulk of a muscle or organ.
  - *Paraplegia* is paralysis of the lower portion of the trunk and both legs.
  - *Paresis* is partial or incomplete paralysis.

  - *Paresthesia* is numbness, tingling, or burning due to injury of the nerve(s) innervating the affected area.
  - *Quadriplegia* is paralysis of all four extremities.
  - *Spasticity* is a motor disorder characterized by increased muscle tone, exaggerated tendon jerks, and clonus.
  - *Tremor* is involuntary quivering movement of a body part.

For guidelines for assessing mobility in the home,

 Go to Chapter 31, **Home Care Box: Home Care Assessment for a Patient with Mobility Concerns,** in Volume 1.

STANDARDIZED LANGUAGE

Selected NOC Outcomes for Energy Maintenance and Mobility

Class: Energy Maintenance	**Class: Mobility**
Activity Tolerance	Ambulation
Endurance	Ambulation: Wheelchair
Energy Conservation	Balance
Psychomotor Energy	Body Positioning: Self-Initiated
Rest	Coordinated Movement
Sleep	Immobility Consequences: Physiological
	Immobility Consequences: Psycho-Cognitive
	Joint Movement: Ankle, Elbow, Fingers, Hip, Knee, Neck, Shoulder, Spine, Wrist (specify)
	Mobility
	Skeletal Function
	Transfer Performance

Source: Moorhead, S., Johnson, M., & Maas, M. (Eds.). (2004). *Nursing outcomes classification (NOC)* (3rd ed.). St Louis: Mosby.

Selected NIC Interventions for Activity and Exercise Management and Immobility Management

Class: Activity and Exercise Management	**Class: Immobility Management**
Body Mechanics Promotion	Bed Rest Care
Energy Management	Cast Care: Maintenance
Exercise Promotion	Cast Care: Wet
Exercise Promotion: Strength Training	Physical Restraint
Exercise Promotion: Stretching	Positioning
Exercise Therapy: Ambulation	Positioning: Wheelchair
Exercise Therapy: Balance	Self-Care Assistance: Transfer
Exercise Therapy: Joint Mobility	Splinting
Exercise Therapy: Muscle Control	Traction/Immobilization Care
Teaching: Prescribed Activity/Exercise	Transport

Source: Dochterman, J.M., & Bulechek, G.M. (Eds.). (2004). *Nursing interventions classification (NIC)* (4th ed.). St Louis: Mosby.

What Are the Main Points in This Chapter?

- The skeletal system includes bones, cartilage, ligaments, and tendons. The skeleton forms the framework of the body and protects the internal organs.

- Movement depends on the interaction between the skeleton and the muscles. The ligaments, tendons, and cartilage serve as the interface between these two systems.

- Contraction of skeletal muscle causes the muscle to shorten, thus causing one bone to move at the joint.

- There are four natural curves to the spine. Proper posture maintains these natural curves.

- For your body to be balanced, your line of gravity must pass through your center of gravity, and your center of gravity must be close to your base of support. In the human body, the center of gravity is below the umbilicus at the top of the pelvis. The feet provide the base of support.

- Range of motion (ROM) is the maxium movement possible at a joint. Active range of motion is defined as the movement of the joint through the entire ROM by the individual.

- Principles of body mechanics are the rules that allow you to move your body without causing injury.

- The surgeon general of the United States recommends 30 minutes or more of moderate-intensity physical activity on all, or most, days of the week.

- A well-rounded exercise program focuses on flexibility, resistance training, and aerobic conditioning.

- Exercise is associated with an overall decrease in mortality in men and women of all ages.

- Factors that influence activity and exercise level include developmental stage, health concerns, nutrition, lifestyle, attitudes, and external factors.

- Severe illness associated with prolonged immoblization causes physiological changes in almost every body system.

- A nursing history focused on activity and exercise assesses usual activity, fitness goals, mobility concerns, underlying health concerns, lifestyle, and external factors.

- Physical assessment that is focused on activity and exercise should include examination of the musculoskeletal system. Other important data include vital signs, height, weight, body mass index, body alignment, joint function, gait, and activity tolerance.

- Patients require a change of position at least every 2 hours to prevent skin breakdown, muscle discomfort, damage to superficial nerves and blood vessels, or contractures.

- Range-of-motion exercises maintain joint mobility and limit the complications of immobility.

- Patients who have been confined to bed for more than a week or who have sustained major injury require conditioning before they are able to resume walking.

- Canes, braces, walkers, and crutches are available to assist a patient to walk. These aids promote stability and independence.

Sexual Health

Overview

Sexuality encompasses physical, emotional, social, and spiritual dimensions. It influences how we feel about ourselves as individuals and how we interact with others and our environment. Both physical and psychological health affect sexuality and sexual functioning.

Because sexual health is challenged by high-risk sexual behaviors, sexually transmitted infections (STIs), negative interpersonal relationships, sexual victimization, and physical and mental health concerns, a sexual history is an important component of the nursing assessment.

A calm, professional approach may help you feel more comfortable and competent as you collect sexual data from your patient. Including sexuality as a routine part of your nursing assessment reinforces the concept that sexuality is an integral part of life. Many patients will not raise the topic of sexuality, so if you do not mention it, you will not meet patient needs. Counseling for sexual problems and teaching about body function and reproduction, self-care, contraception, and prevention of STIs are nursing interventions that can enhance your patient's sexual well-being.

Thinking Critically About Sexual Health

The exercises in the following section allow you to practice the kind of thinking you will use as a full-spectrum nurse. Because these are critical-thinking activities, there is usually no single right answer. Discuss answers with your peers—discussion can stimulate critical thinking. If you have difficulty with any of the questions, consult with your instructor.

Caring for the Garcias

As you may recall, Joe and Flordelisa Garcia are raising their 3-year-old granddaughter, Bettina. Bettina has made friends with Lili, another little girl at preschool. Bettina has asked whether they can play together.

Flordelisa works at the preschool and knows Lili and her family. She is unsure whether she should allow her granddaughter to play with Lili because Flordelisa is uncomfortable with Lili's family. Lili was conceived via artificial insemination and is being raised by a lesbian couple. Her parents are open about the relationship and shared the conception information with Flordelisa voluntarily.

A. Flordelisa calls the clinic to speak with you. She explains the situation and asks you whether you think it would be a problem to allow the girls to play together. She is concerned that being around this family may be a bad influence on Bettina. How would you respond?

B. Flordelisa remains concerned and presses you for more information. She is concerned that Bettina's interest in Lili may indicate that Bettina has homosexual tendencies. How would you address her concerns?

C. Flordelisa admits that Joe does not agree with her. "He told me that sexual orientation is genetic." How would you react to this statement?

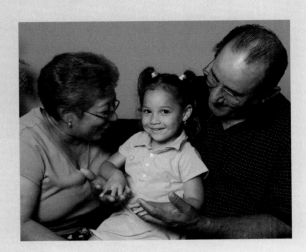

727

1

A 34-year-old married woman is admitted to the hospital following an alleged rape. You are caring for her the next day. She will remain hospitalized for several days because of a head injury she suffered during the rape.

a How can you best approach this woman to establish a positive rapport?

b What fears is this patient likely to express?

c The patient's spouse is coming to visit. What concerns do you think that he may have?

d You begin to feel overwhelmed by this couple's emotions and questions. What can you do to help provide this couple with optimal care?

2

Your 26-year-old male client recently had a spinal cord injury. The doctors have talked to him about the possibility of regaining motor function and perhaps being able to walk again after intense therapy. What he now seems to be most concerned about is his relationship with his 25-year-old fiancée.

a What aspects of their relationship do you think he is concerned about?

b Do you have enough theoretical and patient information regarding his injury to answer all of his concerns?

c As you consider some of the changes in sexual functioning that may follow a spinal cord injury, what suggestions might you share with him?

d What clues might you get that would indicate that talking to the fiancée may be appropriate?

3 You are seeing Jessica, a 14-year-old girl, at the clinic. Her throat culture is positive for gonorrhea. The girl's mother has gone down to the coffee shop. The doctor has left a prescription for antibiotics. You are left to take care of the discharge from the clinic.

a How would you explain the culture results to Jessica?

b Jessica tells you that she cannot possibly have a sexually transmitted infection (STI) because she is a virgin. How would you respond?

c Jessica tells you that she has had oral sex with her boyfriend, but no one else. What education regarding STIs and antibiotics would be appropriate?

d What information would you give the mother when she returns?

4 A 45-year-old married man with young children has just been informed that he is HIV positive. He is shocked by the news. He admits he had an extramarital relationship with a man 7 years ago.

a What concerns is he likely to have? As his nurse, what biases do you have that you will have to put aside to help him?

b What theoretical knowledge would you need at a later time to help him deal with questions about sexual activity?

c What patient information would you need to help him deal with questions about sexual activity?

5 Review the following scenarios from "Meet Your Patients" in Volume 1.

Jocelyn Carter recently underwent a fine-needle aspiration to evaluate a small breast mass that was discovered on a routine screening mammogram. Two days after the procedure, the surgeon informed her that the mass was malignant and recommended surgery. Today, she arrives at the registration area at 6:00 A.M. She tells you that the last week has been a whirlwind of activity. "I had to arrange child care, cancel a business trip, and organize the house so that I could take a few days off to have the surgery. Honestly, I don't know how I am. I haven't had time to think about it." As she waits in the surgery holding area, she begins to cry. You hold her hand and ask whether she would like to talk. She asks you, "Do you think my husband will still want me? I'm afraid he will be turned off when he looks at me now."

Gabriel Thomas comes to the outpatient clinic complaining of a throbbing headache for the last 3 days. He explains that he tried several over-the-counter medicines and has had no relief. You check his blood pressure and measure the reading at 240/130 mm Hg. When you ask whether he has ever been treated for high blood pressure he replies, "Are you another one of these people trying to get me to take drugs that will ruin my sex life?"

Frank Thanee had a mitral valve replacement 3 days ago. He has been transferred to the cardiology floor for an additional day of hospitalization. His partner, Greg, has spent the last 3 days at the hospital and has just left to check on the apartment and feed their cat. Frank confides that he is worried about his parents' expected visit. "I've never been able to tell them about Greg. They would never be able to understand it, never mind approve. I don't know how to handle this. What do you think I should do?"

a Write etiologies for each of the patients. The nursing diagnosis is provided for you in each case.

Jocelyn Carter—Ineffective Sexuality Patterns

Gabriel Thomas—Ineffective Sexuality Patterns

Frank Thanee—Sexual Dysfunction

b For each of the patients, instead of the sexuality diagnosis, identify another nursing diagnosis that you should explore to see whether it fits the situation better. Consult a nursing diagnosis handbook, as needed.

Jocelyn Carter:

Gabriel Thomas:

Frank Thanee:

6 For each of the following concepts, use critical thinking to describe how or why it is important to nursing, patient care, or sexual health. Note that these are *not* to be merely definitions.

Sexual health

Gender

Sexual orientation

Sexual expression

Sexually transmitted infections

Fertility control

Practical Knowledge
knowing how

In this section you will find guidelines to assist you in assessing and planning care related to patients' sexual health.

TECHNIQUES

TECHNIQUE 32–1	**Taking a Sexual History**

1. Provide privacy.
   - Usually it is *not* enough merely to pull the curtains around the bed.
   - Talk to the client alone. At some point, you will probably want to talk with both partners, because the client and partner are a unit. Nevertheless, you should be aware that a patient may prefer to be alone when you take a sexual history. It is one thing to discuss blood pressure in the presence of family, but quite another to discuss sexual health issues, which may threaten the very core of a relationship. For example, a wife is not likely to discuss domestic violence with her abusing husband at her side. An 18-year-old man will probably not admit to having sex with another man when his father is present. An adolescent daughter may not want to discuss her STI in front of her mother.

2. Be relaxed in your approach, and allow the client time to answer your questions fully. Your manner and attitude are critical.

3. Make eye contact. If you are embarrassed or avoid eye contact, your client will be uncomfortable.

4. Avoid communication stoppers, such as:
   - "I'm only asking you these questions because I have to."
   - "I know that you probably won't want to tell me but . . . "
   - "You're not having any sexual problems, are you?"

5. A more inviting opening might be something such as:
   - "Many people are embarrassed when asked questions about their sexuality, but whatever you tell me will remain confidential."

   - "Many people hesitate to talk about sexual problems. However, your sexual health is important to your overall health, and I would like to ask you a few questions about that."

6. Be aware of verbal and nonverbal cues that indicate concerns. Many people will cloak their concerns in comments such as, "I suppose that I won't need to worry about sexy lingerie any longer," or "Sex is for the young. I just have to accept that I'm sick and older now." Your response to such statements either negates or validates their identity as sexual beings. Follow up with comments that encourage the client to provide more details (see Chapter 18 for communication techniques).

7. If the client is uncomfortable, reassure him by letting him know that some information, because of its private nature, may be difficult to discuss.

8. Tell your client to use terminology that he is comfortable with.

9. To help the client feel comfortable, consider statements such as the following:
   - "Most people wonder how this surgery (or illness) may affect their sexual functioning."
   - "Whenever these medications are suggested, there are questions about sexual side effects."
   - "Have you thought about the kinds of adaptations you may have to make in your sex life after this surgery/treatment/illness?"

10. Begin with a less sensitive topic, such as "How is your relationship with your partner (spouse)?" Then you can move into more sensitive areas: "Many older women have some vaginal dryness that creates discomfort during intercourse. Do you have any concerns about this?"

ASSESSMENT GUIDELINES AND TOOLS

This section contains guidelines and questions for taking a sexual history.

Topics to Include in a Sexual History

The topics to include in the sexual history depend on the nature of the patient's concern. The following topics are most commonly included in a sexual history.

- Reproductive history
- Sexual self-concept
- History of sexually transmitted infections
- History of sexual dysfunction
- Present sexual functioning
- Other factors that affect sexuality, such as medications and diseases

- Signs or symptoms of sexual abuse (see Procedure 9–1)
- Knowledge level about sex, reproduction, and contraception

Tailor your assessment to meet the client's needs. For example, Frank Thanee ("Meet Your Patients") is concerned about his family's reaction to his lifestyle and sexual orientation. In his situation, you would focus your assessment on his sexual self-concept, family relationships, present sexual functioning, and specific concerns about his heart and the impending family visit.

Suggested Sexual Health History Questions

Women

Menstrual Cycle

- How old were you when you started your periods?
- When was your last menstrual period?
- How often are your periods? How would you describe the flow? How long does your period last?
- Do you have any problems with your periods, such as cramping, breast pain, or heavy flow?
- What products do you use during your period, such as tampons and pads? Do you ever use douches, either during your period or at other times?

Cancer Screening

- When was your last Pap smear?
- Have you ever had an abnormal Pap smear? If so, how was it treated?
- Do you examine your breasts? If so, how often?
- Have you noticed asymmetry, lumps, or masses in your breasts? If so, describe them and show me where they are.
- When was your last mammogram? What were the results?

Child-Bearing History

- How many living children do you have?
- How many times have you been pregnant?
- Have you ever had a miscarriage? An abortion?

- How many of your births were preterm (prior to 38 weeks)? Term?

Men

Sexual Activity

- Do you have any difficulty achieving or maintaining an erection?

Cancer Screening

- Have you been taught to examine your testicles? Do you practice testicular self-exam?
- Is there a history of testicular cancer in your family?

Both Men and Women

Illnesses and Medications

- What types of illnesses have you been treated for in the past?
- Have you ever been hospitalized? Have you ever had surgery?
- What medications, herbal remedies, or over-the counter medicines do you take?

Family Responsibilities

- Do you have children? If so, how many? How many are still at home? Dependent on you?
- Are you responsible for other children? [This question may reveal whether the person continues to care for an adult disabled child or for grandchildren.]

(continued)

Genitalia

- Have you noticed any redness, swelling, discharge, or odor in your genital area?
- Have you noticed asymmetry, lumps, or masses in the genitals? If so, describe them and show me where they are.
- Have you ever been told you have a hernia?
- Have you ever had trauma to your genitals?
- Are you having any problems urinating?

Sexual Patterns

- Are you sexually active? If not, have you ever been?
- Do you have sex with men, women, or both?
- What types of sexual activity do you engage in? Oral, anal, or genital?
- How many partners do you currently have? How many partners have you had in the last 6 months?
- How would you describe your satisfaction with your current sexual relationship?
- What are your thoughts about how this procedure/illness may affect your sexual relationship?

- Have you experienced any recent changes in your sexual function, in either your level of desire, your sexual activity, participation, or satisfaction?
- Do you have any concerns about your sexual function, including your level of desire, activity, participation, or satisfaction?
- Do you ever feel threatened by your partner?

Contraception (as appropriate)

- Do you use birth control? If so, what type and how often?
- How satisfied are you with your method of contraception?

Sexually Transmitted Infections

- Have you ever been treated for an STI? If so, what type?
- Are you concerned about STIs or HIV?
- Do you take any precautions to avoid infections?

Abuse

- Have you ever been forced to have sex against your will?
- Have you ever been threatened or abused by a partner?

TABLES

Fertility Control Methods

Fertility Control Method	Advantages	Disadvantages
Abstinence—No sexual intercourse	100% effective Cost free	Lack of sexual expression May create stress in relationship
Fertility awareness (natural family planning, rhythm)—Intercourse only when a woman is thought to be in the infertile phase of her menstrual cycle	Cost free May be consistent with religious teachings No physical side effects	Requires cooperation of both partners Menstrual cycle must be regular Relatively high failure rate: Pregnancy may result No protection against STIs
Withdrawal (coitus interruptus)—Removal of the penis from the vagina before ejaculation	Cost free	Requires discipline and mutual cooperation Pre-ejaculatory fluid may contain sperm Relatively high failure rate; pregnancy may result No protection against STIs
Male and female condoms	Obtained without a prescription Relatively inexpensive Protects against STIs	Must be put on prior to penetration; therefore, may diminish spontaneity of intercourse May decrease sensation for both partners Cannot be used if either partner has latex allergy
Spermicides—Jelly, creams, or foams placed in the vagina	Obtained without a prescription More effective when used with a barrier (condom)	Significant pregnancy rate when used without a barrier (condom) No protection against STIs
Oral contraceptives (birth control pills)	Very effective Do not interfere with intercourse Regulate menstrual flow Decrease menstrual cramps	Require a healthcare visit and prescription Significant cost (unless obtained through Planned Parenthood) Must be taken as prescribed to be effective Drug interactions No protection against STIs Carry some undesirable side effects Contraindicated for some women (e.g., those who smoke, who have significant varicose veins)
Depo-Provera injections	Lasts 3 months Highly effective Do not interfere with intercourse	Require a healthcare provider visit Amenorrhea (may be seen as an advantage) No protection against STIs
Intrauterine device (IUD)—A small piece of plastic that also may contain metal or a hormone: placed through the cervix into the uterus by a healthcare provider	Highly effective May remain in place for years Does not interfere with intercourse	Increased risk of pelvic inflammatory disease (PID) Must be inserted by a healthcare provider Increased menstrual flow and cramping No protection against STIs

Fertility Control Methods *(continued)*

Fertility Control Method	Advantages	Disadvantages
Diaphragm—Latex dome-shaped cup with a flexible rim that is inserted in the vagina and fits over the cervix	Few side effects Quite effective if used properly with spermicide	Must be inserted prior to intercourse, thereby compromising spontaneity Must be removed about 6 hours after intercourse Must be used with a spermicide Increased risk of urinary tract infection (UTI) No protection against STIs
Female sterilization (tubal ligation)	Effective Long-term cost-effectiveness May be reversible	Surgical procedure May not be reversible No protection against STIs
Male sterilization (vasectomy)	Effective Long-term cost-effectiveness Does not interfere with sexual performance May be reversible in some cases	Usually not reversible Psychological effects No protection against STIs

STANDARDIZED LANGUAGE

Examples of NOC Outcomes and Goals for Sexuality Problems

NANDA Diagnosis	NOC Outcomes	Examples of Goals Using NOC Indicators
Ineffective Sexuality Patterns	Abuse Recovery: Sexual	(3, moderate) Demonstrates evidence of appropriate same-sex relationships
	Body Image	(4, often positive) Satisfaction with body function
	Child Development: Adolescence (12–17 years)	(4, often demonstrated) Expresses comfort with own sexual identity
	Child Development: Middle Childhood (6–11 years)	(4, often demonstrated) Identifies with same-sex peer group
	Role Performance	(3, moderately adequate) Performance of intimate role behaviors
	Self-Esteem	(4, often positive) Description of self
	Sexual Identity	(4, often demonstrated) Challenges negative images of sexual self
Sexual Dysfunction	Abuse Recovery: Sexual	(4, substantial) Evidence of appropriate opposite-sex relationships
	Physical Aging	(3, moderate deviation from normal range) Sexual functioning
	Risk Control: Sexually Transmitted Diseases	(4, often demonstrated) Notifies sexual partner(s) in event of STD infection
	Sexual Functioning	(4, often demonstrated) Sustains arousal through orgasm

Source: Moorhead, S., Johnson, M., & Maas, M. (Eds.). (2004). *Nursing outcomes classification (NOC).* (3rd ed.). St Louis, Mosby.

Examples of NIC Interventions and Nursing Activities for Sexuality Problems

NANDA Diagnosis	NIC Interventions	Examples of Nursing Activities (NIC)
Ineffective Sexuality Patterns	Body Image Enhancement	Instruct children about the functions of the various body parts, as appropriate.
	Coping Enhancement	Assist the patient in developing an objective appraisal of the event.
	Counseling	Demonstrate empathy, warmth, and genuineness.
	Family Planning: Contraception	Explain reasons for most unplanned pregnancies.
	Role Enhancement	Encourage patient to identify a realistic description of change in role.
	Self-Esteem Enhancement	Explore previous achievements.
	Sexual Counseling	Preface questions about sexuality with a statement that tells the patient that many people experience sexual difficulties.
	Teaching: Safe Sex	Discuss abstinence as a means of birth control, as appropriate.
Sexual Dysfunction	Abuse Protection Support	Refer adult(s) to shelters for abused spouses, as appropriate.
	Behavior Management: Sexual	Identify sexual behaviors that are unacceptable, given the particular setting and patient population.
	Coping Enhancement	Explore with the patient previous methods of dealing with life problems.
	Counseling	Encourage expression of feelings.
	Infection Protection	Teach patient and family members how to avoid infections.
	Risk Identification	Determine compliance with medical and nursing treatments.
	Sexual Counseling	Begin with the least sensitive topics and proceed to the more sensitive.
	Teaching: Safe Sex	Discuss with patient ways to convince partners to use condoms.
	Teaching: Sexuality	Discuss peer and social pressure in relation to sexual activity.

Source: Dochterman, J. M., & Bulechek, G. M. (Eds.). (2004). *Nursing interventions classification (NIC)* (4th ed.). St Louis: Mosby.

What Are the Main Points in This Chapter?

- Sexuality is a broad and complex aspect of the self, with physical, emotional, social, and spiritual dimensions.
- Sexuality involves how we feel about ourselves as individuals and how we interact with others and our environment.
- Gender, gender identity, and sexual orientation contribute to expression of our sexuality throughout the life cycle.
- There are both typical and atypical forms of sexual expression.
- Sexual victimization is a societal and healthcare concern.
- Physical and psychological health status affects sexuality and sexual functioning.

- Sexual health is challenged by high-risk sexual behaviors, sexually transmitted infections (STI), negative interpersonal relationships, and sexual dysfunctions.
- A sexual history is a component of the nursing assessment.
- There are strategies you can use to help you gain comfort and competence in collecting sexual data.
- Sexual well-being may be enhanced through nursing interventions such as counseling for sexual problems, dealing with inappropriate sexual behavior, and teaching about body function and reproduction, self-care, contraception, and prevention of STIs.

Knowledge Map

Sexuality

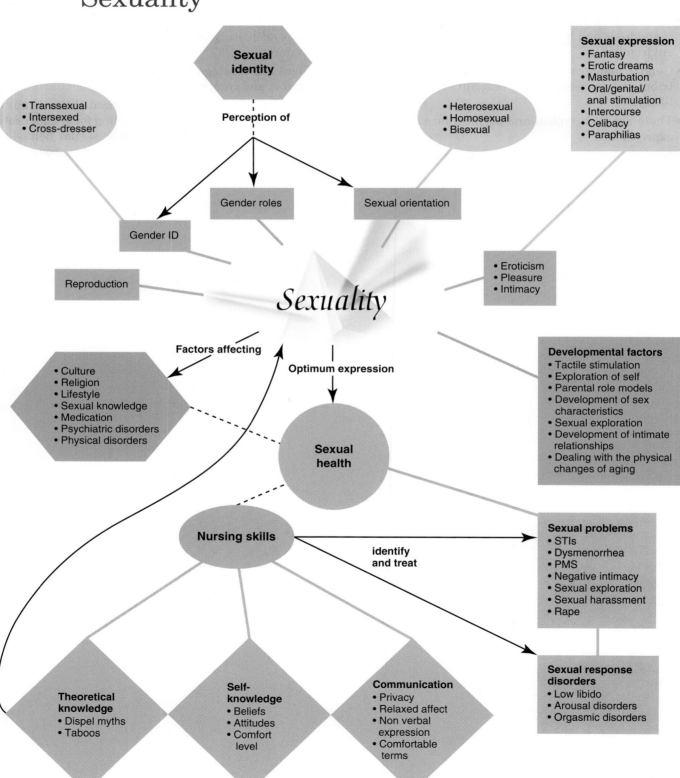

Sexual identity

Perception of

• Transsexual
• Intersexed
• Cross-dresser

• Heterosexual
• Homosexual
• Bisexual

Sexual expression
• Fantasy
• Erotic dreams
• Masturbation
• Oral/genital/
  anal stimulation
• Intercourse
• Celibacy
• Paraphilias

Gender roles

Sexual orientation

Gender ID

Reproduction

• Eroticism
• Pleasure
• Intimacy

Sexuality

Factors affecting

Optimum expression

• Culture
• Religion
• Lifestyle
• Sexual knowledge
• Medication
• Psychiatric disorders
• Physical disorders

Developmental factors
• Tactile stimulation
• Exploration of self
• Parental role models
• Development of sex
  characteristics
• Sexual exploration
• Development of intimate
  relationships
• Dealing with the physical
  changes of aging

Sexual health

Nursing skills

identify
and treat

Sexual problems
• STIs
• Dysmenorrhea
• PMS
• Negative intimacy
• Sexual exploration
• Sexual harassment
• Rape

Theoretical knowledge
• Dispel myths
• Taboos

Self-knowledge
• Beliefs
• Attitudes
• Comfort
  level

Communication
• Privacy
• Relaxed affect
• Non verbal
  expression
• Comfortable
  terms

Sexual response disorders
• Low libido
• Arousal disorders
• Orgasmic disorders

Sleep
& Rest

Overview

Sleep is a basic physiological need. It promotes physical, mental, and spiritual well-being by restoring energy and reducing body demands while the body repairs itself. Illness and pain can interfere with the ability to sleep and rest; conversely, people who suffer from sleep disorders have an increased susceptibility to illnesses.

The hypothalamus and various neuro-transmitters are involved in the physiology of sleep. A person's age also affects how long he or she sleeps. Common sleep disorders include insomnia, sleep apnea, and narcolepsy. Nursing interventions to promote sleep include scheduling nursing care around sleep, creating a restful environment, and supporting bedtime rituals and routines.

Sleep medications, as a rule, should be used only as a temporary measure. Teaching patients and their families about the importance of rest and sleep is an important health promotion intervention.

Thinking Critically About Sleep and Rest

The exercises in the following section allow you to practice the kind of thinking you will use as a full-spectrum nurse. Because these are critical thinking activities, there is usually no single right answer. Discuss answers with your peers—discussion can stimulate critical thinking. If you have difficulty with any of the questions, consult with your instructor.

Caring for the Garcias

Flordelisa Garcia arrives at the clinic accompanied by her husband, Joe. She appears very tired. Joe tells you that she has been sleeping poorly. "She worries so much. She worries about Bettina, our grandchild. She worries about our kids. Now she's worried about my mother. When we were going through that mammogram scare, she was even worse!"

Mrs. Garcia shrugs her shoulders. "I can't help it. I'm like that. I've always been a worrier. But it's gotten worse lately. Now I worry and get so emotional. I lie in bed thinking about all this stuff and end up in tears. Then when I finally get to sleep, I wake up covered with sweat. I've tried extra soy for hot flashes, melatonin from the health food store, herbal tea, and even Benadryl—but nothing seems to work. I'm so tired. But when I get up, I have to deal with all these little kids at work. They're bouncing all over the place and noisy. I just get so short-tempered with them. That's not like me. I can't take this anymore."

A. *Patient data:* Clearly Mrs. Garcia has a sleep problem. Underline the data that are defining characteristics (symptoms) of a sleep problem.

B. *Patient data:* Which data suggest ideas about the etiologies (causes) of Mrs. Garcia's sleep problem?

C. *Nursing diagnosis:* NANDA has two sleep-related nursing diagnoses: Sleep Deprivation and Disturbed Sleep Pattern. You have already identified the

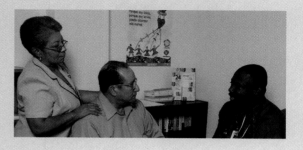

patient's defining characteristics. Now, what *knowledge* do you need to decide which of these NANDA labels to use?

D. How could you obtain this knowledge?

E. Sleep Deprivation is defined as "prolonged periods of time without sleep" and Disturbed Sleep Pattern is defined as "time-limited disruption of sleep." Can you make the diagnosis on the basis of this knowledge? Why or why not?

F. Following are some of the defining characteristics for these two nursing diagnoses:

Disturbed Sleep Pattern	Sleep Deprivation
Verbal complaints of not feeling well rested	Daytime drowsiness
Dissatisfaction with sleep	Decreased ability to function
Excess sleepiness	Tiredness
Emotional lability	Irritability
Decreased ability to function	Hallucinations
Inability to stay asleep	Acute confusion
	Inability to concentrate
	Apathy
	Slowed reactions

Certainly there is some overlap between the two sets of symptoms. Nevertheless, which set seems to be a better fit for Mrs. Garcia? Why?

G. Write a nursing diagnosis for Mrs. Garcia.

1 You are a nurse working on a psychiatric unit. You are assigned to Sheryl, a 23-year-old woman with the diagnosis of anorexia nervosa (a life-threatening eating disorder characterized by an intense fear of weight gain and extremely restrictive food intake). Sheryl attends therapy each day, seems to be taking her medications, and is eating the required amount of food at each meal. But she continues to lose weight. The night nurse reports that Sheryl is unable to sleep at night; seems frightened, almost panicky; paces the hall; and cries. Sheryl is unwilling to talk about her inability to sleep, but you read in her chart that she was sexually abused during the night while she was in a foster home. As you are straightening up in her room, you find several of Sheryl's sleeping pills. Sheryl walks into the room and begs you to be her friend and not to tell anyone. She promises to take her pills that night.

a What do you think may be contributing to Sheryl's inability to sleep? Explain your reasoning.

b How do you *feel* about keeping Sheryl's secret? Why might you want to tell other caregivers about the sleeping pills? What reasons can you think of for *not* telling?

c For you to deal effectively with Sheryl's sleep problem, what theoretical knowledge would you need?

d Now assess your current theoretical knowledge. Do you need more knowledge about certain topics to help Sheryl? If so, where can you find out what you need to know?

2 Imagine that you are a registered nurse at a local nursing home. Gwen, a 74-year-old woman, has captured your heart. Gwen has severe rheumatoid arthritis with pain and joint deformities, so she cannot ambulate or perform activities of daily living independently. Gwen's family visits every weekend, and they always bring cookies or candy, usually chocolate. Gwen likes to eat these treats just before bedtime, right after her bedtime medications. She receives a stool softener, a sleeping pill, and a pain pill for her arthritis. Lately she has been awakening at least twice each night, seeming quite confused. She tells the day shift nurse that she needs another sleeping pill at bedtime because "I'm not sleeping as well as I used to, because I have to get up so many times to go to the bathroom." She also seems more sluggish than usual during the day. You will need to integrate all available information. Don't worry if you do not know much about arthritis or if there are other things you have not yet studied. Just try to reason out the questions based on the knowledge you *do* have.

a If you have not yet studied arthritis and urinary elimination, you may lack some theoretical knowledge you need to answer the following questions. What information do you need? Where would you go to get it?

b What are some reasons that Gwen might be awakening?

c What might be causing her confusion at night?

d Should you address the problem of having chocolate before bed? Why or why not?

e List as many different interventions as you can that you might use to address the problem of eating sweets before bed.

f Consider the consequences. How might her family react if you suggest that they bring something besides sweets?

g What teaching might you do with the family?

3 You are a home health nurse. One of your patients is a 55-year-old man named Grant. He is homebound because of complications of diabetes. He states that he sleeps during the day, taking several naps. His chief complaint today is a pain in his left foot. There are alternative medicine books and bottles of vitamins and minerals all over the house. He believes he can cure his diabetes with herbs. He refuses to take any medications that are prescribed for him by his physician.

a Do you have enough information to conclude that Grant has a sleep problem? Explain your answer.

b Examine the patient situation (context). What factors lead you to suspect that Grant may not be sleeping enough at night?

c What would you do to find out whether Grant is getting enough sleep?

d Imagine how you would *feel* about Grant's decision to forgo his medication and use herbal treatments.

e What personal values and biases do you have that will affect the way you respond to Grant?

4 For each of the following concepts, use critical thinking to describe how or why it is important to nursing, patient care, or sleep and rest. Note that these are *not* to be merely definitions.

Sleep

Rest

Theoretical knowledge about the physiology of sleep

Circadian rhythm

Stages of sleep (e.g., REM sleep)

Sleep apnea

Sedatives

Sleep diary

Practical Knowledge
knowing how

This section will help you learn to give a back massage, assist you in obtaining a sleep history, and provide standardized language to use in planning care for clients with sleep problems.

PROCEDURES

In the not-so-distant past, a relaxing back massage was a part of the evening care routine for every hospitalized patient. In this era of cost containment, this sleep enhancer has become a "nice but not essential" procedure. Massage has therapeutic benefits, however. It promotes circulation, physical and emotional comfort, and sleep. Furthermore, it is an independent nursing activity for which you do not need a medical order (except in very rare circumstances). Try to offer a back rub whenever you can, and teach and encourage UAPs to do so as well. Refer to the following procedure.

PROCEDURE 33–1 Giving a Back Massage

 For steps to follow in *all* procedures, refer to the inside back cover of this book.

critical aspects
- Warm the lotion.
- Raise bed to working height.
- Position the patient comfortably on her side or prone.
- Place lotion on your hands.
- Rub down the length and then up the sides of the back.
- Never rub directly over the spine.
- Apply gentle thumb pressure on either side of the spine at midback, pushing outward for about 2.5 cm (1 inch) along the trapezius muscle.
- Always apply pressure away from the spine, not toward it.
- Go to the spots that felt the tightest or that the patient states are tight. Work in small circles, using gentle thumb pressure.
- Gently shake the scapula.
- Apply horizontal strokes across the scapula, using your thumb.
- Apply circles using the heels of your hands down both sides of the spine.
- Apply horizontal strokes using the heels of your hands across the latissimus dorsi muscle.
- Gently rub your hands up either side of the spine from the base of the back to the base of the neck, and then down the sides of the back.

Equipment
Skin care lotion

Delegation
You can delegate back massage to unlicensed assistive personnel (UAP) if the patient's condition and the UAP's skills

allow. However, giving the back rub yourself provides an excellent opportunity to assess the patient and provide emotional support.

Assessment
Check skin for reddened areas.

PROCEDURE 33–1   **Giving a Back Massage** *(continued)*

Procedural Steps

Step 1 Warm the lotion by placing the bottle in warm water.

Cold lotion can cause muscle contraction; warming the lotion helps relax the muscles.

Step 2 Raise the bed to working height.

Prevents back strain of the nurse.

Step 3 Position patient comfortably on her side or prone.
a. Untie the patient's gown, and expose her back.
b. Raise the siderail on the opposite side of the bed.

Prevents the patient from falling off the bed when your turn her toward the side of the bed away from you.

c. Wash the patient's back with warm water, if needed.

Warm water will help relax the muscles while removing any sweat and soiling.

Step 4 Place lotion on your hands.

Placing the lotion directly on the back may cause the patient's muscles to tighten.

Step 5 Place your hands on either side of the spine at the base of the neck. Using gentle, continuous pressure, rub down the length and then up the sides of the back. ▼

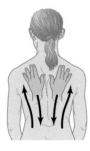

a. Repeat this motion several times.
b. Never rub directly over the spine.

The spine is a vulnerable area.

Step 6 Apply gentle thumb pressure (using the fleshy part of your thumbs) on either side of the spine at the midback, pushing outward for about 2.5 cm (1 inch). ▼

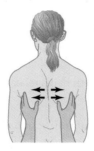

a. Repeat from the midback to the base of the neck in a series of small, outward strokes.

Strokes should be along the muscle length and not across the muscle to help stretch and relax it.

b. Ask the patient whether the amount of pressure is comfortable.

Be careful not to cause the patient discomfort, which might cause further muscle tightness.

c. Always apply pressure away from the spine, not toward it.

This gently stretches the muscles and helps prevent placing pressure on the spine.

d. If you are unable to do both sides at the same time, do one side and then the other.

Work as symmetrically as possible to increase muscle relaxation.

Step 7 Now go to the spots that felt the tightest or that the patient states are tight. Work in small circles, using gentle thumb pressure. ▼

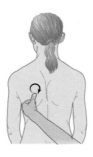

Small circular movements can help release muscle "knots" and relax tightened muscles.

Step 8 Gently shake the scapula. Place your palm on one scapula, and gently shake it by quickly moving your palm back and forth. Repeat on the other side. ▼

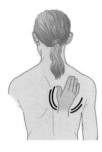

Movement of the scapula decreases when muscles tighten; gently vibrating the scapula helps loosen the muscles.

Step 9 Apply horizontal strokes across the scapula, using your thumb. Using horizontal strokes from near the spine across the bottom of the scapula, push out all the way across the scapula from the spine. Move up and repeat until you have covered the entire scapula and top of shoulder. Repeat on the other side. ▼

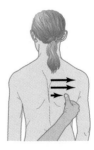

This movement helps loosen the trapezius muscle.

Step 10 If you find tender spots, use the fleshy parts of your fingers in a small circular motion.

➤

PROCEDURE 33–1   Giving a Back Massage *(continued)*

Step 11   Apply pressure in circles using the heels of your hands down both sides of the spine. Beginning at the upper shoulder and working down to the lower back, apply pressure in medium-sized circles down the sides of the spine with the heels of your hands. Be cautious not to apply too much pressure. Assess patient for comfort. ▼

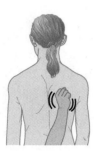

The circular motion helps relax tightened areas in the muscles.

Step 12   Apply horizontal strokes using the heels of your hands across latissimus dorsi muscle. Using horizontal strokes from near the spine below the scapula, push out from the spine across to the ribs, and work down across the lower back with the heels of your hands.

This movement helps relax the latissimus dorsi muscle.

Step 13   Gently rub your hands up either side of the spine from the base of the back to the base of the neck and then down the sides of the back. Repeat several times.

Long strokes to help increase circulation and promote relaxation of the back muscles.

Note: If you are unable to do a complete back massage, ask the patient where she is most uncomfortable, and massage those areas. If the patient has general tightness, use the long strokes down each side of the spine and back up the sides.

Evaluation

Assess:
• Patient's report of comfort, relaxation, and how soon patient falls asleep.

Documentation

This is a routine aspect of care and is usually documented on a flow sheet.

ASSESSMENT GUIDELINES AND TOOLS

Questions for a Brief Sleep History

A brief assessment for all patients should include questions about the following:

Usual Sleeping Pattern

- When do you go to sleep and wake up?
- How many hours do you sleep?
- How often do you waken at night, for example, to go to the bathroom?
- Do you feel adequately rested when you wake up?

Sleeping Environment

- Would you like a night-light?
- What room temperature do you prefer?
- What noise level do you prefer (for example, radio, television, absolute quiet)?

Bedtime Routines/Rituals

- What do you typically do in the hour before bedtime?
- What do you do to help you fall asleep?

Sleep Aids

- Do you need a special pillow or positioning aid?
- Do you take any sleep medications or other drugs that may affect sleep?

Sleep Changes or Problems

- Have your sleep patterns changed?
- Do you have any difficulties sleeping?

If the person reports experiencing satisfactory sleep, that is an adequate assessment, and you merely need to support her usual sleep patterns and rituals. When you suspect a sleep problem, you will perform a more in-depth assessment, such as a detailed sleep history or sleep diary.

Detailed Sleep History

1. How do you sleep at night?
2. What time do you usually retire?
3. How many times do you get up during the night (e.g., to go to the bathroom)?
4. How would you rate the quality of your sleep on a scale of 1 to 10, with 10 meaning "great"?
5. Have there been any recent changes in your sleep patterns? If so, what are they?
6. Is there any physical reason for your sleep problem?
7. Do you feel rested in the morning?
8. What other signs and symptoms do you have when you have difficulty sleeping?
9. Do you snore?
10. Do you have any bedtime rituals?
11. Do you take medication to help you sleep?
12. Describe your sleep environment: dark, quiet, TV on, night-light, music?
13. Do you exercise during the day? What type?
14. Do you take a nap. If you do, for how long?
15. Have you ever kept a sleep diary? If so, have you noted anything that might interfere with your sleep at night?
16. Is there anything that I have not asked that might help you sleep while you are in the hospital (having surgery, receiving home care)?

Sleep Diary

A sleep diary provides specific information on the patient's sleep-wakefulness patterns over a long period. The diary is usually kept for 14 days and may include the following.

1. Time you went to bed:_____
2. What did you eat or drink just before bedtime? _____
3. What mental and physical activities did you engage in the 2 to 3 hours before bedtime?_____
4. Were you worried or anxious about anything when you went to bed?_____
5. Approximate time you fell asleep:_____
6. Times you woke during the night:_____
7. Times you fell back to sleep:_____
8. Time you woke up:_____
9. Sleep medications you have taken:_____
10. Any repeated doses? _____ Times:_____
11. Episodes of "disorientation":_____
12. Frequency of pain medication taken and times:_____
13. Did you feel refreshed in the morning?_____

STANDARDIZED LANGUAGE

Selected NOC Outcomes and NIC Interventions for Sleep Diagnoses

Nursing Diagnosis	NOC Outcomes	NIC Interventions
Readiness for Enhanced Sleep	Rest Sleep Personal Well-Being	Environmental Management: Comfort Sleep Enhancement
Disturbed Sleep Pattern	Rest Sleep Personal Well-Being	Coping Enhancement Energy Management Environmental Management: Comfort Simple Relaxation Therapy Sleep Enhancement
Sleep Deprivation	Rest Sleep Symptom Severity	Coping Enhancement Energy Management Environmental Management: Comfort Simple Relaxation Therapy Sleep Enhancement

Sources: Dochterman, J., & Bulechek, G. (Eds.). (2004). *Nursing interventions classification (NIC)* (4th ed.). St Louis: Mosby; Moorhead, S., Johnson, M., & Maas, M. (Eds.). (2004). *Nursing outcomes classification (NIC)* (3rd ed.). St Louis, Mosby.

What Are the Main Points in This Chapter?

- Sleep is a basic physiological need.
- Sleep and rest promote physical, mental, and spiritual well-being by restoring energy and reducing body demands while the body repairs itself.
- Illness can interfere with the ability to sleep and rest; conversely, people who suffer from sleep disorders have an increased susceptibility to illnesses.
- The hypothalamus and various neurotransmitters are involved in the physiology of sleep.
- Circadian rhythm is a biorhythm that is influenced by both internal and external stimuli, especially the light-dark patterns of day and night.
- During the four stages of NREM sleep, sleep progressively deepens.
- The brain waves produced during REM sleep are similar to those of alert wakefulness. REM is characterized by rapid eye movements and dreaming.
- Duration of sleep varies according to age.

- Factors affecting sleep include developmental needs and stressors, work, exercise, foods, other lifestyle factors, use of medications, illness, pain, and the environment.
- Common sleep disorders include insomnia, sleep apnea, and narcolepsy.
- It is important to obtain information about the patient's usual sleep patterns and rituals; this may require use of a sleep diary.
- Nursing interventions to promote sleep include scheduling nursing care, creating a restful environment, and supporting bedtime rituals and routines.
- Pain is one of the main deterrents to sleep.
- Sleep medications, as a rule, should be used only as a temporary measure.
- Teaching patients and their families about the importance of rest and sleep is an important health promotion intervention.

34 Skin Integrity
& Wound Healing

CHAPTER

Overview

The major functions of the skin are protection of the internal organs, unique identification of an individual, thermoregulation, metabolism of nutrients and metabolic waste products, and sensation. Age, mobility, nutrition, hydration, underlying conditions, medications, and hygiene are factors that influence the ability to maintain intact skin and heal wounds.

Wounds are disruptions in the skin. If there are no breaks in the skin, a wound is described as *closed*. A wound is considered *open* if there is a break in the skin or mucous membranes. Acute wounds may be intentional (e.g., surgical incisions) or unintentional (e.g., from trauma) and are expected to be of relatively short duration. Wounds that exceed the anticipated length of recovery are classified as chronic wounds.

A wound that involves minimal or no tissue loss and has wound edges that approximate heals by primary intention. A wound that involves extensive tissue loss and has margins that cannot be approximated, or is infected, heals by secondary intention. The wound is left open and allowed to heal from the inner layer to the surface. Tertiary intention healing, or delayed primary closure, occurs when two surfaces of granulation tissue are brought together surgically. Initially the wound is allowed to heal by secondary intention.

Healing occurs in three stages: inflammatory, proliferative, and maturation. The *inflammatory phase* lasts from 1 to 5 days and consists of two major processes: hemostasis and inflammation. The *proliferative phase* occurs from days 5 to 21. It is characterized by cell development aimed at filling the wound defect and resurfacing the skin. The *maturation phase* is the final phase of the healing process. It begins in the second or third week and continues until the wound is completely healed.

The RYB color classification system guides wound treatment. Protect a red wound, cleanse a yellow wound, and debride a black wound. The goal of all wound care is to heal a wound in the most rapid and comfortable manner. Dressings and wound treatments must be modified as the wound evolves.

Thinking Critically About Skin Integrity and Wound Healing

The exercises in the following section allow you to practice the kind of thinking you will use as a full-spectrum nurse. Because these are critical-thinking activities, there is usually no single right answer. Discuss answers with your peers—discussion can stimulate critical thinking. If you have difficulty with any of the questions, consult with your instructor.

Caring for the Garcias

Bettina Sanford, Joe and Flordelisa Garcia's 3-year-old grandchild, fell at the neighborhood playground. She has abrasions on her knees, a deep puncture wound on her left hand, and a laceration on her scalp. Mr. and Mrs. Garcia bring her to the clinic for assessment. She is crying loudly and moving all extremities. No treatment has been given.

A. What should be your first course of action?

B. What kind of care will Bettina need at the clinic?

C. You determine that the scalp laceration will need to be sutured. What actions should you take to prepare Bettina for the suturing?

D. One week later Bettina arrives at the clinic with her grandmother to have the sutures removed. The scalp laceration is dried and healed. When you inspect her other wounds, you notice that her left knee is erythematous, warm and painful to touch, and draining a moderate amount of purulent drainage. What assessment questions should you ask?

E. Flordelisa Garcia tells you that Bettina would not allow her to clean or dress the abraded knees. You cleanse the knee and remove several small pieces of gravel from the wound bed. The wound is yellow and malodorous. What kind of care will Flordelisa need to provide to Bettina to heal the left knee?

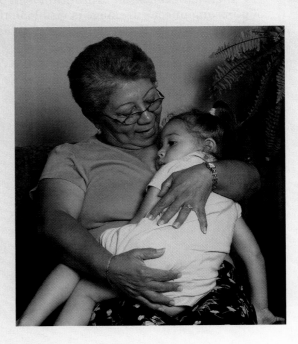

1 You are caring for a 22-year-old man who is paralyzed from the waist down secondary to an automobile accident. He has been admitted to the hospital with a urinary tract infection manifested by a fever of 102°F (39°C) and lethargy. His family reports he has been withdrawn and sits in his wheelchair watching TV all day long.

a What risk factors does this patient have for skin breakdown?

b What locations of his body should you be most concerned about in regard to pressure ulcer formation?

c What actions should you take to decrease the risk of pressure ulcers in this man? What further information do you need?

2 A 63-year-old man is admitted to your unit after an emergency appendectomy. His appendix was ruptured, and the surgeon has left the wound open to heal by secondary intention. A Jackson-Pratt drain is in place in the wound bed. A moderate amount of purosanguineous drainage is visible in the drain. The surgeon has ordered wet-to-damp dressings with normal saline packing every 4 hours.

a What actions should you take as you prepare to do the first dressing change?

b How will you secure the dressing?

3 For the following patients, write a NANDA diagnosis related to skin integrity. Include problem, etiology, and defining characteristics. If you do not have enough data for one of those components, state what additional data you need.

a Mrs. Whitefeather is 95 years old. She has cancer, and she has stopped eating and become very thin. Recently she has become too weak to move about in bed without help. However, her skin is intact with no redness, even over her bony prominences. She has a very low score on the Braden pressure ulcer assessment scale.

b Eddie Allen is 4 years old. He has a severe case of poison ivy, which has made blisters on his skin. He has been scratching his "itchies" and has bleeding, excoriated areas over his limbs, face, and trunk.

c Allie Newton has a stage II pressure ulcer on her left heel.

4 For each of the following concepts, use critical thinking to describe how or why it is important to nursing, patient care, or skin integrity and wound healing. Note that these are *not* to be merely definitions.

Shearing

Friction

Pressure

Wound healing process

Preventing pressure ulcers

RYB color classification

Dressing changes

Practical Knowledge
knowing how

PROCEDURES

As a nurse, you will care for many patients who have wounds or who are at risk for impaired skin integrity. You will need practical knowledge of wound assessment and wound care.

All wounds require a focused assessment. Assessment frequency depends on the condition of the wound, the work setting, the patient's overall condition and underlying disease process, the type of wound, and the type of treatment used for the wound. If you are providing wound care, you will assess the wound with every treatment.

Specific nursing interventions directed at maintaining skin integrity or healing wounds focus on providing wound care and applying heat and cold therapies. In this section, you will find procedures for obtaining wound cultures, cleansing wounds, and dressing wounds. You will also find techniques for placing and removing wound closures, caring for wound drains, applying binders and bandages, and applying local heat and cold therapy.

PROCEDURE 34–1   Obtaining a Wound Culture by Swab

 For steps to follow in *all* procedures, refer to inside back cover of this book.

critical aspects
- Position the patient for easy access to the wound and in a manner that will allow the irrigation solution to flow freely from the wound with the assistance of gravity.
- Don protective equipment: gown, face shield, and clean gloves.
- Remove the soiled dressing, and dispose of gloves and dressing.
- Wearing clean gloves, fill a 35 mL syringe, with attached 19-gauge angiocath, with 0.9% (normal) saline solution.
- Holding the angiocath tip 2 cm from the wound bed, gently irrigate the wound (superior to inferior).
- Press the culture swab against an area of red granulating tissue, and rotate.
- Reinsert the swab into the culturette tube, label the tube, and transport it to the lab.

Equipment
- Three pairs of clean gloves
- Culturette tube
- Sterile 4 × 4 gauze in an impermeable tray or separate 4 × 4 packs and an impermeable barrier
- Sterile 0.9% (normal) saline solution for irrigation, warmed to body temperature when possible

Cold solution lowers temperature of wound bed and slows the healing process.

- 35 mL syringe
- 19-gauge angiocath
- Gown and face shield
- Emesis basin
- Water-resistant disposable drapes

Delegation

This is an invasive procedure that requires knowledge of wound healing. It should be performed by a registered nurse. Do not delegate this skill.

Assessments

Note: If the wound is covered when you begin, you will make these assessments when you remove the soiled dressing *and* after cleansing the wound.

- Assess the amount and type of tissue present in the wound bed.

➤

PROCEDURE 34–1   Obtaining a Wound Culture by Swab *(continued)*

Granulating tissue is beefy red with a velvety appearance. It appears with the growth of new blood vessels and connective tissue. Pale pink tissue may indicate compromised blood supply to the wound bed. Necrotic tissue, which is black, brown, or yellow in appearance, is nonviable and inhibits healing. Only red granulating tissue should be swabbed for a culture.

- Assess the type and amount of exudate.

Exudate may be a sign of infection.

- Assess the wound for odor.

A foul odor may indicate infection. Cleanse wounds before you assess for odor, because some dressings interact with wound drainage to produce an odor.

- Assess the tissue surrounding the wound edge.

Surrounding tissue that is red, warm, and/or edematous may indicate infection.

- Assess for pain.

Wounds may be very painful, and wound irrigation may increase pain. Provide ordered pain medication 30 minutes prior to performing the procedure, as indicated.

- Determine whether the wound requires sterile or clean technique for irrigation.

Sterile technique is used for acute surgical wounds and for wounds that have undergone recent sharp debridement, or when the physician orders it. Chronic wounds are colonized with bacteria and may be irrigated with clean technique. Irrigation using clean technique is presented in this procedure. To perform a sterile wound irrigation, see Procedure 34–3.

Procedural Steps

Step 1 Place the patient in a comfortable position that provides easy access to the wound and will allow the irrigation solution to flow freely from the wound, with the assistance of gravity. Position a water-resistant disposable drape to protect the bedding from any possible runoff.

Drape protects the bedding.

Step 2 After washing and drying hands, apply a gown, face shield, and clean gloves.

Protects against splattering that may occur during wound irrigation.

Step 3 Remove the soiled dressing. Dispose of gloves and soiled dressing in a biohazard bag.

Soiled dressings contain contaminants and should be treated as biohazardous waste.

Step 4 Apply clean gloves.

Step 5 Place an emesis basin at the bottom of the wound to collect irrigation runoff. Avoid touching the wound with the basin.

Prevents contamination of wound from the emesis basin; protects linens from runoff.

Step 6 Attach a 19-gauge angiocath to a 35 mL syringe, and fill with normal saline irrigation solution.

A 19-gauge angiocath with a 35 mL syringe provides 8 psi (pounds per square inch) of pressure and is effective for removing bacteria, necrotic tissue, exudate, and/or metabolic wastes. *Note:* This procedure follows guidelines established by the Agency for Healthcare Research Quality (AHRQ). Commercial irrigation kits containing a piston tip syringe may also be used. Their use is discussed in Procedure 34–3.

Step 7 Holding the angiocath tip 2 cm from the wound bed, gently irrigate the wound with a back-and-forth motion, moving from the superior aspect to the inferior aspect.

Irrigating from top to bottom prevents flow of contaminated solution over the cleansed area. ▼

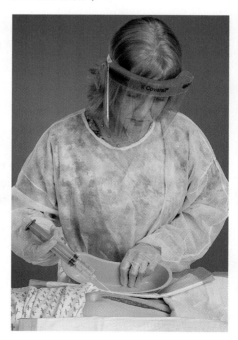

PROCEDURE 34–1   **Obtaining a Wound Culture by Swab** *(continued)*

Step 8 Dispose of the syringe and angiocath in the sharps container, and dispose of the gloves in the biohazard waste.

Prevents contamination and needlestick injury.

Step 9 Obtain a culturette tube, and twist the top of the tube to loosen the swab.

Step 10 Apply clean gloves, and locate an area of red, granulating tissue in the wound bed.

Step 11 Withdraw the swab from the culturette tube. Press the swab against the granulating area, and rotate the swab.
a. Do not allow the swab to touch anything other than the granulating area of the wound.
b. Do not swab culture areas where slough or eschar is present.

These are areas of avascular or necrotic tissue and are contaminated with bacteria. AHRQ does not recommend routine wound cultures of open wounds because they are colonized with bacteria. Swab cultures detect only surface bacteria and are not a reliable means for diagnosing wound infection. ▼

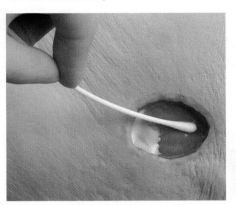

Step 12 Carefully insert the swab back into the culturette tube, making sure it does not make contact with the opening of the tube upon reinsertion. Twist the cap to secure the tube.

Decreases risk of contamination; ensures that any microorganisms that grow in the culture are from the wound and were not introduced from the environment.

Step 13 Crush the ampule of culture medium at the bottom of the tube. (*Note:* Inspect the culture tube to determine whether this step is required.)

The ampule contains medium for growth of organism.

Step 14 Label the culturette tube with the patient's name, birthdate, source of specimen, and date and time of collection.

Ensures obtaining the results for the correct patient.

Step 15 Transport the culture to the lab.

Step 16 Apply a clean dressing to the wound as ordered.

Evaluation
- Determine whether patient remains comfortable. If not, medicate according to orders.
- Monitor lab reports for results of the swab culture.

Documentation
Document the following information (many agencies use a wound/skin flowsheet):
- Appearance and location of the wound, type and amount of exudate, and odor, if present, after irrigation.
- Patient's pain level before you obtained the culture. If the patient was medicated for pain, document the drug and dose used, time given, and patient response.
- Method by which the wound was cleansed before you obtained the swab culture.
- Description of the area where the culture was obtained.
- Dressing reapplied to wound, if applicable.
- Education provided to patient.

➤

PROCEDURE 34–1   **Obtaining a Wound Culture by Swab** *(continued)*

Sample documentation:

> **07/25/07 1000** *Wound irrigation with 0.9% NS to 4 cm X 3 cm*
> *stage IV pressure ulcer on coccyx. Patient*
> *voices no complaints of pain prior to or after*
> *irrigation. Wound bed 50% red, granulating tissue*
> *and 50% yellow slough after irrigation. Scant*
> *amount of serosanguineous drainage from wound.*
> *No purulent drainage or odor noted. Surrounding*
> *tissue slightly red with increased warmth to area.*
> *Swab culture obtained in medial wound edge, from*
> *red, granulating tissue. Culturette transported*
> *to lab. Wound filled with saline-moistened gauze*
> *and covered with Stratasorb as ordered. Pt.*
> *instructed on procedure, reason for culture, and*
> *possible results. Pt. verbalizes understanding.*
> *Will continue to monitor.*———— *S. Robertson RN*

PROCEDURE 34–2   **Obtaining a Needle Aspiration Culture from a Wound**

 For Steps to follow in *all* procedures, refer to the inside back cover of this book.

critical aspects

- Administer pain medication 30 minutes prior to the procedure, if necessary.
- Cleanse the wound with saline-moistened gauze, wiping from the center of the wound toward the edge.
- Draw up 1 mL of 0.9% (normal) saline for injection into a 22-gauge needle attached to a 3 mL syringe.
- Insert the needle 1 to 2 mm into the wound bed, and inject 1 mL of normal saline.
- Aspirate 1 mL of fluid from the wound bed.
- Express the fluid into the culture tube.
- Label the culture tube, and transport it to the lab.
- Apply a clean dressing to the wound as ordered.

PROCEDURE 34–2   Obtaining a Needle Aspiration Culture from a Wound *(continued)*

Equipment

- Two pairs of clean gloves
- Gown and face shield
- 0.9% (normal) saline solution for irrigation, warmed to body temperature when possible

Cold solution lowers temperature of wound bed and slows the healing process.

- Sterile 4 × 4 gauze pads in an impermeable tray
- Vial of 0.9% (normal) saline for injection
- 22-gauge needle
- 3 mL syringe
- Lab tube with culture medium

Delegation

This is an invasive procedure that requires knowledge of wound healing. It should be performed by a registered nurse. Do not delegate this skill.

Assessment

Note: If the wound is covered when you begin, you will make these assessments when you remove the soiled dressing *and* after cleansing the wound.

- Assess the amount and type of tissue present in the wound bed.

Granulating tissue is beefy red with a velvety appearance. It appears with the growth of new blood vessels and connective tissue. Pale pink tissue may indicate compromised blood supply to the wound bed. Necrotic tissue, which is black, brown, or yellow in appearance, is nonviable and inhibits healing.

- Assess the type and amount of exudate.

Exudate may be a sign of infection.

- Assess the wound for odor.

A foul odor may indicate infection. Cleanse wounds before you assess for odor, because some dressings interact with wound drainage to produce an odor.

- Assess the tissue surrounding the wound edge.

Surrounding tissue that is red, warm, and/or edematous may indicate infection.

- Assess for pain.

Wounds may be very painful, and wound irrigation may increase pain. Provide ordered pain medication 30 minutes prior to performing the procedure, as indicated.

Procedural Steps

Step 1 Position the patient so the wound is easily accessible. Position a water-resistant disposable drape under the patient to collect fluid runoff.

Drape protects the linens.

Step 2 After washing and drying your hands, apply a gown, face shield, and clean gloves.

Protects you from splattering.

Step 3 Remove the soiled dressing. Dispose of gloves and soiled dressing in a biohazard bag.

Soiled dressings contain contaminants and should be treated as biohazardous waste.

Step 4 Open a tray of sterile 4 × 4 gauze. Moisten the gauze with normal saline solution for irrigation.

The sterile container tray is impermeable.

Step 5 Attach a 22-gauge needle to a 3 mL syringe, and aspirate 1 mL of sterile normal saline from the vial. Cap the needle, using a one-handed technique (see Procedure 23–10), and place the syringe on the bedside table.

Maintains sterility and prevents needle-stick injury.

Step 6 Apply procedure gloves.

Prevents introducing microorganisms into the wound to be cultured.

Step 7 Gently cleanse the wound with the saline-moistened gauze by lightly wiping a section of the wound from the center toward the wound edge. Discard the gauze in a biohazard receptacle, and repeat in the next section using a new piece of gauze with each wiping pass.

Removes surface bacteria and exudate. ▼

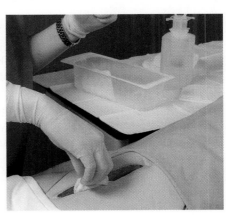

➤

PROCEDURE 34–2

Obtaining a Needle Aspiration Culture from a Wound *(continued)*

Step 8 Uncap the syringe from the bedside table, and insert the needle 1 to 2 mm into the wound bed. Inject 1 mL of normal saline into the wound tissue.

Allows for an adequate amount of culture fluid to be aspirated. ▼

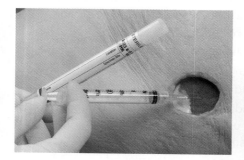

Step 9 Pull back on the syringe plunger to aspirate approximately 1 mL of fluid into the barrel of the syringe. Remove the needle from the wound bed after you have collected the aspirate.

Step 10 Place the collected fluid into a culture tube containing culture medium.

Culture medium supports the growth of microorganisms. ▼

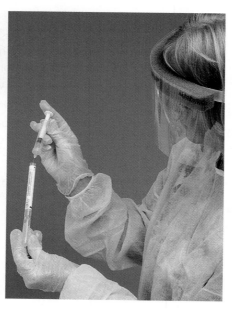

Step 11 Label the culture tube with the patient's name, birthdate, source of specimen, and date and time of collection. (A label may be supplied with the culture kit.)

Ensures obtaining the results for the correct patient.

Step 12 Transport the culture to the lab.

Step 13 Apply a clean dressing to the wound as ordered.

Evaluation

- Determine whether patient remains comfortable. If not, medicate according to orders.
- Monitor the wound bed at the puncture site for evidence of bleeding.
- Monitor lab reports for results of the aspirate culture.

Documentation

Document the following information (many agencies use a wound/skin flowsheet):

- Appearance and location of the wound, type and amount of exudate, and odor, if present, after irrigation.
- Patient's pain level before you obtained the culture. If the patient was medicated for pain, document the drug and dose used, time given, and patient response.
- Method by which the wound was cleansed before you obtained the aspiration culture.

PROCEDURE 34–2

Obtaining a Needle Aspiration Culture from a Wound *(continued)*

- Description of the area where culture was obtained.
- Dressing reapplied to wound, if applicable.
- Education provided to patient.

Sample documentation:

07/25/07	1800	Pt. denies pain at wound site. Central abdominal wound cleansed with saline-moistened gauze. Wound bed 90% yellow slough and 10% red, granulating tissue. Scant amount of serous drainage with no odor noted. Surrounding skin tissue slightly edematous in appearance. Aspiration culture performed with injection of 1 mL of normal saline via 22-gauge needle into 3 o'clock position of wound bed. Aspirated 1 mL for culture. Specimen transported to lab. No bleeding noted at puncture site after aspiration. Wound redressed with saline-moistened gauze. Pt. tolerated procedure well and remains free of pain.————————— L. Burrough, RN

PROCEDURE 34–3   Performing a Sterile Wound Irrigation

For steps to follow in *all* procedures, refer to the inside back cover of this book.

Note: This procedure uses sterile technique. Sterile technique is used for acute surgical wounds, for wounds that have recently undergone sharp debridement, or when the physician has ordered sterile technique.

critical aspects

- Administer pain medication 30 minutes prior to the procedure, if necessary.
- Position the patient for easy access to the wound and in a manner that will allow the irrigation solution to flow freely from the wound with the assistance of gravity.
- Don protective equipment: gown, face shield, and clean gloves.
- Remove the soiled dressing, and dispose of gloves.
- Set up a sterile field with a sterile irrigation kit or a 35 mL syringe and a 19-gauge angiocath, dressing supplies, and irrigation solution.
- Wearing sterile gloves, fill either the syringe and angiocath or the piston-tip syringe with irrigation solution.
- Holding the syringe 2 cm from the wound bed, gently irrigate the wound with a back-and-forth motion, moving from the superior aspect to the inferior aspect.
- Dry the tissue surrounding the wound with sterile gauze.
- Apply a new dressing as ordered.
- Dispose of used equipment and soiled dressings in a biohazard container.
- Reposition the patient.

Equipment

- One pair of clean gloves
- One pair of sterile gloves
- Gown and face shield
- Water-resistant, disposable drapes
- Warmed (body temperature) irrigation solution

Cold solution lowers temperature of wound bed and slows the healing process.

- Sterile gauze
- Dressing supplies
- Biohazardous waste container
- Sterile impermeable barrier
- Sterile bowl

For Variation A:
- Sterile emesis basin
- 35 mL syringe
- 19-gauge angiocath

For Variation B:
- Sterile commercial irrigation kit containing a sterile basin and piston-tip syringe

Delegation

This is an invasive, sterile procedure that requires knowledge of wound healing. It should be performed by a registered nurse. Do not delegate this skill.

Assessment

Note: If the wound is covered when you begin, you will make these assessments when you remove the soiled dressing *and* after cleansing the wound.

- Assess the amount and type of tissue present in the wound bed.

Granulating tissue is beefy red with a velvety appearance. It appears with the growth of new blood vessels and connective tissue. Pale pink tissue may indicate compromised blood supply to the wound bed. Necrotic tissue, which is black, brown, or yellow in appearance, is nonviable and inhibits healing.

- Assess the type and amount of exudate.

Exudate may be a sign of infection.

- Assess the wound for odor.

PROCEDURE 34–3 Performing a Sterile Wound Irrigation *(continued)*

A foul odor may indicate infection. Cleanse wounds before you assess for odor, because some dressings interact with wound drainage to produce an odor.

• **Assess the tissue surrounding the wound edge.**

Surrounding tissue that is red, warm, and/or edematous may indicate infection.

• **Assess for pain.**

Wounds may be very painful, and wound irrigation may increase pain. Assess for pain so you can provide ordered pain medication 30 minutes prior to performing procedure if needed.

• **Determine whether the wound requires sterile or clean technique for irrigation.**

Sterile technique is used for acute surgical wounds, for wounds that have undergone recent sharp debridement, or when the physician has ordered it. Chronic wounds are colonized with bacteria and may be irrigated with clean technique. Irrigation using clean technique is presented in steps 1 through 5 of Procedure 34–1.

Procedural Steps

Step 1 Place the patient in a comfortable position that provides easy access to the wound and will allow the irrigation solution to flow freely from the wound, with the assistance of gravity. Position a water-resistant disposable drape to protect the bedding from any possible runoff.

Drape protects the bedding.

Step 2 After washing and drying your hands, apply a gown, face shield, and clean gloves.

Protect against splattering that may occur during wound irrigation.

Step 3 Remove the soiled dressing. Dispose of gloves and soiled dressing in a biohazard bag.

Soiled dressings contain contaminants and should be treated as biohazardous waste.

Step 4 Set up a sterile field on a clean, dry surface. Add the following supplies to the field:
• Sterile gauze
• Sterile bowl
• Dressing supplies

• *Variation A:* a 19-gauge angiocath, 35 mL syringe, and sterile emesis basin
• *Variation B:* a sterile commercial irrigation kit

Setting up a sterile field at bedside provides easy access to equipment for irrigation. Note: This kit includes a sterile, disposable measuring device for wound assessment. ▼

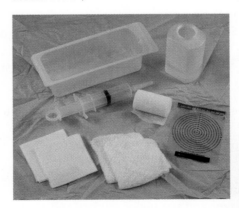

Step 5 Pour the warmed irrigation solution into the sterile bowl.

Step 6 Don sterile gloves.

Maintains sterile technique.

Step 7 Irrigate the wound.
a. Place the sterile basin at the bottom of the wound to collect irrigation runoff.

b. **Variation A** Attach the 19-gauge angiocath to the 35 mL syringe, and fill with the irrigation solution.

A 19-gauge angiocath and 35 mL syringe provides 8 psi of pressure and is effective for removing bacteria, necrotic tissue, exudate and/or metabolic wastes.

Variation B Fill a piston-tip syringe with irrigation solution.

c. Holding the angiocath tip or syringe tip 2 cm from the wound bed, gently irrigate the wound with a back-and-forth motion, moving from the superior aspect to the inferior aspect.

Irrigating from top to bottom prevents flow of contaminated solution over cleansed area. ▼

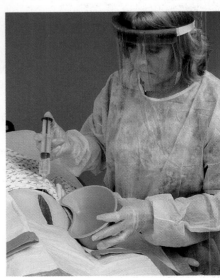

➤

PROCEDURE 34–3   Performing a Sterile Wound Irrigation
(continued)

d. Repeat the irrigation until the solution returns clear.

Removes exudate, debris, and some surface bacteria.

Step 8 Remove the basin or sterile container from the base of the wound.

Step 9 Pat the skin surrounding the wound dry with sterile gauze, beginning at the top of the wound and working downward.

Moisture on the surrounding tissue may lead to maceration and further breakdown of the wound margins.

Step 10 Dress the wound as ordered.

Step 11 Dispose of the contaminated irrigation fluid in appropriate manner.

Contaminated fluid should be disposed of as biohazardous waste.

Step 12 Remove soiled drapes from the patient area.

Makes the patient more comfortable.

Step 13 Remove your gloves, face shield, and gown. Dispose of these items appropriately.

Contaminants from the irrigation may be present on these items, and they should also be considered biohazardous.

Step 14 Wash your hands.

Step 15 Reposition the patient to a comfortable position.

Step 16 Assess patient's pain level and tolerance to the procedure.

Promotes comfort.

Step 17 Answer any questions the patient may have.

Provides for patient understanding.

Step 18 Rewash your hands.

Prevents cross-contamination between patients.

Evaluation

- Determine whether patient remains comfortable. If not, medicate according to orders.
- Reassess the wound at regular intervals.

Patient Teaching

- Teach the patient about the expected healing process.
- Inform the patient and caregiver about signs and symptoms of infection and the need to report these findings.

Home Care

Wound irrigation is commonly done in the home. In most cases, clean technique is used in the home setting.

Documentation

Document the following information (many agencies use a wound/skin flowsheet):
- Appearance and location of the wound, type and amount of exudate, and odor, if present, after irrigation.
- Patient's pain level. If the patient was medicated for pain, document the drug and dose used, time given, and patient response.
- Method by which the wound was cleansed.
- Dressing reapplied to the wound, if applicable.
- Education provided to the patient.

PROCEDURE 34–3   **Performing a Sterile Wound Irrigation**
(continued)

Sample documentation:

07/23/07	0930	Pt. rates pain as 7 on scale of 1 to 10. Medicated with Lortab 5/500 ii tabs by mouth as ordered. Will monitor for effectiveness.————————— R. Bell, RN

07/23/07	1000	Pt. rates pain as 1 on scale of 1 to 10. Wound irrigation procedure explained to pt., who verbalizes understanding. Left leg propped on pillows to allow access and irrigation. 10 cm × 5 cm wound on left calf gently cleansed with 0.9% NS via piston-tip syringe. After cleansing, 60% red granulating tissue and 40% yellow slough present in wound bed, with minimal amount of serous drainage and no foul odor. Surrounding tissues intact. No bleeding or tissue trauma noted after irrigation. Wound filled with saline-moistened gauze. Education regarding wound irrigation reinforced with pt. and pt. verbalizes understanding. Will continue to monitor.———— R. Bell, RN

PROCEDURE 34–4   Removing and Applying Dry Dressings

 For steps to follow in *all* procedures, refer to the inside back cover of this book.

Note: This procedure uses clean technique because wound care is now usually performed using a clean approach rather than sterile technique.

critical aspects

- Administer pain medication 30 minutes prior to the procedure, if necessary.
- Place the patient in a comfortable position that provides easy access to the wound.
- Wearing clean gloves, remove the soiled dressing and discard it in a biohazard receptacle.
- Cleanse the wound with saline-moistened gauze.
- Assess the wound for location, appearance, odor, and drainage.
- Apply a dry dressing.
- Secure the dressing with tape.

Equipment

- Two pairs of clean gloves
- Sterile normal saline solution for irrigation, warmed to body temperature when possible

Cold solution lowers the temperature of wound bed and slows the healing process.

- Tray of sterile 4 × 4 gauze
- Sterile gauze for dressings
- Tape

Delegation

This is a procedure that requires knowledge of wound healing. It should be performed by a registered nurse. Do not delegate this skill.

Assessments

Note: When you begin, the wound will likely be covered with a dressing. You will make these assessments when you remove the soiled dressing *and* after cleansing the wound.

- Assess the type and amount of exudate.

Exudate may be a sign of infection.

- Assess the wound for odor.

A foul odor may indicate infection. Clean wounds before you assess for odor, because some dressings interact with wound drainage to produce an odor.

- Assess the tissue surrounding the wound edge.

Surrounding tissue that is red, warm, and/or edematous may indicate infection.

- Assess for pain.

Wounds may be very painful. Assess for pain and provide ordered pain medication 30 minutes prior to performing procedure if needed.

Procedural Steps for Removing Dry Dressing

Step 1 Place the patient in a comfortable position that provides easy access to the wound.

Provides for patient comfort and proper nurse body mechanics during dressing change.

Step 2 Wash your hands, and apply clean gloves.

Observes universal precautions.

Step 3 Loosen the edges of the tape of the old dressing. Stabilize the skin with your hand as you pull the tape in the opposite direction.

Decreases discomfort and trauma to skin as tape is removed.

Step 4 Beginning at the edges of the dressing, lift the dressing toward the center of the wound. If the dressing sticks, moisten it with normal saline before removing it completely.

Moistening the dressing decreases the risk of bleeding and/or removal of granulating tissue.

PROCEDURE 34–4

Removing and Applying Dry Dressings
(continued)

Step 5 Assess the type and amount of drainage on the soiled dressing.

Allows for evaluation of wound healing. Purulent drainage is sometimes an indication of infection.

Step 6 Dispose of the soiled dressing and gloves in a biohazard bag.

Soiled dressings contain contaminants and should be disposed of as biohazardous waste.

Step 7 Remove the cover of a tray of sterile 4 × 4 gauze. Moisten the gauze with sterile saline.

The sterile container tray is impermeable and allows you to moisten the gauze while maintaining sterility. Gauze will not shed fibers into the wound (as do cotton balls). Fibers and any other foreign bodies in a wound promote inflammation and delay healing.

Step 8 Wash your hands and apply clean gloves.

Step 9 Gently cleanse the wound with the saline-moistened gauze by lightly wiping a section of the wound from the center toward the wound edge. Discard the gauze in a biohazard receptacle, and repeat in the next section using a new piece of gauze with each wiping pass.

Removes surface bacteria and exudate. Prevents transfer of microorganisms from the surrounding skin into the wound.

Step 10 Discard the gloves and soiled gauze into a biohazard bag.

Soiled gauze contains contaminants and should be disposed of as biohazardous waste.

Step 11 Assess wound for location, amount of tissue present, exudate, and odor.

Procedural Steps for Applying Dry Dressing

Step 12 Wash your hands.

Step 13 Open sterile gauze packages on a clean, dry surface.

Maintains sterility of gauze. ▼

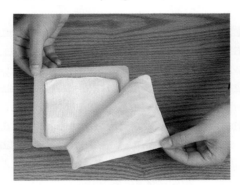

Step 14 Apply clean gloves.

Step 15 Apply a layer of dry dressings over the wound. If drainage is expected, use an additional layer of dressings.

The first layer serves as a wick for drainage. A second layer is needed if increased absorption is required.

Step 16 Place strips of tape at the ends of the dressing and evenly spaced over the remainder of the dressing. Use strips that are sufficiently long to secure the dressing in place. ▼

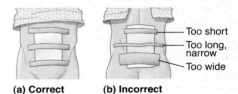

Too short
Too long, narrow
Too wide

(a) Correct　　**(b) Incorrect**

Step 17 Remove gloves, turning them inside out, and discard them in a biohazard receptacle.

Soiled gloves contain contaminants and should be disposed of as biohazardous waste.

Step 18 Assist the patient to a comfortable position.

Evaluation
- Determine whether the dressing is clean, dry, and intact.
- Verify that the patient experienced minimal discomfort during the procedure.

Patient Teaching
- Teach the patient about the expected healing process.
- Inform the patient and caregiver about the signs and symptoms of infection and the need to report these findings.

PROCEDURE 34–4   Removing and Applying Dry Dressings
(continued)

Home Care

- Help the client to store dressings appropriately to keep them clean, for example, in a plastic container with a lid.
- Teach the client or caregivers to dispose of contaminated dressings and gloves by double-bagging them in moisture-proof bags (e.g., plastic grocery bags).
- Advise the client and family whether they can get the wound wet (e.g., during bathing). If it must be kept dry, demonstrate how to cover it with a waterproof barrier (e.g., a plastic bag).

Documentation

Document the following information (many agencies use a wound/skin flowsheet):

- Appearance and location of the wound, type and amount of exudate, and odor, if present, after cleansing.
- Patient's pain level prior to the procedure. If the patient was medicated for pain, document the drug and dose used, time given, and patient response.
- Method of cleansing the wound.
- Type of dressing applied to the wound.
- Education provided to the patient.

Sample documentation:

| 09/27/07   1500 | Pt. with no c/o pain. Gauze dressing removed from lateral aspect of right forearm without difficulty. No drainage noted on gauze. Surrounding skin intact. Abrasion on right, lateral forearm cleansed with normal saline. Sterile gauze dressing reapplied to wound and anchored with cloth tape. Pt. instructed to report any changes noted at wound site, such as bleeding, drainage, or increase in pain. ———— D. Enferma, RN |

PROCEDURE 34–5

Removing and Applying Wet-to-Damp Dressings

➤ For steps to follow in *all* procedures, refer to the inside back cover of this book.

Note: This procedure uses clean technique because wound care is now usually done using a clean approach rather than sterile technique.

critical aspects

- Assess for pain, and medicate 30 minutes prior to procedure, if necessary.
- Place the patient in a comfortable position that provides easy access to the wound.
- Wearing clean gloves, remove the soiled dressing and discard it in a biohazard receptacle.
- Cleanse the wound with saline-moistened gauze.
- Assess the wound for location, appearance, odor, and drainage.
- Apply a single layer of moist, fine-mesh gauze to the wound. Be sure to place gauze in all depressions of the wound.
- Apply a secondary moist layer over the first layer. Repeat this process until the wound is filled with moistened sterile gauze.
- Cover the moistened gauze with a surgipad.
- Secure the dressing with tape or Montgomery straps.

Equipment

- Three pairs of clean gloves
- Sterile solution for irrigation, warmed to body temperature when possible

Cold solution lowers the temperature of wound bed and slows the healing process.

- Water-resistant disposable drapes
- Sterile fine-mesh gauze in a tray for dressing
- Surgipad
- Tape or Montgomery straps

Delegation

This is an invasive procedure that requires knowledge of wound healing. It should be performed by a registered nurse. Do not delegate this skill.

Assessment

Note: When you begin, the wound will likely be covered with a dressing. You will make these assessments when you remove the soiled dressing *and* after cleansing the wound.

- Assess the amount and type of tissue present in the wound bed.

Granulating tissue is beefy red with a velvety appearance. It appears with the growth of new blood vessels and connective tissue. Pale pink tissue may indicate compromised blood supply to the wound bed. Necrotic tissue, which is black, brown, or yellow in appearance, is nonviable and inhibits healing.

- Assess the type and amount of exudate.

Exudate may be a sign of infection.

- Assess the wound for odor.

A foul odor may indicate infection. Clean wounds before you assess for odor, because some dressings interact with wound drainage to produce an odor.

- Assess the tissue surrounding the wound edge.

Surrounding tissue that is red, warm, and/or edematous may indicate infection.

- Assess for pain.

Wounds may be very painful. Assess for pain and provide ordered pain medication 30 minutes prior to performing procedure, if needed.

➤

PROCEDURE 34–5

Removing and Applying Wet-to-Damp Dressings *(continued)*

Procedural Steps for Removing Wet-to-Damp Dressing

Step 1 Place the patient in a comfortable position that provides easy access to the wound.

Provides for patient comfort during dressing change.

Step 2 Wash your hands, and apply clean gloves.

Observes universal precautions.

Step 3 Loosen the edges of the tape of the old dressing. Stabilize the skin with your hand as you pull the tape in the opposite direction.

Decreases discomfort and skin trauma as you remove the tape.

Step 4 Beginning with the top layer, lift the dressing from the corner toward the center of the wound. If the dressing sticks, moisten it with normal saline before completely removing it. Continue to remove layers until you have removed the entire dressing.

Moistening the dressing decreases the risk of bleeding and/or removal of granulating tissue. ▼

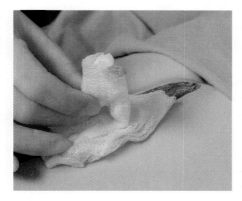

Step 5 Assess the type and amount of drainage present on the soiled dressing.

Type of drainage is an indication of the stage of healing. Purulent drainage is sometimes an indication of infection.

Step 6 Dispose of the soiled dressing and gloves in a biohazard bag.

Soiled dressings contain contaminants and should be disposed of as biohazardous waste.

Step 7 Remove the cover of a tray of sterile 4 × 4 gauze. Moisten the gauze with sterile saline.

The sterile container tray is impermeable and allows you to moisten the gauze while maintaining sterility.

Step 8 Apply clean gloves.

Avoids introducing microorganisms into the wound.

Step 9 Gently cleanse the wound with the saline-moistened gauze by lightly wiping a section of the wound from the center toward the wound edge. Discard the gauze in a biohazard receptacle, and repeat in the next section using a new piece of gauze with each wiping pass.

Removes surface bacteria and exudate. Prevents transfer of microorganisms from the skin to the wound.

Step 10 Discard the gloves and soiled gauze into a biohazard bag.

Soiled gauze contains contaminants and should be disposed of as biohazardous waste.

Step 11 Assess the wound for location, amount of tissue present, exudate, and odor.

Procedural Steps for Applying Wet-to-Damp Dressing

Step 12 Open a sterile gauze pack tray and a surgipad. The amount of gauze you use depends on the size of the wound.

Maintains sterile field and supplies.

Step 13 Moisten sterile gauze with sterile solution for irrigation.

Step 14 Apply clean gloves.

Step 15 Wring out excess moisture from the gauze. Apply a single layer of moist, fine-mesh gauze to the wound. Be sure to place gauze in all depressions or crevices of the wound. You may need to use forceps or a cotton applicator to ensure that you fill deep depressions or sinus tracts with gauze.

Maintains a moist environment for the wound bed. ▼

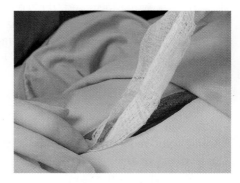

Step 16 Apply a secondary moist layer over the first layer. Repeat this process until the wound is completely filled with moistened sterile gauze—but do not tightly *pack* the gauze into the wound. Avoid extending the moist dressing onto the surrounding skin.

Packing the gauze can restrict blood flow to the area. Moist dressing on the surrounding skin can cause maceration.

PROCEDURE 34–5

Removing and Applying Wet-to-Damp Dressings *(continued)*

Step 17 Cover the moistened gauze with a surgipad.

Protects the wound from external contaminants. ▼

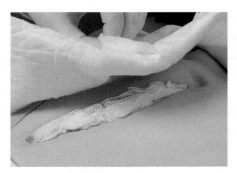

Step 18 Secure the dressing with tape or Montgomery straps.

Montgomery straps are useful when dressings must be frequently changed, because they do not cause trauma to the skin. ▼

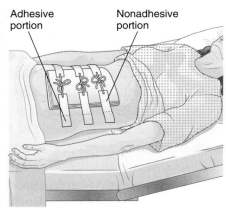

Adhesive portion   Nonadhesive portion

Step 19 Dispose of gloves and materials in the biohazard waste receptacle.

Step 20 Assist the patient to a comfortable position.

Step 21 Provide patient teaching on wound care and expected outcomes.

Evaluation

• Verify that the patient experiences minimal discomfort with procedure.
• Note whether the patient verbalizes understanding of the procedure.

Patient Teaching

• Teach the patient about the expected healing process.
• Inform the patient and caregiver about signs and symptoms of infection and the need to report these findings.

Home Care

• Help the client store dressings appropriately to keep them clean, for example, in a plastic container with a lid.
• Teach the client or caregivers to dispose of contaminated dressings and gloves by double-bagging them in moisture-proof bags (e.g., plastic grocery bags).
• Advise the client and family whether they can get the wound wet (e.g., during bathing). If it must be kept dry, demonstrate how to cover it with a waterproof barrier (e.g., a plastic bag).

Documentation

Document the following information (many agencies use a wound/skin flowsheet):

• Appearance and location of the wound, type and amount of exudate, and odor, if present, after cleansing.
• Patient's pain level prior to procedure. If the patient was medicated for pain, document the drug and dose used, time given, and patient response.
• Method of cleansing the wound.
• Type of dressing applied to the wound.
• Education provided to the patient.

➤

PROCEDURE 34–5 | **Removing and Applying Wet-to-Damp Dressings** *(continued)*

Sample documentation

| 08/31/07 2100 | 100% red granulating tissue noted in wound bed of stage IV pressure ulcer on sacrum. No tunneling or undermining observed. Minimal amount of serosanguineous drainage on old dressing. Wound cleansed with normal saline prior to application of new dressing. Wet-to-damp dressing applied. Pt. tolerated procedure well, with no verbalization of pain throughout procedure. Pt. placed on 2-hour turn schedule and educated on pressure relief. Pt. verbalizes understanding. —W. Earl, RN |

PROCEDURE 34–6 | **Applying a Transparent Film Dressing**

 For steps to follow in *all* procedures, refer to the inside back cover of this book.

critical aspects
- Place the patient in a comfortable position that provides easy access to the wound.
- Remove the soiled dressing, if necessary.
- Cleanse the surrounding skin and wound.
- Assess the condition of the wound.
- Apply the transparent film dressing to the wound by removing the center backing and holding the dressing firmly by the edges.
- Remove the edge liners.

Equipment
- Clean gloves
- Sterile gauze
- Normal saline solution or specified cleansing agent, warmed to body temperature when possible

Cold solution lowers the temperature of wound bed and slows the healing process.
- Scissors (if needed)
- Acetone or alcohol (if needed)
- Transparent film dressing (e.g., Op-Site, Tegederm, Bio-Occlusive)

PROCEDURE 34–6   Applying a Transparent Film Dressing
(continued)

Delegation

Because assessment of the wound and knowledge of clean technique are important, you should not delegate this procedure to unlicensed assistive personnel.

Assessment

• Assess area to determine whether a transparent film dressing is appropriate.

Transparent film dressings are appropriate for stage I and stage II pressure ulcers, for minor skin abrasions, and for securing and preventing contamination of IV sites. Use them only on wounds with minimal exudate.

• Determine the size of the wound.

Allows you to select a dressing of the appropriate size.

Procedural Steps

Step 1 Place the patient in a comfortable position that provides easy access to the wound.

Step 2 If a dressing is present, wash your hands, apply clean gloves, and remove the old dressing.

Step 3 Dispose of the soiled dressing and gloves in the biohazard waste receptacle.

Observe universal precautions.

Step 4 Apply clean gloves, and cleanse the skin surrounding the wound with normal saline or a mild cleansing agent. Be sure to rinse the skin well if you use a cleanser. Allow the skin to dry.

Prepares the skin for application of the dressing. Skin must be dry for the dressing to adhere.

Step 5 If hair is present in the area where you will apply the dressing, clip the hair with scissors.

Provides comfort when the dressing is later removed. Promotes adherence of dressing.

Step 6 If the skin is oily, cleanse the surrounding skin with alcohol or acetone, and allow it to dry.

Alcohol and acetone defat the skin, which allows the dressing to adhere.

Step 7 Cleanse the wound as ordered or according to agency procedure.

Cleansing of wounds removes bacteria and necrotic debris from wound beds.

Step 8 Assess the condition of the wound. Note the size, location, type of tissue present, amount of exudate, and odor.

Step 9 Remove soiled gloves, and reapply clean gloves.

Step 10 Remove the center backing liner from the transparent film dressing. ▼

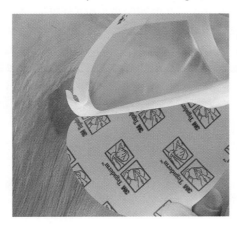

Step 11 Holding the dressing by the edges, apply the transparent film to the wound. To prevent the dressing from wrinkling, maintain a slight stretch on the edges of the dressing.

Results in a comfortable dressing that is wrinkle-free and does not restrict mobility.

Step 12 Remove the edging liner from the dressing.

Allows the dressing to fully adhere to patient's skin.

Step 13 Dispose of soiled equipment, and remove your gloves.

Step 14 Assist the patient to a comfortable position.

Step 15 Provide teaching to the patient about the use of transparent film dressings.

Promotes patient understanding.

➤

PROCEDURE 34–6   Applying a Transparent Film Dressing
(continued)

Evaluation

- Verify that the transparent film dressing is appropriate for the wound.
- Determine whether the dressing adheres comfortably to skin.
- Ensure that patient verbalizes understanding of treatment.

Patient Teaching

- Teach patient about the expected healing process.
- Inform the patient and caregiver about signs and symptoms of infection and the need to report these findings.

Documentation

Document the following information (many agencies use a wound/skin flowsheet):

- Appearance and location of the wound, type and amount of exudate, and odor, if present, after cleansing.
- Patient's pain level prior to procedure. If the patient was medicated for pain, document the drug and dose used, time given, and patient response.
- Method of cleansing the wound and surrounding skin.
- Type of dressing applied to the wound.
- Education provided to the patient.

Sample documentation:

| 10/31/06 | 0600 | Stage I pressure area noted on left heel. Skin is red, nonblanchable on pressure, but intact. Pt. denies pain at site. No drainage noted. Transparent film dressing applied to site for protection. Left heel floated with pillows. Will inform physician and continue to monitor every shift. Pt. instructed on reason for and methods of pressure reduction to affected area. Pt. verbalizes understanding.— R. Jones, RN |

| PROCEDURE 34–7 | Applying a Hydrocolloid Dressing |

 For steps to follow in *all* procedures, refer to the inside back cover of this book.

critical aspects
- Place the patient in a comfortable position.
- Remove the soiled dressing, if necessary.
- Cleanse the wound, if necessary.
- Assess the wound, or other area where hydrocolloid dressing will be applied, for size, location, appearance, exudate, odor, and signs and symptoms of infection.
- Shave the area around the wound if necessary.
- Apply the hydrocolloid dressing.

Equipment
- Gloves
- Normal saline solution (if needed)
- Emesis basin (if needed)
- Sterile gauze for cleansing (if needed)
- Disposable razor (if needed)
- Scissors (if dressing needs to be trimmed)
- Hydrocolloid dressing 3 to 4 cm (1.5 inch) larger in circumference than the wound
- Moisture-proof bag

Delegation
This procedure requires knowledge of wound healing, dressings, and infection control and prevention. You should not delegate this procedure to unlicensed assistive personnel.

Assessment
- Assess area to determine whether a hydrocolloid dressing is appropriate.

A hydrocolloid dressing is appropriate for wounds with minimal drainage. This type of dressing may also be used to protect skin at risk for breakdown. Hydrocolloids autolytically debride necrotic tissue from the wound bed.

- Determine the size of the wound.

Allows you to select a dressing of the appropriate size.

Procedural Steps

Step 1 Place the patient in a comfortable position that provides easy access to the wound.

Provides for patient comfort and proper nurse body mechanics during dressing change.

Step 2 If a dressing is present, wash your hands, apply clean gloves, and remove the old dressing.

Step 3 Dispose of the soiled dressing and gloves in the biohazard waste receptacle.

Step 4 Wash your hands. Apply clean gloves, and cleanse the skin surrounding the wound with normal saline or a mild cleansing agent. Be sure to rinse the skin well if you use a cleanser. Allow the skin to dry. Do not attempt to remove residue that is left on the skin from the old dressing.

Prepares the skin for application of the dressing. Removing residue irritates the surrounding skin.

Step 5 Cleanse the wound as ordered. Wound cleansing may be performed with clean or sterile technique, depending on the type of wound.

Cleansing the wound removes bacteria and necrotic debris from wound bed.

Step 6 Remove soiled gloves, and assess the condition of the wound. Note the size, location, type of tissue present, amount of exudate, and odor.

Granulating tissue is beefy red with a velvety appearance. It appears with the growth of new blood vessels and connective tissue. Pale pink tissue may indicate compromised blood supply to the wound bed. Necrotic tissue, which is black, brown, or yellow in appearance, is nonviable and inhibits healing. A hydrocolloid dressing will interact with ➤

PROCEDURE 34–7   Applying a Hydrocolloid Dressing *(continued)*

wound drainage to produce a thick, yellow gel that may have a foul odor. Clean the wound prior to assessing for exudate and odor.

Step 7 With the backing still intact, cut the hydrocolloid dressing to the desired shape and size. The hydrocolloid dressing should extend 3 to 4 cm (1.5 inches) beyond the wound margin on all sides.

Provides complete coverage of the wound.

Step 8 Apply clean gloves, and remove the backing of the hydrocolloid dressing, starting at one edge. Place the exposed adhesive portion on the patient's skin. Position the dressing to cover the wound. ▼

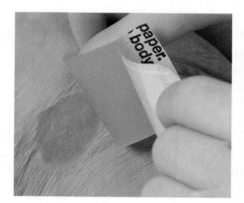

Step 9 Gradually peel away the remaining liner, and smooth the hydrocolloid dressing onto the skin by placing your hand on top of dressing and holding in place for 1 minute.

Warmth enhances adhesion of the dressing to the skin. ▼

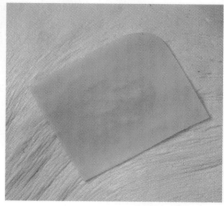

Step 10 Assist the patient to a comfortable position, and remove your gloves. Wash your hands.

Step 11 Provide teaching to the patient about the use of hydrocolloid dressings.

Promotes patient understanding.

Evaluation

- Verify that a hydrocolloid dressing is appropriate for the wound.
- Note whether the dressing adheres comfortably to the skin.
- Ensure that the patient verbalizes understanding of treatment.
- Inspect the dressing daily. Change it if it becomes dislodged, leaks, or wrinkles or if it develops an odor.

Patient Teaching

- Teach the patient about the expected healing process.
- Inform the patient and caregiver about signs and symptoms of infection and the need to report these findings.

Home Care

Hydrocolloid dressings may be required in the home setting. Teach caregivers to change the dressing if it begins to leak, develops an odor, or begins to separate from the skin.

PROCEDURE 34–7   **Applying a Hydrocolloid Dressing** *(continued)*

Documentation

Document the following information (some agencies use wound care flowsheets):

- Appearance and location of the wound, type and amount of exudate, and odor, if present, after cleansing.
- Patient's pain level prior to the procedure. If the patient was medicated for pain, document the drug and dose used, time given, and patient response.
- Method of cleansing the wound and surrounding skin.
- Type of dressing applied to the wound.
- Education provided to the patient.

Sample documentation:

01/30/07 1800	Pt. medicated with Tylenol 650 mg by mouth for mild pain at 1730. Pain rated as 1 on scale of 1 to 10 at this time. Soiled hydrocolloid dressing removed from shear injury to left mid-scapula area. Shear cleansed with normal saline and gauze. After cleansing, shear is 3.5 × 4 cm and covered with 100% yellow slough. Moderate amount of serous drainage with no odor noted. Hydrocolloid reapplied as ordered. Pt. with no complaints of pain. Educated patient on autolytic action of hydrocolloid and expected outcomes. Will continue to monitor. ———————— S. Thanee, RN

TECHNIQUES

TECHNIQUE 34–1   Placing Steri-Strips

1. Cleanse the skin surrounding the wound, pat it dry, and allow it to dry thoroughly. The skin surrounding the wound must be clean and dry in order for the strips to adhere.
2. Apply tincture of benzoin, and allow it to dry (or follow agency procedures). This enhances adhesion of the strips.
3. Apply strips across the wound, drawing the wound edges together. (Steri-strips may be used in conjunction with staples or sutures.)
    a. Place the strips so that they extend at least 2 to 3 cm ($\frac{3}{4}$ to 1 inch) on either side of the wound to ensure closure.
    b. Place the strips 2 to 3 cm ($\frac{3}{4}$ to 1 inch) apart along the wound.
4. Instruct patients not to pull or tug on the strips.
5. Instruct patients that they do not need to keep the strips dry: they can bathe and shower.
6. Adhesive strips are often kept in place until they begin to separate from the skin on their own.

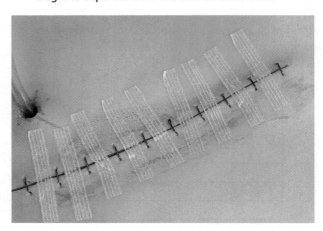

TECHNIQUE 34–2 | Removing Sutures and Staples

Removing Sutures

1. Obtain a suture removal kit.
2. Use the forceps to pick up one end of the suture.
3. Slide the small scissors around the suture, and cut near the skin. This helps you avoid pulling the exposed portion of the suture through the underlying tissue.
4. With the forceps, gently pull the suture in the direction of the knotted side to remove it.

Removing Staples

1. Obtain a staple remover.
2. Place the staple remover under the center of each staple, and slowly close it. This spreads the ends of the staples apart, freeing them from the skin.
3. Remove every other staple, and check the tension on the wound.
4. If there is no significant pull on the wound, remove the remaining staples. Consider placing a piece of gauze nearby so that you have a place to deposit the staples as you remove them.

Suture types

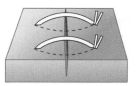

Plain interrupted

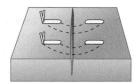

Mattress interrupted

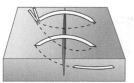

Plain continuous

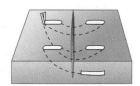

Mattress continuous

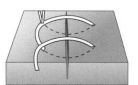

Blanket continuous

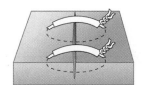

Retention

Removal techniques

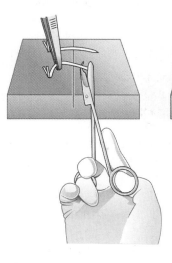

Removing interrupted sutures

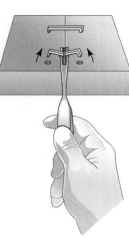

Removing staples

TECHNIQUE 34–3 | Shortening a Drain

1. Wearing procedure gloves, remove wound dressings.
2. Don sterile gloves; use sterile scissors to cut halfway through a sterile gauze dressing (for later use), or use a sterile precut drain dressing.
3. Cleanse the wound, using sterile gauze swabs and the prescribed cleaning solution. In some situations, you may use sterile forceps to manipulate the swabs.
4. If the drain is sutured in place, use sterile scissors to cut the suture.
5. Grasp the full width of the drain at the level of the skin and pull it out by the prescribed amount (e.g., 6 mm, or $\frac{1}{4}$ inch).
6. Insert a sterile safety pin through the drain at the level of the skin. Hold the drain tightly, and insert the pin above your fingers to keep from sticking the client or your fingers.

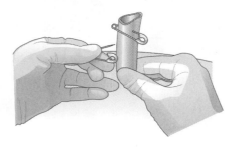

7. Using sterile scissors, cut off the drain at about 2.5 cm (1 inch) above the skin.

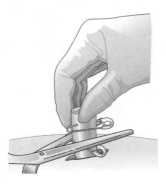

8. Apply precut sterile gauze around the drain; then redress the wound.

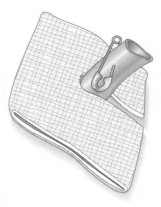

TECHNIQUE 34–4 Emptying a Closed-Wound Drainage System

1. Read the instructions on the drainage device. Procedures vary among manufacturers and different systems.
2. Wear procedure gloves.
3. Open the drainage port, and empty the drainage into a small graduated container.

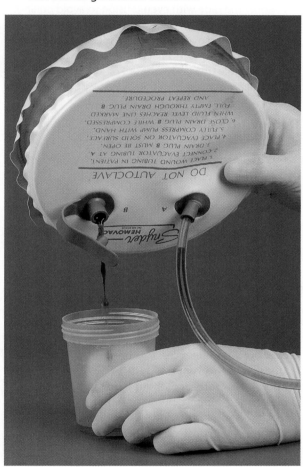

4. With the port still open, place the collection device on a firm, flat surface.
5. Use the palm of one hand to press down on the device and eject air from it. Do not stand directly over the air vent, because it can splash or bubble.

6. Use the other hand to cleanse the port and plug with an alcohol or Betadine swab.

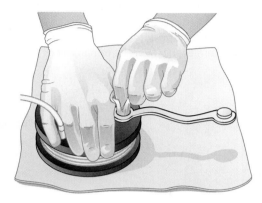

7. Continuing to press down on the device (to create the negative pressure needed to facilitate suction), replace the plug in the port.
8. Measure the drainage in the graduated container; discard drainage in the toilet. Wash the graduated container.
9. Remove your gloves; record the amount of drainage.

TECHNIQUE 34–5 Taping a Dressing

1. Choose the type of tape based on wound size, location, amount of drainage, frequency of dressing changes, patient's activity level, and type of dressings used.
2. Place strips of tape at the ends of the dressing, and space them evenly over the remainder of the dressing.

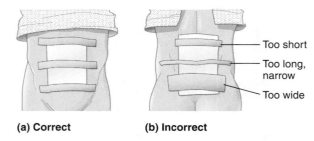

(a) Correct   **(b) Incorrect**

Too short
Too long, narrow
Too wide

3. Choose tape of the width that is appropriate for the size of the dressing. The larger the dressing, the wider the tape needed for securing. For example, a large abdominal dressing may require 3 inch tape, whereas a small incision on an extremity may need only $\frac{1}{2}$ inch tape.
4. Use strips that are sufficiently long to secure the dressing in place.
5. Apply the tape with even tension to avoid pulling the wound.
6. When taping over joints, apply the tape at a right angle to the direction of joint movement, or at a right angle to a body crease. For example, tape a shoulder or knee horizontally, not lengthwise.

Removing Tape

1. Gently pull the tape parallel to the skin toward the center of the wound. This prevents damage to the skin and wound.
2. Apply light traction to the skin while pulling the tape. This minimizes damage to the skin.

TECHNIQUE 34–6 Applying Binders

Before applying a binder, perform the following assessments:
- Assess the condition of the wound (if one is present). Note the amount and type of drainage. A wound must be dressed before it is bandaged; if there is a significant amount of exudate, you will need to apply a secondary dressing.
- Assess for pain, and check the circulation of the underlying body parts before and after applying the binder. Look for cool, pale, or cyanotic skin, tingling, and numbness.
- Determine whether the client or family has the skills to reapply the binder when necessary.

Observe the following guidelines, regardless of the type of binder you use:
- Choose a binder of the proper size. Measure.
- Thoroughly clean and dry the part to be covered. Heat and moisture contribute to skin breakdown.
- Place the body part in its normal position (e.g., with the joint slightly flexed), whenever possible. This prevents strain on ligaments and muscles.

- Pad between skin surfaces (e.g., under the axilla) and over bony prominences. This prevents pressure and abrasion of the skin.
- Apply the binder with enough pressure to provide the needed support, but not too tightly, to ensure that circulation is not interrupted to the area.
- Change binders whenever they become soiled or wet.
- Assess circulation and comfort regularly.

Applying an Abdominal Binder

1. Measure the patient for the abdominal binder.
   a. Place the patient in supine position.
   b. With a disposable measuring tape, encircle the abdomen at the level of the umbilicus. Note the measurement. This is the length of the binder.
   c. Measure the distance from the costal margin to the top of the iliac crests. This is the width of the binder.
   d. Dispose of gloves and measuring tape, and wash your hands.

TECHNIQUE 34–6   Applying Binders *(continued)*

e. Based on the measurements, obtain an abdominal binder.

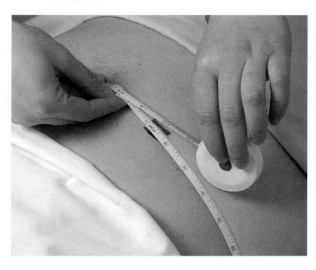

2. Assist the patient to roll to one side. Roll one end of the binder to the center mark. Place the rolled section of the abdominal binder underneath the patient. Position the binder appropriately between the costal margin and iliac crest.
3. Assist the patient to turn to the other side as you unroll the binder from underneath him.
4. Pad any pressure areas or skin abrasions.
5. With your dominant hand, grasp the end of the binder on the side farthest from you, and steadily pull toward the center of the patient's abdomen. With your nondominant hand, grasp the end of binder closest to you, and pull toward the center. Overlap the ends of the binder so that the Velcro enclosures meet.

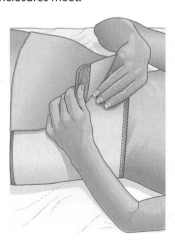

6. Remove the abdominal binder every 2 hours, and assess the underlying skin and dressings. Change wound dressings if they are soiled, or as ordered.

Applying a Triangular Arm Binder

A triangular arm binder or sling is used to support the upper extremities. Obtain a commercial sling (consisting of a sleeve for the arm and a strap to go around the neck) or a triangular piece of fabric. To form a splint from a triangular cloth, follow these steps:

1. Have the patient place the affected arm in a natural position across the chest, elbow flexed slightly.
2. Place one end of the triangle over the shoulder of the uninjured arm, and allow the triangle to fall open so that the elbow of the injured arm is at the apex of the triangle.
3. Move the sling behind the injured arm.
4. Pull up the lower corner of the triangle over the injured arm to the shoulder of the injured arm.
5. Tie the sling with a square knot at the neck on the side of the injured arm.
6. Adjust the injured arm within the sling to ensure patient comfort.

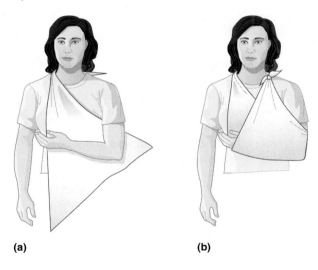

(a)   (b)

TECHNIQUE 34–6 Applying Binders *(continued)*

Applying a T-Binder

A T-binder is used to secure dressings or pads in the perineal area. A single T-binder is often used for women. A double T-binder is most commonly used for men. To apply a T-binder, follow these steps:

1. Position the waist tails under the patient at the natural waistline. Bring the right and left tails together, and secure them at the waist with pins or clips.

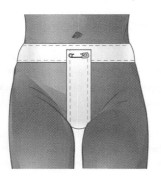

2. For a single T-binder, bring the center tail up between the legs of the patient. Secure the tail at the waist with pins or clips.
3. For a double T-binder, bring the tails up on either side of the penis. Secure the tail at the waist with pins or clips.

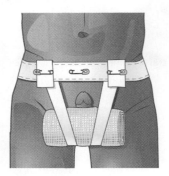

TECHNIQUE 34–7 Applying Bandages

Before applying a bandage, perform the following assessments:

- Determine the body part or area to be bandaged. This allows you to choose the correct width of gauze or elastic bandage to use.
- Assess the condition of the wound (if one is present). Note the amount and type of drainage. A wound must be dressed before it is bandaged; if there is a significant amount of exudate, you will need to apply a secondary dressing.
- Assess for pain, and check the circulation of the underlying body parts before and after applying the bandage. Look for cool, pale, or cyanotic skin, tingling, and numbness.
- Determine whether the client or family has the skills to reapply the bandage when necessary.

Observe the following guidelines, regardless of the type of bandage you use:

- Thoroughly clean and dry the part to be covered. Heat and moisture contribute to skin breakdown.
- Stand facing the patient so that you can wrap the bandage evenly in the proper direction.

- Bandage the body part in its normal position (e.g., with the joint slightly flexed), whenever possible. This prevents strain on ligaments and muscles.
- Always work from distal to proximal (or peripheral to central). This improves venous return and helps prevent edema.
- Pad between skin surfaces (e.g., between the toes) to prevent pressure and abrasion of the skin.
- Apply the bandage with enough pressure to provide the needed support; but do not bandage too tightly. Make sure that circulation to the area is not interrupted.
- If possible, leave the fingers (if you are bandaging an arm) or toes (if you are bandaging a leg or foot) exposed so that you can assess the circulation to the extremity.
- Choose a bandage of the proper width. For example, use a 2.5 cm (1 inch) wide bandage for a finger, a 5 cm (2 inch) wide bandage for an arm, and a wider bandage for a leg.
- Pad bony prominences before bandaging.
- Change bandages whenever they become soiled or wet.
- After bandaging, assess circulation and comfort regularly.

TECHNIQUE 34–7 Applying Bandages *(continued)*

Circular Turns

Use this technique to wrap a finger or toe, or as an anchor at the beginning and end of another wrapping technique.

1. With one hand, hold one end of the bandage in place.
2. With the other hand, encircle the body part several times with the bandage—each wrap should completely cover the previous wrap.
3. If circular turns are not being combined with another technique, secure the bandage with tape or metal clips when you are finished.

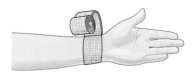

Spiral Turns

Spiral turns are a variation of the circular turn technique. Spiral turns are most commonly used to wrap an extremity.

1. Anchor the bandage by making two circular turns.
2. Continue to wrap the extremity by encircling the body part with each turn angled at approximately 30° so that you are overlapping the preceding wrap by two-thirds the width of the bandage.
3. Complete the wrap by making two circular turns and securing the bandage with tape or metal clips.

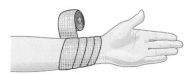

Spiral Reverse Turns

Spiral reverse turns are used to bandage cylindrical body parts that are not uniform in size.

1. Anchor the bandage by making two circular turns.
2. Bring the next wrap up at a 30° angle.
3. Place the thumb of your nondominant hand on the wrap to hold the bandage.

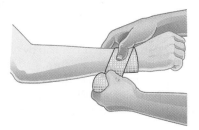

4. Fold the bandage back on itself, and continue to wrap at a 30° angle in the opposite direction.

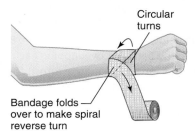

Circular turns

Bandage folds over to make spiral reverse turn

5. Continue to wrap the bandage, overlapping each turn by two-thirds. Align each bandage turn at the same position on the extremity.

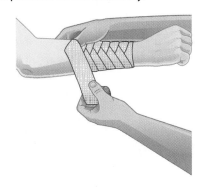

6. Complete the wrap by making two circular turns and securing the bandage with tape or metal clips.

TECHNIQUE 34–7 | **Applying Bandages** *(continued)*

Figure-8 Turns

The figure-8 wrap is used on joints (e.g., ankle, elbow).
1. Anchor the bandage by making two circular turns.
2. Wrap the bandage by ascending above the joint and descending below the joint to form a figure 8. Continue to wrap the bandage, overlapping each turn by two-thirds. Align each bandage turn at the same position on the extremity.

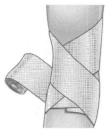

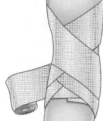

3. Complete the wrap by making two circular turns and securing the bandage with tape or metal clips.

Recurrent Turns

1. Anchor the bandage by making two circular turns.
2. Fold the bandage back on itself; hold it against the body part with one hand. With the other hand, make a half turn perpendicular to the circle turns and central to the distal end being bandaged.

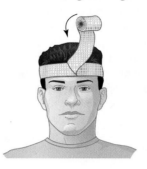

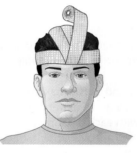

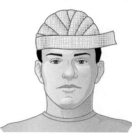

3. Hold the central turn with one hand, and fold the bandage back on itself; bring it over the distal end of the body part to the right of the center, overlapping the center turn by two-thirds the width of the bandage.
4. Next, hold the bandage at the center with one hand as you bring the bandage back over the end to the left of center. Continue holding and folding the bandage back on itself, alternating right and left until the body part is covered. Overlap by two-thirds the bandage width with each turn.
5. Start and return each turn to the midline or center of the body part, and angle it slightly more each time to continue covering the body part.
6. Complete the bandage by making two circular turns and securing the bandage with tape or metal clips.

TECHNIQUE 34–8 Local Application of Heat

Preparation

- Determine whether there are any contraindications to the treatment, such as impaired circulation, bleeding, wound complications, or inability to tolerate the treatment.
- Explain the application and rationale to the patient.

Moist Heat (Irrigations, Compresses, Hot Soaks)

- Soak a washcloth or towel in warm water (105 to 115°F [40 to 46°C]), and wring out the excess before applying to the skin. For open areas, you must use a compress.
- A **compress** is a moist gauze dressing applied to a wound. Soak the gauze in the heated solution (105 to 115°F [40 to 46°C]), and then apply it to the wound. Usually, you will use sterile gloves, gauze, and solution.
- A **soak** involves immersing the affected area. Sterilized tubs are often used for this procedure. Soaking helps cleanse a wound and remove encrusted material.
- Reapply compresses or towels, and change the water frequently to maintain a constant temperature. (Heat disperses quickly.)
- A **bath** is a modification of a soak. A **sitz bath** soaks the patient's perineal area. A special tub or chair may be used. Because of infection control concerns, disposable sitz baths are preferred. Check that the water temperature is from 105 to 110°F (40 to 43°C). Instruct the patient to soak for 15 minutes.

Dry Heat (Electric Heating Pads, Disposable Hot Packs, Hot Water Bags)

- **Aquathermia** pads (also called K-pads) are plastic or vinyl pads that circulate water in the interior. Connect the pad via tubing to the electric heating unit, which constantly exchanges water that has been heated to the specified temperature. Fill the reservoir about two-thirds full of distilled water. Set the temperature control to 98 to 105°F (37 to 40.5°C). Cover the pad, and apply it to the body part.

- For disposable hot packs and hot water bags or bottles, use water that is 115 to 125°F (46 to 52°C). Fill the bag about two-thirds full, expel the air from the bag, and close the top. Tip the bag upside down to test for leaking. Wrap the bag in a towel, and place it on the patient. Hot water bags are common in home use, but not in healthcare agencies because of the danger of burns from improper use.
- When applying electric heating pads, be sure that the body part is dry or that the pad has a waterproof cover. Use pads with a switch that the client cannot turn up; for home use, warn the patient about the danger of burns from high settings. Do not use pins (e.g., to hold a cover in place) or other sharp objects on the pad. The pin could go through a wire and cause an electric shock.

Safety Precautions

- Measure the water temperature with a bath thermometer.
- Tell the client to report any discomfort during the treatment.
- Avoid direct contact with the heating device. Cover the hot pack with a washcloth, towel, or fitted sleeve.
- Do not place the heating device (pad, bag) under the patient; place it over the body part. This helps prevent burns.
- Apply heat intermittently, leaving it on for no more than 15 minutes at a time in an area. This helps prevent tissue injury (e.g., burns, impaired circulation). It also makes the therapy more effective by preventing *rebound phenomenon:* At the time the heat reaches maximum therapeutic effect, the opposite effect begins.
- Check the skin frequently for extreme redness or blistering.
- Assess for hypotension and faintness. If they occur, discontinue the treatment. Have the patient lie down for several minutes. When the faint feeling passes, assist the patient to sit up slowly. Recheck the blood pressure (BP) when the patient is in the sitting position. If the BP remains low, encourage the patient to remain seated. If the patient is ambulatory, have her dangle her feet for several minutes before she gets up.

TECHNIQUE 34–9   Local Application of Cold

Preparation

- Determine whether there are any contraindications to the treatment, such as impaired circulation, bleeding, wound complications, or inability to tolerate the treatment.
- Explain the application and rationale to the patient.
- Assess for indications for cold application (e.g., fever above 104°F [40°C]). Measure the client's temperature.

Cooling Baths

- A cooling bath is often used to treat a high fever (above 104°F [40°C]). It promotes heat loss through conduction and vaporization.
- Prepare a pan of water with a temperature from 65 to 90°F (18 to 32°C).
- You may add a fan to increase heat loss if the temperature is markedly elevated.
- Slowly sponge the face, arms, legs, back, and buttocks with the cool water. Do not dry the areas; cover with a damp towel.
- Take about 30 minutes to complete the bath. Cooling the body too rapidly will cause shivering, which will increase heat production.
- You may also place ice bags or cold packs on the forehead and in the axillae and the groin.
- Assess the patient constantly during a cooling bath. If the patient begins to shiver, his temperature may actually rise.

Cold Compresses

- Apply a cool, damp cloth or towel to the body part.

- Renew the compress or cloth frequently (the temperature of the compress or cloth will rapidly rise toward body temperature).

Ice Collars, Ice Bags, Commercially Prepared Cold Packs, Aquapads

- Fill the ice bag with ice chips or an alcohol-based solution.
- You can make an ice bag out of a procedure glove or small plastic bag by filling it with ice chips and tying a knot in the top.
- Cover ice bags or packs with a towel or soft cover.
- Apply to the skin for a maximum of 15 minutes, then remove. You may reapply the cold pack in 1 hour.

Safety Precautions

- Measure water temperature with a bath thermometer.
- Tell the client to report any discomfort during the treatment.
- Avoid direct contact with the cooling device. Cover the cold pack with a washcloth, towel, or fitted sleeve.
- Apply cold intermittently, leaving it on for no more than 15 minutes at a time in an area. This helps prevent tissue injury (e.g., impaired circulation). It also makes the therapy more effective by preventing *rebound phenomenon:* At the time the cold reaches maximum therapeutic effect, the opposite effect begins. Check the skin frequently for extreme redness or blistering.
- Observe for tissue damage: bluish purple mottled appearance of the skin, numbness, and sometimes blisters and pain.

ASSESSMENT GUIDELINES AND TOOLS

Wound Assessment

Assess all wounds for the following:

- *Location.* Describe the location of the wound in anatomic terms. For example, you would describe an incision from cardiac surgery as a midsternal incision extending from the manubrium to the xiphoid process.

- *Size.* Measure the length and width of the wound in centimeters. To measure wound depth, gently insert a sterile cotton tip applicator into the deepest part of the wound. Measure the applicator from skin level to the tip. If possible, use photo documentation, indicating the dimensions on the photo. This is especially useful in the case of a wound with an irregular border.

- *Appearance.* Your description of the appearance of the wound should be very detailed. You must describe:

  1. *The type of wound (open or closed).* If the wound is sutured, examine the closure. Are the wound edges approximated? Is there tension on any aspect of the wound? Are the stitches intact?

  2. *The color of the wound.* Redness and inflammation for the first 2 to 3 days is normal, but erythema or swelling beyond that time may indicate infection.

  3. *Condition of the wound bed (in an open wound).* A beefy red, moist appearance is evidence of healing. A pale color or dry texture indicates a delay in healing. Examine for necrosis, slough, and eschar. Examine for a tunnel or sinus tract in the wound bed; if there is one, inspect and probe it for depth and characteristics.

- *The skin surrounding the wound.* Observe for skin discoloration, hematoma, or additional injury to the surrounding tissue. Observe for maceration, tunneling, crepitus, blistering, or erythema. Examine the edges of the wound for epithelial tissue and contraction. Look for undermining beneath the wound margins.

- *Drainage.* Determine whether drainage or exudate is present. If so, describe the color, consistency, amount, and odor.

  1. Assess the quantity of wound drainage by weighing dressings before they are applied and again when they have been removed. The change in weight reflects the amount of drainage that they have absorbed.

  2. If a drain is present, measure the amount of fluid in the collection container.

  3. Odor may indicate fistula formation or contamination with bacteria. If a new odor develops, assess carefully for presence of a fistula.

- *Patient responses.* Ask your patients about pain, discomfort, or itching related to the wound or wound care.

Assessing an Untreated Wound

Your assessment should determine what, if any, additional professional support is necessary. Assess the following aspects (the same as for treated wounds):

- Location
- Size
- Appearance
- Description of drainage
- Condition of wound margins
- Condition of surrounding skin
- Effect of the wound on the patient

In addition, assess the following:

- *Bleeding.* If bleeding is profuse, apply direct pressure to the site. If bleeding continues after you apply pressure for 5 minutes or if blood is spurting from the wound, call the physician immediately.

- *Severity of the wound.* A gaping wound, or a deep wound with fat, fascia, or muscle exposed, will need additional care.

- *Last tetanus immunization.* Immunization should be given if (1) the last immunization was 10 years ago or longer, (2) the wound is contaminated with dirt or debris and the tetanus injection was given more than 5 years ago, or (3) it is uncertain when the patient last received an immunization.

- *Whether the wound was caused by a bite.* Determine whether the wound is caused by any type of bite, animal or human. A deep bite wound usually requires additional observation and/or antibiotics.

- *Pain.* Assess for pain. Any wound causing severe pain requires a comprehensive evaluation.

- *Numbness or loss of movement.* If any deficit is detected, the client will need immediate evaluation.

- *Presence of chronic medical conditions.* Examples include diabetes, malnutrition, immunocompromise, or a bleeding disorder. Patients with conditions that affect wound healing will need ongoing evaluation.

DIAGNOSTIC TESTING

Tests for Assessing Wounds

Test	Normal Range	Comments
Leukocyte (WBC) count	4500–10,000/mm^3	Usually done as a part of a complete blood count but may be ordered as an independent test. WBCs may increase when a wound develops; continued elevation may signal infection. A low WBC count may delay wound healing. Leukocytes are responsible for an inflammatory reaction at the wound site, phagocytosis of bacteria and cellular debris, and the creation of antibodies.
Serum protein Serum albumin Serum pre-albumin	6–8 g/dL 3.8–4.6 g/dL 12–42 mg/dL	Low serum levels indicate limited nutritional stores that delay wound healing or place the patient at high risk for pressure ulcers. Serum protein may be monitored as a predictor of the ability to heal a wound or prevent a pressure ulcer. Serum protein and albumin levels are closely related. However, both fluctuate slowly. A more accurate measure of a patient's immediate protein stores is reflected in pre-albumin level.
Coagulation studies: Partial thromboplastin time, activated (aPTT) Prothrombin time (clotting time) International normalized ratio (INR)	Varies with respect to equipment and reagents used. Critical values: > 70 seconds or < 53 seonds Critical values: > 20 seconds (uncoagulated) or 3 times normal control (anticoagulated) A standardized test to evaluate clotting times, considered the gold standard	Prolonged coagulation times may result in excessive blood loss or ongoing bleeding in the wound bed. Shortened coagulation times increase the risk for blood clot formation problems, such as deep vein thrombosis, pulmonary embolus, or stroke. Altered coagulation may result from anticoagulant medications, a concurrent illness, trauma, or reaction to transfusions.
Wound cultures	Negative; no growth of pathogens	Wound cultures may be ordered to determine the types of bacteria present in the wound. Cultures may be obtained by swab, aspiration, or tissue biopsy. A positive culture may not indicate an infection as chronic wounds are colonized with bacteria.
Tissue biopsy	Negative; no growth of pathogens	Wounds are not considered infected unless the bacteria count exceeds 100,000 organisms per gram of tissue. Exception: The presence of beta hemolytic streptococci in any number indicates infection.

STANDARDIZED LANGUAGE

Selected Standardized Outcomes and Interventions for Skin and Wound Diagnoses

Patient Situation (Data/Defining Characteristics)	NANDA Diagnosis	NOC Outcomes	Selected Indicators	Selected NIC Interventions and Specific Activities
Mrs. Whitefeather is 95 years old. She has cancer and has stopped eating and become very thin. Recently she has become too weak to move about in bed without help. However, her skin is intact with no redness, even over her bony prominences. She has a very low score on the Braden pressure ulcer assessment scale.	Risk for Impaired Skin Integrity	Tissue Integrity: Skin & Mucous Membranes *Other outcomes:* *Immobility Consequences: Physiological* *Nutritional Status: Food & Fluid Intake* *Nutritional Status: Nutrient Intake*	(4-not compromised) • Hydration • Tissue Perfusion • Skin Intactness (5-None) • Erythema • Blanching • Skin lesions	Bed Rest Care • Keep bed linen clean, dry, and wrinkle free. • Facilitate small shifts of body weight. Pressure Ulcer Prevention • Monitor any reddened areas closely. • Turn every 1 to 2 hours, as appropriate. • Turn with care (e.g., avoid shearing) to prevent injury to fragile skin. • Post a turning schedule at the bedside, as appropriate. • Avoid massaging over bony prominences. • Utilize specialty beds and mattresses, as appropriate. • Avoid use of "donut" type devices in sacral area. *Other interventions:* Positioning • Pressure Management • Skin Surveillance • Nutrition Management
Eddie Allen is 4 years old. He has a severe case of poison ivy, which has made blisters on his skin. He has been scratching his "itchies" and has bleeding excoriated areas over his limbs, face, and trunk.	Impaired Skin Integrity	Tissue Integrity: Skin & Mucous Membranes *Other outcomes:* *Infection* *Immune Hypersensitivity Response*	(4-mildly compromised) • Skin intactness (4-mild) • Skin lesions • Erythema (5-none) • Purulent drainage • Serosanguineous drainage	Wound Care • Monitor characteristics of the wound, including drainage, color, size, and odor. • Cleanse with normal saline or a nontoxic cleanser, as appropriate. • Apply an appropriate ointment to the skin/lesion, as appropriate. • Instruct patient and family member(s) in wound care procedures and signs of infection. *Other interventions:* Pruritus Management Skin Surveillance Wound Irrigation

Selected Standardized Outcomes and Interventions for Skin and Wound Diagnoses *(continued)*

Patient Situation (Data/Defining Characteristics)	NANDA Diagnosis	NOC Outcomes	Selected Indicators	Selected NIC Interventions and Specific Activities
Allie Newton has a stage II pressure ulcer on her left heel.	Impaired Tissue Integrity	Wound Healing: Secondary Intention *Other outcomes:* *Tissue Integrity: Skin & Mucous Membranes*	(4-substantial) • Granulation • Decreased wound size (4-limited) • Purulent drainage • Surrounding skin erythema • Wound inflammation • Foul wound odor	• Medicate the patient before the irrigation, as needed for pain control. • Maintain a sterile field during the irrigation procedure, as appropriate. • Cleanse and dry the area around the wound after the procedure. • Monitor progress of granulating tissue. • Report any sign of infection and/or necrosis to the physician. *Other interventions:* Wound Care Pressure Management Infection Protection Medication Administration

Sources: NANDA International. (2005). *Nursing diagnoses: Definitions and classification 2005–2006.* Philadelphia: Author; Johnson, M., Bulechek, G., Dochterman, J., Maas, M., & Moorhead, S. (2001). *Nursing diagnoses, outcomes, and interventions: NANDA, NOC, and NIC linkages.* St Louis: Mosby; Johnson, M., Maas, M., & Moorhead, S. (Eds.). (2004). *Nursing outcomes classification (NOC)* (3rd ed.). St Louis: Mosby; and McCloskey, J. & Bulechek, G. (Eds.). (2004). *Nursing Interventions classification (NIC)* (4th ed.). St Louis: Mosby.

What Are the Main Points in This Chapter?

- The major functions of the skin are protection of the internal organs, unique identification of an individual, thermoregulation, metabolism of nutrients and metabolic waste products, and sensation.

- Age, mobility, nutrition, hydration, underlying conditions, medications, and hygiene are factors that influence the ability to maintain intact skin and heal wounds.

- If there are no breaks in the skin a wound is described as *closed*. A wound is considered *open* if there is a break in the skin or mucous membranes.

- Acute wounds may be intentional (e.g., surgical incisions) or unintentional (e.g., from trauma) and are expected to be of short duration.

- Wounds that exceed the anticipated length of recovery are classified as chronic wounds. Chronic wounds include pressure, arterial, venous, and diabetic ulcers. A chronic wound may linger for months or years.

- *Clean wounds* are uninfected wounds with minimal inflammation. *Clean-contaminated wounds* are surgical incisions that enter the gastrointestinal, respiratory, or genitourinary tracts. *Contaminated wounds* include open, traumatic wounds or surgical incisions in which a major break in asepsis occurred. *Infected wounds* are wounds with evidence of infection, such as presence of microorganisms.

- A wound that involves minimal or no tissue loss and has wound edges that approximate heals by primary intention.

- A wound that involves extensive tissue loss and has margins that can not be approximated, or is infected, heals by secondary intention. The wound is left open and allowed to heal from the inner layer to the surface.

- Tertiary intention healing, or delayed primary closure, occurs when two surfaces of granulation tissue are brought together. Initially the wound is allowed to heal by secondary intention. The length of time for secondary healing varies but is usually less than 1 week.

- Healing occurs in three stages: inflammatory, proliferative, and maturation. The *inflammatory phase* lasts from 1 to 5 days and consists of two major processes: hemostasis and inflammation. The *proliferative phase* occurs from days 5 to 21. It is characterized by cell development aimed at filling the wound defect and resurfacing the skin. The *maturation phase* is the final phase of the healing process. It begins in the second or third week and continues until the wound is completely healed.

- Wound closure methods include adhesive strips (Steri-Strips), absorbent sutures, surgical staples, and surgical glue.

- Drainage is the flow of fluids from a wound or cavity. It is often referred to as exudate—fluid that oozes as a result of inflammation.

- Surgical complications include hemorrhage, infection, dehiscence, evisceration, and fistula formation.

- Pressure ulcers are caused by unrelieved pressure over time that compromises blood flow to tissue, resulting in ischemia in the underlying tissue.

- A stage 1 pressure ulcer is as an area of persistent redness. Stage II pressure ulcers involve partial-thickness skin loss of the epidermis, dermis, or both. A stage III pressure ulcer is characterized by full-thickness skin loss involving damage or necrosis of subcutaneous tissue, which may extend down to, but not through, the underlying fascia. The ulcer appears as a deep crater. Stage IV pressure ulcers involve full-thickness skin loss with extensive destruction, tissue necrosis, or damage to muscle, bone, or support structures. Undermining and sinus tracts (blind tracts underneath the epidermis) are common.

- An eschar is a black leathery covering of necrotic tissue. An ulcer covered by an eschar cannot be classified because it is impossible to determine the depth.

- The Braden and Norton scales evaluate risk for problems with skin integrity.

- When assessing a wound, note the following: the type of wound, the color of the wound and surrounding skin, the condition of the wound bed, drainage and odor, and the level of pain associated with the wound or wound care.

- Preventing pressure ulcers focuses on skin care, nutrition, positioning, using therapeutic mattresses and cushions, and patient/family teaching.

- The RYB color classification system guides wound treatment. Protect a red wound, cleanse a yellow wound, and debride a black wound.

- Four types of debridement are used: sharp, mechanical, enzymatic, autolytic.

- Ideal wound irrigation pressures range from 4 pounds per square inch (psi) to 15 psi. Current recommendations are to use a 35 mL syringe attached to a 19-gauge angiocath. This will deliver the solution at approximately 8 psi.

- Heat application promotes vasodilatation, increases tissue metabolism, increases capillary permeability, reduces blood viscosity, and reduces muscle tension.

- The application of cold causes vasoconstriction, local anesthesia, reduced cell metabolism, increased blood viscosity, and decreased muscle tension.

35 Oxygenation

Overview

The structures of the airways, lungs, chest cavity, heart, and blood vessels function together to supply oxygen to the tissues; thus, abnormalities in any of these structures can interfere with tissue oxygenation. Developmental stage, environment, individual characteristics, lifestyle, medications, and pathological factors can interfere with ventilation, circulation, or gas exchange, leading to problems with tissue oxygenation.

Interventions to promote optimal respiratory function include deep, regular breathing, flu and pneumonia immunizations for at-risk individuals, frequent position changes, incentive spirometry, and preventing aspiration. Supplemental oxygen is used to prevent hypoxemia. For patients who cannot maintain their own airway, artificial airways—such as oropharyngeal, nasopharyngeal, and endotracheal—provide an open airway. Airways are suctioned as needed to remove secretions and maintain patency.

Promoting circulation ensures that oxygenated blood reaches tissues and organs and venous blood returns to the heart. Activities that promote venous return and prevent clot formation enhance circulation. Cardiac monitoring is used to identify the patient's baseline rhythm and rate and recognize significant changes and lethal dysrhythmias that require immediate intervention. Chest tubes remove air or fluid from the pleural space so that the lungs can fully expand and the heart can contract without undue pressure.

Thinking Critically About Oxygenation

The exercises in the following section allow you to practice the kind of thinking you will use as a full-spectrum nurse. Because these are critical-thinking activities, there is usually no single right answer. Discuss answers with your peers—discussion can stimulate critical thinking. If you have difficulty with any of the questions, consult with your instructor.

Caring for the Garcias

Katherine Garcia, Joe's 76-year-old mother, has been complaining of fatigue and a persistent cough for approximately 2 weeks. Joe scheduled an appointment for his mother at the family clinic. You are the nurse at the clinic. Katherine appears disheveled. Her clothes are mismatched and rumpled, and her hair is tousled. Normally she appears at the clinic dressed as though she were going out for the evening. She has a hard time signing in at the desk and tells the receptionist she has a 1:00 P.M. appointment, but it is 9:00 A.M. Katherine's vital signs are as follows: BP, 142/90 mm Hg; pulse, 94 bpm and regular; respirations, 24 and labored; temperature, 99.6°F (37.5°C) oral.

A. What additional assessment data would be useful to gather at this time?

B. During her visit at the clinic, you notice that Katherine is extremely confused. Her weight has dropped 7 pounds since her visit last month, her mucous membranes are dry, and she is quite dyspneic with any activity. Katherine is diagnosed with pneumonia. Because of her rapid decline, she is admitted to the hospital to receive antibiotics administered intravenously. At the hospital, her initial pulse oximetry reading is 90%, and she is unable to cough up secretions. Write the most appropriate nursing diagnosis to focus interventions for Katherine.

C. What actions should you anticipate taking?

D. The hospitalist (hospital-based physician) writes orders for IV fluids, antibiotics, suction PRN, and continuous pulse oximetry. What additional orders will you need to provide care for Katherine? What therapy would you suggest?

E. Katherine requires suctioning to help remove secretions. She has a weak cough and crackles and rhonchi throughout all lung fields. There are few secretions in her oropharynx, and she bites down on the catheter. What technique would you use to suction her? Explain your choice.

F. After 4 days in the hospital, Katherine is discharged to home. She asks the hospital nurse, "What can I do to make sure I never get that sick again?" How would you answer this question?

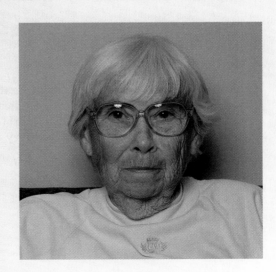

1

Recall the four patients discussed in the "Meet Your Patients" scenario:

- Mary is a 4-year-old girl with a history of asthma. Her mother, Ms Green, has brought her in for an "asthma attack." Mary is sitting in her mother's lap and breathing rapidly through an open mouth. She has a cough that sounds congested and wheezy. The physician has already ordered a nebulized treatment containing albuterol (Proventil) and ipratropium bromide (Atrovent).
- Mr. Chu is a 68-year-old man complaining of cough, sore throat, fatigue, and weakness. His BP is 166/82, pulse is 90, respirations are 26, and temperature is 100.4°F (38.0°C).
- William is a 19-year-old man who has had a sudden onset of right-sided chest pain and shortness of breath. His chest x-ray film revealed a right pneumothorax, and he is currently receiving 35% oxygen by face mask while waiting for an ambulance to transport him to the hospital for further evaluation.
- Ms Saunders is a 45-year-old homemaker. She says she has been extremely tired, easily becomes short of breath, and is unable to complete her chores without frequent rest breaks. She is pale and seems tired. Her vital signs are as follows: BP, 136/78 mm Hg; pulse, 86 bpm; respirations, 24 and unlabored; temperature, 98.4°F (36.7°C); and pulse oximetry 98% on room air. She is now waiting for her lab results, which include a complete blood count (CBC).

a Which patients are experiencing problems with ventilation? Explain your answer.

b Which patient appears to be experiencing problems with hypoxia? Does the problem appear to be related to oxygenation or perfusion? Explain your answers.

c Mr. Chu has smoked two packs of cigarettes per day for 50 years. ABGs reveal a low PO_2 and a high PCO_2 consistent with chronic lung disease. He is diagnosed with an acute exacerbation of chronic bronchitis. He is placed on oral antibiotics and long-acting bronchodilators by metered-dose inhaler (MDI). What teaching could you offer to help Mr. Chu mobilize and expectorate secretions?

d Mary receives her nebulizer treatment and markedly improves. The physician has ordered a variety of take-home medications that you must teach her mother about. The treatment plan includes a protocol based on peak expiratory flow monitoring. Discuss how you might involve Mary in her own care.

e William's chest x-ray film reveals a spontaneous pneumothorax. There is no apparent fluid in the pleural space. What chest tube systems can be used to treat his pneumothorax? Explain your thinking.

f Ms Saunders is diagnosed with severe anemia. She is hospitalized because her hemoglobin is 5.9 g/dL. How will this affect her oxygenation? What interventions would improve her fatigue?

2 You are caring for a 68-year-old woman on the night shift. Earlier today she had an abdominal hysterectomy under general anesthesia. You note that her respiratory rate has steadily risen from 16 to 26 and that she has developed a mild, nonproductive cough. When you listen to her chest, you hear crackles throughout. She has a 40 pack-year cigarette smoking history. Identify an appropriate nursing diagnosis for this patient. Explain the reasons for your choice.

3 For each of the following concepts, use critical thinking to describe how or why it is important to nursing, patient care, or oxygenation. Note that these are *not* to be merely definitions.

Ventilation

Gas exchange

Artificial airways

Suctioning

Negative pressure in the chest

Hypoventilation

Hyperventilation

Perfusion

Supplemental oxygen

Pulse oximetry

Practical Knowledge
knowing how

PROCEDURES

In this section you will find the procedures necessary for supporting oxygenation. As you perform the procedures, apply the theoretical knowledge you obtained in Volume 1. The registered nurse is responsible for assessing patients' oxygenation and their responses to procedures. Some, but not all, of the procedures in this section can be delegated to qualified UAPs. Refer to the delegation notes in the procedures and to agency policies.

PROCEDURE 35–1 Collecting a Sputum Specimen

 For steps to follow in *all* procedures, refer to the inside back cover of this book.

critical aspects

35–1A: For Obtaining an Expectorated Specimen
- Position the patient in high or semi-Fowler's position.
- Caution the patient not to touch the inside of the sterile container or lid.
- Instruct the patient to breathe deeply for three or four breaths, then expectorate the specimen with a deep cough.
- Label the specimen container with the name of the patient, the test, and the collection date and time.
- Place the specimen in a plastic bag labeled with a biohazard label. Follow agency policy.
- Send the specimen to the laboratory immediately. If specimen transport is delayed, consult the lab; refrigeration may be required.

35–1B: For Obtaining a Specimen by Suction
- Position the patient in high or semi-Fowler's position.
- Don protective eyewear.
- Attach the suction tubing to the male adapter of the inline sputum specimen container.
- Don sterile gloves.
- Attach the sterile suction catheter to the rubber tubing on the inline sputum specimen container.
- Lubricate the suction catheter with sterile saline solution.
- Insert the tip of the suction catheter gently through the nasopharynx, endotracheal tube, or tracheostomy tube. Advance the tip into the trachea (see Procedure 35–6 or Procedure 35–7).
- When the patient begins coughing, apply suction for 5 to 10 seconds to collect the specimen.
- If an adequate specimen (5 to 10 mL) is not obtained, allow the patient to rest for 1 minute, and then repeat the procedure. Administer oxygen to the patient at this time, if indicated.
- When an adequate specimen is collected, discontinue suction, and gently remove the suction catheter.
- Label the specimen container with the name of the patient, the test, and the collection date and time.
- Place the specimen in a plastic bag labeled with a biohazard label. Follow agency policy.
- Send the specimen to the laboratory immediately. If specimen transport is delayed, consult the lab; refrigeration may be required.

➤

PROCEDURE 35–1   Collecting a Sputum Specimen *(continued)*

Equipment

Procedure 35–1A: Obtaining an Expectorated Specimen

- Sterile specimen container with lid
- Procedure gloves
- Glass of water
- Emesis basin
- Tissues
- Pillow (if abdominal or chest incision is present)
- Patient identification label
- Completed laboratory requisition form
- Small plastic bag with a biohazard label for delivering the specimen to the laboratory (or container designated by the agency)

Procedure 35–1B: Obtaining a Specimen by Suction

- Sterile suction catheter
- Suction device (portable or wall)
- Sterile gloves
- Protective eyewear
- Inline sputum specimen container or trap
- Sterile saline solution
- Patient identification label
- Completed laboratory requisition form
- Small plastic bag with a biohazard label for delivering the specimen to the laboratory (or container designated by the agency)
- Oxygen therapy equipment, if indicated
- Linen-saver pad or towel

Delegation

You can delegate collection of an expectorated sputum specimen to a UAP who has been adequately trained in performing the skill. Assess the patient's respiratory status first; if the patient's condition is unstable, do not delegate the procedure.

You should not delegate obtaining a specimen obtained by tracheal suctioning.

Assessment

- Assess the patient's comprehension of the procedure.

Understanding allays anxiety and promotes cooperation.

- Assess respiratory status, including breath sounds; respiratory rate, depth, and pattern; skin and nail bed color; and tissue perfusion.

You may need to delay sputum collection if the patient is in respiratory distress.

- Assess ability to deep-breathe, cough, and expectorate.

If the patient is unable to deep-breathe, cough, and expectorate, suctioning may be necessary to obtain an adequate sputum specimen.

- Check when the patient last ate or had a tube feeding.

Specimen collection should be delayed for 1 to 2 hours after eating because the procedure may cause vomiting, which creates a risk for aspiration of stomach contents.

- If suctioning is required to obtain the specimen, check for factors such as anticoagulant therapy, bleeding disorders, or low platelet count.

These factors place the patient at risk for bleeding when the suction catheter is introduced.

Procedural Steps

Step 1 Verify the medical order for type of sputum analysis.

The type of sputum specimen determines the number of specimens required and the time of day the specimen should be collected. For example, specimens to confirm tuberculosis typically require three consecutive morning samples.

Step 2 Position the patient according to the required specimen collection technique.

a. For an expectorated specimen, assist the patient to high or semi-Fowler's position or to a sitting position at the edge of the bed.

These positions promote lung expansion and enhance the patient's ability to cough.

b. For a suctioned specimen, position the patient in high or semi-Fowler's position.

These positions facilitate insertion of the suction catheter and prevent aspiration should the patient vomit during the procedure. They also promote lung expansion.

PROCEDURE 35–1   Collecting a Sputum Specimen *(continued)*

Step 3 Drape a towel or linen-saver pad over the patient's chest.

Protects the patient's gown from soiling during specimen collection.

Step 4 If the patient has an abdominal or chest incision, have the patient splint the incision with a pillow.

Splinting the incision decreases discomfort when the patient coughs.

PROCEDURE 35–1A   Collecting an Expectorated Specimen

Procedural Steps

Follow steps 1 through 4, above.

Step 5 Hand the patient a glass of water and emesis basin, and have him rinse his mouth.

Rinsing the mouth reduces specimen contamination.

Step 6 Provide the patient with the specimen container. Advise the patient to avoid touching the inside of the container.

Prevents inadvertent specimen contamination. ▼

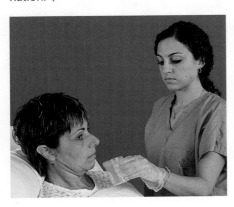

Step 7 Ask the patient to breathe deeply for three or four breaths, and then ask him after a full inhalation to hold his breath and then cough.

Deep breathing opens airways and stimulates the cough reflex. Coughing after a full inhalation creates enough force to mobilize secretions through the airways and into the pharynx.

Step 8 Instruct the patient to expectorate the secretions directly into the specimen container.

Prevents specimen contamination from outside organisms.

Step 9 Tell the patient to repeat deep breathing and coughing until an adequate sample is obtained.

Typically 5 to 10 mL of sputum is required to ensure adequate sputum analysis.

Step 10 Cover the specimen container with the lid immediately after the specimen is collected.

Covering the container immediately prevents inadvertent spread of microorganisms.

Step 11 Label the specimen container with a patient identification label that contains the name of the test and collection date and time.

Correctly identifying the specimen ensures accurate diagnosis and treatment.

Step 12 Place the specimen in a plastic bag labeled with a biohazard label. Attach a completed laboratory requisition form.

Placing the specimen in a plastic bag protects healthcare workers from exposure to microorganisms. Completing the laboratory requisition form ensures proper processing of the specimen.

Step 13 Send the specimen to the laboratory immediately, or refrigerate it if transport might be delayed.

If bacterial cultures are delayed, contaminating organisms may grow, producing false culture results and possibly inappropriate treatment.

➤

PROCEDURE 35–1B   Collecting a Suctioned Specimen

Procedural Steps

Follow Steps 1 through 4, above.

Step 5 Administer oxygen to the patient, if indicated.

Suctioning may cause hypoxemia; providing oxygen prevents hypoxemia.

Step 6 Prepare the suction device, and make sure it is functioning properly.

Adequate suction is necessary to mobilize secretions.

Step 7 Don protective eyewear.

Protects your eyes from splattering of secretions during suctioning.

Step 8 Attach the suction tubing to the male adapter of the inline sputum specimen container.

Provides suction for the specimen container to aspirate sputum directly into the specimen container. ▼

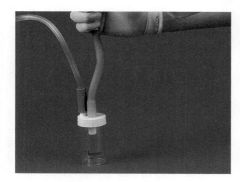

Step 9 Don sterile gloves.

Protects the patient's sterile airways from contamination by outside organisms that might otherwise be introduced during suctioning.

Step 10 Attach the sterile suction catheter to the rubber tubing on the inline sputum specimen container.

Ensures that sputum specimen goes directly into the specimen container instead of the suction tubing. ▼

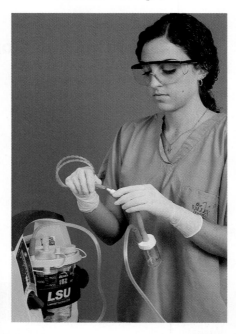

Step 11 Lubricate the suction catheter with sterile saline solution.

Eases insertion and prevents trauma to mucosa.

Step 12 Insert the tip of the suction catheter gently through the nasopharynx, endotracheal tube, or tracheostomy tube. Advance the tip into the trachea (see Procedure 35–6 or Procedure 35–7).

Gently inserting the suction catheter prevents airway trauma.

Step 13 When the patient begins coughing, apply suction by placing your finger over the suction control port for 5 to 10 seconds to collect the specimen.

Applying suction for longer than 10 seconds can cause hypoxia.

Step 14 If an adequate specimen (5 to 10 mL) is not obtained, allow the patient to rest for 1 minute, and then repeat the procedure. Administer oxygen to the patient at this time, if indicated.

Allowing the patient a rest period and administering oxygen prevents hypoxia.

Step 15 When you have collected an adequate specimen, discontinue suction, then gently remove the suction catheter.

Applying suction during catheter removal can damage the airway mucosa.

Step 16 Remove the suction catheter from the specimen container, and dispose of the catheter in the appropriate container.

Prevents the spread of infection.

Step 17 Remove the suction tubing from the specimen container, and connect the rubber tubing on the specimen container to the plastic adapter. ▼

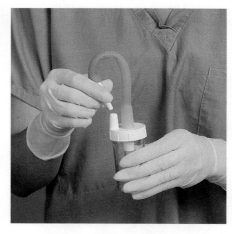

Step 18 If sputum comes in contact with the outside of the specimen container, clean the outside with a disinfectant, according to agency policy.

Prevents spread of infection to staff members who must handle the specimen.

PROCEDURE 35–1B Collecting a Suctioned Specimen *(continued)*

Step 19 Provide the patient with tissues after expectorating, and provide mouth care.

Mouth care promotes patient comfort.

Step 20 Label the specimen container with a patient identification label that contains the name of the test and collection date and time.

Correctly identifying the specimen ensures accurate diagnosis and treatment.

Step 21 Place the specimen in a plastic bag labeled with a biohazard label. Attach a completed laboratory requisition form.

Placing the specimen in a plastic bag protects healthcare workers from exposure to microorganisms. Completing the laboratory requisition form ensures proper processing of the specimen.

Step 22 Send the specimen to the laboratory immediately, or refrigerate it if transport might be delayed.

If bacterial cultures are delayed, contaminating organisms may grow producing false culture results and possibly inappropriate treatment.

Evaluation

- Evaluate the patient's respiratory status during and after the procedure, especially if suctioning was necessary.
- Examine the color, consistency, and odor of sputum specimen.
- Promptly report laboratory results to the physician.
- Evaluate the patient's understanding of the procedure and test results.

Patient Teaching

- Explain proper collection techniques to avoid specimen contamination.
- Show the patient proper coughing techniques to ensure an adequate specimen.
- Explain the importance of avoiding mouthwash before the procedure, as it may alter laboratory results.
- If the patient has an incision, show him how to splint his incision to avoid discomfort during coughing and expectoration.

Home Care

Explain how to collect an expectorated sputum specimen and the importance of sending the specimen to the laboratory immediately after collection.

➤

PROCEDURE 35–1   **Collecting a Sputum Specimen** *(continued)*

Documentation

- Record the date and time the specimen was collected, the method of collection, and the type of specimen ordered.
- Note the amount, color, consistency, and odor of the specimen.
- Document the patient's tolerance to the procedure.

Sample of a narrative note (expectorated specimen):

| 6/5/07 | 0700 | Expectorated specimen collected for culture and sensitivity. Specimen contained 10 mL of thick, green, sweet-smelling sputum. Patient tolerated procedure with no dyspnea, distress, or signs of hypoxia. Specimen sent to the lab immediately after collection.——S. Ryan, RN |

Sample of a narrative note (suctioned specimen):

| 9/2/07 | 2100 | Patient suctioned via tracheostomy, sputum specimen obtained and sent for acid fast bacillus (AFB) analysis. Specimen contained 15 mL of yellow, tenacious, odorless sputum. Patient became short of breath with suctioning. 100% O_2 administered via tracheostomy hood for 10 minutes after suctioning. Shortness of breath abated with treatment. O_2 returned to 40%. ——————S. Ryan, RN |

PROCEDURE 35–2   Monitoring Pulse Oximetry (Arterial Oxygen Saturation)

➤ For steps to follow in *all* procedures, refer to the inside back cover of this book.

critical aspects

- Choose a sensor that is appropriate for the patient's age, size, and weight and for the desired location.
- Attach the probe sensor to the site. Make sure the photodetector and light-emitting diodes on the probe sensor face each other.
- Connect the sensor probe to the oximeter, and turn it on.
- Read the SaO_2 measurement on the digital display when it reaches a constant value, usually in 10 to 30 seconds.
- Set and turn on the alarm limits for SaO_2 and pulse rate, according to the manufacturer's instructions, patient condition, and agency policy if continuous monitoring is necessary.
- Remove the probe sensor, and turn off the oximeter.

Equipment

- Nail polish remover, if necessary
- Oximeter
- Oximeter probe sensor appropriate for patient age, size, weight and for the desired location

Delegation

Because it is noninvasive and simple to perform, you can delegate application of the pulse oximeter probe and measurement of arterial oxygen saturation (SaO_2) to a UAP or LPN who is adequately trained to perform the skill. Inform the UAP or LPN how often to take measurements, and instruct them to notify you immediately if SaO_2 falls below 95%. Patients with underlying pulmonary disease may be accustomed to low oxygen saturation levels, so you may need to adjust the lower limit alarm and the level for notification for these patients.

Assessment

- Assess the patient's need for SaO_2 monitoring: risk factors, such as heart or pulmonary disease; low hemoglobin level; confusion, decreased level of consciousness, or respiratory distress.

SaO_2 monitoring helps detect oxygenation problems early. Monitoring is especially important in patients at risk, such as those with heart and pulmonary disease, those recovering from anesthesia, and those who are ventilator-dependent.

- Assess the patient's respiratory status, including breath sounds; respiratory rate, depth, and pattern; tissue perfusion; and skin and nail bed color.

Assessment findings may suggest a decrease in oxygen saturation and validate oximetry readings.

- Determine the optimal location for the oximeter probe sensor, for example, the finger, earlobe, or bridge of the nose. Check the capillary refill and pulse at the pulse closest to the site.

To ensure accurate monitoring, choose a site that has adequate circulation, is free from artificial nails, and contains no moisture. Technique 35–2 offers suggestions on site placement based on patient factors.

- Assess for factors that may interfere with pulse oximetry measurement, such as hypotension, hypothermia, and tremors.

The sensor requires adequate circulation to recognize hemoglobin molecules that absorb the emitted light. Tremors may produce artifacts that may be misinterpreted by the oximeter, causing false readings.

- Check patient history for allergy to adhesive.

An allergic reaction may occur if an adhesive-backed disposable probe sensor is used in a patient with a history of allergy to adhesives.

- Assess the site every 4 hours if you are using an adhesive probe sensor or every 2 hours if you are using a clip-on probe sensor.

Skin breakdown may occur if continuous monitoring is instituted. Assessment also confirms that the sensor is still in place.

➤

PROCEDURE 35–2

Monitoring Pulse Oximetry (Arterial Oxygen Saturation) *(continued)*

Procedural Steps

Step 1 Choose a sensor appropriate for the patient's age, size, and weight and for the desired location. If the patient is allergic to adhesive, use a clip-on probe sensor. Use a nasal sensor if the patient's peripheral circulation is compromised.

Promotes patient comfort and ensures accurate readings.

Step 2 Prepare the site by cleansing and drying it. If the finger is the desired location, remove nail polish or an acrylic nail, if present.

Dirt and skin oils on the site can interfere with passage of light waves. Nail polish or acrylic nails may interfere with signal transmission, causing inaccurate SaO_2 measurement.

Step 3 Remove the protective backing if you are using a disposable probe sensor that contains adhesive.

Prepares the probe sensor for application.

Step 4 Attach the probe sensor to the chosen site. Make sure that the photodetector and light-emitting diodes on the probe sensor face each other. Most probe sensors contain markings to facilitate correct placement. If you are using a clip-on probe sensor, warn the patient that he may feel a pinching sensation.

Choose the site based on the status of circulation to the extremity and patient movement. Inadequate circulation to the site and artifact caused by motion may alter SaO_2 results. The photodetector and light-emitting diodes must be properly placed to ensure accurate readings. The spring mechanism used to keep the clip-on sensor in place may cause minor discomfort.

Step 5 Connect the sensor probe to the oximeter, and turn it on. Check the pulse rate displayed on the oximeter to see whether it correlates with the patient's radial pulse.

Correlation between the oximeter pulse display and the patient's radial pulse confirms accuracy.

Step 6 Read the SaO_2 measurement on the digital display when it reaches a constant value, usually in 10 to 30 seconds.

The oximeter requires time to register an accurate reading. ▼

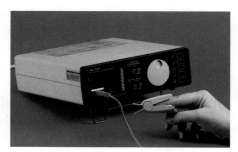

Step 7 Set and turn on the alarm limits for SaO_2 and pulse rate, according to manufacturer instructions, patient condition, and agency policy if continuous monitoring is necessary.

Alarms must be set at appropriate levels to signify when SaO_2 or pulse rate fall below predetermined levels. Alarms help ensure prompt recognition and treatment of hypoxia.

Step 8 Obtain readings as ordered or indicated by the patient's respiratory status.

Some agencies require a physician order for pulse oximetry to ensure reimbursement.

Step 9 Rotate the site every 4 hours if you are using an adhesive probe sensor and every 2 hours if you are using a clip-on probe sensor, if continuous monitoring is indicated.

Probe sensors and prolonged pressure may irritate the skin; rotating the site prevents skin breakdown.

Step 10 Remove the probe sensor, and turn off the oximeter when monitoring is no longer necessary.

Some oximeters are battery-powered; leaving them on after use depletes the battery.

Evaluation

- Evaluate the patient's understanding of the procedure and the obtained values.
- Compare pulse oximetry results with the patient's clinical presentation.
- Evaluate the effectiveness of therapy by comparing SaO_2 results before, during, and after treatment.

Patient Teaching

- Demonstrate the procedure to the patient and caregiver, especially if the patient will be continuing pulse oximetry at home.
- Explain to the patient and caregiver the significance of SaO_2 results.
- Discuss the signs and symptoms of hypoxia (confusion, restlessness, shortness of breath, dyspnea, cyanosis, and somnolence) with the patient and caregiver.

PROCEDURE 35–2   **Monitoring Pulse Oximetry (Arterial Oxygen Saturation)** *(continued)*

Home Care

- Explain to the patient and caregiver where to obtain a pulse oximeter.
- Discuss normal SaO_2 results with the patient and caregiver, and tell them when to notify the physician of abnormal results or signs and symptoms of hypoxia.
- Help the patient identify risk factors that decrease SaO_2 levels.

Documentation

- Record the date and time of each pulse oximetry reading obtained. Most agencies use a flowsheet if frequent monitoring is necessary.
- Document whether readings are intermittent or continuous.
- If readings are continuous, record alarm parameters.
- Chart the patient's vital signs and SaO_2 results, and indicate whether the patient is breathing room air or receiving oxygen therapy. If the patient is receiving oxygen therapy, note the oxygen concentration and the mode of delivery.
- Document acute decreases in SaO_2, any precipitating factors, treatment interventions, and the patient's response.

Sample of a narrative note:

11/14/06	1500	Patient complained of shortness of breath after receiving 500 mL fluid bolus for decreased urine output. Lungs with crackles throughout lung fields. BP 192/96 mm Hg, heart rate 116 beats/minute, respiratory rate 32 breaths/minute, and SaO_2 88% on room air. Patient placed on O_2 at 4 L/minute via nasal cannula. Dr. Illyomade notified. Lasix 40 mg IV given as ordered. ————— L. Reynolds, RN

11/14/06	1600	Patient diuresed 300 mL dilute urine. BP 140/86 mm Hg, heart rate 98 beats/minute, respiratory rate 24 breaths/minute. Respirations regular, nonlabored, breath sounds with bibasilar crackles. SaO_2 98% on O_2 at 4 L/minute via nasal cannula. Patient states breathing is improved. ————— L. Reynolds, RN

PROCEDURE 35–3	**Applying and Caring for a Patient with a Cardiac Monitor**

 For steps to follow in *all* procedures, refer to the inside back cover of this book

critical aspects

- Expose the patient's chest, and identify electrode sites based on the monitoring system and the patient's anatomy.
- With an alcohol pad, clean the areas where electrodes will be placed, and allow them to dry.
- Gently rub the placement sites with a washcloth or gauze pad until the skin reddens slightly.
- Remove the electrode backing, and make sure the gel is moist.
- Apply the electrodes to the sites by pressing firmly.
- Check the patient's ECG tracing on the monitor. If necessary, adjust the gain on the monitor to increase the waveform size.
- Set the upper and lower heart rate alarm limits according to agency policy, and turn them on.
- Obtain a rhythm strip by pressing the "record" button.

Equipment

- Alcohol pads
- Gauze dressing
- Washcloth
- Shaving supplies or scissors, if necessary
- Disposable electrodes

For hardwire monitoring, add:
- Cardiac monitor
- Cable with leadwires
- Safety pin
- 1-inch tape

For telemetry, add:
- Transmitter with leadwires (with a new battery inserted before each use)
- Transmitter pouch
- Pouch to carry transmitter

Delegation

You should not delegate this procedure to the LPN or UAP because it requires knowledge of anatomy, physiology, and advanced assessment techniques.

Assessment

- Assess cardiovascular status, including heart sounds, pulse rate, and blood pressure, and check for the presence of pain.

Assessment findings may indicate the need for cardiac monitoring.

- Assess skin integrity of the chest before applying electrodes.

Skin lesions contraindicate the application of leads to the affected area.

- Assess for dysrhythmias.

Early recognition of dysrhythmias allows for prompt treatment, which improves patient outcomes.

Procedural Steps

Step 1 Prepare the monitoring equipment.

Variation Hardwire Monitoring

a. Plug the cardiac monitor into an electrical outlet, and turn it on.

Allows the monitor to warm up while you prepare the patient for monitoring.

b. Connect the cable with lead wires into the monitor.

The cable and lead wires must be properly connected to the monitor to obtain an accurate ECG tracing.

Variation Telemetry Monitoring

c. Insert a new battery into the transmitter.

A new battery should be inserted with each use to ensure transmitter function.

d. Turn on the transmitter.

Tests the unit to make sure that the battery is functional.

e. Connect the lead wires to the transmitter, if they are not permanently attached. Be sure to attach each one to its correct outlet.

PROCEDURE 35–3

Applying and Caring for a Patient with a Cardiac Monitor *(continued)*

The lead wires must be properly connected to the transmitter to obtain an accurate ECG tracing.

Step 2 Expose the patient's chest, and identify electrode sites based on the monitoring system being used and the patient's anatomy.

The monitoring system will dictate lead placement. Sites over soft tissues or close to bone provide accurate waveforms; sites over bony prominences, thick muscles, and skinfolds can produce artifact. ▼

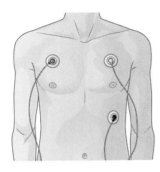

Step 3 If the patient's chest contains dense hair, shave or clip the hair with scissors at each electrode site.

Hair may interfere with electrical contact, preventing accurate ECG waveform transmission.

Step 4 With an alcohol pad, clean the areas chosen for electrode placement, and allow them to dry.

Alcohol removes oil on the skin that may prevent the electrodes from adhering.

Step 5 Gently rub the placement sites with a washcloth or gauze pad until the skin reddens slightly.

Removes dead skin cells and promotes better electrical contact.

Step 6 Remove the electrode backing, and make sure the gel is moist. Discard the electrode if the gel is dry.

A dry electrode will not conduct electrical activity.

Step 7 Apply the electrode to the site by pressing it firmly. Repeat with the remaining electrodes.

Pressing the electrode firmly creates a tight seal, which ensures electrical contact.

Step 8 Attach the lead wires to the electrodes by snapping or clipping them in place.

Step 9 Secure the monitoring equipment.

Variation Hardwire Monitoring

Wrap a piece of 1-inch tape around the cable, and secure it to the patient's gown with a safety pin.

Secures the cable so leads are not inadvertently disconnected with patient movement.

Variation Telemetry Monitoring

Place the transmitter in the pouch, and tie the pouch strings around the patient's neck and waist. Place the transmitter into the patient's robe pocket if a pouch is not available.

Allows the patient independence with ambulation.

Step 10 Check the patient's ECG tracing on the monitor. If necessary, adjust the gain on the monitor to increase the waveform size.

The ECG tracing should be of adequate size to accurately assess all of the waveform components.

Step 11 Set the upper and lower heart rate alarm limits according to agency policy or patient condition, and turn them on.

Step 12 Obtain a rhythm strip by pressing the "record" button.

You must obtain a rhythm strip to document the patient's cardiac rhythm. ▼

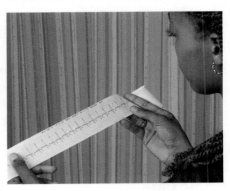

Variation Hardwire Monitoring

Press the "record" button on the bedside monitor.

The "record" button, located on the monitor at the bedside, allows you to print a rhythm strip immediately when cardiac symptoms occur.

Variation Telemetry Monitoring

Press the "record" button on the transmitter of the telemetry unit

The "record" button on the telemetry transmitter allows you or the patient to print a rhythm strip immediately when cardiac symptoms occur.

Step 13 Interpret the rhythm strip, and mount it appropriately (e.g., with transparent tape) in the patient's chart.

Provides a permanent record of the patient's heart activity; identifies abnormalities in the patient's rhythm.

➤

PROCEDURE 35–3 **Applying and Caring for a Patient with a Cardiac Monitor** (continued)

Evaluation

- Evaluate changes in the patient's cardiac rhythm.
- Check skin integrity, and replace the electrodes at least every 24 hours.

Avoids skin irritation at the electrode sites. In addition, the gel begins to dry, so replacement ensures an adequate waveform.

Patient Teaching

- Explain cardiac monitoring to the patient. If the patient is monitored by telemetry, teach him how to record a rhythm strip if he experiences symptoms.
- Tell the patient being monitored by telemetry to remove the transmitter before showering. Ask the patient to inform you before removing it.
- Discuss home telemetry monitoring with the patient and caregiver if the patient requires telemetry monitoring after discharge.

Home Care

- Evaluate the patient and caregiver's ability to continue telemetry monitoring at home with help from an outside agency.
- Help the patient and caregiver arrange for home telemetry monitoring by contacting the monitoring agency.
- Explain to the caregiver and patient that the emergency medical service will be notified by the monitoring agency if a dysrhythmia develops.
- Instruct the caregiver and patient about proper lead placement and the need to rotate electrode sites to prevent skin breakdown.

Documentation

- Document the date and time that monitoring was instituted.
- Note the monitoring lead selected.
- Document a rhythm strip every 8 hours and with changes in the patient's condition according to agency policy. Label the rhythm strip (if the monitor does not label it for you) with the date, time, patient's name, and room number. Indicate on the strip when symptoms and treatment interventions occurred.
- Document the patient's response to treatment.

Sample of a narrative note:

9/18/06	0900	*Patient transferred to CCU after complaining of midsternal chest pain and palpitations. Cardiac monitoring initiated in lead II. Rhythm strip reveals sinus tachycardia at a rate of 105 beats/minute with frequent PVCs [premature ventricular contractions]. SL NTG [sublingual nitroglycerin] 1/150 gr administered for midsternal chest pain, rated a 4 on a 1 to 10 pain scale. Pain relieved in 2 minutes.*
		— S. Exos, RN

PROCEDURE 35–4 Performing Percussion, Vibration, and Postural Drainage

 For steps to follow in *all* procedures, refer to the inside back cover of this book.

critical aspects

- Help the patient assume the appropriate position based on the lung field that requires drainage.
- Keep the patient in the desired position for 10 to 15 minutes.
- Using cupped hands, perform percussion over the affected lung area for 1 to 3 minutes while the patient is in the desired drainage position.
- Next, perform vibration.
- Assist the patient to sit up. Have him cough at the end of a deep inspiration to clear the airways of secretions.
- Repeat postural drainage, percussion, and vibration for each lung field that requires treatment. The entire treatment should not exceed 60 minutes.
- Provide mouth care.

Equipment

- Bed capable of being placed in Trendelenburg's position
- Pillows
- Patient gown
- Facial tissues
- Emesis basin
- Sputum specimen container, if needed
- Suction equipment, if needed
- Stethoscope

Delegation

You should assess the patient to determine the need for the procedure and to evaluate whether the patient can tolerate the procedure. You should perform the initial procedure, but you can delegate subsequent treatments to a respiratory therapist or unlicensed assistive personnel (UAP) who is adequately trained. Instruct the respiratory therapist or UAP to report any changes in the patient's condition immediately.

Assessment

- Check the patient's chest x-ray results.

Identifies which lung fields require treatment.

- Assess the patient's respiratory status, including respiratory rate, depth, and rhythm; breath sounds; color; and pulse oximetry results.

Determines the need for and effectiveness of percussion, vibration, and postural drainage.

- Determine when the patient has last eaten.

Postural drainage should not be performed for at least 2 hours after meals to prevent nausea, vomiting, and aspiration.

- Assess the patient for dysrhythmias, coagulopathy, hypertension, and pain or tenderness in the chest area being treated.

If any of these are present, the procedure should be avoided because it might worsen these conditions.

➤

PROCEDURE 35–4   Performing Percussion, Vibration, and Postural Drainage *(continued)*

Procedural Steps

Step 1 Help the patient assume the appropriate position, based on the lung field that requires drainage.

Helps mobilize secretions in the affected lung field by gravity.

a. *Apical areas of the upper lobes.* If possible, have the patient sit at the edge of the bed. If needed, place a pillow at the base of the spine for support. If the patient is not able to sit at the edge of the bed, place him in high-Fowler's position. ▼

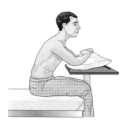

(a)

b. *Posterior section of the upper lobes.* Position the patient in supine position with pillow under her hips and knees flexed. Have the patient rotate slightly away from the side that requires drainage. ▼

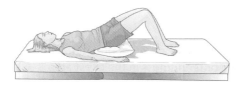

(b)

c. *Middle or lower lobes.* Place the bed in Trendelenburg's position. Position the patient in Sims' position. To drain the left lung, position the patient on his right side. For the right lung, position the patient on his left side. ▼

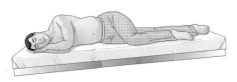

(c)

d. *Posterior lower lobes.* Keeping the bed flat, position the patient prone with a pillow under her stomach. ▼

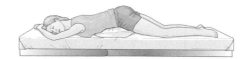

(d)

Step 2 Have the patient remain in the desired position for 10 to 15 minutes.

Allows adequate drainage of secretions by gravity from the desired lung field.

Step 3 Perform percussion over the affected lung area while the patient is in the desired drainage position.

Loosens and mobilizes secretions.

a. Promote relaxation by instructing the patient to breathe deeply and slowly.

Relaxation helps the patient tolerate the procedure.

b. Place a towel over the patient's skin or cover with the patient's gown the area to be percussed.

Protects the skin and promotes patient privacy and comfort.

c. Avoid clapping over bony prominences, female breasts, or tender areas of the chest.

Percussing over these areas may cause discomfort and compromise tissue integrity.

d. Cup your hands, keeping your fingers flexed and your thumbs pressed against your index fingers.

Cupping your hands promotes patient comfort during percussion.

e. Place your cupped hands over the lung area that requires drainage.

f. Percuss the lung area for 1 to 3 minutes by alternately striking your cupped hands rhythmically against the patient. ▼

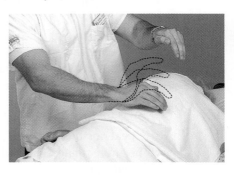

Step 4 Perform vibrations while the patient remains in the desired drainage position. ▼

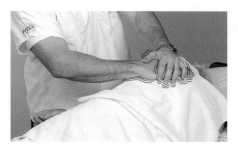

a. Place the flat surface of one hand over the lung area that requires vibration. Place your other hand on top of that hand at a right angle.

Using the flat surfaces of the hands provides a large surface area to transmit vibrations through the chest. Placing one hand on top of the other provides better leverage for vibrating.

b. Instruct the patient to inhale slowly and deeply.

Promotes relaxation.

c. Instruct the patient to make an "fff" or "sss" sound as she exhales.

d. As the patient exhales, press your fingers and palms firmly against the patient's chest wall.

PROCEDURE 35–4 **Performing Percussion, Vibration, and Postural Drainage** *(continued)*

Vibrating during exhalation enhances the downward movement of the rib cage that occurs during exhalation.

e. Push down, and gently vibrate with your hands over the lung area.

Vibration helps mobilize secretions.

f. Continue performing vibrations for three exhalations.

Step 5 After performing postural drainage, percussion, and vibration, allow the patient to sit up. Have her cough at the end of a deep inspiration. Suction the patient if she is unable to expectorate secretions. If a sputum specimen is needed, collect it in a specimen container.

Helps clear the airway of secretions.

Step 6 Repeat steps 1 through 5 for each lung field that requires treatment. The entire treatment should not exceed 60 minutes.

Providing treatment for longer than 60 minutes fatigues the patient.

Step 7 Provide mouth care.

Cleanses the mouth of secretions and promotes patient comfort.

Evaluation

- Evaluate the effectiveness of percussion, vibration, and postural drainage.
- Auscultate breath sounds every 2 to 4 hours, as indicated.
- Monitor pulse oximetry and arterial blood gas results.
- Evaluate the need for further treatment with percussion, vibration, and postural drainage.

Patient Teaching

- Demonstrate percussion, vibration, and postural drainage if the patient will be continuing it at home.
- Reinforce the importance of immediately reporting shortness of breath or any difficulty breathing.
- Explain the importance of drinking fluids to help thin and mobilize secretions.
- Explain coughing and deep-breathing exercises.

Home Care

- Explain to the family and caregiver how to perform percussion, vibration, and postural drainage if the patient requires continued treatment at home.
- Most patients will not have a bed that can be placed in Trendelenburg position. Teach the patient and caregivers how to position the patient with hips elevated on pillows, higher than chest, or, if the patient is able, to assume a knee-chest position.
- Provide the patient and caregiver with contact information of healthcare personnel who can be reached for advice or emergencies.

Documentation

- Document the date and time you performed percussion, vibration, and postural drainage.
- Note the positions used for postural drainage and the length of time the patient maintained each position.
- Note the locations in which you performed percussion and vibration.

➤

PROCEDURE 35–4

Performing Percussion, Vibration, and Postural Drainage *(continued)*

- Document the patient's tolerance to the procedure, as well as any complications and the nursing interventions you used to treat the complication.
- Document the amount, color, odor, and consistency of sputum you obtained during the procedure and whether you sent a sputum specimen to the lab.

Sample of a narrative note:

3/25/07	1300	Patient placed in Trendelenburg position in the left lateral position with a pillow placed between her legs. Postural drainage performed for 10 minutes. Percussion and vibration performed over the right lower lobe. Patient expectorated about 10 mL of thick, yellow, odorless secretions. Specimen sent to the lab. Patient tolerated the procedure without shortness of breath. After the procedure, Sa0$_2$ was 98%, with oxygen at 2 L/minute via nasal cannula, BP 142/78 mm Hg, HR 98 beats/min, and RR 24 breaths/minute. Breath sounds with few fine crackles auscultated over the right lung base.————— J. Simmons, RN

PROCEDURE 35–5

Administering Oxygen by Cannula, Face Mask, or Face Tent

For steps to follow in *all* procedures, refer to the inside back cover of this book.

critical aspects

- Attach the flow meter to the wall oxygen source.
- Assemble and apply the oxygen equipment according to the device prescribed (nasal cannula, face mask, or face tent).
- Turn on the oxygen using the flow meter, and adjust it according to the prescribed flow rate.
- Make sure that the oxygen equipment is set up correctly and functioning properly before you leave the patient's bedside.

Equipment

- Oxygen source
- Flow meter
- Oxygen tubing
- Nasal cannula, oxygen mask, or face tent
- Prefilled humidification device
- Padding

Delegation

You should assess the patient, then initiate oxygen therapy as needed. You can delegate reapplication of oxygen therapy to appropriately trained assistive personnel when necessary.

Assessment

- Assess the patient's comprehension of oxygen therapy.

Understanding allays anxiety and promotes cooperation.

- Assess the patient's respiratory status, including respiratory rate, depth, and rhythm; breath sounds; color; and pulse oximetry results.

Determines the need for and effectiveness of oxygen therapy.

- Assess nares (if a nasal cannula is being used) and ears for signs of skin breakdown.

Procedural Steps

Step 1 Attach the flow meter to the wall oxygen source. If you are using a portable oxygen tank, attach the flow meter to the tank if it is not already connected.

The flow meter regulates the amount of oxygen delivered.

Step 2 Assemble the oxygen equipment. (See the table at the end of this procedure for various oxygen delivery devices.)

Assembling the oxygen equipment readies the equipment for oxygen administration.

Procedure Variation A
Nasal Cannula

Step 3 Attach the humidifier to the flow meter. (Humidification is necessary only for flow rates > 3 L/min.) If you are not using a humidifier, attach the adapter to the flow meter.

Humidification prevents drying of the nasal membranes.

Step 4 Attach the nasal cannula to the humidifier or the adapter.

Step 5 Place the nasal prongs in the patient's nares, and then place the tubing around each ear.

Properly positions the device for successful oxygen delivery.

➤

PROCEDURE 35–5

Administering Oxygen by Cannula, Face Mask, or Face Tent *(continued)*

Step 6 Use the slide adjustment device to tighten the cannula in place under the patient's chin.

The nasal cannula must fit securely to ensure accurate oxygen delivery. ▼

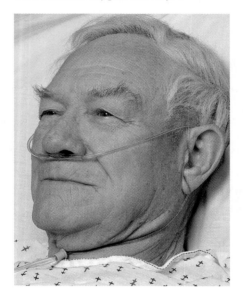

Step 7 Turn on the oxygen using the flow meter, and adjust it according to the prescribed flow rate.

Ensures that oxygen is delivered at the prescribed rate. Oxygen delivered at an incorrect rate can cause patient injury.

Step 8 Make sure that the oxygen equipment is set up correctly and functioning properly before you leave the patient's bedside.

Procedure Variation B
Face Mask

Step 9 Attach the prefilled humidifier to the flow meter.

The humidification device must be attached to the flow meter to ensure delivery of humidified oxygen, which prevents the drying of airways that occurs with high oxygen flow rates.

Step 10 Attach the oxygen tubing connected to the mask to the humidifier.

Prepares the tubing for oxygen delivery.

Step 11 Gently place the face mask on the patient's face, applying it from the bridge of the nose to under the chin.

Fits the mask snugly to the patient's face, preventing oxygen from escaping around the edges of the mask.

Step 12 Secure the elastic band around the back of the patient's head. Make sure the mask fits snugly but comfortably.

The mask must fit snugly so that oxygen cannot escape around the edges of the mask. The mask must also fit comfortably, because a fit that is too tight may cause skin breakdown. ▼

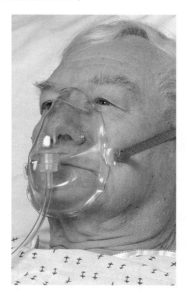

Step 13 Turn on the oxygen, using the flow meter, and adjust it according to the prescribed flow rate.

Ensures that oxygen is delivered at the prescribed rate. Oxygen delivered at an incorrect rate can cause patient injury.

Step 14 Make sure that the oxygen equipment is set up correctly and functioning properly before you leave the patient's bedside.

Procedure Variation C
Face Tent

Step 15 Attach the prefilled humidifier to the flow meter.

Ensures delivery of humidified oxygen, which prevents the drying of the airways that occurs with high oxygen flow rates.

Step 16 Attach the oxygen tubing to the face tent.

Ensures adequate oxygen delivery.

Step 17 Attach the oxygen tubing to the humidifier.

Prepares the tubing for oxygen delivery.

Step 18 Gently place the face tent in front of the patient's face, making sure that it fits under the chin.

Ensures a proper fit.

Step 19 Secure the elastic band around the back of the patient's head.

The elastic band must go around the back of the patient's head to keep the face mask in place. ▼

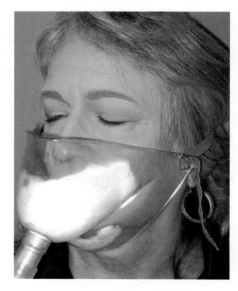

Step 20 Turn on the oxygen using the flow meter, and adjust it according to the prescribed flow rate.

Ensures that oxygen is delivered at the prescribed rate. Oxygen delivered at an incorrect rate can cause patient injury.

Step 21 Make sure that the oxygen equipment is set up correctly and functioning properly before you leave the patient's bedside.

PROCEDURE 35–5

Administering Oxygen by Cannula, Face Mask, or Face Tent *(continued)*

Evaluation

- Auscultate breath sounds every 2 to 4 hours, as indicated.
- Monitor pulse oximetry or arterial blood gas results.
- Evaluate skin areas that come in contact with oxygen delivery system for signs of skin breakdown.

Patient Teaching

- Demonstrate oxygen administration to the patient and caregiver if the patient will be continuing oxygen therapy at home.
- Explain the importance of immediately reporting shortness of breath or any difficulty breathing.

Home Care

- Explain to the family and caregiver where to obtain oxygen equipment and what services are available. Make sure they choose a supplier who has 24-hour emergency services.
- Instruct the patient and caregiver about oxygen therapy and its use, as well as safety measures that they must institute.
- Teach the patient and caregiver to clean the nasal cannula or face mask with soap and warm water when it becomes soiled.
- Provide the patient and caregiver with contact information of healthcare personnel who can be reached for advice or emergencies.
- In the home, liquid oxygen and oxygen concentrators are more commonly used than portable oxygen tanks. Liquid oxygen may be kept in small, portable containers; an oxygen concentrator removes nitrogen from room air and concentrates O_2. It requires a battery pack or electrical outlet for power. Oxygen concentrators can deliver flow up to 4 L/min to create an F_{IO_2} of approximately 36%.

Documentation

- Document the date, time, and reason oxygen therapy was initiated.
- Note the type of oxygen delivery system used, the amount of oxygen administered, and the patient's response to oxygen therapy.
- Document vital signs, pulse oximetry values, breath sounds, skin color, and respiratory effort.

Sample of a narrative note (nasal cannula):

12/24/07	2245	Patient's SaO_2 on room air = 89%. Breath sounds clear to auscultation, respirations unlabored at 24/minute. Dr. Schilling made aware. O_2 applied at 2 L/min via nasal cannula. SaO_2 after oxygen applied = 93%.
		R. Roumalade, RN

PROCEDURE 35–5 **Administering Oxygen by Cannula, Face Mask, or Face Tent** (*continued*)

Sample of a narrative note (face mask):

| 12/25/07 | 2000 | Patient developed acute shortness of breath, RR @ 36 & labored, P = 126, and BP 212/110 mm Hg. Pulse ox. 80% on room air. Crackles and expiratory wheezes auscultated throughout both lung fields. Dr. Chow made aware of patient's condition. Partial rebreather mask @ 10 L/min and Lasix 40 mg IV prescribed and administered. Pulse ox. on partial rebreather = 90%. ————— S. Peters, RN |

Sample of a narrative note (face tent):

| 1/1/07 | 0200 | Patient receiving oxygen via 40% aerosol mask. Patient began complaining that aerosol mask was very uncomfortable. Patient stated, "Isn't there any other way that you can give me this oxygen?" Dr. Sell notified. Patient's oxygen therapy changed to a 40% face tent. Patient tolerating face tent without difficulty. Pulse ox. on face tent 98%. RR= 18 and nonlabored. Breath sounds clear to auscultation. ————— |
| | | ————— T. Smith, RN |

Oxygen Delivery Systems

Delivery Method	F_{IO_2}	Discussion	Nursing Responsibilities
Nasal cannula 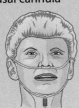	1 L/min = 24% 2 L/min = 28% 3 L/min = 32% 4 L/min = 36% 5 L/min = 40% 6 L/min = 44%	• Relatively comfortable. • Patients can eat, talk, and cough with a nasal cannula in place. • Works best if the patient breathes through his nose.	• Check frequently that the prongs are in the patient's nose. • Assess for dryness of the nasal mucosa. • Humidify flow at rates above 3 L/min (flow rates above 3 L/min are drying)
Simple face mask: A clear, flexible mask that covers the nose and mouth and delivers oxygen flow into the mask. 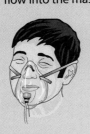	5–10 L/min = 40–60%	• Requires flow rates greater than 5 L/min to prevent accumulation and rebreathing of exhaled CO_2 from within the mask. • Masks are not easily tolerated because they fit tightly and keep heat from radiating from the face, making patients feel hot. • Talking is muffled by the mask, and it must be removed for the patient to eat or drink.	• Place face mask securely over the mouth and nose. • Elastic straps fit around the head to hold the mask in place. Place the straps well above the ears to prevent skin irritation and breakdown. • Place gauze or other soft material beneath the straps to prevent irritation. • Check the skin around the mask frequently. • Check the skin over the ears where the mask strap rubs.
Partial rebreather mask: Uses the reservoir bag to capture some exhaled gas for rebreathing. 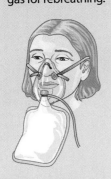	6–15 L/min = 50–90%	• Allows higher F_{IO_2} levels to be delivered because O_2 is collected in the reservoir bag for inhalation. • Exhalation ports allow most exhaled air to escape. • Several types are available. • Can deliver an F_{IO_2} above 50% at flow rates of 6–15 L/min. • Patient rebreathes some exhaled air along with O_2.	• Maintain the flow at a high enough rate to prevent the reservoir bag from collapsing during inhalation.
Nonrebreather mask: A type of reservoir bag mask; a valve keeps exhaled air from entering the reservoir bag. 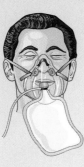	6–15 L/min = 70–100%	• Contains only O_2, which allows higher F_{IO_2} delivery. An F_{IO_2} of 60–100% can be delivered at flow rates of 6–15 L/min. • This mask is the only external device capable of delivering an F_{IO_2} of 100%.	• Maintain the flow at a rate high enough to prevent the reservoir from collapsing during inhalation.

➤

Oxygen Delivery Systems *(continued)*

Delivery Method	F$_{IO_2}$	Discussion	Nursing Responsibilities
Venturi mask: A cone-shaped adapter that serves as a mixing valve to control the amount of O_2 and room air that flows through the mask. 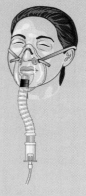	24–50%	• The cone-shaped adapter at the base of the mask allows a precise F$_{IO_2}$ to be delivered. This is very useful for patients with chronic lung disease. • Exhalation ports keep CO_2 buildup to a minimum.	• The adapter indicates the required oxygen flow rate needed to deliver the desired F$_{IO_2}$. Ensure that flow is set at the rate specified to deliver the F$_{IO_2}$ desired.
Face tent: A large, open plastic mask that fits under the chin. It is open at the top and is held in place with an elastic band around the head. 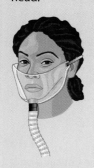	8–12 L/min = 30–55%	• Less reliable than a face mask for delivering precise F$_{IO_2}$ levels. • Does allow moderate- to high-density aerosol delivery for humidification. • Patients who feel claustrophobic in a face mask often tolerate a face tent.	• Check the skin over the ears where the mask strap rubs.
Tracheostomy collar: A small, cup-shaped device that fits over the tracheostomy opening and is held in place with elastic straps around the neck. 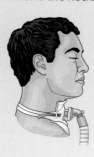	4–10 L/min = 24–100%	• It is possible to deliver both high F$_{IO_2}$ and high humidity with a tracheostomy collar. • Large-bore tubing is used to deliver humidification to the trachea; however, water frequently condenses inside the tubing and can be accidentally drained into the tracheostomy. Usually, a water trap of some sort is placed in the tubing to prevent this problem.	• Watch for water accumulation in the tubing.

Oxygen Delivery Systems *(continued)*

Delivery Method	FIO₂	Discussion	Nursing Responsibilities
T-piece: A T-shaped plastic piece; the bottom of the T fits directly and tightly onto the tracheostomy tube. 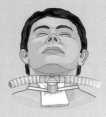	4–10 L/min = 24–100%	• Oxygen and humidity are delivered into one end of the T and exhaled through the other end.	• Take care that the oxygen delivery tubing does not pull on the T-piece, which can dislodge the tracheostomy tube and create an airway emergency.

PROCEDURE 35–6   Performing Tracheostomy Care

 For steps to follow in *all* procedures, refer to the inside back cover of this book.

critical aspects

- No formal recommendation can be made about wearing sterile rather than clean gloves when performing endotracheal care according to the Centers for Disease Control (Tablan, Anderson, Besser, Bridges, and Hajjeh, 2004).
- Position the patient in semi-Fowler's position.
- Suction the tracheostomy (see Procedure 35–9).
- Place the tracheostomy care equipment on the overbed table, and prepare the equipment, using sterile or modified sterile technique, depending on agency policy.
- Remove the oxygen source, if the patient is receiving supplemental oxygen.
- Remove the inner cannula with your nondominant hand, and dispose of it (if it is a disposable cannula) or clean it (if it is a reusable cannula).
- Attach the oxygen source to the outer cannula, if possible.
- Clean the stoma under the faceplate with the cotton-tipped applicators saturated with hydrogen peroxide.
- Clean the top surface of the faceplate and the skin around it with the gauze pads saturated with hydrogen peroxide or half-strength hydrogen peroxide.
- Clean areas using the cotton-tipped applicators and gauze pads saturated with normal saline solution or half-strength hydrogen peroxide.
- Dry the skin around the faceplate and stoma with dry sterile gauze.
- Remove soiled tracheostomy stablizers.
- Have the patient flex his neck, and apply new tracheostomy stabilizers.
- Insert a precut, sterile tracheostomy dressing under the faceplate and new tracheostomy stabilizers.

PROCEDURE 35–6   **Performing Tracheostomy Care** (*continued*)

Equipment

- Tracheostomy suction equipment (see Procedure 35–9)
- Tracheostomy care kit or the following sterile supplies: several cotton-tipped applicators, two basins, a brush, sterile 4 × 4 gauze pads, sterile precut tracheostomy dressing
- Two pairs of sterile gloves and/or procedure gloves
- Disposable inner cannula that is the same size as the tracheostomy, if available
- Normal saline solution
- Hydrogen peroxide
- Roll of twill tape or Velcro tracheostomy holder
- Bandage scissors
- Towel or linen-saver pad
- Overbed table
- Face shield

Caution: Use only the sterile precut dressing, or open and refold a 4 × 4 gauze pad into a V-shape. Do not cut 4 × 4 gauze, and do not use cotton-filled gauze squares, because the patient may aspirate the cotton or gauze fibers.

Important Note: No formal recommendation can be made about whether to wear sterile or clean gloves when performing endotracheal care, according to the Centers for Disease Control (Tablan, Anderson, Besser, Bridges, and Hajjeh, 2004). Although sterile technique has been the typical method used in hospitals, the trend now is toward a modified sterile technique; and clean technique is the usual method for suctioning in the home setting.

If the patient has an increased susceptibility to infection, sterile technique may be advised. Nonsterile, disposable gloves should be worn for the protection of any caregiver that is not a family member and by those concerned about personally acquiring infection.

- **Sterile technique** is the use of a sterile catheter and supplies with sterile gloves.
- **Modified sterile technique** is use of a sterile catheter and supplies, but with nonsterile procedure gloves.
- **Clean technique** is use of a clean catheter and clean hands or nonsterile gloves. The portion of the catheter that will be inserted in the tracheostomy tube is protected to avoid contact with unclean surfaces.

You should follow the procedure used in your organization or school.

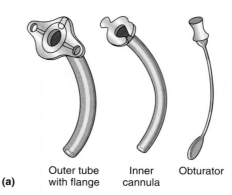

(a)   Outer tube with flange   Inner cannula   Obturator

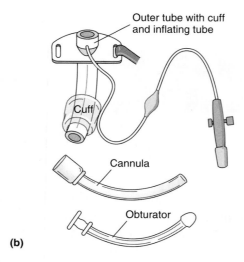

Outer tube with cuff and inflating tube

Cuff

Cannula

Obturator

(b)

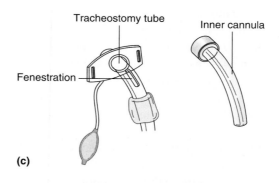

Tracheostomy tube   Inner cannula

Fenestration

(c)

(a) Nondisposable tracheostomy equipment
(b) Disposable tracheostomy equipment
(c) Fenestrated tracheostomy equipment

PROCEDURE 35–6 **Performing Tracheostomy Care** (*continued*)

Delegation

In acute care settings and with new tracheostomies, you should not delegate this procedure to the UAP. For long-standing and well-healed tracheostomies, you can safely delegate care to a UAP or LPN who is adequately trained to perform the skill. The patient who will be discharged with a tracheostomy should also be trained, along with caregivers, to perform the skill.

Assessment

- Assess the patient's respiratory status, including respiratory rate, depth, and rhythm; breath sounds; color; and pulse oximetry results.

Helps determine whether the patient can tolerate tracheostomy care.

- Assess the tracheostomy site for drainage, redness, or swelling.

Drainage, redness, or swelling may indicate infection.

- Assess the need for suctioning to remove airway secretions.

Determination of the need for tracheostomy suction is based on the quality of breath sounds, respiratory effort and rate, patient comfort, tachycardia, and increase in the peak airway pressure if the patient requires mechanical ventilation.

Procedural Steps

Step 1 Position the patient in semi-Fowler's position, and place a towel or linen-saver pad over the patient's chest.

Semi-Fowler's position promotes lung expansion and prevents back strain in the nurse performing the procedure. A towel or linen-saver pad prevents soiling of the patient's gown.
Place a small, rolled towel under the patient's shoulders to expose the neck.

Step 2 Don sterile gloves (alternatively, you may put a sterile glove on your dominant hand and a clean glove on your other hand). Suction the tracheostomy (see Procedure 35–9). Remove and discard the soiled tracheostomy dressing in the appropriate receptacle, and then remove and discard your gloves.

Suctioning clears the tracheostomy of secretions that could occlude the outer cannula after the inner cannula is removed for care.
Although sterile technique has been the typical method of suctioning in the hospital, the trend is toward a modified sterile technique. In the home environment, a clean technique is the usual method for endotracheal suctioning. When using clean technique caregivers vary according to how often to replace and clean a single catheter. Some change the catheter after each suctioning procedure while others change

only every 24 hours or when the catheter becomes contaminated during use.

Step 3 Place the tracheostomy care equipment on the overbed table, and prepare the equipment, using sterile technique.

Helps maintain sterility during tracheostomy care. Preparing the equipment before beginning care ensures efficiency.

a. Pour hydrogen peroxide into one of the sterile solution containers, and pour normal saline solution into the other one. Alternatively, you may mix hydrogen peroxide with normal saline in one container to form a half-strength solution.

Hydrogen peroxide is used to clean the inner cannula (if a disposable inner cannula is not available), faceplate, and tracheostomy site. Normal saline is used to rinse the inner cannula, faceplate, and tracheostomy site after they are cleaned with hydrogen peroxide.

b. Open three 4 × 4 gauze packages. Wet the gauze in one package with hydrogen peroxide, wet the gauze in another package with normal saline solution, and keep the third package dry.

You will use the third package of gauze to dry the skin around the tracheostomy site after cleaning.

c. Open two cotton-tipped applicator packages. Wet the applicators in one

package with normal saline solution, and wet the applicators in the other package with hydrogen peroxide.

Prepares the applicators for cleaning the exposed surface of the outer cannula and the stoma site located under the faceplate of the tracheostomy tube, respectively.

d. Open the package containing a new disposable inner cannula, if available.

Allows for quick replacement of the inner cannula.

e. Open the package of Velcro tracheostomy ties, or cut a length of twill tape long enough to go around the patient's neck two times. Make sure to cut end of the tape on an angle.

Allows for quick stabilization of the tracheostomy tube, preventing dislodgement. Cutting the twill tape on an angle allows for easy insertion through the faceplate eyelets.

Step 4 Don sterile gloves (or a sterile glove on your dominant hand and a clean glove on your nondominant hand); keep the glove on your dominant hand sterile. Handle the sterile supplies with the dominant hand only.

Step 5 With your nondominant hand, remove the oxygen source, if the patient has been receiving supplemental oxygen.

➤

PROCEDURE 35–6 **Performing Tracheostomy Care** *(continued)*

Step 6 Unlock and remove the inner cannula with your nondominant hand, and care for it accordingly.

Variation Disposable Inner Cannula

a. If a disposable inner cannula was in place, dispose of the inner cannula in the biohazard receptacle according to agency policy.

Prevents contamination by bacteria contained in the inner cannula.

Variation Reusable Inner Cannula

b. If a reusable inner cannula was used, place the inner cannula into the basin filled with hydrogen peroxide.

Hydrogen peroxide helps loosen tenacious secretions.

Step 7 Attach the oxygen source to the outer cannula, if possible.

Prevents oxygen desaturation in the patient during the procedure.

Step 8 Care for the inner cannula.

Variation Reusable Inner Cannula

a. Pick up the reusable inner cannula from the container of hydrogen peroxide, and scrub it with the sterile nylon brush, using your dominant hand.

Cleans the inner cannula of secretions. ▼

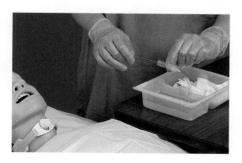

b. Immerse the inner cannula in the container of sterile normal saline solution, and agitate it until it is rinsed thoroughly.

Immersing the inner cannula in normal saline solution and agitating it removes the hydrogen peroxide (which can cause tissue irritation) and debris from the inner cannula.

c. Tap the inner cannula against the side of the container.

Tapping the inner cannula against the side of the container removes excess fluid so the patient does not aspirate it when you reinsert the cannula.

Step 9 Remove the oxygen source, using your nondominant hand (if the patient requires supplemental oxygen), and reinsert the inner cannula into the patient's tracheostomy in the direction of the curvature. Following manufacturer instructions, lock the inner cannula in place securely.

Remember to keep dominant hand sterile. Lock the inner cannula in place securely to prevent it from dislodging.

Step 10 Reattach the oxygen source, if indicated.

Provides the patient with needed oxygen and prevents oxygen desaturation.

Step 11 Clean the stoma under the faceplate with the cotton-tipped applicators saturated with hydrogen peroxide, using a circular motion from the stoma site outward. Use each applicator only once, and then discard it.

Prevents contamination of the cleaned area. ▼

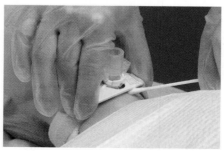

Step 12 Clean the top surface of the faceplate and the skin around it with the gauze pads saturated with hydrogen peroxide. Use each gauze pad only once, and then discard it.

Removes secretions that provide a prime medium for microorganism growth; prevents contamination of cleaned areas.

Step 13 Repeat steps 11 and 12, using the cotton-tipped applicators and gauze pads saturated with normal saline solution.

Removes the hydrogen peroxide and debris that can irritate the skin.

Step 14 Dry the skin and outer cannula surfaces by patting them lightly with the remaining dry gauze pad.

Helps prevent skin breakdown and removes moisture, which can promote bacterial growth around the stoma site.

Step 15 Seek assistance from another staff member to help with changing the tracheostomy stabilizers.

Prevents accidental dislodging should the patient begin coughing during the procedure.

Step 16 Remove soiled tracheostomy stablizers.

Variation Removing a Soiled Velcro Tracheostomy Holder

a. With the assistant stabilizing the tracheostomy tube, disengage the Velcro on both sides of the soiled holder, and remove it gently from the eyes of the faceplate. Discard the Velcro holder in the nearest biohazard receptacle.

Removing the soiled holder promotes hygiene and prevents the spread of infection.

PROCEDURE 35–6   **Performing Tracheostomy Care** *(continued)*

Variation Removing Soiled Twill Tape Tracheostomy Ties

b. With the assistant stabilizing the tracheostomy tube, cut the soiled tracheostomy ties using bandage scissors. Avoid cutting the tube of the tracheostomy balloon. Remove the ties gently from the eyes of the faceplate, and discard them in the nearest biohazard receptacle.

The tracheostomy balloon helps stabilize the tracheostomy in the trachea and prevents an air leak. Cutting the tube to the balloon prevents the balloon from holding air. Removing the soiled holder promotes hygiene and prevents the spread of infection.

Step 17 Have the patient flex his neck, and apply new tracheostomy stabilizers.

Flexing the neck provides the same neck circumference as when the patient coughs and thus helps prevent you from placing the tracheostomy stabilizers in such a way that they would be excessively tight.

Variation Using a Velcro Tracheostomy Holder

a. Unfasten the Velcro. Thread one end of the tracheostomy holder through the eyelet of the faceplate, and fasten the Velcro.

Prepares the holder for insertion through the tracheostomy faceplate.

b. Bring the holder around the back of the patient's neck.

The holder must be placed around the patient's neck to adequately secure the tracheostomy.

c. Thread the remaining end of the tracheostomy holder through the empty eyelet of the faceplate, and

fasten the Velcro, making sure that the holder fits securely.

Secures the tracheostomy. ▼

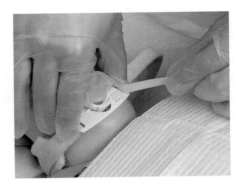

d. Place one finger under the holder to make sure that the holder is securing the tracheostomy effectively but isn't too tight.

Securing the tracheostomy too tightly might place pressure on the jugular veins, interfere with coughing, or cause necrosis at the tracheostomy insertion site.

Variation Using Twill Tape

e. Thread one end of the twill tape into one of the eyelets on the tracheostomy faceplate.

f. Continue to thread the twill tape through the eyelet, bringing both ends of the tape together.

g. Bring both ends of the twill tape around the back of the patient's neck.

The twill tape must be placed around the patient's neck to adequately secure the tracheostomy.

h. Thread the end of the twill tape that is closest to the patient's neck through the back of the eyelet on the faceplate.

Helps secure the tracheostomy.

i. Have your assistant place one finger under the twill tape while you tie the two ends together in a square knot.

Securing the tracheostomy too tightly might place pressure on the jugular veins, interfere with coughing, or cause necrosis at the tracheostomy insertion site.

Step 18 Insert a precut, sterile tracheostomy dressing under the faceplate and new tracheostomy stabilizers or fold a 4 × 4 gauze into a V shape (below). ▼

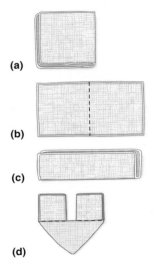

(a)
(b)
(c)
(d)

The new dressing absorbs secretions and prevents skin breakdown under the faceplate. ▼

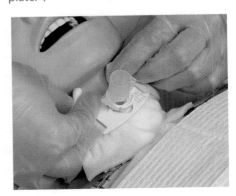

Step 19 Dispose of the used equipment in the appropriate biohazard receptacle according to agency policy.

Properly disposing of used equipment prevents cross-contamination.

PROCEDURE 35–6   **Performing Tracheostomy Care** (continued)

Evaluation

- Assess the area around the stoma site for signs of skin breakdown.
- Evaluate the patient's tolerance of the procedure. Note whether there were any signs of respiratory distress.

Patient Teaching

- Explain to the patient and his family that bloody secretions are normal for 2 to 3 days after tracheostomy insertion or for 24 hours after a tracheostomy change.
- Tell the patient to inform the nurse immediately if the tracheostomy becomes dislodged.
- Teach tracheostomy care to the patient and caregiver if the tracheostomy is expected to remain long term.

Home Care

- Clean technique can be used for tracheostomy care if the tracheostomy is more than 1 month old.
- Instruct the patient and caregiver about home oxygen therapy and suctioning, if necessary.
- Demonstrate tracheostomy care to the caregiver, and ask for a return demonstration.
- Provide the patient and caregiver with information about where to purchase tracheostomy care supplies.
- Supply the patient and caregiver with contact information of healthcare personnel who can be reached for advice or emergencies.

Documentation

- Document the date and time that you performed tracheostomy care.
- Note the color, amount, consistency, and odor of secretions.
- Note the condition of the stoma and skin around the stoma site; note the presence of drainage, redness, or swelling.
- Document respiratory status, including respiratory rate, depth, and pattern; skin color; and breath sounds.
- Note the patient's tolerance of the procedure.
- If problems arose, document any interventions that were necessary.

Sample of a narrative note:

3/25/07	0600	Trach. care performed without difficulty. Patient tolerated procedure without gagging, coughing, or pallor. Scant amount of thin, white, odorless secretions suctioned via trach. Trach site without drainage, redness, or swelling. 8 mm disposable inner cannula replaced. RR = 20; respirations regular, nonlabored; breath sounds clear. Remains on room air, pulse oximetry 98%—
		— E. Jacobs, RN

PROCEDURE 35–7

Performing Oropharyngeal and Nasopharyngeal Suctioning

 For steps to follow in *all* procedures, refer to the inside back cover of this book.

critical aspects

- Position the patient in semi-Fowler's position, with the face turned toward you for oropharyngeal suctioning or the neck hyperextended for nasopharyneal suctioning.
- Turn on the suction, and adjust the pressure regulator according to agency policy (typically 100 to 120 mm Hg for adults, 95 to 110 mm Hg for children, and 50 to 95 mm Hg for infants).
- Prepare the suction equipment. If you are using the nasal approach, open the water-soluble lubricant.
- Pick up the suction catheter with your dominant (sterile) hand, and attach it to the connection tubing.
- Approximate the depth the suction catheter should be inserted.
- Remove the oxygen delivery device.
- If the patient's oxygen saturation is less than 94%, or if he is in any distress, you may need to administer supplemental oxygen before, during, and after suctioning (see Procedure 35–5).
- Lubricate and insert the suction catheter into the mouth or naris.
- Gently advance the catheter the premeasured distance into the pharynx.
- Place a finger over the suction control port of the catheter to engage the suction.
- Apply suction while you withdraw the catheter, using a continuous rotating motion.
- After you withdraw the catheter, clear it by placing the tip into the container of sterile saline and applying suction.
- Lubricate the catheter, and repeat suctioning as needed, allowing 20-second intervals between suctioning.
- Dispose of equipment in a biohazard receptacle.

Equipment

- Portable or wall suction device with connection tubing and a collection canister
- Linen-saver pad or towel
- Sterile suction catheter kit (12 to 18 Fr. for adults, 8 to 10 Fr. for children, and 5 to 8 Fr. for infants). If a kit isn't available, collect the following: sterile gloves, sterile suction catheter of the appropriate size, and a sterile container (If you will suction both the oropharynx and the nasopharynx, you need a separate sterile catheter for each.)
- Pour-bottle of sterile normal saline solution
- Sterile basin or other container for fluids
- Face shield or goggles
- Sterile gloves
- Water-soluble lubricant for nasopharyngeal suctioning
- Sputum trap, if a specimen is needed

Delegation

Do not delegate oropharyngeal and nasopharyngeal suctioning to an LPN or UAP, because these procedures require theoretical knowledge, assessment skills, sterile technique, and problem-solving ability. However, the UAP (and the client or family) can use a Yankauer tube to suction the oral cavity because this is not a sterile procedure.

Assessment

- Assess respiratory status, including respiratory rate, depth, and rhythm; breath sounds; color; and pulse oximetry results.

Determines whether the patient requires suctioning. Suctioning removes oxygen from airways, so it should be done only as necessary.

- Assess for signs that indicate the need for suctioning: gurgling sounds during respiration, restlessness, labored respirations, decreased oxygen saturation, increased heart and respiratory rates, and the presence of adventitious breath sounds during auscultation.

Suctioning should be performed only when necessary to prevent unnecessary tissue trauma.

▶

PROCEDURE 35–7

Performing Oropharyngeal and Nasopharyngeal Suctioning *(continued)*

Procedural Steps

Step 1 Position the patient.

Variation Oropharyngeal Suctioning

a. Position the patient in semi-Fowler's position, with his head turned toward you.

This position facilitates inserting the suction catheter and prevents straining your back.

Variation Nasopharyngeal Suctioning

b. Position the patient in semi-Fowler's position with his head hyperextended, unless contraindicated.

This position facilitates inserting the suction catheter and prevents straining your back.

Step 2 Place the linen-saver pad or towel on the patient's chest.

Prevents soiling of the patient's gown during suctioning.

Step 3 Put on a face shield or goggles.

Protects you from contamination with secretions that may splash during suctioning.

Step 4 Turn on the wall suction or portable suction machine, and adjust the pressure regulator according to agency policy (typically 100 to 120 mm Hg for adults, 95 to 110 mm Hg for children, and 50 to 95 mm Hg for infants).

The suction regulator must be set appropriately to prevent tissue trauma and hypoxia.

Step 5 Test the suction equipment by occluding the connection tubing.

Testing the equipment ensures proper functioning before use.

Step 6 Open the suction catheter kit or, if a kit isn't available, the gathered equipment. If you are using the nasal approach and if the patient does not have a nasal trumpet, open the water-soluble lubricant.

Step 7 Don sterile gloves; consider (and keep) your dominant hand sterile; consider your nondominant hand nonsterile.

Keeping the dominant hand sterile prevents contaminating the upper airways with an unsterile suction catheter.

Step 8 Pour sterile saline into the sterile container, using your nondominant hand.

Sterile saline is necessary to clear the suction catheter of secretions after suctioning. The outside of the saline container is not sterile; it would contaminate your dominant hand.

Step 9 Pick up the suction catheter with your dominant hand, and attach it to the connection tubing (to suction).

Step 10 Put the tip of the suction catheter into the sterile container of normal saline solution, and suction a small amount of normal saline solution through the suction catheter. Apply suction by placing a finger over the suction control port.

Ensures that the suction equipment is functioning properly.

Step 11 Approximate the depth to which you will insert the suction catheter.

Variation Oropharyngeal Suctioning

a. Measure the distance between the edge of the patient's mouth and the tip of the patient's ear lobe.

Determines the proper distance you should insert the suction catheter for oropharyngeal suctioning.

Variation Nasopharyngeal Suctioning

b. Measure the distance between the tip of the patient's nose and the tip of the patient's ear lobe.

Helps determine the proper distance you should insert the suction catheter for nasopharyngeal suctioning.

Step 12 Using your nondominant hand, remove the oxygen delivery device, if present. Have the patient take several slow, deep breaths. If the patient's oxygen saturation is less than 94%, or if he is in any distress, you may need to administer supplemental oxygen before, during, and after suctioning. See Procedure 35–5.

Deep breathing hyperoxygenates the patient and helps prevent hypoxia during suctioning.

Step 13 Lubricate and insert the suction catheter.

Variation Oropharyngeal Suctioning

a. Lubricate the catheter tip with the normal saline solution.

Eases catheter insertion.

b. Using your dominant hand, gently but quickly insert the suction catheter along the side of the patient's mouth into the oropharynx.

Inserting the suction catheter along the side of the mouth prevents gagging. ▼

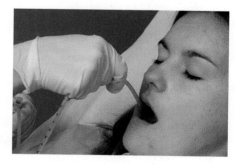

c. Advance the suction catheter quickly to the premeasured distance (usually 7 to 10 cm in the adult), being careful not to force the catheter.

Ensures that the suction catheter will reach the pharynx. Forcing the catheter during insertion may cause tissue trauma.

Variation Nasopharyngeal Suctioning

d. Lubricate the catheter tip with the water-soluble lubricant.

PROCEDURE 35–7

Performing Oropharyngeal and Nasopharyngeal Suctioning *(continued)*

Eases passage of the suction catheter through the naris. Water-soluble lubricant is preferred because it will dissolve if it accidentally enters the lungs, whereas an oil-based lubricant (e.g., petroleum jelly or lotion) will not dissolve in the respiratory tract and causes complications if it enters the lungs.

e. Using your dominant hand, gently but quickly insert the suction catheter into the naris.

Prevents trauma to the nares. ▼

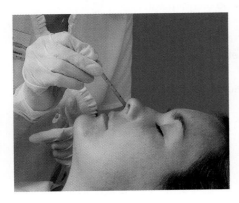

f. Advance the suction catheter, aiming downward to the premeasured distance (usually 13 to 15 cm in the adult) and being careful not to force the catheter. If you meet resistance, you may need to try the other naris.

Advancing the suction catheter the premeasured distance ensures that the suction catheter will reach the pharynx. Forcing the catheter during insertion may cause tissue trauma.

Step 14 Place a finger (e.g., your thumb) over the suction control port of the suction catheter, and start suctioning the patient. Apply suction while you withdraw the catheter, using a continuous rotating motion. Limit suctioning to 5 to 10 seconds.

Using a continuous rotating motion while withdrawing the catheter prevents trauma to any one area of the airway. Limiting suctioning to less than 10 seconds prevents hypoxia.

Step 15 After you withdraw the catheter, clear it by placing the tip of the catheter into the container of sterile saline and applying suction.

Ensures patency of the catheter for repeat suctioning.

Step 16 Lubricate the catheter, and repeat suctioning as needed, allowing at least 20-second intervals between suctioning.

Several passes with the suction catheter may be needed to clear the airway of secretions. Total suctioning time should be limited to 5 minutes, however, to prevent trauma and hypoxia.

Variation Nasopharyngeal Suctioning

Each time you repeat suction, alternate nares.

Alternating nares prevents trauma to one naris.

Step 17 Coil the suction catheter in your dominant hand. Pull the sterile glove off over the coiled catheter. (Alternatively, wrap the catheter around your dominant, gloved hand, and hold the catheter as you remove the glove over it.) Discard the glove containing the catheter in a biohazard receptacle designated by your agency.

Coiling the catheter inside the glove prevents contamination with secretions.

Step 18 Using your nondominant hand, clear the connecting tubing of secretions by placing the tip into the container of sterile saline.

Ensures patency and prepares the equipment for future use.

Step 19 Dispose of equipment in water-resistant waste container/bag, and make sure new suction supplies are readily available for future suctioning needs.

The patient may require suctioning at any time, so equipment must be readily available.

Step 20 Provide mouth care.

Promotes patient comfort and clears the mouth of any secretions the patient may have expectorated.

Step 21 Position the patient in a comfortable position, and allow him to rest.

Promoting comfort and allowing for a period of rest helps the patient recover from suctioning, which may be very tiring.

Evaluation

- Assess the color, consistency, and amount of secretions.
- Evaluate the patient's tolerance of the procedure. Note whether there were signs of respiratory distress during the procedure.
- Evaluate the effectiveness of the procedure by comparing breath sounds, vital signs, and pulse oximetry before and after the procedure.

➤

PROCEDURE 35–7   **Performing Oropharyngeal and Nasopharyngeal Suctioning** *(continued)*

Patient Teaching

- Explain the importance of administering supplemental oxygen to the patient before suctioning.
- Inform the patient that coughing typically increases with suctioning.
- Demonstrate oropharyngeal or nasopharyngeal suctioning to the caregiver, and ask for a return demonstration if suctioning will be required at home.

Home Care

- Instruct the family and caregiver where to obtain suction equipment.
- Provide the patient and caregiver with contact information of healthcare personnel who can be reached for advice or emergencies.
- Explain that the procedure can be performed using clean technique instead of sterile technique in the home setting.
- Instruct the caregiver that suction catheters can be cleaned for reuse by washing them with soapy water and then boiling them for 10 minutes. After they are cleaned, rinse the catheters with normal saline solution or tap water.
- Change the secretion collection container every 24 hours, or clean it according to home care agency guidelines every 24 hours.

Documentation

- Document the date, time, and reason you performed suctioning.
- Note the suction technique you used and the catheter size.
- Note color, consistency, and odor of secretions.
- Document the patient's respiratory status before and after the procedure.
- Document the patient's tolerance of the procedure and any complications that occurred as a result of the procedure, with resulting interventions.

Sample of a narrative note:

3/15/07	2200	Respirations labored, with a rate of 28 breaths/minute. Pulse oximetry on room air 92%. Breath sounds with rhonchi scattered throughout. Gurgling audible in the upper airways. Patient unable to mobilize secretions with coughing. Suctioned by the nasopharyngeal route using a 14 Fr. catheter. Approximately 30 mL of thin, tan, odorless secretions obtained. Respirations nonlabored, with a rate of 20 breaths/minute after suctioning. Lungs clear on auscultation, no gurgling audible. Pulse oximetry 96%. Patient tolerated the procedure without difficulty. ———— W. Earl, RN

| PROCEDURE 35–8 | **Performing Orotracheal and Nasotracheal Suctioning** |

 For steps to follow in *all* procedures, refer to the inside back cover of this book.

critical aspects

- Position the patient in semi-Fowler's position.
- Turn on the wall suction or portable suction machine, and adjust the pressure regulator according to agency policy (typically 100 to 120 mm Hg for adults, 95 to 110 mm Hg for children, and 50 to 95 mm Hg for infants).
- Prepare the suction equipment. If you are using the nasal approach, open the water-soluble lubricant.
- Don sterile glove(s).
- Pick up the suction catheter with your dominant hand, and attach it to the connection tubing.
- Approximate the depth the suction catheter should be inserted.
- Administer supplemental oxygen, if indicated (see Procedure 35–5).
- Insert the catheter in the nose or mouth, and advance it to the pharynx.
- Advance the catheter from the pharynx to the trachea by passing the catheter when the patient inhales.
- Place a finger over the suction control port of the catheter.
- Apply suction while you withdraw the catheter, using a continuous rotating motion. Apply suction for no longer than 10 seconds.
- After you withdraw the catheter, clear it by placing the tip of the catheter into the container of sterile saline and applying suction.
- Lubricate the catheter, and repeat suctioning as needed, allowing intervals of at least 30 seconds between suctioning.
- Replace the oxygen source.
- Coil the suction catheter in your dominant hand. Pull the sterile glove off over the coiled catheter. Discard the glove containing the catheter in a receptacle designated by your agency.
- Dispose of equipment, and make sure new suction supplies are readily available for future suctioning.
- Provide mouth care.

Equipment

- Portable or wall suction device with connection tubing and a collection canister
- Linen-saver pad or towel
- Sterile suction catheter kit (12 to 18 Fr. for adults, 8 to 10 Fr. for children, and 5 to 8 Fr. for infants). If a kit isn't available, collect the following: sterile gloves, sterile suction catheter of the appropriate size, and a sterile container
- Pour-bottle of sterile normal saline solution
- Sterile basin or other container for fluids
- Face shield or goggles
- Water-soluble lubricant for nasotracheal suctioning
- Sputum trap, if a specimen is needed

Delegation

You should not delegate orotracheal and nasotracheal suctioning to an LPN or UAP, because these procedures require theoretical knowledge, assessment skills, and problem-solving ability.

Assessment

- Assess respiratory status, including respiratory rate, depth, and rhythm; breath sounds; color; and pulse oximetry results.

Helps determine whether the patient requires suctioning. Suctioning removes oxygen from airways and should be done only when essential. ➤

PROCEDURE 35–8   Performing Orotracheal and Nasotracheal Suctioning *(continued)*

- Assess for signs that indicate the need for suctioning: gurgling sounds during respiration, restlessness, labored respirations, decreased oxygen saturation, increased heart and respiratory rates, and the presence of adventitious breath sounds during auscultation.

Suctioning should be performed only when necessary to prevent unnecessary tissue trauma.

Procedural Steps

Step 1 Position the patient.

Variation Orotracheal Suctioning

a. Position the patient in semi-Fowler's position, with the head turned to face you.

Facilitates inserting the suction catheter and prevents back strain.

Variation Nasotracheal Suctioning

b. Position the patient in semi-Fowler's position, with his head hyperextended, unless contraindicated.

Facilitates inserting the suction catheter and prevents back strain.

Step 2 Place the linen-saver pad or towel on the patient's chest.

Prevents soiling of the patient's gown during suctioning.

Step 3 Put on a face shield or goggles.

Protects you from contamination with secretions that may splash during suctioning.

Step 4 Turn on the wall suction or portable suction machine, and adjust the pressure regulator according to agency policy (typically 100 to 120 mm Hg for adults, 95 to 110 mm Hg for children, and 50 to 95 mm Hg for infants).

The suction regulator must be set appropriately to prevent tissue trauma and hypoxia.

Step 5 Test the suction equipment by occluding the connection tubing.

Ensures proper functioning before you insert the catheter in the patient's airway.

Step 6 Open the suction catheter kit or, if a kit isn't available, the gathered equipment. If you are using the nasal approach, open the water-soluble lubricant.

Step 7 Don sterile gloves. (Alternatively, put a sterile glove on your dominant hand and a clean procedure glove on your nondominant hand.) Consider your dominant hand sterile and your nondominant hand nonsterile.

Keeping the dominant hand sterile prevents contaminating the upper airways with an unsterile suction catheter.

Step 8 Pour sterile saline into the sterile container, using your nondominant hand.

Sterile saline will be used to clear the suction catheter of secretions after suctioning.

Step 9 Pick up the suction catheter with your dominant hand, and attach it to the connection tubing, maintaining sterility of your hand and the catheter.

Prepares the suction catheter for use.

Step 10 Put the tip of the suction catheter into the sterile container of normal saline solution, and suction a small amount of normal saline solution through the suction catheter. Apply suction by placing a finger over the suction control port of the suction catheter.

Lubricates the catheter and helps ensure that the suction equipment is functioning properly.

Step 11 Using your nondominant hand, remove the oxygen delivery device, if present. If the patient's oxygen saturation is less than 94%, or if he is in any distress, you may need to administer supplemental oxygen before, during, and after suctioning. See Procedure 35–5.

Removing the oxygen delivery device facilitates suctioning.

Step 12 Have the patient take several slow, deep breaths.

Taking several slow deep breaths promotes relaxation and helps hyperoxygenate the patient before suctioning.

Step 13 Approximate the depth you should insert the suction catheter. For adults, insert the catheter about 15 cm for an oral approach and 20 cm for a nasal approach. Be careful not to contaminate the catheter while you measure.

Variation Oral Approach

a. Measure the distance between the edge of the patient's mouth to the tip of the ear lobe and down to the bottom of the neck. ▼

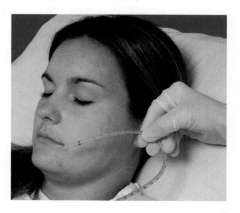

PROCEDURE 35–8

Performing Orotracheal and Nasotracheal Suctioning *(continued)*

Variation Nasal Approach

b. Measure the distance from the tip of the nose to the tip of the ear lobe and down to the bottom of the neck.

Inserting the suction catheter the proper distance prevents trauma and ensures suctioning of the trachea.

Step 14 Lubricate and insert the suction catheter.

Eases passage of the suction catheter.

Variation Orotracheal Suctioning

a. Lubricate the suction catheter tip with the normal saline solution.

Eases insertion.

b. Using your dominant hand, gently but quickly insert the suction catheter along the side of the patient's mouth into the oropharynx.

Prevents gagging.

c. When the patient inhales, advance the suction catheter to the predetermined distance (usually 15 cm in the adult), being careful not to force the catheter.

Advancing the suction catheter when the patient inhales ensures that the catheter enters the trachea rather than the esophagus. Forcing the catheter during insertion may cause tissue trauma.

Variation Nasotracheal Suctioning

d. Lubricate the catheter tip with the water-soluble lubricant.

Eases passage of the suction catheter through the nares. Water-soluble lubricant is preferred because it will dissolve if it accidentally enters the lungs, whereas an oil-based lubricant (e.g., petroleum jelly) won't dissolve in the respiratory tract and causes complications if it enters the lungs.

e. Using your dominant hand, gently but quickly insert the suction catheter into the naris and down to the pharynx.

Prevents trauma to the naris.

f. When the patient inhales, advance the suction catheter, gently aiming downward to the predetermined distance (usually 20 cm in the adult), being careful not to force the catheter.

Ensures that the catheter enters the trachea. Forcing the catheter during insertion may cause tissue trauma.

Step 15 Place a finger (e.g., your thumb) over the suction control port of the catheter. Apply suction while you withdraw the catheter, using a continuous rotating motion. Apply suction for no longer than 10 seconds.

Using a continuous rotating motion while withdrawing the catheter prevents trauma to any one area of the airway. Limiting suctioning to less than 10 seconds prevents hypoxia. ▼

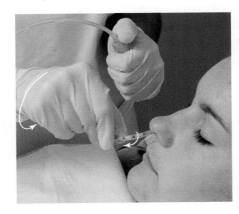

Step 16 After you withdraw the catheter, clear it by placing the tip of the catheter into the container of sterile saline and applying suction.

Ensures patency of the catheter for repeat suctioning. ▼

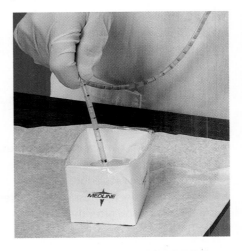

Step 17 Lubricate the catheter, and repeat suctioning as needed, allowing intervals of at least 30 seconds between suctioning. Reapply oxygen between suctioning efforts, if required.

Several passes with the suction catheter may be needed to clear the airway of secretions. Total suctioning time should be limited to 5 minutes, however, to prevent trauma and hypoxia.

Step 18 Replace the oxygen source.

Prevents hypoxia.

Step 19 Coil the suction catheter in your dominant hand (alternatively, wrap it around your dominant hand). Hold the catheter while you pull the sterile glove off over it. Discard the glove containing the catheter in a water-resistant receptacle (e.g., bag) designated by your agency.

Coiling the catheter inside the glove prevents contaminating the environment with secretions.

➤

PROCEDURE 35–8 Performing Orotracheal and Nasotracheal Suctioning *(continued)*

Step 20 Using your nondominant hand, clear the connecting tubing of secretions by placing the tip into the container of sterile saline.

Ensures patency and prepares the equipment for future use.

Step 21 Dispose of equipment, and make sure new suction supplies are readily available for future suctioning.

The patient may require suctioning at any time, so equipment must be readily available.

Step 22 Provide mouth care.

Providing mouth care promotes patient comfort and clears the mouth of any secretions the patient may have expectorated.

Step 23 Position the patient in a comfortable position, and allow him to rest.

Promoting comfort and allowing for a period of rest helps the patient recover from the stress of suctioning.

Evaluation

- Assess the color, consistency, and amount of secretions.
- Evaluate the patient's tolerance of the procedure. Note whether there were signs of respiratory distress during the procedure.
- Evaluate the effectiveness of the procedure by comparing breath sounds, vital signs, and pulse oximetry before and after the procedure.

Patient Teaching

- Explain the importance of administering supplemental oxygen or of taking several deep breaths before suctioning.
- Inform the patient that coughing typically increases with suctioning.
- Demonstrate orotracheal or nasotracheal suctioning to the caregiver, and ask for a return demonstration if suctioning will be required at home.

Home Care

- Instruct the family and caregiver about where to obtain suction equipment.
- Provide the patient and caregiver with contact information of healthcare personnel who can be reached for advice or emergencies.
- Explain that the procedure can be performed using clean technique instead of sterile technique in the home.
- Instruct the caregiver that suction catheters can be cleaned for reuse by washing them with soapy water and then boiling them for 10 minutes. After they are cleaned, rinse the catheters with normal saline solution or tap water.
- Change the secretion collection container every 24 hours, or clean it according to home care agency guidelines every 24 hours.

PROCEDURE 35–8 **Performing Orotracheal and Nasotracheal Suctioning** *(continued)*

Documentation

- Document the date, time, and reason you performed suctioning.
- Note the suction technique you used and the catheter size.
- Note the color, consistency, and odor of secretions.
- Document the patient's respiratory status before and after the procedure.
- Document the patient's tolerance of the procedure and any complications that occurred as a result of the procedure.
- Document any interventions you performed to address complications that occurred.

Sample of a narrative note:

10/8/07	2130	Patient's breath sounds revealed rhonchi throughout both lung fields. Respirations 36 breaths/minute and slightly labored. Pulse ox. 89% on 40% aerosol mask. Nasotracheal suctioning performed using a 14 Fr. catheter. Moderate amount of creamy, yellow, odorless secretions obtained. After suctioning, breath sounds included a few scattered crackles. Respiratory rate 28 breaths/minute and nonlabored. Pulse ox. 93 %. Patient tolerated suctioning without difficulty. —S. Hunter, RN

PROCEDURE 35–9

Performing Tracheostomy or Endotracheal Suctioning

For steps to follow in *all* procedures, refer to the inside back cover of this book.

critical aspects

- Use sterile, modified sterile, or clean technique, according to agency policy and patient status.
- Position the patient in semi-Fowler's position, unless contraindicated.
- Turn on the wall suction or portable suction machine, and adjust the pressure regulator (typically 100 to 120 mm Hg for adults, 95 to 110 mm Hg for children, and 50 to 95 mm Hg for infants).
- Pick up the suction catheter with your dominant hand, and attach it to the connecting tubing. (Consider your dominant hand sterile and your nondominant hand unsterile.)
- Hyperoxygenate the patient according to agency policy and patient need by using the resuscitation bag or the 100% button on the ventilator.
- Insert the suction catheter gently, with suction off, into the endotracheal tube or tracheostomy tube.
- Advance the suction catheter, gently aiming downward and being careful not to force the catheter. Advance the catheter until you meet resistance.
- Apply suction as you withdraw the catheter. Make sure to apply suction for no longer than 10 seconds.
- Repeat suctioning as needed, allowing intervals of at least 30 seconds between suctioning. Make sure to hyperoxygenate the patient between each pass.
- Replace the oxygen source, if you removed the patient from the source during suctioning.
- Provide mouth care.
- Reposition the patient to provide comfort and prevent pressure ulcers.

35–9A: For Using Inline Closed Suctioning Equipment

- Prepare the equipment. You need to perform these steps only once per day:
  1. Open the inline suction catheter, using sterile technique.
  2. Remove the adapter on the ventilator tubing.
  3. Attach the inline suction catheter equipment to the ventilator tubing.
  4. Reconnect the adaptor on the ventilator tubing.
  5. Attach the other end of the inline suction catheter to the connection tubing placed to suction.
- Position the patient in semi-Fowler's position, unless contraindicated.
- Turn on the wall suction or portable suction machine, and adjust the pressure regulator (typically 100 to 120 mm Hg for adults, 95 to 110 mm Hg for children, and 50 to 95 mm Hg for infants).
- Hyperoxygenate the patient according to agency policy.
- Don clean procedure gloves.
- If a lock is present on the suction control port, unlock it.
- Gently insert the suction catheter into the airway by maneuvering the catheter within the sterile sleeve.
- Advance the suction catheter into the airway, being careful not to force the catheter. Advance the catheter until you meet resistance.
- Apply suction while withdrawing the catheter. Make sure to apply suction for no longer than 10 seconds.
- Withdraw the inline suction catheter completely into the sleeve. The indicator line on the catheter should appear through the sleeve.
- Attach the prefilled, 10 mL container of normal saline solution to the saline port located on the inline equipment. Squeeze the 10 mL container of normal saline solution while applying suction. Lock the suction regulator port.

PROCEDURE 35–9

Performing Tracheostomy or Endotracheal Suctioning *(continued)*

Equipment

- Portable or wall suction device with tubing and a collection canister
- Linen-saver pad or towel
- Resuscitation bag connected to oxygen source
- Closed suction system or sterile suction catheter kit (12 to 18 Fr. for adults, 8 to 10 Fr. for children, and 5 to 8 Fr. for infants). If a kit is not available, collect the following: sterile or procedure gloves, a sterile container, and a sterile suction catheter of the appropriate size. As a rule of thumb, use the largest catheter that fits without forcing inside the tracheostomy tube.
- Pour-bottle of sterile, normal saline solution; sterile basin or container for fluids
- Prefilled 10-mL containers of normal saline solution
- Face shield or goggles

Delegation

Typically you should not delegate tracheostomy or endotracheal suctioning to an LPN or UAP, because both procedures require theoretical knowledge, assessment skills, and problem-solving ability. However if the patient has a permanent tracheostomy tube in place and the patient will require long-term care, care can be delegated to assistive personnel.

Assessment

- Assess the patient's respiratory status, including respiratory rate, depth, and rhythm; breath sounds; color; and pulse oximetry results.

Helps determine whether the patient requires suctioning.

- Assess for signs that indicate the need for suctioning: restlessness, labored respirations, decreased oxygen saturation, increased heart and respiratory rates, and the presence of adventitious breath sounds during auscultation.

Suctioning should be performed only when necessary to prevent unnecessary oxygen desaturation and tissue trauma.

Procedural Steps

Step 1 Position the patient in semi-Fowler's position, unless contraindicated.

Promotes lung expansion and oxygenation.

Step 2 Place the linen-saver pad or towel on the patient's chest.

Prevents soiling of the patient's gown during suctioning.

Step 3 Put on a face shield or goggles.

Protects you from contamination with secretions that may splash during suctioning.

Step 4 Turn on the wall suction or portable suction machine, and adjust the pressure regulator according to agency policy (typically 100 to 120 mm Hg for adults, 95 to 110 mm Hg for children, and 50 to 95 mm Hg for infants).

Choosing the appropriate pressure prevents tissue trauma and ensures successful suctioning.

Step 5 Test the suction equipment by occluding the connection tubing.

Ensures proper functioning before you insert suction catheter.

Step 6 Open the suction catheter kit or (if a kit isn't available) the gathered equipment.

Sterile technique is necessary to avoid contaminating the upper airway when you introduce the suction catheter.

Step 7 Don sterile gloves; consider your dominant hand sterile and your nondominant hand nonsterile. Alternately, use clean procedure gloves.

Keeping your dominant hand sterile prevents contamination of the suction catheter.

Step 8 Pour sterile saline into the sterile container, using your nondominant hand.

Sterile saline is used to clear the suction catheter of secretions after suctioning.

Step 9 Pick up the suction catheter with your dominant hand, and attach it to the connection tubing.

Prepares the suction catheter for use.

Step 10 Put the tip of the suction catheter into the sterile container of normal saline solution, and suction a small amount of normal saline solution through the suction catheter. Apply suction by placing a finger over the suction control port of the suction catheter.

Lubricates the catheter and helps ensure that the suction equipment is functioning properly.

Step 11 Hyperoxygenate the patient according to agency policy and patient status.

Helps prevent hypoxia during suctioning. Suctioning clears secretions, but it also removes oxygen from airways.

Variation Patient Requiring Mechanical Ventilation

a. Press the 100% O_2 button on the ventilator, or attach the resuscitation bag to the endotracheal tube or tracheostomy tube and manually hyperoxygenate the patient by compressing the resuscitation bag three to five times as the patient inhales. Remove the resuscitation bag, and place it next to the patient when you are finished.

➤

PROCEDURE 35–9

Performing Tracheostomy or Endotracheal Suctioning *(continued)*

Ventilators typically have a button that, when pushed, allows you to hyperoxygenate the patient for a total of 2 minutes. Once this time period elapses, the ventilator automatically resumes its previous settings. Some agencies require the nurse to manually hyperoxygenate the patient; follow agency policy.

Variation Patient Not Requiring Mechanical Ventilation

b. If the patient does not require mechanical ventilation, attach the resuscitation bag to the tracheostomy or endotracheal tube, and hyperoxygenate the patient by compressing the resuscitation bag three to five times. Remove the resuscitation bag, and place it next to the patient when you are finished.

Hyperoxygenation must be performed manually if the patient does not require mechanical ventilation. ▼

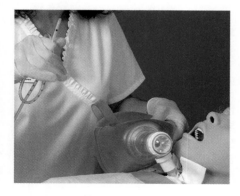

Step 12 Perform suctioning.
a. Lubricate the suction catheter tip with the normal saline solution.

Eases passage of the suction catheter through the endotracheal tube or tracheostomy tube.

b. Using your dominant hand, gently but quickly insert the suction

catheter into the endotracheal tube or tracheostomy tube.

Prevents airway trauma. ▼

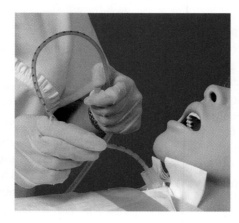

c. Advance the suction catheter, with suction off, gently aiming downward, and being careful not to force the catheter.

Forcing the catheter during insertion may cause tissue trauma.

d. Apply suction while you withdraw the catheter. Make sure to apply suction for no longer than 10 seconds.

Applying suction for longer than 10 seconds causes hypoxia and may cause tissue trauma.

Step 13 Repeat suctioning as needed, allowing at least 30-second intervals between suctioning. Make sure to hyperoxygentate the patient between each pass.

Several passes with the suction catheter may be needed to clear the airway of secretions. Total suctioning time should be limited to 5 minutes, however, to prevent trauma and hypoxia.

Step 14 Replace the oxygen source, if the patient was removed from the source during suctioning.

The oxygen source must be replaced to prevent hypoxia.

Step 15 Coil the suction catheter in your dominant hand (alternatively, wrap it around your dominant hand). Pull the sterile glove off over the coiled catheter. Discard the glove containing the catheter

in a water-resistant receptacle designated by your agency.

Coiling the catheter inside the glove prevents contaminating the environment with secretions.

Step 16 Using your nondominant hand, clear the connecting tubing of secretions by placing the tip into the container of sterile saline.

Clears the tubing, preparing it for later reuse.

Step 17 Provide mouth care.

Clears the mouth of secretions and bacteria, which place the patient at risk for nosocomial pneumonia.

Step 18 Reposition the patient.

Promotes comfort and prevents skin breakdown.

Important Note: No formal recommendation can be made about whether to wear sterile or clean gloves when performing endotracheal suctioning, according to the Centers for Disease Control (Tablan, Anderson, Besser, Bridges, and Hajjeh, 2004). Although sterile technique has been the typical method used in hospitals, the trend now is toward a modified sterile technique; and clean technique is the usual method for suctioning in the home setting.

If the patient has an increased susceptibility to infection, sterile technique may be advised. Nonsterile, disposable gloves should be worn for the protection of any caregiver that is not a family member and by those concerned about personally acquiring infection.

- *Sterile technique* is the use of a sterile catheter and supplies with sterile gloves.
- *Modified sterile technique* is use of a sterile catheter and supplies, but with nonsterile procedure gloves.
- *Clean technique* is use of a clean catheter and clean hands or nonsterile gloves. The portion of the catheter that will be inserted in the tracheostomy tube is protected to avoid contact with unclean surfaces.

You should follow the procedure used in your organization or school.

PROCEDURE 35–9A

Performing Tracheostomy or Endotracheal Suctioning Using an Inline Closed System

Procedural Steps

Step 1 Prepare the equipment. An inline suction unit is available only for patients on a mechanical ventilator. Most agencies require the respiratory therapy department to set up the inline closed suction equipment. If this is not your agency's policy, perform the following to prepare equipment for future use. You need to perform these steps only once per day:

a. Open the suction catheter, using sterile technique.

The inline suction catheter should remain sterile to prevent contamination of the airways.

b. Remove the adapter on the ventilator tubing.

Prepares the tubing for attachment of the inline suction catheter.

c. Attach the closed suction catheter equipment to the ventilator tubing.

d. Reconnect the adapter on the ventilator tubing.

Positions the suction catheter properly for advancing the catheter and suctioning.

e. Attach the other end of the inline suction catheter to the connection tubing placed to suction.

Connects the suction catheter to the suction source. ▼

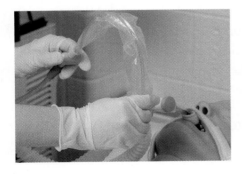

Step 2 Position the patient in semi-Fowler's position, unless contraindicated.

Promotes lung expansion and oxygenation.

Step 3 Turn on the wall suction or portable suction machine, and adjust the pressure regulator according to agency policy (typically 100 to 120 mm Hg for adults, 95 to 110 mm Hg for children, and 50 to 95 mm Hg for infants).

Choosing the appropriate pressure prevents tissue trauma and ensures successful suctioning.

Step 4 Hyperoxygenate the patient according to agency policy.

Hyperoxygenating the patient before suctioning helps prevent hypoxia during suctioning.

Step 5 Don clean procedure gloves.

The suction catheter is now contained within a sterile unit. You do not need to wear sterile gloves.

Step 6 If a lock is present on the suction control port, unlock it.

Readies the suction control port for suctioning.

Step 7 With your dominant hand, pick up the suction catheter contained within the plastic sleeve.

Using the dominant hand improves dexterity.

Step 8 Gently insert the suction catheter into the airway by maneuvering the catheter within the sterile sleeve.

Step 9 Advance the suction catheter into the airway, being careful not to force the catheter. Advance the catheter until you meet resistance.

Forcing the catheter during insertion may cause airway trauma.

Step 10 Apply suction by depressing the button over the suction control port as you withdraw the catheter. Make sure to apply suction for no longer than 10 seconds.

Applying suction for longer than 10 seconds causes hypoxia and may cause tissue trauma.

Step 11 Withdraw the suction catheter completely into the enclosed sleeve. The indicator line on the catheter should appear through the sleeve.

The indicator line is a safety mechanism designed to make sure the suction catheter is withdrawn completely.

Step 12 Attach the prefilled, 10 mL container of normal saline solution to the saline port located on the inline equipment.

Provides a flush solution to clear the suction catheter of secretions.

Step 13 Squeeze the 10 mL container of normal saline solution while applying suction.

Clears the catheter of secretions preparing the catheter for repeat use.

Step 14 Lock the suction regulator port.

Prevents you from inadvertently applying suction.

➤

PROCEDURE 35–9   **Performing Tracheostomy or Endotracheal Suctioning** *(continued)*

Evaluation

- Assess the color, amount, and consistency of secretions.
- Evaluate the patient's tolerance of the procedure. Note whether there were signs of respiratory distress during the procedure.
- Evaluate the effectiveness of the procedure by comparing breath sounds, vital signs, and pulse oximetry before and after suctioning.

Patient Teaching

- Teach the patient and caregiver how to perform suctioning if the patient will be discharged with an artificial airway. Make sure they can successfully provide a return demonstration.
- Teach the caregiver strategies for managing the patient's airway at home.

Home Care

- Instruct the family and caregiver where to obtain suction equipment.
- Provide the patient and caregiver with contact information of healthcare personnel who can be reached for advice or emergencies.
- Provide the patient and caregiver with information about home oxygen therapy.

Documentation

- Document the date, time, and reason you performed suctioning.
- Note the size of the suction catheter you used.
- Note the amount, color, consistency, and odor of secretions.
- Document the patient's respiratory status before and after the procedure.
- Document the patient's tolerance of the procedure.
- Document any complications that occurred as a result of the procedure, and document interventions you made in response.

Sample of a narrative note for patient on ventilator:

9/20/07	0800	Patient coughing on ventilator. Breath sounds with rhonchi throughout. Pulse oximetry 91%. Ventilator settings: TV 650 mL, FiO_2 60%, RR 14, PEEP 5 cm. Patient placed on FiO_2 100% and then suctioned using a 14 Fr. catheter. Patient suctioned for copious amounts of green, foul-smelling secretions. Breath sounds after suctioning reveal few scattered rhonchi. Sputum specimen sent for culture and sensitivity. Dr. Snyder made aware of characteristics of secretions. Portable chest x-ray ordered.

L. Brown, RN

PROCEDURE 35–9   Performing Tracheostomy or Endotracheal Suctioning *(continued)*

Sample of a narrative note for a patient with a tracheostomy:

06/05/07	1350	Patient receiving oxygen via 30% trach collar. Pulse ox 93%, RR 22 breaths/minute, heart rate 90 beats/minute, blood pressure 146/90 mm Hg. Upper airway rhonchi auscultated. Patient hyperoxygenated with 100% oxygen using a resuscitation bag. Patient suctioned for a moderate amount of thick, yellow, odorless secretions using a 12 Fr. suction catheter. Patient tolerated the procedure without signs of distress. Patient returned to 30% trach collar; lungs clear to auscultation. Pulse ox 98%, RR 18 breaths/minute, heart rate 80 beats/minute, blood pressure 126/86 mm Hg. ————————— L. Brown, RN

| PROCEDURE 35–10 | Caring for a Patient on a Mechanical Ventilator |

> For steps to follow in *all* procedures, refer to the inside back cover of this book.

critical aspects

- Prepare the resuscitation bag; keep it at the bedside.
- The respiratory therapy department is responsible for setting up mechanical ventilation in most agencies. If you must assume the responsibility, refer to the manufacturer's instructions.
- Verify ventilator settings with the physician's order.
- Check the ventilator alarm limits. Make sure they are set appropriately.
- Attach the ventilator tubing to the endotracheal tube or tracheostomy tube.
- Prepare the suctioning equipment.
- Check the ventilator tubing frequently for condensation. Drain the condensate into a collection device, or briefly disconnect the patient from the ventilator and empty the tubing into a waste receptacle, according to agency policy. Never drain the condensate into the humidifier.
- Provide the patient with an alternative form of communication, such as a letter board or white board.
- Check ventilator settings regularly.
- Give sedatives or antianxiety drugs as needed; request an order if necessary. Try to determine the cause of anxiety.
- Reposition the patient regularly, being careful not to pull on the ventilator tubing.
- Provide frequent oral care. Moisten the lips with a cool, damp cloth and water-based lubricant.
- Ensure that the call light is always within reach, and answer call light and ventilator alarms promptly.

Ventilator Terminology

Term	Explanation
F_{IO_2}	Fraction of inspired oxygen
Tidal volume	Amount of air delivered with each breath from the ventilator
Assist-control mode—also known as continuous mechanical ventilation (CMV)	The preset number of breaths per minute delivered by the machine. If the patient is able to initiate breaths, the machine will deliver a breath when the patient begins to inspire. If the patient is unable to breathe on his own, the machine will deliver the preset number of breaths in a rhythmic fashion.
Synchronized intermittent mandatory ventilation (SIMV)	A ventilator setting that delivers a minimum number of ventilations per minute if the patient does not ventilate independently. This mode is used for weaning patients from the ventilator.
Pressure support	Provides positive pressure on inspiration to decrease the workload of breathing.
Continuous positive airway pressure (CPAP)	Provides positive pressure during inspiration and expiration to keep alveoli open in a spontaneously breathing patient.
Positive end expiratory pressure (PEEP)	Provides positive pressure on expiration to keep airways open for patients on CMV or SIMV mode ventilation.

PROCEDURE 35–10

Caring for a Patient on a Mechanical Ventilator

(continued)

Equipment

- Two oxygen sources
- Air source that provides 50 psi
- Mechanical ventilator
- Resuscitation bag with oxygen connection tubing
- Humidification device
- Ventilator tubing
- Condensation collection device

Delegation

Care of a mechanically ventilated patient requires advanced knowledge of pulmonary anatomy and physiology and, therefore, should not be delegated to assistive personnel.

Assessment

- Review the patient's medical record to make sure that mechanical ventilation is included in the patient's care options outlined in his advance directive.

Mechanical ventilation may be a care option that the patient does not wish to pursue.

- If the patient's condition allows, assess the patient's comprehension of mechanical ventilation therapy.

Comprehension helps allay the patient's anxiety and promotes cooperation.

- Assess the need for mechanical ventilation by assessing the patient's respiratory status, including respiratory rate, depth, and rhythm; breath sounds; color; and pulse oximetry results.
- After mechanical ventilation is instituted, assess for chest expansion and auscultate for bilateral breath sounds.

Ensures that the patient is being ventilated.

- Assess the patient's tolerance to mechanical ventilation. Check whether the patient is breathing in synchronicity with the ventilator. Assess pulse oximetry and arterial blood gas results.

If the patient is not tolerating mechanical ventilation, she may require a sedative and paralytic agent. Changes in ventilator settings may also increase tolerance.

- Frequently assess the ventilator tubing for kinking.

Kinking of the tubing restricts airflow.

- Assess the patient's readiness for weaning from the ventilator.

Success depends on the patient's readiness to wean.

Procedural Steps

Step 1 Prepare the resuscitation bag.

The resuscitation bag should be readily available to provide ventilation in the event of an emergency. ▼

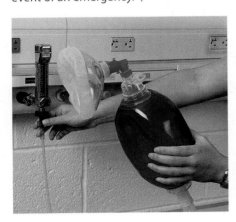

a. Attach a flow meter to one of the oxygen sources.

The flow meter helps regulate oxygen delivery.

b. Attach an adapter to the flow meter, and connect the oxygen tubing to the adapter.

The adapter helps connect the oxygen tubing to the flow meter.

c. Turn on the oxygen, and adjust the flow rate.

The oxygen must be turned on for use; the flow meter adjusts the oxygen flow.

Step 2 The respiratory therapy department is responsible for setting up mechanical ventilation in most agencies. If you must assume the responsibility, refer to the manufacturer's instructions.

The respiratory therapist is specially trained to set up mechanical ventilation.

Step 3 Verify ventilator settings with the physician's order.

Ventilator settings must be individualized according to the patient's size and condition. Incorrect settings may cause harm to the patient. ▼

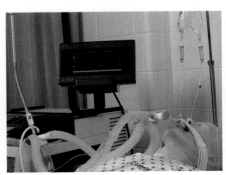

▶

PROCEDURE 35–10 Caring for a Patient on a Mechanical Ventilator
(continued)

Step 4 Check the ventilator alarm limits. Make sure they are set appropriately.

Alarm limits that are not set appropriately could result in patient harm.

Step 5 Attach the ventilator tubing to the endotracheal tube or tracheostomy tube.

Step 6 Place the ventilator tubing in the securing device.

Prevents dislodging the endotracheal tube or tracheostomy when the patient moves.

Step 7 Prepare the suction equipment (see Procedure 35–9).

Suctioning equipment should be readily available when the patient requires suctioning.

Step 8 Check the ventilator tubing frequently for condensation. Drain the fluid into a collection device, or briefly disconnect the patient from the ventilator and empty the tubing into a waste receptacle, according to agency policy. Never drain the fluid into the humidifier.

Condensation in the ventilator tubing can cause resistance to airflow. Moreover, the patient can aspirate it. The fluid should not be drained into the humidifier because the patient's secretions may have contaminated it. ▼

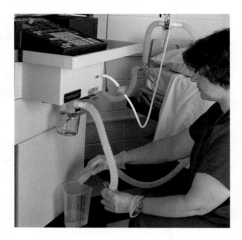

Step 9 Check ventilator settings regularly.

Step 10 Provide the patient with an alternative form of communication, such as a letter board or white board.

The patient on a mechanical ventilator is unable to speak. This can produce extreme anxiety. An alternative method of communication must be used so the patient can express her needs and concerns.

Step 11 Reposition the patient regularly, being careful not to pull on the ventilator tubing.

Pulling on the tubing creates pain. Patient comfort promotes relaxation, which improves the effectiveness of the ventilator.

Step 12 Provide frequent oral care. Moisten the lips with a cool, damp cloth and water-based lubricant.

Step 13 Ensure that the call light is always within reach, and answer call light and ventilator alarms promptly.

Ensures that you will attend immediately to any breathing problem; reassures the patient and thus relieves anxiety.

Evaluation

- Evaluate the patient's tolerance of mechanical ventilation. Verify that the patient is being adequately ventilated and that she is breathing in synchrony with the ventilator.
- Auscultate breath sounds every 2 to 4 hours, according to agency policy.
- Monitor continuous pulse oximetry.

Patient Teaching

- Explain mechanical ventilation to the patient and her family. Include information about the alarms they will hear.
- Demonstrate an alternative form of communication to the patient and family.
- When appropriate, explain the weaning process to the patient and family.
- If the patient requires mechanical ventilation after discharge, make arrangements for a home ventilator, and teach the patient and caregiver how to use it.

PROCEDURE 35–10   **Caring for a Patient on a Mechanical Ventilator**
(continued)

Home Care

- Explain to the family and caregiver where to obtain a home ventilator, resuscitation bag, and oxygen equipment and what services are available. Make sure they choose a supplier who has 24-hour emergency services available.
- Help the patient and caregiver devise a backup plan for ventilating the patient in the event of a power failure.
- Tell the caregiver to notify the utility company and area emergency personnel that the patient is being maintained on a ventilator at home.
- Instruct the patient and caregiver about oxygen therapy and its use as well as safety measures that they must institute.
- Teach the patient and caregiver to clean the ventilator tubing with soap and warm water when it becomes soiled.
- Provide the patient and caregiver with contact information of healthcare personnel who can be reached for advice or emergencies.

Documentation

- Document the date and time mechanical ventilation was initiated.
- Note the type of ventilator used and the prescribed settings.
- Document the patient's response to mechanical ventilation, including vital signs, breath sounds, ease of breathing, pulse oximetry, intake and output, skin color, and arterial blood gas and chest x-ray results.

Sample of a narrative note:

2/26/07	0800	*Patient found difficult to arouse. Dr. Henry made aware. ABG obtained, results included: pH 7.28; PCO$_2$ 78 mm Hg; and PO$_2$ 48 mm Hg. Dr. Henry in to evaluate patient, anesthesia called to intubate patient. Patient medicated with Versed 5 mg IV and intubated orally with a 7.5 Fr. ET tube. Patient placed on mechanical ventilator: TV 700 mL; FiO$_2$ 80%, and RR 14. Portable chest x-ray confirms ideal placement of endotracheal tube as well as white-out of both lung fields. Arterial blood gases to be obtained in 30 minutes. Pulse oximetry 90% since being placed on ventilator. —L. Biello, RN*

PROCEDURE 35–11 — Caring for a Patient with Chest Tubes (Disposable Water-Seal System)

> For steps to follow in *all* procedures, refer to the inside back cover of this book.

critical aspects

- Obtain and prepare the prescribed drainage system.
- Position the patient according to the indicated insertion site.
- As soon as the chest tube is inserted, attach it to the drainage system using a connector.
- Using sterile technique, wrap petroleum gauze around the chest tube insertion site, and dress the site with two precut sterile drain dressings covered by a large drainage dressing (ABD).
- Secure the dressing in place with 2-inch silk tape, making sure to cover the dressing completely.
- Using the spiral taping technique, wrap 1-inch silk tape around the connections. Wrap from top to bottom and bottom to top.
- If suction is prescribed, attach the suction tubing to the suction source. Alternatively, if suction is not prescribed, leave the suction vent on the drainage system open.
- Prepare the patient for a portable chest x-ray exam.
- Keep emergency supplies at the bedside in the event of tube dislodgement or system failure.
- Maintain the chest tube and drainage system by preventing kinks, ensuring patency of the air vent, and keeping the system below the level of the chest tube.

Equipment

- Two disposable drainage systems
- Two rubber-tipped hemostats
- Sterile gloves
- Mask and gown
- Sterile 4 × 4 gauze dressings
- Sterile, precut drain dressings
- Petroleum gauze dressings
- Large drainage dressings (ABD)
- 2-inch silk tape
- 1-inch silk tape

Delegation

Some agencies permit only registered nurses in the critical care units to perform dressing changes. The physician must perform dressing changes on other units. You should not delegate this procedure, because it requires advanced knowledge of pulmonary anatomy and physiology. As needed, teach the LPN and UAP how to safely provide care for the patient with chest tubes. Instruct them to notify a registered nurse immediately if the chest drainage system becomes disconnected, the chest tube becomes dislodged, sudden bleeding occurs, or the patient develops respiratory distress.

Assessment

- Assess the patient's knowledge of chest tube therapy.

Understanding helps allay fears and anxiety.

- Assess respiratory status, including respiratory rate, depth, and rhythm; breath sounds; skin color; and pulse oximetry results.

Provides a baseline for comparison after chest tube insertion. Evaluates chest tube functioning afterward.

- Assess type, color, and amount of chest tube drainage.

Confirms chest tube patency and determines whether bleeding is present.

- Assess for the presence of crepitus and drainage around the chest tube insertion site.

Crepitus is a sign that air is leaking into the subcutaneous tissues. Drainage is a sign that fluid is leaking around the insertion site. Both may indicate a compromise in tube patency.

- Check the disposable chest drainage system for the presence of an air leak.

An air leak indicates that air is leaking from the chest and a tight seal has not yet formed over the site of injury.

PROCEDURE 35–11

Caring for a Patient with Chest Tubes (Disposable Water-Seal System) *(continued)*

Procedural Steps

Step 1 Obtain and prepare the prescribed drainage system. ▼

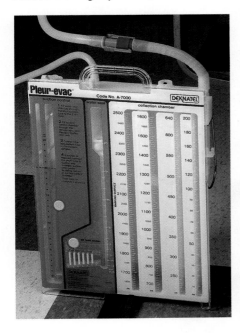

Variation Disposable Water-Seal System Without Suction

a. Remove the cover on the water-seal chamber, and, using the funnel provided, fill the second (water-seal) chamber with sterile water or normal saline. Fill the chamber to the 2 cm mark, or as indicated.

The water-seal chamber allows air to exit from the pleural space during exhalation and prevents air from entering the pleural space during inspiration.

b. Replace the cover on the water-seal chamber.

Protects the chamber from contamination.

Variation Disposable Water-Seal System With Suction

c. Remove the cover on the water-seal chamber, and, using the funnel provided, fill the water-seal chamber

(second chamber) with sterile water or normal saline to the 2 cm mark.

See step 1a.

d. Add sterile water or normal saline solution to the suction control chamber. Add the amount of fluid specified by the physician's order, typically 20 cm.

Suction is regulated by the height of fluid in the suction control chamber.

e. Attach the tubing from the suction control chamber to the connecting tubing attached to the suction source. ▼

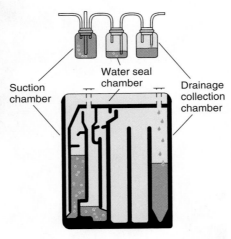

Suction chamber   Water seal chamber   Drainage collection chamber

Step 2 Position the patient according to the indicated insertion site.

A chest tube to remove air is usually inserted in the second intercostal space at the midclavicular line. If the chest tube is indicated for fluid drainage, the physician typically inserts the tube on the midaxillary line in the 5th or 6th intercostal space.

Step 3 Don a mask, gown, and sterile gloves.

Prevents contamination of the surgical site and protects you from splashing.

Step 4 Provide support to the patient while the physician prepares the sterile field, anesthetizes the patient, and inserts and sutures the chest tube. As soon as the chest tube is inserted, attach it to drainage system using a connector.

Immediately attaching the chest tube to the drainage system prevents air from entering the pleural cavity.

Step 5 Using sterile technique, wrap petroleum gauze around the chest tube insertion site.

Petroleum gauze creates a seal that prevents air from leaking around the site.

Step 6 Place a precut, sterile drain dressing over the petroleum gauze.

Absorbs drainage from the insertion site, thereby preventing skin irritation and possible breakdown. ▼

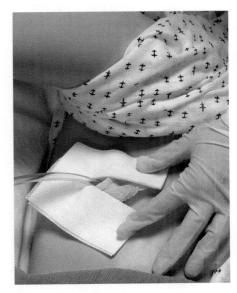

Step 7 Place a second sterile, precut drain dressing over the first drain dressing with the opening facing in the opposite direction from the first.

The second drain dressing helps secure the first drain dressing and provides reinforcement against drainage.

Step 8 Place a large drainage dressing (ABD) over the two precut drain dressings.

The large drainage dressing helps cover the insertion site, protecting it from outside sources of infection.

➤

PROCEDURE 35–11

Caring for a Patient with Chest Tubes (Disposable Water-Seal System) *(continued)*

Step 9 Secure the dressing in place with 2-inch silk tape, making sure to cover the dressing completely.

Protects the chest tube from becoming dislodged and provides a seal over the insertion site, protecting it from outside sources of infection.

Step 10 Date, time, and initial the dressing.

Informs other staff members when the dressing change was completed and by whom.

Step 11 Using the spiral taping technique, wrap 1-inch silk tape around the chest tube, starting above the connector and continuing below the connector. Reverse your wrapping by taping back up the tubing (using the spiral technique) until the wrapping is above the connector.

Ensures a tight connection between the two tubings, thereby preventing an air leak at the connection site. ▼

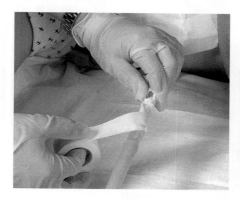

Step 12 Cut an 8-inch-long piece of 2-inch tape. Loop one end around the top portion of the drainage tube, and secure the remaining end of the tape to the chest tube dressing.

Prevents pulling at the chest tube site when the patient moves.

Step 13 If suction is prescribed, adjust the suction source until gentle bubbling occurs in the suction control chamber. (*Note:* Increasing suction at the suction source increases airflow through the system and creates more bubbling, but it does not increase the amount of suction placed on the chest cavity.) If suction is not prescribed, leave the suction tubing on the drainage system open.

If suction is not prescribed, keep the suction tubing open to maintain negative pressure. Gentle bubbling indicates that adequate suction is being applied. ▼

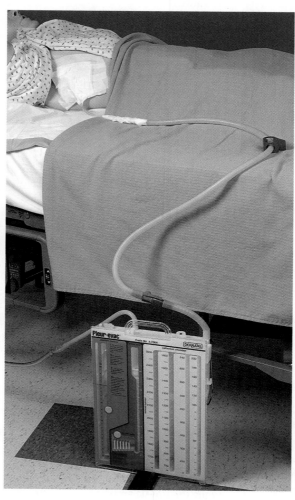

Step 14 Make sure that the drainage tubing lies in a straight line with no kinks from the chest tube to the drainage chamber.

Facilitates drainage and prevents fluid from accumulating in the pleural cavity.

Step 15 Prepare the patient for a portable chest x-ray exam.

A chest x-ray exam should be performed after the chest tube is inserted to ensure proper placement.

PROCEDURE 35–11

Caring for a Patient with Chest Tubes (Disposable Water-Seal System) *(continued)*

Step 16 Institute safety measures.

a. Place two rubber-tipped clamps at the patient's bedside for special situations.

Rubber-tip clamps are used to clamp the chest tube to check for an airleak, to change the drainage system, and to assess whether the chest tube can be safely removed.

b. Place a petroleum gauze dressing at the bedside in case the chest tube becomes dislodged.

If the tube becomes dislodged, place a petroleum gauze dressing over the insertion site to prevent air from entering the pleural cavity.

c. Keep a spare disposable drainage system at the patient's bedside.

To use in case the drainage system in use is accidentally upended or the drainage collection chamber becomes filled. ▼

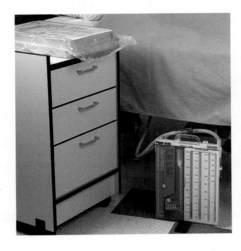

Step 17 Position the patient for comfort, as indicated.

If the patient received a chest tube to relieve a pneumothorax, the preferred position is semi-Fowler's position. Alternatively, if the chest tube was inserted to promote fluid drainage, high-Fowler's position is recommended.

Step 18 Maintain patency of the chest tube and drainage system.

a. Make sure the drainage tubing is free of kinks.

Kinks in the drainage tubing increase pressure in the pleural cavity and prevent fluid drainage.

b. Inspect the air vent in the drainage system to make sure it is patent.

The air vent must remain patent to allow air to escape. If air builds up in the pleural cavity, pneumothorax may occur.

c. Make sure the drainage system is located below the insertion site and anchor the collection device to assure that it remains upright.

If the drainage system is located above the insertion site, fluid may flow back into the pleural cavity, compromising the patient's respiratory status.

Evaluation

- Evaluate the patient's tolerance to the chest tube insertion. Determine whether the patient's respiratory status has changed.
- Auscultate breath sounds every 2 hours.
- Check chest drainage every 15 minutes for the first 2 hours, and then check as prescribed.
- Monitor the chest tube insertion site for drainage and subcutaneous emphysema at least every 4 hours.
- Monitor intake and output every 8 hours.
- Check laboratory values to evaluate blood loss and oxygenation.
- Monitor character of drainage (e.g., color and amount).
- Monitor that the waterseal chamber is bubbling.

Patient Teaching

- Teach the patient and family about chest tube insertion.
- Explain the importance of immediately reporting chest pain, shortness of breath, or tube dislodgement.

➤

PROCEDURE 35–11 **Caring for a Patient with Chest Tubes (Disposable Water-Seal System)** *(continued)*

Home Care

- Explain to the patient and caregiver how to care for the chest tube at home.
- Provide the patient and caregiver with contact information should problems with the chest tube arise.

Documentation

- Document the date and time of the chest tube insertion.
- Document the name of the physician who performed the procedure.
- Note the location of insertion site, the size of the chest tube, the type of drainage system, and the amount of suction applied, if any.
- Note the color and amount of drainage.
- Record the chest tube output on the intake and output portion of the flowsheet (in most agencies).
- Note the presence of subcutaneous emphysema or air leak, if any.
- Document vital signs, breath sounds, and pulse oximetry.
- Document complications and any interventions preformed as a result of the complications.
- Document the results of the chest x-ray exam.

Sample of a narrative note for chest tube insertion:

8/24/07	0230	Patient presented with acute shortness of breath, pulse ox. 84%, respirations 40 breaths/minute and shallow, heart rate 132 beats/minute, and blood pressure 189/100 mm Hg. Breath sounds absent on right side. Patient received morphine sulfate 4 mg IV push. Chest tube placed by Dr. Phan under sterile conditions in the anterior chest, midclavicular line, above the 2nd ICS. Chest tube attached to 20 cm of water pressure. Small air leak present, no crepitus. Portable chest x-ray obtained after the procedure, revealed chest tube in good placement with the right lung expanded. Vital signs post insertion: pulse ox 94%, blood pressure 154/90 mm Hg, heart rate 100 beats/minute, and respiratory rate 24 breaths/minute. Breath sounds audible bilaterally. ——— ——— S. Mays, RN

PROCEDURE 35–11   **Caring for a Patient with Chest Tubes (Disposable Water-Seal System)** *(continued)*

Sample of a narrative note for chest tube maintenance:

9/25/07	1500	Post op day 2, status post left thoracotomy. Chest tube dressing clean and dry. No air leak or subcutaneous emphysema present. Chest tube drainage this shift 100 mL. Vital signs stable, patient remains afebrile. Chest X-ray this a.m. shows left lung expanded with no signs of pneumonia. ——— S. Laurence, RN

PROCEDURE 35–12   **Performing Cardiopulmonary Resuscitation, One- and Two-Person**

 For steps to follow in *all* procedures, refer to the inside back cover of this book.

critical aspects

- Establish whether the patient is unresponsive. (Shake the patient and shout, "Are you OK?")
- Activate the emergency response system immediately if the patient is an adult. If you are alone and the patient is an infant or child, perform CPR for 1 minute, and then activate the emergency response system.
- Carefully place the patient on a hard surface. Logroll the patient if you suspect a cervical spine injury. If the patient is in a hospital bed, place a CPR board under the patient's back.
- Properly position yourself.
- *A—Airway.* Open the patient's airway. Use either the head-tilt–chin-lift maneuver or the jaw-thrust maneuver.
- *B—Breathing.* Check for breathing. (Place your ear over the patient's mouth and nose. Look, listen, and feel for breathing for no longer than 10 seconds.) If the patient is breathing, continue to hold the airway open. If the patient is not breathing, administer two slow breaths.
- *C—Circulation.* Check for signs of circulation. Use the carotid pulse in adults and children, and the brachial or femoral pulse in infants. Assess for a pulse for 5 to 10 seconds. Also check for other signs of circulation, such as movement.
- If signs of circulation are absent, correctly position your hands and begin chest compressions.
- Continue CPR for four cycles, then reassess pulse.
- Stop CPR if the patient responds, regains an adequate pulse, and begins to breathe; if you are too exhausted to continue; or if signs of death are obvious.

Note: CPR technique is frequently updated to reflect new research findings. Please consult the American Heart Association web site for the most recent report.

Equipment

- Resuscitation bag with mask, mouth shield, or face mask with a one-way valve
- Oxygen source, if available
- Chest compression board or hard surface

Delegation

Assistive personnel trained in basic life support can perform cardiopulmonary resuscitation (CPR).

Assessment

- Assess the following
  a. *Airway.* Assess the patient's level of consciousness.

Assessing the patient's level of consciousness prevents administering CPR to a patient who is sleeping or has a depressed level of consciousness.

  b. *Breathing.* Assess for airway patency and breathing.
  c. *Circulation*

Injury can result if CPR is administered on a patient who doesn't require it.

- Determine (preferably in advance of an emergency) whether the patient has an advance directive stating that he does or does not wish to have CPR performed.
- Monitor the effectiveness of chest compressions and ventilations.

Ineffective chest compressions and ventilations can have detrimental effects on the patient.

- Assess the patient's cardiac and respiratory status after cardiac rhythm and respirations are restored.

The patient's condition is typically unstable after an arrest; therefore, careful, frequent assessment of the cardiac and respiratory systems is necessary to quickly detect deterioration in the patient's status.

Procedural Steps

Step 1 Establish whether the patient is unresponsive by shaking him and shouting, "Are you OK?"

Unresponsiveness must be determined to avoid performing CPR on a patient who might be sleeping or have a decreased level of consciousness.

Step 2 Activate the emergency response system immediately if the patient is an adult. If you are alone and the patient is an infant or child, perform CPR for 1 minute, and then activate the emergency response system.

Activating the emergency response system immediately ensures that advanced life support equipment such as a defibrillator, airway management equipment, and IV medications are on the way for use.

Step 3 Carefully place the patient on a hard surface. Logroll the patient if you suspect a cervical spine injury. If the patient is in a hospital bed, place a CPR board under the patient's back.

A hard surface is necessary to provide chest compressions adequately. Log-

rolling the patient maintains stability of the cervical spine should a cervical spine injury be present.

Step 4 Properly position yourself.

Variation One-Person CPR

a. Position yourself on the floor, with your knees parallel to the patient's sternum.

This position requires the least amount of body movement when you switch from compressions to ventilations.

Variation Two-Person CPR

b. Position yourself on the floor, with your knees parallel to the patient's sternum. The second person should position himself on the opposite side of the patient, with his knees parallel to the patient's sternum. If the patient is in a hospital bed, stand with your body parallel to the patient's sternum.

Positioning one person on each side of the patient allows one person to deliver

chest compressions while the other person ventilates the patient.

Step 5 Open the patient's airway.

Variation Head-Tilt–Chin-Lift Maneuver

a. Place one hand on the patient's forehead, and apply firm pressure, tilting the patient's head back.

Tilting the patient's head back helps open the airway. ▼

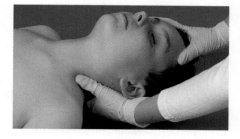

b. Place the fingertips of your other hand under the patient's chin, and lift his chin. Keep the patient's mouth partially open.

This maneuver pulls the base of the tongue away from the back of the throat, maintaining an open airway.

PROCEDURE 35–12

Performing Cardiopulmonary Resuscitation, One- and Two-Person *(continued)*

Variation Jaw-Thrust Maneuver

c. Kneel at the patient's head, with your elbows on the floor. Place your thumbs on his lower jaw near the corners of the mouth.

Placing the thumbs on the lower jaw near the corners of the mouth prepares you to lift the jaw to open the airway.

d. Place your fingers around the lower jaw, and lift the lower jaw with your fingertips.

This maneuver pulls the base of the tongue away from the back of the throat, maintaining an open airway while protecting the cervical spine. ▼

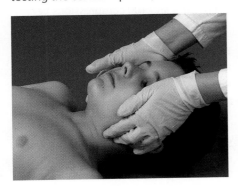

Step 6 While keeping the airway open, check for breathing by placing your ear over the patient's mouth and nose. Look, listen, and feel for breathing for no longer than 10 seconds.

Assesses the patient's ability to move air into and out of the lungs. Cardiac arrest can occur independent of respiratory arrest, at least initially.

Step 7 If the patient is breathing or resumes effective breathing, continue to hold the airway open. Alternatively, if the patient is not breathing, administer two slow breaths.

You should initiate two slow breaths immediately if the patient isn't breathing to provide the patient with much-needed oxygen.

Variation Adult (Adolescent and Older)

a. Pinch the patient's nose with your thumb and fingers. Place your mouth, the mouth shield, or the face mask over the patient's mouth.

Prevents air from escaping through the nares when you deliver a breath.

b. Deliver two breaths into the patient's mouth, allowing 1 second per breath. Move your mouth or mask to allow the patient to exhale between breaths. Deliver subsequent breaths at a rate of 10 to 12 breaths per minute.

Allowing 1 second per breath allows the adult's lungs to expand appropriately and ensures adequate oxygen delivery.

Variation Child (1 to Adolescence)

a. Pinch the child's nose with your thumb and fingers. Place your mouth, the mouth shield, or the face mask over the child's mouth.

Prevents air from escaping through the nares when you deliver a breath.

b. Deliver two breaths into the child's mouth, allowing 1 second per breath. Move your mouth or mask to allow the child to exhale between breaths. Deliver subsequent breaths at a rate of 12–20 breaths per minute.

Delivering two breaths over 1 second per breath allows the child's lungs to expand appropriately and ensures adequate oxygen delivery.

Variation Infant (Less Than 1 Year of Age)

a. Place your mouth over the infant's mouth and nose, forming a seal.

A seal keeps air from escaping through the nares when you deliver a breath.

b. Deliver two breaths (very gentle puffs) into the infant's nose and mouth, allowing 1 second per breath. Allow the infant to exhale between breaths. Deliver subsequent breaths at a rate of 12–20 breaths/minute.

Delivering two breaths over 1 second per breath allows the infant's lungs to expand appropriately and ensures adequate oxygen delivery.

Step 8 Check for signs of circulation, using the carotid pulse in adults and children and the brachial or femoral pulse in infants. Assess for a pulse for 5 to 10 seconds. Also check for other signs of circulation, such as movement.

Lets you know whether chest compressions are indicated. Chest compressions are indicated when the pulse is absent in the adult or is less than 60 beats per minute in the infant. Check the pulse for 5 to 10 seconds, because the pulse may be present but difficult to detect if it is slow, irregular, weak, or rapid.

Step 9 If signs of circulation are absent, correctly position your hands, and begin chest compressions. If a second person is present, the second person should assess the pulse while the first person performs compressions.

Correct hand placement prevents patient injury. Allowing the second person to check for a pulse helps assesses the effectiveness of CPR.

a. Adult:
   (1) Place the heel of one hand over the lower half of the sternum, and place your other hand on top of the first hand, locking them in position. ▼

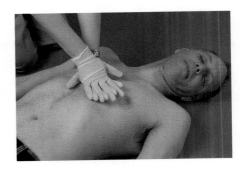

➤

PROCEDURE 35–12

Performing Cardiopulmonary Resuscitation, One- and Two-Person *(continued)*

(2) Compress $1\frac{1}{2}$ to 2 inches at a rate of 100 compressions per minute.

The chest must be compressed $1\frac{1}{2}$ to 2 inches to ensure adequate circulation and prevent patient injury.

b. Child:
(1) Place the heel of one hand over the lower half of the sternum. ▼

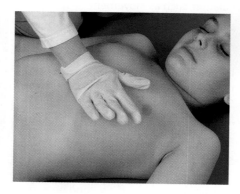

(2) Compress $\frac{1}{3}$ to $\frac{1}{2}$ the depth of the chest at a rate of 100 compressions per minute.

The chest must be adequately compressed to ensure adequate circulation and to prevent injury.

c. Infant:
(1) Place two fingers 1 finger-breadth below the intermammary line. ▼

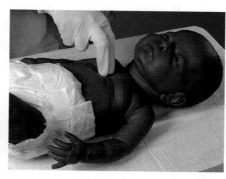

Because the chest is small, fingers are used to prevent compressing too forcefully, as could occur if you used the hand.

(2) Compress $\frac{1}{3}$ to $\frac{1}{2}$ the depth of the chest at a rate of at least 100 compressions per minute, 120 compressions per minute in the newborn.

The chest must be adequately compressed to ensure adequate circulation and to prevent injury.

Step 10 Continue ventilating the patient.

Variation Adult

The second rescuer should administer the ventilations, making sure to deliver the breath as the rescuer administering compressions pauses between compressions.

Note: The ratio for compressions to ventilations is 15:2 for two persons and 30:2

for one person CPR in an adult. The person performing chest compressions must pause momentarily to allow the second person to deliver ventilations.

Pausing to deliver ventilations ensures adequate delivery of ventilations. This technique delivers 10 to 12 breaths per minute and approximately 100 compressions per minute.

Variation Child and Infant

Administer two breaths for every 30 compressions with a single rescuer and 2 breaths per 15 compressions with two rescuers.

This technique delivers about 20 breaths per minute and 100 compressions per minute.

Step 11 Continue CPR for four cycles, and then reassess pulse.

Reassessing pulse prevents administering CPR inadvertently to the patient who doesn't require it.

Step 12 Stop CPR if the patient responds, regains an adequate pulse, and begins to breathe; if you are too exhausted to continue; or if signs of death are obvious.

CPR should be continued only as needed. Part of administering CPR responsibly is knowing when to stop the procedure when the patient's condition becomes hopeless.

Evaluation

- After the airway is opened, monitor for the return of spontaneous respirations.
- Evaluate the effectiveness of ventilations and chest compressions.

PROCEDURE 35–12 **Performing Cardiopulmonary Resuscitation, One- and Two-Person** *(continued)*

Patient Teaching

- Instruct the family and caregivers where they can receive CPR training and certification if the patient is at risk for experiencing cardiopulmonary arrest.
- Explain the importance of keeping emergency phone numbers readily available in the event of an emergency.

Home Care

- Activate the emergency response team by dialing 911 in the community setting or by dialing another designated emergency number if the 911 service is not available.
- Make sure the patient is on a firm surface before administering CPR.

Documentation

- Document the date and time the arrest occurred.
- Document whether the patient experienced cardiac or respiratory arrest or both.
- Record the events surrounding the arrest, such as the location of the patient when the arrest occurred, precipitating factors, who discovered the patient, and whether the arrest was witnessed.
- Document who initiated CPR.
- Record the name of the physician notified.
- Record the length of time in which the patient received CPR.
- Document any complications and the patient's response to CPR.
- Record all information on the designated code record if the arrest occurred within the hospital setting, including medications given and procedures performed.

Sample of a narrative note:

07/05/07	1700	Patient found lying on the bathroom floor. Unresponsiveness established by Jackie Smith, CNA, who called for help and initiated the code response. She opened the patient's airway using the jaw-thrust maneuver. No respirations were detected. 2 breaths were delivered using a face mask. Jim Lyons, RN arrived on the scene and assessed the patient's carotid pulse for 10 seconds—pulse was absent. Chest compressions were initiated at a rate of 100 compressions/minute. ACLS protocol was then initiated. See the code record for details. At 1745 the code was stopped and the patient was pronounced dead by Dr. Polk, who then notified the patient's wife.————— S. Nye, RN

TECHNIQUES

TECHNIQUE 35–1 · Assessing Breathing Patterns

Type	Description	Illustration	Discussion
Eupnea	Normal respirations, with equal rate and depth, 12–20 breaths per minute		Rate is about 12–20 per minute.
Bradypnea	Slow respirations, <10 breaths per minute		May cause poor gas exchange. Caused by sedative and opioid medications and neuromuscular dysfunction.
Tachypnea	Fast respirations, >24 breaths per minute, usually shallow		Generally caused by hypoxemia or increased oxygen demand (e.g., exercise); however, respirations that are rapid but shallow draw limited air into the alveoli and may result in hypoventilation.
Kussmaul's respirations	Respirations that are regular but abnormally deep and increased in rate		A compensatory mechanism for metabolic disorders that lower blood pH, as well as a form of hyperventilation caused by fear, anxiety, or panic.
Biot's respirations	Periods of respirations of equal depth, alternating with periods of apnea (absence of breathing)		Often associated with damage to the medullary respiratory center or high intracranial pressure due to brain injury.
Cheyne-Stokes respirations	Gradual increase in depth of respirations, followed by gradual decrease and then a period of apnea		Often associated with damage to the medullary respiratory center or high intracranial pressure due to brain injury.
Apnea	Absence of breathing		Respiratory arrest requires immediate cardiopulmonary resuscitation.

Most irregular breathing patterns are due to brain injury or the effects of drugs on the brain.

TECHNIQUE 35–2   Tips for Obtaining Accurate Pulse Oximetry Readings

Pulse oximetry is a valuable assessment tool. However, several factors can interfere with the accuracy of the readings. These factors are discussed below.

Patient movement. A fingernail bed is the most common site to place the probe. A tremor, twitch, shivering, or movement in bed can make pulse oximetry reading troublesome. If the patient is unable to cooperate or control his movement, try using an ear probe or nasal sensor to achieve more accurate readings.

Thick acrylic fingernails and nail polish affect pulse oximetry readings. If the patient has acrylic nails, place the probe on a toe or earlobe. Some nail polish dyes also affect pulse oximetry readings, so remove nail polish before placing the probe. Many facilities stock individually packaged nail polish remover pads (similar in size to alcohol prep pads) to remove nail polish.

Poor perfusion of the area where the probe is placed may cause a low reading.

- A bent elbow, for example, may cause a slight decrease in circulation to the finger nail bed. If SaO_2 monitoring is crucial to the patient's plan of care, use the earlobe as the preferred site to minimize the effect of movement on the reading.

- Vasoconstriction due to cool extremities may also limit circulation. Keep the extremities warm to obtain a more accurate reading.
- If poor perfusion is related to a disease process, use the earlobe or nose as the monitoring site.

Bright fluorescent lighting is typical in many health care facilities. Unfortunately it may influence the accuracy of the reading. Dim the lights or cover the probe with bed covers or a towel to reduce error.

Anemia, carbon monoxide, intravascular dyes, and dark skin color are factors you should consider when interpreting oximetry readings. Because these factors cannot be controlled, watch for trend changes in the readings.

Equipment function should be checked:

- *Weak signal or, no signal*—Check the patient's vital signs. If they are satisfactory, check the circulation to the site. If that is satisfactory, check equipment connections.
- *Inaccurate reading suspected*—Check the reading using the equipment on a healthy person. If it seems accurate, check the patient's medications and check for history of circulatory disorders; also check items listed above.

TECHNIQUE 35–3   Guidelines for Preventing Aspiration

To prevent aspiration, follow these guidelines with at-risk patients:

- Position the unconscious patient on his side to protect the airway.
- Position the patient upright for feeding or with the head of bed elevated.
- Be sure the head of bed remains elevated for at least 30 minutes after each feeding. If the patient is receiving continuous tube feedings, the head of bed must remain elevated.
- Request medications in elixir or liquid form.
- Break or crush pills, when appropriate, before you administer them.
- Keep a suction setup available for routine and emergency use.
- If the patient is intubated, keep the endotracheal or tracheostomy cuff inflated, and suction above the cuff before deflating the cuff.
- Do not offer food or fluids if the client is heavily sedated or in the initial recovery phase of anesthesia.

Enteral Feedings

- Check the placement of the nasogastric tube before you administer enteral feedings.
- Check gastric residual volume before administering the next enteral feeding. Hold the feeding if the residual volume is high. (*Note:* The amount of acceptable residual volume depends on the amount and frequency of feedings.)
- Also see Procedure 26–3 for step-by-step instructions for administering feedings through gastric and enteric tubes.

Oral Feedings

- Offer small, frequent meals.
- Avoid thin liquids, or use thickening agents.
- Offer foods or liquids that can be formed into a bolus before they are swallowed.
- Cut food into small pieces.

TECHNIQUE 35–4   Oxygen Therapy Safety Precautions

- Post signs indicating that oxygen is in use.
- Do not permit smoking near oxygen delivery systems.
- Ensure that three-pronged plugs are used for electrical devices (to prevent sparks).
- Allow no open flames (e.g., candles) near oxygen.
- Avoid electrical equipment with frayed wires or loose connections.

- Avoid using petroleum products, aerosol products, and products containing acetone where oxygen is in use. (These are flammable substances that are easily ignited.)
- Secure oxygen tanks to rigid stands.
- Secure portable oxygen cylinders in holders or carriers provided.

TECHNIQUE 35–5   Inserting an Oropharyngeal Airway

Oropharyngeal airways are C-shaped plastic devices available in infant, pediatric, and adult sizes. They should be used only in unconscious patients, because they are likely to trigger gagging, vomiting, or laryngospasm if airway reflexes are intact. To insert an oral airway, follow these steps:

1. Gather the following supplies:
   - A variety of sizes of oral airway (Most adults can accommodate an 80 mm airway)
   - Procedure gloves
   - Suction equipment
   - Tongue blade
2. Select the appropriate size of airway by placing the airway on the outside of the cheek. The length of the airway should extend from the front teeth to the end of the jaw line.
3. Wash your hands, and don clean gloves.
4. Explain the procedure to the patient. Recall that because hearing is the last sense lost, the patient may be able to hear you.
5. Clear the mouth of any debris or secretions. You may need to suction the mouth.
6. Place the patient in supine or semi-Fowler's position. Hyperextend the neck, unless contraindicated.
7. Open the mouth. You may need to hold the tongue down with a tongue blade as you insert the airway.

8. Insert the airway into the mouth in the upside-down position (inner curve of the C faces upward toward the nose).

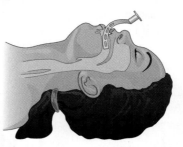

9. Rotate the airway 180° so that the ends of the C turn downward over the back of the tongue. Continue to insert the airway until the front flange is flush with the lips.

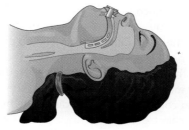

10. Keep the head tilted slightly back and the chin elevated to help the oropharygeal airway function optimally.
11. Verify patency of the airway by auscultating for bilateral breath sounds.
12. Do not tape the airway in place.
13. Continually reassess the need for the airway. Remove it when the patient begins to cough or gag.
14. Keep suction available at the bedside. Suction the oropharynx as needed by inserting the suction catheter alongside the airway.
15. Provide oral hygiene at least every 2 to 4 hours.

TECHNIQUE 35–6 Inserting a Nasopharyngeal Airway

1. Select the appropriate size airway. To measure, hold the airway next to the patient's face. The length of the airway should extend from the nares to the end of the jawline, below the ear. Airways are available in a variety of pediatric and adult sizes. Generally, the larger the internal diameter, the longer the tube.
2. Lubricate the airway with water-soluble lubricant.
3. Tilt the patient's head backward, and gently insert the tip of the airway into the nose.
4. Advance the airway along the floor of the nostril into the posterior pharynx behind the tongue. If you meet resistance, rotate the tube slightly to enhance passage.
5. When the tube is fully inserted, the outer flange of the tube should rest on the nostril, and only the tip of the tube should be visible at the top of the posterior pharynx.
6. Have the patient open her mouth; inspect the pharynx for proper placement of the tube tip.
7. Auscultate the lungs for the presence of bilateral breath sounds.
8. Provide frequent oral and nares care; assess the skin around the nostril.
9. Remove and reinsert the airway in the other naris every 8 hours to prevent mucosal injury.

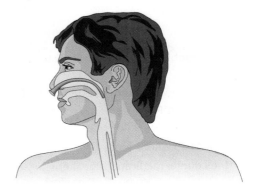

TECHNIQUE 35–7 Caring for Patients with Endotracheal Airways

The following are activities associated with the care of all types of endotracheal airways.
- Secure the endotracheal tube with ties, tapes, or a commercial holder to prevent accidental displacement.
- Inspect skin around tube or tracheal stoma for redness, drainage, or irritation at least every 8 hours.
- Provide skin care around the tube and tape or holder at least daily.
- Change the endotracheal or tracheostomy ties every 24 hours. Secure the orotracheal tube to the opposite side of the mouth with each change of tape or ties to prevent skin erosion and breakdown.
- Inflate the cuff of the tube with a minimal occlusive volume and monitor cuff pressures to prevent pressure necrosis inside the trachea. (This is a joint responsibility with the respiratory therapist.)
- Note the centimeter reference marking on the endotracheal tube to monitor for possible displacement.
- Minimize pulling and traction on the artificial airway by supporting all tubing connected to the airway and using flexible catheter mounts and swivels. If the patient is conscious, remind him not to pull on the airway.
- Use a bite block between the teeth to prevent the patient from occluding an orotracheal tube.
- Have emergency equipment immediately available for reintubation if the tube should become dislodged.
- Provide 100% humidification of inspired air.
- Suction the airway when secretions collect.

ASSESSMENT GUIDELINES AND TOOLS

Questions to Assess Risk for Impaired Oxygenation

Demographic Data

- What is your age?
- Where do you live?
- What is your occupation?

Health History

- What healthcare problems are you currently being treated for?
- Have you ever been hospitalized or had surgery? If so, when and for what reason?
- Do you have a history of allergies or asthma?
- What medications do you currently take?
- What over-the-counter medications or alternative treatments do you use? What do you use them for?

Respiratory History

- Have you ever been diagnosed with a respiratory problem? If so, what was the diagnosis? When was the diagnosis made?
- Have you noticed any changes in your breathing?
- How often do you cough?
- When you do cough, is it productive?
- What do the secretions you cough up look like and smell like?
- How much sputum do you produce?
- How do you treat your cough?
- Do you ever wheeze or feel short of breath?
- What causes you to wheeze or feel short of breath?
- Do body positions affect your breathing pattern?
- What position do you lie in when you sleep? Do you use more than one pillow?
- Do you ever wake up short of breath?

Cardiovascular History

- Have you ever been diagnosed with a heart or circulatory problem?

- Have you ever been told you have high blood pressure or a heart murmur?
- Do you experience cold hands and feet frequently?
- Have you ever had chest pain? If so, describe the circumstances.
- How was the chest pain treated?
- What measures do you take to relieve or prevent the pain?
- Do you easily become fatigued or feel your heart rate is very rapid?

Environmental History

- Are there pets in the house?
- What response, if any, do you have to pets, dust, pollen, or plants?
- Are you exposed to smoke or fumes in the home and workplace?
- Are you exposed to respiratory irritants such as asbestos, chemicals, coal dust, fungus, molds, or soot in the home or workplace?
- What type of heating, air conditioning, or air filtering system do you have in the home or workplace?

Lifestyle

- What is your current stress level? What are your major sources of stress?
- What is you usual diet? Is your current diet typical, or have you recently changed your eating habits?
- What is your usual activity level?
- What level of activity makes you feel short of breath?
- Do you smoke now, or have you ever smoked?
- If you smoke, how many packs per day and for how many years have you smoked?
- Do you smoke marijuana or use other substances?

DIAGNOSTIC TESTING

Tests Related to Oxygenation

Test	Purpose
Angiogram	A contrast dye is injected into a vein, and serial films are taken to assess patency of the vessels.
Arterial blood gas (ABG)	An analysis of arterial blood that evaluates the effectiveness of gas exchange.
Bronchoscopy	Insertion of a flexible endoscope to evaluate the larynx, trachea, and bronchial tree.
Cardiac catherization	A catheter is passed into the heart to assess pressures, blood flow, and the size and patency of chambers.
Chest x-ray study (CXR)	Provides an anterior-posterior or lateral view of the heart and lungs (e.g., to evaluate size, masses, fluid).
CK-MB	The MB isoenzyme is present only in the heart muscle. A serum measurement of the MB band is used to detect a myocardial infarction (MI). Levels rise with an acute MI.
Echocardiogram	An ultrasound evaluation of the heart that examines heart function and blood flow.
Electrocardiogram (ECG)	Electrodes placed on the extremities and chest wall conduct electrical activity from the heart. ECG illustrates heart rate, rhythm, and size and helps evaluate heart damage.
Hemoglobin (Hgb)	A serum measurement that affects the oxygen-carrying capacity of the blood. May be measured separately or as part of a complete blood count.
Holter monitor	A continuous ECG tracing used to correlate symptoms and cardiac activity. Typically the tracing lasts 48 hours to 7 days.
Pulmonary function studies	A series of tests to detect lung volume and capacity.
Sputum culture	A microscopic evaluation of the sputum.
Technetium scan	Technetium 99m Sestamibi is injected intravenously. Approximately 90 to 120 minutes later, the heart is scanned. Areas of myocardial damage appear as "hot spots" on the scan.
Thoracentesis	Insertion of a large-bore needle through the chest wall into the pleural space to obtain fluid specimens, to instill medication, or to drain accumulations of fluid.
Throat culture	A swab of the pharynx or tonsils is performed to assess pathogens present in the pharynx.
Treadmill test	Evaluates the effect of exercise on the heart and circulation via continuous ECG and vital sign monitoring during exercise.
Troponin	A serum evaluation of a complex of proteins is used to detect MI. Levels of these contractile proteins remain elevated for up to 7 days after MI.
Ventilation-perfusion scan	Used to assess for pulmonary embolus, this scan entails injection of a radioactive substance that allows blood flow to the lungs to be evaluated. A second substance is inhaled that maps out oxygen distribution in the lungs.
White blood cell (WBC) count	A serum measure to assess for the presence of infection.

diagnostic testing

Reading a Tuberculin Skin Test Result

Size of Induration	Considered Positive For
>5 mm	• People who have had recent close contact with someone with active TB • People who have HIV or risk factors for HIV • People with previous history of TB
>10 mm	• IV drug users known to be HIV-negative • People with medical conditions that increase the risk of progressing from latent TB to active TB (e.g., diabetes mellitus, use of steroids, chronic renal failure, some malignancies) • Residents and employees of high-risk congregate settings: prisons, skilled nursing facilities (SNFs) and other long-term facilities, healthcare facilities, and homeless shelters • Foreign-born persons recently arrived (i.e., within the last 5 years) from countries having a high incidence of TB • Low-income groups • Children under 4 years of age or exposed to adults in high-risk categories
>15 mm	• People who do not meet any of the above criteria

diagnostic testing

Arterial Blood Gas Values: Evaluating Adequacy of Oxygenation

SaO$_2$	Arterial Po$_2$	Comment
95–100%	80–100 mm Hg	Normal arterial values in healthy people.
90%	60 mm Hg	Po$_2$ > 60 mm Hg is required to sustain life and activity. This level is NOT normal in healthy people.
75%	40 mm Hg	Normal venous values; a LETHAL arterial value in ANYONE.

STANDARDIZED LANGUAGE

Nursing Diagnoses Associated with Impaired Ventilation and Gas Exchange

Nursing Diagnosis	Defining Characteristics	Etiologies
Ineffective Airway Clearance	• Nonproductive or weak/absent cough • Tracheobronchial obstruction (signs of choking, inability to speak, stridor) • Inability to remove airway secretions (changes in respiratory rate, depth, rhythm or pattern, dyspnea) • Copious tracheobronchial secretions	• Ineffective cough secondary to constricted airways, neuromuscular weakness or paralysis, or respiratory muscle fatigue • Poor mucociliary function secondary to anesthesia, sedation, or chemical damage • Thick secretions secondary to dehydration or inhaling dry air
Ineffective Breathing Pattern	• Abnormal respiratory rate, depth, or pattern • Increased breathing effort (nasal flaring, use of accessory muscles, chest retractions) • Dyspnea • Splinted/guarded breathing • Decreased or absent breath sounds • Decreased chest excursion	• Airway irritation, inflammatory or infectious process • Neuromuscular impairment (brain injury, spinal cord injury, neuromuscular disease) • Fatigue • Restricted lung expansion (pain, chest trauma, or pulmonary fibrosis) • Anxiety • Metabolic abnormalities
Impaired Gas Exchange	• Hypoxemia • Hypercarbia • Hypoxia (confusion, somnolence, irritability, organ dysfunction, cyanosis) • Respiratory distress	• Altered oxygen supply (e.g., hypoventilation, airway obstruction, high altitudes) • Alveolar-capillary membrane changes (e.g., atelectasis, inflammation, lung infections, ARDS) • Altered blood flow (e.g., pulmonary embolus, pulmonary vasoconstriction) • Altered blood oxygen carrying capacity (e.g., anemia, carbon monoxide poisoning, hemorrhage)
Impaired Spontaneous Ventilation	• Dyspnea • Increased metabolic rate • Increased P_{CO_2} • Decreased P_{O_2} • Decreased S_{aO_2} • Increased heart rate • Decreased tidal volume • Apprehension • Use of accessory muscles	• Respiratory muscle fatigue or weakness • Metabolic factors • Central nervous system dysfunction
Dysfunctional Ventilatory Weaning Response	*Severe* • Deterioration in ABG levels • Significant increase in baseline heart rate (20 bpm) and respiratory rates • Increase in baseline BP (20 mm Hg) • Cyanosis • Adventitious breath sounds • Decreased level of consciousness • Shallow, gasping breaths • Profuse diaphoresis	• Perceived inability to wean; powerlessness • Anxiety; Fear • Deficient knowledge of weaning process • Insufficient trust in nurse • Uncontrolled episodic energy demands • Adverse environment (e.g., noisy, unfamiliar nursing staff) • History of ventilator dependence greater than 4 or 5 days

➤

Nursing Diagnoses Associated with Impaired Ventilation and Gas Exchange *(continued)*

Nursing Diagnosis	Defining Characteristics	Etiologies
Dysfunctional Ventilatory Weaning Response *(continued)*	*Moderate* • Pallor, mild cyanosis • Use of accessory muscles • Apprehension • Baseline increase in BP (< 20 mm Hg); in respirations (< 5 breaths/min); in heart rate (< 20 bpm) *Mild* • Warmth • Restlessness • Queries about possible machine malfunction • Expresses feelings of increased need for O_2 • Fatigue • Breathing discomfort	• Inadequate nutrition • Disturbed Sleep Pattern • Uncontrolled pain • Ineffective Airway Clearance

Source: NANDA International (2004). *NANDA nursing diagnoses: Definitions and classifications. 2005–2006.* Philadelphia: Author.

Nursing Diagnoses Associated with Impaired Circulation

Nursing Diagnosis	Defining Characteristics	Etiologies
Decreased Cardiac Output	Symptoms vary depending on whether the problem is one of preload or afterload. • Altered heart rate and rhythm: Tachycardia, bradycardia, palpitation, ECG changes • Anxiety, restlessness • Altered preload: Jugular vein distention, fatigue, edema, murmurs, weight gain, changes in central venous pressure • Altered afterload: Cold, clammy skin; dyspnea; oliguria; prolonged capillary refill; weak, thready, or absent peripheral pulses; BP changes; skin color changes • Impaired contractility: Hypotension, crackles, cough, dyspnea, cardiac output greater than 4 L/min, S_3 or S_4 sounds	• Heart abnormalities (e.g., myocardial infarction, valvular heart disease, dysrhythmias, impaired contractility) • Vascular abnormalities (e.g., severe vasodilation, vasoconstriction, or hypertension) • Pulmonary abnormalities • Blood volume abnormalities • Electrolyte imbalance • Drug effects
Altered Tissue Perfusion (Specify: Cardiopulmonary, Cerebral, GI, Peripheral, Renal)	Defining characteristics are signs of organ dysfunction. The organ affected determines the signs you will observe. For example, decreased cerebral perfusion results in restlessness, confusion, lethargy, dizziness, syncope, altered mental status, or motor or sensory deficits.	• Decreased or absent blood flow due to embolus, constriction, shock, or low blood volume • Decreased venous return due to incompetent veins • Vascular spasm • Increased pressure in the tissues (e.g., inflammation, obstruction) • External constriction (e.g., cast, restraints)

Source: NANDA International. (2005). *NANDA nursing diagnoses: Definitions and classifications 2005–2006.* Philadelphia: Author.

Examples of NOC Outcomes and NIC Interventions Linked to Oxygenation Diagnoses

Nursing Diagnoses	NOC Outcomes	NIC Interventions
Ineffective Airway Clearance	Respiratory Status: Airway Patency	Airway Management Airway Suctioning Cough Enhancement Respiratory Monitoring
Ineffective Breathing Pattern	Respiratory Status: Ventilation Vital Signs	Airway Management Respiratory Monitoring
Impaired Gas Exchange	Respiratory Status: Gas Exchange Vital Signs	Airway Management Oxygen Therapy Respiratory Monitoring
Decreased Cardiac Output	Blood Coagulation Cardiac Pump Effectiveness Circulation Status Fluid Balance Fluid Overload Severity Vital Signs	Bleeding Precautions Bleeding Reduction Cardiac Care (all levels) Hemodynamic Regulation Hemorrhage Control Hypovolemia Management Hypervolemia Management Shock Prevention Shock Management
Impaired Tissue Perfusion	Tissue Perfusion: Cardiac, Cerebral, Abdominal Organs, Peripheral, Pulmonary Fluid Balance Electrolyte & Acid/Base Balance	Circulatory Care Circulatory Precautions Cardiac Care (all levels)
Risk for Aspiration	Aspiration Prevention Respiratory Status: Ventilation Swallowing Status	Aspiration Precautions Vomiting Management
Activity Intolerance	Activity Tolerance Energy Conservation Knowledge: Treatment Regimen	Energy Management Teaching: Prescribed Activity/Exercise

Source: Dochterman, J. M., & Bulechek, G. M. (Eds.). (2004). *Nursing interventions classification (NIC)* (3rd ed.). St Louis: Mosby; Johnson, M., Maas, M., & Moorhead, S. (Eds.). (2004). *Nursing outcomes classification (NOC)* (3rd ed.). St Louis: Mosby.

What Are the Main Points in This Chapter?

- The structures of the airways, lungs, chest cavity, heart, and blood vessels function together to supply oxygen to the tissues; thus, abnormalities in any of these structures can interfere with tissue oxygenation.

- Developmental stage, environment, individual characteristics, lifestyle, medications, and pathological factors can interfere with ventilation, circulation, or gas exchange leading to problems with tissue oxygenation.

- A health assessment related to oxygenation includes assessment of ventilation (breathing), circulation (blood flow), and gas exchange (exchange of oxygen and carbon dioxide). The length and focus of the assessment varies with the purpose and urgency of the clinical situation.

- A physical examination related to adequacy of oxygenation includes observations of adequacy of breathing, circulation, and gas exchange.

- Pulse oximetry and arterial blood gases are used to monitor oxygen saturation.

- Small changes in oxygen saturation are associated with large shifts in the amount of oxygen available to the tissues and organs.

- The purposes of cardiac monitoring are to identify the patient's baseline rhythm and rate, recognize significant changes in the baseline rhythm and rate, and recognize lethal dysrhythmias that require immediate intervention.

- Interventions to promote optimal respiratory function include deep regular breathing, flu and pneumonia immunizations for at-risk individuals, frequent position changes, incentive spirometry, and preventing aspiration.

- Deep breathing, coughing exercises, and hydration promote deep inhalation and forceful expulsion of secretions.

- Supplemental oxygen is used to prevent hypoxemia. It may be delivered via a variety of methods.

- Artificial airways provide an open airway for patients who cannot maintain their own airway. The most common artificial airways are oropharyngeal, nasopharyngeal, and endotracheal.

- The airways can be suctioned to remove secretions and maintain patency. Signs that indicate the need for suctioning include gurgling sounds during respiration, restlessness, labored respirations, decreased oxygen saturation, increased heart and respiratory rates, and the presence of adventitious breath sounds during auscultation.

- Chest tubes remove air or fluid from the pleural space so that the lungs can fully expand.

- Promoting circulation ensures that oxygenated blood reaches tissues and organs and venous blood returns to the heart. Activities that promote venous return and preventing clot formation assist with circulation.

- Respiratory medications promote ventilation and oxygenation by their effects on the respiratory system. The major types of respiratory medicines include bronchodilators, corticosteroids, cough preparations, decongestants, antihistamines, and mucolytics.

- Cardiovascular drugs are used to enhance cardiac output, thus providing increased blood flow and oxygenation to organs and tissues. They include vasodilators, beta-adrenergic blocking agents, diuretics, and positive inotropes.

Fluids, Electrolytes,
& Acid-Base Balance

Overview

Body fluid is composed primarily of water, gases, and dissolved solid substances. Intracellular fluid (ICF) is contained within the cells and is essential for cell function and metabolism. Extracellular fluid (ECF) consists of three types of fluid: interstitial, intravascular, and transcellular fluid. ECF carries water, dissolved solids, nutrients, and oxygen to the cells and removes the waste products of cell metabolism. The body loses fluids through urine, skin, insensible losses, and feces. When the body is in a healthy state, fluid losses are equivalent to fluid intake.

Electrolytes are dissolved solids that carry an electrical charge. Potassium and magnesium are the major positively charged electrolytes in the ICF; phosphate and sulfate are the major negatively charged electrolytes. The major electrolytes of ECF are sodium, chloride, bicarbonate, and albumin.

The amount of acid or base present in a solution is measured as pH. A serum pH below 7.35 indicates acidosis. A serum pH above 7.45 indicates alkalosis. Buffer systems maintain serum pH by either absorbing free hydrogen ions or releasing free hydrogen ions. The lungs and kidneys also play an essential role in regulating acid-base balance.

Physical assessment focused on a client's fluid, electrolyte, and acid-base balance examines the skin, mucous membranes, cardiovascular and respiratory systems, and neurological status. The client's intake and output (I & O) are monitored to assess fluid status. Tests used to monitor fluid, electrolyte, and acid-base balance include measurement of serum electrolytes and osmolality, complete blood count, urinalysis, and measurement of arterial blood gases.

Nursing interventions for patients with fluid, electrolyte, or acid-base imbalance address preventing imbalances, modifying oral intake, providing parenteral replacement, and transfusing blood products. You will use a vascular access device to administer parenteral fluids and blood. IV lines may provide access to peripheral or central veins. You are responsible for maintaining the correct rate of flow and for monitoring the client's response to the infusion.

Thinking Critically About Fluids, Electrolytes, and Acid-Base Balance

The exercises in the following section allow you to practice the kind of thinking you will use as a full-spectrum nurse. Because these are critical-thinking activities, there is usually no single right answer. Discuss answers with your peers—discussion can stimulate critical thinking. If you have difficulty with any of the questions, consult with your instructor.

Caring for the Garcias

Joseph Garcia has been prescribed the following medicines:

lisinopril (Prinivil) 20 mg by mouth daily
hydrochlorothiazide (HydroDiuril) 25 mg by
    mouth daily
metformin (Glucophage) 500 mg by mouth BID

Today he had blood drawn for analysis. Following are the electrolyte panel results.

Sodium	136 mEq/L
Potassium	3.0 mEq/L
Chloride	96 mEq/L
Bicarbonate	24 mEq/L
BUN	18 mg/dL
Creatinine	0.8 mg/dL

A. Review the lab results. Compare Joe's lab work with the established norms for these values. Based on the lab results, what kind of assessment questions would be appropriate to ask Joe?

B. Use your pharmacology text to review Joe's medications. Which, if any, of these medicines might be contributing to Joe's lab results?

C. What teaching would be appropriate for Joe?

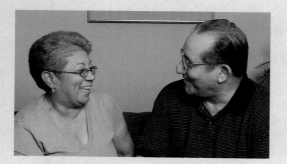

1

Recall the "Meet Your Patients" scenario in Volume 1. When you review Jackson La-Guardia's chart to prepare for clinical day, you find that he is in the emergency department (ED) with four other members of the LaGuardia family. All of them have come to the ED complaining of nausea, vomiting, and diarrhea related to severe gastroenteritis, a viral intestinal disorder. The family members include the following:

8-month-old Jason, grandson of Jackson
26-year-old Susanna, Jackson's daughter and Jason's mother
60-year-old Jackson
58-year-old Gemma, Jackson's wife
82-year-old Martha, Jackson's mother

Jason, Jackson, and Martha are being admitted to the hospital. However, Susanna and Gemma have been asked to follow up tomorrow in the urgent care clinic. The following questions pertain to this scenario.

a Martha LaGuardia's orders call for lactated Ringer's solution with 20 mEq KCl per liter to infuse at 150 mL/hr. After 4 hours of infusion, Martha begins to complain of shortness of breath and develops a cough. What do you suspect may be happening? What actions should you take?

b What theoretical knowledge will you use in caring for Ms LaGuardia's immediate problem?

c Jason LaGuardia has been ordered to receive 250 mL of 0.9% saline solution over 8 hours. What type of equipment should you consider using?

d Calculate the drip rate for Jason's infusion if a gravity flow device is used. What further information do you need to perform this calculation?

e As you may recall, Jackson LaGuardia has end-stage renal disease. His lab work reveals a hemoglobin of 7.6 mg/dL and a hematocrit of 21%. He has been ordered to receive two units of packed red blood cells over 8 hours. Given his condition, for what fluid balance problem is he at risk? What additional parameters should you assess while he is receiving the transfusion?

2   You are asked to administer an antibiotic intravenously via piggyback. You are not familiar with the equipment that this facility uses. As a student, what approach should you take to solve this problem?

3   Identify techniques that you have observed that may contribute to contamination of an IV site.

4   Interpret the following ABG results. Explain your thinking.

a   pH   7.47 P_{CO_2} 45 mm Hg HCO_3^- 32 mEq/L

b   pH   7.32 P_{CO_2} 50 mm Hg HCO_3^- 25 mEq/L

c   pH   7.30 P_{CO_2} 41 mm Hg HCO_3^- 18 mEq/L

d   pH   7.45 P_{CO_2} 30 mm Hg HCO_3^- 22 mEq/L

5 For each of the following concepts, use critical thinking to describe how or why it is important to nursing, patient care or fluids, electrolytes, and acid-base balance. Note that these are *not* to be merely definitions.

Homeostasis

Selectively permeable membranes

Fluid imbalance

Electrolyte imbalances

Acid-base imbalances

Parenteral fluid and electrolyte replacement

Practical Knowledge

knowing how

To prevent, identify, and treat fluid, electrolyte, and acid-base problems, you will need to be skilled at initiating and managing intravenous infusions of fluids and blood, performing focused history and physical assessments, and interpreting arterial blood gas values.

PROCEDURES

| PROCEDURE 36–1 | **Initiating a Peripheral Intravenous Infusion** |

 For steps to follow in *all* procedures, refer to the inside back cover of this book.

critical aspects

- Prepare the intravenous solution and administration set.
- Locate a vein for placing the IV catheter. Select the most distal vein on the hand or arm initially.
- Clip excessive hair at the site with scissors.
- Don procedure gloves.
- Apply the tourniquet, and cleanse the site. Allow the antiseptic to dry on the skin.
- Using your nondominant hand, stabilize the vein, making sure not to contaminate the insertion site.
- Inform the patient that you are about to insert the catheter.
- Open the catheter. Grasp it with the thumb and forefinger of your dominant hand, making sure that the bevel is up.
- Holding the catheter at a 20 to 30° angle, pierce the skin.
- Lower the catheter so that it is parallel to the skin, and advance the catheter.
- Watch for a flashback of blood; then disengage the stylet, and insert the catheter.
- While holding the catheter in place with one hand, release the tourniquet with your other hand.
- Quickly connect the tubing adapter to the IV catheter, using aseptic technique.
- Open the roller clamp, and allow the IV fluid to flush the catheter, and then adjust the flow rate according to the physician's order.
- Cover the insertion site with a sterile, semipermeable, transparent dressing.
- Loop and tape the administration tubing and the connection between the catheter and tubing.
- Label the dressing with the date and time of insertion, catheter size, and your initials.
- If the insertion site is located near a joint, place an arm board under the joint, and secure it with tape.

PROCEDURE 36–1

Initiating a Peripheral Intravenous Infusion
(continued)

Equipment

- Appropriately sized intravenous (IV) catheter
- Scissors
- Linen-saver pad
- Tourniquet
- Antiseptic swabs that contain solutions such as 2% tincture of iodine, alcohol, or chlorhexidine
- Sterile, transparent, semipermeable dressing
- 1-inch nonallergenic tape
- Arm board, if necessary
- Administration set
- IV solution
- Extension tubing, if necessary

Delegation

In some states and agencies you can delegate peripheral IV catheter insertion to a licensed practical nurse (LPN) who is properly trained in the skill.

Assessment

- Assess the patient's need for IV therapy by checking vital signs, laboratory values, urine output, skin turgor, breath sounds, and the condition of mucous membranes.
- Assess the arms and hands for a potential insertion site.

You must carefully assess insertion sites to avoid inserting a catheter in a potentially dangerous site. For example, do not insert an IV catheter in an area that contains a draining wound or in an extremity that contains a dialysis fistula. Generally, IV catheters are not inserted in the legs or feet.

- Monitor the patient's tolerance of IV therapy by auscultating breath sounds and monitoring vital signs, urine output, laboratory values, and neck vein distention.

The presence of crackles, diminished urine output, and distended neck veins signals heart failure, which can be a complication of IV therapy.

- Check for factors such as anticoagulant therapy, bleeding disorders, or low platelet count.

These factors place the patient at risk for bleeding during IV catheter insertion.

Procedural Steps

Note: Maintain scrupulous sterile technique throughout this procedure.

Any microorganisms inadvertently introduced go directly into the bloodstream and can quickly cause sepsis.

Step 1 Prepare the intravenous solution and administration set.

a. Following the six "rights" of medication administration, check the IV solution to make sure that you have the proper solution with the prescribed additives.

IV solutions are considered medications, and you should check them carefully to avoid administration errors.

b. Check the expiration date on the IV solution bag.

Do not use IV solution after the expiration date.

c. Check the IV solution for discoloration or particulate matter.

Solutions that are discolored or contain particulate matter may be contaminated and should not be used.

d. Label the IV solution container with the patient's name, date, and your initials. Place a time tape on the solution container with the prescribed infusion rate, time the infusion began, and the time of completion. ▼

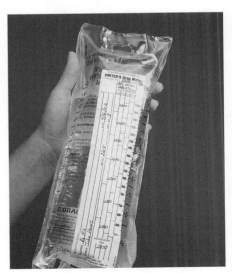

➤

PROCEDURE 36–1 Initiating a Peripheral Intravenous Infusion
(continued)

e. Take the administration set from the package, label the tubing with the date and time, and then close the roller clamp by rolling it downward.

Close the roller clamp so that fluid does not flow through inadvertently after the bag is spiked.

f. Remove the protective cover from the IV solution container port.

g. Remove the protective cover from the spike on the IV administration set, making sure the spike remains sterile. Place the spike into the port of the solution container. If the solution is contained in a glass bottle, clean the rubber stopper on the top of the bottle with an alcohol pad. Then insert the spike of the administration set through the black rubber stopper. ▼

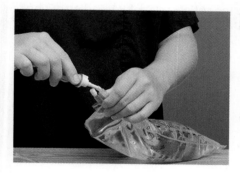

h. Be certain the tubing is clamped. Hang the IV solution container on an IV pole.

i. Lightly compress the drip chamber, and allow it to fill up halfway. If you are using extension tubing, attach it to the end of the administration set. Prime the tubing (remove the air from the tubing) by opening the roller clamp and allowing the fluid to slowly fill the tubing. ▼

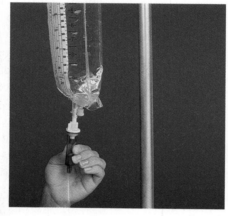

j. Inspect the tubing for air. If air bubbles remain in the tubing, flick the tubing with a fingernail to mobilize the bubbles.

Step 2 Locate a vein for inserting the IV catheter. Select the most distal vein on the hand or arm. Avoid using an arm or hand that contains a dialysis graft or fistula, or the affected arm of a patient who has undergone a mastectomy.

Choose the most distal veins on the hand or arm so that you can perform subsequent venipunctures proximal to the previous site. This preserves veins for long-term therapy and prevents extravasation of fluid and medicines. Avoid extremities in which circulation is impaired.

Step 3 Place a linen-saver pad under the patient's arm.

Protects the bed from soiling during venipuncture.

Step 4 Place the patient's arm in a dependent position.

Gravity helps fill and dilate the vein, making venipuncture easier.

Step 5 Apply a tourniquet 10 to 15 cm (4 to 6 inches) above the selected site. Palpate the radial pulse. If no pulse is present, loosen the tourniquet, and reapply it with less tension.

Occluding the arterial flow diminishes venous filling, making venipuncture difficult.

Step 6 Palpate the vein and press it downward, making sure that it rebounds quickly. If the vein is not adequately dilated, have the patient open and close his fist; apply heat (e.g., a warm towel); lightly tap the vein site; or stroke the extremity from distal to proximal below the selected venipuncture site.

These methods help dilate the vein to ease venipuncture. Heat relaxes the vein wall, and the other methods move blood into the vein.

Step 7 After selecting the vein, gently release the tourniquet. If excessive hair is present at the venipuncture site, clip it with a scissors.

Clipping the hair helps the dressings to adhere after catheter insertion.

Step 8 Apply procedure gloves.

Protects you from inadvertent exposure to blood.

Step 9 Choose an appropriate IV catheter based on the size of the vein and the solution to be infused. Using aseptic technique, open the package.

Reduces the risk of extravasation and phlebitis. Always use the smallest diameter and shortest catheter that will deliver the desired solution flow.

PROCEDURE 36–1

Initiating a Peripheral Intravenous Infusion
(continued)

Step 10 Gently reapply the tourniquet and cleanse the site, using an antiseptic swab that contains 2% tincture of iodine, alcohol, or chlorhexidine (avoid using chlorhexidine in infants under age 2 months). Cleanse the area using a circular motion, starting at the site and working outward several inches.

Removes microorganisms from the skin so that they do not enter the venous system during venipuncture. Working "clean to dirty" avoids moving microorganisms toward the puncture site. ▼

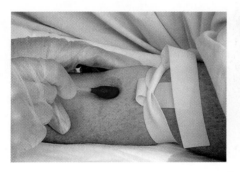

Step 11 Allow the antiseptic to dry on the skin.

Increases the antiseptic's effectiveness; promotes patient comfort on puncture of the skin.

Step 12 Using your nondominant hand, stabilize the vein by stretching the skin over the vein, making sure not to contaminate the insertion site.

Eases insertion and prevents inadvertent damage to the underside of the vein.

Step 13 Inform the patient that you are about to insert the catheter and that it may be uncomfortable.

Keeping the patient informed promotes cooperation and lessens anxiety.

Step 14 Pick up the catheter.

Variation A Wing-Tipped Catheter (Butterfly)

Grasp the catheter by the wings, using the thumb and forefinger of your dominant hand and making sure that the bevel is up. Remove the protective cap from the needle.

Stabilizes the catheter for insertion. Inserting the needle bevel up makes it less likely that you will pierce both vein walls (go "through" the vein). ▼

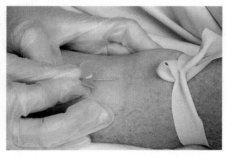

Variation B Over-the-Needle Catheter

Grasp the catheter by the hub, using the thumb and forefinger of your dominant hand and making sure that the bevel is up.

Stabilizes it for insertion. ▼

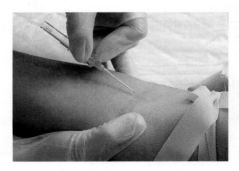

Step 15 Holding the catheter at a 20 to 30° angle, pierce the skin.

Holding the catheter at a 20 to 30° angle allows you to pierce the skin without inadvertently piercing the back of the vein.

Step 16 Lower the catheter so that it is parallel to the skin, and advance the catheter into the vein. Watch closely for a flashback of blood into the chamber of the catheter or the tubing of the winged catheter.

The flashback of blood indicates that the vein has been cannulated.

Step 17 Advance the catheter.

Variation A Wing-Tipped Catheter

Fully advance the needle.

Variation B Over-the-Needle Catheter

Advance the catheter to at least half of its length. Withdraw the needle as you advance the catheter fully into the vein.

Step 18 While holding the catheter in place with one hand, release the tourniquet with your other hand.

Releasing the tourniquet restores full circulation to the patient's extremity and prevents injury.

Step 19 Quickly connect the administration set adapter to IV catheter, using aseptic technique. ▼

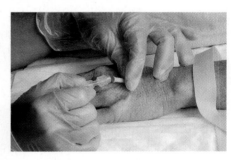

Step 20 Still stabilizing the catheter, slowly open the roller clamp, and allow the IV fluid to flush the catheter. Adjust the flow rate according to the physician's order.

Flushing the blood from the catheter with IV fluid helps maintain patency of the catheter.

➤

PROCEDURE 36–1

Initiating a Peripheral Intravenous Infusion
(continued)

Step 21 Cover the insertion site with a sterile semipermeable transparent dressing. If the site is not clean and dry, first clean the site with an antiseptic swab and allow it to dry. ▼

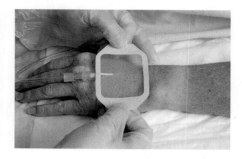

a. Open the package containing the dressing. Using aseptic technique, remove the protective backing from the dressing, making sure not to touch the sterile surface.

b. Cover the insertion site and the hub or winged portion of the catheter with the dressing. Do not cover the tubing of the administration set.

c. Gently pinch the transparent dressing around the catheter hub to secure the hub. Smooth the remainder of the dressing so that it adheres to the skin.

Step 22 Loop the administration tubing, and place a piece of tape over the connection between the catheter and tubing and the looped section of the tubing.

Looping the tubing supplies slack to prevent the IV catheter from becoming dislodged.

Step 23 Label the dressing with the date and time of insertion, catheter size, and your initials.

Peripheral IV catheters should be replaced every 72 to 96 hours to prevent phlebitis. Labeling the dressing with the date and time of insertion helps communicate when catheters should be changed. ▼

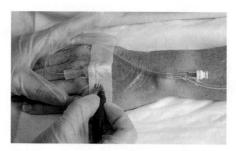

Step 24 If the insertion site is located near a joint, place an arm board under the joint, and secure it with tape.

Using an arm board stabilizes the joint and helps prevent the catheter from becoming dislodged.

Evaluation

- Monitor the IV site and flow rate hourly while IV fluid is infusing. Check for signs of infiltration, extravasation, and phlebitis.
- Evaluate the patient's tolerance to IV therapy.
- Report any signs of fluid overload, such as edema, shortness of breath, jugular vein distention, or hypertension.

Patient Teaching

- Instruct the patient about IV therapy.
- Teach the patient the importance of notifying staff immediately if the catheter or administration set becomes dislodged or if the insertion site becomes tender, red, or swollen.
- Explain the adverse effects of IV therapy, and tell the patient to notify staff if he develops difficulty breathing.
- Teach the patient safety measures to avoid dislodging the catheter.

Home Care

- Explain home IV therapy to the patient and caregiver, and teach them how to identify complications.
- Provide the patient with the name and phone numbers of people to contact in case problems arise with the catheter or site.

PROCEDURE 36–1   **Initiating a Peripheral Intravenous Infusion**
(continued)

Documentation

- Chart the date and time of insertion, the gauge and type of catheter, the number of attempts, and the location of the insertion site.
- Document the type and rate of the IV fluid infusing.
- Note the patient's tolerance to the procedure. Chart any adverse reactions to the insertion or IV therapy and the interventions required.
- Often, IV care is documented on a flowsheet. Fluids infused are documented on the I & O record, as well.

Sample of a narrative note:

6/07/07	0200	20-gauge, winged catheter inserted without difficulty on the first attempt. Site dressed with a transparent, semipermeable dressing. 1 L of D_5/0.9% NSS hung at 125 mL/hour. Patient tolerated venipuncture without difficulty. Instructed patient to notify nursing staff immediately if pain or swelling occurs at the insertion site. Also instructed patient about precautions to take to avoid dislodging IV catheter and importance of notifying staff immediately should catheter become dislodged.
		———S. Lyons, RN

PROCEDURE 36–2   Regulating the IV Flow Rate

For steps to follow in *all* procedures, refer to the inside back cover of this book.

critical aspects
- Check the solution to make sure that you have the proper IV fluid with the prescribed additives.
- Verify the prescribed infusion rate.
- Calculate the drip rate.
- Apply a time tape to the IV solution container. Mark the time the infusion was started.
- Open the roller clamp so that IV fluid begins to flow.
- Using a watch, count the number of drops entering the drip chamber in 1 minute.
- Adjust the roller clamp, increasing or decreasing the flow until you achieve the prescribed drip rate.
- Monitor the infusion rate 15 minutes after you begin the infusion; then monitor the rate hourly.

Equipment
- IV solution hanging on an IV pole and attached to an administration set
- Watch with a second hand
- Time tape

Delegation
Refer to your state nurse practice act regarding delegation of this task to an LPN.

Assessment
- Assess the IV catheter for patency before starting the infusion and then hourly while the IV fluid infuses.

Ensures that the fluid will infuse at the correct rate and without complication.
- Assess the IV site for signs of phlebitis, infiltration, or extravasation.

You must change the IV catheter before regulating the flow rate if any of these complications occur.
- Assess the patient's need for IV therapy by checking laboratory values, urine output, and vital signs and by auscultating breath sounds.

IV therapy creates a risk for fluid overload.

Procedural Steps

Step 1 Follow the six "rights" of medication administration. Check the solution to make sure that you have the proper IV fluid hanging with the prescribed additives. Also verify the infusion rate.

IV solutions are considered medications, and you should check them carefully to avoid administration errors.

Step 2 Calculate the hourly rate if it is not specified in the order. Divide the volume to be infused by the number of hours it is to be infused. For example, if the physician prescribes 1000 mL to run over 4 hours, the infusion rate is 250 mL/hr.

You must carefully calculate the infusion rate to ensure that the patient receives the correct volume of fluid.

Step 3 Calculate the drip rate by multiplying the number of milliliters to be infused in 60 minutes by the drop factor in drops/per milliliter; then divide by 60 minutes:

$$\frac{\text{Hourly rate in mL} \times (\text{drops/mL})}{60 \text{ minutes}} = \text{drip rate}$$

For example, an hourly rate of 100 mL multiplied by 15 drops/mL and divided by 60 minutes equals the drip rate. Therefore, the drip rate equals 25 drops per minute.

Each administration set has a drip factor that is determined by the manufacturer. The drip factor is the number of drops necessary to deliver 1 mL of solution. Microdrip tubing has a drip factor of 60 drops/mL; blood administration tubing

PROCEDURE 36–2   **Regulating the IV Flow Rate** *(continued)*

typically has a drip factor of 10 drops/mL; macrodrip tubing has a drip factor of 15 drops/mL.

Step 4 Verify your calculations.

Having a second person verify your calculations prevents administration errors. If a second person is unavailable, double-check your calculations.

Step 5 Apply a time tape to the IV solution container next to the volume markings. Mark the time tape with the time that the infusion was started. Continue to mark 1-hour intervals on the time tape until you reach the bottom of the container.

The time tape allows all nurses to accurately monitor the rate of administration.

Step 6 Open the roller clamp so that IV fluid begins to flow.

The roller clamp must be opened to allow the flow of fluid.

Step 7 Using a watch, count the number of drops entering the drip chamber in 1 minute.

Timing the drip rate for 1 minute helps accurately achieve the correct drip rate. ▼

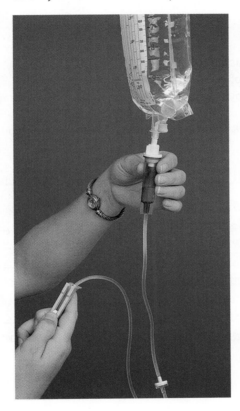

Step 8 Adjust the roller clamp by increasing or decreasing the flow until you achieve the prescribed drip rate.

IV solution is considered a medication and must infuse at the prescribed rate.

Step 9 Monitor the infusion rate 15 minutes after you begin the infusion; then monitor it hourly.

Changes in the patient's position may speed up or slow down the infusion rate; frequent monitoring of the infusion rate ensures that the correct volume of fluid infuses over the correct length of time.

Evaluation

- Evaluate the patient's response to IV therapy by checking for signs of excessive or deficient fluid volume.
- Evaluate the IV site for signs of infiltration, extravasation, and phlebitis.
- Check the appropriate laboratory studies to help evaluate the effectiveness of IV therapy.
- For flow rate problems be sure the drip chamber is above the level of the IV site and there are no kinks in the tubing; raise or lower the bag as needed to achieve the correct rate.

Patient Teaching

- Explain the adverse effects of IV therapy and tell the patient to notify staff immediately if he develops difficulty breathing.
- Discuss the importance of notifying staff immediately if the catheter or administration set becomes dislodged or if the insertion site becomes tender, red, or swollen.
- Teach the patient safety measures if he is permitted to ambulate and the IV is infusing.

➤

PROCEDURE 36–2 **Regulating the IV Flow Rate** *(continued)*

Home Care

- Explain home IV therapy to the patient and caregiver, and teach them how to identify complications.
- Provide the patient and caregiver with the name and phone numbers of people to contact in case problems arise with the catheter or insertion site.

Documentation

- Chart the date and time the infusion was started.
- Document the type of IV fluid, the rate of infusion, and the IV catheter site.
- Note the patient's tolerance of IV therapy. Document any complications of IV therapy and the interventions taken.
- Document the volume infused on the I & O record. Often IV care is documented on a flowsheet.

Sample of a narrative note:

9/18/06	1500	An infusion of $D_5$1/2 NS was started through a 20-gauge catheter, located in the right forearm at a rate of 100 mL/hr. No redness, swelling, or discomfort present at the site. Patient's lungs are clear to auscultation. Urine output greater than 30 mL/hour; see I & O sheet. Patient NPO for a CT scan of the abdomen. Tolerating IV fluid without difficulty. — S. Chen, RN

PROCEDURE 36–3　Setting Up and Using IV Pumps

For steps to follow in *all* procedures, refer to the inside back cover of this book.

critical aspects

- Calculate the infusion rate.
- Attach the IV pump to the IV pole, and plug it into the nearest electrical outlet.
- Take the administration set from the package, label the tubing with the date and time, and close the clamp on the administration set.
- Remove the protective covers, and spike the port of the solution container with the administration set. Hang the IV solution container on the IV pole.
- If a filter is required, attach it to the end of the administration set.
- Compress the drip chamber of the administration set, and allow it to fill halfway.
- Place the electronic eye on the drip chamber between the fluid level and the origin of the drop. (If there is no electronic eye, consult the manufacturer's instructions for setup).
- Prime the administration set with fluid by opening the roller clamp and allowing the fluid to flow slowly through the tubing. Close the clamp.
- Inspect the tubing for the presence of air. If air bubbles remain in the tubing, flick the tubing with a fingernail to mobilize the bubbles.
- Turn on the IV pump, and load the administration tubing into the pump according to the manufacturer's instructions.
- Program the pump with the prescribed infusion rate (hourly rate) and the volume to be infused (usually the total amount in the IV bag). Again, follow the manufacturer's instructions—each pump is different.
- Apply procedure gloves, and connect the administration set adapter to the IV catheter. Take care not to contaminate the adapter hub, the IV catheter, or the insertion site.
- Unclamp the administration set tubing, and press the start button on the IV pump.
- Make sure that the alarms are turned on and audible.
- Check the pump hourly to make sure that the correct volume is infusing.
- At the end of your shift (or at the time specified by your healthcare facility), clear the pump of the volume infused, and record the volume on the patient's I & O form.

Equipment

- IV pump
- Administration set appropriate for IV pump
- IV pole
- IV fluid or medicated solution

Delegation

You can delegate the task of setting up an IV pump to an LPN who is specially trained in IV therapy. Do not delegate this task to UAP. Do, however, instruct the UAP to notify you of any pump alarms that sound.

Assessment

- Assess the patient's need for IV therapy by checking vital signs, laboratory values, urine output, skin turgor, breath sounds, and the condition of mucous membranes.
- Monitor the patient's tolerance of IV therapy by auscultating breath sounds and by monitoring vital signs, urine output, laboratory values, and neck vein distention.

These data help determine the patient's fluid balance.

- Assess the existing IV catheter for patency.

Occlusion of the IV catheter prevents the infusion of IV fluid.

- Assess the IV site hourly for signs of phlebitis, infiltration, and extravasation.

Early detection of these complications allows for prompt intervention and treatment.

➤

PROCEDURE 36–3   **Setting Up and Using IV Pumps** *(continued)*

Procedural Steps

Step 1 Calculate the infusion rate by dividing the volume to be infused by the number of hours it is to be infused. For example, if the order states 1000 mL to run over 8 hours, divide 1000 mL by 8 hours to determine the infusion rate of 125 mL/hr.

You must carefully calculate the infusion rate to ensure that the patient receives the correct dose. Pumps are usually programmed in milliliters per hour instead of drops per minute.

Step 2 Verify your calculations.

Verifying your calculations with a colleague or by recalculating prevents administration errors.

Step 3 Attach the IV pump to the IV pole, and plug it into the nearest electrical outlet.

The IV pump must be stabilized on an IV pole for safe use. It should be plugged into an electrical outlet when in use so that the battery remains charged for transport. ▼

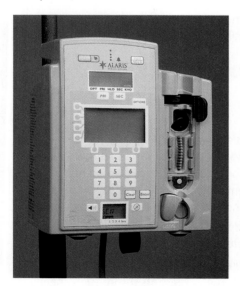

Step 4 Take the administration set from the package, label the tubing with the date and time, and close the clamp on the administration set.

Labeling the administration set with the date and time informs the nursing staff when the administration set should be changed. Close the clamp to prevent inadvertent loss of fluid.

Step 5 Remove the protective covers, and spike the port of the solution container with the administration set. Hang the IV solution container on the IV pole.

Step 6 Compress the drip chamber of the administration set, and allow it to fill halfway. Place the electronic eye on the drip chamber between the fluid level and the origin of the drop. (If there is no electronic eye, consult the manufacturer's instructions for setup.)

Prepares the administration set for priming and prevents air from entering the tubing with the solution. On gravity-type pumps, the electronic eye counts the number of drops to ensure the proper rate. Infusion pumps compress the tubing to move fluid; they measure the amount internally.

Step 7 If a filter is required, attach it to the end of the administration set.

Filters are recommended to filter minute particles from the solution.

Step 8 Prime the administration set with fluid by opening the roller clamp and allowing the fluid to flow slowly through the tubing. Close the clamp.

Removes air from the tubing to prevent air embolus.

Step 9 Inspect the tubing for the presence of air. If air bubbles remain in the tubing, flick the tubing with a fingernail to mobilize the bubbles.

Air bubbles in the administration tubing interrupt flow.

Step 10 Turn on the IV pump, and load the administration tubing into the pump according to the manufacturer's instructions.

This process differs among manufacturers. ▼

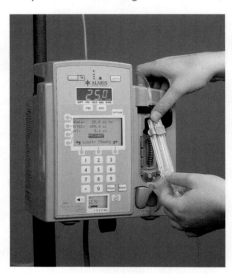

Step 11 Program the pump with the prescribed infusion rate (hourly rate) and the volume to be infused (usually the total amount in the IV bag). ▼

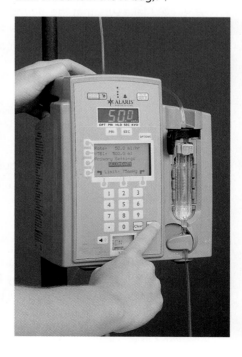

PROCEDURE 36–3   Setting Up and Using IV Pumps *(continued)*

Step 12 Apply procedure gloves, use an antiseptic wipe to cleanse the infusion port, and connect the administration set adapter to the IV catheter or port.

Procedure gloves protect you from exposure to body fluids when you disconnect the tubing from the IV catheter.

Step 13 Unclamp the administration set tubing (open the roller clamp all the way), and press the start button on the IV pump.

Allows the IV fluid to flow through the administration set.

Step 14 Make sure that the alarms are turned on and audible.

The alarms must be functioning so that the pump can alert you of problems, such as kinks, air in the tubing, or catheter occlusion.

Step 15 Check the pump hourly to make sure the correct volume is infusing.

Infusion pumps sometimes malfunction, so frequent monitoring is essential.

Step 16 At the end of your shift (or at the time specified by your healthcare facility), clear the pump of the volume infused and record the volume on the patient's I & O form.

Clearing the pump of the volume infused during your shift helps the oncoming shift accurately monitor the fluid infused during their shift.

Evaluation

- Evaluate the correct functioning of the IV pump hourly.

Patient Teaching

- Explain use of the IV infusion pump to the patient.
- Teach the patient the importance of notifying staff immediately if the infusion pump alarm sounds, the catheter or administration set becomes dislodged, or the insertion site becomes tender, red, or swollen.
- Teach the patient safety measures if he is able to ambulate while the infusion pump is in use.

Home Care

- Explain home IV infusion pump use to the patient and caregiver, and teach them how to identify complications. (Most home infusion pumps are smaller than institutional pumps.)
- Provide the patient with the name and phone numbers of people to contact in case problems arise with the catheter, insertion site, IV infusion pump, or other equipment.

Documentation

- Chart the type and volume of IV fluid infusing along with the infusion rate.
- Record use of the infusion pump, and note the patient's tolerance of IV therapy.
- Document any complications of IV therapy and the interventions taken.
- Document the volume infused on the patient's I & O record. Often, IV care is documented on a flowsheet.

Sample of a narrative note:

7/26/07	0600	*Patient admitted from the ED with dehydration.*
		NSS infusing at 250 mL/hr via infusion pump
		through an 18-gauge catheter. No signs of
		infiltration. No tenderness, redness, or swelling
		at the insertion site. BP 90/46 mm Hg. HR
		118 beats/minute, RR 24 breaths/minute, and
		temp. 102.6 °F rectally. ———— R. Brill, RN

| PROCEDURE 36–4 | **Changing IV Solutions, Tubing, and Dressings** |

> For steps to follow in *all* procedures, refer to the inside back cover of this book.

critical aspects

36–4A: For Changing the IV Solution

- Prepare and label your next container of IV solution 1 hour before the present infusion is scheduled to finish.
- Close the roller clamp on the infusing (empty) administration set.
- Wearing procedure gloves, remove the old IV solution container from the IV pole. Remove the spike from the bag, keeping the spike sterile.
- Spike the new IV solution bag.
- Hang the new IV solution container on the IV pole, and inspect the tubing for air.
- Open the roller clamp, and adjust the drip rate.
- Adhere the time tape to the new IV solution container. Mark the times.

36–4B: For Changing the IV Solution and Tubing

- Prepare the new IV solution and tubing.
- Wearing procedure gloves, carefully remove the tape securing the connection between the catheter and tubing.
- Close the roller clamp on the administration set.
- Remove the protective cover from the distal end of the new administration set.
- Stabilize the IV catheter with your nondominant hand while applying pressure over the vein just above the insertion site.
- Quickly, but gently, disengage the old tubing from the IV catheter, and insert the new tubing into the IV catheter.
- Open the roller clamp, and adjust the drip rate.
- Resecure the IV catheter and tubing connection.

36–4C: For Changing the IV Dressing

- Wearing procedure gloves, stabilize the catheter with your nondominant hand, and carefully remove the dressing.
- Inspect the insertion site. Using a circular motion, cleanse the insertion site with an antiseptic swab containing 2% tincture of iodine, alcohol, or chlorhexidine.
- Allow the antiseptic to dry on the skin.
- Cover the insertion site with a sterile semipermeable transparent dressing.
- Loop and tape the administration tubing and tape the connection between the catheter and tubing and the looped section of the tubing.
- Label the dressing with the date and time of insertion, catheter size, and your initials.

Equipment

- Administration set
- IV solution
- IV pole
- Sterile transparent semipermeable dressing

- Antiseptic swabs that contain solutions such as 2% tincture of iodine, alcohol, or chlorhexidine (chlorhexidine is not recommended in infants under age 2 months)
- 1-inch nonallergenic tape
- Time tape
- Watch with a second hand

PROCEDURE 36–4

Changing IV Solutions, Tubing, and Dressings
(continued)

Delegation

You can delegate the tasks of changing IV solutions, tubing, and dressings to an LPN who is specially trained in IV therapy. The task should not be delegated to UAP. Do, however, instruct the UAP to notify you of any problems that occur with IV therapy, such as the disconnecting of the administration set, catheter dislodging, or complaints of pain, swelling, or redness at the insertion site.

Assessment

- Assess the IV catheter for patency before changing the solution container, administration set, or dressing.
- Assess the IV site for signs of phlebitis, infiltration, or extravasation.

You must change the IV catheter if any of these complications occur; the Centers for Disease Control and Prevention recommends rotating the IV site every 72 to 96 hours to reduce the risk of phlebitis.

PROCEDURE 36–4A

Changing the IV Solution

Procedural Steps

Step 1 Following the six "rights" of medication administration, prepare and label your next container of IV solution 1 hour before the present infusion is scheduled to finish.

Preparing the next IV solution container reduces the risk of the present container running dry and thereby causing clots to form that would occlude the catheter.

Step 2 Close the roller clamp on the administration set.

Prevents air from entering the tubing while the IV solution container is being changed.

Step 3 Wearing procedure gloves, remove the old IV solution container from the IV pole. Remove the spike from the bag, keeping the spike sterile.

The spike must remain sterile to prevent contamination of the new IV fluid. Procedure gloves protect you from inadvertent exposure to body fluids.

Step 4 Remove the protective cover from the new IV solution container port.

Step 5 Place the spike into the port of the new solution container. If the solution is contained in a glass IV bottle, first clean the rubber stopper on the top of the bottle with an alcohol pad; then, insert the spike of the administration set through the black rubber stopper.

Cleansing the stopper removes particulate matter.

Step 6 Hang the IV solution container on the IV pole.

Allows the fluid to infuse by gravity.

Step 7 Inspect the tubing to be sure that it is free of air bubbles and the drip chamber remains half-filled. Flick the tubing with a finger to mobilize the bubbles.

Prevents air from entering the system as the new solution is hung. If the IV solution has completely emptied from the bag, the drip chamber may no longer be half-filled ▼.

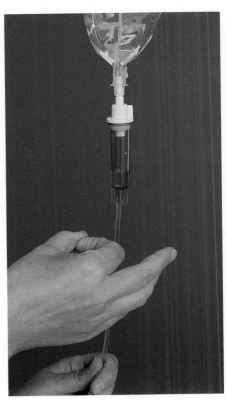

PROCEDURE 36–4

Changing IV Solutions, Tubing, and Dressings
(continued)

Step 8 Open the roller clamp and adjust the drip rate, as prescribed.

IV solution is considered a medication and must infuse at the prescribed rate.

Step 9 Affix the time tape to the new IV solution container. Mark the tape with the time the infusion was started, and continue to mark 1-hour intervals on the time tape until you reach the bottom of the container.

The time tape allows you and other nurses to accurately monitor the rate of administration.

PROCEDURE 36–4B

Changing the IV Administration Tubing and Solution

Procedural Steps

Step 1 Prepare the IV solution and tubing as you would when initiating a new IV. (See Procedure 36–1, step 1)

Step 2 Wearing procedure gloves, carefully remove the tape, securing the connection between the catheter and tubing.

Provides access to the connection.

Step 3 Close the roller clamp on the old administration set.

Stops the flow of fluid from the old container.

Step 4 Hang the new administration set on the IV pole.

Step 5 Remove the protective cover from the distal end of the new administration set.

Cover keeps the distal end sterile until you are ready to connect it to the IV catheter.

Step 6 Stabilize the IV catheter with your nondominant hand while applying pressure over the vein just above the insertion site.

Stabilizing the catheter prevents it from becoming dislodged during the tubing change; applying pressure over the vein stops blood from flowing from the catheter as you change the administration tubing. ▼

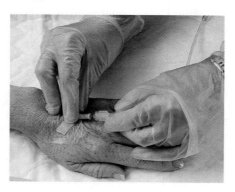

Step 7 Quickly, but gently, disengage the old tubing from the IV catheter, and insert the new tubing into the IV catheter. Use a

hemostat ("mosquito" clamp) to hold the catheter hub if the old tubing does not come loose easily.

IV tubing should be changed every 72 hours. Change it quickly to prevent microorganisms from entering the IV catheter.

Step 8 Open the roller clamp on the new administration set, and allow the IV solution to infuse.

Allowing the solution to infuse clears the IV catheter of blood, preventing catheter occlusion.

Step 9 Using the roller clamp, adjust the flow until you achieve the prescribed rate.

IV solution is considered a medication and must infuse at the prescribed rate.

Step 10 Resecure the IV catheter and tubing connection.

PROCEDURE 36–4C   Changing the IV Dressing

Procedural Steps

Note: This is usually performed at the same time the IV solution and tubing are changed. Most dressings may remain in place for 72 hours and are changed when the insertion site is rotated. However, dressings may be changed at other times if they become soiled or dislodged.

Step 1 Place a linen-saver pad under the patient's arm. Wearing procedure gloves, stabilize the catheter with your nondominant hand, and carefully remove the dressing.

Remove the dressing gently to avoid dislodging the catheter.

Step 2 Inspect the insertion site. Look for erythema, drainage, and tenderness.

If signs of infection, phlebitis, or infiltration are present, you must remove the IV catheter.

Step 3 Using a circular motion, cleanse the insertion site with an antiseptic swab containing 2% tincture of iodine, alcohol, or chlorhexidine (avoid using chlorhexidine in infants under age 2 months). Start at the insertion site, and work outward several inches.

Removes microorganisms from the skin to minimize the risk of their entering the venipuncture site.

Step 4 Allow the antiseptic to dry on the skin.

Increases the antiseptic's effectiveness.

Step 5 Cover the insertion site with a sterile semipermeable transparent dressing.
a. Open the package containing the dressing. Remove the protective backing from the dressing, making sure not to touch the sterile surface.
b. Cover the insertion site and the hub or winged portion of the catheter with the dressing. Do not cover the tubing of the administration set.
c. Gently pinch the transparent dressing around the catheter hub to secure the hub. Smooth the remainder of the dressing so that it adheres to the skin.

Step 6 Loop the administration tubing and place a piece of tape over the connection between the catheter and tubing and the looped section of the tubing.

Looping the tubing supplies slack to prevent the IV catheter from becoming dislodged.

Step 7 Label the dressing with the date and time of insertion, catheter size, and your initials.

Peripheral IV catheters should be replaced every 72 to 96 hours to prevent phlebitis. Labeling the dressing with the date and time of insertion helps communicate to other nurses when to change catheters.

Evaluation
- Evaluate the IV insertion site for signs of infiltration, extravasation, and phlebitis.
- Evaluate the effectiveness of IV therapy by assessing the patient's hydration status.

Patient Teaching
- Explain the adverse effects of IV therapy, and tell the patient to notify staff immediately if he develops difficulty breathing.
- Tell the patient the importance of notifying staff if his IV dressing becomes soiled, dampened, or loosened.
- Discuss the importance of notifying staff immediately if the catheter or administration set becomes dislodged or if the insertion site becomes tender, red, or swollen.

Home Care
- Explain home IV therapy to the patient and caregiver; teach them how to identify complications.
- Make sure the caregiver is able to perform fluid, tubing, and dressing changes when necessary.
- Provide the patient and caregiver with the name and phone numbers of people to contact in case problems arise with the catheter or insertion site.

➤

PROCEDURE 36–4   **Changing IV Solutions, Tubings, and Dressings** *(continued)*

Documentation

- Chart the date and time the IV fluid, tubing and dressing were changed. Document the type of IV fluid and the rate of infusion, as well as the location and condition of the IV catheter insertion site.
- Document any complications of IV therapy and the interventions taken.
- Make sure also to document the IV fluid, tubing, and dressing change on your IV record. Often, IV care is documented on a flowsheet.

Sample of a narrative note:

7/17/07	2300	1 L 0.9% NSS hung at a rate of 100 mL/hr through a 20-gauge angiocath. Tubing and dressing changed. New transparent semipermeable dressing applied over insertion site. Insertion site without redness, tenderness, swelling, or exudate. ———— M. Ramirez, RN

PROCEDURE 36–5   **Converting a Primary Line to a Heparin or Saline Lock**

 For steps to follow in *all* procedures, refer to the inside back cover of this book.

critical aspects

- Assist the client to a comfortable position.
- Place a linen-saver pad under the extremity with the IV catheter.
- Don procedure gloves.
- Remove the IV lock from the package, and flush the adapter with saline or dilute heparin, according to unit policy.
- Carefully remove the IV dressing and the tape that is securing the tubing.
- Close the roller clamp on the administration set.
- With your nondominant hand, apply pressure over the vein just above the insertion site.
- Disengage the old tubing from the IV catheter. Grasp the catheter hub with a hemostat ("mosquito" clamp) if the tubing does not disengage readily.
- Quickly insert the lock adapter into the IV catheter.
- Flush the lock adapter again.
- Apply a sterile transparent semipermeable dressing.
- Discard the used supplies.

PROCEDURE 36-5

Converting a Primary Line to a Heparin or Saline Lock *(continued)*

Equipment

- Peripheral intermittent lock adapter
- Two syringes containing saline or dilute heparin solution
- Linen-saver pad
- Transparent semipermeable dressing
- Alcohol pad

Delegation

You can delegate the task of converting a primary IV line to an intermittent lock device to an LPN who is specially trained in IV therapy. The task should not be delegated to UAP. However, you should instruct the UAP to notify you of any problems with the intermittent lock device, such as dis-lodging of the catheter or client complaints of pain, swelling, or redness at the insertion site.

Assessment

- Assess the patient's fluid status to make sure his condition warrants converting the primary IV line to an intermittent lock.

If the patient is not tolerating oral fluids, his urine output is inadequate, or laboratory test results are abnormal, the patient may still require IV fluids.

- Assess the IV site for signs of phlebitis, infiltration, extravasation, or infection.

If complications are present, you should remove the IV catheter instead of converting it to an intermittent lock.

Procedural Steps

Step 1 Help the client assume a comfortable position that provides access to his IV site.

Promotes cooperation with the procedure and facilitates your ability to perform the procedure.

Step 2 Place a linen-saver pad under the extremity with the IV catheter.

The linen-saver pad protects linens from blood or fluid that might leak during the catheter conversion.

Step 3 Apply procedure gloves. Remove the IV lock from the package, and flush the adapter with the first syringe of saline or dilute heparin, according to unit policy. Replace the cover, or place the adapter back in the sterile package or on a sterile alcohol wipe.

Removes air from the lock. ▼

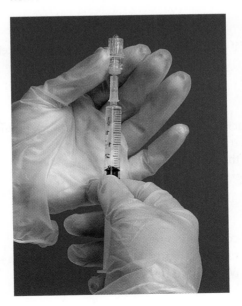

Step 4 Carefully remove the IV dressing and the tape that is securing the tubing.

Provides access to the IV catheter.

Step 5 Close the roller clamp on the administration set.

Prevents loss of IV fluid during the procedure.

Step 6 With your nondominant hand, apply pressure over the vein just above the insertion site.

Applying pressure over the vein stops blood from flowing from the catheter as you change the administration tubing.

Step 7 Gently disengage the old tubing from the IV catheter. If it does not disengage easily, it may help to grip the catheter hub with a hemostat (small "mosquito" clamp).

Prevents the IV catheter from becoming dislodged.

➤

PROCEDURE 36–5

Converting a Primary Line to a Heparin or Saline Lock *(continued)*

Step 8 Quickly insert the lock adapter into the IV catheter.

Insert the adapter quickly to prevent blood from flowing from the IV catheter. ▼

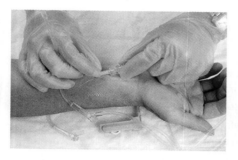

Step 9 Cleanse the injection port of the adapter with an alcohol pad.

Cleaning the port with alcohol helps prevent contamination by microorganisms when the adapter and IV catheter are flushed.

Step 10 Insert a syringe containing saline or dilute heparin into the injection port of the adapter. Flush the catheter gently with the solution.

Ensures patency of the IV catheter. ▼

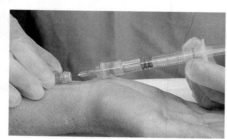

Step 11 Cover the insertion site with a sterile transparent semipermeable dressing. (Refer to Procedure 36–1). Gently pinch the dressing around the lock to secure the hub.

Prevents contamination of the site.

Step 12 Discard the administration set and linen-saver pad in the appropriate receptacle, as designated by your institution. Empty the IV solution container in the nearest sink, and then discard it appropriately.

Discarding used equipment properly keeps the healthcare environment safe.

Evaluation

- Evaluate the patency of the catheter before each use and at least every 8 hours.
- Evaluate the patient's tolerance to intermittent IV therapy.
- Evaluate the insertion site for signs of complications.

Patient Teaching

Explain the importance of notifying staff if the IV site becomes painful, if the catheter becomes dislodged, or the connection is loose.

Home Care

- Explain home use of the intermittent lock to the patient and caregiver. Teach them how to flush the line if they will administer medications through it.
- Provide the patient and caregiver with the name and phone numbers of people to contact in case problems arise with the catheter or insertion site.

Documentation

- Chart the date and time the IV line was converted to an intermittent lock device.
- Note the size and location of the catheter, as well as the type and amount of flush solution used. Record on the I & O record the amount of IV fluid infused.

PROCEDURE 36–5 — Converting a Primary Line to a Heparin or Saline Lock *(continued)*

- Document the condition of the IV site and any complications noted.
- Often, IV care is documented on a flowsheet.

Sample of a narrative note:

| 3/25/07 | 04:00 | Primary IV line located in the right hand changed to a normal saline lock. Catheter flushed with 3 mL of normal saline solution. Site without redness, tenderness, swelling, or drainage. |
| | | — S. Robinson, RN |

PROCEDURE 36–6 — Discontinuing an IV Line

 For steps to follow in *all* procedures, refer to the inside back cover of this book.

critical aspects
- Assist the client to a comfortable position.
- Place a linen-saver pad under the extremity that contains the IV catheter.
- Apply procedure gloves, and close the roller clamp on the administration set.
- Carefully remove the IV dressing and the tape that is securing the tubing.
- Apply a sterile 2 × 2 gauze pad above the IV insertion site and gently remove the catheter, directing it straight along the vein. Do not press on the gauze pad while removing the catheter.
- Apply firm pressure with the gauze pad over the insertion site. Hold pressure for 2 to 3 minutes; hold longer if bleeding persists.
- Remove the soiled 2 × 2 gauze pad, and replace it with a new sterile 2 × 2 gauze pad. Secure it with a piece of 1-inch tape.
- Dispose of the IV catheter, IV supplies, and gloves in the appropriate containers.

Equipment:
- Sterile 2 × 2 gauze dressings
- 1-inch tape
- Linen-saver pad

Delegation
You can delegate the task of discontinuing an IV line to an LPN who is specially trained in IV therapy. The task should not be delegated to UAP. However, you should instruct the UAP to notify you of any bleeding from the insertion site. ➤

PROCEDURE 36–6   **Discontinuing an IV Line** (*continued*)

Assessment

Assess the patient's readiness to have the IV fluid discontinued. For example, determine whether he is tolerating oral fluids and has adequate urine output and whether laboratory values are within normal limits.

If the patient's condition indicates that he still requires IV fluids, notify the physician and do not discontinue the IV line.

Procedural Steps

Step 1 Assist the client to a comfortable position.

Helps ensure patient cooperation with the procedure.

Step 2 Place a linen-saver pad under the extremity that contains the IV catheter.

Protects linens from blood and fluid that might leak from the vessel during catheter removal.

Step 3 Apply procedure gloves, and close the roller clamp on the administration set.

Closing the roller clamp on the administration set prevents IV fluid from spilling onto the bed or client during catheter removal. Procedure gloves protect you from body fluids.

Step 4 Carefully remove the IV dressing and the tape that is securing the tubing.

Step 5 Apply a sterile 2 × 2 gauze pad above the IV insertion site and gently remove the catheter, directing it straight along the vein. Do not press down on the gauze pad while removing the catheter.

Directing the catheter along the vein prevents vein injury while you are removing the catheter. ▼

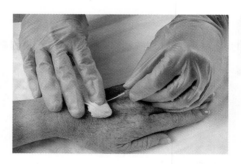

Step 6 Immediately apply firm pressure with the gauze pad over the insertion site. Hold pressure for 2 to 3 minutes; hold longer if bleeding persists.

Holding pressure for 2 to 3 minutes typically stops bleeding.

Step 7 Remove the soiled 2 × 2 gauze pad, and replace it with a sterile 2 × 2 gauze pad. Secure it with a piece of 1-inch tape.

Protects the site from contamination.

Step 8 Dispose of the IV catheter in the appropriate sharps container.

Dispose of the IV catheter properly to prevent the spread of infection and prevent needlestick injury. Even a polyurethane catheter can penetrate the skin.

Step 9 Discard the IV tubing, linen-saver pad, IV solution container, and gloves in the appropriate trash receptacle according to institution policy.

Dispose of used supplies appropriately to promote a safe healthcare environment.

Evaluation

- Evaluate the patient's response after IV therapy is discontinued.
- Evaluate changes in the patient's condition to assess whether IV therapy should be reestablished.

Patient Teaching

- Explain the importance of notifying staff if bleeding or discomfort occurs at the insertion site.
- Instruct the patient about the importance of consuming adequate amounts fluid to prevent dehydration.

PROCEDURE 36–6   **Discontinuing an IV Line** *(continued)*

Documentation

- Chart the date and time that IV therapy was discontinued.
- Note the condition of the site, including the presence of any complications. If complications are present, document your interventions, including physician notification.
- Often you will record this procedure on a flow sheet.

Sample of a narrative note:

12/25/06	2100	RA#2, 22-gauge catheter discontinued. Site without redness, swelling, tenderness, or exudates. Pressure applied to site for 3 minutes. Bleeding stopped and sterile 2 × 2 gauze dressing applied. Informed patient to notify staff if bleeding or discomfort occurs.
		— S. Horowitz, RN

PROCEDURE 36–7	Administering a Blood Transfusion

For steps to follow in *all* procedures, refer to the inside back cover of this book.

critical aspects

- Verify that informed consent has been obtained.
- Verify the physician's order, noting the indication, rate of infusion, and any pretransfusion or post-transfusion medication orders. Administer any pretransfusion medications as prescribed.
- Obtain a blood administration set and IV container of normal saline solution.
- Obtain the blood product from the blood bank according to your institution's policy.
- Recheck the physician's order.
- With another qualified staff member (as deemed by your institution), verify the patient and blood product identification.
- Remove the blood administration set from the package, and label the tubing with the date and time. Then, close the clamps on the administration set.
- Spike the port of the normal saline solution container, and hang the IV solution.
- Compress the drip chamber of the administration set, and prime the tubing with the saline solution.
- Invert the blood filter on the administration set, and prime it with normal saline solution.
- Gently invert the blood product container several times.
- Spike the blood product container through the port, and hang the blood on the IV pole.
- Slowly open the roller clamp closest to the blood product.
- Obtain a set of vital signs.
- Attach the distal end of the administration set tubing to the IV catheter.
- Measure vital signs in 5 minutes, 15 minutes, then 30 minutes, then hourly.
- When the blood has transfused, flush the line with normal saline solution.
- Disconnect the tubing from the IV catheter, and dispose of the blood product container and tubing per agency policy.
- If a second unit of blood is to be transfused, the same administration set may be used.
- Administer any post-transfusion medications ordered.

Procedure Variation: Managing a Transfusion Reaction

- Stop the transfusion immediately. Do not flush the tubing with the normal saline solution.
- Disconnect the administration set from the IV catheter. Obtain vital signs, and auscultate heart and breath sounds.
- Maintain patency of the IV catheter by hanging a new infusion of normal saline solution.
- Notify the physician.
- Place the administration set and blood product container, with the blood bank form attached, inside a biohazard bag. Send the bag to the blood bank immediately.
- Obtain blood (in the extremity opposite the transfusion site) and urine specimens according to your institution's policy.
- Continue to monitor vital signs frequently.
- Administer medications, as prescribed.

PROCEDURE 36–7   Administering a Blood Transfusion *(continued)*

Equipment

- Blood product
- Normal saline IV solution
- Blood administration set
- IV pole
- Watch with a second hand
- Thermometer
- Blood pressure cuff and sphygmomanometer
- Stethoscope

Delegation

Do not delegate this procedure to the LPN or UAP, because blood product administration requires advanced assessment and critical-thinking skills. The LPN and UAP can assist by monitoring vital signs. Instruct both about the complications associated with blood product administration, and instruct them to inform you if any occur.

Assessment

- Assess the patient's need for blood products by assessing vital signs, urine output, and laboratory studies.

Blood products may cause life-threatening complications; therefore, they should be administered only when needed.

- Check the patient's history for previous blood transfusions and reactions.

If the patient has a history of a blood transfusion reaction, precautions must be taken before she receives additional transfusions. For example, she may need premedication with acetaminophen and diphenhydramine, specially treated blood products, and the use of a specialized administration set with greater filtering capabilities.

- Assess the existing IV catheter for patency, and make sure that the catheter is the proper size for blood product administration.

Ideally use an 18-gauge catheter to infuse blood products to prevent hemolysis. A 20-gauge catheter is acceptable. Some authorities believe that a 22-gauge thin-walled catheter can be used without difficulty and without damage to red blood cells (Macklin, 2003); you might consider this if the patient is at high risk for developing phlebitis. However, you will need to follow agency policy on this.

Procedural Steps

Step 1 Verify that an informed consent has been obtained.

Informed consent is required for blood product administration, as for any invasive or risk-bearing procedure.

Step 2 Verify the physician's order, noting the indication, rate of infusion, and any premedication orders. Administer any pretransfusion medications as prescribed.

Verifying the orders helps prevent administration errors.

Step 3 Obtain an IV container of normal saline solution and a blood administration set.

Normal saline solution is the only solution that is compatible with blood products; other IV solutions cause hemolysis of blood cells.

Step 4 Obtain the blood product from the blood bank according to your institution's policy. Wear procedure gloves whenever handling blood products.

Some blood banks require a pick-up slip that verifies the presence of a functioning IV catheter, signed informed consent, and a physician's order, because blood must be discarded after it has been out of refrigeration for 30 minutes.

Step 5 Recheck the physician's order.

Recheck the order to ensure that the proper blood product was dispensed with any special processing that might have been prescribed.

Step 6 With another qualified staff member (as deemed by your institution), verify the patient and blood product identification.

a. Have the patient tell you her full name and date of birth (if she is able), and compare it to the name and date of birth located on the blood bank form.

Allowing the patient to confirm her identity and comparing the information against the blood bank form is a safety measure to ensure that the correct patient is receiving the correct blood product.

b. Compare the patient name and hospital identification number on the patient's identification bracelet with the patient name and hospital identification number on the blood bank form attached to the blood product.

Verifies that the correct patient is receiving the correct blood product.

➤

PROCEDURE 36–7   **Administering a Blood Transfusion** *(continued)*

c. Compare the unit identification number located on the blood bank form with the identification number printed on the blood product container.

Verifies that the blood bank has dispensed the correct blood product. ▼

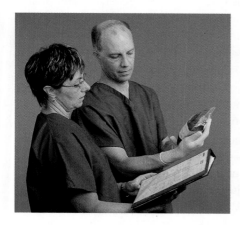

d. Compare the patient's blood type listed on the blood bank form with the blood type listed on the blood product container.

Verifies that the blood type of the product matches the patient's blood type.

e. If all verifications are in agreement, both staff members should sign the blood bank form attached to the blood product container. Contact the blood bank immediately if any discrepancies occur during the identification process. If there are any discrepancies, do not administer the blood product.

Signing the blood bank form confirms that the blood product was identified and verified by two qualified staff members.

f. Document on the blood bank form the date and time that the transfusion was begun.

Blood cannot be infused past the expiration time; documenting the start time alerts the nurse of the expiration time.

g. Make sure that the blood bank form remains attached to the blood product container until administration is complete.

Ensures product identity should a transfusion reaction occur.

Step 7 Remove the blood administration set from the package, and label the tubing with the date and time. Then, close the clamps on the administration set.

Labeling the administration set with the date and time informs the nursing staff when the administration set should be changed.

Step 8 Remove the protective covers from the saline solution container port and from one of the spikes located on the "Y" of the blood product administration set. Place the spike into the port of the solution container.

Step 9 Hang the normal saline solution container on the IV pole.

Facilitates gravity flow.

Step 10 Compress the drip chamber of the administration set, and allow it to fill halfway.

Prevents air from entering the tubing with the solution.

Step 11 Open the roller clamp and prime the administration set tubing with normal saline.

Removes air from the tubing.

Step 12 Depending on the equipment and agency guidelines, attach the blood filter to the administration set and prime it with normal saline solution according to the manufacturer's instructions for use. ▼

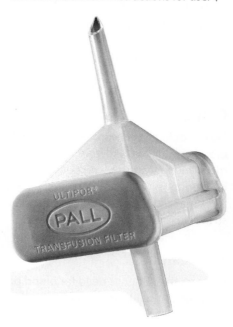

Step 13 Close the roller clamp. Inspect the tubing for the presence of air. If air bubbles remain in the tubing, flick the tubing with a fingernail to mobilize the bubbles.

Air bubbles in the administration tubing can cause an air embolus.

Step 14 Gently invert the blood product container several times.

Mixes the blood product with the preservatives that are added to the container.

PROCEDURE 36–7   Administering a Blood Transfusion *(continued)*

Step 15 Remove the protective covers from the blood filter and the blood product port. Carefully spike the blood product container through the port.

Carefully spiking the blood product container prevents inadvertent puncturing of the container. ▼

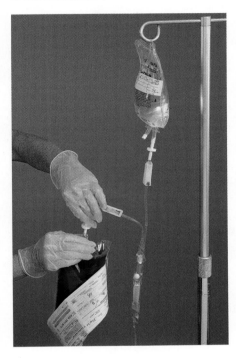

Step 16 Hang the blood product container on the IV pole.

Enables the blood to flow by gravity.

Step 17 Slowly open the roller clamp closest to the blood product.

Allows the blood product to slowly fill that side of the "Y" of the administration set tubing.

Step 18 Obtain and record the patient's vital signs, including temperature, before beginning the transfusion.

Obtaining vital signs establishes a baseline to help monitor for transfusion reactions.

Step 19 Using aseptic technique, attach the distal end of the administration set to the IV catheter.

Using aseptic technique prevents contamination of the IV catheter and administration set.

Step 20 Using the roller clamp, adjust the drip rate, as prescribed. (Keep in mind that blood administration sets have a drip factor of 10 drops/mL.)

A unit of blood cannot hang for more than 4 hours; otherwise, bacterial growth may occur.

Step 21 Remain with the patient during the first 5 minutes, and then obtain vital signs.

Most severe blood transfusion reactions occur during the transfusion of the initial 50 mL of blood.

Step 22 Make sure that the patient's call bell or light is readily available, and have her alert you immediately of any signs or symptoms of a transfusion reaction, such as back pain, chills, itching, or shortness of breath.

To prevent serious complications, the patient should alert you immediately and the transfusion should be stopped.

Step 23 Obtain vital signs in 15 minutes, then again in 30 minutes, and then hourly while the transfusion infuses.

Frequent monitoring alerts you to early signs of transfusion reaction or fluid overload.

Step 24 After the unit has infused, close the roller clamp closest to the blood product container, and open the roller clamp closest to the normal saline solution to flush the administration set with normal saline solution.

Flushing the tubing with normal saline solution clears the tubing of any blood and avoids wasting any of the blood product.

Step 25 Close the roller clamp, and then disconnect the blood administration set from the IV catheter.

Disconnect the administration set if an additional unit of blood has not been prescribed.

Step 26 If another unit of blood is required, you may hang the second unit with the same administration set.

The same administration set can be used for two units of blood.

Step 27 Discard the empty blood container and administration set in the proper receptacle, according to your institution's policy.

Proper disposal of the blood container and administration set promotes a safe healthcare environment.

Procedure Variation
Managing a Transfusion Reaction

Step 1 Stop the transfusion immediately if signs or symptoms of a transfusion reaction occur. Do not flush the tubing with the normal saline solution attached to the blood administration set.

Flushing the tubing with the normal saline solution attached to the blood administration set causes the patient to receive the blood that remains in the tubing.

Step 2 Disconnect the administration set from the IV catheter. Obtain vital signs, and auscultate heart and breath sounds.

Severe transfusion reactions may cause respiratory distress and shock; early recognition and treatment improve patient outcomes.

Step 3 Maintain patency of the IV catheter by hanging a new infusion of normal saline solution, using new tubing.

Maintaining a patent IV catheter with normal saline solution provides IV access in which emergency medication can be administered if necessary.

➤

PROCEDURE 36–7   Administering a Blood Transfusion *(continued)*

Step 4 Notify the physician as soon as you have stopped the blood and assessed the patient.

Step 5 Place the administration set and blood product container, with the blood bank form attached, inside a biohazard bag. Send the bag to the blood bank immediately.

The remainder of the blood must be sent to the blood bank, where it can be analyzed to determine the cause of the reaction.

Step 6 Obtain blood (in the extremity opposite the transfusion site) and urine specimens according to your institution's policy.

Blood banks typically require (1) a specimen for a type and crossmatch to compare with the pretransfusion type and crossmatch, (2) a specimen for free hemoglobin, and (3) a specimen for serum bilirubin level. A urine sample should also be sent to check for hemoglobinurinia, a sign of acute hemolytic reactions.

Step 7 Continue to monitor vital signs frequently.

Obtain vital signs at least every 15 minutes to quickly detect worsening of the patient's condition.

Step 8 Administer medications, as prescribed.

Medications will vary depending on the type of transfusion reaction.

Evaluation

- Evaluate the patient's response to the blood transfusion by checking for signs of fluid imbalance.
- Monitor for signs and symptoms of transfusion reaction,
- Evaluate the IV insertion site for signs of infiltration, phlebitis, or extravasation.
- Check laboratory studies, such as complete blood count, to help evaluate the effectiveness of therapy.

Patient Teaching

- Explain the signs and symptoms of transfusion reactions, and tell the patient to notify staff immediately should they occur.
- Warn the patient to notify staff immediately if tenderness, redness, or swelling occurs at the IV catheter insertion site.
- Explain the importance of notifying staff immediately if the administration set becomes disconnected from the IV catheter or the IV catheter becomes dislodged.

Documentation

- Chart the date, time, and reason the transfusion was started.
- Document transfusion vital signs according to institution policy (some institutions have a special form for transfusion vital signs).

PROCEDURE 36–7   Administering a Blood Transfusion *(continued)*

- Record the amount of blood transfused on the I & O record.
- Chart any complications and the interventions taken.

Sample of a narrative note:

10/22/06 0600	1 unit (250 ml) PRBCs was hung at 0300 and infused through LA#2, 20-gauge catheter for Hgb 8.3 mg/dL. Pretransfusion vital signs: T 98.9° F, BP 100/68 mm Hg, HR 114 beats/minute, and RR 22 breaths/minute. See frequent vital sign sheet for other transfusion vital signs. Breath sounds remained clear throughout the transfusion. No evidence of reaction. Post-transfusion lab due at 1200. — L. Gilmore, RN

TECHNIQUES

TECHNIQUE 36–1   Assessing for Trousseau's and Chvostek's Signs

Positive Trousseau's and Chvostek's signs are signs of hypocalcemia. To check for these signs, follow these guidelines.

Trousseau's Sign

Inflate a syphygomanometer above systolic pressure. Flexion of the wrist and hand constitutes a positive sign.

Chvostek's Sign

Tap the face in front of the ear and below the zygomatic bone. Facial twitching constitutes a positive sign.

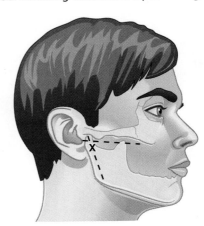

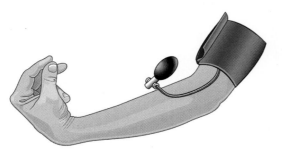

TECHNIQUE 36–2   Interpreting Arterial Blood Gases (ABGs)

Follow these steps to interpret acid-base balance.

Step 1: Examine the pH. A pH value below 7.35 is acidotic. A pH value above 7.45 is alkalotic.

Step 2: Examine the PCO_2 and HCO_3^-. In respiratory disorders, the pH and PCO_2 values move in opposite directions away from the norm. In metabolic disorders, the pH and HCO_3^- values move in the same direction. For example, compare the following values:

pH = 7.30 PCO_2 = 50 mm Hg HCO_3^- = 24 mEq/L
(respiratory acidosis)

pH = 7.50 PCO_2 = 40 mm Hg HCO_3^- = 30 mEq/L
(metabolic alkalosis)

We know the first example is a respiratory disorder because the PCO_2 value is elevated and the pH is low; the values moved in opposite directions. The second example is a metabolic disorder: the pH and HCO_3^- values moved in the same direction. The second example represents metabolic alkalosis.

Step 3: Determine whether there is compensation. In a respiratory problem, the renal system must compensate. In a metabolic problem, the respiratory system compensates. The respiratory system compensates early in the disorder, but it may take up to 3 days for the renal system to compensate fully. The following examples show the effect of compensation on the previous ABGs. Notice that the pH has

begun to move toward the norm as the other system compensates. Both of these examples show partial compensation.

pH = 7.32 PCO_2 = 50 mm Hg HCO_3^- = 28 mEq/L

pH = 7.48 PCO_2 = 32 mm Hg HCO_3^- = 30 mEq/L

Recall that the lungs regulate CO_2 and carbonic acid; the kidneys regulate bicarbonate. In the first example, the bicarbonate has changed: the kidneys are compensating for the respiratory acidosis. In the second example, the PCO_2 has changed: the lungs are compensating for the metabolic alkalosis.

Step 4: Determine the degree of compensation. If the pH is abnormal and only one ABG component is abnormal, no compensation has occurred. The original example in step 2 illustrates ABGs with no compensation (the HCO_3^- is normal). If the pH and one ABG component are abnormal, with the second beginning to change, partial compensation has occurred. This is seen in step 3. Complete compensation occurs when the second component changes sufficiently to return the pH to normal. Continuing with the previous examples, below are ABG results that demonstrate full compensation.

pH = 7.35 PCO_2 = 50 mm Hg HCO_3^- = 30 mEq/L

pH = 7.42 PCO_2 = 30 mm Hg HCO_3^- = 30 mEq/L

ASSESSMENT GUIDELINES AND TOOLS

The following guidelines will help you obtain subjective and objective data about patients' fluid, electrolyte, and acid-base balance.

Nursing History for Fluid, Electrolyte, and Acid-Base Balance

Demographic Data

- Age
- Gender
- Height, weight, BMI

Past Medical History

- Have you ever been hospitalized or had surgery? If so, when and for what reason?
- What healthcare problems are you currently being treated for?
- Have you ever been diagnosed with kidney disease, high blood pressure, diabetes, thyroid, or parathyroid problems?

Current Health Concerns

- What symptoms are you currently experiencing?
- Have you recently experienced any of the following symptoms?

  Excessive thirst
  Excessive perspiration
  Nausea, vomiting, or diarrhea
  Dry skin or mucous membranes
  Dark, concentrated urine
  Limited amounts of urine
  Difficulty breathing
  Swelling of your hands, feet, or ankles
  Dizziness or feeling faint
  Muscle weakness
  Excessive fatigue
  Numbness, tingling, or cramping sensations

- Is your weight stable? Have you had any recent changes in your weight?
- Do you believe you have any problems with fluid loss?

Food and Fluid Intake

- What is your typical fluid intake for a 24-hour period?
- Do you believe you drink adequate amounts of fluid?

- Describe your usual diet.
- Have you recently changed your diet or fluid intake?
- Are you following a special diet?
- Have you ever been placed on a restricted diet?
- Have you experienced any recent changes in your appetite or thirst?
- Do you salt your food?
- Do you ever use salt substitute?

Fluid Elimination

- How often do you urinate in a 24-hour period?
- Have you noticed any recent changes in the amount, frequency, or appearance of your urine?
- How often do you experience vomiting, diarrhea, or constipation? Describe your experience.
- Do you have any wounds? If so, what type, and how much drainage are you experiencing?
- Do you have any breaks in your skin? If so, describe the problem, and show me the area.
- Have you had any unusual fluid losses?

Medications

- What prescribed medications do you currently take?
- What over-the-counter medications or alternative treatments do you use? What do you use them for?
- How often do you take laxatives or anatacids?
- What vitamins or supplements do you take?

Lifestyle

- What is your usual activity level?
- What type of exercise do you engage in? How often?
- How much fluid do you consume before, during, and after exercise?

Physical Assessments for Fluid, Electrolyte, and Acid-Base Balance

Skin

Assess the skin for color, temperature, moisture content, continuity, turgor, and edema.

- *Color and temperature* may be cues to the presence of fever and circulation status.
- *Moisture content* offers some evidence of fluid status. A diaphoretic client is losing fluid at a faster rate than a client with dry skin. Dry, scaling skin may indicate a fluid deficit. Any breaks in the skin are potential areas for fluid loss.
- *Turgor* varies with age, weight, and skin condition but does offer information on fluid status. Pinch the skin over the sternum. Normally skin immediately returns to its normal position. In fluid volume deficit or malnutrition the skin may remain elevated for a period of time before returning to its original position. You must, however, correlate skin turgor with context and other clinical signs. For example, the skin loses elasticity with aging, so clients over age 65 often have decreased turgor.
- *Edema* in dependent areas is a cue for fluid volume excess. In a mobile client, assess the lower extremities and hands. In a bedridden client, edema will shift as the client is turned. Table 19–3 in Chapter 19, Volume 1, demonstrates how to grade edema.

Mucous Membranes

- Inspect the tongue and buccal mucosa. Mouth breathing alone usually does not change these areas.
- Dry, cracked, or dull mucous membranes are signs of fluid volume deficit.

Cardiovascular System

- Assess vital signs (see later section).
- If you suspect fluid volume deficit, assess for *orthostatic hypotension:*

  Assess blood pressure while client is lying or sitting.
  Have the client rise to a seated or standing position, and reassess the blood pressure (BP).
  A drop in systolic BP of greater than 15 mm Hg indicates orthostatic hypotension.

- Check capillary refill. Delayed capillary refill is a sign of fluid volume deficit; rapid capillary refill indicates adequate circulation and volume. If capillary refill is delayed, evaluate feet and hands bilaterally. Delays in just one area indicate impaired circulation to the extremity rather than volume changes.
- Assess venous filling by observing the jugular and hand veins. Flat jugular or hand veins indicate low fluid volume. Distended vessels are a sign of overload.

Respiratory System

- Assess respiratory rate, depth, and pattern. The respiratory system rapidly responds to changes in pH. Similarly, alterations in gas exchange at the alveolar-capillary membrane may trigger pH changes.
- Assess breath sounds. Crackles or moist rales may indicate fluid overload. Areas of consolidation indicate impaired gas exchange.

Neurological System

- Assess level of consciousness and orientation.
- Assess neuromuscular irritability
- Assess energy level and fatigue
- Assess reflexes

For specific neurological cues to alterations in fluid, electrolyte, or acid base balance,

 Go to Chapter 36, **Table 36–5: Electrolyte Imbalances,** and **Table 36–7: Acid-Base Imbalances,** in Volume 1.

Vital Signs

- *Temperature.* An elevated body temperature increases the loss of body fluids.

  In hypernatremia, body temperature elevates because less fluid is available for sweating.
  In uncomplicated fluid volume deficit, body temperature decreases.

- *Pulse:*

  Tachycardia is an early sign of fluid volume deficit.
  Pulse rate is affected by fluid status and some electrolytes (primarily sodium, potassium, calcium, and magnesium).
  Dysrhythmias are seen with potassium and magnesium imbalances.
  The pulse volume is directly affected by fluid status. As fluid volume increases, the pulse volume also increases. Similarly, a drop in fluid volume leads to a drop in pulse volume.

- *Respiratory rate.* Alterations in respiratory rate may cause acid-base imbalances or be associated with compensation for a metabolic disorder.

- *Blood pressure:*

  Blood pressure rises and falls with fluid volume.
  Blood pressure is elevated by hypernatremia and fluid volume excess.
  Respiratory acidosis causes increased heart rate, resulting in BP elevation.
  High potassium intake may lower blood pressure.

Physical Assessments for Fluid, Electrolyte, and Acid-Base Balance

(continued)

Daily Weights

- Use the same balanced scale each day to accurately monitor fluid status.
- Weigh the client at the same time of day, making sure that the client is wearing the same amount of clothing.
- For clients undergoing hemodialysis (blood cleansing through an artificial kidney), weigh the client before and after dialysis treatments.
- You may institute weight monitoring as an independent nursing order.

Fluid Intake and Output

- Measure all fluids consumed or excreted in a 24-hour period.
- I & O are usually tallied at the end of each shift as well as for each 24-hour period. In intensive care units, I & O are often measured hourly.
- Correlate I & O with daily weights to determine fluid status.
- Inform client, family members, and all caregivers that I & O are being monitored.
- Post a sign at the bedside or on the door to the room.
- When possible, have the client assist with monitoring.
- Common fluid measurement equivalents:

  1 fluid ounce = 30 mL
  16 fluid ounces = 1 pint or 480 mL
  5 mL = 1 teaspoon
  15 mL = 1 tablespoon
  Coffee cup = 180 mL
  Coffee mug = 240 mL
  Gelatin or custard = 120 mL
  Juice glass = 120 mL
  Soup bowl = 180 mL

Include the following items as fluid intake:

- *Oral fluids.* Record all fluid items the client consumes, including water or juice taken with medications. If the patient has a water pitcher at the bedside, you will need to monitor the amount consumed each shift.
- *Foods.* Semiliquid foods, such as gelatin, ice cream, sherbert, and custard.
- *Ice chips.* The amount to record is 50% of the volume of the ice. An 8-ounce cup of ice chips is equivalent to 4 ounces of fluid.

- *Parenteral fluids.* Record all IV fluids, including IV infusions, blood products, and fluids used as admixture for IV medications.
- *Enteral feedings.* Record the amount of feeding infused and the amount of fluid used with each flush.
- *Flushing fluids.* If the client receives medications through the feeding tube, record the amount of fluid used to administer the medication and flush the line.
- *Irrigations.* Any irrigation that is instilled and not withdrawn or immediately drained must be recorded as intake. For example, if you are infusing a continuous irrigation through a three-port urinary catheter, record the amount of irrigant instilled in the bladder. Net urine output is actually the total volume drained from the catheter minus the irrigant. However, if you are irrigating an abdominal wound for cleansing purposes, this fluid is not part of the I & O, because it readily drains from the wound.

Fluid output includes the following items:

- *Urine output:*

  Measure the amount of urine drained from a urinary catheter.
  Use a fluid-collecting device to measure urine voided in the bedpan or toilet.
  If fluid status is critical and the client is incontinent, you may need to measure linen or absorbent products. These items must be measured before they are applied and again when they are removed. Each gram of weight change is equivalent to 1 mL of urine.

- *GI fluid loss.* Measure the amount of fluid lost through vomiting or NG suction.
- *Feces.* Measure the amount of fluid in liquid feces. Record the number of BMs and consistency of the stool if the stool is not liquid. When stool is formed, fluid loss in feces is not substantial.
- *Drainage devices.* Record the amount of fluid contained in any drainage device. You will need to empty wound drains or other devices to measure this volume.
- *Wound drainage.* If a wound is draining but the fluid is not collected in a drainage device, you may measure the amount of fluid lost by weighing dressings before and after they are applied. If measuring the exact volume is not crucial, you may be asked to evaluate the degree of saturation of the dressing.

DIAGNOSTIC TESTING

Assessing Fluid, Electrolyte, and Acid-Base Balance

Venous Blood Sample	**Normal Ranges**
Sodium	135–145 mEq/L
Potassium	3.5–5 mEq/L
Chloride	95–105 mEq/L
Bicarbonate	22–26 mEq/L
BUN	10–20 mg/dL
Creatinine	<1.2 mg/dL
Serum osmolality	280–300 mOsm/kg
Urine osmolality	500–800 mOsm/kg
Hematocrit	42–52% in men
	37–47% in menstruating women

Freshly Voided Urine Sample

pH	4.6–8
Specific gravity	1.002–1.028

Arterial Blood Sample

pH	7.35–7.45
P_{CO_2}	35–45 mm Hg
HCO_3^-	22–26 mEq/L

STANDARDIZED LANGUAGE

Selected Nursing Diagnoses, Outcomes, and Interventions for Fluid and Electrolyte Problems

Nursing Diagnoses

Deficient Fluid Volume—Defining characteristics: dry mucous membranes, scant urine output, increased urine concentration, elevated hematocrit, thirst, weakness, weight loss, decreased skin and tongue turgor, decreased blood pressure, and elevated temperature, pulse, and respirations.

Excess Fluid Volume—Defining characteristics: decreased hemoglobin and hematocrit, decreased urine specific gravity, oliguria, restlessness, anxiety, weight gain, edema, venous distention, increased blood pressure, bounding pulse volume, rales and crackles on auscultation, and rapid respirations.

Risk for Deficient Fluid Volume is a potential diagnosis appropriate for a client experiencing vascular, cellular, or intracellular dehydration (recall that this is a loss of total water volume). *Risk factors:* use of diuretic medications, loss of fluid through tubes (e.g., gastric suction), extremes of age, problems affecting access to or swallowing of fluids, and hypermetabolic state.

Risk for Imbalanced Fluid Volume is a potential diagnosis appropriate for a client at risk for increase or decrease of fluids or for rapid fluid shifts in the intravascular, intracellular, or interstitial space. *Risk factors:* Only one has been developed by NANDA: impending major invasive procedures.

Impaired Gas Exchange is an appropriate diagnosis for a client with a disorder affecting gas exchange at the alveolar-capillary membrane. To be certain this diagnosis is accurate, you need information about the patient's arterial blood gas values. Other defining characteristics are those associated with inadequate oxygenation (e.g., confusion, vital signs changes, pallor, hypoxia, hypoxemia).

NOC Outcomes	Selected Indicators
Electrolyte & Acid/Base Balance	Urine specific gravity
	Urine pH
	Serum pH
	Apical heart rate and rhythm
	Respiratory rate and rhythm
	Serum sodium, potassium, chloride, calcium, magnesium
	Serum albumin, creatinine, bicarbonate
	Blood urea nitrogen
	Mental alertness, cognitive orientation
	Muscle strength
Fluid Balance	Blood pressure, mean arterial pressure, central venous pressure, pulmonary wedge pressure
	24-hr I & O balance
	Skin turgor; soft, sunken eyeballs
	Peripheral edema
	Stable body weight
	Hematocrit
	Urine specific gravity
	Adventitious breath sounds
	Thirst
Fluid Overload Severity	Periorbital edema
	Hand edema
	Sacral edema
	Leg edema
	Ascites
	Rales
	Lethargy, confusion
	Decreased urine output, specific gravity

➤

Selected Nursing Diagnoses, Outcomes, and Interventions for Fluid and Electrolyte Problems
(continued)

NOC Outcomes	Selected Indicators
Hydration	Skin turgor Moist mucous membranes Adequate fluid intake Urine output Thirst Decreased blood pressure Rapid, thready pulse

NIC Interventions	Selected Activities
Acid-Base Management (There are specific interventions for each type of acid-base imbalance; for example, Acid-base Management: Metabolic Acidosis)	Maintain patent IV access Monitor ABGs and serum and urine electrolyte levels Monitor respiratory pattern Monitor for worsening electrolyte imbalance with correction of the acid-base imbalance Reduce oxygen consumption (e.g., promote comfort, control fever, and reduce anxiety)
Acid-base Monitoring	Obtain blood for determination of ABG levels, ensuring adequate circulation to the extremity before and after blood withdrawal Monitor for possible causes of HCO_3^- excess, such as vomiting, gastric suction, hyperaldosteronism, diuretic therapy, hypochloremia, and excessive ingestion of medications containing HCO_3^- Monitor for possible causes of carbonic acid deficits and associated hyperventilation, such as pain, CNS lesions, fever, and mechanical ventilation
Electrolyte Management (There is a specific intervention for management of each individual electrolyte, for example, Electrolyte Management: Hypernatremia)	Monitor for abnormal serum electrolyte levels, as available Maintain patent IV access Monitor for loss of electrolyte-rich fluids (e.g., nasogastric suction, ileostomy drainage, diarrhea, wound drainage, and diaphoresis) Attach cardiac monitor, as appropriate
Electrolyte Monitoring	Monitor the serum level of electrolytes Monitor serum albumin and total protein levels, as indicated Monitor for associated acid-base imbalance Monitor for Chvostek and/or Trousseau sign Monitor for signs and symptoms of [specific electrolyte disorders, for example, hyponatremia, hypernatremia]
Fluid Management	Weight patient daily and monitor trends Maintain accurate intake and output record Monitor hydration status (e.g., moist mucous membranes, adequacy of pulses, and orthostatic blood pressure) Give fluids as appropriate
Fluid Monitoring	Determine history of amount and type of fluid intake and elimination habits Determine possible risk factors for fluid imbalance (e.g., hyperthermia, diuretic therapy, renal pathologies, cardiac failure, diaphoresis . . .) Monitor intake and output Restrict and allocate fluid intake as appropriate

(continued)

NIC Interventions	Selected Activities
Fluid Resuscitation	Collaborate with physicians to ensure administration of both crystalloids (e.g., normal saline and lactated Ringer's solution) and colloids (e.g., Hespan and Plasmanate) Obtain and maintain a large-bore IV
Fluid/Electrolyte Management	Obtain laboratory specimens for monitoring of altered fluid or electrolyte levels (e.g., hematocrit, BUN, protein, sodium, and potassium levels) Restrict free water intake in the presence of dilutional hyponatremia with serum sodium level below 130 mEq/L Monitor for signs and symptoms of fluid retention Monitor for fluid loss (e.g., bleeding, vomiting, diarrhea, perspiration, and tachypnea)
Hemodialysis Therapy	Record baseline vital signs: weight, temperature, pulse, respirations, and blood pressure Monitor clotting times and adjust heparin administration appropriately Work collaboratively with patient to adjust diet regulations, fluid limitations, and medications to regulate fluid and electrolyte shifts between treatments
Hypervolemia Management	Weigh patient daily and monitor trends Teach patient the rationale for use of diuretic therapy Monitor changes in peripheral edema as appropriate Monitor respiratory pattern for symptoms of respiratory difficulty Monitor renal function (e.g., BUN and creatinine levels) if appropriate
Hypovolemia Management	Administer hypotonic solutions (e.g., $D_5W/0.45\%$ saline) for intracellular rehydration, if appropriate Administer isotonic solutions (e.g., normal saline and lactated Ringer's solution) for extracellular rehydration, if appropriate Combine crystalloid (e.g., normal saline and lactated Ringer's solution) and colloid (e.g., Hespan and Plasmanate) solutions for replacement of intravascular volume, as prescribed Administer blood products (e.g., platelets and fresh frozen plasma) as appropriate
Intravenous Therapy	Maintain strict aseptic technique Perform IV site checks according to agency protocol Administer IV fluids at room temperature, unless otherwise ordered

Sources: Dochterman, J. M., & Bulechek, G. M. (Eds.). (2004). *Nursing interventions classification (NIC)* (4th ed.). St Louis: Mosby; Moorhead, S., Johnson, M., & Maas, M. (Eds.). (2004). *Nursing outcomes classification (NOC)* (3rd ed.). St Louis: Mosby; NANDA International. (2005). *Nursing diagnoses: Definitions and classification 2005–2006.* Philadelphia: Author.

What Are the Main Points in This Chapter?

- Water is the largest single constituent of the body. Total body water content varies with age, gender, and the number of fat cells.

- Intracellular fluid (ICF) is contained within the cells. It is essential for cell function and metabolism and accounts for approximately 40% of body weight.

- Extracellular fluid (ECF) consists of three types of fluid: interstitial, intravascular, and transcellular fluid. ECF carries water, electrolytes, nutrients, and oxygen to the cells and removes the waste products of cell metabolism. ECF accounts for 20% of body weight.

- Electrolytes that carry a positive charge are called cations. They include sodium (Na^+), potassium (K^+), calcium (Ca^{2+}), and magnesium (Mg^{2+}). Electrolytes that carry a negative charge are called anions.

- Potassium and magnesium are the major cations in the ICF. Phosphate and sulfate are the major anions.

- The major electrolytes of ECF are sodium, chloride, and bicarbonate. Albumin is also present in the ECF.

- Osmosis is a mechanism to maintain homeostasis through the movement of water across a membrane from a less concentrated solution to a more concentrated solution.

- Diffusion is a passive process by which molecules move through a cell membrane from an area of higher concentration to an area of lower concentration.

- Filtration is the movement of both water and smaller particles from an area of high pressure to an area of low pressure.

- Active transport occurs when electrolytes move from an area of low concentration to an area of high concentration. Active transport requires energy expenditure for the movement to occur against a concentration gradient.

- General recommendations for total fluid intake are 2700 mL per day for women and 3700 mL per day for men.

- Fluid loss occurs throughout the day, creating a constant need to replenish fluid. Loss occurs through urine, skin, insensible losses, and feces. When the body is in a healthy state, fluid losses are equivalent to fluid intake.

- Sodium is the major cation in the ECF. Its function is to regulate fluid volume.

- Potassium is the major cation of the ICF. It is a key electrolyte in cellular metabolism.

- Calcium is a vital electrolyte responsible for bone health, neuromuscular function, and cardiac function,

and it is an essential factor in blood clotting. Approximately 99% of body calcium is located in the bones and teeth. The remaining 1% circulates in the blood and is responsible for calcium's actions.

- Magnesium is a mineral used in more than 300 biochemical reactions in the body. As with calcium, only about 1% of magnesium is found in the blood. The remaining 99% is divided between the ICF and combined with calcium and phosphorus in bone.

- Chloride is the most abundant ion in the extracellular fluid. It is usually bound with other ions, especially sodium or potassium. Chloride works with sodium to regulate osmotic pressure between fluid compartments and assists in regulating acid-base balance through the bicarbonate buffer system.

- Phosphate is the most abundant intracellular anion. Most phosphate is found bound with calcium in teeth and bones. Phosphate and calcium levels exist in an inverse relationship.

- Bicarbonate is present in intracellular and extracellular fluids. Extracellular bicarbonate levels are regulated by the kidneys.

- The amount of acid or base present in a solution is measured as pH. The pH is reported on a scale of 1 to 14, with 1 to 6.9 being acidic, 7 being neutral, and 7.1 to 14 being basic, or alkaline.

- A buffer system consists of a weak acid and a weak base. These molecules react with strong acids or bases to keep them from altering the pH by either absorbing free hydrogen ions or releasing free hydrogen ions. The principal buffer system in the ECF is the carbonic acid (H_2CO_3) and sodium bicarbonate ($NaHCO_3^-$) system.

- When the serum pH is too acidic (pH is low), the lungs remove carbon dioxide through rapid, deep breathing. If the serum pH is too alkaline (pH is high), the lungs try to conserve carbon dioxide through shallow respirations.

- The kidneys affect pH by regulating the amount of bicarbonate (base) that is kept in the body.

- Fluid volume deficit occurs when there is a proportional loss of water and electrolytes from the ECF.

- Fluid volume excess involves excessive retention of sodium and water in the ECF.

- When the serum pH falls below 7.35, the patient is acidotic. When the serum pH increases above 7.45, the patient is alkalotic. Arterial blood gases (ABGs) are used to monitor acid-base balance.

- Physical assessment of a client's fluid, electrolyte, and acid-base balance examines the skin, mucous membranes, cardiovascular and respiratory systems, and neurological status. Data are correlated with the nursing history and laboratory studies.

- Intake and output (I & O) are monitored to assess fluid status. To monitor, measure all fluids consumed and excreted in a 24-hour period.

- Tests used to monitor fluid, electrolyte, and acid-base balance include measurement of serum electrolytes and osmolality, complete blood count, urinalysis, and measurement of arterial blood gases.

- Nursing interventions for patients experiencing alterations in fluid, electrolyte, or acid-base balance address preventing imbalances, modifying oral intake, providing parenteral replacement, and transfusing blood products.

- Intravenous fluids are classified as isotonic, hypotonic, and hypertonic solutions, according to how they compare to the osmolality of blood serum.

- Vascular access devices may provide access to peripheral or central veins.

- Intravenous equipment consists of the IV catheter, an administration set, extension tubing, and the IV solution.

- You are responsible for maintaining the correct rate of flow and for monitoring the client's response to the infusion.

- Calculate the drip rate by multiplying the number of milliliters to be infused in 60 minutes (hourly rate) by the drop factor in drops per milliliter and then dividing by 60 minutes. For example, an hourly rate of 100 mL multiplied by 15 drops/mL and divided by 60 minutes equals the drip rate. Therefore, the drip rate equals 25 drops per minute. Use this formula to calculate flow:

$$\frac{\text{Hourly rate in mL} \times (\text{drops/mL})}{60 \text{ minutes}} = \text{drip rate}$$

- Complications at the IV site include infiltration, extravasation, infection, thrombus, and thrombophlebitis. Systemic complications include fluid volume excess, sepsis, and embolus. Systemic complications occur less frequently than local complications but may be life-threatening.

- Blood products are infused when the client has experienced significant blood loss, diminished oxygen-carrying capacity, or a deficiency in one of the blood components.

37 CHAPTER Perioperative Nursing

Overview

Perioperative nursing includes care of patients during the preoperative, intraoperative, and postoperative phases. The focus during the preoperative period is to determine whether the client is physiologically, cognitively, and psychologically prepared for the intraoperative and postoperative phases of surgery. Preoperative care includes teaching the patient about the surgery and expected postoperative care, confirming that surgical consent has been obtained, and physically preparing the patient for surgery.

During the intraoperative phase, nursing care may be delivered by the scrub nurse or first assistant within the sterile field and by the circulating nurse, whose role is to coordinate care within the operative suite. Intraoperative care includes providing skin preparation, positioning the patient for surgery, and carrying out protective measures to ensure patient safety during surgery.

The postoperative phase consists of two parts: the immediate postanesthesia phase and the postoperative recovery phase. Postanesthesia care is delivered in a specialized unit adjacent to the operating room. The patient is carefully monitored and remains in this unit until he has recovered from anesthesia. He is then transferred to a surgical unit or readied for discharge home. Common activities in the postoperative phase include the use of sequential compression devices to help prevent thrombophlebitis and incentive spirometry to help prevent atelectasis and pneumonia.

Thinking Critically About Perioperative Nursing

The exercises in the following section allow you to practice the kind of thinking you will use as a full-spectrum nurse. Because these are critical-thinking activities, there is usually no single right answer. Discuss answers with your peers—discussion can stimulate critical thinking. If you have difficulty with any of the questions, consult with your instructor.

Caring for the Garcias

Katherine Garcia, the 76-year-old mother of Joe Garcia, has been experiencing blurred vision and decreased visual acuity. A local ophthalmologist diagnosed bilateral cataracts. The ophthalmologist has recommended cataract removal in the left eye with insertion of an intraocular lens. He told Mrs. Garcia to schedule the surgery "at your convenience" and explained that the surgery would be performed on an outpatient basis. The ophthalmologist gave Mrs. Garcia a list of activities to prepare for the surgery, containing the following information:

- Schedule a date for your surgery. My receptionist will set up a time for your surgery. All surgeries are performed at Western Medical Center Same-Day Surgery Department.
- Please arrange to be seen by your primary care provider 1 to 2 weeks prior to the surgery to receive clearance for surgery.
- Make an appointment with the Preoperative Center at Western Medical Center Same-Day Surgery Department 1 to 2 days before surgery.
- Arrange to have a ride to and from the surgery.

A. What preoperative testing is Mrs. Garcia likely to undergo? Explain your rationale.

B. The preoperative list states that the client must be seen by the primary care provider to receive clearance for surgery. Why is this an essential part of the preoperative period?

C. What theoretical knowledge do you need to perform preoperative teaching for Mrs. Garcia? How could you obtain that information? (Be specific about your sources.)

D. What content would you include in Mrs. Garcia's preoperative teaching?

E. The ophthalmologist has planned anesthesia via conscious sedation. What factors, if any, might keep Mrs. Garcia from receiving this form of anesthesia? What additional information do you need to answer this question?

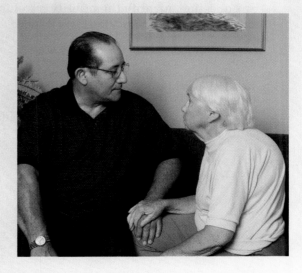

1 You are speaking with several classmates about an upcoming surgical rotation. During the rotation, you will have an opportunity to work with a circulating nurse and a scrub nurse. One of your classmates says that she is very nervous. "I don't know if I will be able to handle this rotation. I'm afraid I might not be able to watch the surgery. I've never really seen anything gross like that before." Another classmate confides that she is worried that she will contaminate everything and put the client at risk. What advice can you give them, and what actions can you take to prepare yourself for your experience in the OR?

2 You are working on a busy surgical unit on the evening shift. There is one UAP on the unit this evening. You are caring for the following clients:

- Mr. Singh ("Meet Your Patient"), who underwent a colon resection and colostomy for colon cancer. He is now in postoperative day 2. Mr. Singh is now complaining of chest pain and shortness of breath.
- Ms Yasmin, a 52-year-old woman admitted to the unit from PACU 1 hour ago after total abdominal hysterectomy and bilateral salpingo-oophrectomy (TAH-BSO—removal of the uterus, ovaries, and fallopian tubes)
- Mr. Stellanski, a 16-year-old with Down syndrome who underwent an emergency appendectomy early this morning.

The PACU calls to inform you that they are ready to transport Mrs. Bauer back to the unit. She is an 87-year-old woman from the local skilled nursing facility who underwent an extensive debridement of a stage IV pressure ulcer on the coccyx. The PACU nurse tells you she is confused and agitated and will need close monitoring.

a What problems does the admission of this new patient present for you? To answer this question, identify the priority nursing activity for each of the three patients you already have, as well as for Mrs. Bauer.

b How will you handle this situation? Identify three options, and explain their advantages and disadvantages.

3 You will be caring for a 23-year-old client who underwent emergency surgery after an automobile accident. He has had no preoperative teaching. What concerns does this raise? How will you address these concerns?

4 For each of the following concepts, use critical thinking to describe how or why it is important to nursing, patient care, or perioperative nursing. Note that these are *not* to be merely definitions.

Preoperative teaching

Preoperative physical preparation

Intraoperative safety measures

Anesthesia

Postoperative complications

Practical Knowledge
knowing how

Perioperative care requires you to use the nursing process to ensure that the patient is in the best possible condition for surgery, is safe during surgery, and has the best possible outcomes postoperatively. Much of perioperative nursing care consists of procedures and techniques designed for prevention and early detection of complications. Recall that full-spectrum nursing involves both thinking and doing—both are equally important.

PROCEDURES

The procedures in this section will help you to prevent postoperative complications. Preoperative teaching of coughing, deep breathing, moving in bed, and leg exercises helps to prevent thrombophlebitis, atelectasis, and pneumonia. Antiembolism stockings and sequential compression devices are designed to promote peripheral circulation and prevent thrombus formation.

| PROCEDURE 37–1 | **Teaching a Patient to Cough, Deep-Breathe, Move in Bed, and Perform Leg Exercises** |

 For steps to follow in *all* procedures, refer to the inside back cover of this book.

critical aspects
- Assess the patient's readiness to learn.
- Ensure that the patient is clear about the difference between coughing and merely clearing the throat.
- Demonstrate how to splint a potential chest or abdominal incision.
- Make sure the patient flexes her knees prior to turning on her side in bed.
- Support the patient who is unable to maintain a side-lying position with pillows.
- Teach the patient to alternately flex and extend the knees.
- Teach the patient to alternately dorsiflex and plantar flex the foot.
- Teach the patient to rotate her ankles in a complete circle.

Equipment

For teaching coughing and deep breathing:
- Folded blanket or a pillow (if teaching will include splinting of a surgical incision site)
- Tissues

For moving in bed:
- Small pillow or folded blanket
- Pillows

Delegation

You or another RN should perform the initial teaching. You may delegate reinforcement of the teaching to an LVN (or LPN) or UAP.

Assessment

- Assess the patient's cognitive level and level of consciousness.

Helps you select the appropriate teaching method and assess the patient's ability to comprehend and follow directions.

PROCEDURE 37–1 Teaching a Patient to Cough, Deep-Breathe, Move in Bed, and Perform Leg Exercises *(continued)*

- Assess the patient's pain level.

Even preoperatively, pain must be well controlled to ensure full patient participation.

- Determine whether the surgical procedure and/or a physical handicap will limit the patient's participation.

For example, a fractured arm that has not yet been repaired in surgery will impair the patient's ability to hold a pillow for splinting.

- Determine whether the surgical procedure may entail special exercises or equipment. In addition, assess for any special equipment, such as braces, slings, or abductor wedges, that may be needed when turning a patient in bed.

Orthopedic surgeries involving the knee and hip often involve special exercises or equipment in the postoperative period. Consult the surgeon before teaching the patient any leg exercises. Spinal and neurological surgeries often limit movement in the postoperative period. For example, some spinal surgeries require the patient to "logroll" (move from head to toe as one unit). Some neurological procedures require limiting the amount of time the patient's head of bed is above 30°. Identify these restrictions preoperatively, and inform the patient and family about them during your teaching session.

- Assess the patient's belief about the ability of the surgical incision to remain intact.

If the patient believes that the incision will not stay together if he coughs or moves, compliance is likely to be low.

Procedural Steps

Teaching a Patient to Deep Breathe and Cough

Deep breathing and coughing expand the lungs, improve ventilation, and help prevent atelectasis and pneumonia.

Step 1 Assist the patient to Fowler's or semi-Fowler's position, with the shoulders relaxed.

Allows for best chest and lung expansion

Step 2 Assist the patient who will have a chest or abdominal incision to practice splinting the site with a folded blanket or pillow.

Counterpressure supports the incision and decreases pain. ▼

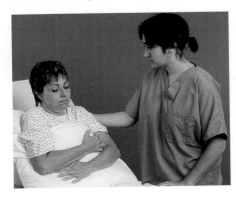

Step 3 Teach the patient diaphragmatic/deep breathing. Tell the patient to:
a. Place her hands anteriorly, along the lower end of the rib cage. The tips of the third fingers should touch at the midline.
b. Slowly take a deep breath in through the nose. Tell the patient that she should feel her chest expanding as the diaphragm moves down.
c. Hold her breath for 2 to 5 seconds

Stimulates surfactant production and helps prevent alveolar collapse.

d. Slowly and completely exhale the breath through her mouth.

Step 4 Teach the patient to cough in conjunction with diaphragmatic breathing. Teach the patient to:
a. Complete two or three cycles of diaphragmatic breathing.
b. On the next breath in, have the patient lean forward and cough rapidly, through an open mouth, using the muscles of the abdomen, thighs, and buttocks. Cough several times on that breath.

Helps patient to distinguish coughing from merely clearing the throat.

Variation Patient Experiencing Weakness

If the patient is too weak to perform this maneuver, have the patient inhale deeply, bend forward slightly, and perform three or four "huffs" against an open glottis to move secretions forward.

Teaching a Patient to Move in Bed

Moving in bed promotes blood circulation, stimulates respiratory function, and helps mobilize gas in the intestines.

Step 5 Start with the patient in the supine position, bedrails up. Then instruct the patient as follows.

Step 6 To turn to the left side: Bend the right leg, sliding the foot flat along the bed and flexing the knee.

Enables the patient to push herself over to the opposite side.

Step 7 Reach the right arm across the chest, and grab the opposite bedrail.

Assists with turning.

➤

PROCEDURE 37–1

Teaching a Patient to Cough, Deep-Breathe, Move in Bed, and Perform Leg Exercises *(continued)*

Step 8 Breathe deeply, and practice splinting any potential abdominal or chest incisions. (Assist the patient to practice as needed.)

Facilitates comfort during movement.

Step 9 Pull on the bedrail while pushing off with the right foot.

Assists patient to turn to the left. ▼

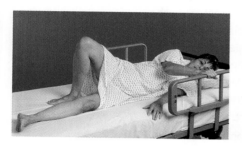

Step 10 If the patient cannot maintain this position independently, place a folded pillow or blanket along her back for support.

Step 11 Change positions every 2 hours, repeating the turning process with the opposite arm and leg. (You will need to assist the patient who needs pillows placed for support.)

Teaching the Patient Leg Exercises

Leg exercises flex and extend the leg muscles to increase peripheral circulation and help prevent thrombus formation. Thrombus formation is a common postoperative complication.

Step 12 Have the patient lie supine in the bed. *Note:* These exercises can be done when the patient is up in a chair, but the effect will be diminished by the effects of gravity.

Step 13 Perform ankle circles. Instruct the patient to:
a. Start with one foot in the dorsiflexed position.
b. Slowly rotate the ankle clockwise.
c. After three rotations, repeat the procedure in a counter-clockwise direction.
d. Repeat this exercise at least three times in each direction, then switch and exercise the other ankle. ▼

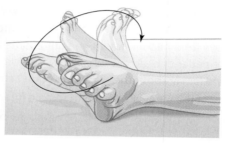

Step 14 Perform ankle pumps. Instruct the patient to:
a. Start with one foot, leg extended.
b. Point the toe until her foot is plantar flexed.
c. Pull the toes back toward her head until the foot is dorsiflexed; at the same time, press the back of the knee into the bed.
d. Make sure she feels a "pull" in the calf.
e. Repeat the alternation between plantar and dorsiflexion several times.
f. Repeat the cycle with the other foot.

Step 15 Perform leg exercises. (*Note:* These exercises may be contraindicated in patients having knee, hip, or back surgery. Check physician orders and/or collaborate with the physical therapist.) Instruct the patient to:
a. Lie supine in the bed.

b. Slowly begin bending the knee, sliding the sole of the foot along the bed until the knee is in a flexed position. ▼

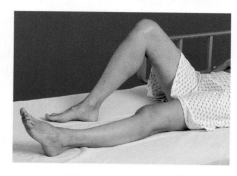

c. Reverse the motion, extending the knee until the leg is once again flat on the bed. ▼

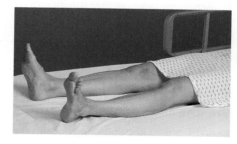

d. Repeat several times.
e. Repeat using the opposite leg.

Evaluation

Make sure that the patient performs correctly a return demonstration of the procedures taught.

PROCEDURE 37–1   **Teaching a Patient to Cough, Deep-Breathe, Move in Bed, and Perform Leg Exercises** *(continued)*

Documentation

In many healthcare facilities, charts have special areas in which you document patient teaching. Documentation should identify the person who completed the teaching, the person to whom the procedures were taught, what procedures were taught, and whether the patient understood the teaching. Also include the name and type of any printed materials given.

Sample documentation:

7/11/06	1530	68 y.o. female scheduled for repair of left tibial fracture in AM. Pt alert and oriented x 3. Rates pain as 1 on scale of 1 to 10. Preoperative instruction given to patient and husband. Instructed about deep breathing and coughing, expectations for preop, intraop, and postop care. Informed pt that she will have a long leg cast. Emphasized the importance of turning and moving in bed. Informed pt and husband that physical therapy will begin on the 1st postoperative day. ———— R. Hayden, RN

PROCEDURE 37–2   **Applying Antiembolism Stockings**

 For steps to follow in *all* procedures, refer to the inside back cover of this book.

critical aspects

- Measure the patient's leg to ensure that you select stockings of the correct size.
- Inspect the legs and feet for edema, abrasions, lesions, open areas, and circulatory changes.
- Elevate the patient's legs for at least 15 minutes prior to applying stockings.
- Turn the stocking inside out to the level of the heel.
- Insert patient's foot into stocking. Gradually unroll and pull the remaining portion of the stocking up and over the leg.
  - Keep knee-high stockings 2.5 to 5 cm (1 to 2 inches) below the joint.
  - Do not apply thigh-high stockings if the thigh circumference is greater than 100 cm (25 inches).
- Make sure the stocking is free of wrinkles and is not rolled at the top or bunched.

➤

PROCEDURE 37–2   Applying Antiembolism Stockings *(continued)*

Equipment

- Measuring tape
- One pair of antiembolism stockings
- Washcloth and towel (if needed to cleanse legs)
- Talcum powder (optional: check manufacturer's recommendations)

Delegation

You can delegate application of antiembolism stockings to unlicensed assistive personnel who have been trained in the task. Instruct the UAP as follows:

- Report the presence of any abnormalities on the lower extremities, such as lesions, sores, or redness, before applying the stockings.
- Have the patient maintain a recumbent position at least 15 minutes before applying the stockings.
- Do not massage the legs.
- Make sure there are no wrinkles in the stockings once they have been applied.

Assessment

- Assess level of consciousness and cognitive ability.

If the patient is unconscious or confused, you will need to obtain assistance to hold and stabilize the lower extremities as you apply the stocking's.

- Assess for signs and symptoms of severe peripheral arterial disease, such as weak or absent pulses, discoloration or cyanosis, or gangrene.

Compression of vessels by antiembolism stockings may further impede arterial flow. They should not be used in clients with any of these findings.

- Assess the condition of the skin. Note the presence of lesions, dermatitis, or major edema, as evidenced by shiny, taut skin.

If skin is overstretched by edema, antiembolism stockings may irritate or worsen skin conditions and cause skin breakdown.

- Note the position of the patient and length of time the patient has been in that position.

Place the patient supine for at least 15 minutes prior to stocking application. This prevents trapping of pooled venous blood.

Procedural Steps

If possible, apply stockings in the morning, before the patient gets out of bed.

Prevents venous distention and edema that occur when the patient is sitting or standing.

Step 1 Measure the patient's lower extremity.

Ensures that you order stockings of the proper size. ▼

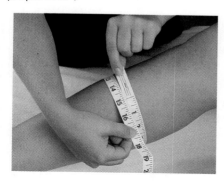

Variation Thigh-High Stockings

a. Measure the circumference of the thigh at the widest section.

The manufacturer of T.E.D. brand stockings recommends that stockings not be applied if the thigh circumference exceeds 100 cm (25 inches).

b. Measure the calf circumference at the widest section.

c. Measure the distance from the gluteal fold to the base of the heel.

Note: If both legs do not measure the same, McConnell (2002) suggests ordering two different sizes, using one from each package to make two pairs.

Variation Knee-High Stockings

a. Measure the circumference of the calf at the widest section.

b. Measure the distance from the base of the heel to the middle of the knee joint.

Step 2 Assist the patient to a supine position, and have him maintain that position

for at least 15 minutes before you apply the stockings. Ideally, apply stockings in the morning, before the patient gets out of bed.

Prevents trapping of pooled venous blood.

Step 3 Cleanse the patient's legs and feet if necessary. Dry well.

Removing surface dirt and/or bacteria will decrease the likelihood of infection and odor.

Step 4 Lightly dust the legs and feet with talcum powder if desired and if recommended by the manufacturer.

Eases the application of the stockings.

Note: Do not use powder if patient is or is likely to become diaphoretic, because perspiration will cause the powder to clump.

Step 5 Holding one stocking at the top cuff in your dominant hand, slide your nondominant arm down and into the stocking until your hand reaches the heel of the stocking.

PROCEDURE 37–2   Applying Antiembolism Stockings *(continued)*

Step 6 Grasp the heel with your hand inside the stocking, and then slowly turn the stocking inside out to the level of the heel with your other hand.

The elastic in the stockings is very strong; this method is the easiest way to fit it over the foot and calf. ▼

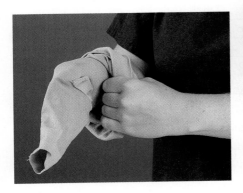

Step 7 Tell the patient to point his toes as you grasp the turned foot of the stocking and ease it onto his foot (like putting on a sock). Center the patient's heel in the heel of the stocking.

Ensures that the pressure of the stocking is over the correct anatomical areas.

Step 8 Pull the remainder of the stocking up and over the leg to 2.5 to 5 cm (1 to 2 inches) below the knee or to the gluteal fold of the thigh (depending on the type of stocking ordered), turning it right side out as you proceed. ▼

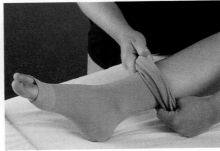

• Be sure the stocking is straight.

Stockings apply varying amounts of compression between ankle, calf, and thigh areas. Keeping the stocking straight ensures that the pressure occurs over the correct areas.

• Keep stockings free of wrinkles and bunching.

Decreases the risk of skin breakdown and areas of inappropriate and potentially dangerous constriction.

Step 9 When using stockings with closed toes, tug gently on the end of the stocking over the toes to create a small space between the end of the toes and the stocking.

Prevents compression of small vessels in the toes, which may impede circulation.

Step 10 Repeat the procedure on the other leg.

Step 11 Remove the stockings and bathe and dry the legs daily.

Step 12 Launder the stockings at least every 3 days; dry them on flat surface.

Soiled stockings can irritate the skin; dry flat to prevent stretching.

Evaluation

• Evaluate patient comfort.

Severe, continuous discomfort may indicate that the stockings are the wrong size.

• Check the stockings for wrinkles and/or rolling down at the top.

Wrinkles and rolling down can cause skin breakdown and areas of constriction.

• Evaluate skin condition.

Elastic stockings should be removed for 20 to 30 minutes every 8 hours to allow for inspection of skin and evaluation of adequacy of circulation.

Home Care

• Teach the patient and/or caregiver to apply the stockings.
• Encourage the patient to have two pairs of stockings on hand so that one pair may be used while the other is being laundered.
• Tell the patient to follow manufacturer's directions for washing the stockings.
• Teach the patient not to roll down the tops of the stockings.

➤

PROCEDURE 37–2   **Applying Antiembolism Stockings** *(continued)*

Documentation

- Document the size of the stockings used and the time and date applied.
- Note the condition of the skin, including any abnormalities.

Sample documentation

> 12/30/06   0930   Pt measured for thigh-high antiembolism stockings: Calf: 11 in. (27.9 cm), Thigh 23 in. (58.4 cm), length 30 in. (76.2 cm). Skin on legs inspected. No open areas or lesions, skin warm & dry, DP and PT pulses palpable. Thigh-high stockings applied, with patient in recumbent position. Use explained to pt and wife, who express understanding. ——— K. Bradsby, RN

PROCEDURE 37–3   **Applying Sequential Compression Devices**

 For steps to follow in *all* procedures, refer to the inside back cover of this book.

critical aspects

- Determine whether elastic stockings are to be used concurrently with the sequential device. If so, apply them (see Procedure 37–2).
- Place the regulating pump for the sequential compression in a location that will ensure patient safety.
- Place the patient in a supine position.
- If you are using SCD and PAS brand thigh-high compression sleeves, measure the thigh.
- Place the lower extremity on the open sleeve, ensuring that the compression chambers are located over the correct anatomical structure (e.g., knee opening is at the level of the joint).
- Leave 1 to 2 fingerbreadths between the sleeve and the extremity.
- Set the regulating pump to the correct pressure, as ordered.
- Instruct the patient to call for assistance in disconnecting the tubing from the sleeve.

Equipment

Note: Sequential compression devices are known by several different brand names, including SCDS (Sequential Compression Decompression Stockings), Flowtrons, and PAS (Pneumatic Air Stockings).

- Compression pump, motor, or machine.
- Connecting tubing, if applicable (In some devices, the tubing is preconnected to the sleeves)
- Compression sleeve (knee-high or thigh-high, depending on the order and the type of device)
- Elastic stockings (if ordered in addition to the sequential compression device)
- Washcloth and towel as needed to cleanse the lower extremities
- Measuring tape

PROCEDURE 37–3   Applying Sequential Compression Devices *(continued)*

Delegation

You may delegate the application of the sequential compression device to the UAP who has had training in that task. As in the application of elastic stockings, instruct the UAP to report any redness, irritation, or open areas on the lower extremities. Instruct the UAP to ensure that all cords and connecting tubing are not in a place that will create a fall risk for the patient or visitors. SCDs should not be removed for long periods of time because they are needed to support the patient's peripheral circulation.

Assessment

• Assess cognitive level and level of consciousness.

Patients with altered cognition may be at higher risk for falls related to the presence of the connecting tubing and attachment to the compression pump. Patients who are unconscious will not be able to report a device that is creating too much pressure.

• Assess signs and symptoms of severe peripheral arterial disease, such as weak or absent pulses, discoloration or cyanosis, or gangrene.

Increased compression of vessels by the sequential device may further impede arterial flow.

• Assess the condition of the skin. Note the presence of lesions, dermatitis, or major edema, as evidenced by shiny, taut skin.

If skin is overstretched by edema, the sequential compression sleeve may irritate or worsen skin conditions and cause skin breakdown.

Procedural Steps

Step 1 Cleanse the lower extremities, if necessary.

Removing surface dirt and/or bacteria will decrease the likelihood of infection and odor.

Step 2 If elastic stockings have been ordered in conjunction with the sequential compression device, apply them, following the steps in Procedure 37–2.

Step 3 For thigh-high sequential compression device sleeves, you must measure the thigh to ensure that the sleeves are of the proper size. Follow the manufacturer's instructions.

Step 4 Place the patient in a supine position.

Prevents venous pooling. Allows for easier application of compression sleeve.

Step 5 Place the compression device pump in a location near an electrical outlet so that the cord will not pose a fall risk. Plug it in. *Note:* Many compression pumps come equipped with hangers so you can hang the device at the bottom of the patient's bed.

Promotes patient safety.

Step 6 Apply the compression sleeve. ▼

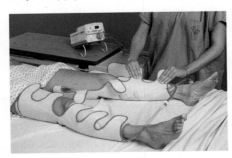

Variation For Flowtron Brand (available in knee-length only):

a. Open the Velcro fasteners on the sleeve.
b. Place the sleeve under the lower leg below the knee, with the "air bladder" side down on the bed.
c. Bring the ends of the sleeve up, and wrap them around the lower leg, leaving 1 to 2 fingerbreadths of space between the leg and the sleeve.

Prevents excess pressure and overcompression.

Variation For SCDS/PAS Brand

a. Open the Velcro fasteners on the sleeve.
b. Place the sleeve under the leg, ensuring that the fastener will close on the anterior surface
For thigh-high sleeves:
Place the opened sleeve under the leg, ensuring that the knee opening is at the level of the knee joint.

Ensures that compression occurs over the correct structures. Prevents decreased range of motion (ROM) of the knee joint.

c. Bring the ends of the sleeve up, and wrap them around the leg, leaving 1 to 2 fingerbreadths of space between the leg and the sleeve.

Prevents excess pressure and overcompression.

Step 7 Connect the sleeve to the compression pump.

Step 8 Turn the pump on and, if applicable, set the compression pressure on the pump device to the manufacturer's recommended setting. *Note:* In some facilities, the compression pressure amount is preset and can be changed only by the central supply/equipment department.

PROCEDURE 37–3   Applying Sequential Compression Devices *(continued)*

Evaluation

After applying the device, make the following ongoing assessments:

- Inflation and deflation of the sleeve

Ensures that the device is actually working.

- Kinking or pinching of the connecting tubing

Would prevent correct inflation of sleeves and may cause overheating or malfunction of the unit.

- Circulation, sensation, and motion of the foot, including skin color, pulses, temperature, capillary refill, motion, and sensation
- Patient comfort

Increasing discomfort may indicate excess or incorrect pressure.

- Skin condition (Remove the compression sleeves at intervals so that you can inspect skin and evaluate the adequacy of circulation. *Note:* If elastic stockings are being used in conjunction with sequential compression device, follow the recommendations in Procedure 37–2.)
- Signs and symptoms of deep-vein thrombosis

Patients having sequential compression device therapy can still develop thrombi.

Patient Teaching

Teach the patient to call for assistance when disconnecting the tubing from the compression pump in order to ambulate.

Prevents patient falls.

Documentation

- Document the date and time you applied the device.
- Note the type and size (if applicable) of the compression sleeve used.
- Document the skin condition, including any abnormalities.

Sample documentation

| 11/11/06 | 1100 | Knee-high SCD applied per order. Skin warm, dry, and intact at time of application. Peripheral pulses palpable. Pt's wife instructed on use of SCD. Pt unresponsive. No evidence of discomfort, no grimace, or movement with application. ———— S. Bee RN |

TECHNIQUES

| TECHNIQUE 37–1 | **Preparing a Room for a Patient's Return from Surgery** |

- Put clean linens on the bed, including pads to protect the linen from drainage.
- Fold the linens back to the end of the bed.
- Raise the bed to stretcher height, and lock the wheels.
- Move furniture and equipment so that the stretcher can be placed directly against the bed.
- Place the following equipment in the room: Stethoscope, manometer, thermometer (to measure vital signs)

IV pole
Emesis basin
Tissues
A clean gown, washcloth, and towel
Extra pillows for positioning the patient
- If needed, set up suction, oxygen, or other special equipment.

| TECHNIQUE 37–2 | **Creating an Operative Field** |

In the intraoperative period, sterile team members are the only persons allowed to enter the sterile field. The sterile field encompasses the client and the area immediately surrounding the client. Creation of the sterile field proceeds as follows:
- Perform a sterile scrub.
- Don sterile gown, gloves, and other surgical attire (e.g., head covering, shoe covers).
- Cleanse the operative site with a surgical prep (e.g., Betadine scrub followed by Betadine paint).

- Cover the area surrounding the operative site with sterile drapes so that only the patient's operative area is exposed.
- Place sterile draping over the remainder of the client's body.
- (In most cases) suspend a vertical drape at neck level so the client's head and airway are accessible to the anesthesiologist or nurse anesthetist (who is not sterile). For neurosurgery, even the head is draped, and the anesthesiologist or nurse anesthetist sits to the side of the head.

ASSESSMENT GUIDELINES AND TOOLS

Preoperative Assessment

Include the following information in your preoperative assessment.

- *Health history.* Discuss current and chronic health problems and prior hospitalizations or surgeries.
- *Physical status.* Identify any mobility concerns, and determine whether the patient uses hearing aids, glasses, or contact lenses.
- *Allergies.* Check allergies to medications, food, tape, soaps, latex, or other substances.
- *Medications.* Ask what prescribed medications and over-the-counter, herbal, or natural remedies the patient takes.
- *Mental status.* Note whether the client is able to respond to questions and offer a health history. Is he oriented? Does he appear anxious?
- *Knowledge and understanding of the surgery and anesthesia.* Ask the client to explain in his own words the planned

surgery and postoperative course. Reinforce accurate statements, and correct misconceptions.

- *Cultural and spiritual factors.* Identify any cultural practices or spiritual beliefs that bring comfort to the client. Discuss how you can integrate these practices into the client's surgical experience.
- *Access to social resources.* Identify the client's support network. Who is available to assist the client after surgery? Whom does the client rely on? Are those people aware of the client's upcoming surgery and condition?
- *Coping strategies.* Have the client identify the strategies he uses to cope with stress.
- *Use of alcohol and drugs.* Inquire about the amount and frequency of alcohol use. Discuss the use of pain medications and recreational drugs. If the client uses these substances, identify the amount and frequency.

Intraoperative Care Questionnaire

Common interview questions include the following:

- What is your name?
- What type of surgery are you going to have today?
- Is someone here with you?
- Are you allergic to any medications?
- When is the last time that you had anything to eat or drink?
- Do you have false teeth, contact lenses, or any other prostheses that need to be removed?

- Have you taken any medications today?
- Do you have any implants, such as metal plates or a pacemaker?
- Do you have any scratches, bruises, or other wounds on your body at this time?
- Are there any parts of your body that are painful, such as a stiff shoulder or leg?

DIAGNOSTIC TESTING

Common Preoperative Screening Tests

Test	Uses
Urinalysis	To detect urinary tract infections (UTIs) and the presence of glucose or protein in the urine, which may indicate poorly controlled diabetes or renal disease
Complete blood count (CBC)	• To detect irregularities in hemoglobin (Hgb) and hematocrit. A low Hgb level is an indication of anemia, which may place the client at risk if significant blood loss occurs. • Measures white blood cell (WBC) count as an indicator of immune function • Measures platelet count, which affects clotting ability
ECG (Electrocardiogram)	To detect cardiac dysrhythmias and other cardiac pathology
Chest x-ray examination	To detect underlying pulmonary disease; also to reveal heart size, as an indicator of heart function
Blood type and crossmatch	To identify blood type in the event that blood transfusion becomes necessary
Serum electrolytes	To detect sodium, potassium, chloride, magnesium, calcium, and pH imbalances, which affect cardiac and other organ function and fluid balance
Fasting blood sugar	To detect diabetes or poorly controlled diabetes
Comprehensive metabolic panel	Includes electrolytes, blood glucose, liver function tests (ALT, AST), serum albumin and protein, and renal function tests (BUN and creatinine); used to detect underlying health problems that may affect surgical risk or outcome

STANDARDIZED LANGUAGE

Selected Standardized Nursing Diagnoses, Outcomes, and Interventions for Preoperative Patients

Nursing Diagnoses	Selected NOC Outcomes and Goals Using NOC Indicators	Selected NIC Interventions and Nursing Activities (Shaded activities are routine nursing measures for all patients)
Anxiety related to change in health status	*NOC outcomes:* Anxiety Level Anxiety Self-Control *NOC goals patient will exhibit:* • (5) No restlessness • (4) Only mild muscle and facial tension • (4) Only mild difficulty concentrating • (5) No increased blood pressure, pulse rate, or respiratory rate • (5) No physical signs of anxiety such as: dilated pupils, sweating, and dizziness • (3) Moderate verbalized anxiety *Individualized goals:* • Identifies symptoms that are indicators of her anxiety • Communicates need for assistance	Anxiety Reduction • Use a calm, reassuring approach • Explain all procedures, including sensations likely to be experienced during the surgical procedure • Seek to understand the patient's perspective of the situation • Provide accurate factual information about the surgery Calming Technique • Maintain eye contact with patient • Encourage slow, purposeful deep breathing Presence • Stay with the patient and provide assurance of safety and security during periods of anxiety • Listen to the patient's concerns • Administer medications as appropriate to reduce anxiety
Fear related to unknown outcome of surgery and fear of pain that may result	*NOC outcomes:* Fear Level Fear Self-Control *NOC goals:* • (5) Exhibits no restlessness or irritability • (5) Reports no difficulty concentrating • (5) No physical signs of fear: increased BP, radial pulse rate, respiratory rate, sweating, dilated pupils, pale skin • (5) No verbalized fear • (5) No crying *Individualized goals:* • Does not exhibit physical signs of fear (e.g., pupil dilation; dry mouth; increased BP, pulse and respiratory rate) • Reports understanding of pain control measures to be used during and after surgery.	Anxiety Reduction • (See Anxiety diagnosis) Coping Enhancement • Assist the patient in developing an objective appraisal of the event • Evaluate the patient's decision-making ability • Encourage the use of spiritual resources, if desired Preparatory Sensory Information • Identify the typical sensations (what will be seen, felt, smelled, tasted, heard) the majority of patients describe as associated with each aspect of the procedure/treatment • Personalize the information by using personal pronouns Security Enhancement • Explain all tests and procedures to patient/family • Assist patient to use coping responses that have been successful in the past

(continued)

Nursing Diagnoses	Selected NOC Outcomes and Goals Using NOC Indicators	Selected NIC Interventions and Nursing Activities (Shaded activities are routine nursing measures for all patients)
Deficient Knowledge of preoperative procedures and postoperative expectations (may be the etiology of other problems, such as Ineffective Management of Therapeutic Regimen, or Risk for Infection)	*NOC outcomes:* Knowledge: Disease Process Knowledge: Treatment Procedure(s) *NOC goals:* Provides: • (3) moderate description of specific disease process • (4) substantial description of treatment procedure(s) • (4) substantial description of precautions related to procedure(s) *Individualized goals:* • Verbalizes rationale for pre- and postoperative interventions • Describes or demonstrates postoperative expectations (i.e., deep breathing, turning/position changes)	Teaching: Preoperative • Inform patient/significant others how long surgery is expected to last • Determine the patient's previous surgical experiences and level of knowledge related to surgery • Provide time for the patient to ask questions and discuss concern • Describe preoperative routines (e.g., anesthesia, diet, bowel preparation, tests/labs, voiding, skin preparation, IV therapy, clothing, family waiting area, transportation to operating room) • Describe any preoperative medications, the effects these will have on the patient, and the rationale for using them • Inform significant others of the place to wait for the results of the surgery • Introduce patient to perioperative staff as appropriate • Discuss possible pain control measures • Describe postoperative routines/equipment (e.g., medications, respiratory treatments, tubes, machines, support hose, surgical dressings, ambulation, diet, family visitation) and explain their purpose • Instruct patient in postoperative deep breathing exercises, splinting incision, coughing • Reinforce information provided by other health care team members, as appropriate • Include the family/significant others [in the teaching-learning process] as appropriate
Disturbed Sleep Pattern related to anxiety about the upcoming surgery	*NOC outcomes:* Sleep *NOC goals:* • (4) Mild interrupted sleep • (5) Hours of sleep (at least 5 hr/24 hr), not compromised • (4) Sleeps through the night, mildly compromised *Individualized goals:* • Reports minimal compromise in hours of sleep and sleep pattern • No difficulty falling and staying asleep reported or observed	Sleep Enhancement • Determine patient's usual sleep-activity pattern • Determine effects of patient's current medications on sleep pattern • Adjust environment (lighting, noise, temperature, etc.) to promote sleep • Demonstrate and explain procedure for progressive muscle relaxation • Administer medication to promote sleep, as appropriate

Sources: Dochterman, J. M., & Bulechek, G. M. (Eds.). (2004). *Nursing interventions classification (NIC)* (4th ed.). St Louis: Mosby; Moorhead, S., Johnson, M., & Maas, M. (Eds.). (2004). *Nursing outcomes classification (NOC)* (3rd ed.). St Louis: Mosby; NANDA International. (2005). *Nursing diagnoses: Definitions and classification 2005–2006*. Philadelphia: Author.

Selected Standardized Nursing Diagnoses, Outcomes, and Interventions for Intraoperative Patients

Nursing Diagnoses (NANDA) and Collaborative Problems	NOC Outcomes and Indicators	NIC Interventions and Activities (*Note:* Shaded interventions are routinely performed for all surgery patients)
Nursing diagnosis: Risk for Aspiration related to depressed respirations and reflexes secondary to anesthesia *Collaborative problem:* Potential Complication of anesthesia: aspiration	*NOC outcome:* Respiratory Status: Airway Patency *NOC goal:* • (5) No choking or adventitious breath sounds	**Artificial Airway Management** • Institute endotracheal suctioning, as appropriate **Aspiration Precautions** • Monitor pulmonary status • Keep suction setup available • Maintain an airway **Sedation Management** • Ensure that emergency resuscitation equipment is readily available, specifically source to deliver 100% O_2, emergency medications, and a defibrillator • Initiate an IV line • Ensure availability of and administer antagonists, as appropriate per physician's order or protocol **Vomiting Management** • Position to prevent aspiration
Nursing diagnosis: Risk for Imbalanced Body Temperature related to exposure in cool environment and administration of cool IV fluids *Collaborative problem:* Potential Complication of surgery and anesthesia: hypothermia	*NOC outcome:* Thermoregulation *NOC goal:* • (5) No hyperthermia • (5) No hypothermia • (4) Mild increased (or decreased) skin temperature	**Temperature Regulation: Intraoperative** • Adjust operating room temperature for therapeutic effect • Apply head covering • Cover exposed body parts • Warm or cool all irrigating, IV, and skin preparation solutions, as appropriate • Continuously monitor patient temperature • Cover patient with heated blanket for transport to postanesthesia care unit **Malignant Hyperthermia Precautions** • Maintain emergency equipment for malignant hyperthermia, per protocol, in operative areas • Notify anesthesiologist and surgeon of patient history • Provide a cooling blanket **Vital Signs Monitoring** • Monitor blood pressure, pulse, temperature, and respiratory status, as appropriate • Monitor skin color, temperature, and moistness
Nursing diagnosis: Risk for Imbalanced Fluid Volume *Collaborative problem:* Potential complication of surgery: fluid and electrolyte imbalance	*NOC outcomes:* Blood Loss Severity Fluid Balance Urinary Elimination Vital Signs	**Fluid Management** • Maintain accurate intake and output record • Insert urinary catheter, if appropriate • Administer IV therapy, as prescribed • Monitor hemodynamic status, including CVP, MAP, PAP, and PCWP, if available

(continued)

Nursing Diagnoses (NANDA) and Collaborative Problems	NOC Outcomes and Indicators	NIC Interventions and Activities (*Note:* Shaded interventions are routinely performed for all surgery patients)
(Clients undergoing surgery are at risk for vascular, cellular, and/or intracellular dehydration [Johnson, Holm, & Godshall, 2000]).	*NOC goals:* • (4) Blood pressure mildly compromised • (5) Mean arterial pressure not compromised • (5) Central venous pressure not compromised • (5) Pulmonary wedge pressure not compromised • (4) Peripheral pulses mildly compromised • (4) 24-hour intake and output balance mildly compromised • (5) Adventitious breath sounds not present • (5) Neck vein distension not present • (5) Peripheral edema not present	• Prepare for administration of blood products (e.g., check blood with patient identification and prepare infusion setup), as appropriate Fluid Monitoring • Determine possible risk factors for fluid imbalance (e.g., … renal pathologies, liver dysfunction …) • Monitor color, quantity, and specific gravity of urine • Monitor for distended neck veins, crackles in the lungs, peripheral edema, and weight gain • Monitor blood pressure, heart rate, and respiratory status • Monitor serum and urine electrolyte values Intravenous (IV) Therapy • Monitor IV flow rate and IV site during infusion • Monitor for IV patency before administration of IV medication
Nursing diagnosis: Risk for Latex Allergy Response or Latex Allergy Response related to multiple previous exposures to latex	*NOC outcomes:* Immune Hypersensitivity Response Symptom Severity *NOC goals:* • (5) No localized inflammatory responses • (5) Respiratory, cardiac, renal, and neurological functions not compromised	Latex Precautions (Intraoperative) • Place allergy band on patient [if not already done preoperatively] • Record allergy or risk in patient's medical record [or check to see that it was done] • Post sign indicating latex precautions • Survey environment and remove latex products • Monitor latex-free environment • Report information to physician, pharmacist, and other care providers, as indicated Preoperative Interventions • Question patient or appropriate other about history of neural tube defect (e.g., spina bifida) or congenital urological condition (e.g., exstrophy of the bladder) • Question patient or appropriate other about systemic reactions to natural rubber latex (e.g., facial or scleral edema, tearing eyes, urticaria, rhinitis, and wheezing) • Question patient or appropriate other about allergies to foods such as bananas, kiwi, avocado, mango, and chestnuts
Nursing diagnosis: Risk for Perioperative Positioning Injury related to patient factors such as edema, emaciation, obesity, and sensory perceptual disturbances secondary to anesthesia	*NOC outcomes:* Circulatory Status Mobility Neurological Status Physical Injury Severity Tissue Perfusion: Peripheral	Circulatory Precautions • Perform a comprehensive appraisal of peripheral circulation (e.g., check peripheral pulses, edema, capillary refill, color, and temperature of extremity)

Selected Standardized Nursing Diagnoses, Outcomes, and Interventions for Intraoperative Patients *(continued)*

Nursing Diagnoses (NANDA) and Collaborative Problems	NOC Outcomes and Indicators	NIC Interventions and Activities (*Note:* Shaded interventions are routinely performed for all surgery patients)
Collaborative problem: Potential complication of surgery: neuromuscular, skeletal, or skin injury	*NOC goals:* • (4) Pao_2 mildly compromised • (4) $Paco_2$ mildly compromised • (4) Skin color not compromised • (5) Joint movement not compromised • (5) Spinal sensory/motor function not compromised • (5) Central motor control not compromised • (5) No burns, bruises, extremity or back sprains, impaired mobility • (4) Capillary refill mildly compromised • (5) Sensation not compromised • (5) All pulses not compromised • (5) Skin integrity not compromised	Positioning: Intraoperative • Use assistive devices for immobilization • Lock wheels of stretcher and operating room bed • Use an adequate number of personnel to transfer patient • Support the head and neck during transfer • Immobilize or support any body part, as appropriate • Maintain patient's proper body alignment • Apply padding to bony prominences • Apply safety strap and arm restraint, as needed • Record position and devices used Surgical Precautions • Verify surgical consent • Verify surgical site • Verify client's blood type • Verify that there is blood on reserve • Verify client's identity • Verify patient's allergies • Check ground isolation monitor • Verify the correct functioning of equipment • Check suction for adequate pressure and complete assembly of canisters, tubing, and catheters • Count sponges, sharps, and instruments before, during, and after surgery, per agency policy; record results of counts • Provide an electrosurgical unit, grounding pad, and active electrode, as appropriate • Verify integrity of electrical cords • Verify proper functioning of electrosurgical unit • Verify that client is not in contact with metal • Check for presence of implants, pacemakers, and metal prostheses pacemakers contraindicating use of electrosurgical cautery • Verify skin integrity at site of [electrocautery] grounding pad • Verify that skin prep solutions are non-flammable • Adjust coagulation and cutting currents, as instructed by physician or per agency policy • Inspect the patient's skin for injury [at conclusion of procedure] • (non-NIC) Monitor sterile technique throughout procedure

Sources: Dochterman, J. M., & Bulechek, G. M. (Eds.). (2004). *Nursing interventions classification (NIC)* (4th ed.). St Louis: Mosby; Moorhead, S., Johnson, M., & Maas, M. (Eds.). (2004). *Nursing outcomes classification (NOC)* (3rd ed.). St Louis: Mosby; NANDA International. (2005). *Nursing diagnoses: Definitions and classification 2005–2006.* Philadelphia: Author.

Selected Standardized Nursing Diagnoses, Outcomes, and Interventions for Postoperative Patients

Nursing Diagnoses	Outcomes and Goals	Nursing Interventions and Activities
Activity Intolerance r/t pain and the surgical procedure and stressors of surgery	*NOC outcomes:* Activity Tolerance Endurance Energy Conservation Psychomotor Energy *NOC goals:* • O$_2$ saturation, heart rate, respiratory rate, systolic and diastolic blood pressure in expected range in response to activity • Respiratory effort in response to activity not compromised • Walking pace and distance not compromised • Reported activities of daily living (ADLs) performance not compromised • Ability to speak while exercising not compromised • Energy restored after rest • Uses naps to restore energy • Exhibits concentration	*NIC interventions:* Activity Therapy Energy Management Exercise Promotion: Strength Training *Nursing activities:* • Collaborate with other disciplines to plan and monitor activity program as appropriate • Assist to choose appropriate activities • Assist to focus on strengths rather than weaknesses • Assist to identify activity preferences • Instruct client, family how to perform desired activities • Refer to community centers, programs as appropriate • Arrange physical activities to reduce competition for oxygen supply to vital body functions (e.g., avoid activity immediately after meals) • Avoid care activities during scheduled rest periods • Assist to sit on side of bed ("dangle"), if unable to transfer or walk • Monitor location and nature of pain during activity • Teach activity organization and time management techniques to prevent fatigue
Acute Pain r/t (1) inflammation or injury in the surgical area, (2) abdominal distention secondary to decreased peristalsis, (3) muscle pain secondary to positioning and tension	*NOC outcomes:* Pain Level Pain Control *NOC goals:* • Rates pain as less than 5 on a 1 to 10 scale • No moaning or crying • No facial expressions of pain • No guarding of incision • Recognizes causal factors • Uses preventive measures • Uses non-analgesic relief measures • Uses analgesics appropriately • Reports symptoms to health care professional	*NIC Interventions:* Analgesic Administration Pain Management Patient-Controlled Analgesia (PCA) Assistance *Nursing activities:* • Assess location, characteristics, onset, duration, frequency, quality, intensity of pain and predisposing factors • Observe for nonverbal discomfort cues • Assure patient of analgesic availability • Consider cultural influences of responses to pain • Utilize developmentally appropriate assessment method • Determine necessary frequency of pain assessment and formulate pain assessment plan • Provide information about the pain, such as causes, anticipated duration • Control environmental factors that may contribute to client's response

➤

Selected Standardized Nursing Diagnoses, Outcomes, and Interventions for Postoperative Patients *(continued)*

Nursing Diagnoses	Outcomes and Goals	Nursing Interventions and Activities
		• Provide information about the pain, such as causes of the pain, how long it will last, and anticipated discomforts from procedures (e.g., teach patient to splint incision when ambulating) • Provide optimal pain relief with analgesics as appropriate • Implement PCA (patient controlled analgesia) as appropriate • Intervene before pain becomes severe • Medicate prior to activity to increase participation • Teach nonpharmacological pain relief measures (e.g., visualization, progressive muscle relaxation) • Utilize multidisciplinary approach to pain management (Dochterman & Bulechek, 2004)
Anxiety r/t change in health status, hospital environment	*NOC outcomes:* Anxiety Level Anxiety Control *NOC goals:* • Uses effective coping strategies • Seeks information to reduce anxiety • Uses relaxation techniques to reduce anxiety • Maintains concentration • Reports absence of physical manifestations of anxiety • Minimal restlessness, hand wringing, muscle tension, facial tension, difficulty concentrating • Minimal changes in vital signs; no dilated pupils, sweating or dizziness • Controls anxiety response	*NIC interventions:* Anxiety Reduction *Nursing activities:* • Use calm, reassuring approach • Observe for verbal and nonverbal signs of anxiety • Explain all procedures and activities • Provide information concerning diagnosis, treatment, prognosis • Administer back rub or neck rub as appropriate • Listen attentively • Create trusting atmosphere • Assist client to identify stressful situations • Assist client to recognize that she is anxious • Assess client's ability to make decisions • Encourage verbalization of feelings, perceptions, and fears related to the surgical procedure • Encourage family visits if these ease client's stress • Support use of appropriate defense mechanisms • Instruct patient in use of relaxation techniques
Nausea r/t manipulation of gastrointestinal tract, decreased peristalsis secondary to anesthesia	*NOC outcomes:* Nausea & Vomiting Control Nausea & Vomiting: Disruptive Effects Nausea & Vomiting Severity Nutritional Status: Food & Fluid Intake *NOC goals:* • No nausea, or intensity only mild. • Minimal retching and vomiting	*NIC interventions:* Nausea Management Medication Management *Nursing activities:* • Encourage to monitor own nausea experience • Encourage to learn strategies for managing own nausea

(continued)

Nursing Diagnoses	Outcomes and Goals	Nursing Interventions and Activities
	• Mild intolerance of odors • Recognizes onset, persistence, severity, frequency, and variation of symptoms of nausea • Uses preventive measures • Uses warning signs to ask for symptom relief • Reports controlling symptoms • Only mild decrease in food and fluid intake • Only mild intolerance of movement	• Perform complete assessment including frequency, duration, severity, and precipitating factors • Observe for nonverbal cues of discomfort • Evaluate past experiences with nausea • Identify strategies that have been successful in relieving nausea • Encourage frequent oral hygiene unless it stimulates nausea • Give cold, clear, odorless foods, as appropriate • Encourage to eat only small amounts of high-carbohydrate and low-fat foods • Control odors and unpleasant visual stimuli in the room • Administer antiemetic medications
Constipation r/t decreased activity, decreased food or fluid intake, decreased peristalsis secondary to anesthesia, pain medication	*NOC outcomes:* Bowel Elimination *NOC goals:* • Elimination pattern normal for patient • Reports ease of stool passage • Ingests adequate fluids • Ingests adequate fiber • Exercises adequate amount • Bloating not present • Bowel sounds present • Passes soft, formed stool in amount appropriate for diet • No pain with passage of stool	*NIC interventions:* Bowel Management Constipation/Impaction Management *Nursing activities:* • Monitor for signs and symptoms of constipation • Note date of last bowel movement • Monitor bowel sounds • Monitor frequency, consistency, shape volume, color of bowel movements • Teach client about specific foods that assist promotion of bowel regularity • Insert rectal suppository, enema, or irrigation, as needed • Evaluate medication profile for GI side effects (e.g., narcotic analgesics) • Give warm liquids after meals • Instruct client in foods high in fiber
Urinary retention r/t anesthesia, preoperative medications (anticholinergics), pain, fear, unfamiliar surroundings, client's position	*NOC outcomes:* Urinary Elimination *NOC goals:* • Empties bladder completely (bladder not palpable; reports subjective feeling of empty bladder) • 24-hour intake and output balanced • Adequate fluid intake • Urine passes without hesitancy	*NIC interventions:* Urinary Retention Care Urinary Catheterization *Nursing activities:* • Perform comprehensive urinary assessment (fluid intake, urinary output, voiding pattern, cognitive function, pre-existing urinary problems) • Provide privacy for elimination • Use power of suggestion (run water, flush toilet) • Provide ample time (at least 10 minutes) for client to empty bladder • Use spirits of wintergreen in bedpan or urinal • Insert urinary catheter as appropriate • Use percussion and palpation to estimate degree of bladder distention • Catheterize for post-voiding residual as appropriate

➤

Selected Standardized Nursing Diagnoses, Outcomes, and Interventions for Postoperative Patients *(continued)*

Nursing Diagnoses	Outcomes and Goals	Nursing Interventions and Activities
Delayed Surgical Recovery (etiologies will vary with pathology)	*NOC outcomes:* Wound Healing: Primary Intention Ambulation Blood Loss Severity Endurance Hydration Infection Severity Nausea & Vomiting Severity Pain Level	*NIC interventions:* Incision Site Care Nutrition Management Pain Management Self-Care Assistance

NOC goals:
- Ready for discharge within prescribed length of stay for surgery performed
- No postoperative complications (e.g., bleeding, infection, delayed wound healing, pneumonia, nausea and vomiting)

Nursing activities:
- Monitor for postoperative complications
- Monitor the healing process in the incision site
- Provide incision care as needed
- Teach patient and family how to care for the incision
- Encourage increased intake of protein, iron, and vitamin C, as appropriate
- Determine, in collaboration with dietician as appropriate, number of calories and type of nutrients needed to meet nutrition requirements
- Select and implement a variety of measures (e.g., pharmacological, nonpharmacological, interpersonal) to facilitate pain relief, as appropriate
- Teach principles of pain management
- Encourage independence, but intervene when patient is unable to perform

Sources: Dochterman, J. M., & Bulechek, G. M. (Eds.). (2004). *Nursing interventions classification (NIC)* (4th ed.). St Louis: Mosby; Moorhead, S., Johnson, M., & Maas, M. (Eds.). (2004). *Nursing outcomes classification (NOC)* (3rd ed.). St Louis: Mosby; NANDA International. (2005). *Nursing diagnoses: Definitions and Classification 2005–2006.* Philadelphia: Author.

What Are the Main Points in This Chapter?

- Perioperative nursing includes care of patients during the preoperative, intraoperative, and postoperative phases.

- Perioperative nursing requires the systematic integration and synthesis of the nursing process with established standards of practice.

- The Association of periOperative Registered Nurses (the AORN) is one of the most highly organized and powerful specialty organizations within the profession of nursing. It is the organization that developed the standards of care that inform perioperative nursing and the standardized language, the Perioperative Nursing Data Set (PNDS).

- Surgeries are commonly categorized according to body system, purpose, degree of urgency, and degree of risk.

- Surgical risk is associated with the type of surgery and the condition of the patient (e.g., age, general health, personal habits).

- During the preoperative period, it is essential to determine whether the client is physiologically, cognitively and psychologically prepared for the intraoperative and postoperative phases of surgery.

- Preoperative care includes assessment, preoperative teaching, confirming that surgical consent has been obtained, and preparing the patient physically for surgery.

- The surgical consent form is a witnessed legal document that ensures that the surgical client has given informed consent for the surgical procedure. The physician is legally responsible for obtaining informed consent; however, the nurse sometimes obtains the patient's signature on the form after verifying that the patient has been informed.

- A great deal of perioperative nursing care is standardized, aimed at preventing potential complications and applicable to all patients having surgery.

- During an operative procedure, there are specific personnel who work within the sterile field and those who work outside the sterile field.

- General anesthesia produces rapid unconsciousness and loss of sensation. Regional anesthesia produces loss of pain sensation without loss of consciousness.

- Intraoperative care includes skin preparation, positioning the patient for surgery, and protective measures to ensure patient safety during surgery.

- The PACU RN integrates knowledge of common complications of surgery, well-established nursing diagnoses for the postoperative client, and data from an individualized comprehensive postoperative assessment to plan and implement appropriate outcomes and interventions for the client during the postoperative stage.

- Assessments during postoperative recovery are the same as those performed in the PACU, but they can be performed less frequently.

- Sequential compression devices may be used to help prevent thrombophlebitis.

- Incentive spirometry may be used to help prevent atelectasis and pneumonia.

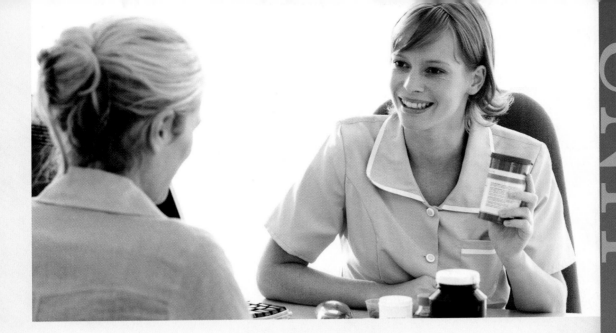

Nursing Functions

38 LEADING & MANAGING

39 NURSING INFORMATICS

40 HOLISTIC HEALING

41 PROMOTING HEALTH

38 CHAPTER

Leading
& Managing

Overview

Leadership is the ability to influence other people. Effective managers possess leadership skills, clinical expertise, and business sense. Although most nurses do not serve in management positions, all nurses must develop management and leadership skills as self-directed, empowered, active participants who work on behalf of quality patient care. Empowerment is the feeling of self-determination, competence, and recognition that your expertise and power within the healthcare system has meaning and positive impact.

Every nurse must develop effective time management skills. Time management includes goal setting and organizing and streamlining your work. In addition, each nurse must understand how to delegate patient care tasks safely and correctly to other healthcare workers. Nurses who work in management positions must also facilitate conflict resolution and, if necessary, function as informal negotiators.

Thinking Critically About Leading and Managing

The exercises in the following section allow you to practice the kind of thinking you will use as a full-spectrum nurse. Because these are critical-thinking activities, there is usually no single right answer. Discuss answers with your peers—discussion can stimulate critical thinking. If you have difficulty with any of the questions, consult with your instructor.

Caring for the Garcias

Katherine Garcia, Joe's mother, is scheduled for outpatient cataract surgery later this week at the local hospital. Joe reports to the clinic wishing to discuss the plan for his mother's surgery "with whoever is the boss." Joe is concerned that his mother will not be staying at the hospital. "She's having surgery. I don't understand this! She's 76 years old. She's going to need help. This doesn't make sense. You have to change things. It won't be safe to do this as planned."

Joe tells you he has discussed his concerns with the ophthalmologist. He tells you that the ophthalmologist told him he was "overreacting. We always do it this way. You just don't understand."

Joe is visibly upset. He believes that his mother is receiving inadequate care. He appeals to you to help him take care of his mother. "This is where Mother gets her care. You know her. You have to change this."

Katherine has been seen at the family clinic several times over the last few years. She takes a medication for osteoporosis and has been counseled about the need for exercise and weight loss. She has also begun to experience problems with "accidents," that is, urine leakage. She has never had surgery in the past, and her only hospitalizations have been for childbirth. Katherine's husband recently passed away, and she has been living alone since then.

A. Devise a plan to resolve this conflict with Joe.

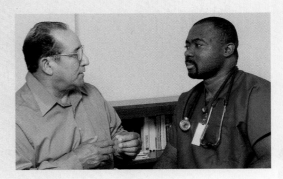

1 Identify a personal or professional change that you would like to see take place, and outline the steps needed to implement the change.

2 Eleanor, an LPN returning to school to obtain her associate's degree in nursing, is faced with a multitude of responsibilities. A wife, a mother of two toddlers, and a full-time staff member at a local hospital, Eleanor suddenly finds herself in a situation in which there just are not enough hours in a day. She is convinced that becoming a registered nurse is an impossible goal. You are Eleanor's mentor. When you ask where she wants to be in 5 years, she answers, "At this moment, I think, on an island in Tahiti!"

a Help Eleanor develop a personal time inventory. To help her determine specifically what to include, make your own personal time inventory to share with her as an example.

b Once Eleanor has finished her time plan, how would you tell her to use it to make better use of her time? Make specific suggestions.

3 What strategies could you use to better manage your time?

4 Why is it important to learn good time management habits while you are a student?

5 This is your first semester in the nursing program. Although you have attended college to complete the prerequisite courses, this seems to be so different. All of a sudden, you have to attend clinical rotations in addition to classes. And you have to prepare ahead of time for the clinical experience, often even going to the hospital the night before to obtain information related to your patients. You feel like you are drowning! What can you do?

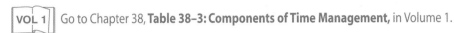 Go to Chapter 38, **Table 38–3: Components of Time Management,** in Volume 1.

Work through the table, asking yourself questions such as the following. Be very specific in your answers; give examples.

a *Prioritizing*

- What tasks do you have to complete on a daily basis? Weekly? During the semester?

- List the tasks in order of importance.

- Which of the tasks do you have control over (e.g., scheduling a haircut or setting aside time to read the next assignment versus taking a test that is scheduled).

b *Assigning priorities:* Assign priorities to the tasks you have identified.

c *Questioning effectiveness, efficiency:* Ask yourself, "How can I accomplish these tasks in the least amount of time but to the best of my ability?"

d *Rechecking:* Review your plan. Mentally and physically recheck the plan. Revise the plan as needed.

e *Self-reliance:* Carry out your plan. Use critical-thinking skills, and adapt the plan as needed so that you "go with the flow."

thinking critically about leading & managing

f   *Treating:* Be good to yourself, but commit yourself to time management and excellence. How can you do that? What treats will you give yourself?

6   For each of the following concepts, use critical thinking to describe how or why it is important to nursing, patient care, or managing or leading. Note that these are *not* to be merely definitions.

Leadership skills

Management skills

Becoming a mentor

Being a mentee

Time management

Resolving conflicts

Delegating appropriately

Understanding the change process

What Are the Main Points in This Chapter?

- Leadership is the ability to influence other people.
- You probably already have many leadership qualities that you can begin demonstrating immediately.
- You will need to begin developing effective management skills while you are in nursing school.
- Effective managers possess a combination of qualities: leadership skills, clinical expertise, and business sense.
- It is never too early in your career to develop a SWOT analysis. Throughout your nursing program, revisit the analysis, and update it as you gain new knowledge and skills.
- Be mindful of nurses who demonstrate strong mentor qualities. Do not be afraid to ask for their support and guidance. Develop mentor qualities of your own, so you can also mentor a new student.
- At times throughout our nursing careers, we will all assume the role of follower.
- Followers need to be self-directing, actively participating experts who work on behalf of the organization.
- Nurses have expertise power and authority over other healthcare workers. It is important that you understand your sources of power and use them wisely.
- Nurses need and want to feel empowered. The nursing shortage has caused healthcare agencies to find methods of empowering nurses.
- Delegation of patient care tasks to other healthcare workers is one of the most important responsibilities of the registered nurse.
- Nurses must understand change and act as change agents within today's healthcare setting.
- Managing change involves recognizing and decreasing resistance.
- Conflict is inevitable, but it does not need to be destructive.
- One of a manager's responsibilities is to facilitate conflict resolution and, if necessary, function as an informal negotiator.
- Effective time management is essential to planning safe, effective patient care and demonstrating management skills.
- Time management includes goal setting and organizing and streamlining your work.

Knowledge Map

Leading and Managing

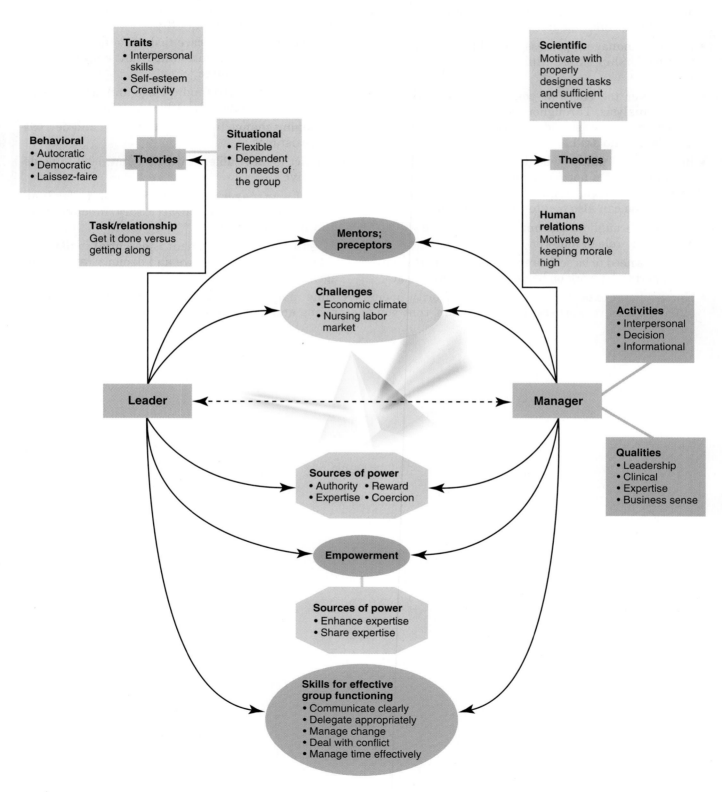

Traits
• Interpersonal skills
• Self-esteem
• Creativity

Behavioral
• Autocratic
• Democratic
• Laissez-faire

Theories

Situational
• Flexible
• Dependent on needs of the group

Task/relationship
Get it done versus getting along

Scientific
Motivate with properly designed tasks and sufficient incentive

Theories

Human relations
Motivate by keeping morale high

Mentors; preceptors

Challenges
• Economic climate
• Nursing labor market

Leader

Manager

Activities
• Interpersonal
• Decision
• Informational

Qualities
• Leadership
• Clinical
• Expertise
• Business sense

Sources of power
• Authority • Reward
• Expertise • Coercion

Empowerment

Sources of power
• Enhance expertise
• Share expertise

Skills for effective group functioning
• Communicate clearly
• Delegate appropriately
• Manage change
• Deal with conflict
• Manage time effectively

Nursing Informatics

Overview

Nurses use vast amounts of data, information, and knowledge daily. Informatics is the processing and management of data, information, and knowledge necessary for making practice decisions.

Electronic health records (EHR) enable an organization to increase productivity and efficiency and facilitate research on which evidence-based practice is founded. Passwords should be used and protected to ensure the privacy of patient records.

Information taken from the Web should be evaluated carefully. CINAHL and MEDLINE are two reliable databases for searching for nursing literature.

Thinking Critically About Nursing Informatics

The exercises in the following section allow you to practice the kind of thinking you will use as a full-spectrum nurse. Because these are critical-thinking activities, there is usually no single right answer. Discuss answers with your peers—discussion can stimulate critical thinking. If you have difficulty with any of the questions, consult with your instructor.

Caring for the Garcias

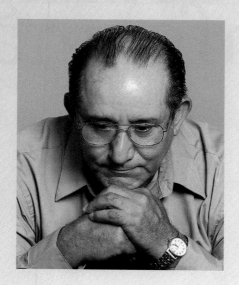

Joe Garcia, a patient you have been caring for at the Family Medicine Center, has been devastated by his recent diagnoses of type II diabetes mellitus and hypertension. "Oh my, this is bad. This stuff kills you. I don't understand what I did to cause this?" he sighs. He is having difficulty following his medication regimen and says he just doesn't understand what he is supposed to do. You have supplied him with information at each of his clinic visits as well as handouts, medication information, and a reminder sheet for his medicines. Joe asks you if there is any information available on the Internet.

A. What advice would you give him about looking up medical information on the Internet?

B. What sources would you recommend to Joe?

1 Refer to the following table. For each of the uses listed, what kind of information do you think the database should provide? That is, what kind of data would you need? For example, look at the first item under "In Nursing Practice" in column 1. For "Literature access and retrieval," you would use a database that contains information about journals, books, reports, and their content, perhaps CINAHL.

Work with your classmates. Share your knowledge and experience to answer these questions. Consult your instructor as needed.

For all of the following, what kind of database would you use? What kind of information would you need?

Use	Type of Information Needed
In Nursing Practice	
Literature access and retrieval (e.g., for evidence-based practice)	*Suggested answer:* CINAHL; information about books, journals, and their content; possibly, the Web
Care planning	*Clues:* What information would you need for care planning? Where would you find it?
Client records (e.g., documenting, order entry, retrieving lab results)	
Telenursing (e.g., in home health)	
Case management	

➤

Use	Type of Information Needed
In Nursing Education	
Literature access and retrieval	
Computer-assisted instruction (CAI) programs	
Classroom technology	
Distance learning	
Testing and grading	
Student records	

Use	Type of Information Needed
In Nursing Administration	
Quality assurance and utilization review	*Clues:* What information would you need to evaluate the quality of care in your institution? Where would you find it?
Employee records (e.g., to track licenses, immunizations)	
Staffing patterns, hiring	
Buildings and facilities management	
Finance and budgets	
Accreditation reviews (e.g., monitoring quality control)	

thinking critically about nursing informatics

Use	Type of Information Needed
In Nursing Research	
Literature review	
Data collection	
Data analysis (both qualitative and quantitative)	
Research dissemination	
Applying for grants	

2 Search for "online nursing journals" on the Web. Make a list of nursing journals that provide full-text articles that are available on the Web, and at no charge. Hint:

 Go to Chapter 39, **Resources for Caregivers and Health Professionals,** on the Electronic Study Guide.

3 For each of the following concepts, use critical thinking to describe how or why it is important to nursing, patients, or nursing informatics. Note that these are *not* to be merely definitions.

Nursing informatics

Data

Knowledge

Wisdom

Evidence-based practice

Computers

Hardware

thinking critically about nursing informatics

Storage media

Connectivity

Listservs

Telehealth

Electronic health records

Standardized nursing language

Literature databases

The World Wide Web

Evaluating web sites

Practical Knowledge
knowing how

STANDARDIZED LANGUAGE

American Nurses Association Recognized Languages for Nursing

Language	Description	Recognition Date
NANDA International	Language includes more than 170 diagnostic labels with etiologies, risk factors, and defining characteristics.	1992
Nursing Interventions Classification (NIC)	The fourth edition contains 486 direct and indirect interventions assigned to one of seven domains and 30 classes. Each intervention includes a concept label, definition, and activities.	1992
Clinical Care Classification (CCC)	Developed by Virginia Saba, this language is used primarily by home health agencies and community settings. This language contains 182 nursing diagnoses and 198 interventions developed to code, index, classify, document, track, and analyze clinical care processes.	1992
Omaha System	This language also documents care in community and home care agencies. This system consists of 42 nursing diagnoses, nursing interventions, and a problem-rating scale for outcomes.	1992
Nursing Outcomes Classification (NOC)	The third edition of NOC consists of 260 outcomes, including seven family unit and six community level outcomes. The NOC is a comprehensive standardized language designed to help clinicians evaluate the effectiveness of nursing interventions.	1997
Nursing Management Minimum Data Set (NMMDS)	This data set describes health care and nursing environment associated with the diagnosis, intervention, and outcome segments from the administrative, management, and resource management perspectives. It is composed of 17 data elements in three categories: environment, nurse resources, and financial recources.	1998
Patient Care Data Set (PCDS)	Judy Ozbolt developed this language, which is composed of a data dictionary, 363 nursing diagnoses, 1357 patient care actions, and 311 patient care goals. The PCDS was developed for multidisciplinary use.	1998
Perioperative Nursing Data Set (PNDS)	The PNDS language describes perioperative nursing practice and consists of 64 nursing diagnoses, 127 nursing interventions, and 29 patient outcomes. This was the first nursing language developed by a nursing specialty.	1999
Statistical Nomenclature of Medicine Reference Terminology (SNOMED RT)	SNOMED RT is a reference terminology that includes clinical concepts used to describe assessment, diagnosis, intervention, and outcome. Although it includes nursing concepts, it is not developed specifically for nursing, but rather for a broad spectrum of healthcare domains.	1999
Nursing Minimum Data Sets (NMDS)	This data collection establishes comparability of nursing data across populations settings, geographic areas, and times. It describes the nursing care of patients or clients and their families in a variety of settings, both institutional and noninstitutional.	1999
International Classification for Nursing Practice (ICNP)	ICNP describes nursing practice in various clinical settings worldwide using common language. It includes nursing phenomena, outcomes, and actions.	2000

➤

American Nurses Association Recognized Languages for Nursing *(continued)*

Language	Description	Recognition Date
ABCcodes	ABCcodes fit into existing data fields on insurance claim forms and in healthcare information systems. The design of ABCcodes supports over 11 million code combinations to describe current and emerging alternative medicine, nursing, and other integrative healthcare practices. Approximately 4200 codes have been assigned to date.	2000
Logical Observation Identifiers Names and Codes (LOINC®)	This is universal terminology for identifying laboratory results (e.g., hemoglobin) and other clinical observations (e.g., vital signs).	2002

What Are the Main Points in This Chapter?

- Whatever their roles—staff nurse, administrator, educator, researcher, primary care provider—nurses use vast amounts of data, information, and knowledge in their daily work.
- Informatics is the processing and management of data, information, and knowledge necessary for making practice decisions.
- A computer has four main functions: input, processing, output, and storage.
- Connectivity is a term referring to the ways in which computers and other hardware communicate and share information.
- Some forms of electronic communication include telephone, videoconferencing, fax, e-mail, Listservs, and telehealth applications.
- Electronic health records (EHR) enable an organization to replace its paper charts with electronic records, thereby increasing productivity and efficiency and facilitating research to improve health care.
- Standardized nursing languages facilitate the inclusion of nursing in the EHR and make visible nursing contributions to health care.
- It is important to use and protect passwords to protect the privacy of patient records.
- Evidence-based practice requires the ability to manage and process a great deal of information to identify a clinical problem, search the literature, evaluate the evidence, and decide on an intervention.
- Information taken from the Web should be evaluated carefully; do not believe everything you see on the Web.
- CINAHL and MEDLINE are two important databases to search for nursing literature.

Knowledge Map

Nursing Informatics

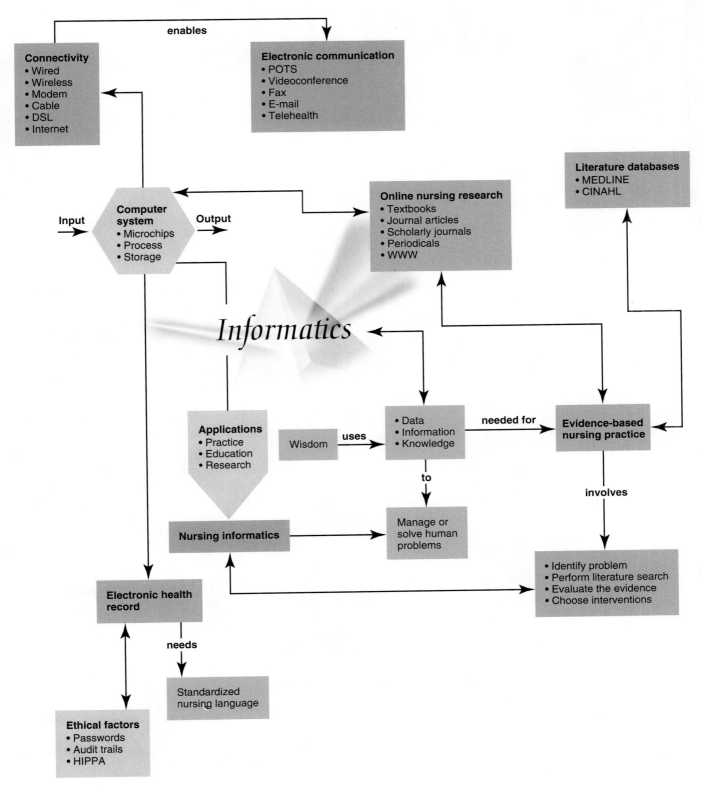

40 Holistic Healing

Overview

Complementary and alternative modalities (CAM) are used in conjunction with or instead of traditional medical care. Many of these modalities predate the traditional Western health system. They include ayurveda, traditional Chinese medicine, acupuncture, homeopathy, and naturopathy. Integrative health care refers to coordinated care that encompasses all treatments and health practices used by a patient. Typically, this care includes traditional and CAM therapies. Women, people with higher educational levels, and people who have been hospitalized in the past year are more likely to use CAM.

CAM therapies can be categorized as mind-body interventions, biologically based therapies, manipulative and body-based therapies, and energy therapies.

- Mind-body interventions enhance health by targeting the mood and reaction to stress. They include prayer, meditation, imagery, humor, yoga, hypnosis, and biofeedback.
- Biologically based therapies include food, herbs, vitamins, and aromatherapy. These therapies are readily available and are often practiced in conjunction with traditional health care and other CAM.
- Manipulative and body-based therapies focus on moving the body to improve health. They include chiropractic, massage, and osteopathy.
- Energy therapies manipulate the energy fields that surround the body. They are among the most widely used forms of CAM. They include therapeutic touch, t'ai chi and Qigong, Reiki, and magnet therapy.

You should assess patients' use of CAM and integrate CAM into your nursing care as appropriate. In addition, you should facilitate communication about CAM between patients and their physicians and use self-care practices to promote your own health and wholeness.

Thinking Critically About Holistic Healing

The exercises in the following section allow you to practice the kind of thinking you will use as a full-spectrum nurse. Because these are critical-thinking activities, there is usually no single right answer. Discuss answers with your peers—discussion can stimulate critical thinking. If you have difficulty with any of the questions, consult with your instructor.

Caring for the Garcias

Several months ago Flordelisa Garcia had a complete physical examination with Jordan Miller, FNP. Flordelisa has been experiencing irregular menses, poor sleep, and hot flashes. Jordan explained that these were common complaints associated with menopause. Flordelisa has chosen to avoid hormone replacement therapy because of all the controversy surrounding its use. Instead she has been experimenting with CAM therapies. Friends have suggested she try wild yam cream and a diet high in soy protein.

A. To know how to advise Flordelisa, what theoretical knowledge do you need?

B. Search the Internet and other CAM resources for information on these treatment modalities. What advice would you offer her about these modalities?

C. Flordelisa is also interested in CAM therapies for her husband, Joe. Several varieties of therapies and supplements are marketed for patients with hypertension and diabetes. Outline the approach you might take when working with Joe and Flordelisa to integrate their interest in CAM therapies with their conventional health care.

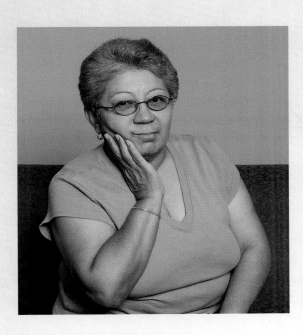

1 Recent health survey research indicates that U.S. healthcare consumers are increasing their use of complementary and alternative modalities (CAM). Consumers often do not inform their primary care providers of such use. Use these findings to identify six implications for nursing practice.

2 As a nurse on a surgical day care unit, you notice how anxious patients are while they await surgery. Describe a simple relaxation technique that you could teach the patients.

3 Describe a simple imagery technique that could be used with all preoperative patients.

4 Patients who use alternative therapies may not disclose their use to conventional practitioners. Create three interview questions that would elicit this information.

5 How can you support a patient's placebo response to enhance healing?

6 What preliminary assessments and interventions should the nurse conduct prior to using aromatherapy with patients in a healthcare setting?

7 A UAP, Maggie, has been helping Janelle Hunt get settled into her room at a long-term care facility. Ms Hunt is very old and too frail to live alone, but she is mentally alert and competent. She says to Maggie, "I have brought my magnet mattress pad with me, and my special pillow. I have bad arthritis, and I have to have those on my bed." The UAP comes to you, visibly annoyed. "That new patient wants me to put her own special mattress on the bed. Now I ask you, what good would that thing do? It will be a pain to change the sheets with that thing on there, not to speak of what happens if she is incontinent on it. Do I really have to do that?" How would you respond to Maggie?

8 For each of the following concepts, use critical thinking to describe how or why it is important to nursing, patient care, or holistic healing. Note that these are *not* to be merely definitions.

Holistic care

Integrative care

Alternative treatment modality

Complementary treatment modality

American Holistic Nurses Association

Practical Knowledge
knowing how

There are three very practical applications of CAM you can use in your practice:

1. You can, and should, facilitate communication about CAM between your patients and their healthcare providers.
2. You can use self-care practices to promote your own health and wholeness.
3. You can, with minimal training, use some of the less complex CAM therapies as independent nursing interventions.

TECHNIQUES

In this section you will find techniques and guidelines for performing some of the less complex CAM therapies. All are NIC standardized interventions (Dochterman & Bulechek, 2004). You can learn to use most of the therapies by doing a little extra reading. For others, such as therapeutic touch, you should probably attend a workshop or find a mentor who will guide you in their use. None of the therapies included here requires credentialing or extensive training.

TECHNIQUE 40–1 **Performing Autogenic Training**

Autogenic Training is assisting with self-suggestions about feelings of heaviness and warmth for the purpose of inducing relaxation (Dochterman & Buleckek, 2004, p. 181). This is one of the many ways to induce relaxation. Follow these steps:

1. Seat the patient in a recumbent position.
2. Place a prepared script to the patient, pausing to give the patient enough time to repeat the script internally.

3. Use statements that elicit feelings of heaviness, lightness, or floating of specific body parts.
4. Instruct the patient to repeat the statements to himself to elicit the feeling within the body part (e.g., say to the patient, "Repeat 'My arm is getting heavy,' while you feel your arm growing heavy.")
5. Rehearse with the script for 15 to 20 minutes.
6. After mastering heaviness sensations, proceed to elicit feelings of warmth.

TECHNIQUE 40–2 **Using Calming Technique**

Calming Technique is "reducing anxiety in a patient experiencing acute distress" (Dochterman & Bulechek, 2004, p. 221). You do not need special preparation for this intervention; you are probably already doing it to some extent. The following are examples of nursing activities involved:

1. Maintain eye contact.
2. Maintain a calm, deliberate manner.
3. Sit and talk with the patient.
4. Encourage slow, purposeful deep breathing.

5. Reassure the patient of her personal safety or security.
6. Reduce or eliminate stimuli that create fear or anxiety.
7. Use distraction as appropriate.
8. Offer a back rub, as appropriate.
9. Offer a warm bath or shower.
10. Offer warm fluids or milk.
11. Hold and comfort an infant or child.
12. Speak softly or sing to an infant or child.
13. Give a pacifier to an infant.

TECHNIQUE 40–3   Using Humor

Humor is helping "the patient to perceive, appreciate, and express what is funny, amusing, or ludicrous in order to establish relationships, relieve tension, release anger, facilitate learning, or cope with painful feelings" (Dochterman & Bulechek, 2004, p. 422). Some healthcare agencies have created "humor rooms" for patients and staff, supplied with humorous books, videotapes, cartoons, and so on. When using humor, you need to be aware of your feelings and those of others and aware of cultural differences in what people see as funny.

1. Determine the types of humor that the patient appreciates.
2. Discuss with the patient advantages of laughter.
3. Avoid content areas about which the patient is sensitive.
4. Make available a selection of humorous games, cartoons, jokes, videos, tapes, books, and so on.
5. Point out humorous incongruity in a situation.
6. Encourage visualization with humor (e.g., picture a forbidding authority figure dressed only in underwear).
7. Encourage silliness and playfulness.
8. Avoid using humor with patients who are cognitively impaired.
9. Respond positively to humor attempts that the patient makes.
10. Monitor patient response, and discontinue the humor strategy if it is ineffective.

TECHNIQUE 40–4   Facilitating Meditation

Meditation Facilitation consists of "facilitating a person to alter his/her level of awareness by focusing specifically on an image or thought" (Dochterman & Bulechek, 2004, p. 498). You will need some theoretical knowledge about meditation, but it is a simple, noninvasive technique that you can use at the bedside.

1. Prepare a quiet environment.
2. Instruct the patient to sit quietly and comfortably.
3. Instruct the patient to close his eyes, if he desires, and to relax all muscles and remain relaxed.
4. Help the patient to select a mental device to repeat during the procedure (e.g., repeating a word, such as "one").
5. Instruct the person to inhale, then say the word silently while breathing out through the nose.
6. Continue with the exercise, focusing on the mental device chosen, for as long as needed.
7. When finished, instruct the patient to sit quietly for several minutes with his eyes open.
8. Have the patient perform the procedure once or twice daily, but not within 2 hours after meals.

TECHNIQUE 40–5 | Performing Simple Guided Imagery

Simple Guided Imagery is "purposeful use of imagination to achieve relaxation and/or direct attention away from undesirable sensations" (Dochterman & Bulechek, 2004, p. 649). This technique is useful for mild to moderate pain and anxiety. You do not need extensive training to use it. Commercial audiotapes are available to guide imagery, or you may guide the patient.

1. Have the patient assume a comfortable position, with eyes closed.
2. Arrange a quiet environment at a time when you will not be interrupted.
3. Have the patient describe an image he has experienced as pleasurable and relaxing, such as lying on a beach, watching a snowfall, floating on a raft, or watching the sun set.
4. Choose a scene that involves as many of the five senses as possible.
5. Use techniques (e.g., rhythmic breathing) to induce relaxation.
6. Using permissive directions, such as "perhaps," and "if you wish," or "you might like," have the patient travel mentally to the scene and help him to describe the setting in detail.
7. Have the patient slowly experience the scene: How does it look, smell, sound, feel, taste?
8. Use words that convey pleasurable images (e.g., floating, melting, releasing).
9. Develop a cleansing or clearing portion of imagery (e.g., "all pain appears as red dust and washes downstream in a creek as you enter").
10. Assist the patient to develop a method of ending the imagery, such as counting slowly while breathing deeply and thinking about being relaxed, refreshed, and alert.
11. Encourage the patient to express his thoughts and feelings after the experience.
12. Prepare the patient for unexpected (but often therapeutic) experiences, such as crying.
13. Follow up to assess the effects of imagery and any resulting changes in sensation and perception.

TECHNIQUE 40–6 | Performing Simple Massage

Simple Massage is "stimulation of the skin and underlying tissues with varying degrees of hand pressure to decrease pain, produce relaxation, and/or improve circulation" (Dochterman & Bulechek, 2004, p. 651). Unlike special massage techniques, simple massage does not require advanced training.

1. Determine the patient's degree of psychological comfort with touch.
2. Screen for contraindications (e.g., poor skin integrity, deep-vein thrombosis).
3. Prepare a warm, comfortable, quiet environment.
4. Apply moist heat before or during massage as indicated.
5. Drape to expose only the area to be massaged.
6. Use warm lotion, oil, or dry powder to reduce friction. Place no oils or lotion on the head or scalp.
7. Massage the hands or feet if other areas are inconvenient or uncomfortable for the patient.
8. Adapt the massage area, technique, and pressure to the patient's comfort and the purpose of the massage.
9. Encourage the patient to breathe deeply, relax, and concentrate on the good feelings of the massage.
10. Avoid lengthy conversation during the massage, unless you use it as a distraction technique.
11. Do not massage over open lesions or tender skin areas.
12. When the message is completed, instruct the patient to rest until he is ready and then to move slowly.

TECHNIQUE 40–7　Performing Simple Relaxation Therapy

Simple Relaxation Therapy is "use of techniques to encourage and elicit relaxation for the purpose of decreasing undesirable signs and symptoms such as pain, muscle tension, or anxiety" (Dochterman & Bulechek, 2004, p. 652). This technique does not require advanced training, but you will need to know various ways to induce relaxation (e.g., music therapy, meditation, and progressive muscle relaxation).

1. Explain to the patient the benefits of relaxation and the various types you can offer.
2. Provide a detailed description of the chosen relaxation intervention.
3. Instruct the patient to assume a comfortable position, with eyes closed.
4. Elicit behaviors that are conditioned to produce relaxation, such as deep breathing, yawning, abdominal breathing, or peaceful imaging.
5. Instruct the patient to relax and let the sensations happen.
6. Use low tone of voice and slow, rhythmical pace of words.

7. Demonstrate and practice the relaxation technique with the patient.
8. Encourage return demonstrations, if possible.
9. Encourage frequent repetition or practice of technique(s) selected.

The following is an example of a relaxation technique you could use at steps 2 and 7.

- Have the patient close her eyes and observe the breathing pattern at her nostrils, where air enters and leaves the body.
- Direct the patient to observe the sensation of the breath at the nostril, consistently staying with this focus point. Tell her that when a thought or feeling arises, she should simply return to breathing awareness.
- You can, at first, guide her breathing by saying, "Breathe in. Breathe out. Focus on the breath at your nostrils." Periodically say, "Focus on your breath at the end of your nose."

TECHNIQUE 40–8　Performing Therapeutic Touch

Therapeutic Touch (Dochterman & Bulechek, 2004, p. 734) requires special training and practice (usually a one- or two-day workshop). If you have had some instruction and someone has demonstrated the technique to you, you may be able to use this intervention effectively. The following NIC activities summarize it.

1. Center yourself.

 Go to Chapter 40, **Box 40–2: Therapeutic Touch,** in Volume 1.

2. Focus on the intention to facilitate wholeness and healing at all levels of consciousness.
3. Place your hands 2.5 to 5 cm (1 to 2 inches) from the patient's body.
4. Begin the assessment of the energy field by moving your hands slowly and steadily over as much of the patient's body as possible, from head to toe and front to back.

5. Note the overall pattern of energy flow, especially any areas of disturbance, such as congestion or unevenness, which you may feel through very subtle cues in your hands. For example, some practitioners feel temperature change or tingling.
6. Focus intention on facilitating symmetry and healing in disturbed areas.
7. Get the energy flowing. Begin by moving the hands in very gentle downward movements through the patient's energy field, thinking of the patient as a unitary whole and facilitating an open and balanced energy flow.
8. Continue the treatment by very gently facilitating the flow of healing energy into areas of disturbance.
9. Finish when you judge that the appropriate amount of change has taken place (i.e., for an infant, 1 to 2 minutes; for an adult, 5 to 7 minutes), keeping in mind the importance of gentleness.

What Are the Main Points in This Chapter?

- Holistic health care is founded on the belief that each person is a whole in constant interaction with the environment. There is no separation between body, mind, or spirit.
- The conventional medical approach is often referred to as *allopathy,* a term used to denote medical practice that is focused on counteracting symptoms.
- A complementary modality is one that is used in conjunction with traditional medical care.
- An alternative modality is one that is used instead of traditional medical care.
- Integrative health care refers to coordinated care that encompasses all treatments and health practices used by a patient.
- In holistic care, treatment outcomes are enhanced if both the practitioner and the patient believe that the treatment will be effective.
- Holism contends that all healing is self-healing.
- Absence of spirituality creates a sense of disconnection from one's true source, a loss of meaning to one's life, and a state of dis-ease.
- Women, people with higher educational levels, and people who have been hospitalized in the past year are more likely to use complementary and alternative modalities (CAM).
- Alternative medical systems predate the traditional Western health system. They include ayurveda, traditional Chinese medicine, acupuncture, homeopathy, and naturopathy.
- Mind-body interventions target the mood and reaction to stress to enhance health. They include prayer, meditation, imagery, humor, yoga, hypnosis, and biofeedback.
- Biologically based therapies include food, herbs, vitamins, and aromatherapy. These therapies are readily available and are often practiced in conjunction with traditional health care and other CAM.
- Manipulative and body-based therapies focus on moving the body to improve health. They include chiropractic, massage, and osteopathy.
- Energy therapies manipulate the energy fields that surround the body. They are among the most widely used forms of CAM. They include therapeutic touch, t'ai chi and Qigong, Reiki, and magnet therapy.
- Holistic nursing practice is a theory-based, relationship-centered, potent solution to a number of problems facing contemporary nursing and health care.
- You should facilitate communication about CAM between patients and their physicians.
- As a holistic healer, you should use self-care practices to promote your own health and wholeness.
- You should assess patients' use of CAM and integrate CAM into your nursing care as appropriate.

Knowledge Map

Holistic Health Care

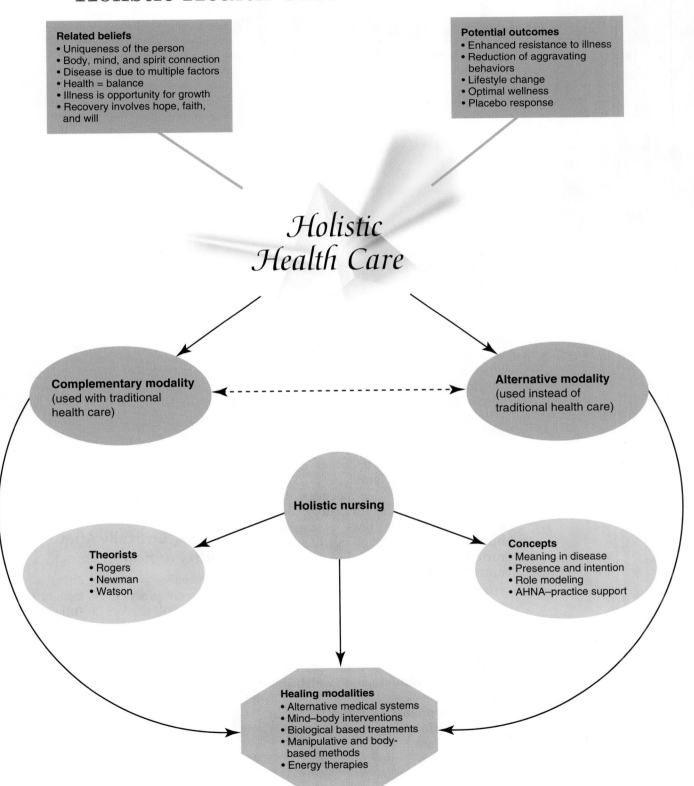

Related beliefs
- Uniqueness of the person
- Body, mind, and spirit connection
- Disease is due to multiple factors
- Health = balance
- Illness is opportunity for growth
- Recovery involves hope, faith, and will

Potential outcomes
- Enhanced resistance to illness
- Reduction of aggravating behaviors
- Lifestyle change
- Optimal wellness
- Placebo response

Holistic Health Care

Complementary modality (used with traditional health care)

Alternative modality (used instead of traditional health care)

Holistic nursing

Theorists
- Rogers
- Newman
- Watson

Concepts
- Meaning in disease
- Presence and intention
- Role modeling
- AHNA–practice support

Healing modalities
- Alternative medical systems
- Mind–body interventions
- Biological based treatments
- Manipulative and body-based methods
- Energy therapies

41 Promoting Health

Overview

Health promotion activities help a person develop a state of physical, spiritual, and mental well-being. Health promotion activities are useful to everyone, whether well or sick, because they encourage optimum function. Health protection activities are motivated by a desire to avoid illness. Both health promotion and health protection involve making changes in individual lifestyle and making choices that affect one's health prospects. However, the motivation that underlies each of these activities is different.

A health promotion assessment involves obtaining a health history, physical examination, fitness assessment, lifestyle and risk appraisal, life stress review, assessment of healthcare beliefs, nutritional assessment, and screening activities. Health screening activities are designed to detect disease at an early stage so that treatment can begin before there is an opportunity for disease to spread or become debilitating. Health screening activities vary based on developmental stage and identified risk factors.

Health promotion activities for all age groups include nutrition, exercise, safety concerns, changing unhealthy lifestyles, immunizations, and screenings. These activities may be conducted in acute care facilities, the workplace, local communities, or schools. There are three levels of activities for health protection: primary, secondary, and tertiary prevention. Primary interventions are designed to prevent or slow the onset of disease. Secondary interventions are designed to detect illnesses in early stages. Tertiary interventions focus on stopping the disease from progressing and on rehabilitation.

Thinking Critically About Health Promotion

The exercises in the following section allow you to practice the kind of thinking you will use as a full-spectrum nurse. Because these are critical-thinking activities, there is usually no single right answer. Discuss answers with your peers—discussion can stimulate critical thinking. If you have difficulty with any of the questions, consult with your instructor.

Caring for the Garcias

Joe and Flordelisa Garcia; their 3-year-old grand-daughter, Bettina; and Katherine, Joe's 76-year old mother, are all patients at the Family Medicine Center. Jordan Miller, the family nurse practitioner at the center, asks you to devise a health promotion program for each member of the family.

A. What information should you gather before you begin?

B. How might you obtain this information?

C. How will each of their plans differ?

D. Review Meet the Garcias on p. 1. Also review the physical exam findings on Joe:

 Go to Chapter 19, **p. 358,** in Volume 1.

What health promotion strategies and health screenings should you recommend to Joe Garcia?

E. How would you begin to organize and priori-tize a health promotion program for Joe?

F. Using therapeutic communication, give exam-ples of appropriate questions to ask Joe about his health beliefs.

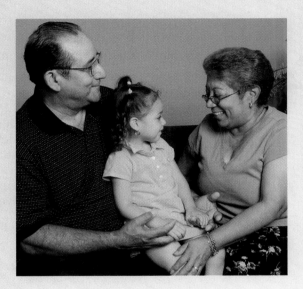

thinking critically about promoting health

1

While working in a physician's office, a 70-year-old woman is referred to you for counseling regarding health promotion activities. She is hypertensive and obese.

a How does her age affect your assessments and communication?

b What types of learning aids might be needed?

c What health screenings are appropriate for this client?

2

Below is a group of clients who wish to enroll in a health-promotion program.

- Jennifer Kaska is 23 years old and was diagnosed with diabetes mellitus at the age of 12 years. She checks her blood sugar and administers insulin as needed. She runs 3 miles, 3 days a week.
- Maurice Rosenthal is 47 years old with no known illness. He is 6 feet tall and weighs 240 pounds. His body mass index (BMI) is 33 kg/m^2, indicating obesity. He takes no routine medication, only acetaminophen for occasional headaches.
- Clara Fenton is 83 years old and has been diagnosed with hypertension, emphysema, and osteoporosis. She takes ten prescription medications daily in addition to a multivitamin and an occasional laxative.

Discuss the pros and cons of providing a group program that includes these three clients.

3 L. F. is a 50-year-old man with heart disease. He had coronary artery bypass surgery 1 month ago. He has stopped going to his prescribed cardiac rehabilitation program because of the distance he must travel to the rehabilitation center. Discuss at least two approaches for working with this client.

4 Cecelia Kent is 32 years old. She takes no medications and has annual physical exams. She walks 4 to 5 miles, 5 days per week, and lifts light weights two to three times per week. She eats a low-fat, low-salt, low-sugar diet. She has never smoked and drinks only limited alcohol.

a She asks you to recommend further health promotion activities. How would you respond?

b How could you incorporate Cecelia into a health promotion class that includes Jennifer Kaska, Maurice Rosenthal, and Clara Fenton (from question 2)?

5 For each of the following concepts, use critical thinking to describe how or why it is important to nursing, patient care, or health promotion. Note that these are *not* to be merely definitions.

Health promotion

Illness prevention

Lifestyle

Hardiness

Health screenings

Health education

ASSESSMENT GUIDELINES AND TOOLS

Health Promotion: Physical Fitness Assessment

Cardiorespiratory Fitness

There are many different modes of testing, such as field tests (walking or running), motor-driven treadmills, stationary bicycles, and step testing.

- *Field tests* for running are good for children. A 9-year-old child should be able to complete a 1-mile run in approximately 10 minutes, and a 17-year-old boy should be able to complete a 1-mile run in approximately $7\frac{1}{2}$ minutes (www.presidentschallenge.org).

- *The step test* is appropriate for most adults. Using a 12-inch bench, instruct the participant to step up and down at a rate of 24 steps per minute for 3 minutes. At the end of 3 minutes, he should check his heart rate. Stop testing immediately if the participant experiences any chest pain, shortness of breath, or lightheadedness. Results depend on age and gender and are available below.

Step Test Evaluation Charts

3-Minute Step Test (Men)

	18–25	26–35	36–45	46–55	56–65	65+
Excellent	<79	<81	<83	<87	<86	<88
Good	79–89	81–89	83–96	87–97	86–97	88–96
Above average	90–99	90–99	97–103	98–105	98–103	97–103
Average	100–105	100–107	104–112	106–116	104–112	104–113
Below average	106–116	108–117	113–119	117–122	113–120	114–120
Poor	117–128	118–128	120–130	123–132	121–129	121–130
Very poor	>128	>128	>130	>132	>129	>130

3-Minute Step Test (Women)

	18–25	26–35	36–45	46–55	56–65	65+
Excellent	<85	<88	<90	<94	<95	<90
Good	85–98	88–99	90–102	94–104	95–104	90–102
Above average	99–108	100–111	103–110	105–115	105–112	103–115
Average	109–117	112–119	111–118	116–120	113–118	116–122
Below average	118–126	120–126	119–128	121–129	119–128	123–128
Poor	127–140	127–138	129–140	130–135	129–139	129–134
Very poor	>140	>138	>140	>135	>139	>134

Muscular Fitness

Muscle strength measures the amount of weight a muscle (or group of muscles) can move at one time. This is recorded as a ratio of weight pushed (or lifted) divided by body weight. For example, a woman weighing 150 pounds who is able to lift 86 pounds will have a ratio of 86 divided by 150, or 0.57.

- Have the participant warm up and stretch prior to the test. Weight benches are ideal sites for testing upper body and leg strength.

- Compare the ratio obtained to normative standards or to previous personal scores to evaluate improvement.

►

Health Promotion: Physical Fitness Assessment *(continued)*

Muscle endurance refers to the ability of a muscle to perform repeated movements. The push-up or curl-up (crunch) test may be performed to evaluate endurance. Ask the participant to perform as many push-ups or curl-ups as possible without pausing. The number of repetitions is the score. Once again, compare scores to norms or previous performance.

Flexibility

Flexibility is the ability to move a joint through its range of motion. *The sit-and-reach test* evaluates low back and hip [trunk] flexion.

- Have the participant sit on a floor mat with legs fully extended and feet flat against a box. Have her extend her arms and hands forward as far as possible and hold for a count of 3.
- Using a ruler, measure the distance in inches that the client can reach beyond the proximal edge of the box. If the client cannot reach the edge, measure the distance of the fingertips from the edge, and report it as a negative number.

Norms for trunk flexion vary among men and women. The desired range for men is +1 to +5 inches, and for women is +2 to +6 inches (Pender, Murdaugh, & Parsons, 2002).

Lifestyle and Risk Assessment

Lifestyle refers to the manner in which a person conducts his life. You can gather this information by interview or by using a variety of questionnaires. A health risk appraisal (HRA) is a questionnaire that evaluates risk for disease based on current demographic data, lifestyle, and health behaviors. The following is an example of an HRA.

Name _____ Age _____ Gender _____

Health View

In general, would you say your present health is?
- ☐ Excellent
- ☐ Very good
- ☐ Good
- ☐ Fair
- ☐ Poor

General Practices

(1) Physical activity. How many days each week do you get at least 30 minutes of physical activity, such as brisk walking, cycling, active gardening, active dance, swimming, jogging, or active sports? _____

(2) Strength exercises. How many days each week do you do strength-building exercises, such as weight lifting or calisthenics? _____

(3) Smoking status. Indicate your present smoking status.
- ☐ Current smoker   ☐ Ex-smoker
- ☐ Nonsmoker, never smoked regularly

Environmental smoke. Do you live with or work with smokers and breathe second-hand smoke regularly?
- ☐ Yes   ☐ No

(4) Alcohol. How many drinks do you typically have on a day you drink? *One drink is a bottle or can of beer (12 oz),*

a glass of wine or wine cooler (3.5 oz), a shot glass of liquor (1.5 oz).
- ☐ Never drink
- ☐ Have no more than one drink in a day
- ☐ Have no more than two drinks in a day
- ☐ Sometimes have 3 or 4 drinks in a day
- ☐ Sometimes have 5 or more drinks in a day

(5) Sleep. How many hours of sleep do you usually get each night? _____

Eating Practices

(6) Breakfast. How many days each week do you usually eat breakfast (more than just coffee and a roll)? _____

(7) Bread/grains. How many servings of whole-grain breads and cereals do you eat daily? *One serving = 1 slice bread, $\frac{1}{2}$ cup dry cereal, $\frac{1}{2}$ cup cooked oatmeal or other whole-grain cereal or brown rice.* _____

(8) Fruits and vegetables. How many servings of fruits and vegetables do you eat daily? *One serving = 1 medium fruit, 6 oz fruit or vegetable juice, 1 cup raw fruit or vegetables, $\frac{1}{2}$ cup cooked fruit or vegetables.* _____

Legumes. How many times a week do you eat legumes (peas, beans, lentils, garbanzos)? *One serving = $\frac{1}{2}$ cup cooked.*
_____

(9) High-fat and high-cholesterol foods. How often do you eat foods high in saturated fat and cholesterol (e.g., steak, hamburger, hot dog, sausage, bacon, cheese, fried chicken, French fries, ice cream, cheesecake, or other rich desserts)?
- ☐ Daily
- ☐ Eat these foods 3 or more times a week
- ☐ Seldom or never eat these foods

(continued)

(10) Nuts/seeds. How many servings of nuts do you usually eat each week? *One serving = 1 oz or a small handful, or 2 tablespoons of natural nut butter.* _____

Refined foods. How often do you eat highly refined foods (soda pop, snack foods, chips, refined cereals, pastry, candy)?

☐ Daily

☐ Eat these foods 3 or more times a week

☐ Seldom or never eat refined foods

Water. How many glasses (8 oz) of water do you typically drink each day? _____

(11) Weight. How many pounds have you gained since you were 21 to 24 (enter 0 if you weigh the same, weigh less, or are less than 21 years. _____

(12) Mental/Social Health

Happiness. How happy have you been during the last month?

☐ Very happy

☐ Pretty happy

☐ Not too happy

☐ Very unhappy

Mood/feelings

1. During the past month, have you often been bothered by feeling down, depressed, or hopeless?
   ☐ Yes   ☐ No

2. During the past month, have you often been bothered by having little interest or pleasure in doing things?
   ☐ Yes   ☐ No

3. Have your feelings in the past month caused you significant distress or impaired your ability to function socially or at work (or school)?
   ☐ Yes   ☐ No

Stress and coping. How much of the time do you feel stressed out and unable to cope with life?

☐ Seldom or never

☐ Occasionally

☐ Much of the time

☐ Most of the time

(13) Social Support

Support. Do you have family or friends you can get help from if needed?
☐ Yes   ☐ No

Social Interaction. Do you have frequent social contact with family or friends?
☐ Yes   ☐ No

(14) Community

Do you meet regularly with a faith community or other group that gives you support, comfort, meaning, and direction in your life?
☐ Yes   ☐ No

(15) Safety

Seat belts. What percent of the time do you wear seat belts when riding in a car? _____

Smoke alarm. Do you have a working smoke alarm on each floor of your home, including the area in which you sleep?
☐ Yes   ☐ No   ☐ Don't know for sure

Helmet. When biking or roller blading, do you always wear a helmet and protective gear?
☐ Yes   ☐ No

Drinking and driving. Do you ever drive soon after drinking or ride with someone who has been drinking?
☐ Yes   ☐ No

(16) Safer Sex

Practice safer sex. Are you in a monogamous relationship, or always use condoms, or abstain from sexual relations?
☐ Always   ☐ Don't always practice safer sex

(17) Preventive Exams

Do you keep current on recommended preventive exams (see list below) and immunizations?
☐ Yes   ☐ No   ☐ Don't know for sure

Recommended Preventive Exams

- Periodic checkup, including blood pressure, height and weight, and cholesterol check as recommended by your doctor.
- PAP tests within last 1 to 3 years, for women 18 or older
- Mammogram within last 2 years, for women 40 or older
- Colorectal cancer screening for all persons 50 or older
- Prostate exam, for men 50 or older
- Flu and pneumonia immunizations, for everyone 65 or older

Height _____

Weight _____

Blood pressure _____

Blood cholesterol _____ (mg/dL)

──────────Scoring──────────

Your score is the number of good health indicators you meet out of the 17 possible listed (below) in this assessment. The higher your score, the healthier your lifestyle. The Average HealthStyle Score is 9.4

►

Lifestyle and Risk Assessment *(continued)*

Health Indicator	Guidelines for Good Health
1. Physical activity	Get 30 or more minutes of physical activity most days of the week.
2. Strength training	Do strength building exercises at least twice per week.
3. Not smoking	Avoid all tobacco use and frequent exposure to second-hand smoke.
4. Alcohol use	Alcohol is not recommended, but if you drink, limit to 1 to 2 drinks in a day.
5. Adequate rest	Get adequate rest, at least 7 to 8 hours of sleep daily for best health.
6. Breakfast daily	Eat a good breakfast daily for optimal physical and mental performance.
7. Whole grains	Choose whole-grain breads and cereals, at least 3 or more servings/per day.
8. Fruits and vegetables	Eat at least 5 servings of fruits and vegetables daily.
9. Fats, cholesterol	Limit fatty meats, whole milk, and butter. Vegetable oils are healthier.
10. Nuts	Nuts contain healthy fats and protect against heart disease.
11. Healthy weight	Maintain a healthy weight by eating well and participating in regular physical activity.
12. Mental health	Develop good coping skills, and maintain a happy, hopeful outlook.
13. Social support	Maintain good social support and frequent contact with family and friends.
14. Community	Participate regularly in a faith community or other group that provides meaning, direction, and support in your life.
15. Safety	Be safety conscious; wear safety belts in the car and helmets when biking.
16. Safer sex	Keep a monogamous relationship, or always use condoms, or abstain.
17. Regular exams	Get regular exams, including age/gender recommended preventive exams.

Source: Hall, D. R. (2004). *Lifestyle check assessment.* Vanderbilt University Health and Wellness.

Life Stress Review

Daily hassles, life events, and other stressors trigger physiological responses that may, over time, induce illness (Selye, 1976; Rahe, 1974). You will find one type of life change events assessment tool in Chapter 25, Assessment Guidelines and Tools, The Holmes-Rahe Social Readjustment Scale. Alternatively, you might want to interview your patient to assess the following:

• His belief in his ability to control the experience (e.g., an impending decision, an illness)

• How deeply involved he feels in the activity that is producing stress (i.e., is it something he can change, or wants to change?)

• Whether he is able to view such a change as a challenge to grow

STANDARDIZED LANGUAGE

Examples of NOC Standardized Health Promotion Outcomes

Outcome and Definition*	Examples of Indicators
Community Health Status—General state of well-being of a community or population	Prevalence of health promotion programs
Community Risk Control: Lead Exposure—Community actions to reduce lead exposure and poisoning	Planning and organization of lead screening programs that include focus on preschools
Family Health Status—Overall health and social competence of family unit	Immunization of members
Family Physical Environment—Physical arrangements in the home that provide safety and stimulation to family members	Dwelling well ventilated
Health Beliefs—Personal convictions that influence health behaviors	Perceived importance of taking action
Health Beliefs: Perceived Ability to Perform—Personal conviction that one can carry out a given health behavior	Perception that health behavior is not too complex
Health Beliefs: Perceived Control—Personal conviction that one can influence a health outcome	Belief that own actions control health outcomes
Health Beliefs: Perceived Resources—Personal conviction that one has adequate means to carry out a health behavior	Perceived adequacy of time
Health Beliefs: Perceived Threat—Personal conviction that a threatening health problem is serious and has potential negative consequences for lifestyle	Perceived threat to health
Health Orientation—Personal commitment to health behaviors as lifestyle priorities	Perception that health is a high priority in making lifestyle choices
Health Promoting Behavior—Personal actions to sustain or increase wellness	Seeks balance among exercise, work, leisure, rest and nutrition
Health Seeking Behavior—Personal actions to promote optimal wellness, recovery, and rehabilitation	Performs self-screening when indicated
Knowledge: Health Behavior—Extent of understanding conveyed about the promotion and protection of health	Description of effective stress management techniques
Knowledge: Health Promotion—Extent of understanding conveyed about information needed to obtain and maintain optimal health	Description of behaviors that promote health
Knowledge: Health Resources—Extent of understanding conveyed about relevant healthcare resources	Description of community resources available for assistance
Leisure participation—Use of relaxing, interesting, and enjoyable activities to promote well-being	Participates in activities other than regular work
Personal Safety Behavior—Personal actions of an adult to control behaviors that can cause physical injury	Practices safe sexual behaviors
Physical Fitness—Performance of physical activities with vigor	Muscle strength Muscle endurance

Source: Moorhead, S., Johnson, M., & Maas, M. (Eds.). (2004). Nursing outcomes classification (NOC) (3rd ed.). St Louis: Mosby.

*All of the outcomes in the Growth & Development class may be used (e.g., Child Development: Preschool; Physical Maturation: Female; Sexual Functioning).

Selected NIC Wellness Interventions

Intervention and Definition	Examples of Activities
Breast Examination—Inspection and palpation of the breasts and related areas	Encourage patient to demonstrate self-palpation during and after clinical breast examination
Community Health Development—Assisting members of a community to identify a community's health concerns, mobilize resources, and implement solutions	Identify health concerns, strengths, and priorities with community partners
Environmental Management: Worker Safety—Monitoring and manipulation of the worksite environment to promote safety and health of workers	Identify applicable OSHA standards and worksite compliance with standards
Environmental Risk Protection—Preventing and detecting disease and injury in populations at risk from environmental hazards	Monitor incidents of illness and injury related to environmental hazards
Exercise Promotion—Facilitation of regular physical activity to maintain or advance to a higher level of fitness and health	Appraise individual's health beliefs about physical exercise
Family Planning: Contraception—Facilitation of pregnancy prevention by providing information about the physiology of reproduction and methods to control conception	Determine ability and motivation of patient and partner to correctly and regularly use contraception
Health Education—Developing and providing instruction and learning experiences to facilitate voluntary adaptation of behavior conducive to health in individuals, families, groups, or communities	Target high-risk groups and age ranges that would benefit most from health education
Health Policy Monitoring—Surveillance and influence of government and organization regulations, rules, and standards that affect nursing systems and practices to ensure quality care of patients	Compare requirements of policies and standards with current practices
Health Screening—Detecting health risks or problems by means of history, examination, and other procedures	Complete appropriate Department of Health or other records for monitoring abnormal results, such as high blood pressure
Health System Guidance—Facilitating a patient's location and use of appropriate health services	Inform the patient of accreditation and state health department requirements for judging the quality of a facility
Immunization/Vaccination Management—Monitoring immunization status, facilitating access to immunizations, and providing immunizations to prevent communicable disease	Determine immunization status at every health care visit (including emergency department and hospital admission), and provide immunizations as needed
Oral Health Promotion—Promotion of oral hygiene and dental care for a patient with normal oral and dental health	Teach and encourage flossing Review dental hygiene facts with parents
Parent Education: Childrearing Family—Assisting parents to understand and promote the physical, psychological, and social growth and development of their toddler, preschool, or school-age child/children (also Parent Education: Adolescent and Parent Education: Infant)	Teach parents and caregivers about expected growth and development
Patient Contracting—Negotiating and agreement with an individual that reinforces a specific behavior change	Encourage the individual to identify own goals, not those he/she believes the healthcare provider expects

(continued)

Intervention and Definition	Examples of Activities
Program Development [Wellness]—Planning, implementing, and evaluating a coordinated set of activities designed to enhance wellness, or to prevent, reduce, or eliminate one or more health problems for a group or community	Assist the group or community in identifying significant health needs or problems
Smoking Cessation Assistance—Helping another to stop smoking	Help patient identify reasons to quit and barriers to quitting
Spiritual Growth Facilitation—Faciliation of growth in patient's capacity to identify, connect with, and call upon the source of meaning, purpose, comfort, strength, and hope in his/her life	Encourage conversation that assists the patient in sorting out spiritual concerns
Sports-Injury Prevention: Youth—Reduce the risk of sports-related injury in young athletes	Monitor proper use and condition of safety equipment
Substance Use Prevention—Prevention of an alcoholic or drug use lifestyle	Conduct programs in schools on the avoidance of drugs and alcohol as recreational activities

Teaching:
    Infant Nutrition
    Infant Safety
    Infant Stimulation
    Toddler Nutrition
    Toddler Safety
    Toilet Training
	Note: Teaching is integral to all health promotion/disease prevention activities, whether or not there is a special intervention label for the particular content

Teaching: Safe Sex—Providing instructions concerning sexual protection during sexual activity	Stress the importance of knowing the partner's sexual history, as appropriate
Values Clarification—Assisting another to clarify her/his own values in order to facilitate effective decision making	Think through the ethical and legal aspects of free choice, given the particular situation, before beginning the intervention
Vehicle Safety Promotion—Assisting individuals, families, and communities to increase awareness of measures to reduce unintentional injuries in motorized and nonmotorized vehicles.	Educate about the importance of proper and regular use of protective devices to decrease risk of injury (e.g., car seats, seat belts, helmets)

Source: Dochterman, J. M., & Bulechek, G. M. (Eds.). (2004). *Nursing interventions classification (NIC)* (4th ed.). St Louis: Mosby.

What Are the Main Points in This Chapter?

- Health promotion refers to helping clients develop an optimal state of health.

- Motive is the difference between health promotion and health protection (illness prevention).

- There are three levels of activities for health protection: primary, secondary, and tertiary prevention. Primary interventions are designed to prevent or slow the onset of disease. Secondary interventions are designed to detect illnesses in early stages. Tertiary interventions focus on stopping the disease from progressing and on rehabilitation.

- The Healthy People 2010 initiative is designed to achieve two overarching goals: increase quality and years of healthy life and eliminate health disparities.

- Pender's Health Promotion Model (HPM) identifies three groups of variables that affect health behavior: (1) individual characteristics and experiences; (2) behavior-specific cognitions and affect; and (3) behavioral outcome.

- A wellness wheel identifies six dimensions of health: emotional, intellectual, physical, spiritual, social/family, and occupational.

- The transtheoretical model of change identifies four stages of change: contemplation, determination, action, and maintenance.

- Health promotion activities for all age groups include nutrition, exercise, safety concerns, changing unhealthy lifestyles, immunizations, and screenings.

- Health promotion activities may be conducted in acute care facilities, the workplace, local communities, or schools.

- A health promotion assessment involves obtaining a health history, physical examination, fitness assessment, lifestyle and risk appraisal, life stress review, assessment of healthcare beliefs, nutritional assessment, and screening activities.

- Health screening activities are designed to detect disease at an early stage so that treatment can begin before there is an opportunity for disease to spread or become debilitating.

- Health screening activities vary based on developmental stage and identified risk factors.

- Nurses promote health through role models, counseling, health education, and providing and facilitating support.

Knowledge Map

Promoting Health

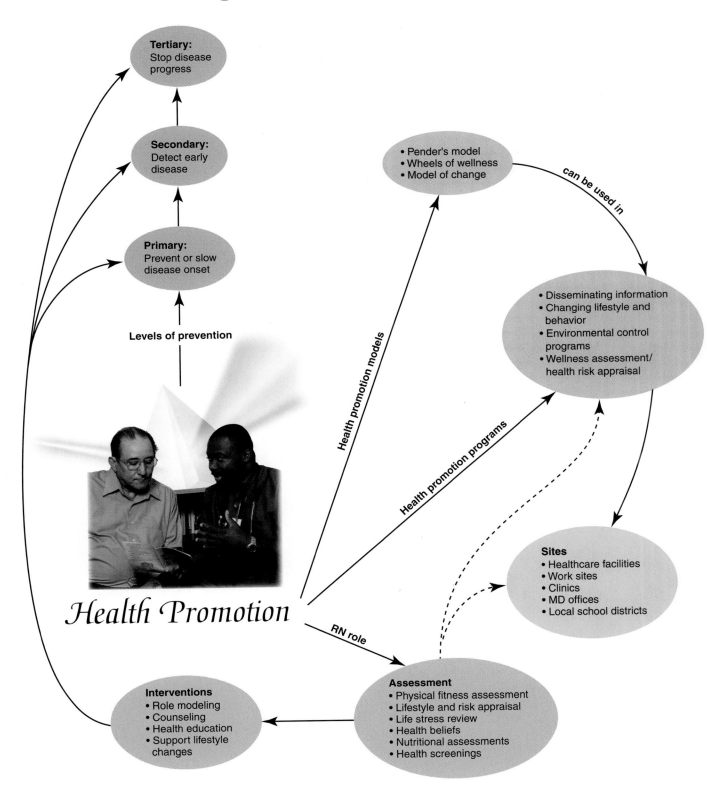

Tertiary:
Stop disease progress

Secondary:
Detect early disease

Primary:
Prevent or slow disease onset

Levels of prevention

• Pender's model
• Wheels of wellness
• Model of change

can be used in

• Disseminating information
• Changing lifestyle and behavior
• Environmental control programs
• Wellness assessment/ health risk appraisal

Health promotion models

Health promotion programs

Sites
• Healthcare facilities
• Work sites
• Clinics
• MD offices
• Local school districts

Health Promotion

RN role

Interventions
• Role modeling
• Counseling
• Health education
• Support lifestyle changes

Assessment
• Physical fitness assessment
• Lifestyle and risk appraisal
• Life stress review
• Health beliefs
• Nutritional assessments
• Health screenings

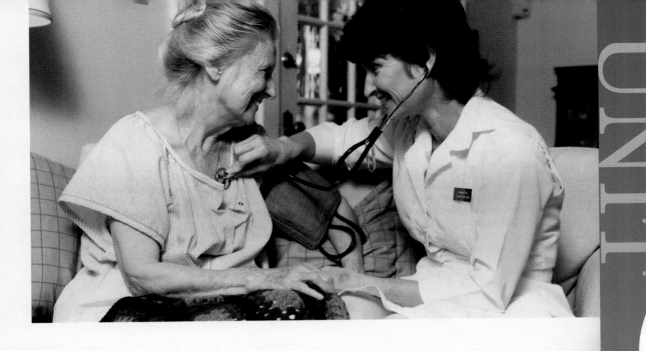

The Context
for Nurses' Work

42 COMMUNITY NURSING

43 NURSING IN HOME CARE

44 ETHICS AND VALUES

45 LEGAL ISSUES

42 Community Nursing

Overview

In the community setting, nurses' roles vary widely, depending on the community and its identified needs. The nursing care is by nature holistic, and it involves large numbers of clients. Community health nurses function as client advocates, educators, collaborators, counselors, and case managers.

Although the terms *community health nursing* and *public health nursing* are often used interchangeably, the two are not identical. Community health nursing focuses on the health of individuals, families, and groups and on how their health affects the community as a whole. Public health nursing focuses on the community at large and the eventual effect of the community's health status on the health of individuals, families, and groups.

Community-based care refers to acute care or rehabilitative services performed in clinics, offices, and other facilities in the community rather than in acute care settings. Common practice areas for community-based nurses include schools, churches, prison systems, disaster relief services, occupational and public health clinics, and international relief organizations. In these settings, nurses function as advocates, educators, collaborators, counselors, and effective communicators. Community-oriented nursing combines components of community and public health. The focus is a comprehensive look at the individual, family, group, and community at large.

A vulnerable population is a population whose members have a higher probability of developing illness than do members of the general population. Because of their increased risks, vulnerable populations are a major focus of community health efforts.

The Omaha classification system is a commonly used documentation system for generating a care plan for a community or an individual within the community setting.

Thinking Critically About Community Nursing

The exercises in the following section allow you to practice the kind of thinking you will use as a full-spectrum nurse. Because these are critical-thinking activities, there is usually no single right answer. Discuss answers with your peers—discussion can stimulate critical thinking. If you have difficulty with any of the questions, consult with your instructor.

Caring for the Garcias

Floredelisa Garcia works as a preschool teacher in her community. She regularly cares for Andre, a 2-year-old boy. Over the last few months, she has noticed that Andre has many bruises and seems withdrawn. She is concerned that Andre might be experiencing child abuse, but she is reluctant to make that accusation, especially because neither her boss nor her co-worker seem to have noticed anything amiss.

Ms Garcia talks to her husband, Joe, about her concerns: "I'm worried about Andre, but I'm afraid to say anything. What if I'm wrong? I'd probably lose my job. But if I'm right and I don't say anything, I could still lose my job, and Andre could be hurt even worse." Joe suggests that she contact the clinic nurse at the Family Medicine Center for confidential advice on how to proceed.

A. Imagine that you are the clinic nurse. Use the full-spectrum nursing model to identify at least ten questions that you would need to answer to further investigate Flordelisa's concerns.

B. *Self-knowledge:* What personal values do you have that would affect the manner in which you handle this situation? Explain.

C. *Ethical knowledge:* What is the most important ethical issue in this situation? That is, what is the most important goal? Note that there may be several moral and legal issues, but you are being asked to identify the *most* important one. Note also that we are not asking you what the nurse *can* do, but rather what the nurse ideally *should* do.

D. You share the questions you have with Flordelisa. She believes that there is a real need to investigate child abuse. You advise her to call the local child protective services (CPS) agency. Based on your knowledge of community and public health nursing, what aspects of the community health role will the nurse from CPS use as she investigates this situation?

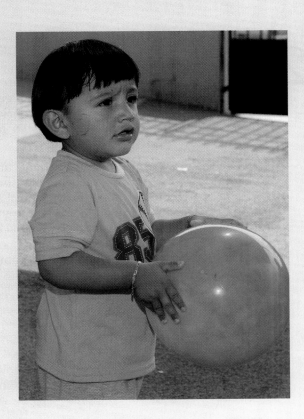

1 You are nearing completion of your fundamentals course. One night while you are preparing for your next clinical, the telephone rings. It is your neighbor, Tanya. Her 5-year-old daughter, Tiffany, attends kindergarten at the local public school. Tiffany came home with a letter from the school nurse stating that another child in the class was ill with chickenpox and that all the students in the class had been exposed to the disease.

Tanya is concerned about the risks to Tiffany and the rest of the family. She does not recall whether Tiffany was vaccinated against chickenpox, and she is unsure whether she herself had the disease when she was a child. Tanya is 4 months pregnant, and the family has no health insurance. She states that because you are a nursing student, she thought you might know what she should do or where she might go for assistance.

What are the key pieces of information (both theoretical knowledge and patient data) you need to solve your neighbor's situation?

2 You are a nurse in a public health clinic providing routine childhood immunizations. A 16-year-old mother comes into the clinic requesting "shots" for her newborn baby as well as a birth control "shot." She indicates that she has no money to pay for the shots because her 20-year-old boyfriend gave her enough only to get to the clinic. Which of the following is your nursing priority for this situation? What will you do next? Explain *how* you have chosen your priority diagnosis. On what did you base your choice?

- Give the newborn the immunizations, and arrange for the client to meet with the social worker regarding securing healthcare insurance.
- Educate the mother about birth control and the fact that it is not an immunization.
- Take the client and child to a private room, and discuss the general health of the newborn and the plans for a physician/clinic to see the child. Also ask about the health needs of the mother.
- Ask the mother whether she is being abused and report the incident if so.

3 Your assignment is to conduct a community assessment of your neighborhood. How will your membership in the community affect your assessment? What activities could you delete from the assessment?

4 You are driving home from your nursing school clinical day and happen on a car over-turned along a deserted country road. You recall what you learned about the "Good Samaritan" laws. Under these circumstances, are you allowed to perform the skills you have learned in lab? What is your best course of intervention?

5 For each of the following concepts, use critical thinking and summarize how or why it is important to nursing, patient care, or community nursing. Note that these are *not* to be merely definitions.

Community

Aggregates

Census tracts

Vulnerable populations

Healthy People 2010

Windshield survey

thinking critically about community nursing

Primary intervention

Secondary intervention

Tertiary intervention

Disaster preparedness

Omaha system

Practical Knowledge
knowing how

Practical knowledge in community nursing requires you to apply the nursing process to both individuals and groups.

STANDARDIZED LANGUAGE

This section provides guidelines for using NANDA, NOC, NIC, and the Omaha system to develop problem statements, goals, and nursing orders to use in planning care for aggregates and communities.

Omaha Problem Classification Scheme

The Omaha system consists of 42 *diagnostic labels* organized into four *domains* (categories), along with two sets of *modifiers*. Refer to the accompanying box for the four Omaha categories, examples of diagnosis (problem) labels, and problem modifiers. As you can see, the problem labels in the environment domain are especially useful in community nursing. For the complete Problem Classification Scheme,

 Go to the **Omaha System web site at www.omahasystem.org**

To create a diagnostic statement, choose an appropriate label, and add a modifier to it from each of the two sets in the accompanying box. For example, a group

Environment diagnosis for workers in a meat-packing plant with lax safety standards might read *"Deficit in Group* Workplace Safety." If only one worker were at risk (perhaps because of her inattention to safety rules), you could write *Potential Deficit in Individual* Workplace Safety.

Domain: Environment

Problems: Income, Sanitation, Residence, and Workplace Safety

Modifiers: (1) Health Promotion, Potential Deficit, or Deficit
 (2) Family, Individual, or Group

Diagnostic Statements:
 Deficit in *Group* Workplace Safety
 Potential Deficit in Individual Workplace Safety

Omaha System: Domains and Examples of Problem Labels

- *Environmental Domain*—The material resources, physical surroundings, and substances both internal and external to the client, home, neighborhood, and broader community
 Problem (Diagnosis) Labels: Income, Sanitation, Residence, Neighborhood/Workplace Safety

- *Psychosocial Domain*—Patterns of behavior, communication, relationships, and development.
 Problem (Diagnosis) Labels: Social Contact, Role Change, Interpersonal Relationships

- *Physiological Domain*—Functional status of processes that maintain life.
 Problem (Diagnosis) Labels: Hearing, Pain, Respiration

- *Health Related Behaviors Domain*—Activities that maintain or promote wellness, promote recovery, or maximize rehabilitation potential.
 Problem (Diagnosis) Labels: Nutrition, Personal Hygiene, Prescribed Medication Regimen

Problem Modifiers

- Set 1—Health Promotion, Potential Deficit, Deficit
- Set 2—Family, Individual, Group*

*Martin and Scheet (1992, p. 67) suggest that *Group* be added to these modifiers

Source: Martin, K. S., & Scheet, N. J. (1992). *The Omaha system: Applications for community health nursing.* Philadelphia: Saunders, pp. 67–74. Used with permission.

Using the NOC and Omaha Systems to Write Aggregate Goals

NOC Outcomes

NOC standardized outcomes in the Community Health domain include the following:

- Community Competence
- Community Disaster Readiness
- Community Health Status
- Community Health Status: Immunity
- Community Risk Control: Chronic Disease
- Community Risk Control: Communicable Disease
- Community Risk Control: Lead Exposure
- Community Risk Control: Violence
- Community Violence Level

You can use these NOC labels to write goals by adding the appropriate NOC indicators and scales (see the Standardized Language section of Chapter 5, in this volume).

Omaha System Outcomes

Using the Omaha system, you will develop goals/outcomes from the words in the nursing diagnosis. Recall that all nursing diagnoses are identified as either *individual, family,* or *group,* so a group nursing diagnosis will automatically indicate a group goal. For example, for the diagnosis Deficit in Group Workplace Safety, you would build the outcomes around the words "Group Workplace Safety." The Omaha system includes a 5-point "Problem Rating Scale for Outcomes" (see the accompanying table) that describes what you expect to achieve in terms of the client's knowledge, behavior, and status.

Omaha Problem Rating Scale for Outcomes

Concept	1	2	3	4	5
Knowledge					
The ability of the client to remember and interpret information	No knowledge	Minimal knowledge	Basic knowledge	Adequate knowledge	Superior knowledge
Behavior					
The client's observable responses, actions, or activities fitting the occasion or purpose	Never appropriate	Rarely appropriate	Inconsistently appropriate	Usually appropriate	Consistently appropriate
Status					
The condition of the client in relation to objective and subjective defining characteristics	Extreme signs/symptoms	Severe signs/symptoms	Moderate signs/symptoms	Minimal signs/symptoms	No signs/symptoms

Source: Martin, K. S., & Scheet, N. J. (1992). *The Omaha system: Applications for community health nursing.* Philadelphia: Saunders, p. 92. Used with permission from Elsevier Science.

Using the table, you would create expected outcomes by applying this scale to Group Workplace Safety, as follows:

Nursing Diagnosis: Deficit in Group Workplace Safety

Rating Scale Concept	Present Status Before Interventions	Expected Outcome
Knowledge	(2) Minimal knowledge of workplace safety	(4) Adequate knowledge of workplace safety
Behavior	(2) Rarely appropriate safety behaviors	(4) Usually appropriate group safety behaviors
Status	(2) Severe signs/ symptoms (e.g., frequent accidents or injuries)	(4) Minimal signs/symp- toms (e.g., few accidents or injuries)

This means that after your interventions, you expect the group to have adequate knowledge of workplace safety, demonstrate usually appropriate behaviors (e.g., usually follow the safety rules), and demonstrate minimal accidents or injuries. To evaluate the client's progress, you would assign a scale number to the group's actual knowledge, behavior, and status *after interventions.*

Using the NIC and Omaha Interventions Labels

The NIC taxonomy includes 16 interventions specifically designed for community health (see the accompanying table).

The Omaha taxonomy provides four "intervention categories" you can use in community-oriented nursing practice:

1. *Health Teaching, Guidance and Counseling.* These primary prevention activities include giving information, anticipating client problems, encouraging client action and responsibility for self-care, and assisting with coping, decision making, and problem solving. As a community-oriented nurse, you should spend most of your time offering this level of intervention.

2. *Treatments and Procedures.* These are secondary interventions directed toward preventing disease, identifying risk factors and early signs and symptoms, and decreasing or alleviating signs and symptoms.

NIC Community Health Classes and Interventions

Class: Community Health Promotion—Interventions that promote the health of the whole community	Class: Community Risk Management—Interventions that assist in detecting or preventing health risks to the whole community
Interventions:	*Interventions:*
Case Management	Community Disaster Preparedness
Community Health Development	Communicable Disease Management
Fiscal Resource Management	Environmental Management: Community
Health Education	Environmental Management: Worker Safety
Health Policy Monitoring	Environmental Risk Protection
Immunization/Vaccination Management	Health Screening
Program Development	Risk Identification
	Surveillance: Community
	Vehicle Safety Promotion

Source: Dochterman, J. M., & Bulecheck, G. M. (Eds.). (2004). *Nursing interventions classification (NIC)* (4th ed). Philadelphia: Mosby, p. 125. Used with permission from Elsevier Science.

3. *Case Management.* Case management is a tertiary intervention that includes coordination, advocacy, and referral. These activities involve facilitating service delivery on behalf of the client, communicating with health and human service providers, promoting assertive client communication, and guiding the client toward appropriate community resources.

4. *Surveillance.* These nursing activities include detection, measurement, critical analysis, and monitoring to indicate client status in relation to a given condition or phenomenon.

To write an intervention statement, you must combine one of those four "categories" of interventions with 63 "targets" (objects of the nursing interventions), such as bowel care and nutrition. Then you must add patient-specific information to individualize the nursing order. See the accompanying table for intervention categories, examples of targets, and intervention statements (nursing orders). To see the entire set of intervention targets,

 Go to the **Omaha System web site at** **www.omahasystem.org/shminter.htm**

You will notice that the targets can be used for individuals as well as groups. It is the designation of the nursing diagnosis as *individual, family,* or *group* that determines this.

Omaha Intervention Categories and Examples of Targets

Categories	**Examples of Targets**
I. Health Teaching, Guidance, and Counseling	Anatomy/physiology
II. Treatments and Procedures	Behavior modification
III. Case Management	Communication
IV. Surveillance	Discipline
	Feeding procedures
	Homemaking
	Substance use
	Wellness
	Examples of aggregate targets:
	Caretaking/parenting skills
	Day-care/respite
	Durable medical equipment
	Education
	Employment
	Environment
	Finances
	Housing
	Legal system
	Transportation
	Other community resource

Examples of Nursing Intervention Statements

Treatments and Procedures (II): Feeding procedures (demonstrate to Mrs. Adams how to feed Mr. Adams at the next visit)

Surveillance (IV): Feeding procedures (After teaching, observe a feeding. Monitor for choking.)

Source: Martin, K. S., & Scheet, N. J. (1992). *The Omaha system: Applications for community health nursing.* Philadelphia: Saunders, p. 82. Used with permission from Elsevier Science.

What Are the Main Points in This Chapter?

- A community can be defined as a place with defined boundaries, a group of people with a common language, rituals, or customs.
- Each community determines the meaning of health and nursing activities to promote health.
- A vulnerable population is defined as an aggregate that is at increased risk of adverse health outcomes. Members of vulnerable groups have a higher probability of developing illness.
- The community nurse assesses three general dimensions of a community: structure, status, and process.
- Common practice areas for community-based nurses include schools, churches, prison systems, disaster relief services, occupational and public health clinics, and international relief organizations.
- Community health nursing focuses on the health of individuals, families, and groups and how their individual health affects the community as a whole.

- Public health nursing focuses on the community at large and the eventual effect of the community's health status on the health of individuals, families, and groups.
- Community-oriented nursing combines components of community and public health. Nurses practicing community-oriented nursing are fluid in their approach. Their focus is a comprehensive look at the individual, family, group, and community at large. Community-based nurses function as advocates, educators, collaborators, counselors, and effective communicators.
- Community-based nurses may provide care at three levels: primary, secondary, and tertiary. The focus is primary prevention.
- The Omaha classification system is a commonly used documentation system for generating a care plan for a community or an individual within the community setting.

Knowledge Map

Community Nursing

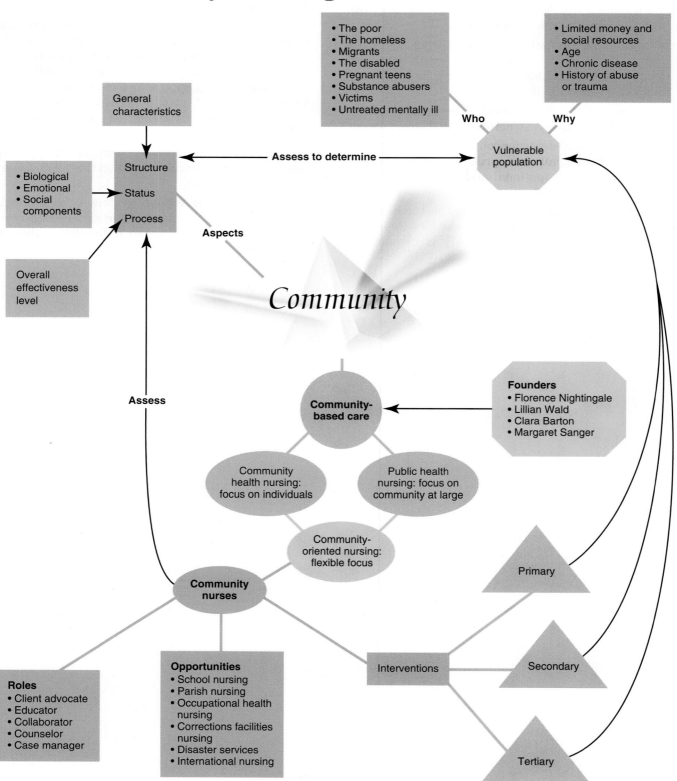

General characteristics

- Biological
- Emotional
- Social components

Structure

Status

Process

Overall effectiveness level

Aspects

Assess to determine

Assess

Community

- The poor
- The homeless
- Migrants
- The disabled
- Pregnant teens
- Substance abusers
- Victims
- Untreated mentally ill

Who

- Limited money and social resources
- Age
- Chronic disease
- History of abuse or trauma

Why

Vulnerable population

Community-based care

Founders
- Florence Nightingale
- Lillian Wald
- Clara Barton
- Margaret Sanger

Community health nursing: focus on individuals

Public health nursing: focus on community at large

Community-oriented nursing: flexible focus

Community nurses

Primary

Interventions

Secondary

Tertiary

Roles
- Client advocate
- Educator
- Collaborator
- Counselor
- Case manager

Opportunities
- School nursing
- Parish nursing
- Occupational health nursing
- Corrections facilities nursing
- Disaster services
- International nursing

Nursing in Home Care

Overview

Home health agencies may be public, voluntary, proprietary, or hospital-based organizations that provide both direct and indirect care. Some agencies specialize in certain types of clients (e.g., maternal-child clients). Home health nursing fosters client and family independence and promotes self-care. Hospice nurses provide care for clients who are dying. They frequently work in home care and focus on providing comfort and managing symptoms.

To prepare for a home visit, obtain information from the referral, identify the purpose of the visit, gather required supplies, and contact the client to arrange the visit. Your goal for the visit is to establish rapport with the client and family, assess their needs, develop and discuss the plan of care and needed services, provide skilled care, and evaluate the need for continued services.

The home health nurse usually works alone during a home visit, without immediate access to other healthcare professionals. In addition, many factors within the home, such as cleanliness and noise, are not within the nurse's control. As a nurse delivering home care, you will need to follow Standard Precautions but recognize how infection control techniques may be modified to the home environment.

Home health care is reimbursed by Medicare, by Medicaid, by private insurance, and through direct payment from the client. To be eligible for continuing care under Medicare and most private insurers, a client must be homebound and require skilled nursing care. Most home-care agencies use the Clinical Care Classification (CCC) system as the basis for providing and documenting care. After a home visit, you must document care, coordinate services for the client, and prepare for future visits.

Thinking Critically About Nursing in Home Care

The exercises in the following section allow you to practice the kind of thinking you will use as a full-spectrum nurse. Because these are critical-thinking activities, there is usually no single right answer. Discuss answers with your peers—discussion can stimulate critical thinking. If you have difficulty with any of the questions, consult with your instructor.

Caring for the Garcias

Katherine Garcia, the 76-year-old mother of Joseph Garcia, has completed 2 weeks of physical therapy at Mercy Care Center (a skilled nursing facility) after her surgery to repair a fractured right hip. She is now able to get out of bed with assistance and requires a walker to ambulate even short distances.

Mrs. Garcia is very unhappy at Mercy Care Center. Some of her friends have entered nursing homes because of health problems, and two have died while at the facilities. Although she realizes that their deaths were related to health problems rather than placement issues, she is very nervous about staying at the center. At a care conference, her family requests that she be discharged home for ongoing therapy. It is determined that she is eligible for Medicare-covered services.

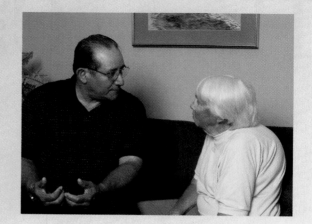

What type of home services will Mrs. Garcia probably need?

1

As a beginning home health nurse, you have been assigned to visit the following clients today:

- Mr. Roland Escobar ("Meet Your Patient" in Volume 1), a 78-year-old man recovering from a cerebrovascular accident (stroke)
- Ms Sally Littlemoon, a 48-year-old woman with diabetes mellitus, blindness, and lower extremity cellulitis (a skin infection)
- Ms Beatrice Wayne, a 67-year-old woman who has undergone elective coronary artery bypass graft surgery (open heart surgery)
- Mr. Kent Churchill, an 80-year-old man with a recent hip fracture and surgical repair
- Ms Chana Padir, a 50-year-old woman with severe pain secondary to breast cancer with extensive metastases. She is receiving hospice care.

a Explore some alternatives for your schedule. How would you prepare to make these five visits in one day? How would you determine how to arrange your schedule?

b The report you receive from the home health supervisor includes the following information:

- Ms Littlemoon and Mr. Churchill require dressing changes.
- Mr. Escobar and Ms Wayne require teaching about their medications.
- Mr. Escobar, Ms Littlemoon, and Mr. Churchill require venipuncture for lab work.
- Ms Padir is having increasing pain.

Based on this information, what else do you need to know and/or do before you begin your visits?

What practical knowledge will you need to provide care for these clients?

c How might the care you deliver to Ms Wayne differ from the care you give to Ms Padir? To answer the question, consider the context for each woman. How are their situations different?

d When visiting Ms Padir, you realize that her husband and children are very fearful of her impending death. They seem overwhelmed by the care she requires. What values and beliefs do you have about death and dying that might influence your care of the Padir family? (Review Chapters 14 and 15 if necessary.)

What must you consider in order to plan your interventions? How might you intervene?

e When you arrive at the home of Ms Wayne, she is dressed and out of bed. She tells you she is able to get out of bed and ambulate about the house independently with very little pain. She can identify the medications she is receiving, their purpose, and their schedule for administration. Her chest wound is healing nicely, and her breath sounds are clear. She informs you that she is planning on going to her cabin in the mountains this upcoming weekend with her husband and children. What actions must you take with regard to continuing her home visits? Why? What rules/guidelines will influence your choice of action?

2   For each of the following concepts, use critical thinking to describe how or why it is important to nurses, patient care, or nursing in home care. Note that these are *not* to be merely definitions.

Delivering health care in the home setting

Skilled services

Caregiver Role Strain

Preparing for the home visit

Developing rapport at the home visit

Assessment of the home environment

Documentation of home healthcare services

Clinical Care Classification system

CONDUCTING A HOME VISIT

Before the Visit

- Gather information from the referral.
- Secure permission to visit.
- Arrange time and date of visit with the client and/or family.

At the Visit

- Build trust.
- Assess the client, family, and community.

- Develop a plan with the client and family.
- Deliver skilled care.
- Identify need(s) for future services.
- Refer to appropriate departments and community services.

After the Visit

- Document assessments and care.
- Evaluate progress toward goals.
- Modify plan as needed.

SAFETY CONSIDERATIONS IN HOME CARE

Before the Visit

- Plan ahead. Know where you are headed. Use a map. Contact the client or family regarding directions if it is unclear where you are headed. File a visit plan with your office each day.
- Dress in appropriate attire as dictated by your agency. Wear a name tag clearly identifying you and the agency. Wear shoes that will allow you to run if necessary.
- Carry a cell phone if possible.
- Do not carry a purse or large sums of money. Instead, use a waist or fanny pack. In the pack, carry enough money for emergency transportation, telephone numbers, and emergency contact information.
- Keep your car in good repair, and always have enough gasoline in the tank. Be prepared for inclement weather, and always carry an emergency car safety pack.
- Observe your surroundings as you drive to the visit. Notice the location of emergency services, local gas stations, and public places if help is required.
- Park as close to your destination as possible. If possible, park your car facing the direction you wish to go when you leave. Avoid dead ends, alleys, and poorly lighted areas.
- Check your surroundings before you leave your car. If you feel unsafe, leave the area and call your office.
- Lock the car. Leave no valuables in sight.

- Prepare your bag while you are still in the car.
- Carry your bag on one arm. In the opposite hand, carry your keys. Always have them ready. You can use keys to defend yourself by placing the pointed ends of the keys between your fingers. They may also be required if you decide to exit quickly.
- Walk directly to the client's house. Walk in the middle of the sidewalk. Use common walkways. Avoid isolated and poorly lighted areas. Do not take shortcuts.
- Knock or ring the doorbell before entering. Never enter without being invited. If there is no answer at the door, call the patient using your cell phone, or return to a secure public pay phone and dial the client.
- If for any reason you feel that the neighborhood is unsafe, do not get out of the car. Instead, leave the neighborhood and phone your agency.

At the Visit

- Introduce yourself and clearly identify your agency. Show your name badge.
- When you enter the home, observe all exits. Sit where you have access to an exit.
- Notice who is present in the home. Request introductions. This information is useful for planning care as well as for ensuring safety.

SAFETY CONSIDERATIONS IN HOME CARE *(continued)*

- Leave immediately if you suspect drug use, drug dealing, or drunken behavior.
- Leave immediately if there is a violent domestic argument. Do not attempt to intervene. When you return to your car, use your cell phone to dial 911, or drive to a phone booth in a safe location and place the call.
- Request that animals be kept in another room while you make your visit.
- If weapons are visible, request that they be put away immediately. Leave the home if this request is not met.
- If household members interfere with the visit, discuss the problem with the client. You may need to arrange a time to visit when they are not present.

After the Visit

- Continue to observe the safety precautions you used when getting to the visit. Do not let down your guard as you return to your car.
- If you are in an unsafe neighborhood or poorly lighted area, do not consult the map for directions to your next visit. Leave immediately and drive to a secure public location, and then consult the map.
- Inform your agency if you believe the home or neighborhood is potentially hazardous. Request an escort service if future visits are required.
- Document your assessments and the care delivered.

STANDARDIZED LANGUAGE

CCC Care Components

A	Activity Component	L	Respiratory Component
B	Bowel Gastric Component	M	Role Relationship Component
C	Cardiac Component	N	Safety Component
D	Cognitive Component	O	Self-Care Component
E	Coping Component	P	Self-Concept Component
F	Fluid Volume Component	Q	Sensory Component
G	Health Behavior Component	R	Skin Integrity Component
H	Medication Component	S	Tissue Perfusion Component
I	Metabolic Component	T	Urinary Elimination Component
J	Nutritional Component	U	Life Cycle Component
K	Physical Regulation Component		

An Example of CCC Nursing Diagnoses and Interventions

A—ACTIVITY COMPONENT **(1 of 21 Care Components)**

01   Activity Alteration **(Main Nursing Diagnosis)**

A01   Activity Care Interventions

Actions performed to carry out physiological or psychological daily activities.

Example: Passive Range of Motion/Teach Family

Subcategories that provide greater definition of the problem

01.1   Activity Intolerance
01.2   Activity Intolerance Risk
01.3   Diversional Activity Deficit
01.4   Fatigue
01.5   Physical Mobility Impairment
01.6   Sleep Pattern Disturbance
01.7   Sleep Deprivation

What Are the Main Points in This Chapter?

- Home health nursing fosters client and family independence and promotes self-care.

- In the home setting, many factors, such as cleanliness and noise level, are not within the nurse's control. In addition, the home health nurse works alone, without immediate access to other healthcare professionals.

- Home health agencies may be public, voluntary, proprietary, or hospital-based agencies. They may provide direct or indirect care and may specialize in certain types of clients.

- As a full-spectrum nurse working in home health care, you will function in the following roles: communicator, direct care provider, client/family educator, client advocate, and case manager.

- Hospice nurses work in hospitals, special hospice facilities, or the homes of patients who are dying. The goal of their care is to provide comfort and manage symptoms.

- Home health care is reimbursed by Medicare, by Medicaid, by private insurance, and through direct payment from the client.

- To be eligible for continuing care under Medicare and most private insurers, a client must be homebound and require skilled nursing care.

- Preparation for a home visit includes obtaining information from the referral, identifying the purpose of the visit, gathering required supplies, and contacting the client to arrange the visit.

- During a home visit, you will establish a rapport with the client and family, assess the needs of the client and caregivers, develop and discuss the plan of care and needed services with the client and caregivers, provide skilled care, and evaluate the need for continued services.

- The Clinical Care Classification (CCC) system is a system of care and documentation used by most home care agencies.

- Interventions to reduce Caregiver Role Strain include providing emotional support and arranging additional home and community services to support the client and caregiver.

- As a nurse delivering home care, you will need to follow Standard Precautions but recognize how infection control techniques may be modified to the home environment.

- After a home visit you must document care, coordinate services for the client, and prepare for future visits.

Knowledge Map

Home Health Care

Increased prevalence due to:
- Reimbursement changes
- Population changes
- Decreasing length of stay

Home Care

Goals
- Promote self-care
- Promote independence
- Complete patient/family teaching

Providers
- Public agencies
- Voluntary agencies
- Proprietary organizations
- Hospital-based agencies
- Hospice organizations

Advantages
- Direct view of client environment
- Direct clues to client strength, resources, motivation

Challenges
- No control of environment
- No immediate assistance
- No stored client information on site
- No other healthcare team members

- Physicians
- Nurses
- Aides:
  PT/ST/OT/RT
- Nutritionists
- Social workers
- Pharmacists
- Chaplains

Nursing roles
- Provider
- Educator
- Advocate
- Care coordinator

Making a home visit
- Determine purpose
- Gather supplies
- Assess/address safety issues
- Develop rapport with client/family; show courtesy and respect
- Verify client data
- Provide care
- Document care

Ethics
& Values

Overview

Ethics is a formal process for deciding right and wrong conduct in situations where issues of values and morals arise. Morals are learned and internalized throughout the life span. Ethical decisions are affected by a person's values, moral frameworks and principles, and professional guidelines. Six important moral principles are autonomy, nonmaleficence, beneficence, fidelity, veracity, and justice.

Nursing ethics refers to ethical questions that arise out of nursing practice. Nursing ethics problems arise from technological advances, the needs of a multicultural population, cost containment efforts in health care, the nature of nursing work, and the nature of the nursing profession.

Several ethical theories guide discussion of ethical issues. Consequentialist theories are moral theories in which the rightness or wrongness of an action depends on the consequences of the act, rather than on the nature of the act itself. Deontological theories consider an action to be right or wrong independent of its consequences. Feminist ethics asserts that focusing too much on deontological principles distracts one from dealing with larger social issues and that objectivity is impossible. An ethics-of-care directs attention to a patient's specific situation viewed within the context of his or her life narrative. It emphasizes feelings, but not at the expense of some conventional ethical principles, such as autonomy or beneficence.

Nurses can obtain ethical guidance from professional codes of ethics, standards of practice, and the American Hospital Association's *Patient Care Partnership*. Specific ethical issues the nurse is likely to encounter may involve AIDS, abortion, allocation of resources, issues of confidentiality, end-of-life issues (e.g., advance directives, DNAR orders, life-sustaining treatments, informed consent, organ transplantation), and reproductive technologies. One method of working through an ethical problem is to perform assessment and diagnosis, as in the nursing process; then use the mnemonic MORAL:

Massage the dilemma
Outline the options
Resolve the dilemma
Act by applying the chosen option
Look back and evaluate

Thinking Critically About Ethics and Values

The exercises in the following section allow you to practice the kind of thinking you will use as a full-spectrum nurse. Because these are critical-thinking activities, there is usually no single right answer. Discuss answers with your peers—discussion can stimulate critical thinking. If you have difficulty with any of the questions, consult with your instructor.

Caring for the Garcias

Katherine Garcia, Joe's mother, has hypertension. She is forgetful about taking her medicines. Since her husband died, she has experienced periods of depression. When asked about her medicines she often replies, "It doesn't really matter since my husband died. If I die, what difference will it make?"

Katherine was scheduled to have lunch with friends but did not arrive. When her friends called the house, they got no answer. At the end of lunch, one of Katherine's friends decided to call Joe to inform him of her concerns about his mother. Joe found his mother unresponsive on the kitchen floor. He dialed 911, and she was brought to the hospital by ambulance. At the hospital, the emergency department (ED) doctor tells Joe that his mother has had a massive stroke brought on by uncontrolled hypertension. He asks Joe whether Katherine has an advance directive or living will. Katherine has neither. The physician asks Joe to consider what level of care to offer his mother. He tells Joe that comprehensive treatment would include intubation, mechanical ventilation, and tube feeding support. He feels it is unlikely that she will experience significant recovery from this stroke.

Joe tells you, "I want everything done for my mother. I lost my father this year, and I'm not going to lose her, too." Flordelisa reminds you that Katherine has been depressed since her husband died and has expressed a desire to die. Because Joe and Flordelisa are not in agreement about the course of action, no decision is communicated. Katherine's condition continues to deteriorate, and the ED physician feels he must intubate her, place her on a ventilator, and admit her to the ICU based on policy.

A. You are aware of Katherine's statements and her poor compliance with treatment. What, if any, concerns do you have about this course of action?

B. Katherine continues to decline. Joe is informed that the "only thing keeping his mother alive is the ventilator and IV medicines." Do you consider this heroic treatment?

C. How would you approach Joe to speak with him about how he is feeling?

D. Joe and Floredelisa have asked to meet with the team providing care to Katherine. They announce that they would like all the "heroic measures to end." They request that Katherine be allowed to die. Could you participate in this care? What actions would you be comfortable with? What actions would you be uncomfortable with?

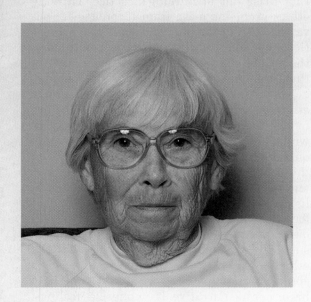

1 Some examples of ethical issues you may encounter are end-of-life issues, abortion or other reproductive issues, breaches of patient confidentiality, and incompetent or illegal practices of colleagues. Stop for a moment and think about a time when you have witnessed an ethical challenge in the clinical area.

a Describe the situation.

b How well equipped did you feel to handle the situation?

c What guided your thoughts and actions?

2 At the beginning of this chapter, Alan ("Meet Your Patients") a teenager, had been injured in a soccer game. Without a blood transfusion, he may die, but because his family is of the Jehovah's Witness faith, Alan's parents have refused to sign permission for his transfusion. Taking each of the abilities required for ethical agency, state whether or not you think these people have the abilities listed below: Alan, Alan's parents, the physician, the nurse. Explain your thinking. An ethical agent must be able to:

a Perceive the difference between good and evil, right and wrong.

Alan

Parents

Physician/surgeon

Nurse

thinking critically about ethics & values

b Understand abstract moral principles.

Alan

Parents

Physician/surgeon

Nurse

c Reason and apply moral principles to make decisions, weigh alternatives, and plan ways to achieve goals.

Alan

Parents

Physician/surgeon

Nurse

d Decide and choose freely.

Alan

Parents

Physician/surgeon

Nurse

e Act according to his choice; this assumes both the power and the capability to act.

Alan

Parents

Physician/surgeon

Nurse

3 Consider Alan's situation again. Analyze the situation (a) using a deontological framework and moral principles, and (b) using a utilitarian framework. Focus on this question: Is it ethical to try hard to influence the parents to consent to allow a blood transfusion?

a Deontology

b Utilitarianism

c Did you reach a different conclusion depending on the framework you selected?

4 You are a busy nurse caring for a team of eight patients. One patient is the mother of the hospital administrator. She had surgery 3 days ago and is progressing nicely, but she is very demanding and requires a great deal of assistance to be repositioned in bed and to move from bed to chair. She has frequent visitors, including children and young grandchildren. In the next room is a young Haitian woman whose bill is paid by Medicaid. She has a history of drug abuse and had surgery just this morning. She speaks little English and seems very anxious. She is experiencing nausea and pain and needs a transfusion of a unit of packed blood cells this evening. Her boyfriend is at the desk requesting to bring her 3-year-old daughter to the unit so that she may see her mother. The visiting policy says that children must be at least 12 years old to visit the unit. Consider what aspects of justice apply to this situation and how it might be most equitably handled. Focus on the principle of justice.

5 An example of the feminist ethical approach arises in deciding whether to allocate federal healthcare resources to younger people (e.g., education, day care, free immunizations) or to older adults (e.g., prescription drug insurance, long-term care). Feminist reasoning would be as follows:

- In the United States more older adults are women than men.
- Older women tend to be poorer and are more likely to be alone than are men.
- Therefore, if health care for older adults were to be rationed, it would negatively affect women more than men.
- Therefore, it would be unfair and unethical to allocate more resources to younger people than to older adults.

a Analyze this decision using a deontological framework. Explain your reasoning, as was done above.

b Analyze this decision using a consequentialist framework. Explain your reasoning.

6 Deception can take different forms, from intentional lying to nondisclosure of information or partial disclosure of information. Think about your duty to tell the truth. Is there ever a time when being completely honest is not the best nursing intervention? Do you consider withholding information the same as lying?

7 Review the following scenario. Examine your self-knowledge, and work through the steps of the values clarification process (choosing, prizing, and acting). An older couple with no other children learn that their unborn child has Down syndrome. The couple need to make a difficult decision because the mother is 18 weeks' pregnant.

a How would you feel about this couple if they chose to have this child and insisted on doing everything possible to keep the baby alive even if it is born with severe handicaps?

b Do you think that your professional relationship with this couple would change if they chose to terminate the pregnancy?

C   How can you help the couple clarify their values?

1. List alternatives.

2. Examine the possible consequences of the alternative choices.

3. Choose freely.

4. Feel good about the choice that has been made.

5. Affirm the choice to others.

6. Act on the choice.

7. Act with a consistent pattern.

Practical Knowledge
knowing how

Practical knowledge in nursing ethics primarily involves communication and problem-solving skills. We have included one model of ethical decision making, as well as guidelines for patient advocacy, for your quick reference in clinical situations.

TECHNIQUES

TECHNIQUE 44–1 Using the MORAL Model for Ethical Decision Making

- **M—Massage the dilemma.** Identify and define the issues in the dilemma. Consider the options of all the major players in the dilemma and their value systems. This includes patients, family members, nurses, physicians, clergy, and other interdisciplinary healthcare members.
- **O—Outline the options.** Examine all the options, including those that are less realistic and conflicting. This stage is designed only for considering options and not for making final decisions.
- **R—Resolve the dilemma.** Review issues and options, applying basic principles of ethics to each option. Decide the best option based on the views of all those concerned in the dilemma.

- **A—Act by applying the chosen option.** This step is usually the most difficult because it requires actual implementation, whereas the previous steps allow only for dialogue and discussion.
- **L—Look back; reflect on the entire process.** Evaluate all steps, including the implementation. No process is complete without thorough evaluation. Ensure that those involved are able to follow through on the final option. If not, a second decision may be required and the process must begin again at the first step.

Sources: Adapted from Yoder-Wise, P. (2003). *Leading and managing in nursing* (3rd ed.). St Louis: Mosby; and Tschundin, V. (2003). *Ethics in nursing: The caring relationship* (2nd ed.). Oxford, England: Butterworth & Heinemann.

TECHNIQUE 44–2 Using Guidelines for Advocacy

The following principles will help you to function effectively as an advocate.

1. Keep the moral principle of patient autonomy always in mind.
2. Know and document the facts of the case.
3. Know the arguments of those who oppose the patient. Use role playing to develop a strategy for responding to the arguments.
4. Have a sound base of support for your actions. Be familiar with any policies or laws that apply.
5. Form a coalition of allies, if you can. Get consultation. Communicate, inform, and clarify their collaborative roles.
6. Intervene high enough in the hierarchy to get the job done. If the difficulty is with a physician or an organizational policy, merely going to the charge nurse will not be enough. You will need to communicate with nurse administrators or other agency administrators.
7. Demonstrate to the system how it is defeating its own goals (e.g., for patient care).
8. Avoid getting into a power contest if possible (use steps 1 through 7 first). If you must, decide how far you need to go and whether you are willing to go that far. You will need to enlist people with more power in the system than you have (e.g., family members, physicians, administrators).
9. Be aware of client vulnerability. When possible, avoid confrontation. If there is risk for the client (as in a power contest), be sure the client is aware of his risks and possible gains; then let him choose how far to take the situation.
10. Have alternative actions. Assess risks realistically. Weigh them against potential gains.

What Are the Main Points in This Chapter?

- Ethics is a formal process for deciding right and wrong conduct in situations where issues of values and morals arise.

- Nursing ethics refers to ethical questions that arise out of nursing practice.

- Morals are learned and internalized throughout the life span. Carol Gilligan proposed that moral development and reasoning are different among men and women.

- Ethical agency is the ability to make ethical choices and to be responsible for one's ethical actions. In practice, nurses sometimes make moral decisions that they are not able to carry out.

- A whistleblower is a person "who identifies an incompetent, unethical, or illegal situation, or actions of others, in the workplace and reports it to someone who may have the power to stop it" (Ahern & McDonald, 2002, p. 314).

- Nursing ethics problems arise from technological advances, the needs of a multicultural population, cost containment efforts in health care, the nature of nursing work, and the nature of the nursing profession.

- Nurses have complex obligations and multiple complex relationships within healthcare organizations (e.g., with employers, physicians, patients, families, and other nurses).

- Ethical decisions are affected by a person's values, moral frameworks and principles, and professional guidelines.

- A value is a belief that you have about the worth of something; a value is highly prized and expressed through behaviors, feelings, and decisions.

- Values are transmitted through social interaction.

- Six important moral principles are autonomy, nonmaleficence, beneficence, fidelity, veracity, and justice.

- Consequentialist theories are moral theories in which the rightness or wrongness of an action depends on the consequences of the act, rather than on the nature of the act itself.

- The principle of utility states that a "good" act is one that produces the greatest good for the greatest number of people.

- Deontological theories consider an action to be right or wrong independent of its consequences.

- Feminist ethics asserts that focusing on deontological principles distracts one from dealing with larger social issues and that objectivity is impossible.

- An ethics of care directs attention to a patient's specific situation viewed within the context of his or her life narrative. It emphasizes feelings, but not at the expense of some conventional ethical principles, such as autonomy or beneficence.

- Nurses can obtain ethical guidance from professional codes of ethics, standards of practice, and the American Hospital Association's *Patient Care Partnership.*

- Specific ethical issues the nurse is likely to encounter may involve AIDS, abortion, allocation of resources, issues of confidentiality, end-of-life issues (e.g., advance directives, DNAR orders, life-sustaining treatments, informed consent, organ transplantation), and reproductive technologies.

- Values clarification is the process of becoming conscious of and naming one's values. Nurses can assist clients with values clarification.

- A full value must be chosen freely, cherished and made known to others, translated into behaviors, and integrated into lifestyle.

- Not all moral problems are dilemmas. A dilemma is a particular kind of moral problem: It is a painful situation in which a choice must be made between two equally undesirable actions. There is no clearly right or wrong option.

- One method of working through an ethical problem is to perform assessment and diagnosis, as in the nursing process; then use the mnemonic MORAL: Massage the dilemma, Outline the options, Resolve the dilemma, Act by applying the chosen option, and Look back and evaluate.

- A good compromise preserves the integrity of all parties when there is disagreement among them in a moral situation.

- Nurses should be patient advocates because (1) their professional role requires it, (2) they have special knowledge that the patient does not have, and (3) they have a special relationship with patients.

- The nurse's role as an advocate is to inform, support, and communicate.

Knowledge Map

Ethics in Nursing

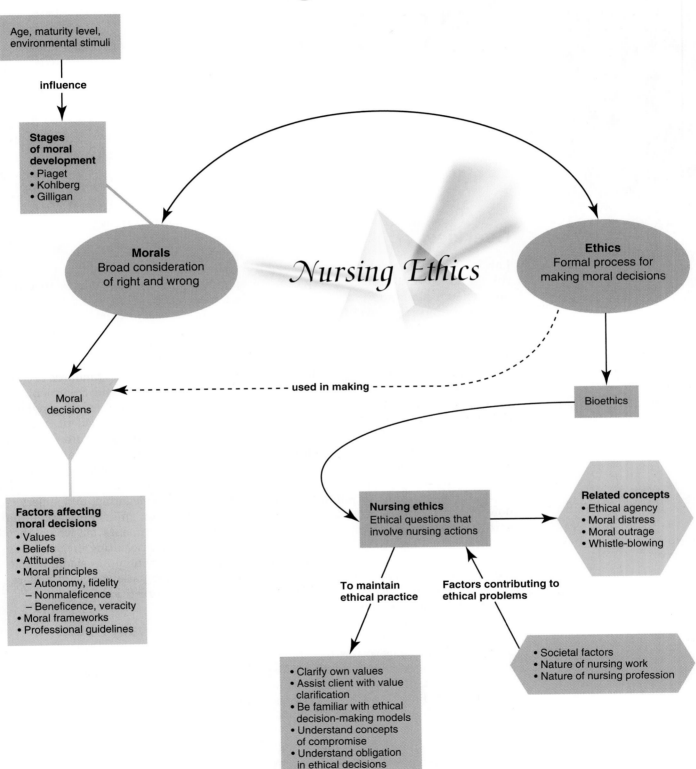

Age, maturity level, environmental stimuli

influence

Stages of moral development
- Piaget
- Kohlberg
- Gilligan

Morals
Broad consideration of right and wrong

Nursing Ethics

Ethics
Formal process for making moral decisions

Moral decisions

- - - **used in making** - - -

Bioethics

Factors affecting moral decisions
- Values
- Beliefs
- Attitudes
- Moral principles
  - Autonomy, fidelity
  - Nonmaleficence
  - Beneficence, veracity
- Moral frameworks
- Professional guidelines

Nursing ethics
Ethical questions that involve nursing actions

Related concepts
- Ethical agency
- Moral distress
- Moral outrage
- Whistle-blowing

To maintain ethical practice

Factors contributing to ethical problems

- Clarify own values
- Assist client with value clarification
- Be familiar with ethical decision-making models
- Understand concepts of compromise
- Understand obligation in ethical decisions

- Societal factors
- Nature of nursing work
- Nature of nursing profession

Legal Issues

Overview

Law is a set of enforceable principles and rules established to protect society. State laws affecting nursing practice include mandatory reporting laws, Good Samaritan laws, and safe harbor laws. In most states, nurses are obligated legally to report suspected or actual patient abuse and also to report impaired health professionals.

State boards of nursing, under the state's nurse practice act, are responsible for licensing, credentialing, and disciplinary procedures involving nurses and nursing. Standards of care look to what a reasonable and prudent nurse would do in the same or similar situation. They are based on mandatory standards (e.g., in nurse practice acts) and voluntary standards (e.g., standards set by professional organizations such as the American Nurses Association).

Federal and state courts develop common law. Common law may be classified as civil or criminal law. Criminal law deals with wrongs or offenses against society. Civil law deals with wrongs to individuals. Negligence is a wrong committed against an individual by one who has failed to use ordinary care. Malpractice is negligence committed against an individual by a licensed professional, involving a duty, breach of that duty, an injury, and damages. Nursing malpractice claims, in general, result from failure to maintain the standard of practice. Such claims include failure to assess, diagnose, plan,

implement, and evaluate patient responses to care. A nurse may be involved in a malpractice claim as a defendant, a fact witness, or an expert witness.

Nurses can help reduce their legal risks by developing open, honest, respectful, caring relationships with patients and families; observing standards of care; avoiding medication and treatment errors; reporting and documenting patient care properly; filing incident reports properly; being sure to obtain informed consent; attending to patient safety; maintaining confidentiality and privacy; providing patient education and counseling; assigning, delegating, and supervising according to guidelines; accepting only those assignments for which they are qualified; participating in continuing education; observing professional boundaries; reporting patient abuse; and reporting unsafe practitioners.

Thinking Critically About Legal Issues

The exercises in the following section allow you to practice the kind of thinking you will use as a full-spectrum nurse. Because these are critical-thinking activities, there is usually no single right answer. Discuss answers with your peers—discussion can stimulate critical thinking. If you have difficulty with any of the questions, consult with your instructor.

Caring for the Garcias

Joe and Flordelisa Garcia have requested an appointment with you, the nurse at the Family Medicine Clinic, to discuss advance directives. Their experience with Joe's mother, Katherine, has created concerns about end-of-life care.

A. Joe asks you, "Do you think it's appropriate to create an advance directive at my age?" How would you respond?

B. Joe tells you that he believes in "natural death." He states, "I don't want extraordinary measures, and I never want to be resuscitated." Flordelisa responds that she is extremely uncomfortable with blanket statements about treatment. "If he got hit by a car or had some accident, I would want you to do everything in your power to treat him.

I couldn't carry out his wishes," she states. What actions should you take to help Joe and Flordelisa resolve this discrepancy?

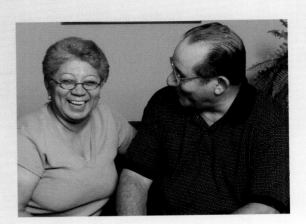

1 Imagine that you are the nurse in the "Meet Your Nurse Role Model" in Volume 1 scenario. You are a nurse employed by a temporary agency assigned to a nursing home for a 12-hour shift. On arrival, you discover that the registered nurse assigned for the previous shift suddenly quit, leaving two unlicensed professional assistants (UAPs) to provide patient care and complete the narcotics check. The UAPs inform you that you will be assigned to 20 patients requiring heavy care, with one UAP for the 12-hour shift. The nursing supervisor will not arrive for one hour, and the administrator for another hour and a half. You make a decision to not accept the assignment, to report the decision and reasons to your agency supervisor, and to leave the nursing home immediately.

Use the critical-thinking model to identify questions to ask yourself in reflecting and deciding what to do.

VOL 1   Go to Chapter 2, **Table 2–2,** in Volume 1.

a What questions do you need to ask about context?

b What questions do you need to ask about credible sources?

c What questions do you need to ask about considering alternatives?

d What questions do you need to ask about analyzing your assumptions?

e What questions do you need to ask about reflecting and deciding?

2 Analyze this passage from Volume 1:

> The Health Care Quality Improvement Act of 1986 (HCQIA), implemented in 1990, created the National Practitioner Data Bank (NPDB). The NPDB collects and provides information related to (1) medical malpractice payments made on behalf of healthcare providers; (2) adverse actions taken against clinical privileges of physicians, osteopaths, and dentists; and (3) actions by professional societies adversely affecting membership. This law is designed to protect patients by providing knowledge of practitioners who have been sanctioned for not meeting legal standards of care in the past. Reporting of this information to the NPDB is mandatory, and failure to do so will result in fines and penalties (Fedorka & Resnick, 2000, pp. 105–106). (*Note:* This applies only to advanced practice nurses.)

• How do you think the HCQIA functions?

• What rights does it help protect?

3 Imagine that you are working in a large medical center in an area where there have been several robberies and assaults in the past 6 months, mostly late at night. Although the parking lot is nearly a block from the employees' exit and is not well lighted, there is only one security guard on duty outside the hospital after 10:00 P.M. Despite protests from employees, all the way up the chain of command, no efforts are being made to improve lighting or to hire more security guards. What standards and laws might be helpful to the employees?

4 George Agnew, 75 years old, is admitted to the emergency department after being involved in a serious car accident. His wife is with him, and she is very upset—to the point of being hysterical. It is likely that Mr. Agnew will die, but physicians are considering whether to place him on a ventilator in the next hour or so. You need to know Mr. Agnew's wishes on this issue, but he is not conscious. The charge nurse tells you not to ask Mrs. Agnew because it will just upset her more.

a What is going on in the situation that may influence the outcome?

b What factors may influence your behavior and others' behavior in this situation?

c What values or biases do you have that influence your behavior in this situation?

d Where might you get the information you need instead of asking Mrs. Agnew?

e What would you do? What legal support, if any, do you have?

5 For each of the following concepts, use critical thinking to describe how or why it is important to nurses, patients, or legal issues. Note that these are *not* to be merely definitions.

Civil law

The U.S. Constitution Bill of Rights and the *Patient Care Partnership*

The ANA Code of Ethics; the ANA Standards of Practice; and the ANA Bill of Rights for Registered Nurses

Patient advocacy

Battery

Vicarious liability

Practical Knowledge
knowing how

TECHNIQUES

TECHNIQUE 45–1 | **Using Equipment Safely**

The following will help you to ensure proper and safe use of equipment:
1. Obtain appropriate training on equipment use.
2. Follow the healthcare agency's protocols, policies, and procedures on the use of the equipment.
3. Follow the manufacturer's operating instructions.
4. Be sure that the medical equipment has been properly inspected.
5. Perform safety checks regularly and before use.

6. Position and use equipment properly during treatment.
7. Know how the equipment functions; be alert to signs that it is not working properly.
8. Make sure that rooms are not cluttered with equipment.
9. Follow agency policies regarding equipment brought from the patient's home (e.g., hair dryers, electric shavers, radios); usually these should be inspected for proper grounding and safe cords.

TECHNIQUE 45–2 | **Tips for Avoiding Malpractice**

- Develop open, honest, respectful, caring relationships with patients and families. Patients are less likely to sue if they feel that you were caring and professional. Angry patients who feel mistreated are more likely to bring suit.
- Second to communication and relationships, careful, thorough documentation is the best defense should a lawsuit occur:
  1. Use and document all steps of the nursing process.
  2. Thorough documentation is especially important for patients who will not comply with treatments or who complain a lot.
  3. Courts assume that if care is not documented, it was not given.
- Know and follow applicable laws: (1) federal laws, (2) your state's nurse practice act (perform only the activities within your scope of practice and competence).
- Know and follow agency policies and procedures.
- Know and follow standards of care set forth in the state nurse practice act, professional organizations

in your area of practice, literature, agency policy, and so on.
- Follow the "six rights" of medication administration (see Chapter 23).
- Perform falls risk assessments, document, and take measures to ensure patient safety.
- Recognize "problem" patients. Try to identify the basic problem or complaint and intervene to resolve it.
- Follow medical orders, but clarify them as needed. Do not implement a questionable order or one you do not understand.
- Don't blame or criticize other healthcare providers in the presence of patients (e.g., "Sorry you didn't get your pain medication. The night shift was a little short-staffed last night.")
- Maintain patient privacy and confidentiality.
- Don't make statements that may appear to be an admission of guilt (e.g., "Omigosh, I forgot to shut off that IV!").

▶

TECHNIQUE 45–2   Tips for Avoiding Malpractice *(continued)*

- Stay competent in your area of practice; for example, attend continuing education and inservice programs to improve your knowledge and skills.
- Don't accept a clinical assignment that you think you are not competent to perform. Evaluate your assignment with your supervisor if there is a question.
- Recognize significant assessment cues, and notify primary care providers of changes in the patient's condition or patient complaints.
- Document the time and content of telephone conversations with other healthcare providers.

- Send copies only, never originals, of records and reports requested by other professionals.

Sources: Aiken, T. D. (2004). *Legal, ethical, and political issues in nursing* (2nd ed.). Philadelphia: F. A. Davis Company; Carson, W. Y. (2001). Nursing malpractice: Protect yourself. *American Journal of Nursing, 101*(8), 81; Chitty, K. K. (1993). *Professional nursing: Concepts and challenges* (2nd ed.). Philadelphia: Saunders; Croke, E. M. (2003). Nurses, negligence, and malpractice. *American Journal of Nursing, 103*(9): 54–63; and Eskreis, T. R. (1998). Seven common legal pitfalls in nursing. *American Journal of Nursing, 98*(4), 34–40.

TECHNIQUE 45–3   Guidelines for Documenting Care

To be considered accurate and complete, your reporting and documentation of patient care must address the following:

1. Patient status (e.g., symptoms and responses to treatments)
2. The nursing care given
3. Orders of physicians, dentists, or podiatrists
4. Medications and treatments
5. Patient responses
6. Consultations with other members of the healthcare team regarding patient status

You might find helpful the FACT mnemonic for documenting care. When documenting care, you must be:
   Factual
   Accurate
   Complete
   Timely

Source: Helm, A. (2003). *Nursing malpractice: Sidestepping legal minefields.* Philadelphia: Lippincott, Williams & Wilkins, pp. 1–33.

What Are the Main Points in This Chapter?

- Law is a set of enforceable principles and rules established to protect society. Laws derive from the Constitution and from federal and state sources.

- Federal and state legislatures develop statutes.

- Some federal laws that provide protection for nurses and patients include the following: Emergency Medical Treatment and Active Labor Act (EMTALA), the Health Care Quality Improvement Act of 1986 (HCQIA), the Americans with Disabilities Act (ADA), the Patient Self-Determination Act (PSDA), the U.S. Department of Health and Human Services (DHHS) "Privacy Rule" (2004), the Newborns' and Mothers' Health Protection Act of 1996 (NMHPA), and the National Labor Relations Act of 1935 (NLRA).

- State laws affecting nursing practice include mandatory reporting laws, Good Samaritan laws, and safe harbor laws.

- In most states, nurses are obligated legally to report suspected or actual patient abuse and also to report impaired health professionals.

- State boards of nursing, under the state's nurse practice act, are responsible for licensing, credentialing, and disciplinary procedures involving nurses and nursing.

- Standards of care look to what a reasonable and prudent nurse would do in the same or similar situation. They are based on mandatory standards (e.g., in nurse practice acts) and voluntary standards (e.g., those set by professional organizations such as the American Nurses Association).

- Federal and state courts develop common law.

- Common law may be classified as civil or criminal law.

- Criminal law deals with wrongs or offenses against society.

- Civil law deals with wrongs to individuals.

- Intentional torts include assault and battery, false imprisonment, fraud, and invasion of privacy.

- Negligence is a wrong committed against an individual by one who has failed to use ordinary care.

- Malpractice is negligence committed against an individual by a licensed professional involving a duty, breach of that duty, an injury, and damages.

- Malpractice claims, in general, result from failure to maintain the standard of practice, including failure to assess, diagnose, plan, implement, and evaluate patient responses to care.

- A nurse may be involved in a malpractice claim as a defendant, a fact witness, or an expert witness.

- Nurses can help reduce their legal risks by developing open, honest, respectful, caring relationships with patients and families and observing standards of care.

Knowledge Map

Legal Issues in Nursing

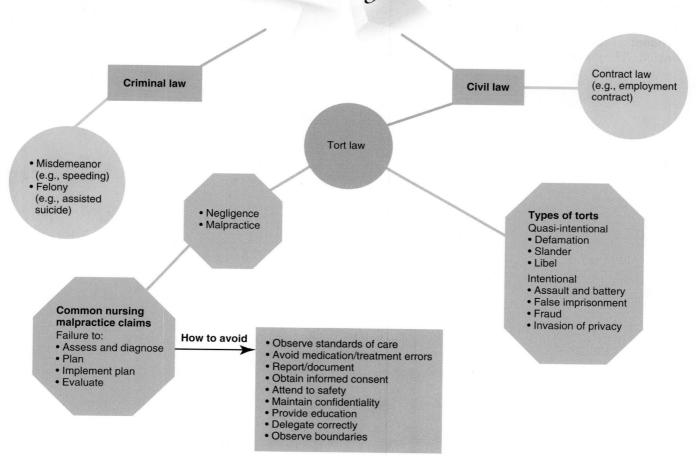

State laws
- Mandatory reporting
- Good Samaritan
- Nurse Practice Acts
  – Credentialing
  – Licensing
  – Discipline

Standards of practice
- What a reasonable and prudent nurse would do
- Mandatory = Nurse Practice Act
- Voluntary = ANA

Federal laws
- Bill of Rights
- EMTALA
- National Practitioner Data Bank
- ADA
- Patient Self-Determination Act
- HIPPA
- Newborn/Mothers Protection Act
- National Labor Relations Act

Other guidelines
- Agency policies and procedures
- Nursing Code of Ethics
- Patient Care Partnership
- ANA Bill of Rights for Nurses

Laws and Regulations

Criminal law

Civil law

Contract law (e.g., employment contract)

Tort law

- Misdemeanor (e.g., speeding)
- Felony (e.g., assisted suicide)

- Negligence
- Malpractice

Types of torts
Quasi-intentional
- Defamation
- Slander
- Libel

Intentional
- Assault and battery
- False imprisonment
- Fraud
- Invasion of privacy

Common nursing malpractice claims
Failure to:
- Assess and diagnose
- Plan
- Implement plan
- Evaluate

How to avoid →
- Observe standards of care
- Avoid medication/treatment errors
- Report/document
- Obtain informed consent
- Attend to safety
- Maintain confidentiality
- Provide education
- Delegate correctly
- Observe boundaries

Critical-Thinking Model

Process	Definition	Questions for Focusing
Contextual awareness (deciding what to observe and consider)	This includes an awareness of what's happening in the context of the situation, including values, cultural issues, and environmental influences.	• What is going on in the situation that may influence the outcome? • What factors may influence my behavior and others' behavior in this situation? • What about this situation have I seen before? What is different? • Who should be involved in order to improve the outcome? • What else was happening at the same time that affected me in this situation? • What happened just before this incident that made a difference? • What emotional responses influenced how I reacted in this situation? • What changes in behavior alerted me that something was wrong?
Inquiry (based on credible sources)	This involves applying standards of good reasoning to your thinking when analyzing a situation and evaluating your actions.	• How do I go about getting the information I need? • What framework should I use to organize my information? • Do I have enough knowledge to decide? If not, what do I need to know? • Have I used a valid, reliable source of information (e.g., patient, other professionals, references)? • Did I (do I need to) validate the data (e.g., with the client)? • What else do I need to know? What information is missing? • Are the data accurate? Precise? • What's important and what's not important in this situation? • Did I consider professional, ethical, and legal standards? • Have I jumped to conclusions?
Considering alternatives	This involves exploring and imagining as many alternatives as you can think of for the given situation.	• What is one possible explanation for [insert what is happening or what happened]? • What are other explanations for what is happening? • What is one thing I could do in this situation? • What are two more possibilities/alternatives? • Are there others who might help me develop more alternatives? • Of the possible actions I am considering, which one is most reasonable? Why are the others not as reasonable? • Of the possible actions I am considering, which one is most likely to achieve the desired outcomes?
Analyzing assumptions	This involves recognizing and analyzing assumptions you are making about the situation, and examining the beliefs that underlie your choices.	• What have I (or others) taken for granted in this situation? • Which beliefs/values are shaping my assumptions? • What assumptions contributed to the problem in this situation? • What rationale supports my assumptions? • How will I know my assumption is correct? • What biases do I have that may affect my thinking and my decisions in this situation?
Reflecting skeptically and deciding what to do	This involves questioning, analyzing, and reflecting on the rationale for your decisions.	• What aspects of this situation require the most careful attention? • What else might work in this situation? • Am I sure of my interpretation in this situation? • Why is (was) it important to intervene? • What rationale do I have for my decisions? • In priority order, what should I do in this situation and why? • Having decided what was wrong/happening, what is the best response? • What might I delegate in this situation? • What got me started taking some action? • What priorities were missed? • What was done? Why was it done? • What would I do differently after reflecting on this situation?

Sources: Model based on Brookfield, S. D. (1991). *Developing critical thinkers.* San Francisco: Jossey-Bass; McDonald, M. E. (2002). *Systematic assessment of learning outcomes: Developing multiple-choice exams.* Boston: Jones and Bartlett Publishers; Paul, R. W. (1993). *Critical thinking: What every person needs to survive in a rapidly changing world* (3rd ed.). Santa Rosa, CA: Foundation for Critical Thinking; Raingruber, B. & Haffer, A. (2001). *Using your head to land on your feet.* Philadelphia: F. A. Davis Company; and Wilkinson, J. M. (2001). *Nursing process and critical thinking* (3rd ed.). Upper Saddle River, NJ: Prentice Hall.

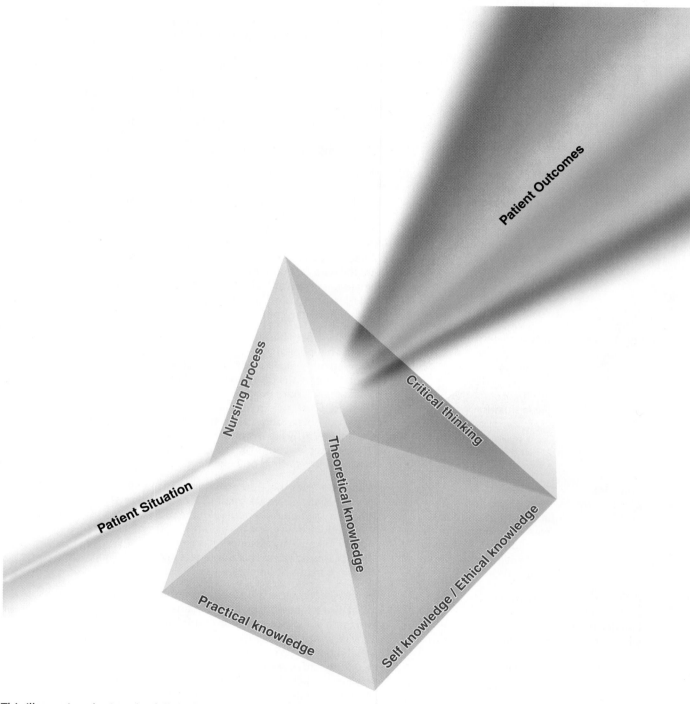

This illustration depicts the full-spectrum model of nursing used throughout this learning package. A full-spectrum nurse uses critical thinking and the nursing process to apply various types of knowledge (theoretical, practical, ethical, and self-knowledge) to the patient situation to bring about desired health outcomes. Truly, thinking and doing.

Bibliography

CHAPTER 1

Aiken, L. H. (1990). Charting the future of hospital nursing. *Image: Journal of Nursing Scholarship* 22, no. 2: 72–78.

Alberta Association of Registered Nurses. (1998). *Bylaws.* Edmonton, Alberta, Canada: Author.

American Association for the History of Nursing. (2001). *Nursing history in the curriculum: Preparing nurses for the 21st century.* Philadelphia: Author.

American Hospital Association (2002). *Hospital Statistics, 2002.* Chicago: AHA.

American Nurses Association. (1980). Nursing's social policy statement. Washington, DC: Author.

American Nurses Association (1991). *Nursing's agenda for health care reform,* Kansas City, Mo. The Association.

American Nurses Association. (1995). Nursing's social policy statement. Washington, DC: Author.

American Nurses Association. (1998). *Managed care: Challenges and opportunities for nursing. www.nursingworld.or/readroom/fsmgdcar.htm*

American Nurses Association. (2001). *Code of ethics for nurses.* Working draft#10A. Washington, DC: Author. Retrieved October 10, 2002, from: *http://nursingworld.org/ethics/chcode10.htm#9_1*

American Nurses Association. (2002). *Nursing's agenda for the future.* Washington, D.C.: The Association.

American Nurses Association. (2004). *Standards of clinical nursing practice* (3rd ed.). Washington, DC: American Nurses Publishing.

Anthony, M. K., Standing, T. S., & Hertz, J. E. (2001). Nurses' beliefs about their abilities to delegate within changing models of care. *Journal of Continuing Education in Nursing, 32*(5), 210–215.

Association for Registered Nurses in Newfoundland and Labrador. (2002). *Standards for nursing practice.* St John's, NF: Author.

Benner, P. (1984). *From novice to expert: Excellence and power in clinical nursing practice.* Menlo Park, CA: Addison-Wesley.

Benner, P., & Wrubel, J. (1989). *The primacy of caring.* Menlo Park, CA: Addison-Wesley.

Bodenheimer, T. S., & Grumbach, K. (2004). *Understanding health policy: A clinical approach.* Stamford, CT: Appleton and Lange.

Bright, M. A. (2002). *Holistic health and healing.* Philadelphia: F. A. Davis Company.

Brush, B. L., & Capezuti, E. (2001). Historical analysis of siderail use in American hospitals. *Journal of Nursing Scholarship, 33*(4), 381–385.

Brush, B., Lynaugh, J. E., Boschma, G., Rafferty, A. M., Stuart, M., & Tomes, N. J. (1999). *Nurses of all nations: A history of the International Council of Nurses, 1899–1999.* Hagerstown, MD: Lippincott Williams & Jenkins.

Buerhaus, P. I. 1997. How changes in payment systems are affecting nurses. In McCloskey, J. C., Grace, H. K., ed. *Current issues in nursing,* 5th ed. St. Louis: C.V. Mosby.

Canadian Nurses Association. (1987). *A definition of nursing practice. Standards for nursing practice.* Ottawa, Ontario, Canada: Author.

Canadian Nurses Association. (1993). *The scope of nursing practice: A review of issues and trends.* Ottawa, Ontario, Canada: Author.

Carnegie, M. E. (1995). *The path we tread: Blacks in nursing 1854–1994* (3rd ed.). New York: National League for Nursing.

Chambers, P. (1958). *A doctor alone: A biography of Elizabeth Blackwell, the first woman doctor.* London: Abelard-Schuman.

Christy, T. (1975). The methodology of historical research: A brief foundation. *Nursing Research, 24*(3), 189–192.

College of Nurses of Ontario. (1996). *Professional standards for registered nurses and registered practical nurses in Ontario.* Toronto, Ontario, Canada: Author.

Curran, C. (1997). The future of academic health centers in a cost-driven market. In McCloskey, J. C. and Grace, H. K. editors. *Current issues in nursing,* 5th ed. St. Louis: Mosby.

Department of Health and Human Services (DHHS). (2003). Annual update of the HHS poverty guidelines: *http://aspe.os.dhhs.gov/povertyh/poverty.htm*

Department of Health and Human Services (DHHS). (2003). Healthy People 2010: *http://dhhs.gov*

Dietz, L. D., & Lehozky, A. R. (1967). *History and modern nursing.* Philadelphia: F. A. Davis Company.

Dock, L. L., & Stewart, I. M. (1938). *A short history of nursing* (4th ed.). New York: Putnam.

Donahue, M. P. (1985). *Nursing: The finest art. An illustrated history.* St. Louis: C. V. Mosby.

Donaldson, S. K., & Crowley, D. (1978). The discipline of nursing. *Nursing Outlook, 26*(2), 113–120.

Fuchs, V. R. 1993. *The future of health policy.* Cambridge, MA: Harvard University Press.

Griffin, G. J., & Griffin, J. K. (1973). *History and trends of professional nursing* (7th ed.). St. Louis: C. V. Mosby.

Health Care Financing Agency (HCFA). (1998). *National health expenditures projections: 1998–2008. www.hcfa.gov/stats/nhe%2Dproj/proj1998/hilites.htm*

Health Resources and Services Administration. (2001). *The registered nurse population: Findings from the national sample survey of registered nurses.* Washington, DC: Bureau of Health Professions.

Henderson, V. (1966). *The nature of nursing.* New York: Macmillan.

Hicks, L. L. and Boles, K. E. 1984. Why health economics? *Nursing Economic$ 2*(3): 175–180.

Huntington, J. A. (1997). Glossary for managed care. *On-line Journal of Issues in Nursing. www.nursingworld/ojin/tpc2 gls.htm*

International Council of Nurses. (2003). *ICN definition of nursing.* Retrieved December 5, 2003, from: *http://www.icn.ch/definition.htm*

Jameton, A. (1984). *Nursing practice: The ethical issues.* Englewood Cliffs, NJ: Prentice Hall.

Joint Commission on Accreditation of Healthcare Organizations. (2000). *Manual of hospital accreditation: 2000 standards.* Chicago: The Commission.

Jonas, S., & Kovner, A. R. (2002). *Healthcare delivery in the U.S.* (7th ed.). New York: Springer.

Kalisch, B., & Kalisch, P. (1995). *The advance of American nursing* (3rd ed.). Philadelphia: Lippincott.

Mahaffey, E. H. (2002). The relevance of associate degree nursing education: Past, present, future. *Online Journal of Issues in Nursing, 7*(2), 3.

Meadus, R. J. (2000). Men in nursing: Barriers to recruitment. *Nursing Forum, 3* 35(3), 5.

Meleis, A. I. (1991). *Theoretical nursing: Development and progress.* Philadelphia: Lippincott.

Nemmers, E. E. (1970). *Dictionary of economics and business.* Totowa, JH: Littlefield, Adams and Co.

Nightingale, F. (1860). *Notes on nursing: What it is, and what it is not*. New York: D. Appleton and Company.

Nightingale, F. (1876). *Notes on nursing for the labouring classes*. London: Harrison.

Northwest Territories Registered Nurses Association. (1995). *Standards of practice for registered nurses*. Yellowknife, Northwest Territories, Canada: Author.

Nurses Association of New Brunswick. (1998). *Standards for nursing practice*. Fredericton, New Brunswick, Canada: Author.

Office of National Cost Estimates: Revisions to the national health accounts and methodology. *Health Care Financing Review* 11 (4): 42–54. HCFA Pub. No. 03298. Office of Research and Demonstrations. Health Care Financing Administration. Washington, U.S. Government Printing Office, Summer 2000.

Pew Health Professions Commission. 1995. *Critical challenges: Revitalizing the health professions for the twenty-first century* (3rd report). Durham, NC: Author.

Pew Health Professions Commission. (1998). *Twenty-one competencies for the twenty-first century*. Durham, NC: Author.

Rasmussen, E. (2001). Picture imperfect. *Nurseweek*, May 7, 2001, 1–3.

Registered Nurses Association of British Columbia. (1998). *Standards for nursing practice in British Columbia*. Vancouver, British Columbia, Canada: Author.

Registered Nurses Association of Nova Scotia. (1996). *Standards for nursing practice*. Halifax, Nova Scotia, Canada: Author.

Reverby, S. (1987). *Ordered to care: The dilemma of American nursing 1850–1945*. Cambridge: Cambridge University Press.

Rosenberg, C. (1987). *The care of strangers*. New York: Basic Books.

Safriet, B. J. (1994). Impediments to progress in healthcare workforce policy: License and practice laws. *Inquiry, 31*(3), 310–317.

Shapiro, S. E. (2002). Viewpoint: In favor of the bachelor's degree. *American Journal of Nursing, 102*(10), 11.

Starr, P. (1982). *The social transformation of American medicine*. New York: Basic Books.

Schorr, T., & Kennedy, M. S. (1999). *100 years of American nursing: Celebrating a century of caring*. Hagerstown, MD: Lippincott Williams & Wilkins.

Stewart, I. M., & Austin, A. L. (1962). *A history of nursing* (5th ed.). New York: G. P. Putnam's Sons.

Takase, M., Kershaw, E., & Burt, L. (2002). Does public image of nurses matter? *Journal of Professional Nursing, 18*(4), 196–205.

Thomka, L. A. (2001). Graduate nurses' experiences of interactions with professional nursing staff during transition to the professional role. *Journal of Continuing Education in Nursing, 32*(1), 15–19.

U.S. Department of Commerce, International Trade Administration (2002) Health and Medical Services. *U.S. Industrial Outlook 2002*. Washington, D.C: U.S. COC.

Venes, D., & Thomas, C. L. (Eds.). (2001). *Taber's cyclopedic medical dictionary*. Philadelphia: F. A. Davis Company. Retrieved November 15, 2003, at *http://www.tabers.com/default.jsp*

Watson, J. (1981). Socialization of the nursing student in a professional nursing education programme. *Nursing Papers, 13*, 19–24.

White, W. D. (1990). The Corporatization of U.S. Hospitals: What Can We Learn from the Nineteenth Century Industrial Experience? *International Journal of Health Services* 20:85–113.

Wilkinson, J. M. (1996). The C Word. A Curriculum for the Future. *N&HC: Perspectives on Community, 17*(2), 72–77.

World Health Organization. (1984). *Health promotion: A discussion document on the concepts and principles*. Geneva, Switzerland: Author.

CHAPTER 2

Alberta Association of Registered Nurses. (1999). *Nursing: Scope and standards of practice*. Retrieved August 27, 2002, from *http://nurses.ab.ca/profconduct/npa.html*

American Nurses Association. (2004). *Nursing: Scope and standards of practice* (3rd ed.). Washington, DC: Author.

Assessment Technologies Incorporated. (1998). *Critical thinking exam* [On-line]. Retrieved from *http://www.atitesting.com/CriticalThinking.asp*

Broadbear, J. T., & Keyser, B. B. (2000). An approach to teaching for critical thinking in health education. *Journal School Health, 70*(8), 322–326.

Brookfield, S. D. (1991). *Developing critical thinkers*. San Francisco: Jossey-Bass.

Burton, A. J. (2000). Reflection: Nursing's practice and education panacea? *Journal of Advanced Nursing, 31*(5), 1009–1017.

Canadian Nurses Association. (1987). *CNA: A definition of nursing practice. Standards for nursing practice*. Ottawa, Ontario, Canada: Author.

Ennis, R. H. (2000). A super-streamlined conception of critical thinking. [On-line]. Retrieved from *http://www.criticalthinking.net/SSConcCTApr3.html*

Frauman, A. C., & Skelly, A. H. (1999). Evolution of the nursing process. *Clinical Excellence in Nursing Practice, 3*(4), 238–244.

Girot, E. A. (2000). Graduate nurses: Critical thinkers or better decision makers? *Journal of Advanced Nursing, 31*(2), 288–297.

Greenwood, J. (2000). Critical thinking and nursing scripts: The case for the development of both. *Journal of Advanced Nursing, 31*(2), 428–436.

Greenwood, J., Sullivan, J., Spence, K., & McDonald, M. (2000). Nursing scripts and the organizational influences on critical thinking: Report of a study of neonatal nurses' clinical reasoning. *Journal of Advanced Nursing, 31*(5), 1106–1114.

Heaslip, P. (1992). Creating the thinking practitioner: Critical thinking in clinical practice. Unpublished Manuscript. (ERIC Document Reproduction Service No. ED 354 822).

Hicks, F. D. (2001). Research issues. Critical thinking: Toward a nursing science perspective. *Nursing Science Quarterly, 14*(1), 14–21.

McDonald, M. E. (2002). *Systematic assessment of learning outcomes: Developing multiple-choice exams*. Boston: Jones and Bartlett Publishers.

Miller, L., & Connelly, M. (1996). *Critical thinking core concepts*. (Critical Thinking across the Curriculum Project). Lee's Summit, MO: Longview Community College.

Moore, B. N., & Parker, R. (2001). *Critical thinking* (6th ed.). Columbus, OH: McGraw-Hill.

North American Nursing Diagnosis Association. (1999). *NANDA nursing diagnoses: Definitions and classification, 1999–2000*. Philadelphia: Author.

Paul, R. W. (1988). *What, then, is critical thinking? The Eighth Annual and Sixth International Conference on Critical Thinking and Educational Reform*. Rohnert Park, CA: Center for Critical Thinking and Moral Critique, Sonoma State University.

Paul, R. W. (1990). *Critical thinking*. Rohnert Park, CA: The Center for Critical Thinking and Moral Critique, Sonoma State University.

Paul, R. W. (1993). *Critical thinking: What every person needs to survive in a rapidly changing world* (3rd ed.). Santa Rosa, CA: Foundation for Critical Thinking.

Paul, R. W., Ennis, R. H., & Norris, S. (1996). In B. Fowler (Ed.), *Critical thinking definitions*. (Critical Thinking across the Curriculum Project). Lee's Summit, MO: Longview Community College.

Platzer, H., Blake, D., & Ashford, D. (2000). An evaluation of process and outcomes from learning through reflective practice groups on a post-registration nursing course. *Journal of Advanced Nursing, 31*(3), 689–695.

Raingruber, B., & Haffer, A. (2001). *Using your head to land on your feet*. Philadelphia: F. A. Davis Company.

Registered Nurses Association of British Columbia. (2000). *Standards for nursing practice in British Columbia*. Pub. No. 128. Vancouver, British Columbia, Canada: Author.

Smith, K. V., & Godfrey, N. S. (2002). Being a good nurse and doing the right thing: A qualitative study. *Nursing Ethics, 9*(3), 301–312.

Smith-Blair, N., & Neighbors, M. (2000). Use of the Critical Thinking Disposition Inventory in critical care orientation. *Journal of Continuing Education in Nursing, 31*(6), 251–256.

Stahl, N., & Stahl, R. (1991). We can agree after all! Achieving consensus for a critical thinking component of a gifted program using the Delphi Technique. *Roeper Review, 14*(2), 79–88.

Tanner, C. A. (2000). Critical thinking: Beyond nursing process. *Journal of Nursing Education, 39*(8), 338–339.

Wilkinson, J. M. (2001). *Nursing process and critical thinking* (3rd ed.). Upper Saddle River, NJ: Prentice Hall.

CHAPTER 3

Acute Pain Management Guideline Panel. (1992). *Acute pain management in adults: Operative procedures, quick reference guide for clinicians.* (AHCPR Publication No. 92-0019). Rockdale, MD: Author.

American Nurses Association. (2001). *Code of ethics for nurses—Provisions* [Electronic version]. Retrieved March 7, 2003, from *http://nursingworld.org/ethics/chcode.htm*

American Nurses Association. (2004). *Nursing: Scope and standards of practice* (3rd ed.). Washington, DC: ANA.

Carnevali, D. L., & Thomas, M. D. (1993). *Diagnostic reasoning and treatment decision making in nursing.* Philadelphia: J. B. Lippincott.

Dochterman, J. M., & Jones, D. A. (Eds.). (2003). *Unifying nursing languages: The harmonization of NANDA, NIC, and NOC.* Washington, DC: American Nurses Association, *NursesBooks.org*

Galanti, G. A. (1991). *Caring for patients from different cultures: Case studies from American hospitals.* Philadelphia: University of Pennsylvania Press.

Giger, J. N., & Davidhizar, R. E. (1999). *Transcultural nursing: Assessment and intervention.* St. Louis: Mosby.

Gordon, M. (1994). *Nursing diagnosis: Process and application* (3rd ed.). St. Louis: C. V. Mosby.

Gorman, L. M., Raines, M. L., & Sultan, D. F. (2002). *Psychosocial nursing for general patient care* (2nd ed.). Philadelphia, F. A. Davis Company.

Joint Commission on Accreditation of Healthcare Organizations. (2000). *Comprehensive accreditation manual for hospitals: The official handbook.* Oakbrook Terrace, IL: Author.

Joint Commission on Accreditation of Healthcare Organizations. (2002). *Hospital accreditation standards: Accreditation policies standards and intent statements.* Oakbrook Terrace, IL: Author.

Karnofsky, D. A., & Burchenal, J. H. (1949). The clinical evaluation of chemotherapeutic agents in cancer. In MacLeod, C. M. (Ed.). *Evaluation of chemotherapeutic agents.* New York: Columbia University Press. Also available at *http://palliative.info/pages/karnofsky.htm*

Katz, S., Ford, A. B., Moskowitz, R. W., et al. (1963). Studies of illness in the aged. The index of the ADL: A standardized measure of biological and psychosocial function. *Journal of the American Medical Association, 185,* 914–919.

Lawton, M. P. (1969). *Lawton instrumental activities of daily living.* The Philadelphia Geriatric Center, Philadelphia, PA. Retrieved on May 25, 2003, from *www.acsu.buffalo.edu/~drstall/assessmenttools.html*

McCaffery, M., & Pasero, C. (1999). *Pain clinical manual* (2nd ed.). St. Louis: Mosby.

NANDA International. (2005). *NANDA nursing diagnoses: Definitions and classification 2005–2006.* Philadelphia: Author.

National Council of State Boards of Nursing. (1997). *Delegation decision-making grid.* Retrieved on March 6, 2003, from *http://nursingworld.org/snas/ia/grid.htm*

National Council of State Boards of Nursing. (2002). *Model nursing practice act.* Retrieved on March 6, 2003, from *http://www.ncsbn.org/public/reguation/nursing_practice_model_practice_act.htm*

Maslow, A. H. (1970). *Motivation and personality* (2nd ed.). New York: Harper & Row.

Orem, D. (1991) *Nursing: Concepts of practice* (4th ed.). St. Louis: Mosby-Year Book.

Pender, N. J., Murdaugh, C. L., & Parsons, M. A. (2002). *Health promotion in nursing practice* (4th ed.). Upper Saddle River, NJ: Prentice Hall.

Purnell, L. D., & Paulanka, B. J. (2003). *Transcultural health care: A culturally competent approach* (2nd ed.). Philadelphia: F. A. Davis Company.

Roy, C., & Andrews, H. (1991). *The Roy adaptation model: The definitive statement.* Norwalk, CT: Appleton & Lange.

Spector, R. E. (2000a). *Cultural care: Guides to heritage assessment and health traditions* (2nd ed.). Upper Saddle River, NJ: Prentice Hall.

Spector, R. E. (2000b). *Cultural diversity in health and illness* (5th ed.). Upper Saddle River, NJ: Prentice Hall.

Stewart, M. J. (1993). *Integrating social support in nursing.* Newbury Park, CA: Sage.

Wilkinson, J. M. (2001). *Nursing process and critical thinking* (3rd ed.). Upper Saddle River, NJ: Prentice Hall.

Williams, S. R., & Schlenker, E. D. (2003). *Essentials of nutrition and diet therapy* (8th ed.). St. Louis: Mosby.

CHAPTER 4

Abdellah, F. (1957). Methods of identifying covert aspects of nursing problems. *Nursing Research, 6*(1), 4–23.

Alberta Association of Registered Nurses. (1999). *Nursing practice: Professional conduct: Nursing practice standards.* Retrieved January 17, 2003, from *http://nurses.ab.ca/profconduct/npa.html*

American Medical Association. (2003). *Current procedural terminology: CPT 2003.* Chicago: Author.

American Nurses Association. (1980). *ANA social policy statement.* Washington, DC: Author.

American Nurses Association. (2004). *Nursing: Scope and standards of practice* (3rd ed). Washington, DC: Author.

American Psychiatric Association. (2000). *Diagnostic and Statistical Manual of Mental Disorders* (4th rev. ed.). Arlington, VA: Author.

Barton, A. J., Gilbert, L., Erickson, V., Baramee, J., Sowers, D., & Robertson, K. (2003, May/June). A guide to assist nurse practitioners with standardized nursing language. *CIN: Computers, Informatics, Nursing, 21*(3), 128–133.

Beyea, S. (1999). Standardized language—Making nursing practice count. *AORN Journal, 70*(5), 831–832, 834, 837, 838.

Beyea, S. (2000). Standardized nursing vocabularies and the perioperative nursing data set: Making clinical practice count. *CIN Plus, 3*(2), 1, 5, 6.

Carpenito, L. J. (2002). *Nursing diagnosis: Application to clinical practice* (9th ed.). Philadelphia: Lippincott.

Craft-Rosenberg, M. (1999). NDEC guidelines for development and evaluation of diagnoses. *Nursing Diagnosis, 10*(2), 84–85.

Delaney, C., Herr, K., Maas, M., & Specht, J. (2000). Reliability of nursing diagnoses documented in a computerized nursing information system. *Nursing Diagnosis, 11*(3), 121–134.

Fry, V. (1953). The creative approach to nursing. *American Journal of Nursing 98*(6), 44–47.

Gebbie, K. (1976). Development of a taxonomy of nursing diagnosis. In J. Walter, et al., *Dynamics of problem-oriented approaches: Patient care and documentation.* Philadelphia: J. B. Lippincott.

Gordon, M. (1994). *Nursing diagnosis: Process and application* (3rd ed.) St Louis: C. V. Mosby.

Green, P. M., & Slade, D. S. (2001). Environmental nursing diagnoses for aggregates and community. *Nursing Diagnosis, 12*(1), 5–13.

Henderson, V. (1964). The nature of nursing. *American Journal of Nursing, 64*(8), 62–68.

Johnson, M. (2002). Criteria for standardized nursing language. *Outcomes Management, 6*(1), 1–3.

Johnson, M., Bulechek, G., Dochterman, J. M., Maas, M., & Moorhead, S. (2001). *Nursing diagnoses, outcomes, and interventions: NANDA, NOC, and NIC linkage.* St Louis: Mosby.

Kalish, R. (1983). *The psychology of human behavior* (5th ed.). Monterey, CA: Brooks/Cole.

Maslow, A. H. (1970). *Motivation and personality.* (2nd ed.). New York: Harper & Row.

NANDA International. (2003). *NANDA Nursing diagnoses: definitions & classification 2003–2004.* Philadelphia: Author.

NANDA International. (2005). *NANDA Nursing diagnoses: definitions & classification 2005–2006.* Philadelphia: Author.

North American Nursing Diagnosis Association. (2001). *Nursing diagnosis: Definitions and classification 2001–2002.* Philadelphia: Author.

Parris, K. M., Place, P. J., Orellana, E., Calder, J., Jackson, K., Karolys, A., et al. (1999). Integrating nursing diagnoses, interventions, and outcomes in public health nursing practice. *Nursing Diagnosis, 10*(2), 49–56.

Smith, H. K., & Donald, J. G. (2002). Thinking processes used by nurses in clinical decision making. *Journal of Nursing Education, 41*(4), 145–153.

Thoroddsen, A., & Thorsteinsson, H. (2002). Nursing diagnosis taxonomy across the Atlantic Ocean: Congruence between nurses' charting and the NANDA taxonomy. *Journal of Advanced Nursing, 37*(4), 372–381.

Wilkinson, J. M. (2001). *Nursing process and critical thinking* (3rd ed.). Upper Saddle River, NJ: Prentice Hall.

World Health Organization. (1992). *Manual of the international classification of diseases and related health problems* (10th rev. ed.). Geneva, Switzerland: Author.

CHAPTER 5

Agency for Health Care Policy and Research. (1993). *Clinical practice guideline development, AHCPR program note.* AHCPR Publication Number 93-0023. Last modified 7/31/95. Washington, DC: Author.

American Medical Association. (2002). *CPT 2003 standard edition.* Chicago: AMA Press.

American Nurses Association/Nursing Information & Data Set Evaluation Center. (2002, January 23). *Recognized languages for nursing.* Retrieved September 1, 2002, from *http://nursingworld.org/ nidsec/classlst.htm*

American Nurses Association. (2004). *Nursing: Scope and standards of practice* (3rd ed.). Washington, DC: Author.

Beyea, S. (2000). Standardized nursing vocabularies and the perioperative nursing data set: Making clinical practice count. *Computers in Nursing, 3*(2), 1,5,6.

Bull, M. J., Hansen, H. E., & Gross, C. R. (2000). Differences in family caregiver outcomes by their level of involvement in discharge planning. *Applied Nursing Research, 13*(2), 76–82.

Dochterman, J. M., & Bulechek, G. M. (Eds.).(2004). *Nursing interventions classification (NIC)* (4th ed.). St Louis: Mosby.

Harris, B. L. (1990). Becoming deprofessionalized: One aspect of the staff nurse's perspective on computer-mediated nursing care plans. *Advances in Nursing Science, 13*(2), 63–74.

Head, B., Maas, M., & Johnson, M. (1997). Outcomes for home and community nursing in integrated delivery systems. *Caring, 16*(1), 50–56.

Healthy People 2010. (2000). Volumes I and II. Washington, DC: U.S. Department of Health and Human Services.

Johnson, M., Bulechek, G. M., McCloskey Dochterman, J., Maas, M., & Moorhead, S. (2002). *Nursing diagnoses, outcomes, and interventions: NANDA, NOC, and NIC linkages.* St Louis: Mosby.

Malijanian, R., Effken, J. A., and Kaerhle, P. (2000). Design and implementation of an outcomes management model. *Outcomes Management for Nursing Practice, 4*(1), 19–25.

Martin, K. S., & Scheet, N. J. (1992). *The Omaha system: Applications for community health nursing.* Philadelphia: W. B. Saunders. Retrieved September 1, 2002, from *http://www .omahasystem.org/shminter.htm*

McCloskey, J. C., & Bulechek, G. M. (Eds.). (1992). *Nursing interventions classification (NIC).* St Louis: Mosby.

Moorhead, S., Johnson, M., & Maas, M. (Eds.). (2004). *Nursing outcomes classification (NOC)* (3rd ed.). St Louis: Mosby.

Mueller, A., Johnston, M., & Bligh, D. (2001). Mind-mapped care plans, a remarkable alternative to traditional nursing care plans. *Nurse Educator, 26*(2), 75–80.

Mueller, A., Johnston, M., & Bligh, D. (2002). Viewpoint: Joining mind mapping and care planning to enhance student critical thinking and achieve holistic nursing care. *Nursing Diagnosis: The International Journal of Nursing Language and Classification, 13*(1), 24–27.

Parlocha, P. K., & Henry, S. G. (1998). The usefulness of the Georgetown Home Health Care Classification system for coding patient problems and nursing interventions in psychiatric home care. *Computers in Nursing, 16*(1), 45–52.

A practical guide to improving patient outcomes. (2000). *Orthopedic Nursing, 19*(Suppl.), 22–28.

Saba, V. K. (1995). Home Health Care Classifications (HHCCs): Nursing diagnoses and nursing interventions. In *An emerging framework: Data system advances for clinical nursing practice.* ANA Publication No. NP-94. Washington, DC: American Nurses Association. Retrieved September 1, 2002, from *http://www.sabacare.com/nursinginterventions.html*

Saba, V. K. (1997). Why the Home Health Care Classification is a recognized nursing nomenclature. *Computers in Nursing, 15*(92), 69–76.

Saba, V. K. (2003). Clinical Care Classification System. Retrieved November 27, 2004, from *http://www.sabacare.com*

Schuster, P. M. (2000). Concept mapping: Reducing clinical care plan paperwork and increasing learning. *Nurse Educator, 24*(2), 76–81.

Schuster, P. (2002). *Concept mapping: A critical-thinking approach to care planning.* Philadelphia: F. A. Davis Company.

Wilkinson, J. M. (2001). *Nursing process and critical thinking* (3rd ed.). Upper Saddle River, N.J.: Prentice Hall.

Zander, K. (1998). Historical development of outcomes-based care delivery. *Critical Care Nursing Clinics of North America, 10*(1), 1.

CHAPTER 6

Acton, G. J., & Winter, M. A. (2002). Interventions for family members caring for an elder with dementia. *Annual Review of Nursing Research, 20,* 149–179.

Agency for Healthcare Research and Quality, National Institutes for Health. (2002). Clinical practice guideline. Pressure ulcer formation: Skin care and early treatment. Retrieved August 30, 2002, from *http://hstat.nlm.nih.gov/hq/Hquest/screen/TextBrowse/t/ 1030737344857/s/58838* Also available from *http://www .ahrq.gov*

American Medical Association. (2002). *CPT 2003 standard edition.* Chicago: AMA Press.

American Nurses Association/Nursing Information & Data Set Evaluation Center. (2002, January 23). *Recognized languages for nursing.* Retrieved September 1, 2002, from *http://nursingworld .org/nidsec/classlst.htm*

American Nurses Association. (2004). *Nursing: Scope and standards of practice* (3rd ed.) Washington, DC: American Nurses Publishing.

Association of Women's Health, Obstetric and Neonatal Nurses. (2001a). *Education and practice resources: Evidence-based clinical practice guidelines: Neonatal Skin Care* (2001). Retrieved August 30, 2002, from *http://www.awhonn.org/awhonn/? pg50-873-5580*

Association of Women's Health, Obstetric and Neonatal Nurses. (2001b). *Promotion of emotional well-being during midlife* (2001). Retrieved August 30, 2002, from *http://www.awhonn.org/ awhonn/?pg50-873-5580*

Bowker, G. C., Star, S. L., & Spasser, M. A. (2001, March). Classifying nursing work. *Online Journal of Issues in Nursing.* Retrieved September 9, 2002, from *http://www.nursingworld.org/ ojin/tpc7/tpc7_6.htm*

Burgener, S. C., & Twigg, P. (2002). Interventions for persons with irreversible dementia. *Annual Review of Nursing Research, 20,* 89–124.

Cronenwett, L. R. (2002, February 19). Research, practice and policy: Issues in evidence based care. *Online Journal of Issues in*

Nursing. Available from *http://www.nursingworld.org/ojin/keynotes/speech_2.htm.*

Dochterman, J. M., & Bulechek, G. M. (Eds.). (2004). *Nursing interventions classification (NIC)* (4th ed.). St Louis: Mosby.

Evidence-based guidelines. (2002). *Evidence-Based Practice, 5*(2), 12, insert 2p.

Frisch, N. C. (2001, May 31). Nursing as a context for alternative/complementary modalities. *Online Journal of Issues in Nursing, 6*(2), 2. Retrieved August 30, 2002, from *http://www.nursingworld.org/ojin/topic15/tpc15_2.htm*

Griens, A. M. G., Goossen, W. T. F., & Van der Kloot, W. S. (2001). Exploring the Nursing Minimum Data Set for the Netherlands using multidimensional scaling techniques. *Journal of Advanced Nursing, 36*(1), 89–101.

Harris, R. M. (1998, June 10). Advanced nursing practice in the 21st century: Do we want to be right or do we want to win? *Online Journal of Issues in Nursing.* Retrieved September 5, 2002, from *http://www.nursingworld.org/ojin/tpc6/tpc6_2.htm*

Iowa Intervention Project. (2001). Determining cost of nursing interventions: A beginning. *Nursing Economics, 19*(4), 146–160.

Institute of Medicine. (1992). *Guidelines for clinical practice: From development to use.* In M. J. Field & K. N. Lohr (Eds.). Washington, DC: National Academy Press.

Johnson, M., Bulechek, G. M., McCloskey Dochterman, J., Maas, M., & Moorhead, S. (2002). *Nursing diagnoses, outcomes, & interventions: NANDA, NOC, and NIC linkages.* St Louis: Mosby.

Lavin, M. A., Meyer, G., Krieger, M., McNary, P., Carlson, J., Perry, A., et al. (2002). Viewpoint. Essential differences between evidence-based nursing and evidence-based medicine. *International Journal of Nursing Terminologies and Classifications, 13*(3), 101–106.

Martin, K. S., & Scheet, N. J. (1992). *The Omaha system: Applications for community health nursing.* Philadelphia: W. B. Saunders. Retrieved September 1, 2002, from *http://www.omahasystem.org/shminter.htm*

McCloskey, J. C., & Bulechek, G. M. (Eds.). (1992). *Nursing interventions classification (NIC).* St Louis: Mosby

McCloskey, J. C., & Bulechek, G. M. (Eds.). (2000). *Nursing interventions classification (NIC)* (3rd ed.). St Louis: Mosby. Also available at *http://coninfo.nursing.uiowa.edu/nic/index.htm* (Revised November 15, 2001; retrieved September 1, 2002).

Newman, D., & Palmer, M. (Eds.). (2003, March [Suppl.]). State of the science on urinary incontinence. Supplement. *American Journal of Nursing.*

O'Connor, N. A., Kershat, W., & Hameister, A. D. (2001). Documenting patterns of nursing interventions. *Journal of Nursing Measurement, 9*(1), 73–90.

Parlocha, P. K., & Chafetz, L. (1999). Planning home care for elderly patients with major depressive disorder: Limits of diagnosis-based critical paths. *Home Health Care Management and Practice, 11*(4), 27–37.

Parris, K. M., Place, P. J., & Orellana, E. (1999). Integrating nursing diagnoses, interventions, and outcomes in public health nursing practice. *Nursing Diagnosis, 10*(2), 49–56.

Pravikoff, D. S., Pierce, S., & Tanner, A. (2003). Are nurses ready for evidence-based practice? *American Journal of Nursing, 103*(5), 95–96.

Rew, L. (2000). Possible outcomes of holistic nursing interventions. *Journal of Holistic Nursing, 18*(4), 307–309.

Saba, V. K. (1995). Home Health Care Classifications (HHCCs): Nursing diagnoses and nursing interventions. In: *An emerging framework: Data system advances for clinical nursing practice.* ANA Publication No. NP-94. Washington, DC: American Nurses Association. Retrieved September 1, 2002, from *http://www.sabacare.com/nursinginterventions.html*

Standardized treatment cuts pneumonia deaths: Guidelines also help lower admission rates. (2001). *Quality Improvement/Total Quality Management, 11*(6), 65–67.

Systems to rate the strength of scientific evidence. (2002, April). File Inventory, Evidence Report/Technology Assessment Number 47.

AHRQ Publication No. 02-E016. Rockville, MD: Agency for Healthcare Research and Quality. Retrieved September 5, 2002, from *http://www.ahrq.gov/clinic/strevinv.htm*

Titler, M. G., Mentes, J. C., Rakel, B. A., Abbott, L., & Baumler, S. (1999). From book to bedside: Putting evidence to use in the care of the elderly. *Joint Commission Journal of Quality Improvement, 25,* 545–556.

Venes, D., & Thomas, C. L. (Eds.). (2004). *Taber's cyclopedic medical dictionary.* Philadelphia: F. A. Davis Company. Available from *http://www.tabers.com/default.jsp*

Wake, M., & Coenen, A. (1999). The International Classification for Nursing practice (ICNP): Toward the beta version. In M. J. Rantz, & P. LeMone (Eds.), *Classification of nursing diagnoses. Proceedings of the Thirteenth Conference. North American Nursing Diagnosis Association.* Glendale, CA: CINAHL Information Systems

Wilkinson, J. M. (2001). *Nursing process and critical thinking.* (3rd ed.). Upper Saddle River, NJ: Prentice Hall.

CHAPTER 7

Alberta Association of Registered Nurses. (1999). *Nursing practice: Professional conduct: Nursing practice standards.* Retrieved August 27, 2002, from *http://nurses.ab.ca/profconduct/npa.html*

American Nurses Association. (1992a). Position statements. *Registered nurse education relating to the utilization of unlicensed assistive personnel.* Washington, DC: Author. Retrieved September 8, 2002, from *http://nursingworld.org/readroom/position/uap/uapuse.htm*

American Nurses Association. (1992b). Position statements. *Registered nurse utilization of unlicensed assistive personnel.* Washington, DC: Author. Retrieved September 8, 2002, from *http://nursingworld.org/readroom/position/uap/uaprned.htm*

American Nurses Association. (1996). *Registered professional nurses and unlicensed assistive personnel* (2nd ed.). Washington, DC: Author.

American Nurses Association. (1999). *Nursing quality indicators: Guide for implementation* (2nd ed). Washington, DC: Author.

American Nurses Association. (2001). *Code of ethics for nurses with interpretive statements.* Washington, DC: Author.

American Nurses Association. (2004). *Scope and standards of practice.* Washington, DC: Author.

Baldridge criteria spur ongoing change. (2001). *Quality Improvement/Total Quality Management, 11*(8), 89.

Baldridge National Quality Program. (2002). *Health care criteria for performance excellence.* Retrieved December 10, 2002, from *www.quality.nist.gov*

Barter, M. (1999). Delegation and supervision outside the hospital. *American Journal of Nursing, 99*(7), 24A–B, 24D.

Batsie, C. (1999). Patient call system provides efficient delegation. *Nursing Management, 30*(1), 50.

Bentley, J. (2001). Promoting patient partnership in wound care. *British Journal of Community Nursing, 6*(10), 493–4, 496, 498, 500.

College of Registered Nurses of Manitoba. (2001). *Standards of practice for registered nurses.* Retrieved December 11, 2002, from *http://222.crnm.mb.ca/standards.htm*

Davidson, S. G., & Scott, R. (1999). Professional practice: Thinking critically about delegation. *American Journal of Nursing, 99*(6), 61–62.

Dochterman, J. M., & Bulechek, G. M. (Eds.). (2004). *Nursing interventions classification (NIC)* (4th ed.). St Louis: Mosby.

Dowding, D. (2001). Examining the effects that manipulating information given in the change of shift report has on nurses' care planning ability. *Journal of Advanced Nursing, 33*(6), 836–846.

Elliott, K. (2001). Implementing nursing clinical indicators. *Professional Nurse, 16*(6), 1158–1161.

Fisher, M. (2000). Do you have delegation savvy? *Nursing 2000, 30*(12), 58–59.

Gibberd, R., Pathmeswaran, A., & Burtenshaw, K. (2000). Using clinical indicators to identify areas for quality improvement. *Journal of Quality in Clinical Practice, 20* (4), 136–144.

Gould, D., Gammon, J., Donnelly, M., Batiste, L., Ball, E., Carneiro de Melo, A. M. S., et al. (2000). Improving hand hygiene in community healthcare settings: The impact of research and clinical collaboration. *Journal of Clinical Nursing, 9*(1), 95–102.

Hamill, C. T., & Luchok, J. (1999). Commission/URAC. Best practices: A necessity in modern health care. *Case Manager, 10*(5), 23–25.

Hopkins, D. L. (2002). Evaluating the knowledge deficits of registered nurses responsible for supervising nursing assistants. A learning needs assessment tool. *Journal of Nurses Staff Development, 18*(3), 152–156.

Joint Commission on Accreditation of Healthcare Organizations (JCAHO). (2002). *Hospital accreditation standards: Accreditation policies standards and intent statements.* Oakbrook Terrace, IL: Author.

ISO 9000: A system-oriented approach to quality management. (2002). *Quality Improvement/Total Quality Management, 12*(1), 1–5.

Kummeth, P., de Ruiter, H., & Capelle, S. (2001). Developing a nursing assistant model: Having the right person perform the right job. *Medical-Surgical Nursing Journal, 10*(5), 255–263.

London, F. (1998). Improving compliance. What you can do. *RN, 61*(1), 43–46.

Malloch, K. (1999). The Performance Measurement Matrix: A framework to optimize decision making. *Journal of Nursing Care Quality, 13*(3), 1–12.

Meyer, G. S., & Massagli, M. P. (2001). The forgotten component of the quality triad: Can we still learn something from "structure"? *Joint Commission Journal on Quality Improvement, 27*(9), 484–493.

National Council of State Boards of Nursing (NCSBN). (1995a). *Delegation: Concepts and decision-making process.* National Council Position Paper. Chicago: Author. Retrieved December 11, 2002, from *http://www.ncsbn.org/files/files/publications/positions/Delegation*

National Council of State Boards of Nursing (NCSBN). (1995b). *Role development: Clinical components of delegation curriculum outline.* Chicago: Author.

National Council of State Boards of Nursing (NCSBN). (1997a). *Delegation decision-making grid.* Chicago: Author. Retrieved September 8, 2002, from *http://www.ncsbn.org/files/uap/delegationgrid.pdf*

National Council of State Boards of Nursing (NCSBN). (1997b). *Delegation decision-making tree.* Chicago: Author. Retrieved September 8, 2002, from *http://www.ncsbn.org/files/uap/delegationtree.pdf*

National Council of State Boards of Nursing (NCSBN). (1997c). *The five rights of delegation.* Chicago: Author. Retrieved September 8, 2002, from *http://www.ncsbn.org/files/uap/fiverights.pdf*

National Council of State Boards of Nursing (NCSBN). (1998). *The continuum of care framework: Roles of the licensed nurse and assistive personnel (AP) in relation to the client.* Chicago: Author. Retrieved September 8, 2002, from *http://www.ncsbn.org/public/res/uap/contcaregrid.pdf*

Oermann, M., & Huber, D. (1999). Patient outcomes: A measure of nursing's value. *American Journal of Nursing, 99*(9), 40–48.

Page, C. K. (1999). Performance improvement integration: A whole systems approach. *Journal of Nursing Care Quality, 13*(3), 59–70.

Parsons, L. C. (1999). Building RN confidence for delegation decision-making skills in practice. *Journal of Nurses Staff Development, 15*(6), 263–269.

Pelletier, L. R. (2000). Error-free healthcare: Mission possible! *Journal for Healthcare Quality, 22*(2), 2, 9.

Pelletier, L. R., Beaudin, C. L., & van Leeuwen, D. (1999). The use of a prioritization matrix to preserve quality resources. *Journal for Healthcare Quality, 21*(5), 36–38.

Poole, L. (2001). PEPP: Collaborating to improve quality. *Journal of the American Health Information Management Association, 72*(4), 43–47.

Rantz, M.J., Popejoy, L., Petroski, G. F., Madsen, R. W., Mehr, D. R., Zwygart-Stauffacher, M., et al. (2001). Randomized clinical trial of a quality improvement intervention in nursing homes. *The Gerontologist, 41*(4), 525.

Registered Nurses' Association of Nova Scotia. (1997). Standards for nursing practice. Retrieved December 11, 2002, from *http://www.crnns.ca/*

Spencer, S. A. (2001). Education, training, and use of unlicensed assistive personnel in critical care. *Critical Care Nursing Clinics of North America, 13*(1), 105–118.

Thomas, L. (1999). Is delegation the answer? *Elder Care, 11*(4), 1.

Wilkinson, J. (2001). *Nursing process and critical thinking* (3rd ed.). Upper Saddle River, NJ: Prentice Hall.

Wilson, L. (2000). Quality is everyone's business: Why this approach will not work in hospitals. *Journal of Quality in Clinical Practice, 20*(4), 131–135.

Woodring, B. C. (2000). If you have taught—have the child and family learned? *Pediatric Nursing, 26*(5), 505–509.

CHAPTER 8

Abdellah, F. G., Beland, I. L., Martin, A., & Matheney, R. V. (1960). *Patient-centered approaches to nursing.* New York: Macmillan.

American Nurses Association. (1981). *Guidelines for the investigative functions of nurses.* Washington, D.C: Author.

American Nurses Association Commission on Nursing Research. (1980). Generating a scientific basis for nursing practice: Research priorities for the 1980s. *Nursing Research, 29,* 219.

Anderson, M. A. (2001). *Nursing leadership, management, and professional practice.* Philadelphia: F. A. Davis Company.

Ball, J., & Bindler, R. (1999). *Pediatric nursing.* Norwalk, CT: Appleton & Lange.

Benner, P. (1984). *From novice to expert: Excellence and power in clinical nursing practice.* Menlo Park, CA: Addison-Wesley.

Benner, P., & Wrubel, J. (1989). *The primacy of caring: Stress and coping in health and illness.* Menlo Park, CA: Addison-Wesley.

Brockopp, D. Y., & Hastings-Tolsma, M. T. (2003). *Fundamentals of nursing research* (3rd ed.). Sudbury, MA: Jones and Bartlett.

Brown, S. S. (1992). Meta-analysis of diabetes patient education research: Variation in intervention effects across studies. *Research in Nursing and Health, 16*(6), 409–419.

Burns, N., & Grove, S. K. (2003). *The practice of nursing research: Conduct, critique, and utilization* (4th ed.). Philadelphia: W. B. Saunders.

Chinn, P., & Kramer, M. (1999). *Theory and nursing: Integrated knowledge development* (5th ed.). St. Louis: Mosby.

Cook, P. R., & Cullen, J. A. (2003). Caring as an imperative for nursing education. *Nursing Education Perspectives, 24*(4), 293–197.

Dochterman, J. M., & Bulechek, G. M. (Eds.). (2004). *Nursing interventions classification (NIC)* (4th ed.) St Louis: Mosby.

Dossey, B. M. (1999). *Florence Nightingale: Mystic, visionary, healer.* Springhouse, PA: Springhouse.

Fain, J. A. (1999). *Reading, understanding, and applying nursing research.* Philadelphia: F. A. Davis Company.

Feil, N. (1993). *Validation therapy.* Cincinnati, OH: Feil Productions.

Flaskerud, J. H., & Halloran, E. J. (1980). Areas of agreement in nursing theory development. *Advances in Nursing Science, 3*(1), 1–7.

Goode, C., Butcher, L., Cipperley, J., et al. (1996). *Research utilization: A study guide* (2nd ed.) Ida Grove, IA: Horn Video Productions.

Haller, K. B., Reynolds, M. A., & Horsley, J. A. (1979). Developing research-based innovation protocols: Process, criteria and issues. *Research in Nursing and Health, 2,* 45–51.

Henderson, V. (1966). *The nature of nursing: A definition and its implications for practice, research, and education.* New York: Macmillan.

Hornberger, C. (2002). M. Rogers and the science of unitary human beings. Washburn University. Retrieved September 16, 2003, from *http://www.washburn.edu/sonu/rogers1.htm*

Horsley, J. A., Crane, J., & Bingle, J. D. (1978). Research utilization as an organizational process. *Journal of Nursing Administration, 4–6.*

Horsley, J. A., Crane, J., Crabtree, M. K., & Wood, D. J. (1983). *Using research to improve practice.* Orlando, FL: Grune & Stratton.

International Consortium of Parse Scholars. (n.d.). Retrieved July 18, 2003, from *http://www.humanbecoming.org/index.html*

Johnson, D. E. (1968). Theory in nursing: Borrowed and unique. *Nursing Research, 11,* 206.

Johnson, D. E. (1980). The behavioral system for nursing. In J. P. Riehl & C. Roy (Eds.), *Conceptual models for nursing practice* (2nd ed.) (pp. 207–216). New York: Appleton-Century-Crofts.

King, I. M. (1971). *Toward a theory for nursing: General concepts of human behavior.* New York: Wiley.

Kolcaba, K. Y. (1994). A theory of holistic comfort for nursing. *Journal of Advanced Nursing, 19,* 1178–1184.

Leininger, M. M. (1978). *Transcultural nursing: Concepts, theories and practices.* New York: John Wiley & Sons.

Leininger, M. M. (1984). *Care: The essence of nursing and health.* Thorofare, NJ: Charles B. Slack.

Levine, M. E. (1967). The four conservation principles of nursing. *Nursing Forum, 6,* 45–59.

Levine, M. E. (1969). *Introduction to clinical nursing.* Philadelphia: F. A. Davis Company.

Marriner-Tomey, A., & Raile-Alligood, M. (2002) *Nursing theorists and their work* (5th ed.). St. Louis: Mosby.

Maslow, A. H. (1970). *Motivation and personality* (2nd ed.). New York: Harper & Row.

Maslow, A. (1971). *The farther reaches of human nature.* New York: Viking Press.

Maslow, A., & Lowery, R. (Eds.). (1998). *Toward a psychology of being* (3rd ed.). New York: Wiley & Sons.

Mayo, A. (1997) Orem's self-care model: A professional nursing practice model. Retrieved July 16, 2003, from *http://members.aol.com/annmrn/nursing_portfolio_I_index.html*

McCalla, C. (1998). University of Western Ontario Faculty of Nursing, Hildegard Peplau Nursing Theorist Home Page. Retrieved July 18, 2003, from *http://publish.uwo.ca/%7Ecforchuk/peplau/hpcb.html*

Merskey, H., & Bogduk, N. (1994). *Classification of chronic pain: Descriptions of chronic pain syndromes and definitions of pain terms.* Seattle, WA: IASP (International Association for the Study of Pain) Press.

National Heart, Lung, and Blood Institute, National Institutes of Health. (2002). *Framingham heart study.* Retrieved July 24, 2003, from *http://www.nhlbi.nih.gov/about/framingham/index.html*

National Institutes of Health. (2002). The NIH almanac—Organization. National Institute of Nursing Research. Retrieved July 24, 2003, from *http://www.nih.gov/about/almanac/organization/NINR.htm*

National Institute of Nursing Research. (2003a). Research themes for the future. Retrieved July 24, 2003, from *http:www.nih.gov/ninr/researach/dea/PARFApage.html*

National Institute of Nursing Research. (2003b). 2004 areas of research opportunity. Retrieved July 24, 2003, from *http:www.nih.gov/ninr/researach/dea/2004AoRO.html*

Neuman, B. M., & Young, R. J. (1972). A model for teaching total person approach to patient problems. *Nursing Research, 21,* 264–269.

Neumann College. (2000). Academics. Division of Nursing & Health Sciences: Neuman systems model. Retrieved July 18, 2003, from *http://www.neumann.edu/academics/undergrad/nursing/model.html*

Newman, M. (n. d.). Health as expanding consciousness. Available at *http://www.healthasexpandingconsciousness.org/*

Nieswiadomy, R. M. (2002). *Foundations of nursing research* (4th ed.). Upper Saddle River, NJ: Prentice Hall.

Nightingale, F. (1859/1992). *Notes on nursing: What it is and what it is not.* Philadelphia: Lippincott.

NurseScribe. (2003). Nursing theory page. Retrieved July 16, 2003, from *http://www.enursescribe.com/nurse_theorists.htm*

Orlando, I. J. (1961). *The dynamic nurse-patient relationship: Function, process, and principles.* New York: G. P. Putnam's Sons.

Parker, M. (2001). *Nursing theories and nursing practice.* Philadelphia: F. A. Davis Company.

Pender, N. J. (2001). *Health promotion in nursing practice* (4th ed.) Upper Saddle River, NJ: Prentice Hall.

Peplau, H. E. (1952). *Interpersonal relations in nursing.* New York: G. P. Putnam's Sons.

Polit, D. F., & Beck, C. T. (2003). *Nursing research: Principles and methods* (7th ed.). Philadelphia: Lippincott.

Rigdon, I. S., Clayton, B. D., & Dimond, M. (1987). Toward a theory of helpfulness for the elderly bereaved: An invitation to a new life. *Advances in Nursing Science, 9*(2), 32–43.

Rogers, M. (1970). *An introduction to the theoretical basis of nursing.* Philadelphia: F. A. Davis Company.

Roy, C. (2003). The Roy adaptation model. Retrieved July 18, 2003, from *http://www2.bc.edu/%7Eroyca*

Schiavenato, M. (2003). VSU College of Nursing, Florence Nightingale Page. Retrieved July 15, 2003, from *http://www.valdosta.edu/nursing/history_theory/florence.html*

Selye, H. (1993). *Neuroendocrinology and stress.* New York: New York Academy of Science.

Transcultural Nursing Society. (1998–2003). Dr. Leininger's Web pages. Retrieved July 16, 2003, from *http://www.tcns.org/menu/menu22.shtml*

University of Kentucky Chandler Medical Center. (1999). The nun study. Retrieved July 24, 2003, from *http://www.nunstudy.org*

von Bertalanffy, L. (1976). *General system theory: Foundations, development and applications* (Rev. ed.). New York: George Braziller.

Watson, J. (1988). *Nursing: Human science and human care. A theory of nursing.* Publication No. 15-2236. New York: National League for Nursing Press.

Watson, J. (2000). University of Colorado Health Sciences Center, School of Nursing. Watson's caring theory. Retrieved July 16, 2003, from *http://www2.uchsc.edu/son/caring/content*

Weaver, D., & Weaver, J. (2001). Findings from the nun study. Retrieved July 24, 2003, from *http://www.centeredpendulum.org/Nun.htm*

Wiedenbach, E. (1964). *Clinical nursing: A helping art.* New York: Springer.

Wilson, H. S. (1993). *Introducing research in nursing* (2nd ed.). Redwood City, CA: Addison-Wesley Nursing.

CHAPTER 9

American Academy of Pediatrics. (1990). *Textbook of neonatal resuscitation.* Elk Grove Village, IL: Author.

American Heart Association. (2002). Obesity and overweight children. Retrieved April 25, 2003, from *http://www.americanheart.org.*

American Obesity Association. (2003). Childhood obesity. Retrieved October 1, 2003, from *http://www.obesity.organization/subs/childhood/prevalence.shtml*

Bonjour, J. (2001). Invest in your bones: How diet, life styles and genetics affect bone development in young people. Retrieved October 10, 2003, from *http://www.osteofound.org/invest_in_your_bones.pdf*

Brazelton, T., & Nugent, J. (1996). Neonatal behavioral assessment scale (3rd ed.). London: MacKeith.

Centers for Disease Control and Prevention (CDC). (2001a). Prevalence of overweight and obesity among adults: United States, 1999–2000. Retrieved October 1, 2003, from *http://www.cdc.gov/nchc/products/pubs/pubd/hestats/obese/obese99.htm*

Centers for Disease Control and Prevention (CDC). (2001b). Youth risk behavior surveillance system: Alcohol/other drug use. Retrieved October 1, 2003, from *http://www.cdc.gov/GraphV*

Centers for Disease Control and Prevention (CDC). (2001c). Youth tobacco surveillance—United States, 2000: *MMWR* highlights. Retrieved October 1, 2003, from *http://www.cdc.gov/tobacco/research_data/youth/ss50.04.highlts.htm*

Centers for Disease Control and Prevention (CDC). (2002a). Child passenger safety. Retrieved April 25, 2003, from *http://www.cdc.gov/safeusa/move/childpassenger.htm*

Centers for Disease Control and Prevention (CDC). (2002b). National vital statistics report. Vol. 50, No. 16, Sept. 16, 2002. Rockville, MD: U.S. Department of Health and Human Services.

Centers for Disease Control and Prevention (CDC). (2002c). Summary health statistics for U.S. adults: National health interview survey, 1998. Series 10, No. 209, Dec. 2002. Rockville, MD: U.S. Department of Health and Human Services.

Cummings, E., & Henry, E. (1961). *Growing old: The process of disengagement.* New York: Basic Books.

Eliopoulos, C. (2001). *Gerontological nursing* (5th ed.). Philadelphia: Lippincott.

Environmental Protection Agency. (2003). Asthma and indoor environments. Retrieved October 1, 2003, from *http://www.epa.gov/asthma/introduction.html#Who Gets Asthma?*

Erikson, E. H. (1963). *Childhood and society* (2nd ed.). New York: W.W. Norton.

Folstein, M. F., Folstein, S., & McHugh P. R. (1975). Mini mental state: A practical method for grading the cognitive state of patients for the clinician. *Journal of Psychiatric Research, 12,* 189–198.

Fowler, J. W. (1981). *Stages of faith: The psychology of human development and the quest for meaning.* New York: Harper & Row.

Freud, A. (1966). *The ego and the mechanisms of defense.* New York: International Universities Press.

Gilligan, C. (1982). *In a different voice: Psychological theory and women's development.* Cambridge, MA: Harvard University Press.

Hart, T. A., & Heimberg, R. G. (2001). Presenting problems among treatment-seeking gay, lesbian, and bisexual youth. *Journal of Clinical Psychology, 57*(50), 615–627.

Havighurst, J. (1963). Successful aging. In R. H. Williams, C. Tibbitts, & W. Donahue (Eds). *Processes of aging.* New York: Atherton Press.

Havighurst, R. J. (1971). *Developmental tasks and education* (3rd ed.). New York: Longman.

Hudson, S., Thompson, D., & Mack, M. (1999). The prevention of playground injuries. *Journal of School Nursing, 156*(3), 30–33.

Ignatavicius, D., & Workman, M. (2002). *Medical-surgical nursing: Critical thinking for collaborative care.* Philadelphia: W.B. Saunders.

Kammerling, S. (2002). Airbags and children: Making correct choices in child passenger restraints. *Maternal Child Nursing, 27*(5), 264–273.

Klingman, L. (1999a). Assessing the female reproductive system. *American Journal of Nursing, 99*(8), 37–43.

Klingman, L. (1999b). Assessing the male genitalia. *American Journal of Nursing, 99*(7), 47–50.

Kohlberg, L. (1968). Moral development. In *International encyclopedia of social science.* New York: Macmillan.

Liu, X., Dietrich, K. N., Radcliffe, J., Ragan, N. B., Rhoads, G. G., & Rogan, W. J. (2002). Do children with falling lead levels have improved cognition? *Pediatrics, 110*(4), 787–791.

National Campaign to Prevent Teen Pregnancy. (2002). United States birth rates for teens 15–19. Retrieved September 22, 2002, from *www.teenpregnancy.org*

National Center for Health Statistics. (1999). *Infant mortality rates vary by race and ethnicity.* (News release). Hyattsville, MD: Author.

National Center for Health Statistics. (2002a). New birth report shows more moms get prenatal care. Retrieved May 6, 2003, from *www.cdc.gov/nchstp/dstd/StatsTrends*

National Center for Health Statistics. (2002b). National vital statistics: Death. Retrieved May 6, 2003, at *www.cdc.gov/NVSR*

National Center for Injury Prevention and Control (NCIPC). (1999). Facts on adolescent injury. Retrieved May 6, 2003, from *www.cdc.gov/nchs*

National Center for Injury Prevention and Control (NCIPC). (2003). Fatal firearm injuries in the United States, 1962–1998. Violence surveillance summary series, No. 3. Retrieved May 6, 2003, from *www.cdc.gov/nchs*

Ogden, C., Kuczmarski, R. J., Flegal, K. M., Mei, Z., Guo, S., Wei, R., et al. (2002). Centers for Disease Control and Prevention 2000 growth charts for the United States: Improvements to the 1977 National Center for Health Statistics version. *Pediatrics, 109*(1), 45–60.

Piaget, J. (1952). *The origins of intelligence in children.* New York: International Universities Press.

Piper, E. (2002). Faith development: A critique of Fowler's model and a proposed alternative. *The Journal of Liberal Religion, 3*(1), 2–8.

Polan, E., & Taylor, D. (2003). *Journey across the life span* (2nd ed.). Philadelphia: F. A. Davis Company.

Preventing teenage pregnancy. (2002). Washington, DC: US Department of Health and Human Services.

Press Release. Retrieved October 10, 2003, from *www.hhs.gov/news/press/2002pres/teenpreg.html*

Sadock, B., & Sadock, V. (2003). *Kaplan & Sadock's synopsis of psychiatry* (9th ed.). Philadelphia: Lippincott Williams & Wilkins.

Singer, L., Arendt, R., Minnes, S., Farkas, K., Salvator, A., Kirchner, H. L., et al. (2002). Cognitive and motor outcomes of cocaine-exposed infants. *Journal of the American Medical Association, 287*(15), 1952–1960.

Tanner, J. (1962). *Growth at adolescence* (2nd ed). Oxford: Blackwell Scientific Publications.

Townsend, M. (2003). *Psychiatric mental health nursing concepts of care* (4th ed.). Philadelphia: F. A. Davis Company.

Tuttle, J., Melnyk, B., & Loveland-Cherry, C. (2002). Adolescent drug and alcohol use: Strategies for assessment, intervention, and prevention. *Nursing Clinics of North America, 37*(3), 443–460.

U.S. Census Bureau. (2000). *United States Census 2000.* Washington, DC: Author.

U.S. Department of Health and Human Services. (2000). *Healthy people 2010* (Conference ed., 2 volumes). Washington, DC: Author.

Wilkinson, J. (2005). *Nursing diagnosis handbook.* (8th ed.). Upper Saddle River, NJ: Prentice Hall.

Wong, D., & Hockenberry-Eaton, M. (2001). *Wong's essentials of pediatric nursing* (6th ed.). St. Louis: Mosby.

Wong, D., Perry, S., & Hockenberry, M. (2002). *Maternal child nursing care.* St Louis: Mosby.

CHAPTER 10

Albom, M. (1997). *Tuesdays with Morrie.* New York: Doubleday.

Benner, P., & Wrubel, J. (1989). *The primacy of caring.* Menlo Park, CA: Addison-Wesley.

Bettelheim, B. (1979). *Surviving and other essays.* New York: Alfred A. Knopf.

Centers for Disease Control and Prevention (CDC). (2003a). Cigarette smoking: Related mortality. Retrieved October 8, 2003, from *http://www.cdc.gov/tobacco/research_data/health_consequences/mortali.htm*

Centers for Disease Control and Prevention (CDC). (2003b). Carbon monoxide poisoning. Retrieved October 8, 2003, from *http://www.cdc.gov/nceh/airpollution/carbonmonoxide/health_tips.htm*

Cheng, N. (1986). *Life and death in Shanghai.* New York: Grove Press.

Cousins, N. (1979). *Anatomy of an illness*. New York: W. W. Norton.

Dossey, B. M., Keegan, L., & Guzetta, C. E. (2003). *Holistic nursing: A handbook for practice* (3rd ed.). Sudbury, MA: Jones & Bartlett.

Dossey, L. (2001). *Healing beyond the body: Medicine and the infinite reach of the mind*. New York: Random House.

Dunn, H. L. (1959). High level wellness for man and society. *American Journal of Public Health, 49*(6), 786–788.

Frankl, V. (1959, 1962, 1984). *Man's search for meaning*. New York: Washington Square Press.

Glod, C. A. (1998). *Contemporary psychiatric-mental health nursing: The brain-behavior connection*. Philadelphia: F. A. Davis Company.

Gonzales, S. (1991). One woman's story of rape. *The Kansas City Star,* Aug. 4, pp. A1, A16, A17.

Gorin, S. S., & Arnold, J. (1998). *Health promotion handbook*. St Louis: Mosby.

Joint Commission on Accreditation of Healthcare Organizations (JCAHO). (2000). *Pain assessment and management: An organizational approach*. Library of Congress Catalog Number: 00-102701.

Kapleau, P. (1997). *The Zen of living and dying*. Boston: Shambhala.

Krishnamurti, J. (1956). *Commentaries on living*. Ojai, CA: Krishnamurti Foundation of America.

Lewis, C. S. (1961). *A grief observed*. London: Faber and Faber.

Lifton, R., & Olson, E. (1974). *Living and dying*. New York: Praeger Publishers.

Lusseyran, J. (1987). *And there was light*. (E. R. Cameron, Trans.). New York: Parabola Books.

Moltman, J. (1983). *The power of the powerless*. San Francisco: Harper & Row.

Myers, J., Sweeney, T., & Witmer, J. (2000). The wheel of wellness counseling for wellness: A holistic model for treatment planning. *Journal of Counseling & Development, 78*(3), 251–267.

Neuman, B. (1995). The Neuman systems model. In B. Neuman, *The Neuman systems model* (3rd ed.) (pp. 3–61). Norwalk, CT: Appleton and Lange.

Nightingale, F. (1859/1992). *Notes on nursing: What it is, and what it is not*. Philadelphia: Lippincott.

Reeve, C. (1998). *Still me*. New York: Random House.

Seigel, B. (1986). *Love, medicine and miracles*. New York: Harper & Row.

Smith, P. (1992). *Living the disrupted life: A symphony of survival*. University of Kansas: unpublished dissertation.

Suchman, E. A. (1972). Stages of illness and medical care. In E. G. Jaco (Ed.), *Patients, physicians, and illness* (2nd ed.). New York: Free Press.

Thompson, J., & Manore, M. (2004). *Nutrition*. San Francisco: Benajmin/Cummings.

Valladares, A. (1986). *Against all hope: The prison memoirs of Armando Valladares*. (A. Hurley, Trans.). New York: Ballantine Books.

Vanauken, S. (1977). *A severe mercy*. New York: Bantam Books.

Watson, J. (1979). *Nursing: The philosophy and science of caring*. Boston: Little, Brown and Company, 2nd printing 1985, boulder, CO: University Press of Colorado.

Wilber, K. (1991). *Grace and grit: Spirituality and healing in the life and death of Treya Killam Wilber*. Boston: Shambhala.

World Health Organization (WHO). (1948). Preamble to the Constitution of the World Health Organization as adopted by the International Health Conference, New York, 19–22 June 1946 and entered into force on 7 April 1948.

CHAPTER 11

Albom, M. (1997). *Tuesdays with Morrie*. New York: Doubleday.

American Psychiatric Association. (2000). *Diagnostic and statistical manual of mental disorders* (4th ed., text revision). Washington, DC: Author.

Association of Saskatchewan Home Economists. (n.d.). Help your child develop a positive body image. Retrieved August 26, 2003, from *http://www.homefamily.net/familyindex.html*

Balon, R. (2001). Anxiety across the life span: Epidemiological evidence and treatment data. *Depression and Anxiety, 13,* 184–189.

Baumeister, R. F. (1987). How the self became a problem: A psychological review of historical research. *Journal of Personality and Social Psychology, 52*(1), 163–176.

Beck, A. T., Brown, G., & Berchick, R. J. (1990). Relationship between hopelessness and ultimate suicide: A replication with psychiatric outpatients. *American Journal of Psychiatry, 147,* 190–195.

Bigler, M., Neimeyer, G. J., & Brown, E. (2001). The divided self revisted: Effects of self-concept clarity and self-concept differentiation on psychological adjustment. *Journal of Social and Clinical Psychology, 20*(3), 396–415.

Bourne, E. J. (2002). *The anxiety and phobia workbook* (2nd ed.). Oakland, CA: New Harbinger Publications.

Bracken, B. A. (Ed.). (1996). *Handbook of self-concept*. New York: Wiley.

Branden, N. (1994). *Six pillars of self-esteem*. New York: Bantam.

Breggin, P. R., & Stern, E. M. (Eds.). (1996). *Psychosocial approaches to deeply disturbed persons*. New York: Haworth Press.

Brigham and Women's Hospital. (2001). *Depression: A guide to diagnosis and treatment*. Boston: Author.

Coleman, J. C., Morris, C. G., & Glaros, A. G. (1990). *Contemporary psychology and effective behavior* (7th ed.). Glenview, IL: Scott, Foresman.

Coopersmith, S. (1967). *The antecedents of self-esteem*. San Francisco: W. H. Freeman.

Dickstein, E. (1977). Self and self-esteem: Theoretical foundations and their implications for research. *Human Development, 20,* 129–140.

Ellemers, N., Spears, R., & Doosje, B. (2002). Self and social identity. *Annual Review of Psychology, 53,* 161–186.

Erikson, E. (1963). *Childhood and society* (2nd ed.). New York: Norton.

Fauerbach, J. A., Heinberg, L. J., Lawrence, J. W., Munster, A. M., Palombo, D. A., Richter, D. B. S., et al. (2000). Effect of early body image dissatisfaction on subsequent psychological and physical adjustment after disfiguring injury. *Psychosomatic Medicine, 62*(4), 576–582.

Finelli, L. A. (2001). Revisiting the identity issue in anorexia. *Journal of Psychosocial Nursing, 39*(8), 23–29.

Ghosh, T. B., & Victor, B. S. (1994). Suicide. In R. E. Hales, S. C. Yudofsky, & J. A. Talbott (Eds.). *The American Psychiatric Press textbook of psychiatry* (2nd ed.). Washington, DC: American Psychiatric Press.

Glod, C. A. (1998). *Contemporary psychiatric-mental health nursing*. Philadelphia: F. A. Davis Company.

Goldberg, R. J., & Tull, R. M. (1983). *The psychosocial dimensions of cancer: A practical guide for health care providers*. New York: Free Press.

Gregory, J. (1996). *The psychosocial education of nurses: The interpersonal dimension*. Aldershot, Hampshire, England: Avebury Ashgate Publishing.

Haber, J., Krainovich-Miller, B., McMahon, A., & Price-Hoskins, P. (1997). *Comprehensive psychiatric nursing* (5th ed.). St. Louis: Mosby.

Hattie, J. (1992). *Self concept*. Hillsdale, NJ: Erlbaum Bacon.

Hillman, J. (1975). *Re-visioning psychology*. New York: Harper & Row.

Himmelhoch, J., Levine, J., & Gershon, S. (2001). Historical overview of the relationship between anxiety disorders and affective disorders. *Depression and Anxiety, 14,* 53–66.

International Society for Mental Health Online (ISMHO). (2001). *All about depression*. Retrieved September 5, 2003, from *http://www.allaboutdepression.com/gen_01.html#3*

Jamison, K. R. (1997). *An unquiet mind: A memoir of moods and madness.* London: Picador.

Johnson, M., Bulechek, G., Dochterman, J., Maas, M., & Moorhead, S. (2001). *Nursing diagnoses, outcomes, and interventions: NANDA, NOC, and NIC linkages.* St. Louis: Mosby.

Kearney-Cooke, A. (n.d.). Develop a positive body image. Retrieved August 26, 2003, from *http://www.local6.com/health/1032675/detail.html*

Kessler, R. C. (1997). The effects of stressful life events on depression. *Annual Review of Psychology, 48,* 191–214.

King, K. A. (1997). Self-concept and self-esteem: A clarification of terms. *Journal of School Health, 67*(2), 68–70.

Kleinman, A., & Good, B. (1985). *Culture and depression.* Berkeley, CA: University of California Press.

Levine, J., Cole, D. P., Chengappa, R., & Gershon, S. (2001). Anxiety disorders and major depression, together or apart. *Depression and Anxiety, 14,* 94–104.

Marsh, H. W. (1988). *Self-description questionnaire I.* San Antonio, TX: Psychological Corporation.

Marsh, H. W. (1989). *Self-description questionnaire III (SDQIII) manual.* Sydney, Australia: University of Western Sydney.

Marsh, H. W. (1991). *Self-description questionnaire II: Manual and research monograph.* San Antonio, TX: Psychological Corporation.

Maslow, A. (1968). *Toward a psychology of being* (2nd ed.). New York: Van Nostrand-Reinhold.

Mead, M. (1934). *Mind, self and society.* Chicago: University of Chicago Press.

Menninger, K. (1963). *The vital balance.* New York: Viking Press.

Morris, C., & Coleman, J. (1997). *Contemporary psychology and effective behavior,* (7th ed.). Upper Saddle River, NJ: Pearson Addison-Wesley.

Murdock, M. (1990). *The heroine's journey.* Boston: Shambhala.

NANDA International. (2005). *Nursing diagnoses: Definitions and classification 2005–2006.* Philadelphia: Author.

National Guideline Clearinghouse. (1996/2002). Major depression, panic disorder and generalized anxiety disorder in adults in primary care. Department of Health and Human Services 1998–2003. Retrieved August 29, 2003, from *http://www.guideline.gov/summary/summary.aspx?doc_id=3350*

Newell, R., & Gournay, K. (Eds.). (2000). *Mental health nursing: An evidence-based approach.* London: Churchill Livingstone.

Parker, G. (2002). *Dealing with depression: A commonsense guide to mood disorders.* Australia: Allen & Unwin.

Peplau, H. (1963). A working definition of anxiety. In S. Burd & M. Marshall (Eds.), *Some clinical approaches to psychiatric nursing.* New York: Macmillan.

Reeve, C. (1998). *Still me.* New York: Random House.

Rund, D. A., & Hutzler, J. C. (1983). *Emergency psychiatry.* St Louis: Mosby.

Stice, E., & Shaw, H. (2003). Prospective relations of body image, eating, and affective disturbances to smoking onset in adolescent girls: How Virginia slims. *Journal of Consulting and Clinical Psychology, 71*(1), 129–135.

Stokes, R., & Frederick-Recascino, C. (2003). Women's perceived body image: Relations with personal happiness. *Journal of Women & Aging, 15*(1), 17–29.

Stuart, G. W., & Laraia, M. T. (2001). *Principles and practice of psychiatric nursing* (7th ed.). St Louis: Mosby.

Townsend, M. C. (2003). *Essentials of psychiatric mental health nursing* (2nd ed.). Philadelphia: F. A. Davis.

U.S. Preventive Services Task Force. (2002). Screening for depression: Recommendations and rationale. *Annals of Internal Medicine, 136*(10), 760–764.

Videbeck, S. L. (2001). *Psychiatric mental health nursing.* Philadelphia: Lippincott.

Walker, L., Timmerman, G. M., Kim, M., & Sterling, B. (2002). Relationships between body image and depressive symptoms during postpartum in ethnically diverse, low income women. *Women Health, 36*(3), 101–121.

Wingood, G. M., DiClemente, R. J., Harrington, K., & Davies, S. L. (2002). Body image and African American females' sexual health. *Journal of Women's Health and Gender Based Medicine, 11*(5), 433–439.

Winter, A. L., deGuia, N. A., Ferrence, R., & Cohen, J. E. (2002). The relationship between body weight perceptions, weight control behaviours and smoking status among adolescents. *Canadian Journal of Public Health, 93*(5), 362–365.

Zigmond, A. S., & Snaith, R. P. (1983). The hospital anxiety and depression scale. *Acta Psychiatrica Scandinavica, 67,* 361–370.

CHAPTER 12

Allen, K. A., Fine, M. A., & Demo, D. H. (2000). An overview of family diversity: Controversies, questions, and values. In D. H. Demo, K. A. Allen, & M. A. Fine (Eds.), *Handbook of family diversity,* pp. 1–14. New York: Oxford University Press.

American Medical Association (2002). *AMA health policy publishes new proposal for expanding health insurance coverage.* Retrieved October 7, 2003, from *http://www.ama-assn.org/ama/pub/category/3373.html*

Baumann, S. L. (2000). Family nursing: Theory-anemic, nursing theory-deprived. *Nursing Science Quarterly, 13*(4), 285–290.

Centers for Disease Control. (2000). Entry into prenatal care—United States, 1987–1997. *Morbidity and Mortality Weekly Report, 49*(18), 393–398. Retrieved October 7, 2003, from *http://www.cdc.gov/epo/mmwr/preview/mmwrhtml/mm4918a1.htm*

Clancy, C. M., & Bierman, A. S. (2000). Quality and outcomes of care for older women with chronic disease. *Women's Health Issues, 10*(4), 178–191.

Denham, S. (2003). *Family health: A framework for nursing.* Philadelphia: F. A. Davis Company.

Dochterman, J. M., & Bulechek, G. M. (Eds.). (2004). *Nursing interventions classification (NIC)* (4th ed.). St. Louis: Mosby.

Friedman, M. M. (1992). *Family nursing: Theory and practice* (3rd ed.). Norwalk, CT: Appleton & Lange.

Friedman, M. M., Bowden, V. R., & Jones, E. G. (2003). *Family nursing: Research, theory, and practice* (5th ed.). Upper Saddle River, NJ: Prentice Hall.

Gillis, C. L., Highley, B. L., Roberts, B. M., & Martinson, I. M. (1989). *Toward a science of family nursing.* Menlo Park, CA: Addison-Wesley.

Hanna, D. R., & Roy, C. (2001). Roy adaptation model and perspective on the family. *Nursing Science Quarterly, 14*(1), 9–12.

Hanson, S. M. (2001). *Family health care nursing: Theory, practice, and research* (2nd ed.). Philadelphia: F. A. Davis Company.

International Child Abuse Network. (2003). Statistics: Child abuse. Retrieved May 13, 2004, from *http://www.yesican.org/statisticsCA.html*

Johnson, B. S. (2000). Mothers' perceptions of parenting children with disabilities. *Maternal Child Nursing: American Journal of Maternal-Child Nursing, 25*(3), 127–132.

Larson, E. A. (2000). The orchestration of occupation: The dance of mothers. *American Journal of Occupational Therapy, 54*(3), 269–280.

Leahy, J. M., & Kizilay, P. A. (Eds.). (1998). *Foundations of nursing practice: A nursing process approach.* Philadelphia: W. B. Saunders.

McGoldrick, M., & Carter, E. (1985). The stages of the family life cycle. In J. Henslin (Ed.), *Marriage and family in a changing society.* New York: Free Press.

Moorhead, S., Johnson, M., & Maas, M. (Eds.). (2004). *Nursing outcomes classification (NOC)* (3rd ed.). St. Louis: Mosby.

Parsons, T., & Bales, R. F. (1955). *Family socialization and interaction process.* New York: Free Press.

Population Reference Bureau. (2003). Types of U.S. married-couple households, 2002. Retrieved November 3, 2003, from *http://www.ameristat.org/Traditional_Families_Account_for_Only_7_Percent_of_U_S_Households.html*

Primeau, L. (2000). Divisions of household work, routines, and child care occupations in families. *Journal of Occupational Science, 7*(1), 19–28.

Schroeder, M., & Affara, F. (Eds.). (2001). *The family nurse: Frameworks for practice.* Geneva, Switzerland: International Council of Nurses.

Schwartz, A. N. (1979). Psychological dependency: An emphasis on the later years. In P. Ragan (Ed.), *Aging parents.* Los Angeles: Andrus Gerontology Center, University of Southern California.

Winstead-Fry, P. (2000). Rogers' conceptual system and family nursing. *Nursing Science Quarterly, 13*(4), 278–280.

Wright, L. M., & Leahey, M. (1984). *Nurses and families: A guide to family assessment and intervention.* Philadelphia: F. A. Davis Company.

CHAPTER 13

American Nurses Association. (1997). *Position statements: Cultural diversity in nursing practice.* Retrieved January 12, 2003, from *http://www.nursingworld.org/readroom/position/ethics/etcldv.htm*

Andrews, M. M., & Boyle, J. S. (2003). *Transcultural concepts in nursing care* (4th ed.). Philadelphia: Lippincott.

Campinha-Bacote, J. (2002). The process of cultural competence in the delivery of healthcare services: A model of care. *Journal of Transcultural Nursing, 13*(3), 181–184.

Canadian Census. (2003). *Canada's ethnocultural portrait: The changing mosaic.* Retrieved March 7, 2003, from *http://www12.statcan.ca/english/census01/products/analytic/companion/etoimm/tables/canada/ethnic.cfm#*

Carballeira, N. (1997). The LIVE and LEARN model for cultural competent family services. *Continuum, 7*–12.

Cross, T., Bazron, B., Dennis, K., & Issacs, M. (1989). *Towards a culturally competent system of care: Vol. I.* Washington, DC: Georgetown University Child Development Center, CASSP Technical Center.

Dochterman, J. M., & Bulechek, G. M. (Eds.). (2004). *Nursing interventions classification (NIC)* (4th ed.). St. Louis: Mosby.

Dozier, W. L. (2003). Race: Anthropologists say divisions were made by man. *The Gazette.* Retrieved August 5, 2003, from *http://www.gazette.net/200018/frederickcty/state/10106-1.html*

Fong, C. (1985). Ethnicity and nursing practice. *Topics in Clinical Nursing, 7*(3), 1–10.

Geissler, E. M. (1991). Transcultural nursing and nursing diagnosis. *Nursing and Health Care, 12*(4), 190–203.

George, T. B. (2000). Defining care in the culture of the chronically mentally ill living in the community. *Journal of Transcultural Nursing, 11*(2), 102–110.

Giger, J. N., & Davidhizar, R. (2002). The Giger and Davidhizar transcultural assessment model. *Journal of Transcultural Nursing, 13*(3), 185–188.

Giger, J. N., & Davidhizar, R. (2004). *Transcultural nursing: Assessment and intervention* (4th ed.). St Louis: Mosby.

Graham-Garcia, J., Raines, T. L., Andrews, J. O., & Mensah, G. A. (2001). Race, ethnicity, and geography: Disparities in heart disease in woman of color. *Journal of Transcultural Nursing, 12*(1), 56–67.

Healthy People 2010. (2002). *Healthy people 2010 documents.* Retrieved April 20, 2003, from *http://www.healthypeople.gov/document/*

Helman, C. (2000). *Culture, health and illness* (4th ed.). Woburn, MA: Butterworth-Heinemann.

Leininger, M. (1978). *Transcultural nursing: Concepts, theories, and practices.* New York: John Wiley & Sons.

Leininger, M. (Ed.). (1991). *Culture care diversity and universality: A theory of nursing.* New York: National League for Nursing Press.

Leininger, M. (1995). *Transcultural nursing: Concepts, theories, and practices* (2nd ed.). New York: McGraw-Hill.

Leininger, M. (2002a). Cultural care theory: A major contribution to advance transcultural nursing knowledge and practice. *Journal of Transcultural Nursing, 13*(3), 189–192.

Leininger, M. (2002b). Founder's focus: Linguistic clichés and buzzwords in the culture of nursing. *Journal of Transcultural Nursing, 13*(4), 334.

Leininger, M. M., & McFarland, M. R. (2002). *Transcultural nursing: Concepts, theories and practices.* New York: McGraw-Hill.

Leppa, C. (2000). Transcultural communication within the health care subculture. In J. Luckmann, *Transcultural communication in health care* (pp. 74–83). Albany, NY: Delmar.

Lipson, J., & Meleis, A. (1985). Culturally appropriate care: The case of immigrants. *Topics in Clinical Nursing, 7*(3), 48–56.

Luckmann, J. (2000). *Transcultural communication in health care.* Albany, NY: Delmar.

Lustig, M. W., & Koester, J. (2003). *Intercultural competence: Interpersonal communication across cultures* (4th ed.). Boston: Pearson Education.

Mechanic, D. (1963). Religion, religiosity, and illness behavior: The special case of the Jews. *Human Organization, 22,* 202–208.

Purnell, L. (2000). A description of the Purnell model for cultural competence. *Journal of Transcultural Nursing, 11,* 40–46.

Purnell, L. (2002). The Purnell model for cultural competence. *Journal of Transcultural Nursing, 13*(3), 193–196.

Purnell, L. D., & Paulanka, B. J. (2003). *Transcultural health care: A culturally competent approach* (2nd ed.). Philadelphia: F. A. Davis Company.

Reynolds, C. L., & Leininger, M. (1993). *Madeleine Leininger: Cultural care diversity and universality theory.* Newbury Park: Sage.

Spector, R. (2000). *Cultural care guides to heritage assessment and health traditions* (2nd ed.). Upper Saddle River, NJ: Prentice Hall.

Spector, R. E. (2002). Cultural diversity in health and illness. *Journal of Transcultural Nursing, 13*(3), 197–199.

Spector, R. E. (2004). *Cultural diversity in health and illness* (6th ed.). Upper Saddle River, NJ: Prentice Hall.

Spratley, E., Johnson, A., Sochalski, J., Fritz, M., & Spencer, W. (2000). *The registered nurse population: Findings from the national sample survey of registered nurses.* Washington, DC: U.S. Department of Health and Human Services, Health Resources and Service Administration, Bureau of Health Professions, Division of Nursing.

Suchman, E. A. (1964). Sociomedical variations among ethnic groups. *American Journal of Sociology, 70,* 319–331.

Suchman, E. A. (1965). Social patterns of illness and medical care. *Journal of Health and Human Behavior, 6,* 2–16.

Tripp-Reimer, T. (1985). Expanding four essential concepts in nursing theory: The contribution of anthropology. In J. McCloskey & H. Grace (Eds.), *Current issues in nursing.* Boston: Blackwell.

Wilkinson, J. M. (2001). *Nursing process and critical thinking* (3rd ed.). Upper Saddle River, NJ: Prentice Hall.

U.S. Bureau of the Census. (2003a). *U.S. census data.* Retrieved January 20, 2003, from *http://www.census.gov*

U.S. Bureau of the Census. (2003b). *U.S. projections of resident populations by race and Hispanic origin.* Retrieved July 20, 2003, from *http://www.census.gov/population/projections/nation/summary/np-t5-b.txt*

U.S. Department of Health and Human Services, OPHS, Office of Minority Health. (2001). *National standards for culturally and linguistically appropriate services in health care: Executive summary.* Washington, DC: Author. Retrieved August 5, 2003, from *http://www.haa.omhrc.gov/HAA2pg/whatsnew10.htm*

Zborowski, M. (1952). Cultural components in responses to pain. *Journal of Social Issues, 8,* 16–30.

Zborowski, M. (1969). *People in pain.* San Francisco: Jossey-Bass.

Zola, I. K. (1966, October). Culture and symptoms: An analysis of patients presenting complaints. *American Sociological Review, 31,* 615–630.

CHAPTER 14

Ameling, A. (2000). Prayer: An ancient healing practice becomes new again. *Holistic Nursing Practice, 14*(3): 40–48.

American Nurses Association. (2004). *Code for nurses.* Washington, DC: American Nurses Publishing.

Aspen Publishers. (2002). *Palliative care: Patient and family counseling manual* (2nd ed.). New York: Author.

American Psychiatric Association. (1994). *Diagnostic and statistical manual of mental disorders* (4th ed). (*DSM-IV*). Washington, DC: Author.

Battaglia, B. (1998). Cultural views on death and dying: Part 3. *Cross Cultural Connection, 3,* 1–4.

Beck, S. E., & Goldberg, E. K. (1996). Jewish beliefs, values and practices: Implications for culturally sensitive nursing care. *Advance Practice Nursing Quarterly, 2*(2), 15–22.

Book of Common Prayer. (1979). New York: Oxford University Press.

Borelli, J. (1990). Buddhism. In J. A. Komonchak, M. Collins, & D. A. Lane (Eds.), *The new dictionary of theology* (pp. 144–147). Collegeville, MN: Liturgical Press.

Boyd, D. (1974). *Rolling thunder.* New York: Random House.

Bradshaw, A. (1996). The legacy of Nightingale . . . spiritual care. *Nursing Times, 92*(6), 42–43.

Bradshaw, A. (1997). Teaching spiritual care to nurses: An alternative approach. *International Journal of Palliative Nursing, 3*(1), 51–57.

Broten, P. J. (1997). Spiritual care documentation: Where is it? *Journal of Christian Nursing, 14*(2), 29–31.

Broussat, F., & Broussat, M.A. (1996). *Spiritual literacy: Reading the sacred in everyday life.* New York: Simon & Schuster.

Brown-Saltzman, K. (1997). Replenishing the spirit by meditative prayer and guided imagery. *Seminars in Oncology Nursing, 13*(4), 255–259.

Byrne, M. (2002). Spirituality in palliative care: What language do we need? *International Journal of Palliative Nursing, 8*(2), 67–74.

Carrigg, K. C., & Weber, R. (1997). Development of the spiritual care scale. *Image: The Journal of Nursing Scholarship, 29*(3), 293.

Cavendish, R., Luise, B., Horne, K., Bauer, M., Gallo, M., Medefindt, J., et al. (2000). Opportunities for enhanced spirituality relevant to well adults. *Nursing Diagnosis: International Journal of Nursing Language and Classification, 11*(4), 151–163.

Cavendish, R., Konecny, L., Mitzeliotis, C., Russo, D., Luise, B., Lanza, M., et al. (2003). Spiritual care interventions of nurses using Nursing Interventions Classification (NIC) labels. *International Journal of Nursing Terminologies and Classifications, 14*(4), 113–124.

Cenkner, W. (1990). Hinduism. In J. A. Komonchak, M. Collins, & D. A. Lane (Eds.), *The new dictionary of theology* (pp. 466–469). Collegeville, MN: Liturgical Press.

Dickenson, C. (1975). The search for spiritual meaning. *American Journal of Nursing, 75*(10), 1789–1793.

Dochterman, J. M., & Bulechek, G. M. (Eds.). (2004). *Nursing interventions classification* (4th ed.). St Louis: Mosby.

Dolan, J. A., Fitzpatrick, H. L., & Hermann, E. K. (1983). *Nursing in society: A historical perspective.* Philadelphia: W. B. Saunders.

Dombeck, M. (1997). Healing the fractured self. In M. S. Roach (Ed.), *Caring from the heart: The convergence of caring and spirituality* (pp. 50–67). Mahwa, NJ: Paulis & Press.

Donahue, M. P. (1985). *Nursing: The finest art. An illustrated history.* St Louis: Mosby.

Dunn, K., & Horgas, A. (2000). The prevalence of prayer as a spiritual self-care modality in elders. *Journal of Holistic Nursing, 18*(4), 337–351.

Elfried, S. (1998). Helping patients find meaning: A caring response to suffering. *International Journal for Human Caring, 2*(1), 33–39.

Emblen, J., & Pesut, B. (2001). Strengthening transcendent meaning. A model for the spiritual nursing care of patients experiencing suffering. *Journal of Holistic Nursing, 19*(1), 42–56.

Esposito, J. L. (1990). Islam. In J. A. Komonchak, M. Collins, & D. A. Lane (Eds.), *The new dictionary of theology* (pp. 527–529). Collegeville, MN: Liturgical Press.

Folta, R. (1996). Bible study: God's gifts are for giving (how to use my talent to help my patients). *Christian Nurse International, 12*(2/3), 15.

Fox, M. (1983). *Meditations with Meister Eckhart.* Santa Fe, NM: Bear & Company.

Friedemann, M., Mouch, J., & Racey, T. (2002). Nursing the spirit: The Framework of Systemic Organization. *Journal of Advanced Nursing, 39*(4), 325–332.

George, L. K., Ellison, C. G., & Larson, D. B. (2002). Exploring the relationships between religious involvement and health. *Psychological Inquiry, 13,* 190–200.

Gilbert, T. (2002). The spiritual art of working with dreams. *Journal of Holistic Nursing, 20*(3), 305–310.

Goldberg, B. (1998). Connection: An exploration of spirituality in nursing care. *Journal of Advanced Nursing, 27*(4), 836–842.

Granstrom, S. L. (1985). Spiritual nursing care for oncology patients. *Topics in Clinical Nursing, 4,* 39–45.

Grey, R. (1996). The psychosocial spiritual care matrix: A new paradigm in hospice care-giving. *American Journal of Hospice and Palliative Care, 13*(4), 19–25.

Harris, W., Gowda, M., Kilb, J., Strychacz, C., Vacek, J., Jones, P., et al. (1999). A randomized, controlled trial of the effects of remote, intercessory prayer on outcomes in patients admitted to the coronary care unit. *Archives of Internal Medicine, 159*(19), 2273–2278.

Highfield, M. E. F. (1992). Spiritual healing of oncology patients: Nurse and patient perspectives. *Cancer Nursing, 15*(1), 1–8.

Highfield, M. E. F. (2000). Providing spiritual care to patients with cancer. *Clinical Journal of Oncology Nursing, 4*(3), 115–120.

Highfield, M. E. F., & Cason, C. (1983). Spiritual needs of patients: Are they recognized? *Cancer Nursing, 6*(3), 187–192.

Hill, P. C., & Pargament, K. I. (2003). Advances in the conceptualization and measurement of religion and spirituality: Implications for physical and mental health research. *American Psychologist, 58*(1), 64–74.

Humphreys, J. (2000). Spirituality and distress in sheltered battered women. *Journal of Nursing Scholarship, 32*(3), 273–278.

Hungelmann, J., Kenkel-Rossi, E., Klassen, L., & Stollenwerk, L. (1996). Focus on spiritual well-being: Harmonious interconnectedness of mind-body-spirit—use of the JAREL spiritual well-being scale. *Geriatric Nursing, 17*(6), 262.

Johnson, C. (2001). An Islamic understanding of health care: What can it teach us? *Accident and Emergency Nursing, 9*(1), 38–45.

Joint Commission on the Accreditation of Healthcare Organizations. (2002). *2002 hospital accreditation standards.* Oakbrook Terrace, IL: Author.

Keegan, L. (2000). A comparison of the use of alternative therapies among Mexican Americans and Anglo-Americans in the Texas Rio Grande Valley. *Journal of Holistic Nursing, 18*(3): 280–295.

Kinney, A., Emery, G., Dudley, W., & Croyle, R. (2002). Screening behaviors among African American women at high risk for breast cancer: Do beliefs about God matter? *Oncology Nursing Forum, 29*(5), 835–843.

Kirkwood, N. A. (1993). *A hospital handbook on multiculturalism.* Harrisburg, PA: Morehouse Publishing.

Kluckhohn, C., & Leighton, D. (1962). *The Navajo.* Garden City, NY: Doubleday.

Kociszewski, C. (2003). A phenomenological pilot study of the nurses' experience providing spiritual care. *Journal of Holistic Nursing, 21*(2), 131–148.

Koenig, H. G., McCollough, M. E., & Larson, D. B. (2001). *Handbook of religions and health.* New York: Oxford University Press.

Krishnamurti, J. (1989). *Think on these things.* New York: Harper Perennial.

Lane, J. (1987). The care of the human spirit. *Journal of Professional Nursing, 3*(6), 332–337.

Kuuppelomaki, M. (2002). Spiritual support for families of patients with cancer: A pilot study of nursing staff assessments. *Cancer Nursing, 25,* 209–218.

Large, J. E. (1965). *The church and healing.* New York: Forward Movement Publications.

Larson, D. B., Pattison, E. M., Blazer, D. G., Omran, A. R., & Kaplan, B. H. (1986). Systematic analysis of research on religious variables in four major psychiatric journals, 1978–1982. *American Journal of Psychiatry, 143,* 329–334.

Larson, D. B., Swyers, J. P., & McCollough, M. E. (1998). *Scientific research on spirituality and health: A report based on the Scientific Progress in Spirituality Conferences.* Bethesda, MD: National Institute for Health Care Research.

le Gallez, P., Dimmock, S., & Bird, H. (2000). Spiritual healing as adjunct therapy for rheumatoid arhtritis. *British Journal of Nursing, 9*(11), 695–700.

Leininger, M. (1997). Transcultural spirituality: A comparative care and health focus. In M. S. Roach (Ed.), *Caring from the heart: The convergence of caring and spirituality* (pp. 99–118). Mahwah, NJ: Paulis & Press.

Levoy, G. (1997). *Callings: Finding and following an authentic life.* New York: Harmony Books.

Lewis, C. S. (1961). *A grief observed.* New York: Seabury Press.

Lo, R. (2003). The use of prayer in spiritual care. *Australian Journal of Holistic Nursing, 10*(1), 22–29.

Lukoff, D. (2002). Internet guided learning: DSM-IV religious and spiritual problems. Retrieved August 20, 2003, from *http://www.internetguides.com/dsm4/lesson1_1.html*

Macquarrie, J. (1977). *Principles of Christian theology* (2nd ed.). New York: Scribner.

Macrae, J. (1995). Nightingale's spiritual philosophy and its significance for modern nursing. *Image: Journal of Nursing Scholarship, 27*(1), 8–10.

Marler, K. I., & Hadaway, C. K. (2002). "Being religious" or "being spiritual" in America: A zero-sum proposition? *Journal for the Scientific Study of Religion, 41,* 289–300.

Matthews, W., Conti, J., & Sireci, S. (2001). The effects of intercessory prayer, positive visualization, and expectancy on the well-being of kidney dialysis patients. *Alternative Therapies in Health and Medicine, 7*(5), 42–52.

Matthews, D., Marlowe, S., & MacNutt, F. (2000). Effects of intercessory prayer on patients with rheumatoid arthritis. *Southern Medical Journal 93*(12), 1177–1186.

McCollough, M. E., Hoyt, W. T., Larson, D. B., Koenig, H. B., & Thoresen, C. (2000). Religious involvement and mortality: A meta-analytic review. *Health Psychology, 19,* 211–222.

McSherry, W. (1998). Nurses' perception of spirituality and spiritual care, *Nursing Standard, 13*(4), 36–40.

Moberg, D. (1982). Spiritual well-being of the dying. In G. Lesnoff-Carabaglia (Ed.), *Aging and the human condition.* Springfield, IL: Human Sciences Press.

Money, M. (2001). Shamanism as a healing paradigm for complementary therapy. *Complementary Therapy and Nurse Midwifery, 7*(3), 126–131.

Moorhead, S., Johnson, M., & Maas, M. (Eds.). (2004). *Nursing outcomes classification (NOC)* (3rd ed.). St. Louis: Mosby.

NANDA International. (2005). *Nursing diagnoses: Definitions and classification 2005–2006.* Philadelphia: Author.

Narayanasamy, A. (2003). Spiritual coping mechanisms in chronically ill patients. *British Journal of Nursing, 11*(22), 1461–1470.

Newlin, K., Knafl, K., & Melkus, G. (2002). African-American spirituality: A concept analysis. *ANS Advances in Nursing Science, 25*(2), 57–70.

O'Brien, M. E. (1999). *Spirituality in nursing: Standing on holy ground.* Sudbury, MA: Jones and Bartlett.

Olson, T. (2003). Buddhism, behavior change, and OCD. *Journal of Holistic Nursing, 21*(2), 149–162.

Orchard, H., & Clark, D. (2001). Tending the soul as well as the body: Spiritual Care in nursing and residential homes. *International Journal of Palliative Nursing, 7*(11), 541–546.

Pawlikowski, J. (1990). Judaism. In J. Komonchak, M. Collins, & D. A. Lane (Eds.), *The new dictionary of theology* (pp. 543–548). Collegeville, MN: Liturgical Press.

Plante, T. G., & Sherman A. C. (Eds.). (2001). *Faith and health: Psychological perspectives.* New York: Guilford Press.

Reeve, C. (1998). *Still me.* New York: Random House.

Reeve, C. (2002). *Nothing is impossible: Reflections on a new life.* New York: Random House.

Roberts, L., Ahmed, I., & Hall, S. (2000). Intercessory prayer for the alleviation of ill health. *Cochrane Database Systems Review (2):* CD000368.

Robinson-Smith, G. (2002). Prayer after stroke: Its relationship to quality of life. *Journal of Holistic Nursing, 20*(4), 352–366.

Ryan, P. (1992). Perception of the most helpful nursing behaviors in a home-care hospice setting: Care-givers and nurses. *American Journal of Hospice and Palliative Care, 9*(5), 22–31.

Satterly, L. (2001). Guilt, shame, and religious and spiritual pain. *Holistic Nursing Practice, 15*(2), 30–39.

Sellers, S., & Haag, B. (1998). Spiritual nursing interventions. *Journal of Holistic Nursing, 16*(3), 338–354.

Seybold, K. S., & Hill, P. C. (2001). The role of religion and spirituality in mental and physical health. *Current Directions in Psychological Science, 10,* 21–24.

Shelley, J., Miller, A., & Fish, S. (1995). Praying with patients: Why, when and how. *Journal of Christian Nursing, 12*(1), 9–13, 28.

Simpson, R. (2002). Healing health care, healing nursing in the 21st century. *Nursing Administration Quarterly, 26*(5), 94–98.

Sodestrom, K., & Martin, I. M. (1987). Patients' spiritual coping strategies: A study of nurse and patient perspectives. *Oncology Nursing Forum, 14*(2), 41–46.

Sparber, A., Bauer, L., Curt, G., Eisenberg, D., Levin, T., Parks, S., et al. (2000). Use of complementary medicine by adult patients participating in cancer clinical trials. *Oncology Nursing Forum, 27*(6), 887–888.

Stepnick, A., & Perry, T. (1992). Preventing spiritual distress n the dying patient. *Journal of Psychosocial Nursing, 30*(1), 17–24.

Stiles, M. (1990). The shining stranger: Nurse-family spiritual relationship. *Cancer Nursing, 13*(4), 235–245.

Sumner, C. (1998). Recognizing and responding to spiritual distress. *American Journal of Nursing, 98* (Nurse Pract. Extra Edition), 26–31.

Taylor, E. (2001). Spirituality, culture, and cancer care. *Seminars in Oncology Nursing, 17*(3): 197–205.

Taylor, E., & Outlaw, F. (2002). Use of prayer among persons with cancer. *Holistic Nursing Practice, 16*(3), 46–60.

Terkel, S. (2003). *Hope dies last: Keeping the faith in difficult times.* New York: New Press.

Theis, S., Biordi, D., Coeling, H., Nalepka, C., & Miller, B. (2003). Spirituality in caregiving and care receiving. *Holistic Nursing Practice, 17*(1), 48–55.

Van Dover, L., & Bacon, J. (2001). Spiritual care in nursing practice: A close-up view. *Nursing Forum, 36*(1), 18–30.

Walker, S., Tonigan, J., Miller, W., Corner, S., & Kahlich, L. (1997). Intercessory prayer in the treatment of alcohol abuse and dependence: A pilot investigation. *Alternative Therapies in Health and Medicine, 3*(6), 79–86.

White, G. (2000). An inquiry into the concepts of spirituality and spiritual care. *International Journal of Palliative Nursing, 6*(10), 479–484.

Widerquist, J. G. (1992). The spirituality of Florence Nightingale. *Nursing Research, 41*(1), 49–55.

Woodard, E., & Richard, S. (2001). God in control: Women's perspectives on managing HIV infection. *Clinical Nursing Research, 10*(3), 233–250.

Wright, M. C. (2002). The essence of spiritual care: A phenomenological enquiry. *Palliative Medicine, 16*(2), 125–132.

Wright, S. G. (2002). Examining the impact of spirituality on nurses and health-care provision. *Professional Nurse, 17*(12), 709–711.

Zuckoff, M. (1995, April 18). More and more claiming American Indian heritage. *Boston Globe.*

CHAPTER 15

American Association of Colleges of Nurses. (1997). *A peaceful death: Recommended competencies and curricular guides to end-of-life care.* (Report from the Robert Wood Johnson End-of-Life Care Roundtable). Washington, DC: Author.

American Nurses Association. (1991). *Position statement: Assisted suicide and euthanasia.* Washington, DC: Author. Retrieved September 12, 2003, from *www.nursingworld.org/readroom/position/ethics/etsuic.htm*

American Nurses Association. (1992). *Position statement: Nursing care and do-not-resuscitate decisions.* Retrieved September 12, 2003, from *www.nursingworld.org/readroom/position/ethics/etdnr.htm*

American Nurses Association. (1994). *Position statement: Active euthanasia.* Retrieved September 12, 2003, from *www.nursingworld.org/readroom/position/ethics/eteuth.htm*

Banura, D., Fender, M., Roesler, M., & Pacquiao, D. (2001). Culturally congruent end-of-life care for Jewish patients and their families. *Journal of Transcultural Nursing, 12*(3), 211, 220.

Bednash, G., & Ferrell, B. (2000). *The end-of life nursing education consortium (2000). The ELNEC curriculum.* Washington, D.C.: American Association of Colleges of Nursing and City of Hope National Medical Center.

Bowlby, J. (1982). *Attachment and loss.* 3 vols. New York: Basic Books.

Boyle, J. S., Bunting, S. M., Hodnicki, D. R., & Ferrell, J. A. (2001). Critical thinking in African American mothers who care for adult children with HIV: A cultural analysis. *Journal of Transcultural Nursing, 12*(3), 193–202.

Corr, C., Nabe, C., & Corr, D. (2003). *Death and dying—Life and living.* Belmont, CA: Thomson-Wadsworth Press.

Davis, C., Wortman, C., Lehman, D., & Silver, R. (2000) Searching for meaning in loss: Are clinical assumptions correct? *Death Studies, 24,* 497–540.

DeSpelder, L., & Strickland, A. (1996). *The last dance.* Mountain View, CA: Mayfield.

Dochterman, J. M., & Bulechek, G. M. (Eds.). (2004). *Nursing interventions classification (NIC)* (4th ed.). St. Louis: Mosby.

Doka, K. (1989). *Disenfranchised grief: Recognizing hidden sorrow.* New York: Lexington Books.

Dworkind, M., & Karnes, B. (2003). *Common stages of the dying process.* Montreal: Jackson Memorial Hospital. Retrieved November 5, 2003, from *http://umjmh.org/HealthLibrary/Miscellaneous/About_Death.htm*

Egan, K. A., & Arnold, R. L. (2003). Grief and bereavement care. *American Journal of Nursing, 103*(9), 42–52.

Engel, G. L. (1964). Grief and grieving. *American Journal of Nursing, 64,* 93–98.

Erikson, E. (1963). *Childhood and society* (2nd ed.). London: Faber and Faber.

Erikson, E. (1968). *Identity, youth and crises.* New York: Norton.

Fallowfield, L., Jenkins, V., & Beveridge, H. (2002). Truth may hurt but deceit hurts more: Communication in palliative care. *Palliative Medicine, 16*(4), 297–303.

Family Hospice Association. (2003). *Choosing a hospice.* Retrieved November 7, 2003, from *http://www.familyhospice.com/html/choose/choose_history.htm*

Ferrell, B., & Coyle, N. (Eds.). (2001). *Textbook of palliative care nursing.* Oxford, England: Oxford University Press.

Ferrell, B. & Coyle, N. (2002). An overview of palliative care nursing. *American Journal of Nursing, 102*(5): 26–32.

Ferrell, B., Grant, M., & Virani, R. (1999). Strengthening nursing education to improve end-of-life care. *Nursing Outlook, 47*(6), 252.

Furman, J. (2002). What you should know about chronic grief: Learn to deal with your own lingering emotions when a patient dies. *Nursing, 32*(2), 56.

Gambles, M., Crooke, M., & Wilkinson, S. (2002). Evaluation of a hospice based reflexology service: A qualitative audit of patient perceptions. *European Journal of Oncology Nursing, 6*(1), 37–44.

Griffie, J., Nelson-Marten, P., & Muchka, S. (2004). Acknowledging the "elephant": Communication in palliative care. *American Journal of Nursing, 104*(1), 48–58.

Hall, J. (1996). *Nursing ethics and law.* Philadelphia: W. B. Saunders.

Hall, P., Shcroder, C., & Weaver, L. (2002). The last 48 hours of life in long-term care: A focused chart audit. *Journal of the American Geriatrics Society, 50*(3), 501–506.

Howard, S. (1989, January). How do I ask? Requesting tissue or organ donations from bereaved families. *Nursing 89,* 70–73.

Johnstone, P., Polston, G., Niemtzow, R., & Martin, P. (2002). Integration of acupuncture into the oncology clinic. *Palliative Medicine, 16*(3), 235–239.

Kübler-Ross, E. (1969). *On death and dying.* New York: Macmillan.

Lindemann, E. (1944). Symptomatology and management of acute grief. *American Journal of Psychiatry, 101,* 141–48.

Manzanec, P., & Tyler, M. K. (2003). Cultural considerations in end-of-life care. *American Journal of Nursing, 103*(3), 50–59.

Matzo, M., & Sherman, D. (2001). *Palliative care nursing.* New York: Springer.

Matzo, M., Sherman, D., Sheehan, D., Ferrell, B., & Penn, B. (2003). Teaching strategies from the ELNEC curriculum. *Nursing Education Perspectives, (24)*1, 176–183.

Moorhead, S., Johnson, M., & Maas, M. (Eds.). (2004). *Nursing outcomes classification (NOC)* (3rd ed.). St. Louis: Mosby.

NANDA International. (2005). *NANDA nursing diagnoses: Definitions and classification 2005–2006.* Philadelphia: Author.

Norton, S., & Bowers, B. (2002). Working toward consensus: Providers' strategies to shift patients from curative to palliative treatment choices. *Research in Nursing and Health, 24*(4), 258–269.

O'Connor, L., & Lunney, M. (1998). Care of the caregiver—Family member with a chronic illness. *Nursing Diagnosis, 9*(4), 152.

Parkes, C. M. (2001), *Bereavement: Studies of grief in adult life* (3rd ed.). New York: Routledge.

Pitorak, E. (2003). Care at the time of death. *American Journal of Nursing, (103)*7, 42–52.

Poor, B., & Poirrier, G. (2001). *End of life nursing care.* Boston: Jones & Bartlett and the National League for Nursing.

President's Commission for the Study of Ethical Problems in Medicine and Biomedical and Behavioral Research. (1981). *Defining death: A report on the medical, legal, and ethical issues in the determination of death.* Washington, DC: U.S. Government Printing Office.

Purnell, L. D., & Paulanka, B. J. (2003). *Transcultural health care: A culturally competent approach* (2nd ed.). Philadelphia: F. A. Davis Company.

Rando, T. (1984) *Grief, dying and death: Clinical interventions for caregivers.* Champaign, IL: Research Press.

Rando, T. (1986), *Loss and anticipatory grief.* Lexington, MA: Lexington Books.

Rando, T. (1991). *How to go on living when someone you love dies.* New York: Bantam.

Rando, T. (1993). *Treatment of complicated mourning.* Champaign, IL: Research Press.

Rando, T. (2000). *Clinical dimensions of anticipatory mourning: Theory and practice in working with the dying, their loved ones, and their caregivers.* Champaign, IL: Research Press.

Schneider, J. (1984). *Stress, loss, and grief.* Baltimore: University Park Press.

Schwartz, J. (2003). Understanding and responding to patients' requests for assistance in dying. *Journal of Nursing Scholarship, 35*(4), 377–383.

Shahar, D., Schultz, R., Shahar, A., & Wing, R. (2001). The effect of widowhood on weight change, dietary intake, and eating behavior in the elderly population. *Journal of Aging and Health, 13,* 186–199.

Sloman, R. (2002). Relaxation and imagery for anxiety and depression control in community patients with advanced cancer. *Cancer Nursing, 25*(6), 432–435.

Steinhauser, K., Christakis, N., Clipp, E., McNeilly, M., Grambow, S., Paarker, J., & Tulsky, J. (2001). Preparing for the end of life: Preferences of patients, families, physicians, and other care providers. *Journal of Pain and Symptom Management, 22*(3), 727–737.

Sulmasy, D. (2001). Addressing the religious and spiritual needs of dying patients. *Western Journal of Medicine, 175,* 251–254.

Teno, J. M., Casey, V. A., Welch, L. C., & Edgman-Levitan, S. (2001). Patient-focused, family-centered end-of-life medical care: Views of the guidelines and bereaved family members. *Journal of Pain and Symptom Management, 22,* 738–751.

Thompson, E., & Reilly, D. (2002). The homeopathic approach to symptom control in the cancer patient: A prospective observational study. *Palliative Medicine, 16*(3), 227–233.

Tilden, V. (2000). Advance directives: Meaningful existence and appropriate care at the end of life. *American Journal of Nursing, 100*(12), 49, 51.

Wildiers, H., & Menten, J. (2002). Death rattle: Prevalence, prevention and treatment. *Journal of Pain and Symptom Management, 23*(4), 310–317.

Worden, J. W. (2002). *Grief counseling and grief therapy: A handbook for the mental health practitioner* (3rd ed.). New York: Springer.

CHAPTER 16

American Nurses Association. (2004). *Nursing: Scope and standards of practice* (3rd ed). Washington, DC: Author.

Brooks, J. T. (1998). An analysis of nursing documentation as a reflection of actual nurse work. *Medsurg Nursing, 7*(4), 189–196.

Charting made incredibly easy (2nd ed.). (2002). Springhouse, PA: Lippincott Williams & Wilkins.

Charting tips: Watch your (charting) language. (2001). *Nursing, 131*(5), 67.

Currie, J. (2002). Improving the efficiency of patient handover. *Emergency Nurse, 10*(3), 24–28.

Dumple, H., James, M., & Phillips, T. (1999, June/July). Charting by exception. *California Nurse,* 9–10.

Handling verbal orders safely: Learn how to instill a measure of safety into those "whispering down the lane" verbal orders. (2001). *Nursing, 31*(12), 43.

Helleso, R., & Ruland, C. (2001). Developing a module for nursing documentation integrated in the electronic patient record. *Journal of Clinical Nursing, 10*(6), 799–805.

Joint Commission on the Accreditation of Healthcare Organizations (JCAHO). (2002). JCAHO establishes annual patient safety goals. *Joint Commission Perspectives, 22*(5), 1–3.

Joint Commission on the Accreditation of Healthcare Organizations (JCAHO). (2004). "Do not use" list required in 2004. Retrieved April 8, 2004, from *http://www.jcaho.org/accredited+organizations/patient+safety/04+npsg/04_faqs.htm*

Keenan, G. M. (1999). Use of standardized nursing language will make nursing visible. *Michigan Nurse, 72*(2), 12–15.

Lampe, S. (1985). Focus charting: Streamlining documentation. *Nurse Manager, 16*(7), 43–46.

Legal questions. (2002). *Nursing, 32*(1), 66.

Martin, A., Hinds, C., & Felix, M. (1999). Documentation practices of nurses in long-term care. *Journal of Clinical Nursing, 8,* 345–352.

Pearson, A. (2003). The role of documentation in making nursing work visible. *International Journal of Nursing Practice, 9*(5), 280–284.

Smith, L. (2002). How to chart by exception. *Nursing, 32*(9), 30.

Squires, A. (2003). Documenting surgical incision care. *Nursing, 33*(1), 74.

Triplett, L. (2002). Electronic supportive documentation: Welcome to the future. *Nursing Home Long Term Management, 51*(12), 40–41.

Trossman, S. (2002). The documentation dilemma. *Tar Heel Nurse, 64*(3), 10.

Trossman, S. (2003). Protecting patient information. *American Journal of Nursing, 103*(1). Retrieved November 19, 2003, from *http://nursingworld.org/ajn/2003/feb/issues.htm*

Waggoner, M., & Grindel, M. Oasis: Measuring outcomes in home care. *Medsurg Nursing, 8*(3), 214–216.

Wise, L., Mersch, J., Racioppi, J., Crosier, J., & Thompson, C. (2000). Evaluating the reliability and utility of cumulative intake and output. *Journal of Nursing Care Quality, 3*(14), 37–42.

CHAPTER 17

American Heart Association. (2002). AHA Medical/Scientific Statement. *Human blood pressure determination by sphygmomanometry,* by D. Perloff et al. (1993). Product Code #88:2460-2467. Retrieved January 9, 2003, from *http://216.185.112.5/presenter.jhtml?identifier=3000894*

American Nurses Association. (2004). *Nursing: scope and standards of practice* (3rd ed). Washington, DC: Author.

Blazys, D. (2000). Does taking an orthostatic blood pressure include taking the pulse? *Journal of Emergency Nursing, 26*(5), 479–480.

Boxer, E., & Kluge, B. (2000). Essential clinical skills for beginning registered nurses. *Nurse Educator Today, 20*(4), 327–335.

Campbell, N. R., Burgess, E., Choi, B. C., Taylor, G., Wilson, E., Cleroux, J., et al. (1999). Lifestyle modifications to prevent and control hypertension. 1. Methods and an overview of the Canadian recommendations. Canadian Hypertension Society, Canadian Coalition for High Blood Pressure Prevention and Control, Laboratory Center for Disease Control at Health Canada, Heart and Stroke Foundation of Canada. *Canadian Medical Association Journal, 160*(9 Suppl), S1–6.

Erickson, R. S., & Yount, S. T. (1991, March/April). Comparison of tympanic and oral temperatures in surgical patients. *Nursing Research, 40,* 90–93.

Frazier, L. (2000). Factors influencing blood pressure: Development of a risk model. *Journal of Cardiovascular Nursing, 15*(1), 62–79.

Guyton, A. C., & Hall, J. E. (2000). *Textbook of medical physiology* (10th ed.). Philadelphia: Saunders.

Hwu, Y. J., Coates, V. E., & Lin, F. Y. (2000). A study of the effectiveness of different measuring times and counting methods of human radial pulse rates. *Journal of Clinical Nursing, 9*(1), 146–152.

Jensen, B. N., Jensen, F. S., Madsen, S. N., & Lossl, K. (2000). Accuracy of digital tympanic, oral, axillary, and rectal thermometers compared with standard rectal mercury thermometers. *European Journal of Surgery, 166*(11), 848–851.

Joint National Committee on Detection, Evaluation, and Treatment of High Blood Pressure. (1997). *The sixth report of the Joint National Committee on Detection, Evaluation, and Treatment of High Blood Pressure.* NIH Publication No. 98-4080. Bethesda, MD: National Institutes of Health.

Joint National Committee on Prevention, Detection, Evaluation and Treatment of High Blood Pressure. (2003). *JNC 7 Express: The seventh report of the Joint National Committee on Prevention, Detection, Evaluation, and Treatment of High Blood Pressure.* NIH Publication No. 03-5233. U. S. Department of Health and Human Services, National Institutes of Health, National Heart, Lung, and Blood Institute, National High Blood Pressure Education Program. Bethesda, MD: National Institutes of Health.

Retrieved May 22, 2003, from *http://www.nhlbi.nih.gov/guidelines/hypertension/index.htm*

Kocoglu, H., Goksu, S., Isik, M., Akturk, Z, & Bayazit, Y. A. (2002). Infrared tympanic thermometer can accurately measure the body temperature in children in an emergency room setting. *International Journal of Pediatric Otorhinolaryngology, 65*(1), 39–43.

Lance, R., Link, M. E., Padua, M., Clavell, L. E., Johnson, G., & Knebel, A. (2000). Comparison of different methods of obtaining orthostatic vital signs. *Clinical Nursing Research, 9*(4), 479–491.

Latman, N. S., Hans, P., Nicholson, L., DeLee Zint, S., Lewis, K., & Shirey, A. (2001). Evaluation of clinical thermometers for accuracy and reliability. *Biomedical Instrumentation and Technology, 35*(4), 259–265.

McCance, K. L., & Huether, S. E. (1998). *Pathophysiology: The biologic basis for disease in adults and children* (3rd ed.). St Louis: Mosby.

Modell, J. G., Katholi, C. R., Kumaramangalam, S. M., Hudson, E. C., & Graham, D. (1998). Unreliability of the infrared tympanic thermometer in clinical practice: A comparative study with oral mercury and oral electronic thermometers. *Southern Medical Journal, 91*(7), 737–738.

Moser, M. (1999). World Health Organization–International Society of Hypertension guidelines for the management of hypertension—Do these differ from the U.S. recommendations? Which guidelines should the practicing physician follow? *Journal of Clinical Hypertension (Greenwich), 1*(1), 48–54.

National Institutes of Health. (1996). *National Heart, Lung, and Blood Institute update on the task force report (1987) on high blood pressure in children and adolescents.* Bethesda, MD: Author.

O'Connor, P. J., Quiter, E. S., Rush, W. A., Wiest, M., Meland, J. T., & Ryu, S. (1999). Impact of hypertension guideline implementation on blood pressure control and drug use in primary care clinics. *The Joint Commission Journal on Quality Improvement, 25*(2), 68–77.

Perloff, D., Grim, C., Flack, J., Frohlich, E. D., Hill, M., McDonald, M., et al. (1993). *Human blood pressure determination by sphygmomanometry.* AHA Medical/Scientific Statement, Product Code: 88:2460-2467. Dallas: American Heart Association.

Prentice, D., & Moreland, J. (1999). A comparison of infrared ear thermometry with electronic predictive thermometry in a geriatric setting. *Geriatric Nursing, 20*(6), 314–317.

Scanlon, V., & Sanders, T. (2003). *Essentials of anatomy and physiology* (4th ed.). Philadelphia: F. A. Davis Company.

Scisney-Matlock, M., Watkins, K. W., & Colling, K. B. (2001). The interaction of age and cognitive representations in predicting blood pressure. *Western Journal of Nursing Research, 23*(5), 476–489.

Sganga, A., Wallace, R., Kiehl, E., Irving, T., & Witter, L. (2000). A comparison of four methods of normal newborn temperature measurement. *MCH: American Journal of Maternal Child Nursing, 25*(2), 76–79.

St. John, R. E., & Thomson, P. D. (1999). Noninvasive respiratory monitoring. *Critical Care Nursing Clinics of North America, 11*(4), 423–435.

U.S. Environmental Protection Agency. (2002). Software for environmental awareness: Mercury in medical facilities. Retrieved September 26, 2002, from *http://www.epa.gov/seahome/mercury.html*

Valle, P. C., Kildahl-Andersen, O., & Steinvoll, K. (2000). Infrared tympanic thermometry compared to mercury thermometers. *Tidsskrift forden Norske Laegeforening (OSLO) 120*(1), 15–17.

Vital signs. (1999). *Best Practice: Evidence Based Practice Information Sheets for Health Professionals, 3*(3), 1–6.

CHAPTER 18

Alberti, R. E., & Emmons, M. *Your perfect right* (Revised ed.). San Luis Obispo, CA: IMPACT, 1990.

Avila, D. L. & Combs, A. W. (1985). *Helping relationships and the helping professions: Past, present, and future.* Boston: Allyn & Bacon.

Baker, L. H., Reifsteck, S. W., & Mann, W. R. (2003). Connected: Communication skills for nurses using the electronic medical record. *Nursing Economics, 21*(2), 85–88.

Black-Schaffer, R. M. (2002). Communication among levels of care for stroke patients. *Topics in Stroke Rehabilitation, 9*(3), 26–28.

Bosek, M. S. D. (2002). Ethics in practice. Effective communication skills: The key to preventing and resolving ethical situations. *JONA's Healthcare Law, Ethics, and Regulation, 4*(4), 93–97.

Bruderle, E. (n.d.). Communication in nursing. Retrieved September 6, 2003, from *http://www06.homepage.villanova.edu/elizabeth.bruderle/1103/communication.htm*

Bryan, K., Axelrod, L., Maxim, J., Bell, L., & Jordan, L. (2002). Working with older people with communication difficulties: An evaluation of care worker training. *Aging and Mental Health 6*(3), 248–254.

Buckman, R. (2002). Communication and emotions. *British Medical Journal, 325*(7366), 672.

Carroll, H. (2003). Improving patients' health: Words matter. *Patient Care Manager, 19*(7), 1–2.

Cohen, S. (2003). Manager's forum: Communicating important news to the staff. *Journal of Emergency Nursing, 29*(3), 278.

Dickerson, S. S., Stone, V. I., Panchura, C., & Usiak, D. J. (2002). The meaning of communication. Experiences with augmentive communication devices. *Rehabilitation Nursing 27*(6), 215–220.

Elliot, R., & Wright, L. (1999). Verbal communication: What do critical care nurses say to their unconscious or sedated patients? *Journal of Advanced Nursing, 29*(6), 1412–1420.

Forchuk, C. (2002). People with enduring mental health problems described the importance of communication, continuity of care, and stigma. *Evidence-Based Nursing, 5*(3), 93.

Hall, E. T. (1969). *The hidden dimension.* Garden City, NJ: Doubleday.

Hemsley, B., Sigafoos, J., Balandin, S., Forbes, R., Taylor, C., Green, V. A., et al. (2001). Nursing the patient with severe communication impairment. *Journal of Advanced Nursing, 35*(6), 827–835.

Hillard, J. (2000). Communication skills are vital in all we do as educators and clinicians. *Education for Health: Change in Learning and Practice, 13*(2), 157.

Hughes, J. P. (2003). Confidentiality. Careless comments: Communicating respect. *Nursing, 33*(7), 81.

Karhila, P., Kettunen, T., Poskiparta, M., & Liimatainen, L. (2003). Negotiation in type 2 diabetes counseling: From problem recognition to mutual acceptance during lifestyle counseling. *Qualitative Health Research, 13*(9), 1205–1224.

Kettunen, T., Poskiparta, M., & Gerlander, M. (2002). Nurse-patient power relationship: Preliminary evidence of patients' power messages. *Patient Education Counseling, 47*(2), 101–113.

Kevan, F. (2003). Challenging behavior and communication difficulties. *Journal of Learning Disabilities, 31*(2), 12–16.

Leininger, M. M., & MacFarland, M. R. (2002). *Transcultural nursing: Concepts, theories, research, and practices* (3rd ed.). New York: McGraw-Hill.

McConnell, E. (2001). Myths and facts . . . about communicating clearly. *Nursing 2001, 31*(4), 74.

Pitorak, P. F. (2003). Palliative nursing: Care at time of death. *American Journal of Nursing, 103*(7), 42–53.

Poskiparta, M., Liimatainen, L., Kettunen, T., & Karhila, P. (2001). From nurse-centered health counseling to empowermental health counseling. *Patient Education Counseling, 45*(1), 69–79.

Richardson, J. (2002). Health promotion in palliative care: The patients' perception of therapeutic interaction with the palliative nurse in the primary care setting. *Journal of Advanced Nursing, 40*(4), 432.

Soldwicsh, S. (2003). In our unit, accept no less than caring behaviors. *Critical Care Nurse, 23*(4), 95–96.

Street, A., & Blackford, J. (2001). Communication issues for the interdisciplinary community palliative care team. *Journal of Clinical Nursing, 10*(5), 643–651.

Stewart, L. A. (2002). The importance of effective communication during a labor action. *Patient Care Staff Report, 2*(5), 7–9.

Summers, L. C. (2002). Mutual timing: An essential component of provider/patient communication. *Journal of American Academy of Nursing Practitioner, 14*(1), 19.

Tannen, D. (1990). *You just don't understand: Women and men in conversation.* New York: Random House.

Teutsch, C. (2003). Patient-doctor communication. *Medical Clinics of North America, 87*(5), 1115–1145.

Travaline, J. M. (2002). Communication in the ICU: An essential component of patient care: Strategies for communicating with patients and their families. *Journal of Critical Illness, 17*(11), 451–460.

Venes, D. (2005). *Taber's Cyclopedic Medical Dictionary,* (20th ed.). Philadelphia, F. A. Davis.

Wells, T. (2002). Should we always get the words right? *Lancet, 359*(9307), 720.

CHAPTER 19

Bates, B. (1999). *A guide to physical examination* (7th ed.). Philadelphia: Lippincott, Williams & Wilkins.

Dillon, P. M. (2003). *Nursing health assessment: A critical thinking, case studies approach.* Philadelphia: F.A. Davis Company.

Goldsmith, L. A., Lazarus, G. S., & Tharp, M. D. (1997). *Adult and pediatric dermatology: A color guide to diagnosis and treatment.* Philadelphia: F. A. Davis Company.

Goroll, A., & Mulley, A. (2000). *Primary care medicine* (4th ed.). Philadelphia: Lippincott, Williams & Wilkins.

Green, B., & Taplin, S. (2003). Breast cancer screening controversies. *Journal of the American Board of Family Practice, 16*(3), 233–241.

Hackshaw, A., & Paul, E. (2003). Breast self-examination and death from breast cancer: A meta-analysis. *British Journal of Cancer, 88*(7), 1047–1053.

Kösters, J., & Gøtzsche, P. (2003). Regular self-examination or clinical examination for early detection of breast cancer. *Cochrane Database Systems Review, 2,* CD003373.

Purnell, L., & Paulanka, B. (2003). *Transcultural health care: A culturally competent approach* (2nd ed.). Philadelphia: F. A. Davis Company.

Scanlon, V. C., & Sanders, T. (2003). *Essentials of anatomy and physiology* 4th ed.). Philadelphia: F. A. Davis Company.

Schnell, Z. B., Van Leeuwen, A. M., & Kranpitz, T. R. (2003). *Davis's comprehensive handbook of laboratory and diagnostic tests with nursing implications.* Philadelphia: F. A. Davis Company.

Staying healthy at 50+. (2000). Washington, DC: U.S. Department of Health and Human Services, Public Health Service, Agency for Healthcare Research and Quality.

Taylor, R.B. (Ed.). (2002). *Family medicine: Principles and practice* (6th ed.). New York: Springer-Verlag.

Thomas, D., Gao, D., Ray, R., Wang, W., Allison, C., Chen, F., et al. (2002). Randomized trial of breast self-examination in Shanghai: Final results. *Journal of the National Cancer Institute, 94*(19), 1445–1457.

Venes, D. (Ed.). (2001). *Taber's cyclopedic medical dictionary* (19th ed.). Philadelphia: F. A. Davis Company.

Weiss, N. S. (2003). Breast cancer mortality in relation to clinical breast examination and breast self-examination. *Breast Journal, 9* (Supplement 2), S86–89.

Wong, D., & Hockenberry-Eaton, M. (2001). *Wong's essentials of pediatric nursing* (6th ed.). Philadelphia: Mosby.

CHAPTER 20

Adams, K., & Corrigan, J. M. (Eds.). (2003). *Priority areas for national action: Transforming health care quality.* Washington, DC: National Academies Press. Also available at *http://www.nap.edu/books/0309085438/html/*

American Nurses Association. (2003). *Standards of clinical nursing practice* (3rd ed.). Washington, DC: American Nurses Publishing.

Andersen, B. M., Lindemann, R., Bergh, K., Nesheim, B., Syversen, G., Solheim, N., et al. (2002). Spread of methicillin-resistant *Staphylococcus aureus* in a neonatal intensive unit associated with understaffing, overcrowding and mixing of patients. *Journal of Hospital Infection, 50*(1), 18–24.

Bachmaier, K., Le, J., & Penninger, J. M. (2000). "Catching heart disease": Antigenic mimicry and bacterial infections. *Nature Medicine, 6*(8), 841–842.

Bauman, R. W. (2004). *Microbiology.* San Francisco: Benjamin Cummings.

Bayuga, S., Zeana, C., Sahni, J., Della-Latta, P., El-Sadr, W., & Larson, E. (2002). Prevalence and antimicrobial patterns of *Acinetobacter baumannii* on hands and nares of hospital personnel and patients: The iceberg phenomenon again. *Heart & Lung: Journal of Acute & Critical Care, 31*(5), 382–390.

Blom, A. W., Gozzard, C., Heal, J., Bowker, K., & Estela, C. M. (2002). Bacterial strike-through of re-usable surgical drapes: The effect of different wetting agents. *Journal of Hospital Infection, 52*(1), 52–55.

Bolyard, E. A., Tablan, O. C., Williams, W. W., Pearson, M. L., Shapiro, C. N., Deitchman, S. D., et al. (1998). Guideline for infection control in health care personnel, 1998. *Infection Control and Hospital Epidemiology, 19,* 407–463.

Boyce, J. M., Pittet, D., Healthcare Infection Control Practices Advisory Committee, & the HICPAC/SHEA/APIC/IDSA Hand Hygiene Task Force. (2002, October 25). Guideline for hand hygiene in health-care settings. *Morbidity and Mortality Weekly Report, 51*(RR16), 1–44.

Braunschweig, C., Gomez, S., & Sheean, P. M. (2000). Impact of declines in nutritional status on outcomes in adult patients hospitalized for more than 7 days. *Journal of the American Dietetic Association, 100*(11), 1316–1324.

Buchanan, J., McCabe, L., & Fitzsimons, D. (2001). Using research to improve infection control practice. *Professional Nurse, 16*(5), 1091–1094.

Calil, R., Marba, S. T., von Nowakonski, A., & Tresoldi, A. T. (2001). Reduction in colonization and nosocomial infection by multiresistant bacteria in a neonatal unit after institution of educational measures and restriction in the use of cephalosporins. *American Journal of Infection Control, 29*(3), 133–138.

Capitano, B., Leshem, O. A., Nightingale, C. H., & Nicolau, D. P. (2003). Cost effect of managing methicillin-resistant *Staphylococcus aureus* in a long-term care facility. *Journal of the American Geriatrics Society, 51*(1), 10–16.

Cavanaugh, B. M. (1999). *Nurses manual of laboratory and diagnostic tests.* Philadelphia: F. A. Davis Company.

Chudleigh, J., & Buckingham, C. D. (1999). A comparison of soap, alcohol and glove use during the nappy-changing procedure in a special care baby unit . . . including commentary by D. Anthony. *Neonatal Research, 5*(6), 437–450.

Clark, A. M. (2003). "It's like an explosion in your life . . .": Lay perspectives on stress and myocardial infarction. *Journal of Clinical Nursing, 12*(4), 544–553.

Cousins, N. (1979). *Anatomy of an illness.* New York: Bantam.

Dochterman, J. M., & Bulechek, G. M. (Eds.). (2004). *Nursing interventions classification (NIC)* (4th ed.). St. Louis: Mosby.

Faure, O., Fricker-Hidalgo, H., Lebeau, B., Mallaret, M. R., Ambroise-Thomas, P., & Grillot, R. (2002). Eight-year surveillance of environmental fungal contamination in hospital operating rooms and haematological units. *Journal of Hospital Infection, 50*(2), 155–160.

Fendler, E. J., Ali, Y., Hammond, B. S., Lyons, M. K., Kelley, M. B., & Vowell, N. A. (2002). The impact of alcohol and sanitizer use on infection rates in an extended care facility. *American Journal of Infection Control, 30*(4), 226–233.

Fouad, F. M., Mamer, O., Sauriol, F., Khayyal, M., Lesimple, A., & Ruhenstroth-Bauer, G. (2004). Cardiac heart disease in the era of sucrose polyester, *Helicobacter pylori* and *Chlamydia pneumoniae. Medical Hypotheses, 62*(2), 257–267.

Franco, G. P., de Barros, A. L., Nogueira-Martins, L. A., & Michel, J. L. (2003). Stress influence on genesis, onset and maintenance of cardiovascular diseases: Literature review. *Journal of Advanced Nursing, 43*(6), 548–554.

Gardner, S. E., Frantz, R. A., & Doebbeling, B. N. (2001). The validity of the clinical signs and symptoms used to identify localized chronic wound infection. *Wound Repair & Regeneration, 9*(3), 178–186.

Gardner, S. E., Frantz, R. A., Troia, C., Eastman, S., MacDonald, M., Buresh, K., et al. (2001). A tool to assess clinical signs and symptoms of localized infection in chronic wounds: Development and reliability. *Ostomy Wound Management, 47*(1), 40–47.

Garner, J. S., & Hospital Infection Control Practices Advisory Committee. (1996, updated 2002). Guideline for isolation precautions in hospitals. *American Journal of Infection Control, 24,* 24–52. Retrieved November 9, 2002, from *http://www.cdc.gov/ncidod/hip/isolat/isolat.htm*

Guyton, A. & Hall, J. (2000). *Textbook of medical physiology.* Philadelphia: Saunders.

Hugonnet, S., Perneger, T. V., & Pittet, D. (2002). Alcohol-based handrub improves compliance with hand hygiene in intensive care units. *Archives of Internal Medicine, 162*(9), 1037–1043.

Iwata, K., Smith, B. A., Santos, E., Polsky, B., & Sordillo, E. M. (2002). Failure to implement respiratory isolation: Why does it happen? *Infection Control & Hospital Epidemiology, 23*(10), 595–599.

Jamulitrat, S., Narong, M. N., & Thongpiyapoom, S. (2002). Trauma severity scoring systems as predictors of nosocomial infection. *Infection Control & Hospital Epidemiology, 23*(5), 268–273.

Karchmer, T. B., Durbin, L. J., Simonton, B. M., & Farr, B. M. (2002). Cost-effectiveness of active surveillance cultures and contact/droplet precautions for control of methicillin-resistant *Staphylococcus aureus. Journal of Hospital Infection, 51*(2), 126–132.

Kyne, L., Sougioultzis, S., McFarland, L. V., & Kelly, C. P. (2002). Underlying disease severity as a major risk factor for nosocomial *Clostridium difficile* diarrhea. *Infection Control & Hospital Epidemiology, 23*(11), 653–659.

Larson, E. L., Early, E., Cloonan, P., Sugrue, S., & Parides, M. (2000). An organizational climate intervention associated with increased handwashing and decreased nosocomial infections. *Behavioral Medicine, 26*(1), 14–22.

Lazarus, R., Kleinman, K., Dashevsky, I., Adams, C., Kludt, P., DeMaria, A., Jr., et al. (2002 August). Use of automated ambulatory-care encounter records for detection of acute illness clusters, including potential bioterrorism events. *Emerging infectious diseases* [serial online]. Retrieved March 24, 2003, from *http://www.cdc.gov/ncidod/EID/vol8no8/02-0239.htm*

Loh, W., Ng, W., & Holton, J. (2000). Bacterial flora on the white coats of medical students. *Journal of Hospital Infection, 45*(1), 65–68.

Mahgoub, S., Ahmed, J., & Glatt, A. E. (2002). Underlying characteristics of patients harboring highly resistant *Acinetobacter baumannii. American Journal of Infection Control, 30*(7), 386–390.

Makris, A. T., Morgan, L., Gaber, D. J., Richter, A., & Rubino, J. R. (2000). Effect of a comprehensive infection control program on the incidence of infections in long-term care facilities. *American Journal of Infection Control, 28*(1), 3–7.

Manangan, L. P., Banerjee, S. N., & Jarvis, W. R. (2000). Association between implementation of CDC recommendations and ventilator-associated pneumonia at selected U.S. hospitals. *American Journal of Infection Control, 28*(3), 222–227.

Manangan, L. P., Pugliese, G., Jackson, M., Lynch, P., Sohn, A. H., Sinkowitz-Cochran, R. L., et al. (2001). Infection control dogma: Top 10 suspects. *Infection Control & Hospital Epidemiology, 22*(4), 243–247.

National Institute of Allergy and Infectious Diseases. (2001). *Microbes in sickness and health.* Washington, DC: National Institutes of Health.

Perry, C., Marshall, R., & Jones, E. (2001). Bacterial contamination of uniforms. *Journal of Hospital Infection, 48*(3), 238–241.

Richmond, J. Y., & McKinney, R. W. (Eds.). (1999). *Biosafety in microbiological and biomedical laboratories* (4th ed.). Washington, DC: U.S. Government Printing Office.

Salemi, C., Canola, M. T., & Eck, E. K. (2002). Hand washing and physicians: How to get them together. *Infection Control & Hospital Epidemiology, 23*(1), 32–35.

Spearing, N. M., Jensen, A., McCall, B. J., Neill, A. S., & McCormack, J. G. (2000). Direct costs associated with a nosocomial outbreak of *Salmonella* infection: An ounce of prevention is worth a pound of cure. *American Journal of Infection Control, 28*(1), 54–57.

Vandenberghe, A., Laterre, P., Goenen, M., Reynaert, M., Wittebole, X., Simon, A., et al. (2002). Surveillance of hospital-acquired infections in an intensive care department—the benefit of the full-time presence of an infection control nurse. *Journal of Hospital Infection, 52*(1), 56–59.

Weber, J. M., Sheridan, R. L., Schulz, J. T., Tompkins, R. G., & Ryan, C. M. (2002). Concise communications: Effectiveness of bacteria-controlled nursing units in preventing cross-colonization with resistant bacteria in severely burned children. *Infection Control & Hospital Epidemiology, 23*(9), 549–551.

Zafar, A. B., Sylvester, L. K., & Beidas, S. O. (2002). *Pseudomonas aeruginosa* infections in a neonatal intensive care unit. *American Journal of Infection Control, 30*(7), 425–429.

Zimmerman, S., Gruber-Baldini, A. L., Hebel, J. R., Sloane, P. D., & Magaziner, J. (2002). Nursing home facility risk factors for infection and hospitalization: Importance of registered nurse turnover, administration, and social factors. *Journal of the American Geriatrics Society, 50*(12), 1987–1995.

CHAPTER 21

Abrahamsen, C. (2001). 2002 guidelines to new technology—patient restraints: JCAHO and HCFA issue new restraint guidelines. *Nursing Management, 32*(12), 69–72.

Accident facts. (1998). Itasca, IL: National Safety Council.

American Academy of Pediatrics. (2004). *Moving kids safely.* Retrieved January 10, 2004, from *http://www.aap.org/family/cps.htm*

American Heart Association (2005). Heimlich maneuver. AHA recommendation. Retrieved February 16, 2005, from *http://www.americanheart.org/presenter.jhtml?identifier=4605*

American Heart Association (2005). Relief of choking in children. Retrieved February 16, 2005 from *http://www.americanheart.org/presenter.jhtml?identifier=3025002*

American Nurses Association. (2003). *Nursing facts: Needlestick injury.* Retrieved May 8, 2003, from *http://www.needlestick.org/readroom/fsneedle.htm*

Brush, B., & Capezuti, E. (2001). Historical analysis of siderail use in American hospitals. *Journal of Gerontological Nursing, 25,* 26–34.

Bureau of Labor Statistics. (2000a). *Occupational industries and illnesses: Industry data.* Retrieved May 28, 2003, from *http://data.bls.gov/cgi-bin/drsrv*

Bureau of Labor Statistics. (2000b). *Table R6: Incidence rates for nonfatal occupational injuries and illnesses involving days away from work per 10,000 full-time workers by industry and selected parts of body affected by injury or illness.* Retrieved May 28, 2003, from *http://www.bls.gov/iif/oshwc/osh/case/ostb1039.pdf*

Capezuti, E., Talerico, K., Sturmpf, N., & Evans, L. (1998). Individualized assessment and intervention in bilateral siderail use. *Geriatric Nursing, 19*(6), 322–330.

Chandra, N., & Hazanski, M. (Eds.). (1997). *Textbook of basic life support for healthcare providers.* Dallas: American Heart Association.

Children's Environmental Health Network. (1999). *Training manual on pediatric environmental health: Putting it into practice.* Retrieved March 2, 2003, from *http://www.cehn.org*

de Castro, A. B. (2003). Health and safety: Barriers to reporting a workplace injury. *American Journal of Nursing, 103*(8), 112.

Department of Health and Human Services, centers for Medicare and Medicaid Services (2003). "Medicare/Medicaid Hospital Surveyor Worksheet," Form CMS-1537 (11/03). Retrieved 6/11/05 from *http://www.cms.hhs.gov/forms/cms1537.pdf*

Dochterman, J. M., & Bulecheck, G. M. (Eds.). (2004). *Nursing interventions classification (NIC)* (4th ed.). St Louis: Mosby.

Farah, M., Simon, H., & Kellerman, A. (1999). Firearms in the home: Parental perception. *Pediatrics, 104* (5), 1059–1063.

Fitzroy, N. (2001). Scale permits early risk assessment. *Australian Nursing Journal, 9*(5), 18–20.

Fortin, J., Yeaw, E., Campbell, S., & Jameson, S. (1998). An analysis of risk assessment tolls for falls in the elderly. *Home Healthcare Nurse, 16*(9), 624–629.

Gilmore-Hall, A. (2003). Health and safety: Eliminating mercury in health care facilities. *American Journal of Nursing, 103*(7), 120.

Grossman, D., Cummings, P., Koepsell, T., Marshall, J., D'Ambrosio, L., Thompson, R., et al. (2000). Firearm safety counseling in primary care pediatrics: A randomized, controlled trial. *Pediatrics, 106*(1), 22–26.

Grossman, V. (2003). Gang members in the ED. *American Journal of Nursing, 103*(2), 52–53.

Health Care Financing Administration. (2000, June). Quality of care-standards. Hospital conditions of patients' rights: Interpretive guidelines. Retrieved November 10, 2002, from *http://www.hcfa.gov/quality/4b2htm*

Hospitals for Healthy Environment. (2002). *Why waste is a problem in healthcare.* Retrieved May 28, 2003, from *http://www.h2e-online.org/about/waste.htm*

Johnson, M., Bulechek, G., McCloskey Dochterman, J., Maas, M., & Moorhead, S. (2001). *Nursing diagnoses, outcomes, and interventions: NANDA, NOC, and NIC linkages.* St Louis: Mosby.

Joint Commission for Accreditation of Healthcare Organizations. (2002). *2002 hospital accreditation standards.* Oakbrook Terrace, IL: Author.

Kakkuri, M. (2000). Home safety checklist. Retrieved May 30, 2003, from *http://www.nsc.org/pubs/fsh/archive/spr00/homecheck.htm*

Karlsson, S., Bucht, G., Rasmussen, B., & Sandman, P. (2000). Restraint use in elder care: Decision making among registered nurses. *Journal of Clinical Nursing, 9*(6), 842–850.

Kennedy-Malone, L., Fletcher, K., & Plank, L. (2004). *Management guidelines for nurse practitioners working with older adults* (2nd ed.). Philadelphia: F. A. Davis Company.

Kirkpatrick, C. (2003, April 21). Safety first: The JCAHO introduces new patient safety goals. *NurseWeek,* 19–21.

Krieger, J., & Higgins, D. (2002). Housing and health: Time again for public health action. *American Journal of Public Health, 92*(5), 758–768.

Lewis, S., Heitkemper, M., & Dirksen, S. (2005). *Medical surgical nursing: Assessment and management of clinical problems* (6th ed.) St Louis: Mosby.

Manoguerra, A. S., Cobaugh, D. J., and the Members of the Guidelines for the Management of Poisonings Consensus Panel. (2004). Guideline on the use of ipecac syrup in the out-of-hospital management of ingested poisons. In *Guidelines for the management of poisonings.* Washington, D.C.: American Association of Poison Control Centers.

Moorhead, S., Johnson, M., & Maas, M. (Eds.). (2004). *Nursing outcomes classification (NOC)* (3rd ed.). St Louis: Mosby.

Morse, J. (1997). *Preventing patient falls.* Thousand Oaks, CA: Sage Publications. California.

Morse, J. (2001). Preventing falls in the elderly. *Reflections on Nursing Leadership,* First Quarter, 26–27.

Mott, J., Wolfe, M., Alverson, C., & Macdonald, S. (2002). National vehicle emissions policies and practices and declining U.S. carbon monoxide–related mortality. *Journal of the American Medical Association, 288,* 988–995.

NANDA International. (2005). *NANDA nursing diagnoses: Definitions and classification 2005–2006.* Philadelphia: Author.

National Ag Safety Database (NASD). (2003). Protect your children from poisons at home. Retrieved November 13, 2003, from *http:www.cdc.gov/nasd/documents/d0001501-d001600/d001584/d0001584.html*

National Center for Injury Prevention and Control. (2000, November 13). *Fact sheet. Falls and fractures among older adults.* Retrieved February 13, 2003, from *http://www.cdc.gov/ncipc/factsheets/falls.htm*

National Center for Injury Prevention and Control. (2003). *National child passenger safety week February 9–15, 2003.* Retrieved January 10, 2004, from *http://www.cdc.gov/ncipc/duip/spotlite/childseat.htm*

National Fire Protection Association. (2001, September / October). *Catastrophic fires of 2000.* Retrieved March 7, 2003, from *http://www.nfps.org*

National Institute for Occupational Safety and Health (NIOSH). (2003). Protect your family: Reduce contamination at home. DHHS (NIOSH) Publication No. 97-125. Retrieved November 17, 2003, from *www.cdc.gov/niosh/thttext.html*

National Safety Council. (2001a). *National Vital Statistics Report, 2001.* Retrieved February 15, 2003, from *www.nsc.org/index.htm*

National Safety Council. (2001b). *Report on injuries in America, 2001.* Itasca, IL: Author. Retrieved February 12, 2003, from *http://www.nsc.org/library/rept2000.htm#top*

National Safety Council. (2001c). *Baby-proofing your home.* Itasca, IL: Author. Retrieved November 17, 2003, from *http://www.nsc.org/library/babyprf.htm*

Nelson, A., Fragala, G., & Menzel, N. (2003). Myths and facts about back injuries in nursing. *American Journal of Nursing, 103*(2), 32–40.

Owen, B., & Garg, A. (1992). Four methods for identification of most back stressing tasks performed by nursing assistants in nursing homes. *International Journal of Industrial Ergonomics, 9,* 213–220.

Parmet, S. (2002). Carbon monoxide poisoning. *Journal of the American Medical Association, 288,* 1036–1044.

Phipatanakul, W., Eggleston, P. A., & Wright, R. A. (2000). Mouse allergen, II: The relationship of mouse allergen exposure to mouse sensitization and asthma morbidity in inner-city children with asthma. *Journal of Allergy Clinical Immunology, 106,* 1075–1080.

Polan, E., & Taylor, D. (2003). *Journey across the lifespan* (2nd ed.). Philadelphia: F. A. Davis Company.

Ray, W., Tay, J., Meador, K., Thapa, P., Grown, A., Kajihara, et al. (1997). A randomized trial of a consultation service to reduce falls in nursing homes. *Journal of the American Medical Association, 278*(7), 557–562.

Rosenstreich, D. L., Eggleston P., & Kattan, M. (1997). The role of cockroach allergy and exposure to cockroach allergen in causing morbidity among inner-city children with asthma. *New England Journal of Medicine, 336,* 1356–1363.

Shaner, H., & Botter, M. (2003). Pollution: Health care's unintended legacy. *American Journal of Nursing, 103*(3), 79, 81, 83–84.

Talerico, K., & Capezuti, E. (2001). Myths and facts about side rails. *American Journal of Nursing, 101*(7), 43–48.

Trapasso, L., & Owens, G. (1996). Eye to the sky: Understanding the danger of thunderstorms and lightning. *Parks & Recreation, (31)*8, 221–226.

Tyson, S. (1999). *Gerontological nursing care.* Philadelphia: Saunders.

U.S. Department of Health and Human Services. (2000). *Healthy people 2010.* (Conference Edition, in Two Volumes). Washington, DC: Author.

U.S. Department of Labor, Occupational Safety and Health Administration (OSHA). (2003a). Frequently asked questions. Retrieved May 29, 2003, from *www.osha.gov/needlesticks/needlefaq.html*

U.S. Department of Labor, Occupational Safety and Health Administration (OSHA). (2003b). How to file a complaint with OSHA. Retrieved May 29, 2003, from *www.osha.gov/as/opa/worker/complain.html*

U.S. Environmental Protection Agency. (1996, September). *The consumer's handbook for reducing solid waste.* EPA #530-K-96-003. Retrieved May 29, 2003, from *http://www.epa.gov/epaoswer/non-hw/reduce/catbook.htm*

U.S. Environmental Protection Agency. (1998, April 28). *Mosquitos: How to control them.* Retrieved May 29, 2003, from *http://www.epa.gov/pesticides/factsheets/mosquito.htm*

U.S. Environmental Protection Agency. (2002). Software for environmental awareness: Mercury in medical facilities. Retrieved September 26, 2002, from *http://www.epa.gov/seahome/mercury.html*

U.S. Environmental Protection Agency. (2003, January 6). *Wastes: your home and community.* Retrieved February 13, 2003, from *http://www.epa.gov/epaoswer/osw/citizens.htm*

U.S. Food and Drug Administration, Center for Food Safety and Applied Nutrition. (2004). Consumer advice on food safety, nutrition, and cosmetics. Last updated 3/17/04. Retrieved July 11, 2004, from *http://www.fda.gov*

Walker, B. (1998). Preventing falls. *Registered Nurse, 61*(5), 40–42.

Whitman, G., Davidson, L., Sereika, S., & Rudy, E. (2001). Stuffing and pattern of mechanical restraint use across a multiple hospital system. *Nursing Research, 50*(6), 356–362.

Wilburn, S. (2003). Health and safety: The needlestick law. *American Journal of Nursing, 103*(2), 104.

Wong, D., & Hockenberry-Eaton, M. (2001). *Wong's essentials of pediatric nursing* (6th ed.). St Louis: Mosby.

Wong, D., Perry, S., & Hockenberry, M. (2002). *Maternal child nursing* (2nd ed.). St Louis: Mosby.

World Health Organization (WHO). (1997). *The world health report 1997: Conquering suffering, enriching humanity.* Geneva, Switzerland: Author.

Worthington, K. (2001). Take-home toxins. *American Journal of Nursing, 101*(9), 88.

Zeitz, P., Orr, M., & Kaye, W. (2002). Public health consequences of mercury spills: Hazardous substances emergency events surveillance system, 1993–1998. *Environmental Health Perspectives, 110*(2), 129–132.

CHAPTER 22

American Academy of Orthopedic Surgeons. (2001). 85% of women changed shoe-wear habits due to foot problems. *Newswise.* Retrieved September 1, 2004, from *http:www.newswise.com/articles/view/26033/*

Andrews, M. M., & Boyle, J. S. (2003). *Transcultural concepts in nursing care* (4th ed.). Philadelphia: Lippincott.

Better elder care: A nurse's guide to caring for older adults. (2002). Springhouse, PA: Springhouse Publications.

Brawley, E. C. (2002). Bathing environments: How to improve the bathing experience. *Alzheimer's Care Quarterly, 3*(1), 38–41.

Centers for Disease Control and Prevention. (2002). Guideline for hand hygiene in health-care settings. *Morbidity and Mortality Weekly Report, RR-26,* 1–47.

Dochterman, J. M., & Bulechek, G. M. (Eds.). (2004). *Nursing interventions classification (NIC)* (4th ed.). St Louis: Mosby.

Dunn, J., Thiru-Chelvam, B., & Beck, C. (2002). Bathing: Pleasure or pain? *Journal of Gerontological Nursing, 28*(11), 6–13.

Frankowski, B. L., & Weiner, L. B. (2002). Head lice. *Pediatrics, 110*(3), 638–643.

Hansel, P. (2000). The challenges of choosing a pediculocide. *Public Health Nursing, 17,* 300–304.

Kovach, C. R., & Meyer-Arnold, E. A. (1996). Coping with conflicting agendas: The bathing experience of cognitively impaired older adults. *Scholarly Inquiry in Nursing Practice, 10*(1), 23–36.

Lucas, L. J., & Matthews-Flint, L. J. (2001). Sound advice about hearing aids. *Nursing 2001, 2,* 59–61.

McFarland, G. K., & McFarlane, E. A. (1997). *Nursing diagnosis and intervention: Planning for patient care* (3rd ed.). St Louis: Mosby.

McNeill, H. E. (2000). Biting back at poor oral hygiene. *Intensive and Critical Care Nursing, 16*(6), 367–372.

Moorhead, S., Johnson, M., & Maas, M. (Eds.). (2004). *Nursing outcomes classification (NOC)* (3rd ed.). St Louis: Mosby.

NANDA International. (2005). *NANDA nursing diagnoses: Definitions and classification, 2005–2006.* Philadelphia: Author.

Nightingale, F. (1860). *Notes on nursing: What it is and what it is not.* New York: D. Appleton and Co. Reprint, 1969. New York: Dover Publications, Inc.

Rakow, P. L. (2000). Perspective on contact lenses. What lens is that new patient wearing? Identifying, inspecting, and verifying the parameters of rigid and soft contact lenses. *Journal of Ophthalmic Nursing and Technology, 19*(6), 304–310.

Ramponi, D. R. (2001). Eye on contact lens removal. *Nursing 31*(8), 56–57.

Rasin, J., & Barrick, A. L. (2004). Bathing patients with dementia. *American Journal of Nursing, 104*(3), 30–33.

Rawlins, C. A., & Trueman, I. W. (2001). Effective mouth care for seriously ill patients. *Professional Nurse, 16*(4), 1025–1028.

Roberts, S. S. (2001). Top ways to prevent dental problems. *Diabetes Forecast, 54*(4), 71–72.

Robles, R., Corcoles, G., Torres, L., de la Cuesta, Y., Arias, R., Parra, M., et al. (2002). Frequency of the adverse events during the hygiene of the critical patients [Spanish]. *Enfermia Intensiva, 13*(2), 47–56.

Schwartz, M. (2000). The oral health of the long-term care patient. *Annals of Long Term Care, 8*(12), 41–46.

Sheppard, C. M., & Brenner, P. S. (2000). The effect of bathing and skin care practices on skin quality and satisfaction with an innovative product. *Journal of Gerontological Nursing, 26*(10), 36–45, 55–56.

Sommer, S. K., & Sommer, N. W. (2002). When your patient is hearing impaired. *RN, 65*(12), 23–32.

Spector, R. (2004). *Cultural diversity in health and illness* (6th ed.). Upper Saddle River, NJ: Prentice Hall Health.

Stieffel, K., Damron, S., Sowers, N., & Velez, L. (2001). Improving oral hygiene for the seriously ill patient: Implementing research-based practice. *Medical-Surgical Nursing Journal, 9* (1), 40–43.

Talerico, K. A., & Capezuti, E. (2001). Myths and facts about side rails. *American Journal of Nursing, 10*(7), 43–48.

Walton, J. C., Miller, J., & Tordecilla, L. (2001). Elder assessment and care. *MEDSURG Nursing, 10*(1), 37–44.

Wilkinson, J. M. (2005). *Nursing diagnosis handbook with NIC interventions and NOC outcomes* (8th ed.). Upper Saddle River, NJ: Prentice Hall Health.

CHAPTER 23

Abrams, A. (2000). *Clinical drug therapy: Rationales for nursing practice.* Philadelphia: Lippincott Williams & Wilkins.

AJN Reports. (2002). Health and safety. *AJN, 102*(12),100.

AJN Reports. (2003). Using technology to address medication errors. *American Journal of Nursing, 103*(4), 25.

American Diabetes Association. (2003). Position statement: Insulin administration, *Diabetes Care, 26,* S121–124. Retrieved June 14, 2004, from *http://care.diabetesjournals.org/cgi/content/full/26/suppl_1/s121*

Aschenbrenner, D., & Venable, S. (2002). *Drug therapy in nursing.* Philadelphia: Lippincott Williams & Wilkins.

Atkinson, W., Pickering, L., Schwartz, B., Weniger, B., Iskander, J., & Watson, J. (2002). General recommendations on immunization. *Morbidity and Mortality Weekly Report, 51,* 1–36.

Austin, S. A safe standard of care for medication administration. (2001). *Nursing Management, 32*(9), 12.

Beacon Health. (2004). Tips for keeping CVADs open. Retrieved June 30, 2004, from *http://www.beaconhealth.org/archived_articles/up033tips.html*

Beers, M. H., & Berkow, R. (Eds.). (1999). Drug therapy and the elderly. In *The Merck manual of diagnosis and therapy* (17th ed.). Whitehouse Station, NJ: Merck. Retrieved May 20, 2003, from *www.merck.com/pubs/mmanual_home/sec22/chapter304e.htm*

Beers, M. H., & Berkow, R. (Eds.). (1999). Drug toxicity. In *The Merck manual of diagnosis and therapy* (17th ed.). Whitehouse Station, NJ: Merck. Retrieved May 20, 2003, from *www.merck.com/pubs/mmanual_home/sec22/chapter302d.htm*

Beers, M. H., & Berkow, R. (Eds.). (1999). Factors affecting drug response. In *The Merck manual of diagnosis and therapy* (17th ed.). Whitehouse Station, NJ: Merck. Retrieved May 20, 2003, from *www.merck.com/pubs/mmanual_home/sec22/chapter301b.htm*

Berkow, R., & Beers, M. H. (Eds.). (2000a). Drug administration, distribution, and elimination. In *The Merck manual of medical information—home edition*. Whitehouse Station, NJ: Merck. Retrieved May 20, 2003, from *www.merck.com/pubs/mmanual_home/sec2/6.htm*

Berkow, R., & Beers, M. H. (Eds.). (2000b). Overview of drugs. In *The Merck manual of medical information—home edition*. Whitehouse Station, NJ: Retrieved May 20, 2003, *www.merck.com/pubs/mmanual_home/sec2/5.htm*

Beyea, S., & Nicoll, L. (1995). Administration of medications via the intramuscular route: An integrative review of the literature and research base protocol for procedure. *Applied Nursing Research, 8*(1), 23–33.

Beyea, S., & Nicoll, L. (1996). Back to basics: Administering IM injections the right way. *American Journal of Nursing, 96*(1), 34–35.

Buckley, T., Dudley, S., & Donowitz, L. (1994). Defining unnecessary disinfection procedures for single-dose and multiple dose vials. *American Journal of Critical Care 3*(6), 448.

Carroll, P. (2003). Medication errors: The bigger picture. *RN, 66*(1), 52–58.

Chiodini, J. (2001). Best practice in vaccine administration. *Nursing Standard, 16*(7), 35–38.

Cleveland, L., Aschenbrenner, D., Venable, S., & Yensen, J. (1999). *Nursing management in drug therapy.* Philadelphia: Lippincott, Williams & Wilkins.

Clinical Practice Committee. (2002). *Policies and procedures for infusion nurses.* (2nd ed.). Norwood, MA: Infusion Nurses Society

Cohen, H., Scott, P., & McCallum, T. (2003). Managers forum: Preventing drug errors. *Journal of Emergency Nursing, 29*(3), 274–276.

Cohen, M. R. (2003). Medication errors. *Nursing 2003, 33*(7), 14.

Cox, J. (2000). Students' corner: Quality medication administration. *Contemporary Nurse, 9*(3/4), 308–313.

Curren, A., & Munday, L. (2005). *Math for meds: Dosage and solutions* (9th ed.). Clifton Park, NY: Delmar Learning.

Deglin, J., & Vallerand, A. (2002). *Davis' drug guide for nurses.* Philadelphia: F. A. Davis Company.

Dochterman, J., & Bulecheck, G. (Eds.). (2004). *Nursing interventions classification (NIC)* (4th ed.). St Louis: Mosby.

Engstrom, J., Giglio, N., Takacs, S., Ellis, M., & Cherwenka, D. (2000). Procedures used to prepare and administer intramuscular injections: A study of infertility nurses. *Journal of Obstetric, Gynecologic, and Neonatal Nursing, 29*(2), 159–168.

Fiesta, J. (1998). Legal aspects of medication administration. *Nursing Management, 29*(1), 22–23.

Fleming, D. R. (1999). Challenging traditional insulin injection practices. *American Journal of Nursing, 99*(2), 72–74.

Ford, N. A., Drott, H. R., & Cieplinski-Robertson, J. A. (2003). Administration of IV medications via Soluset. *Pediatric Nursing, 29*(4), 283–286, 319.

Gahart, B., & Nazareno, A., (2004). *Intravenous medications* (21st ed.). St Louis, C. V. Mosby.

Glazer, G. (2002). Medication administration interventions that must be performed by a registered nurse. *Online Journal of Issues in Nursing, 7*(2), 4.

Hall, C. (2002). *Special considerations for the geriatric population. Critical Care Nursing Clinics of North America, 14*(4), 427–434.

Howard, A., Mercer, P., Nataraj, H.C., & Kang, B.C. (1997, June). Bevel-down superior to bevel-up in intradermal skin testing. *Annals of Allergy, Asthma, & Immunology, 78,* 594–596.

Ignatavicius, D., & Hausman, K. (2005). *Clinical companion for medical–surgical nursing: Critical thinking for collaborative care.* Philadelphia: W. B. Saunders.

Infusion Nurses Society (2000). *Infusion nursing standards of practice.* Norwood, MA: Gardner Foundation.

JCAHO sets patient safety goals for 2003. (2003). *Nursing Spectrum Metro Edition, 3*(8), 25MW.

Joint Commission for Accreditation of Healthcare Organizations (JCAHO). (2002). *2002 hospital accreditation standards.* Oakbrook Terrace, IL: Author.

Karch, A. M., & Karch, F. E. (2003). Practice errors: Not so fast! IV push drugs can be dangerous when given too rapidly. *American Journal of Nursing, 103*(8), 71.

Karow, H. S. (2002). Creating a culture of medication administration safety: Laying the foundation for computerized provider order entry. *Joint Commission Journal on Quality Improvement, 28*(7), 396–402.

Kaushal, R., & Bates, D. W. (2002). Information technology and medication safety: What is the benefit? *Quality & Safety in Health Care, 11*(3), 261–265.

Lacy, C., Armstrong, L., & Goldman, M. (2003). *Drug information handbook 2003–2004.* (11th ed.). Chicago: Lexi-Comp.

Lassetter, J. H., & Warnick, M. L. (2003). Medical errors, drug-related problems, and medication errors: A literature review on quality of care and cost issues. *Journal of Nursing Care Quality, 18*(3), 175–183.

LeDuc, K. (1997). Efficacy of normal saline solution versus heparin solution for maintaining patency of peripheral intravenous catheters in children. *Journal of Emergency Nursing, 23*(4), 306–309.

Lehns, R. (2000). *Pharmacology for nursing care.* Elsevier—Health Sciences Division.

LeMone, P., & Burke, K. (1999). *Medical-surgical nursing: Critical thinking in client care* (4th ed.). Upper Saddle River, NJ: Prentice Hall.

Lilley, L., Harrington S., & Snyder, J. (2004). *Pharmacology and the nursing process.* St Louis: C. V. Mosby.

Lundgren, A., Ek, A., & Wahren, L. (1998). Handling and control of peripheral intravenous lines. *Journal of Advanced Nursing, 27*(5), 897–904.

Martinez De Castillo, S., Castillo, S., & Werner-McCullough, M. (2002). *Calculating drug dosages.* Philadelphia: F. A. Davis Company.

McConnell, E. A. (2002). Administering medication through a gastrostomy tube. *Nursing, 32*(12), 22.

McDonnell, P. J., & Jacobs, M. R. (2002). Hospital admission resulting from preventable adverse drug reactions. *Annals of Pharmacotherapy, 36,* 1331–1336.

Moore, L. A., & Blount, K. A. (2002). Medications and the elderly in the critical care setting. *Critical Care Nursing Clinics of North America, 14*(1), 111–119.

Moorhead, S., Johnson, M., & Maas, M. (2004). *Nursing outcomes classification (NOC)* (3rd ed.). St Louis: Mosby.

Morrison-Karch, A., & Karch, A. (2002). *Focus on nursing pharmacology.* Philadelphia: Lippincott Williams & Wilkins.

Mudge, B., Forcier, D., & Slarrert, M. J. (1998). Patency of 24-gauge peripheral intermittent infusion devices: A comparison of heparin and saline flush solutions. *Pediatric Nursing, 24*(2), 142–149.

National Center for HIV, STD, and TB Prevention, Division of Tuberculosis Elimination. Mantoux tuberculosis skin test facilitator guide. Part one: Administering the Mantoux tuberculin skin test. Retrieved May 25, 2005, from *http://www.cdc.gov/nchstp/tb/pubs/Mantoux/part1.htm*

Pape, T. M. (2003). Applying airline safety practices to medication administration. *Medsurg Nursing, 12*(2), 77–94.

Peragallo-Dittko, V. (1997). Rethinking subcutaneous injection technique. *American Journal of Nursing, 97*(5), 71.

Phillips, D. (2001). *Manual of IV therapeutics* (3rd ed.). Philadelphia: F. A. Davis Company.

Polifroni, E., McNulty, J., & Allchin, N. (2003). Medication errors: More basic than a system issue. *Journal of Nursing Education, 42*(10), 41.

Rodger, M., & King, L. (2000). Drawing up and administering intramuscular injections: A review of the literature. *Journal of Advanced Nursing, 31*(3), 574–582.

Saari, T., & the Committee on Infectious Diseases. (2003). Clinical report: Immunization of preterm and low birth weight infants. *Pediatrics, 112*(1), 193–198. Retrieved January 10, 2004, from *http://www.aap.org/policy/s030131.html*

Skokal, W. (2000). IV push at home? *RN, 63*(20), 26–29.

Smetzer, J. (2001). 2002 guide to new technology medication management: Safer medication management. *Nursing Management, 32*(12), 44–48.

Staten, P. A. (2003). Medication management update. *Nursing Management, 34*(5), 14.

Torrance, C. (1989). Intramuscular injection, part 2. *Surgical Nurse, 2*(6), 24–27.

U.S. Department of Health and Human Services, Centers for Disease Control and Prevention, National Immunization Program. (2002). 2002 general recommendations on immunizations: Aspiration before injection. Retrieved August 16, 2003, from *http://www.cdc.gov/nip/publications/GenRecs.htm#6*

U.S. Department of Health and Human Services, National Institute of Occupational Safety and Health. (1999). Preventing needlestick injuries in health care settings. DHHS (NIOSH) Publication No. 2000–108. Cincinnati, OH: NIOSH—Publications Dissemination.

U.S. Department of Labor, Occupational Safety & Health Administration (OSHA). (1999). How to prevent needlestick injuries. Publication 361. Washington, DC: Author. Retrieved January 5, 2004, from *http://www.osha.gov/SLTC/etools/hospital/hazards/sharps/sharps.html#HandlingandDisposalofNeedles*

Williams, P. N., & Moody, M. L. (2004). Safety in the preparation and use of flush syringes. Retrieved June 30, 2004, from *http://www.baxter.com/doctors/iv_therapies/education/iv_therapy_ce/flush.html#peripheral*

Wolf, Z. R. (2001). Continuing education: Understanding medication errors. *Nursing Spectrum Midwest, 2*(5), 29–34.

Wong, D., & Hockenberry-Eaton, M. (2001). *Wong's essentials of pediatric nursing*. Philadelphia: Mosby.

Workman, B. (1999). Safe injection techniques. *Nursing Standard, 13*(39), 47–53.

Wright, D. (2002). Swallowing difficulties protocol: Medication administration. *Nursing Standard, 17*(14/15), 43.

Zurlinden, J. (2003, January 27). Overwork contributes to a growing number of medication errors. *Nursing Spectrum (Greater Philadelphia/Tri-State Edition), 12*(2), 14.

CHAPTER 24

American Hospital Association. (1992). *A patient's bill of rights*. Chicago, IL: Author. This is a revision of the original that was adopted in 1973.

American Hospital Association. (2003). *The patient care partnership*. Chicago, IL: Author. Retrieved August 18, 2003, from *http://www.hospitalconnect.com:80/aha/ptcommunication/partnership/partnership/index.html*.

American Nurses Association. (2001). *Code of ethics for nurses with interpretive statements*. Washington, DC: American Nurses Publishing.

American Nurses Association. (2004). *Nursing: Scope and standards of practice* (3rd ed.). Washington, DC: American Nurses Publishing.

Anonymous. (2000). Pictorial patient teaching. *Nurse Practitioner, 25*(6), 105.

Bastable, S. B. (2003). *Nurse as educator*. Boston: Jones and Bartlett.

Bloom, B. S., Mesia, B. B., & Krathwohl, D. R. (1964). *Taxonomy of educational objectives* (Vol. 1: *The Affective Domain* and Vol. 2: *The Cognitive Domain*). New York: David McKay.

Bloom B. S., & Krathwohl, D. R. (1956). *Taxonomy of educational objectives: The classification of educational goals. Handbook I: Cognitive domain*. New York: Longmans, Green.

Christman, L. (2000). Patient and family education in managed care and beyond: Seizing the teachable moment. *Nursing Administration Quarterly, 25*(1), 155–156.

Dochterman, J. M., & Bulechek, G. M. (Eds.). (2004). *Nursing interventions classification (NIC)* (4th ed.). St Louis: Mosby.

Fenner, P. C. (2002). Understanding the role of practice in learning for geriatric individuals. *Topics in Geriatric Rehabilitation, 17*(4), 11–32.

Friesen, P., Pepler, C., & Hunter, P. (2002). Interactive family learning following a cancer diagnosis. *Oncology Nursing Forum, 29*(6), 981–987.

Grimes, V. (2002, March-April). Comparing the effect of a skills checklist on teaching time required to achieve independence in administration of infusion medication. *Journal of Infusion Nursing, 25*(2), 109–120.

Henderson, A., & Zernike, W. (2001). A study of the impact of discharge information for surgical patients. *Journal of Advanced Nursing, 35*(3), 435–441.

Hilgenberg, C., & Schlickau, J. (2002). Building transcultural knowledge through intercollegiate collaboration. *Journal of Transcultural Nursing, 13*(3), 241–247.

Holmes, T., & Rahe, R. (1967). The social readjustment and rating scale. *Journal of Psychosomatic Research 11, 213–218*.

Joint Commission on Accreditation of Healthcare Organizations (JCAHO). (2000). *Accreditation manual for hospitals 2000*. Chicago: Author.

Knowles, M. S. (1990). *The adult learner: A neglected species* (4th ed.). Houston: Gulf Publishing.

Lazarus, H. (1999). *Stress and emotion: A new synthesis*. New York: Springer.

Lazarus, H., & Folkman, S. (1948). *Stress appraisal and coping*. New York: Springer.

Lee, D. S., & Lee, S. S. (2000). Pre-operative teaching: How does a group of nurses do it? *Contemporary Nurse, 9*(1): 80–88.

Leininger, M. (1994). Transcultural nursing education: A world-wide imperative. *Nursing & Health Care, 15*(5), 254–257.

Leino-Kilpi, H., Solante, S., & Katajisto, J. (2001). Problems in the outcomes of nursing education create challenges for continuing education. *The Journal of Continuing Education, 32*(4), 183–193.

London, F. (1999). *No time to teach*. Philadelphia: Lippincott.

Marcum, J., Ridenour, G., Hammons, M., & Taylor, M. (2002). A study of professional nurses' perceptions of patient education. *The Journal of Continuing Education in Nursing, 33*(3), 112–121.

Mayer, G. G. (2002). Writing easy-to-read teaching aids. *Nursing, 32*(3), 48–49.

McCaffery, M. (2002). Teaching your patient to use a pain rating scale. *Nursing, 32*(8), 17–20.

Monat, A., & Lazarus, R. (Eds.) (1991). *Stress and coping* (3rd ed.). St Louis: Mosby.

Moorhead, S., Johnson, M., & Maas, M. (Eds.). (2004). *Nursing outcomes classification (NOC)* (3rd ed.). St Louis: Mosby.

NANDA International. (2005). *NANDA nursing diagnoses: Definitions and classification 2005–2006*. Philadelphia: Author.

National Center for Education Statistics. (1996/2003). *National adult literacy survey*. Updated January 2003. Retrieved March 12, 2004 from *http://nces.ed.gov/nadlits/*

Nightingale, F. (1860/1992). *Notes on nursing: What it is and what it is not*. Philadelphia: Lippincott.

Oermann, M., Masserang, M., Maxey, M., & Lange,P. (2002). Clinic visit and waiting: Patient education and satisfaction. *Med/Surg Nursing, 11*(5), 247–257.

PEW Health Professions Commission. (1998). *Recreating health professional practice for a new century: Fourth report*. San Francisco: UCSF Center for the Health Professions.

Piaget, J. (1966). *Origins of intelligence in children*. New York: Norton.

Rankin, S. H., & Stallings, K. D. (2001). *Patient education principles and practice*. (4th Ed.). Philadelphia: Lippincott.

Schrecengost, A. (2001). Do humorous preoperative teaching strategies work? *AORN Journal, 74*(5), 683–689.

Selye, H. (1974). *Stress without distress*. Philadelphia: J. B. Lippincott (classic).

Selye, H. (1976). *The stress of life. (Revised edition)*. New York: McGraw-Hill.

U.S. Department of Education, Office of Educational Research and Improvement, National Center for Education Statistics. (1999). National assessment of adult literacy: Work statement. Retrieved November 4, 2004, from *http://www.ed.gov/searchResults.jhtml*

Wykurz, G., & Kelly, D. (2002). Developing the role of patients as teachers: Literature review. *British Medical Journal, 325*(7368), 818–821.

CHAPTER 25

Al-Hassan, M., & Sagr, L. (2002). Stress and stressors of myocardial infarction patients in the early period after discharge. *Journal of Advanced Nursing, 40*(2), 181–188.

American Psychiatric Association (1994). *Diagnostic and statistical manual of mental disorders* (4th ed.). Washington, DC: Author.

Benson, H. (1976). *The relaxation response*. New York: Avon Books.

Blau, G., Tatum, D. S., & Ward-Cook, K. (2003). Correlates of work exhaustion for medical technologists. *Journal of Allied Health, 32*(3), 148–157.

Brammer, L. M., & MacDonald, G. (1998). *The helping relationship: Process and skills*. Upper Saddle River, NJ: Prentice Hall.

Brennan, B. (1987). *Hands of light: A guide to healing through the human energy field*. New York: Bantam Books.

Cericola, S. A. (2000). Stress: A self-management approach and nursing care plan for nurses. *Plastic Surgery Nursing, 20*(1), 29–33, 40.

Clark, A. M. (2003). "It's like an explosion in your life . . .": Lay perspectives on stress and myocardial infarction. *Journal of Clinical Nursing, 12*(4), 544–553.

Cousins, N. (1979). *Anatomy of an illness*. New York: Bantam Books.

DePew, C. L., Gordon, M., Yoder, L. H., & Goodwin, C. W. (1999). The relationship of burnout, stress, and hardiness in nurses in a military medical center: A replicated descriptive study. *Journal of Burn Care Rehabilitation, 20*(6), 515–522.

Dochterman, J. M., & Bulechek, G. M. (Eds.). (2004). *Nursing interventions classification (NIC)* (4th ed.). St Louis: Mosby.

Fontaine, K. L., & Fletcher, J. S. (2003). *Mental health nursing* (5th ed.). Upper Saddle River, NJ: Pearson.

Franco, G. P., de Barros, A. L., Nogueira-Martins, L. A., & Michel J. L. (2003). Stress influence on genesis, onset and maintenance of cardiovascular diseases: Literature review. *Journal of Advanced Nursing, 43*(6), 548–554.

French, S. E., Lenton, R., Walters, V., & Eyles, J. (2000). An empirical evaluation of an expanded Nursing Stress Scale. *Journal of Nursing Measurement, 8*(2), 161–178.

Gates, D. M. (2001). Stress and coping: A model for the workplace. *AAOHN Journal, 49*, 390–398.

Gilbar, O. (1998). Relationship between burnout and a sense of coherence in health social workers. *Social Work in Health Care, 26*(3), 39–49.

Grieve, R. J. (2002). Day surgery preoperative anxiety reduction and coping strategies. *British Journal of Nursing, 11*, 670–673, 676–678.

Holmes, T., & Rahe, R. (1967). The social readjustment and rating scale. *Journal of Psychosomatic Research, 11*, 213–218.

Johnson, M., Bulechek, G., Dochterman, J., Maas, M., & Moorhead, S. (2001). *Nursing diagnoses, outcomes & interventions: NANDA, NOC, and NIC linkages*. St Louis: Mosby.

Johnson, P. (2002). The use of humor and its influences on spirituality and coping in breast cancer survivors. *Oncology Nursing Forum, 29*(4), 691–695.

Keegan, L. (2003). Therapies to reduce stress and anxiety. *Critical Care Nursing Clinics of North America, 15*(3), 321–327.

Krieger, D. (1993). *Accepting your power to heal*. Santa Fe, NM: Bear & Company.

Lazarus, R. (1999). *Stress and emotion: A new synthesis*. New York: Springer.

Lazarus, R., & Folkman, S. (1984). *Stress appraisal and coping*. New York: Springer.

Leiter, M. P., Harvie, P., & Frizzell, C. (1998). The correspondence of patient satisfaction and nurse burnout. *Social Science in Medicine, 47*(10), 1611–1617.

McEwen, B. S. (1998). Protective and damaging effects of stress mediators. *New England Journal of Medicine, 338*(3), 171–179.

McEwen, B. S. (2000). The neurobiology of stress from serendipity to clinical relevance. *Brain Research, 88*(6), 172–189.

McGowan, B. (2001, July 4–10). Self-reported stress and its effects on nurses. *Nursing Standard, 15*(42), 33–38.

Mitchel, A. M., Kameg, K., & Sakraida, T. J. (2003). Post-traumatic stress: Clinical implications. *Disaster Management Response, 1*(1), 14–18.

Moorhead, S., Johnson, M., & Maas, M. (Eds.). (2004). *Nursing outcomes classification (NOC)* (3rd ed.). St Louis: Mosby.

NANDA International. (2005). *Nursing diagnoses: Definitions and classification 2005–2006*. Philadelphia: Author.

Neeb, K. (2001). *Fundamentals of mental health nursing* (2nd ed.). Philadelphia: F. A. Davis Company.

Olson, R. (1987). Definitions of biofeedback. In M. S., Schwartz, et al. (Eds.), *Biofeedback: A practitioner's guide*. New York: Guilford Press.

Phipps, S. (2002). Reduction of distress associated with paediatric bone marrow transplant: Complementary health promotion interventions. *Pediatric Rehabilitation, 5*(4), 223–234.

Robinson, F. P., Mathews, H. L., & Witek-Janusek, L. (2000). Stress reduction and HIV disease: A review of intervention studies using a psychoneuroimmunology framework. *Journal of the Association of Nurses in AIDS Care, 11*(2), 87–96.

Schafer, W. (2000). *Stress management for wellness* (4th ed.). Stamford, CT: International Thomson Publishing.

Selye, H. (1974). *Stress without distress*. Philadelphia: Lippincott.

Selye, H. (1976). *The stress of life. (Revised edition)*. New York: McGraw-Hill.

Sneed, N. V., Olson, M., Bubolz, B., & Finch, N. (2001). Influences of a relaxation intervention on perceived stress and power spectral analysis of heart rate variability. *Progress in Cardiovascular Nursing, 16*(2), 57–64, 79.

Stuart, B., & Sundeen, S. (1998). *Nurse-client interaction: Implementing the nursing process* (6th ed.). St Louis: Mosby.

Thompson, J., & Manore, M. (2004). *Nutrition and health: An applied approach*. San Francisco: Benjamin Cummings.

U.S. Department of Health and Human Services. (2000). *Healthy people 2010*. Washington, DC: Author.

Weckman, H. (2001). Moving from distress to de-stress: Some suggestions on managing the stress in your life. *SCI Nurse, 18*(3), 148–149.

Wilkinson, J. (2005). *Nursing diagnosis handbook with NIC interventions and NOC outcomes* (8th ed.). Upper Saddle River, NJ: Prentice Hall.

Zink, K. A., & McCain, G. C. (2003). Post-traumatic stress disorder in children and adolescents with motor vehicle-related injuries. *J Spec Pediatr Nurs, 8*(3), 99–106.

Zook, R. (1998). Learning to use positive defense mechanisms. *American Journal of Nursing, 98*(3), 16B, F, H.

CHAPTER 26

Ackley, B. J., & Ladewig, G. B. (2002). *Nursing diagnosis handbook: A guide to planning care* (5th ed.). St Louis: Mosby.

American Academy of Pediatrics. (1994). Infant feeding practices and their possible relationship to the etiology of diabetes mellitus (RE9430). *Pediatrics, 94*(5), 752.

American Academy of Pediatrics, Committee on Nutrition. (1999). Iron fortification of infant formula. *Pediatrics 104*(1), 119–123.

American Gastrointestinal Association. (1995). American Gastroenterological Association medical position statement: Guidelines for the use of enteral nutrition. Retrieved March 11, 2004, from *http://www3.us.elsevierhealth.com/gastro/policy/v108n4p1280.html*

American Heart Association. (2004). Fat substitutes. Retrieved March 10, 2004, from *http://www.americanheart.org/presenter.jhtml?identifier=4633*

Barone, L., Milosavljevic, M., & Gazibarich, B. (2003). Assessing the older person: Is the MNA a more appropriate nutritional assessment tool than the SGA? *Journal of Nutritional Health Aging, 7*(1), 13–17.

Boyle, M. (2001). *Personal nutrition* (4th ed.). Belmont, CA: Wadsworth.

Canada's Food Guide to Healthy Eating. (1997). Ottawa, Ontario: Canadian Government Publishing, Minister of Public Works and Government Services, Canada.

Center for Nutrition Policy and Promotion. (2000). *Dietary guidelines for Americans, 1980–2000.* Washington, DC: United States Department of Agriculture.

Dochterman, J. C., & Bulechek, G. M. (Eds.). (2004). *Nursing interventions classification (NIC)* (3rd ed.). St Louis: Mosby.

Examples of Revised Nutrition Facts Panel Listing Trans Fat. (2003) U.S. Food and Drug Administration, Center for Food Safety and Applied Nutrition. Retrieved 3/25/06 from *http://www.cfsan.fda.gov/~dms/labtr.html*

Food and Nutrition Board, National Academy of Science, Institute of Medicine. (2002). *Dietary reference intakes for energy, carbohydrate, fiber, fat, fatty acids, cholesterol, protein, and amino acids.* Washington, DC: National Academy Press.

Geronimus, A. T., et al. (1993, February). Age patterns of smoking and vitamin C status in adults. *American Journal of Public Health, 79,* 158.

Guenter, P., Ericson, M., & Jones, S. (1997). Enteral nutrition therapy. *Nursing Clinics of North America, 32*(4), 651.

Institute of Medicine. (2000). Dietary intakes of vitamin C, vitamin E, selenium, and carotenoids. *Pharmacist's Letter, 16*(5), 26–27. Washington, DC: The National Academy Press.

Moorhead, S., Johnson, M., & Maas, M. (Eds.). (2004) *Nursing outcomes classification (NOC)* (3rd ed.). St Louis: Mosby.

Kidd, P. S., & Wagner, K. D. (2001). *High acuity nursing* (3rd ed.). Upper Saddle River, NJ: Prentice Hall.

Matarese, L. E., & Gottschlich, M. M. (1998). *Contemporary nutrition support practice: A clinical guide.* Philadelphia: W. B. Saunders.

McCallum, P. D. (2000). Patient generated subjective global assessment. In P. D. McCallum & C. G. Polisena (Eds.). *The clinical guide to oncology nutrition.* Chicago, IL: American Dietetics Association.

Metheney, N., Wehrle, A., Wiersema, L., & Clark, J. (1998a). Testing feeding tube placement: Auscultation vs. pH method. *American Journal of Nursing, 98*(5), 37–42.

Metheney, N., Smith, L., Wehrle, M., Wiersema, L., & Clark, J. (1998b). pH, color, and feeding tubes. *RN, 61*(1), 25–27.

Murphy, M. C., & Brooks, C. N. (2000). The use of the Mini Nutritional Assessment tool in elderly orthopedic patients. *European Journal of Clinical Nutrition, 54*(7), 555–562.

NANDA International. (2005). *NANDA nursing diagnoses: Definitions and classification 2005–2006.* Philadelphia: Author.

National Academy of Sciences. (2000). *Dietary reference intakes: Applications in dietary assessment.* Washington, DC: National Academy Press.

National Heart, Lung, and Blood Institute. (1998). *Clinical guidelines on the identification, evaluation, and treatment of overweight and obesity in adults: The evidence report.* Washington, DC: U. S. Department of Health and Human Services.

National Institute of Health; National Institute of Diabetes and Digestive and Kidney Diseases (NIDDH); National Digestive Diseases Information Clearing house (2003, March). Lactose intolerance. Retrieved April 25, 2005, from *http://digestive.niddk.nih.gov/ddiseases/pubs/lactoseintolerance/NIHPub.No.03-2751.*

Nutritional Screening Initiative. (1995). Washington, DC. Retrieved August 5, 2003, from *http://www.universityhospital.org/geriatric_education/nutrition.html*

Nutrition Screening Initiative. (2003). *Determine your nutritional health.* Washington, DC: National Council on Aging.

Oddy, W. H. (2002). The impact of breastmilk on infant and child health. *Breastfeed Review, 10*(3), 5–18.

Pai, M. P., & Paloucek, F. P. (2000). The origin of the "ideal" body weight equations. *Annals of Pharmacotherapy, 34,* 1066–1069.

Rombeau, J. L., & Rolandelli, R. H. (Eds.). (1997). *Enteral feeding and tube feeding.* Philadelphia: W. B. Saunders.

Russell, R., Rasmussen, H., & Lichtenstein, A. (1999). Modified food guide pyramid for people over seventy years of age. *Journal of Nutrition, 129*(3), 751–753.

Schnell, Z. B., Van Leeuwen, A. M., & Kranpitz, T. R. (2003). *Davis' comprehensive handbook of laboratory and diagnostic tests with nursing implications.* Philadelphia: F. A. Davis Company.

Severson, K., & Burke, C. (2003). *The trans fat solution: Cooking and shopping to eliminate the deadliest fat from your diet.* Berkeley, CA: Ten Speed Press.

Thompson, J., & Manore, M. (2005). *Nutrition and health: An applied approach.* San Francisco: Benjamin Cummings.

United States Department of Agriculture. (2005). *Dietary guidelines for Americans 2005.* Retrieved April 26, 2005, from *www.healthierus.gov/dietaryguidelines.*

U.S. Preventive Services Task Force (USPSTF). (2003). Routine vitamin supplementation to prevent cancer and cardiovascular disease: Recommendations and rationale. Retrieved February 18, 2004, from *http://www.guideline.gov/summary/summary.aspx?doc_id=3698&nbr=2924&string=HEALTHY+AND+DIET.*

U.S. Department of Health and Human Services. (2000). *Healthy people 2010: Understanding and improving health* (2nd ed.). Washington, DC: U.S. Government Printing Office. Retrieved March 1, 2004, from *http://www.healthypeople.gov/Document/HTML/Volume2/19Nutrition.htm.*

Vellas, B., et al (1999). The Mini Nutritional Assessment (MNA) and its use in grading the nutritional status of elderly patients. *Nutrition, 15*(2), 116–122.

Wardlaw, G. M., Hampl, J. S., & DiSilvestro, R. A. (2004). *Perspectives in nutrition* (6th ed.). New York: McGraw-Hill.

Williams, S. R., & Schlenker, E. (2003). *Essentials of nutrition and diet therapy* (8th ed.). St Louis: Mosby.

CHAPTER 27

Archer, C. L., & Foote, J. E. (2000). Urinary incontinence in the elderly female. *Urologic Nursing, 20,* 301–305.

Association of Women's Health, Obstetric and Neonatal Nurses (AWHONN). (2000). *Evidence-based clinical practice guideline: Continence for women.* Washington, DC: Author.

Bates, F., & Porter, G. (2002). The role of the nurse continence advisor in a urology wellness clinic. *Urologic Nursing, 22*(1), 23–26.

Clean intermittent self-catheterization. (2002). Retrieved April 18, 2004, from *http://health.allrefer.com/health/clean-intermittent-self-catheterization-info.html*

Clean intermittent self-catheterization (2004). Retrieved April 17, 2004, from *www.nlm.nih.gov/medlineplus/ency/article/003972.htm*

Cooper, G., & Watt, E. (2003). An exploration of acute care nurses' approach to assessment and management of people with urinary incontinence. *Journal of Wound, Ostomy, & Continence Nursing, 30*(6), 305–313.

Cravens, D. D., & Zweig S. (2000). Urinary catheter management. *American Family Physician, 61*(2), 369–376.

Dillon, P. M. (2003). *Nursing health assessment: A critical thinking, case studies approach.* Philadelphia: F. A. Davis Company.

Dougherty, M. C., Dwyer, J. W., Pendergast, J. F., Boyington, A. R., Tomlinson, B. U., Coward, R. T., et al. (2002). Urinary incontinence in older rural women. *Research in Nursing & Health, 25,* 3–13.

Engberg, S. J., Bender, M. A., & Stilley, C. S. (2003). Bladder matters: Kegels and communication. *American Journal of Nursing, 103*(7), 93–94.

External catheter systems. Retrieved April 5, 2004, from *www.seekwellness.com/incontinence*

Fantl, J.A., Newman D. K., Colling, J., DeLancey, J., Keeys, C., Loughery, R., et al. (1996, January). *Managing acute and chronic urinary incontinence.* Clinical Practice Guideline. Quick Reference Guide for Clinicians, No. 2, 1996 Update. Rockville, MD: U.S. Department of Health and Human Services, Public Health Service, Agency for Health Care Policy and Research. AHCPR Pub. No. 96–0686.

Fultz, N. H., & Herzog, A. R. (2001). Self-reported social and emotional impact of urinary incontinence. *Journal of the American Geriatric Society, 49*(7), 892–899.

Gray, M. (2000). Physiology of voiding. In D. Doughty (Ed.), *Urinary and fecal incontinence: Nursing management.* St Louis: Mosby.

Gray, M., Ratliff, C., & Donovan, A. (2002). Tender mercies: Providing skin care for an incontinent patient. *Nursing, 32*(7), 51–54.

Jirovec, M. M., & Templin, T. (2001). Predicting success using individualized scheduled toileting for memory-impaired elders at home. *Research in Nursing & Health, 24*(1), 1–8.

Johansson, I., Athlin, E., Frykholm, L., Bolinder, H., & Larsson, G. (2002). Intermittent versus indwelling catheters for older patients with hip fractures. *Journal of Clinical Nursing, 11*(5), 651–656.

Kelleher, M. M. B. (2002). Removal of urinary catheters: Midnight vs. 0600 hours. *British Journal of Nursing, 11,* 84, 86, 88–90.

Lekan-Rutledge, D. (2000). Diffusion of innovatin: A model for implementation of prompted voiding in long-term care settings. *Journal of Gerontological Nursing, 26*(4), 25–33.

Lewis, L. (2003). Managing incontinence at home. *American Journal of Nursing, 3*(suppl.), 41.

Logan, K. (2003). Indwelling catheters: Developing an integrated care pathway package. *Nursing Times, 99*(44), 49–51.

Maki, D. G., & Tambyah, P. A. (2001). Engineering out the risk of infection with urinary catheters. *Emerging Infectious Diseases, 7*(2), 1–6.

McConnell, E. A. (2000). New catheters decrease nosocomial infections. *Nursing Management, 31*(6), 51, 55.

McConnell, E. A. (2001). Clinical do's and don'ts: Applying a condom catheter. *Nursing, 31*(1), 70.

Morkved, S., & Bo, K. (2000). Effect of postpartum pelvic floor muscle training in prevention and treatment of urinary incontinence: A one-year follow up. *BJOG: An International Journal of Obstetric and Gynaecology, 107*(8), 1022–1028.

NANDA International. (2005). *Nursing diagnoses: Definitions and classification 2005–2006.* Philadelphia: Author.

Newman, D. K., & Giovanni, D. (2002). The overactive bladder: A nursing perspective. *American Journal of Nursing, 102*(6), 36–46.

Newman, D. (2002). *Managing and treating urinary incontinence.* Baltimore: Health Professions Press.

Newman, D. K., & Palmer, M. H. (Eds.). (2003). State of the science on urinary incontinence. *American Journal of Nursing, 3*(suppl.), 1–5.

Nyman, M., Schwenk, N., & Silverstein, M. (1997). *Management of urinary retention: Rapid versus gradual decompression and risk of complications.* Mayo Clinical Proceedings, 951–956.

Ord, J., Lunn, D., & Reynard, J. (2003). Bladder management and risk of bladder stone formation in spinal cord injured patients. *Journal of Urology, 170*(5), 1734–1737.

Pagana, K., & Pagana, T. (1998). *Mosby's manual of diagnostic and laboratory tests.* St Louis: Mosby.

Polan, E., & Taylor, D. (2003). *Journey across the lifespan* (2nd ed.). Philadelphia: F. A. Davis Company.

Pomfret, I. (2000). Urinary catheters: Selection, management and prevention of infection. *British Journal of Community Nursing, 5*(1), 6–8, 10–13.

Riley, K. E. (1997). Evaluation and management of primary nocturnal enuresis. *Journal of the American Academy of Nurse Practitioners, 9*(1), 33.

Robinson, J. (2000). Managing urinary incontinence in the nursing home: Residents' perspectives. *Journal of Advanced Nursing, 31*(1), 68–77.

Scanlon, V. C., & Sanders, T. (2003). *Essentials of anatomy and physiology.* Philadelphia: F. A. Davis Company.

Schnelle, J. F., Cadogan, M. P., Grbic, D., Bates-Jensen, B. M., Osterweil, D., Yoshii, J., et al. (2003). A standardized quality assessment system to evaluate incontinence care in the nursing home. *Journal of the American Geriatric Society, 51*(12), 1754–1761.

Shultz, J. M. (2002). Urinary incontinence: Solving a secret problem. *Nursing, 32*(11), 53–55.

Simpson L. (2001). Indwelling urethral catheters. *Nursing Standard, 15*(46), 47–53.

State of the Science on Urinary Incontinence (2003a, March). State of the science on urinary incontinence: executive summary. *American Journal of Nursing, 3*(suppl.), 4–8.

State of the Science on Urinary Incontinence. (2003b, March). Discussion and recommendations: Overcoming barriers to nursing care of people with urinary incontinence. *American Journal of Nursing, 3*(suppl.), 47–53.

Tambyah, P. A., Knasinski, V., & Maki, D. G. (2002). The direct costs of nosocomial catheter-associated urinary tract infections in the era of managed care. *Infection Control and Hospital Epidemiology, 23,* 27–31.

Taylor, P. (2001). Choosing the right stoma appliance for a urostomy. *Community Nurse, 7*(2), 35–36.

Ten tips for Foley catheter use and care. (2004). Retrieved April 21, 2004, from *http://nursing.about.com/cs/renalandurologic/a/aafoleycath.htm*

Thompson, J., Manore, M. (2005). *Nutrition and health: An applied approach.* San Francisco: Benjamin Cummings.

Urine sample. (2001, December 9). Retrieved April 5, 2004, from *www.nlm.nih.gov/medlineplus/ency/imagespages/10011.htm*

U.S. Department of Health and Human Services, Centers for Medicare and Medicaid Services. (2000). Nursing home data compendium. Retrieved July 10, 2004, from *http://www.cms.hhs.gov/Medicaid/survey-cert/datacomp.asp*

Watson, N. M., Brink, C. A., Zimmer, J. G., & Mayer, R. D. (2003). Use of the Agency for Health Care Policy and Research Urinary Incontinence Guideline in nursing homes. *Journal of the American Geriatric Society, 51*(12), 1810–1812.

Webber-Jones, J. (1991). Performing clean intermittent self-catheterization. *Nursing 1991, 21*(8), 56.

Wilde, M. H. (2002). Urine flowing: A phenomenological study of living with a urinary catheter. *Research in Nursing & Health, 25*(1), 14–24.

Wong, E. (2004). Guidelines for prevention of catheter-associated urinary tract infections. Retrieved April 19, 2004, from *www.cdc.gov/ncidod/hip/GUIDE/uritract.htm*

Wound, Ostomy, and Continence Nurses Society. (2003). Identifying and treating reversible causes of urinary incontinence. *Ostomy/Wound Management, 49*(12), 28–33.

Wyman, J. F. (2003). Treatment of urinary incontinence in men and older women. *American Journal of Nursing, 103*(3)Supple., 26–35.

CHAPTER 28

Addison, R., Ness, W., Abulafi, M., & Swift, I. (2000). How to administer enemas and suppositories. *Nursing Times, 96*(6), 3–4.

American College of Physicians. (1997). Suggested techniques for fecal occult blood testing and interpretation in colorectal cancer screening. *Annals of Internal Medicine, 126*(5), 808.

Annells, M., & Koch, T. (2002). Faecal impaction: Older people's experiences and nursing practice. *British Journal of Community Nursing, 7*(3), 118, 120–122, 124–126.

Ball, E. M. (2000). A teaching guide for continent ileostomy, *RN, 63*(12), 35–36, 38, 40.

Bryant, D., & Fleischer, I. (2000). Changing an ostomy appliance. *Nursing 2000, 30*(11), 51.

Cavanaugh, C. (2004). How to give yourself an enema. Retrieved April 24, 2004, from *www.geocities.com/valerie_cct/enemas/html*

Christer, R., Robinson, L., & Bird, C. (2003). Constipation: Causes and cures. *Nursing Times 99*(25), 26–27.

Cleveland Clinic. What is colostomy irrigation? Retrieved July 11, 2004, from *www.webmd.com/content/article/45/1811_50433.htm*

Colostomy irrigation procedure. Retrieved July 11, 2004, from *www.dmerc.com/COLO.htm*

Dochterman, J. M., & Bulechek, G. M. (Eds.). (2004). *Nursing interventions classification (NIC)* (4th ed.) St Louis: Mosby.

Erwin-Toth, p. (2001). Caring for a stoma is more than skin deep. *Nursing 2001, 31*(5), 6.

Fecal impaction. (2000, January 12). Retrieved July 11, 2004, from *www.cancersourcern.com*

Garrigues, V., Galvez, C., Ortiz, V., Ponce, M., Nos, P., & Ponce, J. (2004). Prevalence of constipation: Agreement among several criteria and evaluation of the diagnostic accuracy of qualifying symptoms and self-reported definition in a population-based survey in Spain. *American Journal of Epidemiology, 159*(5), 520–526.

He, J., Streiffer, R. H., Muntner, P., Krousel-Wood, M. A., & Whelton, P. K. (2004). Effect of dietary fiber intake on blood pressure: A randomized, double-blind, placebo-controlled trial. *Journal of Hypertension 22*(1), 73–80. Retrieved December 18, 2003, from Ovid.

Hinrichs, M. D., & Huseboe, J. (2001). Research-based protocol: Management of constipation. *Journal of Gerontological Nursing, 27*(2), 17–28.

Hyland, J. The basics of ostomies. *Gastroenterology Nursing, 25*(6), 241–244.

Johnson, M., Bulechek, G., Dochterman, J. M., Maas, M., & Moorhead, S. (2001). *Nursing diagnoses, outcomes, and interventions: NANDA, NOC, and NIC linkages.* St Louis: Mosby.

Kenny, K. A., & Skelly, J. M. (2001). Dietary fiber for constipation in older adults: A systematic review. *Clinical Effectiveness in Nursing, 5*(3), 120–128.

Koch, T., & Hudson, S. (2000). Older people and laxative use: Literature review and pilot study report. *Journal of Clinical Nursing, 9*, 516–525.

Lembo, A., & Camilleri, M. (2003). Chronic constipation. *New England Journal of Medicine, 349*(14):1360–1368.

Leonard, L. (1999). Colostomy irrigation. Retrieved July 11, 2004, from *World Ostomy Resource, http://homepage.powerup.com .au/~takkeno/Col_Irig.htm*

Long, M. (2002). *Crash course: Gastrointestinal system* (2nd ed.). St Louis: Mosby.

McConnell, E. (2002). Changing an ostomy appliance. *Nursing 2002, 32*(3), 17.

Medline Plus. Fecal impaction. Retrieved July 11, 2004, from *www.nlm.nih.gov/medlineplus*

Merchant, M. (2003). Laxatives should be the last resort in constipation. *Nursing Times, 99*(37), 35.

Moorhead, S., Johnson, M., & Maas, M. (Eds.). (2004). *Nursing outcomes classification (NOC)* (3rd ed.). St Louis: Mosby.

Muchoney, M. (2002). Ask the ostomy nurse. *Ostomy Quarterly.* Retrieved July 11, 2004, from *www.voa.org*

NANDA International. (2005). *NANDA nursing diagnoses: Definitions and classification 2005–2006.* Philadelphia: Author.

National Institute of Allergy and Infectious Diseases (NIAID). (2003, May). Food allergy and intolerances: NIAID fact sheet. Retrieved August 2003, from *http://www.niaid.nih.gov/factsheets/food.htm*

Peate, I. (2003). Nursing role in the management of constipation: Use of laxatives. *British Journal of Nursing, 12*(19), 1130–1136.

Pereira, M. A., O'Reilly, E., Augustsson, K., Fraser, G. E., Goldbourt, U., Heitmann, B. L., et al. (2004). Dietary fiber and risk of coronary heart disease: A pooled analysis of cohort studies. *Archives of Internal Medicine, 164*(4), 370–376.

Pillitteri, A. (1999). *Child health nursing: Care of the child and family.* Philadelphia: Lippincott.

Plaisance, L., & Ellis, J. A. (2002). Opioid-induced constipation. *American Journal of Nursing, 102*(3), 72–73.

Rushing, J. (2003). Administering an enema to an adult. *Nursing 2003, 33*(11), 28.

Salcido, R. (2000). Bowel problems in older adults. *Topics in Geriatric Rehabilitation, 16*(1), 92.

Schmelzer, M., Case, P., Chappell, S. M., & Wright, K. B. (2000). Colonic cleansing, fluid absorption, and discomfort following tap water and soapsuds enemas. *Applied Nursing Research, 13*, 83–91.

Schnell, Z. B., Leeuwen, A. M., & Kranpitz, T. R. (2003). *Davis's comprehensive handbook of laboratory and diagnostic tests with nursing implications.* Philadelphia: F. A. Davis Company.

Schnelle, J. F., & Leung, F. W. (2004). Urinary and fecal incontinence in nursing homes. *Gastroenterology, 126*(1 Suppl 2), S41–S47.

Sears, W., & Sears, M. (1999). *The family nutrition book.* Boston: Little, Brown and Company.

Thompson, J. (2000). A practical ostomy guide. *RN, 63*(11), 61–64, 66, 68, 71–73.

Thompson, M. J., Boyd-Carson, W., Trainor, B., & Boyd, K. (2003). Management of constipation. *Nursing Standard, 18*(14–16), 41–42.

University of Pittsburgh Medical Center. Managing your colostomy. Retrieved July 11, 2004, from *www.upmc.com*

Wilkinson, J. (2005). *Nursing diagnosis handbook with NIC interventions and NOC outcomes* (8th ed.). Upper Saddle River, New Jersey: Prentice Hall.

CHAPTER 29

Baily, J. D. (1995). Sense-ability. *Health Facilities Management, 8*(11).

Buckle J. (2001). The role of aromatherapy in nursing care. *Nursing Clinics of North America, 36*(1), 57–72.

Deglin, J. H., & Vallerand, A. G. (2003). *Davis's drug guide for nurses* (8th ed.). Philadelphia: F. A. Davis Company.

Dochterman, J. M., & Bulechek, G. M. (Eds.). (2004). *Nursing interventions classication (NIC)* (4th ed.). St Louis: Mosby.

Dyson, M. (1999). Intensive care unit psychosis, the therapeutic nurse-patient relationship and the influence of the intensive care setting: Analysis of interrelating factors. *Journal of Clinical Nursing, 8*(3), 284–290.

Espmark, A. K., Rosenhall, U., Erlandsson, S., & Steen, B. (2002). The two faces of presbycusis: Hearing impairment and psychosocial consequences. *International Journal of Audiology, 41*(2), 125–135.

Herz, R. S. (2004). A naturalistic analysis of autobiographical memories triggered by olfactory visual and auditory stimuli. *Chemical Senses, 29*(3), 217–224.

Hooker, S. D., Freeman, L. H., & Stewart, P. (2002). Pet therapy research: A historical review. *Holistic Nursing Practice, 17*(1), 17–23.

Johnson, M., Bulechek, G., Dochterman, J., Maas, M., & Moorhead, S. (2001). *Nursing diagnoses, outcomes, and interventions: NANDA, NOC, and NIC linkages.* St Louis: Mosby.

Kee, C. C. (1990). Sensory impairment: Factor X in providing nursing care to the older adult. *Journal of Community Health Nursing, 7*(1), 45–52.

Kennedy-Malone, L., Fletcher, K., & Plank, L. (2004). *Management guidelines for nurse practitioners working with older adults* (2nd ed.). Philadelphia: F. A. Davis Company.

Lang, M. M. (2001). Screening for cognitive impairment in the older adult. *Nurse Practitioner, 26*(11), 32–37.

McElligott D., Holz, M. B., Carollo, L., Somerville, S., Baggett, M., Kuzniewski, S., et al. (2003). A pilot feasibility study of the effects of touch therapy on nurses. *Journal of the New York State Nurses Association, 34*(1), 16–24.

Meehan, T., Vermeer, C., & Windsor, C. (2000). Patients' perceptions of seclusion: A qualitative investigation. *Journal of Advanced Nursing, 31*(2), 370–377.

Meehan, T., Vermeer, C., & Fjeldsoe, J. (2004). Staff and patient perceptions of seclusion: Has anything changed? *Journal of Advanced Nursing, 47*(1), 33–38.

Miller, K. E., Zylstra, R. G., & Standridge, J. B. (2000). The geriatric patient: A systematic approach to maintaining health. *American Family Physician, 61*(4), 1089–1104.

Moorhead, S., Johnson, M., & Maas, M. (Eds.). (2004). *Nursing outcomes classification (NOC)* (3rd ed.). St Louis: Mosby.

Moss, M., Cook, J., Wesnes, K., & Duckett, P. (2003). Aromas of rosemary and lavender essential oils differentially affect cognition and mood in healthy adults. *International Journal of Neuroscience, 113*(1), 15–38.

NANDA International. (2005). *Nursing diagnoses: Definitions and classification 2005–2006.* Philadelphia: Author.

Neal, R. (2001, April 20). First domino falls in touch research. *Focus: News from Harvard Medical, Dental & Public Health Schools,* p. 2.

Nightingale, F. (1866; 1932). *Notes on nursing.* London: Camelot Press, Ltd.

Nusbaum, N. J. (1999). Aging and sensory senescence. *Southern Medical Journal, 92*(3), 267–275.

Polan, E., & Taylor, D. (2003). *Journey across the life span: Human development and health promotion* (2nd ed.). Philadelphia: F. A. Davis Company.

Remington, R. (2002). Calming music and hand massage with agitated elderly. *Nursing Research, 51*(5), 317–323.

Running, A., & Berndt, A. (2003). *Management guidelines for nurse practitioners working in family practice.* Philadelphia: F. A. Davis Company.

Sininger, Y. S., Doyle, K. J., & Moore, J. K. (1999). The case for early identification of hearing loss in children. *Pediatric Clinics of North America, 46*(1), 1–14.

Schofield, P., & Davis, B. (1998). Sensory deprivation and chronic pain: A review of the literature. *Disability and Rehabilitation, 20*(10), 357–366.

Taber's Cyclopedic Medical Dictionary (20th ed.). (2005). Philadelphia: F. A. Davis Company.

Tullmann, D. F., & Dracup, K. (2000). Creating a healing environment for elders. *AACN Clinical Issues, 11*(1), 34–50.

Wilkinson, J. M. (2005). *Prentice Hall nursing diagnosis handbook* (8th ed.). Upper Saddle River, NJ: Prentice Hall Health.

Williams, L. S., & Hopper, P. D. (2003). *Understanding medical surgical nursing* (2nd ed.). Philadelphia: F. A. Davis Company.

Zervakis, J., & Schiffman, S. (2004). Adverse taste side effects of cardiovascular medications. *Geriatric Times, 5*(1), 405–413.

CHAPTER 30

Acello, B. (2000). Meeting JCAHO standards for pain control. *Nursing 2000, 30*(3), 52–54.

Agency for Health Care Policy and Research (AHCPR). (1992). *Acute pain management: Operative or medical procedures and trauma.* AHCPR Publication No. 92-0032. Rockville, MD: U.S. Department of Health and Human Services.

Agency for Health Care Policy and Research (AHCPR). (1994). *Management of cancer pain: Adults. Quick reference guide for the clinicians.* AHCPR Publication No. 94-0593. Rockville, MD: U.S. Department of Health and Human Services.

Agency for Healthcare Research and Quality (AHRQ). (2000). *Guidelines for the use of adjunct measures: Quick reference guide for clinicians.* Rockville, MD: Author.

American Pain Society. (1992). *Principles of analgesic use in the treatment of acute pain and cancer pain* (3rd ed.). Shobie, IL: Author.

Astedt-Kurki, P., & Isola, A. (2001). Humor between nurse and patient, among staff: Analysis of nurses diaries. *Journal of Advanced Nursing, 35*(3), 452–458.

Benedetti, C., & Butler, S. H. (1990). Systemic analgesics. In J. J. Bonica (Ed.), *The management of pain* (2nd ed.) (pp. 1640–1675). Philadelphia: Lea & Febiger.

Berdine, H. J. (2002). The fifth vital sign: Cornerstone of a new pain management strategy. *Disease and Management Outcomes, 10*(3), 155–156.

American Academy of Pediatrics, *Committee on Psychological Aspects of Child and Family Health and American Task Force on Pain in Infants, Children, and Adolescents.* (2001). The assessment and management of acute pain in infants, children and adolescents. *Pediatrics, 108*(3), 793–797.

Cohen, M. (2003). Pushing for safe pain relief. *Nursing 2003, 33*(11), 10.

Collins, P. (1999). Improving pain management in your healthcare organization. *Journal of Nursing Quality, 13*(4), 73–82.

Cornock, M. (1996). Psychological approaches to cardiac pain. *Nursing Standard, 11*(12), 34–38.

Cousins, M. (1994). Acute postoperative pain. In R. Mezack & P. Wall (Eds.), *Textbook of pain* (3rd ed.) (pp. 357–385). New York: Churchill Livingstone.

Crook, R., Rideout, E., & Browne, G. (1984). The prevalence of pain complaints in a general population. *Pain, 18,* 299–314.

Davis, B. (2000). *Caring for people in pain.* New York: Taylor & Francis Books.

Donovan, M., & Miaskowski, C. (1992). Striving for a standard of pain relief. *American Journal of Nursing, 92*(3), 106–107.

Eifried, S. (2003). Bearing witness to suffering: The lived experience of nursing students. *Journal of Nursing Education, 42*(2), 59–67.

Eliopoulos, C. (1999). Using complementary and alternative therapies wisely. *Geriatric Nursing, 20*(3), 139–143.

Evans, D. (2002). The effectiveness of music as an intervention for hospital patients: A systematic review. *Journal of Advanced Nursing, 37*(1), 8–18.

Evans, F. J. (1974). The placebo response in pain reduction. *Advances in Neurology, 4,* 289–296. New York: Raven Press.

Fields, H. (1987). *Pain.* New York: McGraw-Hill.

Germann, W. J., & Stanfield, C. L. (2002). *Principles of human physiology.* San Francisco: Benjamin Cummings.

Gloth, M. (2001, February). Pain management in older adults: Prevention and treatment. *Journal of American Geriatrics Society, 49*(2), 188–189.

Hagle, M., Lehr, V., Brubakken, K., & Shippee, A. (2004). Respiratory depression in adult patients with intravenous patient-controlled analgesia. *Orthopedic Nursing 28*(1), 18–25.

Hamza, M., White, P., Craig, W., Ghoname, E., Ahmed, H., Proctor, T., et al. (2000). Percutaneous electrical nerve stimulation: A novel analgesic therapy for diabetic neuropathic pain. *Diabetes Care, 23*, 365–370.

Heidrich, D. (2002). The Indiana State Nurses Association by special arrangements with the Ohio Nurses Foundation presents: The physiological basis for pain medications: Independent study. *Indiana State Nurses Association Bulletin, 28*(3), 23–27.

Herr, K. (2002). Pain assessment in cognitively impaired older adults. *American Journal of Nursing, 102*(12), 65–66, 68.

Joint Commission on Accreditation of Healthcare Organizations (JCAHO). (2000). *Pain assessment and management: An organizational approach*. Oakbrook Terrace, IL: Author.

Institute for Safe Medicine Practice (ISMP). (2002, May 29). More on avoiding opiate toxicity with PCA by proxy: Too much of a good thing. *ISMP Medication*.

Kaptchuk, T. (2002). Acupuncture: Theory, efficacy, and practice. *Annals of Internal Medicine, 136*(5), 374–385.

Kehlet, H. (1999). Modification of responses to surgery by neural blockade. In M. J. Cousins & P. O. Bridenbaugh (Eds.), *Neural blockade*. Philadelphia: Lippincott-Raven.

Krieger, D. (1993) *Accepting your power to heal: The personal practice of therapeutic touch*. Sante Fe, NM: Bear and Co.

Krieger, D. (1999). Therapeutic touch in hospice care. *American Journal of Nursing, 99*(4), 46.

Kingsley, C. (2001). Epidural analgesia: Your role. *RN, 64*(3), 53–58.

Lyke, E. M. (1992). *Assessing for nursing diagnosis: A human needs approach*. Philadelphia: Lippincott.

Lynch, M. (2001). Pain as the fifth vital sign. *Journal of Intravenous Nursing, 24*(2), 85–94.

The management of persistent pain in older persons. (2002). *Journal of the American Geriatric Society, 50*(6 Suppl), S205–224.

Marders, J. (2004). PCA by proxy: Too much of a good thing. *Nursing 2004, 34*(4), 24.

Mayer, D., Torma, L., Byock, I., & Norris, K. (2001). Speaking the language of pain. *American Journal of Nursing, 101*(2), 44–50.

McCaffery, M. (1989). *Pain: Clinical manual for nursing practice*. St Louis: Mosby.

McCaffery, M. (2003). Pain control: Switching from IV to PO. *American Journal of Nursing, 103*(5), 62–63.

McCaffery, M., & Parero, C. (1999). *Pain clinical manual* (2nd ed.). St Louis: Mosby.

McCreaddie, M., & Davidson, S. (2002). Pain management in drug users. *Nursing Standard, 16*(19), 20.

McQuay, H., Moore, A., & Justins, D. (1997). Fortnightly review: Treating acute pain in hospital. *British Medical Journal, 314* (7093), 1531–1535.

Melzack, R., & Wall, P. (1965). Pain mechanisms: A new theory. *Science, 150*, 971–979.

Melzack, R., & Wall, P. (1996). The challenge of pain (2nd ed.). London: Penguin.

Mersky, H., & Bogduk, N. (Eds.). (1994). *Classification of chronic pain* (2nd ed.). Seattle, WA: International Association for the Study of Pain.

Nichols, R. (2003). Pain management in patients with addictive disease. *American Journal of Nursing, 103*(3), 87–88.

Norred, C. (2000). Minimizing preoperative anxiety with alternative caring-healing therapies. *AORN Journal, 72*(5), 838, 840, 842–843.

O'Mathuna, D. (2000). Evidence-based practice and reviews of therapeutic touch. *Journal of Nursing Scholarship, 32*(3), 279–285.

Panke, J. (2002). Difficulties in managing pain at the end of life. *American Journal of Nursing, 102*(7), 26–34.

Pasero, C. (1997). Pain ratings: The fifth vital sign. *American Journal of Nursing, 97*(2), 15–16.

Portenoy, R. (1996). *Basic mechanisms: Pain management theory and practice*. Philadelphia: F. A. Davis Company.

Reiff, P., & Niziolek, M. (2001). Trouble-shooting tips for PCA. *RN, 64*(4), 33–37.

Richardson, J. (2001). Post-operative epidural analgesia: Introducing evidence-based guidelines through education and assessment process. *Journal of Clinical Nursing, 10*(3), 238–245.

Safety alert. Retrieved May 5, 2004, from www.ismp.org/msaarticles/pcaprint.htm

Slaughter, A., Pasero, C., & Manworren, R. (2002). Unacceptable pain levels: Approaches to pain relief. *American Journal of Nursing, 102*(5), 75–77.

Soderhamn, O., & Idvall, E. (2003). Nurses' influence on quality of care in postoperative pain management: A phenomenological study. *International Journal of Nursing Practice, 9*(1), 26–32.

Taddio, A., Katz, J., Hersich, A., & Koren, G. (1997). Effects of neonatal circumcision on pain response during subsequent routine vaccination. *The Lancet, 349*, 599–603.

Van Nostrand, J., Furner, S., & Suzman, R. (eds.). (1993). *Health data on older Americans: United States, 1992*. Hyattsville, MD: National Center for Health Statistics.

Verhaak, P. (1998). Prevalence of chronic pain disorders among adults: A review of the literature. *Pain, 77*, 231–239.

Vicker, A., & Zollman, C. (1999). ABC of complementary medicine: Hypnosis and relaxation therapies. *British Medical Journal, 319*(7221), 1346–1349.

Warren, D. (1996). Practical use of rectal medications in palliative care. *Journal of Pain Symptom Management, 11*(6), 378–387.

Wilson, M. (2002). Overcoming the challenges of neuropathic pain. *Nursing Standard, 16*(33), 47–53.

Wright, R., & Bell, S. (2001). Nurses' retention of pain management knowledge. *Journal of Staff Development, 17*(6), 309–313.

CHAPTER 31

American College of Sports Medicine (ACSM). (2000). *ACSM guidelines for exercise testing and prescription* (6th ed.). Philadelphia: Lippincott Williams & Wilkins.

American Nurses Association (ANA). (2003). Position statement on elimination of manual patient handling to prevent work-related musculoskeletal disorders. Retrieved April 1, 2005, from *http://www.nursingworld.org/readroom/position/workplac/pathand.htm*

American Nurses Association (ANA). (2004). *ANA handle with care*. Retrieved April 4, 2005, from *www.NursingWorld.org/handlewithcare*

American Nurses Association (ANA). (2005). New ANA ergonomics brochure outlines how to adopt a successful safe-patient handling program. Retrieved April 4, 2005, from *www.nursingworld.org/handlewithcare/*

Astrand, P. O. (2003) *Textbook of work physiology: Physiological basis of exercise* (5th ed.). Stockholm, Sweden: Human Kinetics.

Bailey, C. (1977). *Fit or fat?* Boston: Houghton Mifflin Company.

Blair, S. N., Cheng, Y., & Holder, J. S. (2002). Exercise adherence and 10-year mortality in chronically ill older adults. *Journal of the American Geriatric Society, 50*(12), 1929–1933.

Borg, G. (1998). *Borg's perceived exertion and pain scales*. Stockholm, Sweden: Human Kinetics.

Converso, A., & Murphy, C. (2004). Winning the battle against back injuries. *RN, 67*(2), 52–57.

Dochterman, J. M., & Bulechek, G. M. (Eds.). (2004). *Nursing interventions classification (NIC)* (4th ed.). St Louis: Mosby.

Fletcher, G. F., Balady, G. J., & Amsterdam, E. A. (2001). Exercise standards for testing and training: A statement for healthcare professionals from the American Heart Association. *Circulation 106*(14), 1694–740.

Forman, D. E. & Farquhar, W. (2002). Cardiac rehabilitation and secondary prevention programs for elderly cardiac patients. *Clinics in Geriatric Medicine 16*(3), 619–629.

Foster, C. (2004). "Talk test" measures exercise intensity. *Medicine & Science in Sports & Exercise, 36*(9), 1632–1636.

Gielen, S. Schuler, G., & Hambrecht, R. (2001). Benefits of exercise training for patients with chronic heart failure. *Clinical Geriatrics 9*(4), 32,36,38.

Gregg, E. W., Gerzoff, R. B., Caspersen, C. J., Williamson, D. F., & Narayan, K. M. (2003). Relationship of walking to mortality among U.S. adults with diabetes. *Archives of Internal Medicine, 163*(12), 1440–1447.

Jakicic, J. M., Marcus, B. H., Gallagher, K. I., Napolitano, M., & Lang, W. (2003). Effect of exercise duration and intensity on weight loss in overweight, sedentary women: A randomized trial. *Journal of the American Medical Association, 290*(10), 1323–1330.

Lee, I. M., Sesso, H. D., Oguma, Y., & Paffenbarger, R. S. (2003). Relative intensity of physical activity and risk of coronary heart disease. *Circulation, 107*(8), 1110–1116.

Manson, J. E. & Bassuk, S. S. (2003). Obesity in the United States: A fresh look at its high toll. *Journal of the American Medical Association, 289*(2), 229–230.

Manson, J. E., Greenland, P., LaCroix, A. Z., Stefanick, M. L., Mouton, C. P., Oberman, A., et al. Walking compared with vigorous exercise for the prevention of cardiovascular events in women. *New England Journal of Medicine, 347*(10), 716–725.

Metules, T. J. (2001). Occupational hazards. Watch your back! *RN, 64*(6), 65–66, 82.

Moorhead, S., Johnson, M., & Mass, M. (Eds.). (2004). *Nursing outcomes classification (NOC)* (3rd ed.). St Louis: Mosby.

Nelson, A., Fragala, G., & Menzel, N. (2003). Myths and facts about back injuries in nursing. *American Journal of Nursing, 103*(2), 32–40.

Nelson, A., Lloyd, J. D., Menzel, N., & Gross, C. (2003). Preventing nursing back injuries. *American Association of Occupational Health Nursing Journal, 51*(3), 126–134.

Pagliarulo, M. A. (Ed.). (2001). *Introduction to physical therapy.* St Louis, Mosby.

Simkin, B. S. & Simkin, M. A. (2002). Maximizing the benefits of exercise in the elderly. *Family Practice Recertification, 24*(1), 38–40.

U.S. Department of Health and Human Services. (1996). *Physical activity and health: A report of the surgeon general.* Washington, D.C.: Author.

U.S. Department of Health and Human Services. (2001). *Overweight and obesity: What you can do. Being physically active can help you attain a healthy weight.* Washington, D.C.: Author.

U.S. Department of Health and Human Services. (2004). Healthy people 2010: Understanding and improving health. Retrieved April, 2005, from *www.healthypeople.gov*

CHAPTER 32

Alan Guttmacher Institute. (2002). Sexual and reproductive health: Women and men. *Facts in brief.* Washington, DC: Author.

American Psychiatric Association. *Diagnostic and statistical manual of mental disorders* (4th ed.), Text Revision. (2000). Washington, D.C.: Author.

Annon, J. (1974). *The behavioral treatment of sexual problems.* Honolulu: Enabling Systems.

Basson, R. (2001). Using a different model for female sexual response to address women's problematic low sexual desire. *Journal of Sex and Marital Therapy, 27*, 395–403.

Brady, J. M. (1998). Female genital mutilation. *Nursing, 28*(9), 50–51.

Centers for Disease Control and Prevention. (2001). *Sexually transmitted disease surveillance, 2000.* Atlanta: U.S. Department of Health and Human Services.

Davidson, M. R. (2004). Sexually transmitted infections: Screening and counseling. *Clinician Reviews, 14*(6), 56–62.

Deeks, A. (2002). Sexual desire: Menopause and its psychological impact. *Australian Family Physician, 31*(5), 433–439, 455–456.

Dimmock, P. W., Wyatt, K. M., Jones, P. W., & O'Brien, P. M. (2000). Efficacy of selective serotonin-reuptake inhibitors in premenstrual syndrome: A systematic review. *Lancet, 356*, 1131–1136.

Dunn, M. E., & Culter, N. (2000). Sexual issues in older adults. *AIDS Patient Care and STDs, 14*, 67–69.

EngenderHealth. (2004). Sexual response and sexual practices: Normal changes in response with aging. *Sexuality and Sexual Health: An Online MiniCourse.* Retrieved September 2, 2004, from *http://www.engenderhealth.org/res/onc/sexuality/response/miw/pg5.html*

Frankel, D. (1994). U.S. surgeon general forced to retire. *Lancet, 34*, 1695.

Hordern, A. (2000). Intimacy and sexuality for the woman with breast cancer. *Cancer Nursing, 23*(3), 230–236.

Hughes, M. K. (2000). Sexuality and the cancer survivor: A silent coexistence. *Cancer Nursing, 23*(6), 477–482.

Hyde, J. S., & DeLamater, J. D. (2003). *Understanding human sexuality* (8th ed.). Boston: McGraw-Hill.

Iannacchione, M. A. (2004). The vagina dialogues: Do you douche? *American Journal of Nursing, 104*(1), 40–46.

ITPeople. (2004). Intersexed. Retrieved August 26, 2004, from *www.itpeople.org/intersexed.php*

Jacobson, D. S. (2000). The sexuality and disability unit: Applications for group training. *Sexuality and Disability, 18*(3), 175–177.

Jacoby, S. (1999, September-October). Great sex: What's age got to do with it? *Modern Maturity,* 40–45, 91.

Johns Hopkins Children's Center. (2004). Syndromes of abnormal sex differentiation: A guide for patients and their families. Baltimore: Johns Hopkins University.

Johnson, B. K. (1996). Older adults and sexuality: A multidimensional perspective. *Journal of Gerontological Nursing, 22*(2), 6.

Johnson, M., Bulechek, G., McCloskey-Dochterman, J., Maas, M., & Moorhead, S. (2001). *Nursing diagnoses, outcomes, and interventions: NANDA, NOC, and NIC linkages.* St Louis: Mosby.

King, B. M. (2002). *Human sexuality today* (4th ed.). Upper Saddle River, NJ: Prentice Hall.

Knowles, J. (revised by Johnsen, J.). (2004). *Sexually transmitted infections.* Retrieved August 30, 2004, from *http://www.plannedparenthood.org/sti/sex-safer.htm*

Masters, W. H. & Johnson, V. E. (1966). *Human sexual response.* Philadelphia. Lippincott, Williams & Wilkins.

McCann, E. (2000). The expression of sexuality in people with psychosis: Breaking the taboos. *Journal of Advanced Nursing, 32*(1), 132–138.

Moorhead, S., Johnson, M., & Maas, M. (Eds.) (2004). *Nursing outcomes classification (NOC)* (3rd ed.). St. Louis, Mosby.

Rennison, C. M., & Rand, M. R. (2003). Crime victimization, 2002: Findings from the National Crime Victimization Survey. Washington, D.C.: Bureau of Justice Statistics, U.S. Department of Justice.

Rodgers, J. E. (2001). *Sex: A natural history.* New York: Times Books.

Silverman, H. M. (Ed.). (2000). *The pill book* (9th ed.). New York: Bantam Books.

Stehle, B. F. (1985). *Incurably romantic.* Philadelphia: Temple University Press.

Steiner, M. (2000). Premenstrual syndrome and premenstrual dysphoric disorder: Guidelines for management. *Journal of Psychiatry & Neuroscience, 25*, 459–468.

Wilkinson, J. M. (2005). *Nursing diagnosis handbook with NIC interventions and NOC outcomes* (8th ed.). Upper Saddle River, NJ: Prentice Hall Health.

World Health Organization. (2002). Gender and reproductive rights. WHO draft working definition, October 2002. Retrieved May 20, 2004, from *http://www.who.int/reproductive-health/gender/glossary.html*

Writing Group for the Women's Health Initiative Investigators. (2002). Risks and benefits of estrogen plus progestin in healthy postmenopausal women: Principal results from the Women's Health Initiative randomized controlled trial. *Journal of the American Medical Association, 288,* 321–333.

Zucker, K. J. (2000). Gender identity disorder. In A. J. Sameroff, et al. (Eds.), *Handbook of developmental psychopathology.* (2nd ed.). (pp. 671–686). New York: Plenum Publishers.

CHAPTER 33

Acello, B. (2000). *Basic skills for the health care provider: Restorative care.* Albany, NY: Delmar Publishers.

American Academy of Pediatrics. (2004). *Guide to your child's symptoms.* Retrieved March 30, 2004, from *www.aap.org/pubserv/fears.htm*

American Sleep Apnea Association. (2004). *What is sleep apnea?* Retrieved March 30, 2004, from *www.sleepapnea.org/geninfo.html*

Better elder care: A nurse's guide to caring for older adults. (2001). Springhouse, PA: Springhouse.

Cmiel, C., Karr, D., Gasser, O., Oliphant, L., & Neveau, A. (2004). Noise control: A nursing team's approach to sleep promotion. *American Journal of Nursing, 104*(2), 40–48.

Cohen, B. J., & Wood, D. L. (2000). *Memmler's human body in health and disease* (9th ed.). Philadelphia: Lippincott, Williams and Wilkins.

Dochterman, J. M., & Bulechek, G. M. (Eds.). (2004). *Nursing interventions classification (NIC)* (4th ed.). St Louis: Mosby.

Earley C. J., Heckler, D., Allen, R. P. (2004). The treatment of restless leg syndrome with intravenous iron dextran. *Sleep Medicine, 5*(3), 231–235.

Eliopoulos, C. (2001). *Gerontological nursing.* Philadelphia: Lippincott Williams and Wilkins.

Ferrara, M., & DeGennaro, L. (2001). How much sleep do we need? *Sleep Medicine Review, 5*(2), 155–179.

Germann, W. J., & Stanfield, C. L. (2002). *Principles of human physiology.* San Francisco: Benjamin Cummings.

Goldberg, B. (2002). *Alternative medicine: The definitive guide* (2nd ed.). Berkeley, CA: Celestial Arts.

Harrison, Y., & Horne, J. A. (2000). The impact of sleep deprivation on decision making: A review. *Journal of Experimental Psychology: Applied, 6*(3), 236–249.

Guyton, A. C., & Hall, J. E. (2000). *Textbook of medical physiology* (10th ed.). Philadelphia: Saunders.

McCance, K. L., & Huether, S. E. (2002). *Pathophysiology: The biologic basis for disease in adults and children* (4th ed.). St Louis: Mosby.

McQuarrie, H. G. (2000). Lifestyle tips for insomnia. *Health tracks: A practical guide to managing your health.* Public Employees Health Program, Utah. Retrieved April 24, 2004, from *www.pehp.org/phc/healthtracks/index.html*

Moorhead, S., Johnson, M., & Maas, M. (Eds.). (2004). *Nursing outcomes classification (NOC)* (3rd ed.). St Louis: Mosby.

National Sleep Foundation. (2002). *Sleep poll executive summary.* Retrieved July 24, 2003, from *www.sleepfoundation.org/img/2002SleepInAmericaPoll.pdf*

Oswald, I. (1984). Good, poor, and disordered sleep. In R. G. Priest (Ed.), *Sleep: An international monograph.* London: Update Books.

Polan, E., & Taylor, D. (2003). *Journey across the life span* (2nd ed.). Philadelphia: F. A. Davis Company.

Sorrentino, S. A. (2000). *Mosby's textbook for nursing assistants* (5th ed.). St Louis: Mosby.

Sun, E. R., et al., (1998). Iron and the restless leg syndrome. *Sleep, 21*(4), 371.

Tate, J., & TaSota, F. (2002). More than a snore: Recognising the danger of sleep apnea. *Nursing 2002, 32*(8), 46.

Tuller, D. (2004, March 30). Poll finds even babies don't get enough rest. *New York Times.*

CHAPTER 34

Agostini, J. V., Baker, D. I., & Bogardus, S. T. Prevention of pressure ulcers in older patients. Retrieved December 5, 2002, from *www.ahcpr.gov./clinic/ptsafety/chp27.htm*

Armstrong, D., Bortz, P., & Halter, M. J. (2001). An intergrative review of pressure relief in surgical patients. *AORN Journal, 73,* 645–674.

Autio, L., & Olsen, K. K. (2002). The four S's of wound management: Staples, sutures, steri-strips, and sticky stuff. *Holistic Nursing Practice, 16*(2), 80–88.

Ayello, E. A., & Braden, B. (2002). How and why to do a pressure ulcer risk assessment. *Advances in Skin & Wound Care, 15*(3), 125–131.

Ayello, E. A., Cuddigan, J., & Kerstein, M. D. (2002). Skip the knife: Debriding wounds without surgery. *Nursing, 32*(9), 58–64.

Bergstrom, N., Bennett, M., Carlson, C., Frantz, R., Garber, S., Kaminski, M., et al. (December 1994). *Pressure ulcer treatment: Quick reference guide for clinicians, No. 15.* Rockville, MD: U.S. Department of Health and Human Services, Public Health Service, Agency for Health Care Policy and Research. AHRQ Pub. No. 95-0653.

Bergstrom, N., Bennett, M., Carlson, C., Frantz, R., Garber, S., Jackson, B., et al. (December 1994). *Treatment of pressure ulcers: Clinical Practice Guideline, No. 15.* Rockville, MD: U. S. Department of Health and Human Services. Public Health Service, Agency for Health Care Policy and Research. AHRQ Pub. No. 95-0652.

Bergstrom, N., Braden, B., Kemp, M., Champagne, M., & Ruby, E. (1998). Predicting pressure ulcer risk: A multisite study of the predictive validity of the Braden scale. *Nursing Research, 47,* 261–269.

Bowler, P. G., Duerden, B. I., & Armstrong, D. G. (2001). Wound microbiology and associated approaches to wound management. *Clinical Microbiology Reviews, 14,* 244–269.

Branom, R. (2002). Is this wound infected? *Critical Care Nursing Quarterly, 25*(1), 55–62.

Bryant, R. A., & Rolstad, B. S. (2001). Examining threats to skin integrity. *Ostomy Wound Management, 47*(6), 18–27.

Burdette-Taylor, S. R., & Kass, J. (2002). Heel ulcers in critical care units: A major pressure problem. *Critical Care Nursing Quarterly, 25*(2), 41–53.

Buss, I. C., Halfens, R. J. G., & Abu-Saad, H. H. (2002). The most effective time interval for repositioning subjects at risk of pressure sore development: A literature review. *Rehabilitation Nursing, 27*(2), 59–63.

Calhoun, J. H., Overgaard, K. A., Stevens, M., Dowling, J. P., & Mader, J. T. (2002). Diabetic foot ulcers and infections: Current concepts. *Advances in Skin & Wound Care, 15*(1), 31–42.

Campton-Johnston, S. M., & Wilson, J. A. (2001). Infected wound management: Advanced technologies, moisture-retentive dressings, and die-hard methods. *Critical Care Nursing Quarterly, 24*(2), 64–77.

Cervo, F., Cruz, A., & Posillico, J. (2000). Pressure ulcers analysis of guidelines for treatment and management. *Geriatrics, 55,* 55–60.

Clark, J. J. (2002). Wound repair and factors influencing healing. *Critical Care Nursing Quarterly, 25*(1), 1–12.

Cuddigan, J., Berlowitz, D. R., & Ayello, E. A. (Eds.). (2001). Pressure ulcers in America: Prevalence, incidence, and implications for the future. An executive summary of the National Pressure Ulcer Advisory Panel Monograph. *Advances in Skin & Wound Care, 14*(4), 208–215.

DeFloor, T., & Grypdonck, M. H. (2000). Do pressure relief cushions really relieve pressure? *Western Journal of Nursing Research, 22,* 335–350.

Demling, R. H., & DeSanti, L. (2002). Protein-energy malnutrition and the nonhealing cutaneous wound. Retrieved April 4, 2004, from *www.medscape.com/viewprogram/714-pnt*

Ferguson, J., Olsen, C. L., Tomaselli, N., & Goldberg, M. (2002). Wounds: Nursing care and product selection. Parts I & II. Retrieved December 5, 2002, from *http://nsweb.nursingspectum.com/cc/ce/ce80.htm?AFFILATE=medismart*

Gibson, M. C., Keast, D., Woodbury, M. G., Black, J., Goettl, L., Campbell, K., et al. (2004). Educational intervention in the management of acute procedure-related wound pain: A pilot study. *Journal of Wound Care, 13*(5), 187–190.

Goldberg, M. T., & Tomaselli, N. L. (2002). Management of pressure ulcers and fungating wounds. In A. Berger, R. K. Portnoy, & D. E. Weissman (Eds.). *Principles and practice of palliative care and supportive oncology* (periodicals) (2nd ed.). Philadelphia: Lippincott Williams & Wilkins.

Graff, M. K., Bryant, J., & Beinlich, N. (2000). Preventing heel breakdown. *Orthopedic Nursing, 19*(5), 63–69.

Gray, M., Ratliff, C., & Donovan, A. (2002). Perineal skin care for the incontinent patient. *Advances in Skin & Wound Care, 15*(4), 120–175.

Hall, C. (1997). Wound dressings: Use and selection: With new technology and wide selection in wound care products, nurses have an increased role in decision making. *Geriatric Nursing, 18*(6), 266–267.

Harding, K. G., Morris, H. L., & Patel, G. K. (2002). Healing chronic wounds. *British Medical Journal, 324*(7330), 160–163.

Hess, C. T (2001). Managing a pressure ulcer. *Nursing, 31*(1), 68.

Howard-Ruben, J. (2002). People who pierce—and the nurses who care for (and about) them. *American Journal of Nursing, 3*(8), 29–30.

Kravitz, S. R, McGuire, J., & Shanahan, S. D. (2003). Physical assessment of the diabetic foot. *Advances in Skin & Wound Care, 16*(2), 68–75.

LaMorte, W. W. (2003). Basics of wound closure and healing. Retrieved April 21, 2003, from *www.bumc.bu.edu/Departments/PageMain.asp?Page6067&DepartmentID=69*

Leininger, S. M. (2002). The role of nutrition in wound healing. *Critical Care Nursing Quarterly, 25*(1), 13–21.

Mangram, A. J., Horan, T. C., Pearson, M. L., Silver, L. C., & Jarvis, W. R. (1999). Guideline for prevention of surgical site infection. *Infection Control and Hospital Epidemiology, 20*(4), 247–278.

McGuckin, M., Goldman, R., Bolton, L., & Salcido, R. (2003). The clinical relevance of microbiology in acute and chronic wounds. *Advances in Skin & Wound Care, 16*(1), 12–23.

NANDA International. (2005). *Nursing diagnoses: Definitions and classification 2005–2006.* Philadelphia: Author.

National Pressure Ulcer Advisory Panel. (2002). PUSH Tool. Retrieved August 16, 2004, from *www.npuap.org/pushins.htm*

Nelson, D. B., & Dilloway, M. A. (2002). Principles, products, and practical aspects of wound care. *Critical Care Nursing Quarterly, 25*(1), 33–54.

Nutritional support in wound care. (2004). *Novartis Medical Nutrition U.S.* Fremont, MI. Retrieved August 16, 2004, from *www.novartisnutrition.com/us/articleDetail?id=30*

Ovington, L. G. (2002). Hanging wet-to-dry dressings out to dry. *Advances in Skin & Wound Care, 15*(2), 79–84.

Panel for the Prediction and Prevention of Pressure Ulcers in Adults. (1992, May). *Pressure ulcers in adults: Prediction and prevention. Clinical Practice Guideline, No. 3.* AHRQ Pub. No. 92–0047. Rockville, MD: Agency for Health Care Policy and Research, Public Health Service, U. S. Department of Health and Human Services.

Pedianni, R. (2001). What has pain relief to do with acute surgical wound healing? Retrieved December 22, 2002, from *www.worldwidewounds.com/2001/march/Pediani/pain-reliefsurgical-wounds.html*

Phipps, W. J., Monahan, F. D., Sands, J. K., Marek, J. F., Neighbors, M., & Green, C. J. (2003). *Medical-surgical nursing: Health and illness perspectives* (7th ed.). St Louis: Mosby.

Pierce, G. F., Mustoe, T. A., Altrock, B. W., Deuel, T. F., & Thomason, A. (1991). Role of platelet-derived growth factor in wound healing. *Journal of Cell Biochemisty, 45*(4), 319–326.

Porth, C. M. (2002). *Pathophysiology: Concepts of altered health states.* Philadelphia: Lippincott Williams & Wilkins.

Romanelli, M., Gaggio, G., Piaggesi, Coluccia, M., & Rizzello, F. (2002). Technological advances in wound bed measurements. *Wounds, 14*(2), 58–66.

Rosenberg, C. J. (2002). New checklist for pressure ulcer prevention. *Journal of Gerontological Nursing, 28*(8), 7–12.

Rudolph, D. M. (2002). Why won't this wound heal? Understanding the causes of and interventions for chronic wounds. *American Journal of Nursing, 102*(2), 24dd–24hh.

Serralta, V. W., Harrison-Balestra, C., Cazzaniga, A. L., Davis, S. C., & Mertz, P. M. (2001). Lifestyles of bacteria in wounds: Presence of biofilms? *Wounds, 13*(1), 29–34.

Smith, D. (1995, September 15). Pressure ulcers in the nursing home. *Annals of Internal Medicine, 123*(6), 433–438.

Stone, J. T., Wyman, J. F., Salisbury, S. A., & Chenitz, C. (1999). *Clinical gerontological nursing: A guide to advanced practice.* Philadelphia: Saunders.

Sussman, C., & Bates-Jensen, B. M. (2001). *Wound care* (2nd ed.). Gaithersburg, MD: Aspen.

Thompson, J. (2000). A practical guide to wound care. *RN, 63*(1), 48–53.

U.S. Department of Health and Human Services. (2000). *Healthy people 2010: Understanding and improving health* (Conference edition), Volume 1. Washington, D.C.: U. S. Government Printing Office.

Viejo, A., Puntillo, K. A., White, C., Morris, A. B., Perdue, S. T., et al (2001). Patients' perceptions and responses to procedural pain: Results from thunder project II. *American Journal of Critical Care, 29*(4), 238–249.

Vowden, K., & Vowden, P. (2002) Wound bed preparation. Retrieved December 22, 2002, from *www.worldwidewounds.com/2002/April/Vowden/Wed-Bed-Preparation.html*

Walker, D. (1996). Back to basics: Choosing the correct wound dressing. *American Journal of Nursing, 96*(9), 35–39.

Whitney, J. D., & Heitkemper, M. M. (1999). Modifying perfusion, nutrition, and stress to promote wound healing in patients with acute wounds. *Heart and Lung, 28*(2), 123–133.

Wysocki, A. B. (2002). Evaluating and managing open skin wounds: Colonization versus infection. *AACN Clinical Issues: Advanced Practice in Acute Critical Care, 13*(3), 383–397.

CHAPTER 35

Allender, J. A., & Spradley, B. W. (2001). *Community health nursing: Concepts and practice* (5th ed.). Philadelphia: Lippincott.

American Association of Respiratory Care. (1993). *Respiratory Care.* AARC Clinical Practice Guidelines: Endotracheal suctioning of mechanically ventilated adults and children with artificial airways, *38*(5), 500–504. Retrieved from *http://www.rcjournal.com/cpgs/etscpg.html* on June 1, 2007.

American Association of Respiratory Care. (1999). *Respiratory Care.* AARC Clinical Practice Guidelines: Suctioning of the patient in the home, *44*(1), 99–104. Retrieved from *http://www.rcjournal.com/cpgs/etscpg.html* on June 1, 2007.

American Head and Neck Society. (X) Tracheostomy care. Retrieved at *http://www.headandneckcancer.org/patienteducation/docs/tracheostomy.php* on May 27, 2007.

American Heart Association. (2002). Medications commonly used to treat heart failure. Retrieved July 4, 2004, from *www.americanheart.org/presenter.jhtml?identifier=118*

American Lung Association. (2002a). The asthma handbook. Retrieved July 4, 2004, from *www.alaw.org/childhood_asthma/asthma_handbook/cigarette_smoke.html*

American Lung Association. (2002b). Facts about secondhand smoke. Retrieved July 4, 2004, from *www.alaw.org/tobacco_control/secondhand_smoke/secondhand_smoke.html*

American Thoracic Society. (2000). *American Journal of Respiratory and Critical Care Medicine. 161*(1), pp. 297–308. Retrieved from *http://ajrccm.atsjournals.org/cgi/content/full/161/1/297#SEC4* on May 28, 2007.

American Thoracic Society. (2007). Suctioning. Retrieved at *http://www.thoracic.org/sections/education/care-of-the-child-*

with-a-chronic-tracheostomy/components-of-tracheostomy-care/ on May 19, 2007.

Centers for Disease Control and Prevention, Office on Smoking and Health. (2002). OSH Summary 2002: Targeting tobacco use: The nation's leading cause of death. Retrieved July 4, 2004, from *www.cdc.gov/tobaco/overview/oshsummary02.htm*

Cleveland Clinic. (2005). Tracheal suctioning guidelines. Retrieved at *http://www.clevelandclinic.org/health/health-info/docs/0600/0633.asp?index=4673&src=newsp* on May 28, 2007.

Cummins, R. O. (2005). *Advanced cardiac life support (ACLS) provider manual.* Dallas, TX: American Heart Association.

D'Allessandro, D., & Huth, L. (2002). Colds (upper respiratory tract infections/URI). *Pediatrics: Common questions, quick answers.* Virtual Children's Hospital. Retrieved September 30, 2004, from *www.vh.org/pediatric/patient/pediatrics/cqqa/colds.html#8*

Dochterman, J. M., & Bulechek, G. M. (Eds.). (2004). *Nursing interventions classification (NIC)* (4th ed.). St Louis: Mosby.

Eliopoulos, C. (2001). *Gerontological nursing* (5th ed.). New York: Lippincott.

Elliott, N. (2000). Chest tubes and drainage systems. Available online: *www.nursewise.com/courses/chestube_obj.htm.*

Gulanick, M., Myers. J. L., Klopp, A., Galanes, S., Fradishar, D., & Puzas, M. K. (2003). *Nursing care plans: Nursing diagnosis and intervention* (5th ed.). St Louis: Mosby.

Guyton, A. C., & Hall, J. E. (2000). *Textbook of medical physiology* (10th ed.). New York: Saunders.

Hunt, S. A., Baker, D.W., Chin, M. H., Cinquegrani, M. P., Feldman, A. M., Francis, G. S., et al. (2001). ACC/AHA guidelines for the evaluation and management of chronic heart failure in the adult: Executive summary: A report of the American College of Cardiology/American Heart Association Task Force on Practice Guidelines (Committee to revise the 1995 guidelines for the Evaluation and Management of Heart Failure). *Circulation, 104,* 2996–3007.

Jarvis, C. (2003). *Physical examination and health assessment* (4th ed.). Philadelphia: Saunders.

Johnson, M., Maas, M, & Moorhead, S. (Eds.). (2004). *Nursing outcomes classification (NOC)* (3rd ed.). St Louis: Mosby.

Kidd, P. S., & Wagner, K. D. (2001). *High acuity nursing* (3rd ed.). Upper Saddle River, NJ: Prentice Hall.

Lackner, T. E., Hamilton, G., Hill, J., Davey, C., & Guay, D. R. (2003). Pneumococcal polysaccharide revaccination: Immunoglobulin G seroconversion, persistence, and safety in frail, chronically ill older subjects. *Journal of the American Geriatric Society, 51*(2), 240–245.

Lehne, R. A. (2001). *Pharmacology for nursing care* (4th ed.). New York: Saunders.

Lewis, S. M., Heitkemper, M. M., & Dirksen, S. R. (2004). *Medical surgical nursing: Assessment and management of clinical problems.* St Louis: Mosby.

Lilley, L. L., & Aucker, R. S. (2001). *Pharmacology and the nursing process* (3rd ed.). St Louis: Mosby.

Lindell, K., & Reinke, L. (1999). *Nursing strategies for smoking cessation. ANA continuing education independent study module,* American Nurses Association.

Lipkus, I. M., McBride, C. M., Pollak, K. I., Schwartz-Bloom, R. D., Tilson, E., & Bloom, P. N. (2004). A randomized trial comparing the effects of self-help materials and proactive telephone counseling on teen smoking cessation. *Health Psychology, 23*(4), 397–406.

McCance, K. L., & Huether, S. E. (2002). *Pathophysiology: The biologic basis for disease in adults and children* (4th ed.). St Louis: Mosby.

Medela Medical Supply Company. (2005). Procedure for suctioning a tracheostomy tube: Clean technique. Retrieved from *http://www.tracheostomy.com/resources/pdf/TrachHandbk.pdf* on June 1, 2007.

Mulvihill, M. L., Zelman, M., Holdaway, P., Tompary, E., & Turchaney, J. (2001). *Human diseases: A systematic approach* (5th ed.). Upper Saddle River, NJ: Prentice Hall.

Murry, R. B., & Zentner, J. P. (2001). *Health promotion strategies through the life span* (7th ed.). Upper Saddle River, NJ: Prentice Hall.

NANDA International. (2005). *Nanda nursing diagnoses: Definitions and classifications 2005–2006.* Philadelphia: Author.

National Guidelines Clearinghouse. (2007). Retrieved at *http://www.guideline.gov/summary/summary.aspx?doc_id=6514&nbr=004083&string=tracheostomy* on June 7, 2007.

National Institute of Health Panel. (2001). Third report of the National Cholesterol Education Program (NCEP) Expert Panel on Detection, Evaluation, and Treatment of High Cholesterol in Adults (Adult Treatment Panel III). NIH Publication No. 01-3670. Bethesda, MD: National Institutes of Health.

Porth, C. M. (2002). *Pathophysiology: Concepts of altered states* (6th ed.). New York: Lippincott, Williams, and Wilkins.

Ramsay, J., & Hoffmann, A. (2004). Smoking cessation and relapse prevention among undergraduate students: A pilot demonstration project. *Journal of American College Health, 53*(1), 11–18.

Reiss, B. S., Evans, M. E., & Broyles, B. E. (2002). *Pharmacological aspects of nursing care* (6th ed.). Albany, NY: Delmar.

Scanlon, V. C., & Sanders, T. (2003). *Essentials of anatomy and physiology* (4th ed.). Philadelphia: F. A. Davis Company.

Sierpina, V. S. (2001). *Integrative health care: Complimentary and alternative therapies for the whole person.* Philadelphia: F. A. Davis Company.

Smith, S. F., Duell, D. J., & Martin, B. C. (2002). *Photo guide of nursing skills.* Upper Saddle River, NJ: Prentice Hall.

Tablan, O. C., Anderson, L. J., Besser, R., Bridges, C., Hajjeh. R. (2004). Guidelines for preventing health-care—associated pneumonia: Recommendations of CDC and the Healthcare Infection Control Practices Advisory Committee. *MMWR, 53*(3): 1–36. Retrieved at *http://www.cdc.gov/mmwr/preview/mmwrhtml/rr5303al.htm* on June 12, 2007.

Endorsers:

American College of Chest Physicians

American Health Care Association

Association for Professionals in Infection Control and Epidemiology, Inc.

Infectious Diseases Society of America

Society for Healthcare Epidemiology of America

Society of Critical Care Medicine

The Joanna Briggs Institute for Evidence-Based Nursing and Midwifery. (2000). Best Practice Information Sheet ISSN. Retrieved from *http://www.joannabriggs.edu.au/pdf/BPISEng_4_4.pdf* on May 28, 2007.

United States Department of Health and Human Services. (2000). *Healthy people 2010* (conference edition in two volumes). Washington, DC: U.S. Government Printing Office.

University of Kentucky. (2003). Home tracheostomy care: Patient education. Retrieved at *http://www.tracheostomy.com/resources/pdf/university_kentucky.pdf* on June 1, 2007.

University of North Carolina. (2005). Tracheostomy care without inner cannula. Retrieved at *https://www.unchealthcare.org/site/Nursing/nurspractice/procedures/procedures/proceduret4.pdf/* on May 28, 2007.

Wilson, S. F., & Giddens, J. F. (2001). *Health assessment and nursing practice* (2nd ed.). St Louis: Mosby.

Wong, D. L. (1999). *Whaley & Wong's nursing care of infants and children* (6th ed.). St Louis: Mosby.

Wong, D. L., Perry, S. E., & Hockenberry M. F. (2002). *Maternal-child nursing care* (2nd ed.). St Louis: Mosby.

CHAPTER 36

Ainsman, S. (2003, September 19). *Emergency clinical guide: ABGs.* Retrieved November 1, 2004, from *www.anisman.com/ecg/abg.htm*

American Association of Blood Banks (AABB). (2004). Facts about blood and blood banking. Retrieved November 8, 2004, from *www.aabb.org/All_About_Blood/FAQs/aabb_faqs.htm*

Centers for Disease Control and Prevention. (2002). Guidelines for the prevention of intravascular catheter-related infections. *Morbidity and Mortality Weekly Report, 51*(RR10), 1–32.

Horne, C., & Derrico, D. (1999). Mastering ABGs. *American Journal of Nursing, 99*, 26–33.

Infusion Nurse's Society. (2002). Policies and procedures for infusion nurses (2nd ed.) Infusion Nurses Society Clinical Practice Committee, Norwood. MA: Author.

Institute of Medicine (IOM). (2004). *Dietary reference intakes for electrolytes and water.* Washington, D.C.: National Academies Press.

Intravenous Nursing Society (INS). (2000). Intravenous nursing standards of practice. *Journal of Intravenous Nursing, 21,* S35–45, 72.

Josephson, D. (1999). *Intravenous infusion therapy for nurses: Principles and practice.* Albany, NY: Delmar Publishers.

Kee, J., & Paulanka, B. (1999). *Fluid and electrolytes with clinical applications* (6th ed.). Albany, NY: Delmar Publishers.

Macklin, D. (2003). Phlebitis. *American Journal of Nursing, 103*(2), 55–60.

NANDA International. (2005). *Nursing diagnoses: Definitions and classifications 2005–2006.* Philadelphia: Author.

National Institutes of Health (NIH). (1994). *NIH Consensus Development Conference: Statement on optimal calcium intake.* Washington, D.C.: Author.

Niesen, K. M., Harris, D. Y., Parkin, L. S., & Henn, L. T. (2003). The effects of heparin versus normal saline for maintenance of peripheral intravenous locks in pregnant women. *Journal of Obstetrics, Gynecology, & Neonatal Nursing, 32*(4), 503–508.

Phillips, L. D. (2005). *Manual of IV therapeutics* (4th ed.). Philadelphia: F. A. Davis Company.

Preston, R. A. (2002). *Acid-base, fluids, and electrolytes made ridiculously simple.* Miami: Medmaster.

Rosenthal, P. PICC line. Retrieved December 1, 2004, from: *http://health.discovery.com/diseasesandcond/encyclopedia/3017.html*

Rowlands, A. V., Ingledew, D. K., Powell, S. M., & Eston R. G. (2004). Interactive effects of habitual physical activity and calcium intake on bone density in boys and girls. *Journal of Applied Physiology, 97*(4), 1203–1208.

Saladin, K. *Anatomy and physiology: The unity of form and function* (2nd ed.). available: *www.mhhe.com/biosci/ap/saladin2e/student/olc/chap24studoutline.mhtml*

Scanlon, V. C., & Sanders, T. (2003). *Essentials of anatomy and physiology* (4th ed.). Philadelphia: F. A. Davis.

Schnell, Z., Van Leeuwen, A., & Kranpitz, T. (2003). *Davis's comprehensive handbook of laboratory and diagnostic tests with nursing implications.* Philadelphia: F. A. Davis Company.

Springhouse Corporation. (2000). *Nursing 2000 drug handbook.* Springhouse, PA: Author.

Transport across cell membranes. Retrieved December 1, 2004, from: *http://users.rcn.com/jkimball.ma.ultranet/BiologyPages/D/Diffusion.html*

U.S. Department of Health and Human Services. (2004). *Bone health and osteoporosis: A report of the surgeon general.* Rockville, MD: Author.

Venes, D. (2005). *Taber's cyclopedic medical dictionary* (20th ed.). Philadelphia: F. A. Davis Company.

Wong, F. (1999). A new approach to ABG interpretation. *American Journal of Nursing, 99*, 34–36.

CHAPTER 37

American Association of Nurse Anesthetists (AANA). (2003). Questions and answers: A career in nurse anesthesia. Retrieved July 23, 2004, from *www.aana.org*

Bernier, M. J., Sanares, D. C., Owen, S. V., & Newhouse, P. L. (2003). Preoperative teaching received and valued in a day surgery setting. *AORN Journal, 77*(3), 563–572, 575–578, 581–582.

Dale, A., Rothrock, J. C. & McEwen, D. R. (Eds.). (2003). *Alexander's care of the patient in surgery* (12th ed.). St Louis: Mosby.

DeFazio Quinn, D. M., & Schick, L. (2004). *Perianesthesia nursing core curriculum* (4th ed.). Philadelphia: Saunders.

Dochterman, J. M., & Bulechek, G. M. (Eds.). (2004). *Nursing interventions classification (NIC)* (4th ed.). St Louis: Mosby.

Fortunato, N. H. (Ed.). (2000). *Berry and Kohn's operating room technique* (9th ed.). St Louis: Mosby.

Gilmartin, J. (2004). Day surgery: Patients' perceptions of a nurse-led preadmission clinic. *Journal of Clinical Nursing, 13*(2), 243–250.

JCAHO sets patient safety goals for 2003. (2003). *Nursing Spectrum Metro Edition, 3*(8), 25MW.

Johnson, M., Maas, M., & Moorhead, S. (Eds.). (2004). *Nursing outcomes classification (NOC)* (3rd ed.). St Louis: Mosby.

Johnson, T. K., Holm, C. D., & Godshall, S. D. (2000). Next-generation strategies for physicians and hospitals. *Healthcare Financial Management, 54*(1), 48–51.

Lobb, L. (2003). *Standards, recommended practices, and guidelines: With official AORN statements.* Denver, CO: AORN.

McConnell, E. (2002). Applying antiembolism stockings. *Nursing 2002, 32*(4), 17.

T. E. D. antiembolism stockings, one pair large/regular. Retrieved July 16, 2004, from *www.costco.com/Browse/Product.aspx?Prodid=10044982&whse=&topnav=&cat=488.*

Zeckuhr, M. T. (1999). Nursing practice, nursing standards, nursing process. In K. Litwack (Ed.), *Core curriculum for perianesthesia nurse* (4th ed.), (pp. 9–19). Philadelphia: Saunders.

CHAPTER 38

American Nurses Association. (2002). *Position Statements: Registered nurse utilization of unlicensed assistive personnel.* Washington, D.C.: Author.

American Nurses Association. (2004). *ANA standards of nursing practice.* Washington, DC: Author.

Araujo Group. (n.d.). A compilation of opinions of experts in the field of the management of change. Unpublished report.

Arnold, E., & Boggs, K. (1995). *Interpersonal relationships* (2nd ed.). Philadelphia: Saunders.

Baldwin, F. D. (2002, March). Making do with less. *Healthcare Informatics,* 1–7.

Barker, A. M. (1992). *Transformational nursing leadership: A vision for the future.* New York: National League for Nursing Press.

Barraclough, R. A., & Stewart, R. A. (1992). Power and control: Social science perspectives. In V. P. Richmond & J. C. McCroskey (Eds.), *Power in the classroom: Communication, control and concern.* Hillsdale, NJ: Erlbaum.

Bass, B. M., & Avolio, B. J. (1993). Transformational leadership: A response to critique. In M. M. Chemers & R. Ayman (Eds.), *Leadership theory and research: Perspectives and directions.* San Diego: Academic Press.

Bennis, W., Spreitzer, G. M., & Cummings. (2001) *The future of leadership.* San Francisco: Jossey-Bass.

Bilchik, G. S. (2002, May). Are you the problem? *Hospitals & Health Networks Magazine,* 38–42.

Blais, K. B., Hayes, J. S., Kozier, B., & Erb, G. (2002). *Professional nursing practice: Concepts and perspectives* (4th ed.). Upper Saddle River, NJ: Prentice Hall.

Blake, R. R., Mouton, J. S., & Tapper, M. (1981). *Grid approaches for managerial leadership in nursing.* St Louis: Mosby.

Bos, C. S., & Vaughn, S. (1998). *Strategies for teaching students with learning and behavioral problems* (4th ed.). Boston: Allyn & Bacon.

Browne, M. M., & Kelley, S. M. (1994). *Asking the right questions: A guide to critical thinking.* Englewood Cliffs, NJ: Prentice Hall.

Carroll, L. (1865–1965). *Alice's adventures in wonderland.* New York: Airmont Books. (Original work published 1865.)

Chappel, E. D. (1970). *Culture and biological man: Exploration in behavioral anthropology*. New York: Holt, Rinehart, & Winston. (Reprinted as *The biological foundations of individuality and culture*. Huntingdon, NY: Robert Krieger, 1979.)

Dent, H. S. (1995). *Job shock: Four new principles transforming our work and business*. New York: St. Martin's Press.

Drath, W. (2001). *The deep blue sea*. San Francisco: Jossey-Bass.

Ellis, M. (1999). Self-assessment: Discovering yourself and making the best choices for you! *Black Collegian, 30*(1), 30, 3p, 1c.

Farrell, K., & Broude, C. (1987). *Winning the change game: How to implement information systems with fewer headaches and bigger paybacks*. Los Angeles: Breakthrough Enterprises.

First Consulting Group for the American Hospital Association. (2001). The healthcare workforce shortage and its implications for America's hospitals. Retrieved August 1, 2005, from *www.aha/org/aha/key_issues/workforce/resources/Content/FcgWorkforceReport.pdf*

Feldman, D. A. (2002). *Critical thinking: Strategies for decision making*. Menlo Park, CA: Crisp Publications.

Fitton, R. A. (1997). *Leadership: Quotations from the world's greatest motivators*. Boulder, CO: Westview Press.

Fontaine, K. L., & Fletcher, J. S. (2002). *Mental health nursing* (5th ed.). Redwood City, CA: Prentice Hall.

Fralic, M. F. (2000). What is leadership? *Journal of Nursing Administration, 30*(7/8), 340–341.

Gahar, A. (2000). Programming for college students with learning disabilities. (Grant No.: 84-078C) Retrieved February, 16, 2000, from *www.csbsju.edu*

Grossman, S., & Valiga, T. (2000). *The new leadership challenge*. Philadelphia: F. A. Davis Company.

Hansten, R., & Washburn, M. (1998). *Clinical delegation skills*. Boston: Jones & Bartleff.

Haslan, S. A. (2001). *Psychology in organizations*. Thousand Oaks, CA: Sage Publications.

Heifetz, R. A. & Linsky, M. (2002, June). A survival guide for leaders. *Harvard Business Review*, 65–74.

Heller, R. (1998). *Managing change*. New York: DK Publishing.

Holman, L. (1995). *Eleven lessons in self-leadership: Insights for personal and professional success*. Lexington, KY: A Lessons in Leadership Book.

Kotter, J. P. (1999). Leading change: The eight steps to transformation. In J. A. Conger, G. M. Spreitzer, & E. E. Lawler (Eds.), *The leader's change handbook*. San Francisco: Jossey-Bass.

Lansdale, B. M. (2002). *Cultivating inspired leaders*. West Hartford, CT: Kumarian Press.

Lapp, J. (2002, May). Thriving on change. *CARING Magazine*, 40–43.

Lee, J. A. (1980). *The gold and the garbage in management theories and prescriptions*. Athens, OH: Ohio University Press.

Lewin, K. (1951). *Field theory in social science: Selected theoretical papers*. New York: Harper & Row.

Lichiello, P., & Madden, C. W. (1996). Context and catalysts for change in health care markets. *Health Affairs, 15*(2), 121–129.

Locke, E. A. (1982). The ideas of Frederick Taylor: An evaluation. *Academy of Management Review, 7*(1), 14.

Lukes, S. (1986). *Power*. New York: New York University Press.

Maslow, A. H. (1970). *Motivation and personality*. New York: Harper & Row.

Matejka, J. K., & Dunsing, R. J. (1988). Time management: Changing some traditions. *Management World, 17*(2), 6–7.

McGregor, D. (1960). *The human side of enterprise*. New York: McGraw-Hill.

McNichol, E. (2000). How to be a model leader. *Nursing Standard, 14*(45), 24.

Mintzberg, H. (1989). *Mintzberg on management: Inside our strange world of organizations*. New York: Free Press.

Mondros, J. B., & Wilson, S. M. (1994). *Organizing for power and empowerment*. New York: Columbia University Press.

Moshovitz, R. (1993). *How to organize your work and your life*. New York: Doubleday.

Mulholland, J. (1991). *The language of negotiation: A handbook of practical strategies*. London: Rutledge.

National Council of State Boards of Nursing. (1995, December). Delegation: Concepts and decision-making process. *National Council position paper, 1995*. Retrieved August 1, 2005, from *www.ncsbn.org/resources/complimentary_ncsbn_Delegation.asp*

Navuluri, R. B. (2001). Our time management in patient care. *Research for Nursing Practice, 3*(1). Retrieved August 1, 2005, from *www.graduateresearch.com/NavuTime.htm*

Nelson, M. (2002, May 31). Educating for professional nursing practice: Looking backward into the future. *Online Journal of Issues in Nursing*. Retrieved May 27, 2002, from *www.nursingworld.org/ojin/topic18/tpc18_3.htm*

Parkman, C. A. (1996). Delegation: Are you doing it right? *American Journal of Nursing, 96*(2), 43–48.

Pavitt, C. (1999). Theorizing about the group communication-leadership relationship. In L. R. Frey, (Ed.), *The handbook of group communication theory and research*. Thousand Oaks, CA: Sage Publications.

Pratt, C. (1994). Successful job-search strategies for the 90's. In College Placement Council (Ed.), *Planning job choices* (pp. 15–18). Philadelphia: College Placement Council.

Ritter-Teitel, J. (2002). The impact of restructuring on professional nursing practice. *Journal of Nursing Administration, 32*(1), 31–41.

Sanon-Rollins, G. (2000). Surviving conflict on the job. In *Nursing Spectrum Career Fitness Guide*. Barrington, IL: Gannett.

Scheetz, L. J. (2000). *Nursing faculty secrets*. Philadelphia: Hanley & Belfus.

Shingleton, J. (1994). The job market for '94 grads. In *College Placement Council* (Ed.), *Planning job choices* (pp. 19–26). Philadelphia: College Placement Council.

Simonetti, J., & Ariss, S. (1999). Through the top with mentoring. *Business Horizons, 42*(6), 56–62.

Smialek, M. A. (2001). *Team strategies for success*. Lanham, MD: Scarecrow Press.

Smith, H. W. (1994). *The ten natural laws of successful time and life management: Proven strategies for increased productivity and inner peace*. New York: Warner Books.

Spradley, E., Johnson, A., Sochalski, J., Fritz, M., & Spencer, W. (2000). The registered nurse population, March 2000. Findings from the national sample survey of registered nurses. U.S. Department of Health and Human Services, Health Resources and Service Administration, Bureau of Health Professions Division of Nursing. Retrieved August 1, 2005, from *http://bhpr.hrsa.gov/healthworkforce/reports/rnsurvey/mss1.htm*

Spreitzer, G. M., & Quinn, R. E. (2001). *A company of leaders*. San Francisco: Jossey-Bass.

Tappen, R. M. (2001). *Nursing leadership and management: Concepts and practice* (4th ed.). Philadelphia: F. A. Davis Company.

Tappen, R., Weiss, S., & Whitehead, D. (2004). *Essentials of nursing leadership and management* (3rd ed.). Philadelphia: F. A. Davis Company.

Thomas, D. O. (1995). Speak up! We need good followers too. *Medical Economics, 58*(9), 72.

Thompson, L., & Fox, C. R. (2001). Negotiation within and between groups in organizations: Levels of analysis. In M. E. Turner (Ed.), *Groups at work* (pp. 221–266). Mahwah: Erlbaum.

Trinh, H. Q., & O'Connor, S. J. (2002). Helpful or harmful? The impact of strategic change on the performance of U.S. urban hospitals. *Health Services Research, 37*(1), 145–171.

Trofino, J. (1995). Transformational leadership in health care. *Nursing Management, 26*(8), 42–27.

Ulrich, D. L., & Glendon, K. J. (1999). *Interactive group learning: Strategies for nurse educators*. New York: Springer.

Upenieks, V. (2002). What constitutes successful nurse leadership? *Journal of Nursing Administration, 32*(12), 622–632.

Walsh, B. (1996, June 3). When past perfect isn't. *Forbes ASAP,* 18.

White, R. K., & Lippitt, R. (1960). *Autocracy and democracy: An experimental inquiry.* New York: Harper & Row.

CHAPTER 39

AJN Reports. (2003). Using technology to address medication errors. *American Journal of Nursing, 103*(4), 25.

American Nurses Association. (2004). *Scope and standards of nursing informatics practice.* ANA Pub. #NIP21. Washington, DC: American Nurses Publishing/American Nurses Foundation.

American Nurses Association. (2004). *Nursing: Scope and standards of practice.* Washington, DC: ANA/American Nurses Publishing/American Nurses Foundation.

Ammenwerth, E., Mansmann, U., Iller, C., & Eichstadter, R., (2003). Factors affecting and affected by user acceptance of computer-based nursing documentation: Results of a two-year study. *Journal of the American Medical Informatics Association, 10,* 69–84.

Bech, S. (1997). Evaluation criteria. *The Good, the Bad & The Ugly: or, Why It's a Good Idea to Evaluate Web Sources.* Retrieved March 3, 2003, from *http://lib.nmsu.edu/instruction/evalcrit.html*

Beyea, S. (2000, May). Standardized nursing vocabularies and the perioperative nursing data set: Making clinical practice count. *CIN Plus, 3*(2), 1,5,6.

Bonsor, K. (2002). How nanotechnology will work. Retrieved November 25, 2002, from *www.howstuffworks.com/nanotechnolgy1.htm*

Bradshaw, C., & Dale, C. (1999). Informed choice. *Nursing Management, 6*(3), 8–12.

Checklist to evaluating web sites. (2003). University Libraries, University of Maryland, College Park, MD. Retrieved March 3, 2003, from *www.lib.umd.edu/UES/webcheck.html*

eHealth Ethics Initiative. (2000). Retrieved March 25, 2003, from *www.ihealthcoalition.org/ethics/ehcode.html*

Five criteria for evaluating Web pages. (1998). Retrieved March 3, 2003, from *www.library.cornell.edu/okuref/webcrit.html*

Graves, J., & Corcoran, S. (1989). The study of nursing informatics. *Image: The Journal of Nursing Scholarship, 21*(4), 227–230.

Institute of Medicine. (2000). *To err is human: Building a safer health system.* Washington, DC: National Academy of Sciences.

Kapoun, J. (1998, July/August). Teaching undergrads WEB evaluation: A guide for library instruction. *C & RL News,* 522–523.

The Leapfrog Group. (2000). Patient safety. [Online]. Retrieved June 6, 2001, from *www.leapfroggroup.org/safety1.htm*

Krumsieg, K., & Baehr, M. (2000). *Foundations of learning* (3rd ed.). Corvallis, OR: Pacific Crest.

Low, D. K., & Belcher, J. V. R. (2002). Reporting medication errors through computerized medication administration. *CIN: Computers, Informatics, Nursing, 20*(5), 178–183.

Martin, E. M., Coyle, M. K., Warden, D. L., & Salazar, A. (2003). Telephonic nursing in traumatic brain injury. *American Journal of Nursing, 103*(10), 75–76, 78, 81.

Masys, D. R. (2002). Effects of current and future information technologies on the health care workforce. *Health Affairs, 21*(5), 33–41.

Nelson, R., & Joos, I. (1989, Fall). On language in nursing: From data to wisdom. *PLN Visions,* 6,7.

Pennell, M. M. (2001, May 10). Outpatient errors common in outpatient setting. [online]. Retrieved May 10, 2001, from *http://dailynews.yahoo.com/h/nm/20000510/hl/prescriptions_3.html*

Smith, A. G. (1997). Testing the surf: Criteria for evaluating Internet information resources. *The Public-Access Computer Systems Review, 8*(3). Retrieved March 3, 2003, from *http://info.lib.uh.edu/pr/v8/n3/smith8n3.html*

Spielberg, A. R. (2000). On call and online. *Yearbook of Medical Informatics 2000,* 147–153.

Stevens, K. R. (2001, June). Incorporating evidence based practice into nursing practice. Retrieved July 26, 2004, from *http://www.stti.iupui.edu/lobrary/ojksn/e_iebpnp.html*

University of California–Berkeley. (2002). Evaluating Web pages: Techniques to apply and questions to ask. In *Finding information on the Internet: A tutorial.* Retrieved March 3, 2003, from *www.lib.berkeley.edu/TeachingLib/Guides/Internet/Evaluate.html*

U.S. Department of Health and Human Services. (2001). Standards for privacy of individually identifiable health information. [45 CFR Parts 160 and 164]. Retrieved March 25, 2003, from *www.hhs.gov/ocr/hipaa/*

Watzlaf, V. J. (2002). The impact of clinical terminologies and structured vocabularies. *Proceedings of the Healthcare Information and Management Systems Society, 89,* 1–12.

Weinstein, A. (2001, May). The bandwagon is outside waiting. *Health Management Technology.* [online]. Retrieved May 4, 2001, from *www.healthmgttech.com/cgi-bin/arttop.asp?Page=hopo1bandwagon.htm*

CHAPTER 40

American Heart Association. (2004). Questions and answers about chelation therapy. Retrieved August 27, 2004, from *www.americanheart.org/presenter.jhtml?identifier=3000843*

Astin, J. A. (1998). Why patients use alternative medicine: Results of a national study. *Journal of the American Medical Association, 279*(19): 1548–1553.

Astin, J. A., Shapiro, S. L., Eisenberg, D. M., & Forys, K. L. (2003). Mind-body medicine: State of the science, implications for practice. *Journal of the American Board of Family Practice, 16*(2), 131–147.

Barrett, B., Marchand, L., Scheder, J., Appelbaum, D., Plane, M. B., Blustein, J., et al. (2004). What complementary and alternative medicine practitioners say about health and health care. *Annals of Family Medicine, 2*(3), 253–259.

Bendit, L. J., & Bendit, P. D. (1977). *The etheric body of man: The bridge of consciousness.* Wheaton, IL: Quest.

Bohm, D. (1980). *Wholeness and the implicate order.* New York: Routledge.

Bright, M. A. (2002). *Holistic health and healing.* Philadelphia: F. A. Davis Company.

Buckle, J. (2002). Clinical aromatherapy: Therapeutic uses for essential oils. *Advances in Nursing Practice, 10*(5), 67–68, 88.

Burkhardt, M. A. (1998). Reintegrating spirituality into health care. *Alternative Therapies in Health and Medicine, 4*(2), 127–128.

Burton Goldberg Group. (1994). *Alternative medicine: The definitive guide.* Puyallup, WA: Future Medicine Publishing Co.

Carson, R. (1994). *Silent spring.* Boston: Houghton Mifflin.

Cousins, N. (1979). *Anatomy of an illness.* New York: Bantam.

Cassidy, C. M. (1994). Unraveling the ball of string: Reality, paradigms, and the study of alternative medicine. *Advances: The Journal of Mind-Body Health, 10*(6), 58–92.

Dochterman, J. M., & Bulechek, G. M. (Eds.). (2004). *Nursing interventions classification (NIC)* (4th ed.). St Louis: Mosby.

Dossey, B. M., Keegan, L., & Guzetta, C. E. (Eds.). (2000). *Holistic nursing: A handbook for practice* (3rd ed.). Gaithersburg, MD: Aspen.

Eisenberg, D. M., Davis, R. B., Ettner, S. L., Appel, S., Wilkey, S., Van Rompay, M., et al. (1998). Trends in alternative medicine use in the United States, 1990–1997: Results of a follow-up national survey. *Journal of the American Medical Association, 280*(18), 1569–1575.

Eisenberg, D. M., Kessler, R. C., Foster, C., Norlock, F. E., Calkins, D. R., & Delbanco, T. L. (1993). Unconventional medicine in the United States: Prevalence, costs, and patterns of use. *The New England Journal of Medicine, 328*(4), 246–252.

Ernst, R. (2000). Chelation therapy for coronary heart disease: An overview of all clinical investigations. *American Heart Journal, 140*(1), 139–141.

Fontaine, K. (2000). *Absolute beginner's guide to alternative medicine.* Calumet, IL: Que Publishing.

German Federal Institute for Drugs and Medical Devices. (1998). *Complete German Commission E monographs: The therapeutic guide to herbal medicines.* Boston: Integrative Medical Communications.

Goldberg, B., Anderson, J. W., & Trivieri, L. (2002). *Alternative medicine: The definitive guide* (2nd ed.). Berkeley: Ten Speed Press.

Johnson, P. (2002). The use of humor and its influences on spirituality and coping in breast cancer survivors. *Oncology Nursing Forum, 29*(4), 691–695.

Kabat-Zinn, J. (1994). *Wherever you go, you are there: Mindfulness meditation in everyday life.* New York: Hyperion.

Kreiger, D. (1993). *Accepting your power to heal: The personal practice of therapeutic touch.* Santa Fe: Bear & Company.

Levine, S. (1984). *Healing into life and death.* New York: Doubleday.

Macy, J., & Young, M. Y. (1998). *Coming back to life: Practices to reconnect ourselves, our world.* Stony Creek, CT: New Society.

McCaffrey, A. M., Eisenberg, D. M., Legedza, A. T., Davis, R. B., & Phillips, R. S. (2004). Prayer for health concerns: Results of a national survey on prevalence and patterns of use. *Archives of Internal Medicine, 164*(8), 858–862.

Moorhead, S., Johnson, M., & Maas, M. (2004). *Nursing outcomes classification (NOC)* (3rd ed.). St Louis: Mosby.

NANDA International. (2005). *Nursing diagnoses: Definitions and classification 2005–2006.* Philadelphia: Author.

National Center for Complementary and Alternative Medicine. (2002). Get the facts: 10 things to know about evaluating medical resources on the web. Retrieved September 9, 2004, from *http://nccam.nih.gov/health/webresources/*

National Center for Complementary and Alternative Medicine. (2004). Understanding complementary and alternative medicine. Retrieved August 18, 2004, from *http://nccam.nih.gov/news/images/campractice.htm*

National Institutes of Health. (1997). *National institutes of health consensus development statement on acupuncture, revised draft, November 5, 1997.* Washington, DC: Author.

Perry, R., & Dowrick, C. F. (2000). Complementary medicine and general practice: An urban perspective. *Complementary Therapies & Medicine, 8*(2), 71–75.

Phipps, S. (2002). Reduction of distress associated with paediatric bone marrow transplant: Complementary health promotion interventions. *Pediatric Rehabilitation, 5*(4), 223–234.

Ratterman, R., Secrest, J., Norwood, B., & Ch'ien, A. P. (2002). Magnet therapy: What's the attraction? *Journal of the American Academy of Nurse Practitioners, 14*(8), 347–353.

Richardson, J. (2004). What patients expect from complementary therapy: A qualitative study. *American Journal of Public Health, 94*(6), 1049–1053.

Steinberg, E. M. (2002). *The balance within: The science of connecting health and emotions.* New York: Freeman.

Wolsko, P. M., Eisenberg, D. M., Davis, R. B., & Phillips, R. S. (2004). Use of mind-body medical therapies. *Journal of General Internal Medicine, 19*(1), 43–50.

Wolsko, P. M., Eisenberg, D. M., Simon, L. S., Davis, R. B., Walleczek, J., Mayo-Smith, M., et al. (2004). Double-blind placebo-controlled trial of static magnets for the treatment of osteoarthritis of the knee: Results of a pilot study. *Alternative Therapies in Health & Medicine, 10*(2), 36–43.

CHAPTER 41

Abbott, A. (2002). Health care challenges created by substance abuse: The whole is definitely bigger than the sum of its parts. *Health & Social Work, 27*(3), 162–165.

American Cancer Society. (2002). Cancer prevention and early detection. Retrieved February 25, 2003, from *www.cancer.org*

American College of Sports Medicine (ACSM). (2000). *ACSM'S guidelines for exercise testing and prescription* (6th ed.). New York: Lippincott Williams & Wilkins.

American Heart Association. (n.d.). How do I know if I have high blood pressure? Retrieved March 11, 2003, from *www.americanheart.org*

Bartone, P., Ursano, R., Wright, K., & Ingraham, L. (1989). The impact of a military air disaster on the health of assistance workers. *Journal of Nervous and Mental Disease, 177,* 317–328.

Brosse, A., Sheets, E., Lett, H., & Blumenthal, J. (2002). Exercise and the treatment of clinical depression in adults: Recent findings and future directions. *Sports Medicine, 32*(12), 741–760.

Brown, K., Weaver, M., Artz, L., & Hilyer, J. (1999). Health promotion and disease prevention at the work site. In J. M. Raczynski & R. J. DiClemente (Eds.), *Handbook of health promotion and disease prevention* (pp. 459–474). New York: Kluwer Academic/Plenum Publishers.

Cassidy, T. (2000). Stress, healthiness and health behaviours: An exploration of the role of life events, daily hassles, cognitive appraisal and the coping process. *Counseling Psychology Quarterly, 13*(3), 293–311.

Centers for Disease Control and Prevention (CDC). (2002, April 12) Annual smoking-attributable mortality, years of potential life lost, and economic costs—United States, 1995–1999. *Morbidity and Mortality Weekly Report, 51*(14), 300–303.

Centers for Disease Control and Prevention (CDC). (2003, March 14). *National Vital Statistics Reports, 51*(5). Retrieved March 27, 2003, from *www.cdc.gov*

Centers for Disease Control and Prevention (CDC). Leading causes of death. *National Vital Statistics Reports, 50*(16). Retrieved February 25, 2003, from *www.cdc.gov*

Davis, K., Cokkinides, V., Weinstock, M., O'Connell, M., & Wingo, P. (2002). Summer sunburn and sun exposure among U.S. youths ages 11 to 18: National prevalence and associated factors. *Pediatrics, 110*(1), 27–35.

DiClemente, R., & Cobb, B. (1999). Adolescent health promotion and disease prevention. In J. M. Raczynski & R. J. DiClemente (Eds.), *Handbook of health promotion and disease prevention* (pp. 491–520). New York: Kluwer Academic/Plenum Publishers.

Engle, M., & Kratt, P. (1999). Health promotion in health care settings. In J. M. Raczynski & R. J. DiClemente (Eds.) *Handbook of health promotion and disease prevention* (pp. 443–457). New York: Kluwer Academic/Plenum Publishers.

Erikson, E. (1963). *Childhood and society* (2nd ed.). New York: Norton.

Gilliland, M. J., & Taylor, J. (1999). Planning community health interventions. In J. M. Raczynski & R. J. DiClemente (Eds.), *Handbook of health promotion and disease prevention* (pp. 427–441). New York: Kluwer Academic/Plenum Publishers.

Green, B., & Taplin, S. (2003). Breast cancer screening controversies. *Journal of the American Board of Family Practice, 16*(3), 233–241.

Haber, D. (2002). Wellness general of the United States: A creative approach to promote family and community health. *Family Community Health, 25*(3), 71–82.

Hackshaw, A., & Paul, E. (2003). Breast self-examination and death from breast cancer: A meta-analysis. *British Journal of Cancer, 88*(7), 1047–1053.

Halls, C., & Rhodes, J. (2002, September). Employee wellness and beyond at Appleton Papers Inc. *Athletic Therapy Today,* 46–47.

Harris, R., & Lohr, K. (2002). Screening for prostate cancer: An update of the evidence for the U.S. Preventive Services Task Force. *Annals of Internal Medicine, 137,* 917–929.

Hermon, D., & Hazler, R. (1999). Adherence to a wellness model and perceptions of psychological well-being. *Journal of Counseling & Development, 77,* 339–343.

Hettler, W. (1984). Wellness: Encouraging a lifetime pursuit of excellence. *Health Values: Achieving High Level Wellness, 8,* 13–17.

Hooper, L., Summerbell, C., Higgins, J., Thompson, R., Capps, N., Smith, G., et al. (2001). Dietary fat intake and prevention of cardiovascular disease: Systematic review. *British Medical Journal, 332*(31), 757–763.

James, S., Ashwill, J., & Droske, S. (2002). *Nursing care of children: Principles and practice.* Philadelphia: Saunders.

Kobasa, S. (1979). Stressful life events, personality, and health: An inquiry into hardiness. *Journal of Personality and Social Psychology, 37*(1), 1–11.

Kocakulah, M. C., & Joseforsky, H. (2002). Wellness programs: A remedy for reducing healthcare costs. *Hospital Topics, 80*(2), 26–31.

Kodali, V., Kodavanti, M., Tripuraribhatla, P., Ram, T., Eswaran, P., & Krishnaswamy, K. (1999). Dietary factors as determinants of hypertension: A case control study in an urban Indian population. *Asia Pacific Journal of Clinical Nutrition, 8*(3), 184–189.

Kosaka, M. (1996). Relationship between hardiness and psychological stress response. *Journal of Performance Studies, 3,* 35–40.

Kösters, J., & Gøtzsche, P. (2003). Regular self-examination or clinical examination for early detection of breast cancer. *Cochrane Database Systems Review, 2,* CD003373.

Lazarus, R. S. (1966). *Psychological stress and the coping process.* New York: McGraw-Hill.

Leavell, H., & Clark, E. (1965). *Preventive medicine for doctors in the community.* New York: McGraw-Hill.

Lu, W., Resnick, H., Jablonski, K., Jones, K., Jain, A., Howard, J., et al. (2003). Non-HDL cholesterol as a predictor of cardiovascular disease in type 2 diabetes: The strong heart study. *Diabetes Care, 26*(1), 16–24.

Manson, J., Greenland, P., LaCroix, A., Stefanick, M., Mouton, C. Oberman, A., et al. (2002). Walking compared with vigorous exercise for the prevention of cardiovascular events in women. *New England Journal of Medicine, 347,* 716–725.

McGinnis, J. M. (1992). The public health burden of a sedentary lifestyle. *Medicine, Science, Sports, and Exercise, 24*(6 Suppl), S196–200.

McGinnis, J. M. (2003). A vision for health in our new century. *American Journal of Health Promotion, 18*(2), 146–150.

McGinnis, J. M., & Foege, W. H. (1994). Actual causes of death in the United States. *Journal of the American Medical Association, 270,* 2207–2211.

Miller, W. (2001). Effective diet and exercise treatments for overweight and recommendations for intervention. *Sports Medicine, 31*(10), 717–724.

Murray, S., McKinney, E., & Gorrie, T. (2002). *Foundations of maternal-newborn nursing* (3rd ed.). New York: Saunders.

Myers, J., Sweeney, T., & Witmer, J. (2000). The wheel of wellness counseling for wellness: A holistic model for treatment planning. *Journal of Counseling & Development, 78*(3), 251–267.

NANDA International. (2005). *Nursing diagnosis: Definitions and classifications 2005-2006.* Philidelphia: Author.

National Institutes of Health. (2001, May). Third report of the National Cholesterol Education Program (NCEP) expert panel on detection, evaluation, and treatment of high blood cholesterol in adults (adult treatment panel III). NIH publication No. 01–3670. Washington, DC: Author.

National Safety Council. (2001). Preventing slips and falls in the home. Retrieved March 1, 2003, from *www.nsc.org/library/facts/eldfalls*

Neuman, B. (1995). *The Neuman systems model* (3rd ed.). Stamford, CT: Appleton & Lange.

Paul, L., & Weinert, C. (1999). Wellness profile of midlife women with a chronic illness. *Public Health Nursing, 16*(5), 341–350.

Pender, N., Murdaugh, C., & Parsons, M. (2002). *Health promotion in nursing practice* (4th ed.). Upper Saddle River, NJ: Prentice Hall.

Platen, P. (2001). The importance of sport and physical exercise in the prevention and therapy of osteoporosis. [Electronic version]. *European Journal of Sport Science, 1*(3).

Prochaska, J., & DiClemente, C. (1982). Transtheoretical therapy: Toward a more integrative model of change. *Psychotherapy: Theory, Research and Practice, 19*(3), 276–288.

Rahe, R. (1974). Life change and subsequent illness reports. In E. K. Gunderson & R. H. Rahe (Eds.), *Life stress and illness.* Springfield, IL: Thomas Books.

Reynolds, K., Pass, M., Galvin, M., Winnail, S., Harrington, K., & Diclemente, R. (1999). Schools as a setting for health promotion and disease prevention. In J. M. Raczynski & R. J. DiClemente (Eds.), *Handbook of health promotion and disease prevention.* New York: Kluwer Academic/Plenum Publishers.

Rowe, M. (1999). Teaching health-care providers coping: Results of a two-year study. *Journal of Behavioral Medicine, 22*(5), 511–527.

Ruiz, R., & Fullerton, J. (1999). The measurement of stress in pregnancy. *Nursing and Health Sciences, 1,* 19–25.

Selye, H. (1976). *The stress of life.* New York: McGraw-Hill.

Soinio, M., Laakso, M., Lehto, S., Hakala, P., & Ronnemaa, T. (2003). Dietary fat predicts coronary heart disease events in subjects with type 2 diabetes. *Diabetes Care, 26*(3), 619–624.

Spector, R. (2000). *Cultural diversity in health and illness* (5th ed.). Upper Saddle River, NJ: Prentice Hall.

Task Force on Community Preventive Services. (2002). Recommendations to increase physical activity in communities. *American Journal of Preventive Medicine, 22*(4S), 67–72. Retrieved November 16, 2004, from *http://222.thecommunityguide.org/home_f.html*

Thomas, D., Gao, D., Ray, R., Wang, W., Allison, C., Chen, F., et al. (2002). Randomized trial of breast self-examination in Shanghai: Final results. *Journal of the National Cancer Institute, 94*(19), 1445–1457.

United States Department of Agriculture. (n.d.). *Home and garden bulletin, number 252.* Washington, DC: Author.

U.S. Department of Health and Human Services. (2000). *Healthy people 2010: Understanding and improving health* (2nd ed.). Washington, DC: U.S. Government Printing Office.

U.S. Department of Health and Human Services, Office of the Assistant Secretary for Planning and Evaluation. (2002, June 20). Physical activity fundamental to preventing disease. Retrieved March 14, 2003, from *www.cdc.gov*

Vallee, M., Maccari, S., Dellu, F., Simon, H., Le Moal, M., & Mayo, W. (1999). Long-term effects of prenatal stress and postnatal handling on age-related glucocorticoid secretion and cognitive performance: A longitudinal study in the rat. *European Journal of Neuroscience, 11,* 2906–2916.

Walker, S., Sechrist, K., & Pender, N. (1987). The health-promoting lifestyle profile: Development and psychometric characteristics. *Nursing Research, 36*(2), 76–81.

Wallston, K. A., Wallston, B. S., & DeVellis, R. (1978). Development of the multidimensional health locus of control (MHLC) scales. *Health Education Monographs, 6,* 160–170. (MHLC scales available at Vanderbilt University, Multidimensional health locus of control scales. Retrieved November 17, 2004, from *www.vanderbilt.edu/nursing/kwallston/mhlcscales.htm.* Last modified on December 2, 2003.)

Wasylkiw, L., & Fekken, C. (1999). The dimensionality of health behaviors. *Journal of Social Behavior and Personality, 14*(3), 585–596.

Watson, J. (1979). *Nursing: The philosophy and science of caring.* Boston: Little, Brown and Company.

Weiss, N. S. (2003). Breast cancer mortality in relation to clinical breast examination and breast self-examination. *Breast Journal, 9* Suppl. 2, S86–89.

Witmer, J., & Sweeney, T. (1992). A holistic model for wellness and prevention over the life span. *Journal of Counseling & Development, 71,* 140–148.

World Health Organization (WHO). 1948. Preamble to the constitution of the World Health Organization as adopted by the International Health Conference, New York, 19–22 June, 1946;

signed on 22 July 1946 by the representatives of 61 states (Official Records of the World Health Organization, no. 2, p. 100) and entered into force on 7 April 1948.

World Health Organization (WHO). 1986. Ottawa charter for health promotion. First International Conference on Health Promotion, Ottawa, 21 November 1986. Retrieved March 5, 2003, from *www.who.int/hpr/archive/docs/ottawa*

CHAPTER 42

American Nurses Association (ANA). (1986). *Standards of community health nursing practice.* Washington, DC: American Nurse Publishers.

American Nurses Association (ANA). (2001a). *Nursing bill of rights.* Washington, DC: American Nurse Publishers.

American Nurses Association (ANA). (2001b). *Revised code of ethics of the American Nurses Association.* Washington, DC: American Nurse Publishers.

Beech, B. M., Myers, L., & Beech, D. (2002). Hepatitis B and C infections among homeless adolescents. *Family Community Health, 25*(2), 28–36.

Bodenheimer, T. S., & Grumbach, K. (2005). *Understanding health policy: A clinical approach* (4th ed.). New York: Lange Medical Books/McGraw-Hill Publishing.

Bowles, K. H. (2000). Application of the Omaha system in acute care. *Research in Nursing, 23,* 93–105.

Broadway, R. L. (2002, July). Anthrax threat intensifies focus on disaster preparedness. *Healthcare Financial Management,* 28–31.

Chasey, D. (1999, Winter). Body and soul. *Minority Nursing,* 12–16.

Dossey, B. (1999). An interview with Barbara Dossey and holistic nursing. *Creative Nursing, 5*(3), 7–10.

Gaylord, N. (2002). A community and nursing partnership to meet Healthy People 2010 goals. *Pediatric Nursing, 28*(1), 54–56.

Greene, J. (2002, October). JCAHO's approach to disaster. *Material Management in Health Care,* 14–15.

Martin, K. S., & Norris, J. (1996). The Omaha system: A model for describing practice. *Holistic Nursing Practice, 11*(1), 75–83.

Hemstrom, M., Ambrose, M., Donahue, G., Glick, L., Lai., H. L., Preechawong, S. (2002). The clinical specialist in community health nursing: A solution for the 21st century. *Public Health Nursing, 17*(5), 386–391.

Herdman, E. (2001). The illusion of progress in nursing. *Nursing Philosophy, 2,* 4–13.

Hiemstra, R. (2000). The educative community defined. [Available online.] Retrieved December 23, 2002, from *www.learnativity.com/community.html#def*

Larsson, L. S., & Butterfield, P. (2002). Mapping the future of environmental health and nursing: Strategies for integrating national competencies into nursing practice. *Public Health Nursing, 19*(9), 301–308.

Martin, K. S. (1999). The Omaha system: Past, present and future. *Online Journal of Nursing Informatics, 3*(1). [Available online.] Retrieved September 26, 2002, from *www.cac.psu.edu/~dxm12/art1v3n1art.html*

Martin, K., S., & Scheet, N. J. (1992). *The Omaha system: Applications for community health nursing.* Philadelphia: Saunders. Retrieved March 7, 2003, from *www.omahasystem.org/shminter.htm*

Martin, K., & Scheet, N. (1995). The Omaha system: Nursing diagnoses interventions and outcomes. In N. Lang (Ed.), *Nursing data systems: The emerging framework.* Washington, DC: American Nurses Association Publishing.

Maslow, A. H. (1970). *Motivation and personality* (2nd ed.). New York: Harper and Row.

McClelland, G. M., Teplin, L. A., Abram, K. M., & Jacobs. N. (2002). HIV and AIDS risk behaviors among female jail detainees: Implications for public health policy. *American Journal of Public Health, 92*(5), 818–825.

Mistral, W., & Hollingworth, M. (2001). The supervised methadone and resettlement team nurse: An effective approach with opi-ate-dependent, homeless people. *International Nursing Review, 48,* 122–128.

Nightingale, F. (1860/1969). *Notes on nursing: What it is, and what it is not.* New York: Dover Publications.

Pope, A. M., Snyder, M. A., & Mood, L. H. (Eds.). (1995). *Nursing, health and environment.* Washington, DC: Institute of Medicine, National Academy Press.

Pryor, E. (1987). *Clara Barton: Professional angel.* Philadelphia: University of Pennsylvania Press.

Rowan, J. (1999). Ascent and descent in Maslow's theory. *Journal of Humanistic Psychology, 39*(3), 125–133.

Siegel, B. (1983). *Lillian Wald of Henry Street.* New York: Macmillan.

Substance Abuse and Mental Health Services Administration. (1999). *Mental health: A report of the surgeon general.* Rockville, MD: U.S. Department of Health and Human Services, National Institutes of Health.

U.S. Bureau of the Census. (2002). United States census 2000 facts. [Available online.] Retrieved January 3, 2003, from *www.census .gov*

U.S Department of Health and Human Services. (1999a). Achievements in public health, 1900–1999: Family planning. *Morbidity and Mortality Weekly Report, 48*(47), 1073–1080.

U.S. Department of Health and Human Services. (1999b). Ten great public health achievements—United States, 1900–1999. *Morbidity and Mortality Weekly Report, 48*(50), 1141–1146.

U.S. Department of Health and Human Services. (2002). Healthy People 2010 fact sheet. [Available online.] Retrieved January 4, 2003, from *www.healthypeople.gov/About/hpfact.htm*

Valanis, B. (1999). *Epidemiology in health care* (3rd ed.). Stamford, CT: Appleton & Lange.

CHAPTER 43

Alcock, D., Angus, D., Diem, E., Gallagher, E., & Medves, J. (2002). Home care or long-term care facility: Factors that influence the decision. *Home Health Care Services Quarterly, 21*(2), 35–48.

American Nurses Association. (1999). *Scope and standards of home health nursing practice.* Washington, DC: Author.

Ayers, M., Bruno, A., & Langford, R. W. (1999). *Community-based nursing care: Making the transition.* St Louis: Mosby.

Bonner, C., & Boyd, B. (1997). Managed care: Threat or opportunity for home health? *Online Journal of Issues in Nursing.* Retrieved December 16, 2002, from *www.nursingworld.org/ojin/tpc2/tpc2_5.htm*

Collopy, B., Dubler, N., & Zuckerman, C. (1990). The ethics of home care: Autonomy and accommodation. *Hastings Center Report, 20*(2), S1–16.

Dochterman, J. M., & Bulechek, G. M. (Eds). (2004). *Nursing interventions classification (NIC)* (4th ed.). St Louis: Mosby.

Goodman, C., Woolley, R., & Knight, D. (2003). District nurses' experiences of providing care in residential care home settings. *Journal of Clinical Nursing, 12*(1), 67–76.

Gill, T. M., Baker, D. I., Gottschalk, M., Peduzzi, P. N., Allore, H., & Byers, A. (2002). A program to prevent functional decline in physically frail, elderly persons who live at home. *New England Journal of Medicine, 347*(14), 1068–1074.

Handy, J., Quinn, J., Ryan, M. A., & Weiner, J. (2000). Predictions: Long term care in the decade. *Caring 19*(6), 16–18.

Head, B., Maas, M., & Johnson, M. (1997). Outcomes for home and community nursing in integrated delivery systems. *Caring 16*(1), 50–56.

Humphrey, C. J. (1998). *Home care nursing handbook* (3rd ed.). Gaithersburg, MD: Aspen Publications.

Lee, T., & Mills, M. E. (2000). Analysis of patient profile in predicting home care resource utilization and outcomes. *Journal of Nursing Administration, 30*(2), 67–75.

Madigan, E. A. (2002). The scientific dimensions of OASIS for home care outcome measurement. *Home Healthcare Nurse, 20*(9), 579–583.

Madigan, E. A., Tullai-McGuinness, S., & Neff, D. F. (2002). Home health services research. *Annual Review of Nursing Research, 20*, 267–291.

Moorhead, S., Johnson, M., & Maas, M. (Eds.). (2004). *Nursing outcomes classification (NOC)* (3rd ed.). St Louis: Mosby.

National Association for Home Care (NAHC). (1996). What is home care? Retrieved December 17, 2002, from *www.nahc.org/Consumer/wihc.html*

National Association for Home Care (NAHC). (2001). Basic statistics about home care. Retrieved February 23, 2004, from *www.nahc.org/Consumer/hcstats.html*

Navarra, T., & Ferrer, M. (1997). *An insider's guide to home health care*. Thorofare, NJ: Slack.

Keepnews, D. (1999). Home health payments—Turbulent times. *Nursing Trends & Issues, 4*(9).

Russo, H. E. (2000). Home care in the 21st century. *Caring, 19*(11), 44–45.

Saba, V. K. (1995). Home Health Care Classifications (HHCCs): Nursing diagnoses and nursing interventions. In *An emerging framework: Data system advances for clinical nursing practice*. ANA Publication No. NP-94. Washington, DC: American Nurses Association. Retrieved December 10, 2002, *www.sabacare.com/nursinginterventions.html*

Saba, V. K. (1992a). The classification of home health care nursing diagnoses and interventions. *Caring, 10*(3), 50–57.

Saba, V. K. (1992b). Home health care classification. *Caring, 10*(5), 58–60.

Saba, V. (2002). Nursing classifications: Home health care classification system (HHCC): An overview. *Online Journal of Issues in Nursing*. Retrieved December 10, 2002, from *http://nursingworld.org/ojin/tpc7/tpc7_7htm*

Stackhouse, J. C. (1998). *Into the community: Nursing in ambulatory and home care*. Philadelphia: Lippincott.

Shaughnessy, P. W., Crisler, K., & Schlenker, R. E. (1997). Medicare's OASIS: Standardized outcome and assessment information set for home health care—OASIS-B. National Association for Home Care report.

Sullivan, C. (2000). Canadian study shows promising results on home care cost-effectiveness. *Caring 19*(6), 42–45.

Todero, C. M., LaFramboise, L. M., & Zimmerman, L. M. (2002). Symptom status and quality-of-life outcomes of home-based disease management program for heart failure patients. *Outcomes Management, 6*(4), 161–168.

Warrington, D., Cholowski, K., & Peters, D. (2003). Effectiveness of home-based cardiac rehabilitation for special needs patients. *Journal of Advanced Nursing, 41*(2), 121–129.

Yehle, K. T., & Baird, C. L. (2002). Going home: Introducing adult nursing students to community care. *Nurse Educator, 27*(5), 210–211.

CHAPTER 44

Ahern, K., & McDonald, S. (2002). The beliefs of nurses who were involved in a whistleblowing event. *Journal of Advanced Nursing, 38*(3), 303–309.

Aiken, T. D. (2003). *Legal, ethical and political issues in nursing* (2nd ed). Philadelphia: F. A. Davis Company.

Altun, I. (2002). Burnout and nurses' personal and professional values. *Nursing Ethics, 9*(3), 269–278.

American Colleges of Nursing Association. (1998). *The essentials of baccalaureate education for professional nursing practice*. Washington, DC: Author.

American Hospital Association. (2004). *Patient care partnership*. Retrieved September 5, 2005, from *www.aha.org/aha/ptcommunication/partnership/index.html*

American Nurses Association (ANA). (1988a). *Ethics in nursing: Position statements and guidelines*. Kansas City, MO: Author.

American Nurses Association (ANA). (1988b). *Nursing and the human immunodeficiency virus: A guide for nursing's response to AIDS*. Kansas City, MO: Author.

American Nurses Association (ANA). (1992). *Position statement: Nursing care and do-not-resuscitate decisions*. Retrieved September 12, 2003, from *www.nursingworld.org/readroom/position/ethics/etdnr.htm*

American Nurses Association (ANA). (1995). American Nurses Association: Position statement on assisted suicide. *Health Care Law Ethics, 10*(1–2), 125–127.

American Nurses Association (ANA). Miscellaneous (1998, March/April). ANA supports rights of HIV positive. Retrieved March 26, 2004, from *http://nursingworld.org/tan/98marapr/miscell.htm*

American Nurses Association (ANA). (2001). *Code of ethics for nurses with interpretive statements*. Washington, DC: American Nurses Publishing. Retrieved September 10, 2005, from *www.nursingworld.org/ethics/chcode.htm*

American Nurses Association (ANA). (2004). *Nursing: Scope and standards of practice* (3rd ed.). Washington, DC: Author.

Aroskar, M., Gadow, S., Neuman, E., & Giovinco, G. (1979, April). ANS open forum: The most pressing ethical problems faced by nurses in practice. *Advances in Nursing Science*, 89–99.

Atlantic Information Services. (2002). Nurse interaction with family, friends requires different approach under HIPPA. Retrieved March 15, 2003, from *www.AISHealth.com*

Austin, W. Nursing ethics in an era of globalization. *Advances in Nursing Science, 24*(2), 1–18.

Bandman, E., & Bandman, B. (2002). *Nursing ethics through the life span* (4th ed.). Upper Saddle River, NJ: Prentice Hall.

Barr, P. (1992). The unknown fear—moral distress. *Nebraska Nurse, 15*(1), 13–14.

Bayles, M. (1984). *Reproductive ethics*. Englewood Cliffs, NJ: Prentice-Hall.

Beauchamp, T. L., & Childress, J. F. (2001). *Principles of biomedical ethics*. New York: Oxford University Press.

Becker, P. T., & Grunwald, P. C. (2000). Contextual dynamics of ethical decision making in NICU. *Journal of Perinatal and Neonatal Nursing, 14*(2), 58–73.

Beckwith, F. J., & Peppin, J. F. (2000). Physician value neutrality: A critique. *Journal of Law, Medicine, and Ethics, 28*(1), 67–75.

Benner, P. (2000). The roles of embodiment, emotion, and lifeworld for rationality and agency in nursing practice. *Nursing Philosophy 1*, 5–19.

Benner, P. (2002a). Caring for the silent patient. *American Journal of Critical Care, 11*(2), 480–482.

Benner, P. (2002b). Creating compassionate institutions that foster agency and respect. *American Journal of Critical Care, 11*(2), 164–167.

Benner, P. (2002c). Ethics, ethical comportment, and etiquette. *American Journal of Critical Care, 11*(1), 76–80.

Benner, P. (2003a). Avoiding ethical emergencies. *American Journal of Critical Care, 12*(1), 71–72.

Benner, P. (2003b). Reflecting on what we care about. *American Journal of Critical Care, 12*(2), 165–166.

Bishop, A., & Scudder, J. (2001). *Nursing ethics: Therapeutic caring presence*. Sudbury, MA: Jones & Bartlett.

Blair, P. D. (2001). Report impaired practice—stat. *Nursing Management, 56*(12), 24–25.

Bolmsjo, I., & Hermeren, G. (2003). Conflicts of interest: Experiences of close relatives of patients suffering from amyotrophic lateral sclerosis. *Nursing Ethics, 10*(2), 186–198.

Bortoff, J., Steele, R., Davies, B., Porterfield, P., Garossino, C., & Shaw, M. (2000). Facilitating day-to-day decision making in palliative care. *Cancer Nursing, 23*(2), 141–150.

Botes, A. (2000). An integrated approach to ethical decision making in the health team. *Journal of Advanced Nursing, 32*(5), 1076–1082.

Brier-Mackie, S. (2001). Patient autonomy and medical paternity: Can nurses help doctors to listen to patients? *Nursing Ethics, 8*(6), 510–521.

Brown, C. L. (1999). Ethics and health policy: Introduction. *Image: Journal of Nursing Scholarship, 31*(4), 394–396.

Burkhardt, M., & Nathaniel, A. (2002). *Ethics and issues in contemporary nursing* (2nd ed.). Albany, NY: Delmar Publishing.

Cahn, M. T. (1987). The nurse as moral hero: A case for required dissent. *Dissertation Abstracts International, 50*(3). (University Microfilms International #88-22134).

Cameron, B. (2004). Ethical moments in practice: The nursing "how are you" revisited. *Nursing Ethics, 11*(1), 53–62.

Cameron, M. (2002). Older persons' ethical problems involving their health. *Nursing Ethics, 9*(5), 537–556.

Cameron, M., Schaffer, M., & Park, H. (2001). Nursing students' experience of ethical problems and use of ethical decision-making models. *Nursing Ethics, 8*(5), 432–447.

Canadian Nurses Association (CNA). (1998). *Advance directives: The nurse's role.* Ottawa: Author. Retrieved August 24, 2004, from *http://www.cna-nurses.ca/pages/ethics/ethicsframe.htm*

Canadian Nurses Association (CNA). (1999). *I see and I am silent/I see and speak out: The ethical dilemma of whistle-blowing.* Ottawa: Author. Retrieved August 24, 2004, from *http://www.cna-nurses.ca/pages/ethics/ethicsframe.htm*

Canadian Nurses Association (CNA). (2000). *Working with limited resources: Nurses' moral constraints.* Ottawa: Author. Retrieved August 24, 2004, from *http://www.cna-nurses.ca/pages/ethics/ethicsframe.htm*

Canadian Nurses Association (CNA). (2001). *Futility presents many challenges for nurses.* Ottawa: Author. Retrieved August 24, 2004, from *http://www.cna-nurses.ca/pages/ethics/ethicsframe.htm*

Canadian Nurses Association (CNA). (2002). *Code of ethics for registered nurses.* Ottawa: Author. Retrieved August 24, 2004, from *http://www.cna-nurses.ca/pages/ethics/ethicsframe.htm*

Catalano, J. T. (2003). Ethics in nursing. In J. Catalano (Ed.), *Nursing now!* (3rd ed.). Philadelphia: F. A. Davis Company.

Catanzaro, A. M. (2002). Beyond the misapprehension of nursing rituals. *Nursing Forum, 37*(2), 17–27.

Childress, S. B. (2001). Enhance end-of-life care. *Nursing Management, 32*(10), 32–35.

Chilver, K. (2002). Should we give palliative care to all those that need it? *International Journal of Palliative Nursing, 8*(2), 75–77.

Chinn, P. (2001). Nursing and ethics: The maturing of a discipline. *Advances in Nursing Science, 24*(2), v–vi.

Christensen, A., & Frank-Stromborg, M. (2001). The protection of privacy in a high-tech era. *Journal of Nursing Law, 8*(1), 17–20.

Cochran, M. (1999). The real meaning of patient-nurse confidentiality. *Critical Care Quarterly, 22*(1), 42–49.

Cogliano, J. F. (1999). The medical futility controversy: Bioethical implications for the critical care nurse. *Critical Care Nursing Quarterly, 22*(3), 81–88.

Corley, M. C. (2002). Nurse moral distress: A proposed theory and research agenda. *Nursing Ethics, 9*(6), 636–650.

Corley, M. C. & Minick, P. (2002). Moral distress or moral comfort. *Bioethics Forum, 18*(1–2), 7–14.

Cortis, J. D., & Kendrick, K. (2003). Nursing ethics, caring and culture. *Nursing Ethics, 10*(1), 636–650.

Coverston, C., & Rogers, S. (2000). Winding roads and faded signs: Ethical decision making in a postmodern world. *Journal of Perinatal and Neonatal Nursing, 14*(2), 1–10.

Curtin, L. (2000a). On being a person of integrity—or ethics and other liabilities. *The Journal of Continuing Education in Nursing, 31*(2), 55–58.

Curtin, L. (2000b). The first ten principles for the ethical administration of nursing services. *Nursing Administration Quarterly, 25*(1), 7–14.

Curtin, L., & Flaherty, J. (1982). *Nursing ethics: Theories and pragmatics.* Bowie, MD: Robert J. Brady.

Davis, A. (1999). Global influence of American nursing: Some ethical issues. *Nursing Ethics, 6*(2), 118–125.

Davis, A., Aroskar, M., Liaschenko, J., & Drought, T. (1997). *Ethical dilemmas and nursing practice* (4th ed.). Stanford: CT: Appleton & Lange.

Dawes, B. S. G. (2001). Establishing ethical practices and eliminating "gray." *AORN Journal, 74*(4), 456–459.

DePalma, J., Ozanich, E., Miller, S., & Yancich, L. (1999). "Slow" code: Perspectives of a physician and critical care nurse. *Critical Care Quarterly, 22*(3), 89–96.

DesJardin, K. (2001). Political involvement in nursing—politics, ethics, and strategic action. *AORN Journal, 74*(5), 614–627.

Doane, G. H. (2001). In the spirit of creativity: The learning and teaching of ethics in nursing. *Journal of Advanced Nursing, 39*(6), 521–528.

Doane, G. H. (2002). Am I still ethical? The socially-mediated process of nurses' moral identity. *Nursing Ethics, 9*(6), 623–635.

Doane, G. H., Pauly, B., Brown, H., & McPherson, G. (2004). Exploring the heart of ethical nursing practice: Implications for ethics education. *Nursing Ethics, 11*(3), 240–253.

Donahue, M. P. (2000). Nursing values: A look back, a view forward. *Creative Nursing, 6*(3), 5–10.

Drevdahl, D., Kneipp, S., Canales, M., & Dorcy, K. S. (2001). Reinvesting in social justice: A capital idea for public health nursing? *Advances in Nursing Science, 24*(2), 19–31.

Durham, M. (2002). How research will adapt to HIPAA: A view from within the healthcare delivery system. *American Journal of Law & Medicine, 28,* 491–502.

Eby, M. (2000). Withdrawing or withholding artificial hydration and nutrition. *Nursing Ethics, 7*(5), 374–375.

Erlen, J. (2000). When the family asks, "What happened?" *Orthopaedic Nursing, 19*(6), 68–73.

Erlen, J. (2001a). Moral distress: A pervasive problem. *Orthopaedic Nursing, 20*(2), 76–82.

Erlen, J. (2001b). The nursing shortage, patient care, and ethics. *Orthopaedic Nursing, 20*(6), 61–66.

Erlen, J. (2002a). Adherence revisited: The patient's choice. *Orthopaedic Nursing, 21*(2), 79–83.

Erlen, J. (2002b). When there are limits on health care resources. *Orthopaedic Nursing, 21*(4), 69–74.

Erlen, J. (2004). Wanted—nurses: Ethical issues and the nursing shortage. *Orthopaedic Nursing, 23*(4), 289–292.

Farr, B. (2000). Protecting long-term care patients from antibiotic resistant infections: Ethics, cost-effectiveness, and reimbursement issues. *Journal of American Geriatrics Society, 48*(10), 1340–1342.

Fenton, M. T. (1987). Ethical issues in critical care: A perceptual study of nurses' attitudes, beliefs and ability to cope. Unpublished master's thesis, University of Manitoba, Winnipeg.

Fenton, M. T. (1988). Moral distress in clinical practice: Implications for the nurse administrator. *Canadian Journal of Nursing Administration, 1*(3), 8–11.

Foster, R. (2000). Building ethics of nursing inquiry as we build the science. *Journal of the Society of Pediatric Nurses, 5*(3), 107–111.

Fredrikson, L., & Eriksson, K. (2003). The ethics of the caring conversation. *Nursing Ethics, 10*(2), 138–149.

Fry, S. (2002). *Ethics in nursing practice: A guide to ethical decision making.* Malden, MA: Blackwell Science.

Fry, S., Cunningham, D., Fajkowski, J., McCormick-Gendzel, M., & Day, C. (2001). Evolution of a home health ethics committee. *Home Healthcare Nurse, 19*(9), 565–570.

Fry, S., & Veatch, R. (2000). *Case studies in nursing ethics* (2nd ed.). Sudbury, MA: Jones & Bartlett.

Gamlin, R. (2002). Do not attempt resuscitation: Issues and policies. *International Journal of Palliative Nursing, 8*(7), 361.

Gastmans, C. (1999). Care as a moral attitude in nursing. *Nursing Ethics, 6*(3), 214–223.

Georges, J. J., & Grypdonck, M. (2002). Moral problems experienced by nurses when caring for terminally ill people: A literature review. *Nursing Ethics, 9*(2), 155–178.

Gilligan, C. (1993). *In a different voice.* Cambridge, MA: Harvard University Press.

Gilligan, C. (1995). Hearing the difference: Theorizing connection. *Hypatia, 10*(2), 120–127.

Glen, S. (1999). Educating for interpersonal collaboration: Teaching about values. *Nursing Ethics, 6*(3), 202–213.

Guido, G. W. (2001). *Legal and ethical issues in nursing* (3rd ed.). Upper Saddle River, NJ: Prentice Hall.

Han, S., & Ahn, S. (2000). An analysis and evaluation of student nurses' participation in ethical decision-making. *Nursing Ethics, 7*(2), 115–123.

Hanna, D. R. (2004). Moral distress: The state of the science. *Research and Theory for Nursing Practice, 18*(1), 73–93.

Harris, J. (1999). Biomedical ethics and the role of the nurse: A case study and discussion. *Dermatology Nursing, 11*(3), 196–104.

Hayes, C. (2000). Strengthening nurses' moral agency. *Critical Care Nurse, 20*(3). Retrieved July 27, 2004, from *www.certcorp.org/certcorp/certcorp.nsf/0/2d0b83af2b4ec626882569bb00706821?OpenDocument*

Hicks, T. (2000). Ethical implications of pain management in a nursing home: A discussion. *Nursing Ethics, 7*(5), 392–398.

Holly, C. M. (1993). The ethical quandaries of acute care. *Journal of Professional Nursing, 9*(2), 110–115.

Homer, P. M. (1993). Transmission of human values: A cross cultural investigation of generational and reciprocal. *Genetic: Social and General Psychology Monographs, 119*(3), 345–368.

Hoonaard, W. C. (2001). Is research-ethics review a moral panic? *The Canadian Review of Sociology and Anthropology, 38*(1), 19–36.

How ethical are you? Part I. (1983a, January-February). *Nursing Life, 3,* 25–83.

How ethical are you? Part II. (1983b March–April). *Nursing Life, 3,* 46–56.

Hubert, J. (1999). The thought experiment as a pedagogical device in nursing ethics education. *Journal of Nursing Education, 38*(8), 374–376.

Hunter, S. (2000). Determination of moral negligence in the context of the undermedication of pain by nurses. *Nursing Ethics, 5,* 379–391.

Husted, J., & Husted, G. (1999). Agreement: The origin of ethical action. *Critical Care Quarterly, 22*(3), 12–17.

Husted, G. L., & Husted, J. H. (2001). *Ethical decision making in nursing and healthcare* (3rd ed.). New York: Springer.

Huycke, L., & All, A. (2000). Quality in health care and ethical principles. *Journal of Advanced Nursing, 32*(3), 562–571.

Hyland, D. (2002). An exploration of the relationship between patient autonomy and patient advocacy: Implications for nursing practice. *Nursing Ethics, 9*(5), 472–482.

Ingram, J. E., Buckner, E., & Rayburn, A. (2002). Critical care nurses' attitudes and knowledge related to organ donation. *Dimensions of Critical Care Nursing, 21*(6), 249–255.

International Council of Nurses (ICN). (2000). The ICN code of ethics for nurses. Geneva, Switzerland: Author. Retrieved July 13, 2004, from *www.icn.ch/ethics.htm*

Jacobson, G. (2002). Maintaining professional boundaries: Preparing nursing students for the challenge. *Journal of Nursing Education, 41*(6), 279–281.

Jameton, A. (1984). *Nursing practice: The ethical issues.* Englewood Cliffs, NJ: Prentice Hall.

Jeffers, B. R. (2002). Continuing education in research ethics for the clinical nurse. *The Journal of Continuing Education in Nursing, 33*(6), 265–269.

Johns, C. (1999). Unraveling the dilemmas within everyday nursing practice. *Nursing Ethics, 6*(4), 287–298.

Johnstone, M. (1999). *Bioethics: A nursing perspective* (3rd ed.). Orlando, FL: Harcourt-Saunders.

Karel, M. J. (2000). The assessment of values in medical decision-making. *Journal of Aging Studies, 14*(4), 403–423.

Keay, T. J. (1999). Palliative care in the nursing home. *Generations, 23*(1), 96–98.

Kelly, C. (2000). *Nurse's moral practice: Investing and discounting self.* Indianapolis, IN: Sigma Theta Tau.

Kendrick, K., & Robinson, S. (2002). "Tender loving care" as a relational ethic in nursing practice. *Nursing Ethics, 9*(3), 292–300.

Kenny, G. (2002). The importance of nursing values in interprofessional collaboration. *British Journal of Nursing, 11*(1), 65–68.

Killen, A. (2002). Stories from the operating room: Moral dilemmas for nurses. *Nursing Ethics, 9*(4), 405–415.

Kohlberg, L. (1968). Moral development. In *International encyclopedia of social science.* New York: Macmillan.

Kohlberg, L. (1981). *Essays on moral development.* Volumes 1–3. San Francisco: Harper & Row.

Kuhse, H. (1999). *Caring: Nurses, women, and ethics.* Maldon, MA: Blackwell Publishers.

Kupperschmidt, B. (2000). The invitational conference: A strategy for exploring ethical issues. *Nursing Forum, 35*(2), 25–31.

Lagana, K. (2000). The "right" to a caring relationship: The law and ethic of care. *Journal of Perinatal and Neonatal Nursing, 14*(2), 12–25.

Landry, H., & Landry, M. (2002). Nursing ethics and legal issues: An integrative approach in nursing education. *Journal of Nursing Education, 41*(8), 363–364.

Lark, J., & Gatti, C. (1999). Compliance with advance directives: Nursing's view. *Critical Care Nursing Quarterly, 22*(3), 65–71.

Ledbetter-Stone, M. (1999). Family intervention strategies when dealing with futility of treatment issues: A case study. *Critical Care Nursing Quarterly, 22*(3), 45–50.

Lee, S., & Kristjanson, L. (2003). Human research ethics committees: Issues in palliative care research. *International Journal of Palliative Nursing, 9*(1), 13–18.

Leininger, M. (1988). Leininger's theory of nursing: Cultural care diversity and universality, *Nursing Science Quarterly, 1*(4), 152–150.

Levine, M. E. (1989). Beyond dilemma. *Seminars in Oncology Nursing, 5*(2), 124–128.

Liaschenko, J. (1999). Can justice coexist with the supremacy of personal values in nursing practice? *Western Journal of Nursing Research, 21*(1), 35–50.

Maier-Lorentz, M. (2000). Creating your own ethical environment. *Nursing Forum, 35*(5), 25–29.

Marr, S. (2002). Protect your practice: Informed consent. *Plastic Surgical Nursing, 22*(4), 180–182.

Matheny, M. (1999). Nursing's 21st century values. *Creative Nursing, 5*(3), 5–6.

Mathes, M. M. (2000). Ethical challenges and nursing. *MedSurg Nursing, 9*(1), 44–48.

Mathes, M. M. (2001). Withholding and withdrawing nutrition and hydration by medical means: Ethical perspective. *MedSurg Nursing, 10*(2), 96–102.

McHale, J., & Gallagher, A. (2003). *Nursing and human rights.* New York: Butterworth-Heinmann.

McLaughlin, K., Miller, J., & Wooten, C. (1999). Ethical dilemmas in critical care: Nurse case manager's perspective. *Critical Care Nursing Quarterly, 22*(3), 51–64.

Meyers, J. L. (1994). Working in the grey zone: The moral suffering of critical care nurses. Unpublished master's thesis, Gonzaga University, Spokane, WA.

Michael, J. E. (2002). DNR orders: Proceed with caution. *Nursing Management, 33*(6), 22–23.

Milton, C. (2000a). Beneficence: Honoring the commitment. *Nursing Science Quarterly, 13*(2), 111–115.

Milton, C. (2000b). Informed consent: Process or Outcome? *Nursing Science Quarterly, 13*(4), 291–292.

Milton, C. (2001). Advanced directives: Living with certainty-uncertainty—A nursing perspective. *Nursing Science Quarterly, 14*(3), 195–198.

Milton, C. (2002). Ethical implications for acting faithfully in the nurse-person relationship. *Nursing Science Quarterly, 15*(1), 21–24.

Miracle, V. (2003). Critical care visitation. *Dimensions of Critical Care Nursing, 22*(1), 48–49.

Miriam, M. S., Braunschweig, H., & Rubinstein, R. L. (2002). Terminal care for nursing home residents with dementia. *Alzheimer's Care Quarterly, 3*(3), 233–247.

Mitchell, C. (1982). Integrity in interprofessional relationships. In G. Agich (Ed.), *Responsibility in health care*. Dordrecht, Holland: D. Reidel.

Moore, M. L. (2000). Ethical issues for nurses providing perinatal care in community settings. *Journal of Perinatal and Neonatal Nursing, 14*(2), 25–36.

Mula, C. (2002). The dilemmas of resource allocation. *International Journal of Palliative Nursing, 8*(4), 160.

National Student Nurses Association (NSNA). (2001). *Code of academic and clinical conduct*. National Student Nurses Association. Retrieved May 4, 2004, from *www.nsna.org*.

Noddings, N. (2003). *Caring: A feminine approach to ethics and moral education* (2nd ed.). Berkeley, CA: University of California Press.

Oberle, K., & Tenove, S. (2000). Ethical issues in public health nursing. *Nursing Ethics, 7*(5), 425–438.

O'Keefe, M. E. (Ed.). (2000). *Nursing practice and the law: Avoiding malpractice and other legal risks*. Philadelphia: F. A. Davis Company.

Pask, E. (2003). Moral agency in nursing: Seeing value in the work and believing that I make a difference. *Nursing Ethics, 10*(2), 165–174.

Pearson, L. J. (2003). Our ethical boundaries and dilemmas. *The Nurse Practitioner, 28*(2), 4.

Pellegrino, E. D. (2000). Commentary: Value neutrality, moral integrity, and the physician. *Journal of Law, Medicine, and Ethics, 28*(1), 78–81.

Peter, E., Macfarlane, A., & O'Brien-Pallas, L. (2004). Analysis of the moral habitability of the nursing work environment. *Journal of Advanced Nursing, 47*(4), 356–364.

Peter, E., & Morgan, K. P. (2001). Explorations of a trust approach for nursing ethics. *Nursing Inquiry, 8*(1), 3–10.

Peternelj-Taylor, C. (2003). Whistleblowing and boundary violations: Exposing a colleague in the forensic mileu. *Nursing Ethics, 10*(5), 526–540.

Piaget, J. (1932). *The moral development of a child*. New York: Free Press.

Pinch, W. E. (2000). Confidentiality: Concept analysis and clinical application. *Nursing Forum, 35*(2), 5–21.

Pinquart, M., & Silbereisen, R. K. (2004) Transmission of values from adolescents to their parents: The role of value content and authoritative parenting. *Adolescence, 39*(153), 83–100.

Proot, I. (2001). Autonomy in the care of stroke patients in nursing homes. *Nursing Ethics, 8*(1), 79–80.

Ptacek, J. T., & Ellison, N. M. (2000). Health care providers' perspectives on breaking bad news to patients. *Critical Care Nursing Quarterly, 23*(2), 51–59.

Puntillo, K. A., Drought, T., Drew, B., Stannard, D., Rushton, C., Scanlon, C., White, C. (2001). End-of-life issues in intensive care units: A national random survey of nurses' knowledge and beliefs. *American Journal of Critical Care, 10*(4), 216–219.

Purtilo, R. (1999). *Ethical dimensions in the health professions*. Philadelphia: Saunders.

Raholm, M. B., & Lindholm, L. (1999). Being in the world of the suffering patient: A challenge to nursing ethics. *Nursing Ethics, 6*(6), 528–539.

Randers, I., Olson, T., & Mattiasson, A. C. (2002). Confirming older adult patients' views of who they are and would like to be. *Nursing Ethics, 9*(4), 416–431.

Raths, L., Harmin, M., & Simon, S. (1978). *Values and teaching*. Columbus, OH: Merrill.

Redman, B. K., & Fry, S. T. (2000). Nurses' ethical conflicts: What is really known about them? *Nursing Ethics, 7*(4), 361–366.

Rogers, A., Karlson, S., & Addington-Hall, J. (2000). "All the services were excellent. It is when the human element comes in that things go wrong": Dissatisfaction with hospital care in the last year of life. *Journal of Advanced Nursing, 31*(4), 768–774.

Rokeach, M. (1973). *The nature of human values*. New York: Free Press.

Rumbold, G. (1999). *Ethics in nursing practice* (3rd ed.). Philadelphia: Harcourt, Brace & Company.

Russo, H. (2001). HIPAA: Creating privacy *protection* that works. *Caring, 20*(5), 12–16.

Sahlberg-Blom, E., Ternestedt, B. M., & Johansson, J. E. (2000). Patient participation in decision making at the end of life as seen by a close relative. *Nursing Ethics, 7*(4), 296–313.

Salladay, S. A. (2002). Ethics committee. *Nursing, 32*(8), 76–77.

Sarikonda-Woitas, C., & Robinson, J. H. (2002). Ethical health care policy: Nurses' voice in allocation. (On the scene). *Nursing Administration Quarterly, 26*(4), 72–81.

Savett, L. A. (2000). Values and dealing with change: We define ourselves by the choices we have made. *Creative Nursing, 6*(3), 11–15.

Scanlon, C. (1998). Assisted suicide: How nurses should respond. *International Nursing Review, 45*(5), 152–154.

Scanlon, C. (2000). A professional code of ethics provides guidance for genetic nursing practice. *Nursing Ethics, 7*(3), 262–268.

Schroeter, K. (1999). Ethical perception and resulting action in perioperative nurses. *AORN Journal, 69*(5), 991–1001.

Schwartz, E. (2000). Thinking about moral questions. *Creative Nursing, 6*(3), 10–11.

Scott, R. S. (1985). When it isn't life or death. *American Journal of Nursing, 85*(1), 19–20.

Seedhouse, D. (2000). *Practical nursing philosophy: The universal code*. New York: Wiley.

Severinsson, E. (2003). Moral stress and burnout: Qualitative content analysis. *Nursing and Health Sciences, 5*(1), 59–66.

Simmons, F. M. (1999). The Jehovah's Witness orthopaedic trauma patient: An ethical challenge. *Orthopaedic Nursing, 18*(5), 28–38.

Sloan, A. J. (1999). Whistleblowing: There are risks! *RN, 62*(7), 65–66.

Smith, K. V. & Godfrey, N. (2002) Being a good nurse and doing the right thing: A qualitative study. *Nursing Ethics, 9*(3), 301–312.

Smith, S. P. (2000). Are you protecting your patient's confidentiality? *Nursing Economic$, 18*(6), 294–299.

Spector, R. (2000). *Cultural diversity in health and illness*. Philadelphia: Temple University Press.

Spetz, J. (1999). Victor Fuchs on health care, ethics and the role of nurses. *Image: Journal of Nursing Scholarship, 31*(3), 255–263.

Steele, S. M., & Harmon, V. M. (1979). *Values clarification in nursing*. New York: Appleton-Crofts.

Steele, S. M., & Harmon, V. M. (1983) *Values clarification in nursing* (2nd ed.). New York: Appleton-Crofts.

Tapp, D. M. (2000). The ethics of relational stance in family nursing: Resisting the view of "nurse as expert." *Journal of Family Nursing, 6*(1), 69–91.

Thibault-Prevost, J., Jenson, L., & Hodgins, M. (2000). Critical care nurses' perceptions of DNR status. *Journal of Nursing Scholarship, 32*(3), 259–260.

Thiroux, J. (1977). *Ethics, theory and practice*. Philadelphia: MacMillan.

Thompson, E. (2000). A foundation of uncompromised ethics. *Modern Healthcare, 30*(7), 40–43.

Thompson, I., Melia, K., & Boyd, K. (2000). *Nursing ethics* (4th ed.). London: Churchill-Livingstone.

Tong, R. (1997). *Feminist approaches to bioethics: Theoretical reflection and practical applications*. Boulder, CO: Westview Press.

Tschudin, V. (2003a). *Approaches to ethics: Nursing beyond the boundaries*. New York: Butterworth-Heinemann.

Tschudin, V. (2003b). *Ethics in nursing: The caring relationship* (3rd ed.). New York: Butterworth-Heinemann.

Turkoski, B. (2000). Home care and hospice ethics: Using the code for nurses as a guide. *Home Healthcare Nurse, 18*(5), 308–316.

United States Department of Health and Human Services. (2002). HHS issues first major protections for patient privacy. Retrieved March 15, 2003, from *www.hhs.gov/news/press/2002pres/200020809a.html*

Van Hooft, S. (1999). Acting from the virtue of caring in nursing. *Nursing Ethics, 6*(3), 189–201.

Veronesi, J. (1999). Ethical issues in computerized medical records. *Critical Care Nursing Quarterly, 22*(3), 75–80.

Volbrecht, R. M. (2002). *Nursing ethics: Community in dialogue.* Upper Saddle River, NJ: Prentice Hall.

Volicer, L., Warden, V., & Morris, J. (1999). Fluid deprivation and research ethics. *Journal of the American Geriatrics Society, 47*(10), 1269–1270.

Watson, J. (1981, Summer). Socialization of the nursing student in a professional nursing education programme. *Nursing Papers, 13,* 19–24.

Watson, J. (1988). *Nursing: Human science and human care. A theory of nursing.* New York: National League for Nursing.

White, G. B. (1983). Philosophical ethics and nursing: A word of caution. In P. L. Chinn (Ed.), *Advances in nursing theory development.* Rockville, MD: Aspen Systems.

Wilkinson, J. M. (1987/88). Moral distress in nursing practice: Experience and effect. *Nursing Forum, 23,* 16–29.

Wilkinson, J. M. (1997). Toward a context-sensitive theory of nursing ethics: Classification and comparison of nurses' narratives from four time periods (1934, 1979, 1989 & 1995). Doctoral dissertation, University of Kansas, Kansas City, KS.

Williams, T. (2002). Patient empowerment and ethical decision-making. *Dimensions of Critical Care Nursing, 21*(3), 100–104.

Wilmot, S. (2000). Nurses and whistleblowing: The ethical issues. *Journal of Advanced Nursing, 32*(5), 1051–1057.

Whitbeck, L. B., & Gecas, V. (1988). Value attributions and value transmission between parents and children. *Journal of Marriage and the Family, 50,* 829–840.

Woods, A. (2001). Dealing with medical futility. *Dimensions of Critical Care Nursing, 20*(1), 56.

Woods, M. (1999). A nursing ethic: The moral voice of experienced nurses. *Nursing Ethics, 6*(5), 423–433.

Yoder-Wise, P. (2003). *Leading and managing in nursing.* St Louis: Mosby.

Ziel, S. (2002). Get on board with HIPAA privacy regulations. *Nursing Management, 33*(10), 28–29.

Ziel, S. E., & Gentry, K. L. (2003). Ready? HIPPA's here: Once the HIPPA privacy rule takes effect on April 14, you'll have to exert even more care than usual in guarding the confidentiality of patient information. *RN, 66*(2), 67–72.

CHAPTER 45

Aiken, T. (2004). *Legal, ethical, and political issues in nursing* (2nd ed.). Philadelphia: F. A. Davis Company.

American Hospital Association. (1992). *A patient's bill of rights.* Chicago: Author.

American Nurses Association. (1991). *Position statement: Assisted suicide and euthanasia.* Washington, DC: Author. Retrieved May 20, 2004, from *www.nursingworld.org/readroom/position/ethics/etdnr.htm*

American Nurses Association. (1992a). *Position statement: Registered nurse education relating to the utilization of unlicensed assistive personnel.* Washington, DC: Author. Retrieved September 8, 2002, from *http://nursingworld.org/readroom/position/uap/uapuse.htm*

American Nurses Association. (1992b). *Position statement: Registered nurse utilization of unlicensed assistive personnel.* Washington, DC: Author. Retrieved September 8, 2002, from *http://nursingworld.org/readroom/position/uap/uaprned.htm*

American Nurses Association (1996). *Registered professional nurses and unlicensed assistive personnel* (2nd ed.). Washington, DC: Author.

American Nurses Association. (1998b, February 12). ANA supports treatment rights of HIV-positive dental patient in case pending before U.S. Supreme Court. Retrieved March 26, 2004, from *http://nursingworld.org/pressrel/1998/amicus.htm*

American Nurses Association. (1998a, March/April). ANA supports rights of HIV positive. Retrieved March 26, 2004, from *http://nursingworld.org/tan/98marapr/miscell.htm*

American Nurses Association. (2000). Support for professional practice. *The American Nurse.* Retrieved November 24, 2004, from *http://nursingworld.org/tan/01julaug/hod.htm*

American Nurses Association. (2001). *Code of ethics for nurses with interpretive statements.* Washington, DC: American Nurses Publishing. Retrieved March 19, 2004, from *www.nursingworld.org/ethics/chcode.htm*

American Nurses Association. (2002, November/December). The American Nurses Association's bill of rights for registered nurses. *The American Nurse, 16.*

Barbus, A. J. (1975). The dying person's bill of rights. *American Journal of Nursing, 75*(1), 99.

Barnett, R. E. (2003). The proper scope of the police power. *Notre Dame Law Review, 79. http://ssrn.com/abstract=437201.* Retrieved November 20, 2004, from *www.bu.edu/law/faculty/papers.*

Beckstead, J. W. (2002). Modeling attitudinal antecedents of nurses' decisions to report impaired colleagues. *Western Journal of Nursing Research, 24*(5), 537–551.

Berry, V., & Mackay, T. R. (2001). In M. O'Keefe (Ed.), Advanced practice nursing. *Nursing practice and the law: Avoiding malpractice and other legal risks* (pp. 301–316). Philadelphia: F. A. Davis Company.

Cammuso, B. S., Madden, B. P., & Wallen, A. J. (2001). Forensic nursing. In M. O'Keefe (Ed.), *Nursing practice and the law: Avoiding malpractice and other risks* (pp. 397–415). Philadelphia: F. A. Davis Company.

Canadian Nurses Association. (2002). *Code of ethics for registered nurses.* Ottawa, Ontario: Author. [Online] Retrieved May 21, 2004, from *www.cna-nurses.ca/pages/ethics/ethicsframe.htm*

Colorado Nurse Health Program. (n.d.). The impaired nurse provider profile. Retrieved March 27, 2004, from *http://ouray.cudenver.edu/~eaengelk/CNHP/*

Columbia University. (2000). *The Columbia Encyclopedia* (6th ed.). Columbia University Press. Retrieved January 6, 2004, at *www.columbiaencyclopedia.edu.*

Croke, E. M. (2003). Nurses, negligence, and malpractice. *American Journal of Nursing, 103*(9), 54–63.

Equal Employment Opportunity Commission. (2002). Guidelines on discrimination because of sex. (Section 1604.11, Sexual harassment. Code of Federal Regulations, Title 29, Vol. 4). Retrieved March 27, 2004, from *www.eeoc.gov/types/sexual_harassment.* Last modified January 6, 2004.

Eskreis, T. R. (1998). Seven common legal pitfalls in nursing. *American Journal of Nursing, 98*(4), 34–40.

Fedorka, P., & Resnick, L. K. (2001). Defining nursing practice. In M. O'Keefe (Ed.), *Nursing practice and the law: Avoiding malpractice and other legal risks* (pp. 97–117). Philadelphia: F. A. Davis Company.

Georgia Nurses Association. (1982). Nurse Advocate Program. The impaired nurse: Checklist for detecting potential chemical dependence in an employee. Retrieved March 27, 2004, from *www.georgianurses.org/impaired_nurse.htm#tin*

Hall, J. K. (2001). Vicarious liability for nursing negligence. In M. O'Keefe (Ed.), *Nursing practice and the law: Avoiding malpractice and other legal risks* (pp. 150–162). Philadelphia: F. A. Davis Company.

Hall, J. K., & Hall, D. (2001). Negligence specific to nursing. In M. O'Keefe (Ed.), *Nursing practice and the law: Avoiding malpractice and other legal risks* (pp. 132–149). Philadelphia: F. A. Davis Company.

Helm, A. (2003). *Nursing malpractice: Sidestepping legal minefields.* Philadelphia: Lippincott, Williams & Wilkins.

Helm, A., & Kihm, N. C. (2001). Is professional liability insurance for you? Before you say no, weigh these considerations. *Nursing, 31*(1), 48–49.

Holloway, R. (2001). Patient rights. In M. O'Keefe (Ed.), *Nursing practice and the law: Avoiding malpractice and other legal risks* (pp. 189–198). Philadelphia: F. A. Davis Company.

Lunsford vs. Board of Nurse Examiners, 648 S.W. 2nd. 391 (Tex. App.—Austin 1983).

Marchand, D. V. (2001). American jurisprudence. In M. O'Keefe (Ed.), *Nursing practice and the law: Avoiding malpractice and other legal risks* (pp. 3–22). Philadelphia: F. A. Davis Company.

Mathews, M. D. (2001). In M. O'Keefe (Ed.), *Nursing practice and the law: Avoiding malpractice and other legal risks* (pp. 42–57). Philadelphia: F. A. Davis Company.

National Council of State Boards of Nursing (NCSBN). (1997a). Delegation decision-making grid. Retrieved September 8, 2002, from *www.ncsbn.org/files/uap/delegationgrid.pdf*

National Council of State Boards of Nursing (NCSBN). (1997b). Delegation decision-making tree. Retrieved September 8, 2002, from *www.ncsbn.org/files/uap/delegationtree.pdf*

National Council of State Boards of Nursing (NCSBN). (1997c). The five rights of delegation. Retrieved September 8, 2002, from *www.ncsbn.org/files/uap/fiverights.pdf*

National Council of State Boards of Nursing (NCSBN). (1998). The continuum of care framework: Roles of the licensed nurse and assistive personnel (AP) in relation to the client. Retrieved September 8, 2002, from *www.ncsbn.org/public/res/uap/contcaregrid.pdf*

O'Keefe, M. E. (Ed.). (2001). *Nursing practice and the law: Avoiding malpractice and other legal risks*. Philadelphia: F. A. Davis Company.

Pozzi, C. (2001). Violence in nursing. In M. O'Keefe (Ed.), *Nursing practice and the law: Avoiding malpractice and other legal risks* (pp. 431–457). Philadelphia: F. A. Davis Company.

Sosin, J. (2002). Legally speaking: Careful with that equipment, *RN, 65*(2), 59–62.

Trinkoff, A. M., Zhou, Q., Storr, C. L., & Soeker, K. L. (2000). Workplace access, negative proscriptions, job strain, and substance use in registered nurses. *Nursing Research, 49*(2), 83–90.

U.S. Department of Health and Human Services (2001). Standards for privacy of individually identifiable health information. [45 CFR Parts 160 and 164]. Retrieved March 25, 2003, from *www.hhs.gov/ocr/hipaa/*

U.S. Department of Health and Human Services, Centers for Medicare and Medicaid Services (2003). Emergency Medical Treatment & Labor Act (EMTALA) resource. Retrieved November 20, 2004, from *www.cms.hhs.gov/providers/emtala/default.asp*. Last updated 11/04/04.

Willmann, J. (1999). *Annotated Guide to the Texas Nursing Practice Act* (4th ed.). Austin, TX: Texas Nurses Association.

CHAPTER 46

Advisory Committee on Health Human Resources. (2000). *The nursing strategy for Canada*. Ottawa: Health Canada.

Advisory Committee on Health Human Resources. (2002). *Our health, our future: Creating quality workplaces for Canadian nurses. Final report of the Canadian Nursing Advisory Committee*. Ottawa: Health Canada.

Advisory Committee on Population Health. (1996). *The report on the health of Canadians*. Ottawa: Health Canada.

Advisory Committee on Population Health. (1999). *Toward a healthy future: Second report on the health of Canadians*. Ottawa: Health Canada.

Baumann, A., O'Brien-Pallas, L., Armstrong-Stassen, M., Blythe, J., Bourbonnais, R., Cameron, S., et al. (2001). *Commitment and care: The benefits of a healthy workplace for nurses, their patients and the system. A policy synthesis*. Ottawa: Canadian Health Services Research Foundation & the Change Foundation.

Broughton, H. (2001). *Nursing leadership: Unleashing the power*. Ottawa: Canadian Nurses Association.

Browne, G. (2001). *Key findings from the system-linked research unit on health and social service utilization*. Presented to the Advisory Committee on Health Human Resources Working Group on Nursing and Unregulated Healthcare Workers. Ottawa, October 24, 2001.

Browne, G., Roberts, J., Byrne, C., Gafni, A., Weir, R., & Majumdar, B. (2001). Translating research—The costs and effects of addressing the needs of vulnerable populations: Results of 10 years of research. *Canadian Journal of Nursing Research, 33*(1), 65–76.

Building the Future: An integrated strategy for nursing human resources in Canada. (2003). Retrieved November 4, 2004, from *www.buildingthefuture.ca*

Buresh, B., & Gordon, S. (2000). *From silence to voice: What nurses know and must communicate to the public*. Ottawa: Canadian Nurses Association.

Canadian Association of Occupational Therapists. (2003). *2001–2002 annual report*. Retrieved November 4, 2004, from *www.caot.ca*

Canadian Federation of Nurses Unions. (1991). *Funding health care*. Ottawa: Canadian Federation of Nurses Unions.

Canadian Federation of Nurses Unions. (1993). *Human rights*. Ottawa: Canadian Federation of Nurses Unions.

Canadian Federation of Nurses Unions. (1998). *Privatization of health care position statement*. Ottawa: Canadian Federation of Nurses Unions.

Canadian Federation of Nurses Unions. (2003). Mission statement. Available at *www.nursesunions.ca/about/ms.shtml*

Canadian Health Services Research Foundation. (2003). *Nursing research fund*. Retrieved November 4, 2004, from *www.chsrf.ca/nrf/index_e.shtml*

Canadian Institute for Health Information. (2001). *Canada's health care providers*. Ottawa: Author.

Canadian Institute for Health Information. (2002a). *Health indicators*. Ottawa: Author.

Canadian Institute for Health Information. (2002b). *Supply and distribution of registered nurses in Canada, 2001 report*. Ottawa: Author.

Canadian Institute for Health Information. (2003). *Health care in Canada*. Ottawa: Author.

Canadian Nurse. (2000). Nursing policy: Making the talk matter. Interview with Judith Shamian. *Canadian Nurse, 96*(10), 16–20.

Canadian Nurses Association. (1998). *The quiet crisis in health care: A submission to the House of Commons Standing Committee on Finance and the Minister of Finance*. Ottawa: Author.

Canadian Nurses Association. (2000a). *The environment is a determinant of health*. Ottawa: Author.

Canadian Nurses Association. (2000b). *Framework for Canada's health system*. Ottawa: Author.

Canadian Nurses Association. (2000c). *International trade and labour mobility*. Ottawa: Author.

Canadian Nurses Association. (2000d). *The primary health care approach*. Ottawa: Author.

Canadian Nurses Association. (2001a). *Financing Canada's health system*. Ottawa: Author.

Canadian Nurses Association. (2001b). *Privacy of personal health information*. Ottawa: Author.

Canadian Nurses Association. (2001c). *Reducing the use of tobacco products*. Ottawa: Author.

Canadian Nurses Association. (2001d). *The role of the nurse in telepractice*. Ottawa: Author.

Canadian Nurses Association. (2001e). What is nursing informatics and why is it so important? *Nursing Now: Issues and Trends in Canadian Nursing*. September (No. 11) Ottawa: Author.

Canadian Nurses Association. (2002a). *2001 annual report*. Ottawa: Canadian Nurses Association.

Canadian Nurses Association. (2002b). Demystifying the electronic health record. *Nursing Now: Issues and Trends in Canadian Nursing*. April (No. 13) Ottawa: Author.

Canadian Nurses Association. (2002c). *The nurse practitioner.* Ottawa: Author.

Canadian Nurses Association. (2002d). *Registered nurses 2001 statistical highlights.* Ottawa: Author.

Canadian Nurses Association. (2002e). *Supporting self-care: A shared initiative, 1999–2002.* Ottawa: Author.

Canadian Nurses Association. (2003a). *Clinical nurse specialist.* Ottawa: Canadian Nurses Association.

Canadian Nurses Association. (2003b). *Peace and security.* Ottawa: Canadian Nurses Association.

Canadian Nurses Association & Canadian Medical Association. (2000). *Joint CNA/CMA position statement on environmentally responsible activity in the health sector.* Ottawa: Canadian Nurses Association.

Canadian Nurses Association & College of Family Physicians of Canada. (2001). *Joint CFPC/CNA position statement on physical activity.* Ottawa: Canadian Nurses Association.

Canadian Occupational Health Nurses Association. *About us.* (2003). Retrieved September 15, 2005, from *www.cohnaaciist .ca /english/*

Canadian Physiotherapy Association. (2003). *2001–2002 annual report.* Retrieved September 16, 2004, from *http://www .physiotherapy.ca/annual_report.htm*

Care, W. D., Gregory, D., Whittaker, C., & Chernomas, W. (2003). Nursing, technology, and informatics: An easy or uneasy alliance? In M. McIntyre & E.Thomlinson (Eds.), *Realities of Canadian nursing: Professional, practice, and power issues* (pp. 243–261). Philadelphia: Lippincott Williams & Wilkins.

Clarke, H. (2003). Health and nursing policy: A matter of politics, power, and professionalism. In M. McIntyre & E. Thomlinson, (Eds.), *Realities of Canadian nursing: Professional, practice, and power issues* (pp. 60–82). Philadelphia: Lippincott Williams & Wilkins.

Clarke, H., Lashinger, H. S., Giovannetti, P., Shamian, J., Thomson, D., & Tourangeau, A. (2001). Nursing shortages: Workplace environments are essential to the solution. *Hospital Quarterly, 4*(4), 50–57.

Commission on the Future of Health Care in Canada. (2002). *Building on values: The future of healthcare in Canada—Final report.* [Commissioner Roy. J. Romanow]. Saskatoon, SK: Author.

Coster, G., & Buetow, S. (2001). *Quality in the New Zealand health system: Background paper to the National Health Committee.* Auckland, NZ: National Health Committee.

Dault, M., Lomas, J., & Barer, M. (2004). *Listening for direction II: National consultation on health services and policy issues for 2004–2007.* Ottawa: Canadian Health Services Research Foundation.

Decter, M., & Villeneuve, M. (2001). Repairing and renewing nursing workplaces. *Hospital Quarterly, 5*(1), 46–49.

Department of Justice Canada. (2003a). Canada Health Act. Retrieved June 7, 2004, from *http://laws.justice.gc.ca/en/C-6/15995.htm*

Department of Justice Canada. (2003b). Indian Act. Retrieved June 7, 2004, from *http://laws.justice.gc.ca/en/I-5/73349.html*

Duncan, S., Hyndman, K., Estabrooks, C., Hesketh, K., Humphrey, C., Wong, J., et al. (2003). Nurses' experiences of violence in Alberta and British Columbia hospitals. *Canadian Journal of Nursing Research, 32*(4), 57–78.

EKOS Research Associates. (2002). *Report on the future of health care in Canada: General public survey.* Ottawa: Author.

First Ministers' Meeting. (2000). *First Ministers' meeting communiqué on health.* September 11, Ottawa. Ottawa: Canadiian Intergovernmental Conference Secretariat.

First Ministers' Meeting. (2002). *Provinces pave the way for the future of health care.* Provincial-territorial premiers' meeting, January 24–25, Vancouver. Ottawa: Canadian Intergovernmental Conference Secretariat.

First Ministers' Meeting. (2003). *Health care renewal accord.* Retrieved July 10, 2004, from *www.hc-sc.gc.ca/english/hca2003/*

Fletcher, M. (2003). Be vigilant, nurses warned. *Canadian Nurse, 99*(4), 21.

Fooks, C., & Lewis, S. (2002). *Romanow and beyond: A primer on health reform issues in Canada.* Discussion Paper No. H/05. Ottawa: Canadian Policy Research Network.

Gagnon, D., & Menard, M. (2001). *Listening for direction: A national consultation on health services and policy issues.* Ottawa, ON: Advisory Committee on Health Services of the Conference of the Federal/Provincial/Territorial Deputy Ministers of Health, Canadian Coordinating Office of Health Technology Assessment, Canadian Health Services Research Foundation, Canadian Institute for Health Information, Institute of Health Services and Policy Research of the Canadian Institutes of Health Research.

Government of Alberta. (2001). *A framework for reform. Report of the Premier's Advisory Council on Health.* [D. Mazankowski, Chair]. Edmonton, AB: Premier's Advisory Council on Health.

Government of Alberta. (2003). Cancer Program of 1984. Retrieved September 16, 2005, from *www.gov.ab.ca/home/index.cfm*

Government of British Columbia. (2002). B.C. nursing graduates to meet new national standards. News release retrieved August 9, 2004, from *http://os8150.pb.gov.bc.ca/4dcgi/nritem?5541.*

Government of British Columbia. (2003). Health Authorities Act, 1996. Retrieved September 16, 2005, from *www.gov.bc.ca*

Government of Canada. (1986). *Achieving health for all: A framework for health promotion.* Ottawa: Health and Welfare Canada.

Government of Canada. (2002). *The health of Canadians—The federal role. Final report on the state of the health care system in Canada. Volume six: Recommendations for reform.* [M. J. L. Kirby, Chair]. Ottawa: Standing Senate Committee on Social Affairs, Science and Technology.

Government of Manitoba. (2003). CancerCare Manitoba Act, 2001. Retrieved September 16, 2005, from *www.gov.mb.ca*

Government of New Brunswick. (2002). *Health renewal by the Premier's Health Quality Council, Province of New Brunswick, 2000–2002.* Fredericton, NB: Government of New Brunswick.

Government of New Brunswick. (2003). Mental Health Act. Retrieved September 16, 2005, from *www.gnb.ca*

Government of New South Wales. (1999). *A framework for managing the quality of health services in New South Wales.* NSW, Australia: Author.

Government of Saskatchewan. (2001a). *Healthy people, a healthy province: An action plan for health in Saskatchewan.* Regina, SK: Author.

Government of Saskatchewan. (2001b). *SchoolPlus: A vision for children and youth.* Final Report of the Task Force and Public Dialogue on the Role of the School. Regina, SK: Government of Saskatchewan.

Government of Saskatchewan. (2003). Vital Statistics Act, 1995. Retrieved September 16, 2005, from *www.gov.sk.ca*

Grinspun, D., Virani, T., & Bajnok, I. (2001–2002). Nursing best practice guidelines: The RNAO (Registered Nurses Association of Ontario) project. *Hospital Quarterly,* Winter, *5*(2), 56–60.

Haley, L. (2003). Students take on native recruitment. *Medical Post, 39*(20).

Hall, E. M. (1964). Royal Commission on Health Services. Ottawa: Government of Canada.

Hall, E. M. (1980). *Canada's national-provincial health program for the 1980's: A commitment for renewal.* Justice E. M. Hall, Special Commissioner. Ottawa: Department of National Health and Welfare.

Hart Wasekeesikaw, F. (2003). Challenges for the new millennium: Nursing in First Nations communities. In M. McIntyre & E. Thomlinson, (Eds.), *Realities of Canadian nursing: Professional, practice, and power issues* (pp. 447–469). Philadelphia: Lippincott Williams & Wilkins.

Health Canada. (2001a). *Canada Health Act Annual Report 2000–2001.* Ottawa: Author.

Health Canada. (2001b). *Tactical plan for a pan-Canadian health infostructure. 2001 Update.* Federal-Provincial-Territorial Advisory Committee on Health Infostructure. Ottawa: Office of Health and the Information Highway.

Health Canada. (2003). Canada Health Act. Retrieved August 9, 2004, from *www.hc-sc.gc.ca/medicare/chaover.htm*

Health Canada. (2004). Public Health Agency of Canada. Retrieved August 9, 2004, from *www.hc-sc.gc.ca/english/*

Health Services Restructuring Commission. (1999). *Primary health care strategy.* Toronto: Health Services Restructuring Commission.

Ibbitson, J. (2003, May 22). Let the national health council games begin. Retrieved August 10, 2004, from *www.theglobeandmail.com*

Indian and Northern Affairs Canada. (2003). Treaty No. 6. Retrieved September 15, 2004, from *www.ainc-inac.gc.ca/sm/a-z/t_e.html*

Institute of Medicine. (1999, November). *To err is human.* Washington, DC: National Academy Press.

Institute of Medicine. (2001). *Crossing the quality chasm: A new health system for the 21st century.* Washington, DC: National Academy Press.

Joint Provincial Nursing Committee. (2001). *Good nursing, good health: A good investment.* Toronto: Government of Ontario.

Kouri, D., Chessie, K., & Lewis, S. (2002). *Regionalization: Where has all the power gone? A survey of Canadian decision makers in health care regionalization.* Saskatoon, SK: Canadian Centre for Analysis of Regionalization and Health.

Kulig, J., Thomlinson, E., Curran, F., MacLeod, M., Stewart, N., & Pitblado, R. (2002). *Recognizing and addressing the challenges: The impact of policy on rural and remote nursing practice.* Documentary analysis interim report: Policy analysis for the nature of rural and remote nursing practice in Canada. Lethbridge, AB: University of Lethbridge.

Lalonde, M. (1974). *The Lalonde Report.* Ottawa: Health and Welfare Canada.

Laschinger, H., Finegan, J., Shamian, J., & Almost, J. (2001). Testing Karasek's demands control model in restructured health care settings: Effects of job strain on staff nurses. *Nursing Administration, 31*(5), 233–243.

Lemire Rodger, G. (2003). Canadian Nurses Association. In M. McIntyre & E. Thomlinson (Eds.), *Realities of Canadian nursing: Professional, practice, and power issues* (pp. 124–142). Philadelphia: Lippincott Williams & Wilkins.

Mawandonan Consulting. (2002). *Aboriginal awareness workshop.* Prepared for Saskatchewan Health. Regina, SK: Mawandonan Consulting.

Margoshes, D. (1999). *Tommy Douglas: Building the new society.* Montreal: XYZ Publishing.

McIntyre, M. (2003). The workplace environment. In M. McIntyre & E. Thomlinson (Eds.), *Realities of Canadian nursing: Professional, practice, and power issues* (pp. 304–321). Philadelphia: Lippincott Williams & Wilkins.

McIntyre, M., & McDonald, C. (2003). Unionisation: Collective bargaining in nursing. In M. McIntyre & E. Thomlinson (Eds.), *Realities of Canadian nursing: Professional, practice, and power issues* (pp. 322–337). Philadelphia: Lippincott Williams & Wilkins.

McIntyre, M., & Thomlison, E. (2003). Introduction to nursing issues: Implications for the nursing profession. In M. McIntyre & E. Thomlinson (Eds.), *Realities of Canadian nursing: Professional, practice, and power issues* (pp. 2–16). Philadelphia: Lippincott Williams & Wilkins.

Metis National Council. (2003). Who Are the Metis? Retrieved September 15, 2004, from *www.metisnation.ca/who/indey.html*

National Association of Pharmacy Regulating Authorities. (2003). Available at *www.napra.org*

National Forum on Health Care. (1997). *Canada health action: Building on the legacy. Final report of the National Forum on Health.* Ottawa: Health Canada.

National Steering Committee on Patient Safety. (2002). *Building a safer system:* A national integrated strategy for improving patient safety in Canadian health care. Ottawa: National Steering Committee on Patient Safety.

National Task Force on Recruitment and Retention Strategies. (2002). *Against the odds: Aboriginal nursing.* Ottawa: Health Canada.

Natural Resources Canada. (2003). Historical Indian Treaties Map. Retrieved August 18, 2004, from *http://atlas.gc.ca/site/english/maps/historical/indiantreaties/historicaltreaties*

Ontario Health Services Restructuring Commission. (2000). *Looking back, looking forward: A legacy report from the Ontario Health Services Restructuring Commission, 1996–2000.* Toronto: Author.

Quebec Commission d'etude sure les services de sante et les service sociaux. (2001). *Emerging solutions: Report and recommendations.* [M. Clair, Chairman]. Quebec: Ministere de la Sante et des Services Sociaux.

Regina Qu'Appelle Health Region. (2003). *Improving first nations and Metis health outcomes: A call to action.* Final Report of the Regina Qu'Appelle Health Region's Working Together Towards Excellence Project. Regina, SK: Author.

Registered Psychiatric Nurses Association of Saskatchewan, Saskatchewan Association of Licensed Practical Nurses, & Saskatchewan Registered Nurses Association. (2000). *Nursing in collaborative environments.* Regina, SK: Saskatchewan Health.

Ryten, E. (1997). *A statistical picture of the past, present and future of registered nurses in Canada.* Ottawa: Canadian Nurses Association.

Ryten, E. (2002). *Planning for the future: Nursing human resource projections.* Ottawa: Canadian Nurses Association.

Saskatchewan Commission on Medicare. (2001). *Caring for Medicare: Sustaining a quality system.* [K. J. Fyke, Commissioner]. Regina, SK: Saskatchewan Health.

Saskatchewan health legislation. Last updated 2003. Retrieved September 15, 2005, from Saskatchewan Health web site.

Saskatchewan Health Quality Council. (2003). *Room for improvement: Setting priorities for making Saskatchewan health care better.* Saskatoon, SK: Author.

Shamian, J., Skelton-Green, J., & Villeneuve, M. (2003). Policy is the lever for effecting change. In M. McIntyre & E. Thomlinson, (Eds.), *Realities of Canadian nursing: Professional, practice, and power issues* (pp. 83–104). Philadelphia: Lippincott Williams & Wilkins.

Smadu, M. (2003). Building professional practice environments through policy development. Presentation at the Nursing Leadership Conference, February 10, 2003, Ottawa, ON.

Statistics Canada. (2002). *Annual demographic statistics 2001.* Ottawa: Statistics Canada.

Storch, J. (2003). The Canadian health care system and Canadian nurses. In M. McIntyre & E. Thomlinson (Eds.), *Realities of Canadian nursing: Professional, practice, and power issues* (pp. 34–59). Philadelphia: Lippincott Williams & Wilkins.

Way, D., Jones, L., & Busing, N. (2000). *Implementation strategies: Collaboration in primary care—Family doctors and nurse practitioners delivering shared care.* Toronto: Ontario College of Family Physicians.

Woolhandler, S., & Himmelstein, D. U. (2002). Paying for national health insurance—and not getting it. *Health Affairs, 21*(4), 88–98.

World Health Organization. (1978). *Declaration of Alma-Ata.* International Conference on Primary Health Care, Alma-Ata, USSR, 6–12 September.

World Health Organization. (1986). *Ottawa charter for health promotion: An international conference on health promotion.* November 17–21, 1986.

World Health Organization. (2002). *The world health report.* Geneva, Switzerland: Author.

Text, Photo & Illustration Credits

Text Credits

Note: Unless cited below, text credits appear within the text.

CHAPTER 3

Nursing admission data form, p. 27: North Broward Hospital District, Ft. Lauderdale, FL.

CHAPTER 4

NANDA Taxonomy II, pp. 39–41: NANDA International (2003). NANDA Nursing Diagnoses: Definitions and classification 2003–2004.

CHAPTER 6

Table, p. 55: Adapted from McCloskey & Bulechek (2000). *Nursing Interventions Classification,* 3rd ed, Five intervention labels and definitions. Elsevier Science.

Johnson, Mass, and Moorhead. *Nursing Outcomes Classification,* 2nd ed.

Photo and Illustration Credits

Except as noted below, photos in procedures are by Ted Clow, photos of the Garcia family (Caring for the Garcias) are by Barbara Proud, and illustrations are by Imagineering STA Media Services.

Author Photo, Karen Van Leuven: Richard Friedman

UNIT 1

Photodisc Green/Getty Images

UNIT 2

©Royalty-Free/Corbis

UNIT 3

David Buffington/Photodisc Green at Getty Images

CHAPTER 17

Procedure 17–1, equipment; p. 191 Dillon, P. (2003). *Nursing Health Assessment.* Philadelphia: F. A. Davis Company.

CHAPTER 19

All art and photos except those noted below:

Dillon, P. (2003). *Nursing Health Assessment.* Philadelphia: F. A. Davis Company.

Procedure 19–1, equipment table Ted Clow (except thermometers)

Procedure 19–1, BMI chart Imagineering STA Media Services

Procedure 19–2, documentation Imagineering STA Media Services

Procedure 19–2, Anatomy Atlas, jaundice Centers for Disease Control and Prevention

Procedure 19–2, Anatomy Atlas, petechiae, Procedure 19–16, Anatomy Atlas, rheumatoid arthritis Custom Medical Stock Photo

Procedure 19–4, healthy nail bed Imagineering STA Media Services

Procedure 19–6, cardinal fields Imagineering STA Media Services

Procedure 19–11, Imagineering STA Media Services

Procedure 19–13, step 2 Imagineering STA Media Services

CHAPTER 22

Procedure 22–8, step 3 Courtesy of Sage Products, Inc., Cary, IL.

Procedure 22–9, equipment Procedure 22–9, step 9, Home Care box Courtesy of EZ-Access, 1704B Street NW, Bldg E, Suite 110, Auburn, WA.

UNIT 4

Brand X Pictures/PictureQuest

CHAPTER 28

Procedure 28–5, ostomy equipment Williams, L. & Hopper, P. (2003). *Understanding Medical Surgical Nursing,* 2nd edition, p. 528. Philadelphia: F. A. Davis Company.

CHAPTER 31

Procedure 31–1A, Step 3 Williams, L. & Hopper, P. (2003). *Understanding Medical Surgical Nursing,* 2nd edition, fig. 28–16, p. 424. Philadelphia: F. A. Davis Company.

CHAPTER 35

35.TB1–1, 35.TB1–2, 35.TB1–3, 35.TB1–4, 35.TB1–5, 35.TB1–6, 35.TB1–7 adapted from WVL Vol. 1, ch. 17 table 3

CHAPTER 36

36.P06.EQ.03 adapted from Williams, L. & Hopper, P. (2003). *Understanding Medical Surgical Nursing,* 2nd edition, fig. 26–19, p. 419. Philadelphia: F. A. Davis Company.

Technique 26–1 Dillon, P. (2003). *Nursing Health Assessment,* fig 6–4, Philadelphia: F. A. Davis Company.

Technique 26–2 Dillon, P. (2003). *Nursing Health Assessment,* p. 116, Philadelphia: F. A. Davis Company.

UNIT 5

Stockbyte Platinum at Getty Images

UNIT 6

Image Ideas/PictureQuest

Index

Abbreviations: *b* = box; *ESG* = electronic study guide; *ESG9* = electronic study guide, Chapter 9; *ESG46* = electronic study guide, Chapter 46; *f* = figure; *p* = procedure; *t* = table; *tb* = technique box

A

Abbreviations
  in health care, *(V2) 185*
  in medication order, *(V1) 493*, *(V1) 493b*
  medication-related, *(V2) 522–524*
Abdomen
  assessment of, *(V1) 395p*, *(V2) 293p–299p*
  distention of, *(V1) 947t*
  four quadrants of, *(V1) 383*, *(V1) 383f*
  movement of, *(V1) 325–326*
  variation in contour of, *(V1) 384f*
Abdominal flat plate, *(V2) 666–667*
Abduction
  assessment of, *(V2) 305p–306p*
  as movement, *(V1) 727f*
Ablative surgery, *(V1) 924*
Abnormal anxiety, *(V1) 199*
Aboriginal population
  challenges to health and healthcare, *(ESGV1) 27*
  healthcare delivery system, *(ESGV1) 7*, *(ESGV1) 11–12*
Abrasion, *(V1) 449*, *(V1) 815t*
Abscess, *(V1) 815t*
Absent, bowel sounds as, *(V1) 383–384*
Absorbent dressing, *(V1) 839–840*
Absorption
  blood flow affecting absorption, *(V1) 484*
  of drug in blood, *(V1) 486f*
  of drugs in children and adult, *(V1) 487t*
  factors affecting drug, *(V1) 479*, *(V1) 483*
  pH and ionization affecting drug, *(V1) 483–484*
Abuse
  assessment for, *(V2) 89p–92p*, *(ESG9) 16p*
  child, *(ESG9) 17*
  of elderly, *(ESG9) 37*
  flow chart identifying, *(V2) 88*
  reporting, *(V1) 1087*
Acanthous nigrican, *(V2) 277*
Acceptance
  communication and, *(V1) 181*
  promotion in children, *(V1) 198*
Accessibility, *(ESGV1) 4t*, *(ESGV1) 5*
Accident
  equipment-related, *(V1) 433*
  motor vehicle, *(V1) 428–429*
Accommodation
  as cognitive development competency, *(V1) 167*
  as phase of grieving, *(V1) 266*
  of pupils, *(V1) 371*
Accountable
  of delegated activities, *(V1) 126*
  nurse as, *(V1) 105–106*
Accreditation, *(V1) 1075*
Acculturation, *(V1) 227*
Accuracy, assessment data, *(V1) 57*

Acetaminophen
  for fever, *(V1) 314*
  for pain relief, *(V1) 712*, *(V1) 713*
Achievement, self-concept and, *(V1) 189–190*
Achieving Health for All: A Framework for Health Promotion, *(ESGV1) 28*
Achondroplasia, *(V1) 737*
Acid, *(V1) 895*
Acid-base balance
  ABG to assess, *(V1) 899t*
  assessment of, *(V2) 906–908*
  assessment of imbalance, *(V1) 901*
  history of, *(V2) 905*
  imbalance of, *(V1) 898–899*, *(V1) 900t*
  interpretation of, *(V1) 899*
  overview of, *(V2) 871*
  regulation of, *(V1) 895*
Acidosis, *(V1) 895*, *(V1) 898*
Acne, *(V1) 449*, *(V2) 245*
Acquired immunodeficiency syndrome (AIDS)
  as family health challenge, *(V1) 215–216*
  nursing education for, *(V1) 15*
Acromegaly, *(V1) 370*
Active dying, *(V1) 284*
Active euthanasia, *(V1) 275*
Active immunity, *(V1) 405*
Active involvement, learning, *(V1) 532*
Active listening behavior
  FOLK, *(V1) 49*
  as therapeutic communication, *(V1) 349–350*
Active range of motion (AROM), *(V1) 385*, *(V1) 757*
Active resistance, *(V1) 964*
Active transport
  energy requirement, *(V1) 889*
  process of, *(V1) 890*, *(V1) 890t*
Activities of daily living (ADLs)
  care plan document, *(V1) 85*
  elder assessment for, *(ESG9) 37–38*
  as exercise, *(V1) 757*
  grooming hair, *(V1) 369*
  mobility and, *(V1) 741*
  questions for assessment of, *(V1) 43b*
  self-care of, *(V1) 442*
Activity
  health promotion and restoration, *(V1) 19–20*
  history questions, *(V2) 721*
  importance of leisure, *(V1) 568*
  as intervention, *(V1) 105*
  knowledge and ability to perform, *(V1) 122*
  locating appropriate NIC, *(V1) 114*
  management of, *(V2) 724*
  of nurse in NIC intervention, *(V1) 114*
  nursing
    contributing to battle-ax image, *(V1) 7*
    dependent and independent, *(V1) 6t*

overview of, *(V2) 696*
  patient feedback, *(V1) 123*
  physical assessment of, *(V2) 722–723*
  tolerance of, *(V1) 747*
Activity theory, *(ESG9) 35*, *(ESG9) 37*
Actual loss, *(V1) 264*
Actual nursing diagnosis, *(V1) 61–62*, *(V1) 62f*
Acupoints, *(V1) 993*
Acupressure, *(V1) 710*
Acupuncture
  benefits of, *(V1) 993–994*
  needles for, *(V1) 994f*
  for pain relief, *(V1) 710*
  for stress management, *(V1) 570*
Acute care setting, assessment in, *(V1) 42*
Acute illness, *(V1) 180*
Acute infection, *(V1) 401*
Acute pain
  anxiety and, *(V1) 704*
  duration of, *(V1) 700*
  outcomes and interventions for, *(V2) 695*
  reaction to, *(V1) 705*
Acute renal failure (ARF), *(V1) 633b*
Acute wound, *(V1) 814*
Adaptation
  as cognitive development competency, *(V1) 167*
  definition of, *(V1) 551*, *(ESG9) 5*
  failure of
    organic response to, *(V1) 562–563*
    psychological responses to, *(V1) 563–564*
    somatoform disorders, *(V1) 563*
  knowledge map of, *(V2) 556*
  overview of, *(V2) 542*
  to stress/stressors, *(V1) 553–554*
Adaptation Model, *(V1) 51b*
Adaptive coping, *(V1) 553*
Addiction
  of opioids, *(V1) 713*
  pain management with, *(V1) 719*
Adduction
  assessment of, *(V2) 305p–306p*
  as movement, *(V1) 727f*
A-delta fiber, *(V1) 701–702*, *(V1) 702f*, *(V1) 703f*
Adenosine triphosphate (ATP), *(V1) 285*
Adequate Intakes (AI), *(V1) 586*
Adhesive strips (Steri-Strips), *(V1) 818*
Adjustable bed, *(V1) 748*
Adjuvant analgesic, *(V1) 716*
ADL. *See* Activities of daily living
Administration
  provincial/territorial healthcare insurance and, *(ESGV1) 4*
  public, *(ESGV1) 4*
  role of, *(V1) 479*

Administration set (IV infusion), *(V1) 909,*
    (V1) 909f
Administrative agency, *(V1) 1072*
Administrative law, *(V1) 1072*
Admission forms, *(V1) 293, (V2) 27–30*
Admission nursing database, *(V1) 293*
Adolescence
    assessment of, *(V1) 364, (ESG9) 29*
    death of, *(V1) 268*
    development of, *(ESG9) 26–28*
    developmental task theory, *(ESG9) 4t*
    grief and development, *(V1) 267*
    hair of, *(V2) 248*
    health problems, *(ESG9) 28–29*
    health promotion and screenings,
        (V1) 1010t
    immunization schedule, *(ESG9) 19f*
    milestones of, *(ESG9) 28b*
    nutritional needs, *(V1) 596*
    puberty, *(ESG9) 27*
    safety of, *(V1) 421*
    sensory stimulation needs, *(V1) 682*
    sexual development, *(V1) 769*
    sexual orientation of, *(ESG9) 28b*
    skin, *(V1) 812*
    sleep
        patterns of, *(V1) 799*
        requirements for, *(V1) 795t*
    stressors of, *(V1) 552b*
    suicide of, *(V1) 422*
    teeth development, *(V1) 459, (V1) 459f*
Adoptive family, *(V1) 211*
Adrenocorticotropic hormone (ACTH),
        (V1) 555
Adult
    assessment of, *(V1) 364*
    body fluid of, *(V1) 888t*
    breathing rhythm of, *(V1) 325–326*
    chest size and shape, *(V1) 378*
    developmental task theory, *(ESG9) 4t*
    drug therapy for, *(V1) 487t*
    fremitus of, *(V2) 284*
    grief and development, *(V1) 267–268*
    health promotion and screenings,
        (V1) 1011t
    learning, principles of, *(V1) 535b*
    minerals: DRI, *(V1) 585t–586t*
    nutritional needs, *(V1) 596*
    oxygenation of, *(V1) 855*
    restless leg syndrome (RLS), *(V1) 801*
    safety of, *(V1) 421*
    sensory stimulation needs, *(V1) 682*
    sexuality, *(V1) 769–770*
    skin of, *(V1) 812, (V2) 242*
    sleep
        patterns of, *(V1) 799*
        requirements for, *(V1) 795, (V1) 795t*
    stressors of, *(V1) 552b*
    teeth development, *(V1) 459, (V1) 459f*
    vitamins: DRI, *(V1) 583t–584t*
    See also Elderly
Adult, middle
    assessment of, *(ESG9) 34*
    development of, *(ESG9) 32–33*
    health problems, *(ESG9) 33–34*
    intervention for, *(ESG9) 34*
    transition of, *(ESG9) 33*
Adult, young
    development of, *(ESG9) 31–32*
    health problems, *(ESG9) 32*
    young, assessment of, *(ESG9) 32*
Advance directive, *(V1) 273*

Advanced practice nurse (APN)
    diagnosis and treatment of medical
        problems, *(V1) 59*
    education for, *(V1) 15*
    increased use of, *(V1) 22*
Adventitious breath sounds, *(V1) 380*
Adverse reaction, *(V1) 489*
Advisory Committee on Health Human
        Resources (ACHHR), *(ESGV1) 26–27*
Advisory Committee on Population Health,
        (ESGV1) 28
Advocacy
    guidelines for, *(V2) 1013tb*
    for patient, *(V1) 1048, (V1) 1068–1069*
Aerobic conditioning, *(V1) 732*
Aerobic exercise, *(V1) 731*
Aerosol sprayer, *(V1) 505*
Affective goal, *(V1) 133t*
Affective learning, *(V1) 530, (V1) 531t*
African American
    hair care for, *(V1) 465–466*
    healing system of, *(V1) 234t*
    marriage rate, *(V1) 771*
    statistics in nursing, *(V1) 10t*
    types of folk healers, *(V1) 230t*
Age
    blood pressure and, *(V1) 328*
    changes by, *(ESG9) 36t*
    foot problems increasing with, *(V1) 455*
    as health factor, *(V1) 173–174*
    intervention, as factor influencing, *(V1) 28*
    modification of assessment for,
        (V1) 363–364
    of mother, teratogenic effect on fetus,
        (ESG9) 12
    pharmacokinetics and, *(V1) 487*
    pulse rate, *(V1) 317*
    respiration and, *(V1) 323*
    sensory function and, *(V1) 682, (V1) 683t*
    sleep patterns, *(V1) 799*
    as surgical risk factor, *(V1) 924–925*
Ageism, *(ESG9) 38*
Agency for Healthcare Policy and Research
        (AHCPR), *(V1) 707b*
Agency for Healthcare Research and Quality
        (AHRQ), *(V1) 108, (V1) 709–710*
Agglutination, *(V1) 403*
Aggregate
    definition of, *(V1) 1022*
    Omaha System for, *(V1) 115*
    writing goals for, *(V2) 992*
Aging
    healthcare delivery factor, *(ESGV1) 11*
    I.Q. test for, *(ESG9) 38b*
    theory of, *(ESG9) 35*
Agonist-antagonist, *(V1) 713*
AIDS. *See* Acquired immunodeficiency
        syndrome
Airborne infections, *(V1) 412*
Airborne precautions, *(V1) 412*
Airborne transmission, *(V1) 400*
Air embolus
    as IV therapy complication, *(V1) 917t*
Air pollution, *(V1) 431, (V1) 856*
Air travel, infection and, *(V1) 400*
Airway
    artificial, *(V1) 877–879*
    resistance, *(V1) 848*
    structures of, *(V1) 845–847*
    suctioning of, *(V1) 879*
Alarm stage, of GAS, *(V1) 555–556, (V1) 555f*
Alberta Cancer Program Act, *(ESGV1) 8*

Albinism, *(V1) 369*
Albumin, *(V1) 605*
Alcohol
    adolescence and, *(ESG9) 28*
    fetal alcohol syndrome, *(ESG9) 15*
    as health risk factor, *(V1) 174*
    oxygenation and, *(V1) 858*
    sexual function and, *(V1) 774t*
    sleep and, *(V1) 800*
    teratogenic effect on fetus, *(ESG9) 9*
Alcoholics Anonymous, *(V1) 1018*
Alcott, Louisa May, *(V1) 8*
Aldosterone
    effects of, *(V1) 556f*
    promoting fluid retention, *(V1) 555*
    regulation of, *(V1) 891*
Alginate, *(V1) 839–840*
Algorithm, *(V1) 971*
Algor mortis, *(V1) 285*
Alkali, *(V1) 894*
Alkalosis, *(V1) 895, (V1) 898*
Allen's test, *(V2) 292*
Allergic response, *(V1) 856*
Allergy
    definition of, *(V1) 856*
    as surgical risk factor, *(V1) 925*
Allopathic therapy, *(V1) 47*
Allopathy, *(V1) 989*
Alopecia areata, *(V1) 369, (V2) 334*
Alpha-linoleic acid (omega-3), *(V1) 580*
Alpha wave, *(V1) 796, (V1) 796f*
ALS (Amyotrophic lateral sclerosis), *(V1) 175*
Alternative health care
    modality of, *(V1) 989*
    types of, *(V1) 231*
    See also Complementary/Alternative
        modalities (CAM); Holistic care
Alternative medical system
    acupuncture, *(V1) 993–994*
    Ayurveda, *(V1) 992*
    naturopathy, *(V1) 995*
    traditional Chinese medicine (TCM),
        (V1) 992–993
Alternative medicine, *(V1) 235*
Alternative modality, *(V1) 989*
Alternatives
    considering, *(V1) 30t, (V1) 31*
    considering for intervention selection,
        (V1) 112
    model of critical thinking, *(V1) 31f,*
Altitude, *(V1) 856*
Altruism, *(V1) 1052t*
Alveolar-capillary membrane, *(V1) 847,*
        (V1) 853
Alveolar cell, *(V1) 847, (V1) 847f*
Alveoli, *(V1) 847*
AMB (as evidenced by), *(V1) 75*
Ambularm, *(V1) 434*
Ambulation
    assisting with, *(V1) 755p, (V1) 757, (V1)*
        758f, (V2) 712p–715p
    physical conditioning for, *(V1) 757, (V2)*
        718tb
Ambulatory clinic, *(V1) 293–294*
American Association of Nursing
        Anesthetists (AANA), *(V1) 937*
American Baptist nursing home system, *(V1) 5*
American Heart Association (AHA)
    CPR certification, *(V1) 885*
    DNR and DNAR orders, *(V1) 273*
    fat substitutes, *(V1) 611*
    normal blood pressure, *(V1) 327*

American Hospital Association, (V1) 312, (V1) 529, (V1) 1061–1062, (V1) 1061b, (V1) 1077
American Nurses Association (ANA)
  Bill of Rights for Nurses, (V1) 1077
  Clinical Care Classification (CCC), (V2) 44, (V2) 53
  Code for Nurses, (V1) 16, (V1) 247
  code of ethics, (V1) 1059, (V1) 1060b
  concern over activities of UAP, (V1) 126
  data collection, (V1) 50
  definition of nursing, (V1) 11
  DNAR order recommendations, (V1) 275, (V1) 275b
  evaluation requirements, (V1) 129
  language for nursing, (V2) 957–958
  Nursing: Scope and Standards of Practice, (V1) 1061
  nursing diagnosis, (V1) 58
  Nursing Intervention Classification (NIC), (V2) 53
  Nursing Outcomes Classification (NOC), (V1) 97, (V2) 44
  nursing process, (V1) 31
  Omaha System, (V2) 44, (V2) 53
  Patient Self-Determination Act (PSDA), (V1) 1073
  professional standards for
    assessment, (V1) 39, (V1) 40b
    diagnosing, (V1) 57b
    planning outcomes, (V1) 83b
  recipients for nursing care, (V1) 19
  research priorities, (V1) 154–155
  responsibilities of teaching, (V1) 529
  standardized vocabularies, (V1) 113
  standards of
    care, (V1) 1061
    practice, (V1) 16, (V1) 17t
    professional performance, (V1) 1061b, (V1) 1076b
  support for cultural diversity and competence, (V1) 235
  vocabulary and taxonomy, (V2) 44
American Pain Society, (V1) 707
American Psychiatric Association (APA), (V1) 70, (V1) 200
American Red Cross, (V1) 8
American Society of Perianesthesia Nurses (ASPAN), (V1) 943
Americans with Disabilities Act (ADA), (V1) 1072–1073
Amino acid
  essential and nonessential, (V1) 577, (V1) 578t
  structural formula for, (V1) 577f
Ammonia (NH₃), (V1) 578
Amphiarthroses, (V1) 726
Ampule
  drawing medication up from, (V1) 509, (V1) 523p, (V2) 475p–476p
  injury prevention, (V1) 509f
Amyotrophic lateral sclerosis (ALS), (V1) 175
Anabolism, (V1) 577
Anaerobic exercise, (V1) 731
Analgesic
  adjuvant, (V1) 716
  nonopioid, (V1) 712–713
  opioid, (V1) 713–716, (V1) 717t
Anal intercourse, (V1) 777–778
Anal sphincter, (V1) 653, (V1) 654f
Anal stage, (ESG9) 20–21
Anal stimulation, (V1) 777–778

Analytic reading, (V1) 159–161
Analyzing
  assumption, (V1) 30t, (V1) 31
  assumption for intervention selection, (V1) 112
  biases affecting goal achievement, (V1) 136
  data, (V1) 63
  problem areas for research, (V1) 158–159
Anaphylactic reaction, (V1) 490
Andrews and Boyle transcultural nursing assessment, (V1) 239
Androgyny, (V1) 766
Androphase, (ESG9) 33
Anemia
  hematocrit level and, (V1) 328
  oxygenation and, (V1) 861
Aneroid manometer, (V1) 329–330
Anesthesia
  local and topical, (V1) 717
  peristalsis and, (V1) 656
  recovery from, (V1) 942–949, (V1) 944b
  types of, (V1) 937–939
  urination and, (V1) 625
Anesthesiologist, (V1) 937
Angel-nurse, (V1) 4
Angel of mercy, (V1) 4–5
Anger
  handling patients with, (V2) 549tb
  management of, (V1) 570
  response to stressor, (V1) 561–562
Angina pectoris, (V1) 860
Angiotensin II, (V1) 891
Anhedonia, (V1) 201
Anilingus, (V1) 777–778
Anion, (V1) 888
Anisocoria, (V1) 371
Ankle-brachial index (ABI), (V2) 292
Ankle ROM, (V1) 745t
Ankylosing spondylitis, (V1) 737–738
Ankylosis, (V1) 739
Anorexia nervosa, (V1) 190, (ESG9) 29
Anosmia, (V1) 687
Antacid, peristalsis and, (V1) 656
Antagonistic drug relationship, (V1) 491
Anterior triangle, (V1) 376
Anthropometric measurement, (V1) 602
Antianxiety agent, (V1) 774t
Antibiotics
  early availability of, (V1) 5
  increasing surgical risk, (V1) 926b
  peristalsis and, (V1) 656
Antibody, (V1) 403
Anticholinergic, (V1) 935t
Anticholinergic effect, urine and, (V1) 625
Anticipatory grief, (V1) 269, (V2) 173
Anticoagulant, (V1) 926b
Anticonvulsant, (V1) 774t
Antidepressant medication, (V1) 202, (V1) 774t
Antidiuretic hormone (ADH)
  effects of, (V1) 556f
  promoting fluid retention, (V1) 555
  regulation of, (V1) 891
Antiembolism stockings (TED hose)
  application of, (V1) 934p, (V2) 920p–924p
  as compression device, (V1) 883
  purpose of, (V1) 935f
  surgery preparation, (V1) 935
Antigen, (V1) 402
Antigen-avoidance diet, (V1) 601

Antihistamine
  as preoperative medication, (V1) 935t
  as respiratory medication, (V1) 884
  sexual function and, (V1) 774t
Antihypertensive medication, (V1) 774t, (V1) 926b
Anti-incontinence device, (V1) 648
Antimicrobial spectrum, (V1) 411b
Antipyretic medication, (V1) 314–315
Antiseptic agents, hand-hygiene, (V1) 411t
Antitussive, (V1) 884
Anuria, (V1) 633b
Anus
  assessment of, (V1) 396p, (V2) 330p–331p
  examination of, (V1) 392
  rectum and, (V1) 653
Anxiety
  acute pain and, (V1) 704
  assessment of, (V1) 48
  complementary and alternative medicine (CAM), (V1) 207
  coping with, (V1) 200
  definition of, (V1) 199, (V1) 203
  as an emotional response, (V1) 59
  as factor of urinary retention, (V1) 637
  holistic comfort, (V1) 145
  levels of, (V1) 199–200
  nursing care for, (V1) 202–204
  outcomes and interventions, (V2) 114
  overview of, (V2) 100
  reducing, (V1) 204
  relieving, (V1) 568
  response to stressor, (V1) 558–559
Anxiolytic, (V1) 935t
AORN. See Association of periOperative Registered Nurses (AORN)
The AORN Standards, Recommended Practices and Guidelines, (V1) 923
Aorta, (V1) 853f
Apex, of heart, (V1) 851
Apgar scoring system, (ESG9) 15, (ESG9) 16t
Aphthous ulcer, (V1) 375
Apical pulse
  assessment of, (V1) 311f, (V2) 208p–209p
  locations for, (V1) 320f
  reasons for using, (V1) 319
Apical-radial pulse
  assessment of, (V1) 311f, (V2) 210p–211p
  reasons for using, (V1) 319–320
Apnea
  at birth, (ESG9) 13
  toleration of, (V1) 324
Apothecary system
  conversion of, (V2) 520–521
  for medication dosage, (V1) 492, (V2) 518–519
  metric and household equivalents, (V2) 521
Appeal, (V1) 1081
Appearance, self-concept and, (V1) 189–190
Appendix, (V1) 653
Appetite, improving, (V1) 612–613
Aquapad, (V1) 843f
Arbitration, civil claims, (V1) 1081
Arcus senilis, (V1) 371
Arm exercises, (V1) 757
Army Nursing Service, (V1) 8
Aromatherapy
  common treatments, (V1) 998b
  for disturbed energy field, (V1) 1002
  essential oils, (V1) 687, (V1) 998
Arousal disorder, (V1) 780

Arousal mechanism, (V1) 681–682
Arterial blood gas (ABG)
    acid-base balance, assessment of,
        (V1) 898, (V1) 899t
    adequacy of oxygenation, (V2) 866
    interpretation of, (V1) 899, (V2) 904p
    measurement of, (V1) 868–869
    oxygen and carbon dioxide levels,
        (V1) 326
Arterial oxygen saturation, (V1) 326,
        (V2) 809p–811p
Arterial ulcer, (V1) 815t
Arteriole, (V1) 852
Artery, (V1) 382, (V1) 852
Articular cartilage, (V1) 726
Articulation, of bones, (V1) 726
Artificial airway, (V1) 877–879
Artificial eye, (V1) 467–468, (V1) 468f,
        (V2) 430t
Artificial hypothermia, (V1) 856
Ascending colon, (V1) 653
Ascorbic acid, (V1) 813
Asepsis
    definition of, (V1) 398
    medical, (V1) 408–413
    overview of, (V2) 337
    surgical, (V1) 413–416
As evidenced by (AMB), (V1) 75
Asian/Pacific Islander
    healing system of, (V1) 234t
    sexuality, (V1) 771
    statistics in nursing, (V1) 10t
    types of folk healers, (V1) 230t
ASKED, (V1) 237
Asphyxiation, preventing, (V1) 427
Aspiration
    NIC intervention, (V1) 115t
    precautions for, (V1) 874
    prevention of, (V2) 861tb
Aspiration pneumonia, (V1) 945t
Aspirin
    increasing surgical risk, (V1) 926b
    for pain relief, (V1) 712
    peristalsis and, (V1) 656
Assault and battery, (V1) 1078
Assertiveness
    characteristics of, (V1) 350b
    as communication style, (V1) 350
Assessment
    for abuse, (ESG9) 18p
    of adolescence, (ESG9) 29
    of adult, (ESG9) 32
    age-related changes for, (ESG9) 36t
    of anxiety, (V1) 202–203
        guide for, (V2) 111
        overview of, (V2) 100
    at birth, (ESG9) 15–16
    of blood pressure, (V1) 329–331, (V1) 333
    body composition, (V1) 602–604
    bowel elimination, (V1) 659, (V2) 665
    checklist for, (V1) 294, (V1) 295f
    of child, (ESG9) 26
    collaborative care and, (V1) 39
    collaborative problems, (V1) 61
    of communication, (V1) 348–349
    community-based, (V1) 1029
    computer screen capture of data, (V1) 54f
    concepts of, (V1) 51b, 43
    content and methods of, (V1) 45f
    critical reflection about, (V1) 52–54
    cultural, (V1) 238–239
    database for, (V1) 39

data documentation, (V1) 50, (V1) 52
definition of, (V1) 38
delegation of, (V1) 39–41
of depression, (V2) 100
discharge planning, (V1) 84
documentation of physical findings,
        (V1) 392–393
for dying and grieving, (V1) 276
of elderly, (ESG9) 37–38
of eyes, (V1) 466
for family health status diagnoses,
        (V1) 217–218
fever, (V1) 314–315
flow sheet for, (V1) 53f, (V1) 294,
        (V2) 187
fluid, electrolyte and acid-base
        imbalance, (V1) 901
forms for
    Lawton Instrumental Activities of Daily
        Living, (V2) 26
    Nursing Admission Data Form,
        (V2) 27–30
full-spectrum nursing and, (V1) 34–35
graphic record for, (V1) 53f, (V1) 294
growth and development, (ESG9) 39
guidelines for recording, (V1) 52
of head (HEENT), (V1) 370
health promotion, (V1) 1009,
        (V1) 1012–1013
of hearing, (V1) 373–374
holistic, (V1) 1001
home health care visit, (V1) 1039
of home safety, (V1) 438
of hygiene, (V1) 444
impaired oxygenation, (V1) 861–863
of infant, (ESG9) 18
for infection, (V1) 406–407
intraoperative/postoperative surgery
        phase, (V1) 927
learning, (V1) 537
medical diagnosis, (V1) 59–60
medication-related, (V1) 495
of memory during interview, (V1) 54
of middle adult, (ESG9) 34
Minimum Data Set for Residential
        Assessment and Care Screening
        (MDS), (V1) 299
of mobility and activity, (V1) 740–747
modifying for age groups, (V1) 363–364
musculoskeletal system, (V1) 384–385
of nails, (V1) 369, (V1) 458
nursing diagnosis, (V1) 59
nursing interview, (V1) 46–49
nursing process
    knowledge map of, (V2) 32
    model of, (V1) 31f
    overview of, (V2) 20
nursing process and, (V1) 32, (V1) 32f
nutrition-related problems, (V1) 602
observation, (V1) 44, (V1) 45b
of oral cavity/mouth, (V1) 461
organization of data, (V1) 50
of pain, (V1) 707, (V1) 707b
pain management, (V1) 720–721
peripheral pulse, (V2) 203p–207p
physical, (V1) 44tb–45tb, (V1) 357,
        (V1) 359
for pinworms, (V1) 661
postoperative nursing care, (V1) 943–944
pregnancy, (ESG9) 12
preoperative, (V1) 940
preoperative form for, (V1) 928f–929f

of preschooler, (ESG9) 23–24
professional standards, (V1) 39, (V1) 40b
of pulse, (V1) 318–321
reflecting critically about, (V1) 52–54
relating to other phases of nursing
        process, (V1) 38
of respiration, (V1) 324–326
review of, (V1) 135–136
self-concept and self-esteem, (V1) 193
sensory perception, (V1) 689–690
sexual health, (V1) 781
of skin, (V1) 448–449, (V2) 239p–243p
skin cancer, (V1) 368
sleep patterns, (V1) 804
spiritual
    guidelines for, (V2) 151–152
    overview of, (V2) 147
    tools for, (V1) 256
of stoma, (V1) 671–672, (V1) 671f
of stress, (V1) 564–565
of teeth, (V1) 375
temperature, (V1) 310–314, (V2)
        198p–199p
of toddler, (ESG9) 21
tools for recording, (V1) 52
types of, (V1) 42–44
urinary elimination, (V1) 626
using to promote health, (V1) 181–182
validation of data, (V1) 49–50
of vital signs (VS), (V1) 305
of wounds, (V1) 825–826
Assessment continuum, depression,
        (V1) 205f
Assessment data, (V1) 132
Assimilation, (V1) 167, (ESG9) 5
Assisted suicide, (V1) 273, (V1) 275,
        (V1) 1077
Associate degree (AD), (V1) 14, (V1) 155
Association of periOperative Registered
        Nurses (AORN), (V1) 923
    development of PNDS, (V1) 926–927
    patient-focused model, (V1) 927f
    preoperative assessment for,
        (V1) 928f–929f
Assumption
    analyzing, (V1) 30t, (V1) 31
        biases affecting goal achievement,
        (V1) 136
        for intervention selection, (V1) 112
    as component of theory, (V1) 141
    model of critical thinking, (V1) 31f,
Asthma
    in child, (ESG9) 25
    definition of, (V1) 856
    fungus and mold, (V1) 857
    peak flow meter, (V1) 870f
Astigmatism, (V1) 685b
Asystole (cardiac standstill), (V1) 273
Atelectasis
    as postoperative collaborative problem,
        (V1) 945t
    pulmonary system and, (V1) 860
    respiratory distress syndrome and,
        (V1) 854
Atherosclerosis, obesity and, (V1) 857
Atmospheric pressure, (V1) 856
Atomizer, (V1) 504
Atria, (V1) 851
Atrial natriuretic factor (ANF), (V1) 891
Atrio-ventricular (AV) node, (V1) 852
Atrophy, (V1) 740b
Attachment, (ESG9) 15

Attitude
  in critical thinking, (V1) 27
  definition of, (V1) 1051
Attorney, durable power of, (V1) 273,
    (V1) 1073
Attuning, (V1) 181, (V1) 182
Audiovisual material, (V1) 544–545
Auditory deficit, intervention, (V1) 695
Audit trail, EHR ethics and, (V1) 981
Auscultation
  of abdomen, (V1) 383
  of blood pressure, (V1) 331, (V1) 331f
  cardiac sites for, (V1) 381f
  of client for physical examination,
      (V1) 363
  of major arteries, (V1) 384
  physical assessment, (V1) 45
  for physical assessment, (V2) 230t
  physical assessment, (V2) 234t
  pulse rate assessment, (V1) 318
  using palpation with, (V1) 333
Auscultatory gap, (V1) 333
Authentic, (V1) 153
Authoritarian leadership, (V1) 954
Authority, gaining knowledge by, (V1) 155
Autocratic leadership, (V1) 954
Autogenic training, (V2) 964tb
Autoimmune reaction theory, (ESG9) 35
Autolysis, (V1) 836
Automated dispensing system, (V1) 478,
    (V1) 478f
Automatic stop dates, (V1) 494
Autonomic nervous system
  cardiovascular function and,
      (V1) 853–854
  respiration regulation, (V1) 322
  sympathetic and parasympathetic, (V1) 728
Autonomy
  of an activity, (V1) 105
  definition of, (V1) 1052t
  in nursing, (V1) 22
  principle of, (V1) 1055
  shame and doubt versus, (V1) 167
Autonomy model, (V1) 1068
Autopsy, (V1) 275
Avoidance
  as phase of grieving, (V1) 266
  psychological defense mechanism,
      (V1) 560t
Axillae, assessment, (V2) 275p–279p
Axillary crutch, (V1) 759
Axillary temperature, (V1) 313
Ayurveda
  as complementary and alternative medi-
      cine (CAM), (V1) 235
  core belief, (V1) 992
  defining health, (V1) 171b
Ayurvedic medicine, (V1) 252

B
Babinski reflex, (ESG9) 14
Baby-bottle tooth decay, (V1) 459
Baccalaureate degree, (V1) 14, (V1) 155
Back
  injury to, (V1) 437
  massage of, (V1) 455, (V1) 806p, (V2)
      748p–750p
  preventing injury, (V1) 748
"Back to Sleep" campaign, (ESG9) 18f
Bacteremia, (V1) 401
Bacterial infection, (V1) 399
Bag bath, (V1) 452

Baha'i, (V1) 252
Balance
  achievement of, (V1) 729–730
  assessment of, (V1) 385
  Ayurveda and, (V1) 992
  traditional Chinese medicine (TCM),
      (V1) 992–993
Balanitis, (V1) 780
BALI, for culturally competent care, (V1) 243
Ball-and-socket joint, (V1) 728t, (V1) 745t
Bandage
  application of, (V2) 788tb–790tb
  types of, (V1) 842
Barbiturates
  as preoperative medication, (V1) 935t
  as sleep aid, (V1) 808
Bargaining, collective, (V1) 21
Barium enema (BE), (V2) 667
Baroreceptor, (V1) 854
Barotrauma, (V1) 880
Barton, Clara, (V1) 8, (V1) 1025
Basal metabolic rate (BMR)
  calculation of, (V1) 593b
  definition of, (V1) 592
  factors affecting, (V1) 592–593
  factors influencing, (V1) 308
  overweight and obesity, (V1) 609
Base
  of heart, (V1) 851
  hydrogen ions, binding with, (V1) 895
  of support, (V1) 730, (V1) 730f
Basic needs
  as document in care plan, (V1) 86
  of patient at discharge, (V1) 85
Basic one-part statement, (V1) 74t, (V1) 75
Basic three-part statement, (V1) 74t, (V1) 75
Basic two-part statement, (V1) 74t, (V1) 75
Basophil, (V1) 403t
Bathing
  as activity of daily living (ADL), (V1) 43b
  bed bath, (V2) 384p–395p
  as NIC intervention, (V1) 114b
  packaged bath, (V2) 397p–398p
  patients with dementia, (V1) 454–455
  rationale for, (V1) 450
  self-care deficit, (V1) 445, (V2) 434
  shower or tub, (V2) 429tb
  skin integrity, (V1) 814
  towel bath, (V2) 396p–397p
  types of, (V1) 450–454
Battery, (V1) 1078
Battle-ax, (V1) 7
B cell lymphocyte
  function of, (V1) 402, (V1) 403t
  secretion of immunoglobins, (V1) 403
Beard care, (V1) 465, (V2) 418p–419p
Bed
  adjustable, (V1) 749
  alarm, (V1) 434
  bath, (V1) 450
  bathing procedure, (V2) 384p–395p
  dangling patient at side of, (V2) 709p
  mattress replacement, (V1) 832–833
  monitoring device, (V2) 369p–371p
  moving in, teaching patient,
      (V2) 918p–921p
  occupied, making, (V2) 427p–428p
  positioning patient in, (V1) 750t–752t,
      (V1) 752–753, (V2) 699p–704p
  logrolling, (V2) 703p–704p
  moving and turning, (V2) 699p–702p
  scheduled changes in, (V1) 832b

specialized, (V1) 833
  transferring patient, (V1) 754–756,
      (V2) 704p–711p
  to chair, (V2) 709p–710p
  to stretcher, (V2) 706p–708p
  unoccupied, making, (V2) 424p–426p
Bedpan, (V1) 662p, (V2) 643p–645p
Bedwetting
  management of, (V1) 648
  overview of, (V1) 623, (V1) 637
  as parasomnia, (V1) 803
Behavior
  active listening, (V1) 49, (V1) 349–350
  assessment of low self-esteem, (V1) 193
  avoiding maladaptive, (V1) 568
  belief, values and experience affecting
      nurse, (V1) 68–69
  general survey of client, (V1) 365
  grief and, (V1) 269t
  illness and, (V1) 179–180
  instincts of, (V1) 166–167
  moral, (V1) 1045
  in nursing, (V1) 16b
  pain and, (V1) 706b
  pain influencing, (V1) 704
  professional values and, (V1) 1052t
  response to stressor, (V1) 565
  risk-taking, (V1) 214, (ESG9) 26
  sexual, inappropriate, (V1) 790–791
  stress-related, (V1) 559b
  substance abuse, (V1) 719
  of transformational leadership, (V1) 955t
Behavioral psychiatric diagnosis, (V1) 195
Behavioral theory, (V1) 954
Belief
  affecting nurse behavior, (V1) 68–69
  definition of, (V1) 227, (V1) 1051
  of North American healthcare system,
      (V1) 233t
  refuting currently held, (V1) 964
Belief system, health, (V1) 231
Bell's palsy, (V2) 252
Beneficence, principle, (V1) 1055
Benevolence, (V1) 259
Benner, Dr. Patricia, (V1) 15, (V1) 140,
      (V1) 146–147
Benzodiazepines, (V1) 807
Bereavement
  mourning and adjustment time for,
      (V1) 265
  theory about, (V1) 145
Bertalanfly, Ludwig von, (V1) 151
Beside urine testing, (V1) 634
Beta-adrenergic agent, (V1) 884
Beta-adrenergic blocking agent, (V1) 859
Beta-blocker, (V1) 800
Beta endorphins, (V1) 702
Beta wave, (V1) 796, (V1) 796f
Bhagavad Gita, (V1) 252
Bias
  as barrier to culturally competent care,
      (V1) 237
  definition of, (V1) 69
  NANDA nursing diagnosis with potential
      for, (V1) 240b
  personal, (V1) 254
Bible, (V1) 251
Bicarbonate (HCO₃⁻), (V1) 893t
Bicultural, (V1) 224
Bier intravenous block, (V1) 938–939
Bilateral equality, (V1) 321

Bile salts, (V1) 654
Bilirubin, (ESG9) 15
Bill of Rights, patient, (V1) 529, (V1) 1061, (V1) 1072
Bill of Rights for Nurses, (V1) 1077, (V1) 1087
Bimanual exam, (V2) 329
Binder, application of, (V2) 786tb–788tb
Binge drinking, (ESG9) 28
Bioelectrical impedance, (V1) 603
Bioelectromagnetic therapy, (V1) 999
Bioethics, (V1) 1046
Biofeedback
    for disturbed energy field, (V1) 1002
    for stress management, (V1) 570
    technique for, (V1) 996
    for urinary incontinence, (V1) 647
Biofield therapy, (V1) 999
Biographical data, (V1) 46
Biological agent, outbreak prevention, (V1) 417
Biological half-life, of medication, (V1) 486
Biological integrity, threat to, (V1) 167
Biologically based therapy, (V1) 996–998
Biological variations
    culture care etiquette, (V1) 242t
    as culture specific influencing health, (V1) 229
Biomedical healthcare system, (V1) 231
Biopsy, renal, (V2) 633
Biopsychosocial, (V1) 187, (V1) 188f
Biorhythms, (V1) 795
Bioterrorism, preventing, (V1) 417
Biotransformation, (V1) 485
Birth
    assessment of newborn, (ESG9) 15–16
    health promotion and screenings, (V1) 1010t
    injuries, (ESG9) 15
    premature, (ESG9) 13
    sexual development, (V1) 768
    vaginal, (ESG9) 13
Birth control. See Contraception
Birth defect, (ESG9) 15
Birth rite, (V1) 227
Bisexuality, (V1) 768
Blackwell, Elizabeth, (V1) 6
Bladder
    infection of (cystitis), (V1) 623, (V1) 635–636
    irrigation of, (V1) 644, (V1) 645
        continuous, (V2) 613p–615p
        intermittent, (V2) 610p–612p
    storing urine, (V1) 621–622
Blastocyst, (ESG9) 8
Blended family, (V1) 210
Blister, (V2) 244
Blood
    clot prevention, (V1) 154
    crossmatching and typing, (V1) 919, (V1) 919t
    flow of, (V1) 328, (V1) 484
    loss and pulse rate, (V1) 318
    types of, (V1) 919, (V1) 919t
    viscosity of, (V1) 328
    volume of, (V1) 328
Bloodborne pathogen, exposure to, (V1) 416–417
Blood-brain barrier, (V1) 484
Blood glucose, (V1) 605, (V2) 563p–566p
Blood pressure (BP)
    accurate measurement of, (V2) 217tb
    assessment of, (V1) 311f, (V2) 214p–217p

    auscultation of, (V1) 331, (V1) 331f, (V1) 333
    bladder size of cuff, (V1) 332t
    cuff size, (V1) 330–331, (V1) 331f,
    equipment for assessment, (V1) 329–331
    factors influencing, (V1) 328–329
    measurement of, (V1) 326–327
    normal reading for, (V1) 306t, (V1) 327
    overview of, (V2) 191
    palpation of, (V1) 333
    regulation of, (V1) 328
    self-monitoring, (V1) 332
    sites for measurement of, (V1) 331
    as vital sign (VS), (V1) 305
Blood product
    replacement of, (V1) 918
    types of, (V1) 919–920
Blood transfusion
    administration of, (V1) 914p, (V2) 898p–903p
    initiation of, (V1) 920
    reactions from, (V1) 920–921, (V1) 920t
Blood urea nitrogen (BUN)
    normal ranges for, (V2) 631–632
    protein metabolism and, (V1) 605
    renal function and hydration, (V1) 635
Blood vessel
    immobility, effects on, (V1) 739
    pulmonary and systemic, (V1) 852
    size affecting blood flow, (V1) 328
Bloom's domains of learning, (V1) 531t
Board of registered nursing (BRN)
    continuing education requirements, (V1) 15
    responsibilities of, (V1) 16
Body alignment, (V1) 729
Body appearance
    changes in, (V1) 191
    as component of self-concept, (V1) 191
    general survey of client, (V1) 365
    reassessment of, (V1) 133tb
    shape and symmetry of, (V1) 384–385
    water for, (V1) 582
Body-based therapy, (V1) 998
Body composition
    analysis of, (V1) 594, (V1) 602–604
    measuring circumference, (V2) 579tb
Body fluid
    compartments of, (V1) 887–888
    composition of, (V1) 888
    distribution in body, (V1) 888f
    function of, (V1) 887
    imbalance of, (V1) 896, (V1) 904
    movement of, (V1) 889
    overview of, (V2) 871
    See also Fluid
Body function
    drug absorption, (V1) 484
    pain and, (V1) 706, (V1) 706b
    pain reaction, (V1) 705
    prolonging, (V1) 273
    reassessment of, (V1) 133tb
    reproduction and, (V1) 788
    self-concept and, (V1) 191
    stressor response, (V1) 555–556
    temperature regulation, (V1) 307
Body image
    assessment of, (V2) 108
    disturbed, (V1) 195
    as etiology, (V1) 195–196
    ideal and perceived, (V1) 190
    influence on health, (V1) 191

    as problem, (V1) 195
    promotion of positive, (V1) 197–198
Body language, (V1) 350–351
Body mass, (V1) 487
Body mass index (BMI)
    calculation of, (V1) 603b
    chart for, (V2) 239
    of child, (ESG9) 26
    classification of, (V2) 586
    definition of, (V1) 366
    ranges and values, (V1) 603
Body mechanics
    components of, (V1) 729–730
    guidelines for, (V1) 730–731
Body mechanics, principles of, (V2) 716tb
Body surface area (BSA), (V2) 521
Body system
    client review, (V1) 47
    disease affecting mobility, (V1) 738–739
    growth and function of, (V1) 166
    surgery classification, (V1) 924–925
    vital signs (VS) of, (V1) 305
Body system approach, (V1) 359–360
Body systems framework, (V1) 50
Body temperature. See Temperature
Bolus, (V1) 519, (V1) 615
Bone
    characteristics of, (V1) 725–726, (V1) 726f
    formation abnormalities, (V1) 737
    immobility, effects on, (V1) 739
    integrity of, (V1) 738
    tumor of, (V1) 738
Bone density scan (DEXA test), (ESG9) 34
Borg Rate of Perceived Exertion Scale, (V1) 732b
Boundary, geopolitical, (V1) 1022, (V1) 1022f
Bowel diversion
    conditions requiring, (V1) 657
    intervention for, (V1) 672
    locations for, (V1) 658f
    overview of, (V2) 636
    patient care, (V1) 671–672
Bowel elimination
    assessment of, (V1) 659, (V2) 665
    diagnostic testing for, (V1) 660–661
    outcomes and interventions for, (V2) 669–670
    overview of, (V2) 636
    process of, (V1) 654
Bowel incontinence
    care map for, (V1) 674–675
    management of, (V1) 670–671
    nursing care plan for, (V1) 673–675
    outcomes and interventions for, (V2) 669
Bowel movement (BM), (V1) 654, (V2) 636
Bowel sounds, (V1) 383, (V1) 659
Bowel training, (V1) 671
Bowlby, John, (V1) 266, (V1) 266t
Bowleg (genu verum), (V2) 301
Bowman's capsule, (V1) 620
Brace, for walking, (V1) 759
Brachial artery, (V1) 319, (V1) 319f, (V2) 205
Braden scale, (V1) 823, (V1) 824f
Bradycardia, (V1) 320
Bradykinin, tissue damage, (V1) 701
Bradypnea, (V1) 324
Brain
    hypothalamus of, (V1) 307
    respiratory centers in, (V1) 322
    sensory areas, (V1) 681f
Brain stem, (V1) 270, (V1) 854

Brain wave, (V1) 796, (V1) 796f
Brand name, (V1) 474
Break-through pain, (V1) 713
Breastfeeding
    ineffective, (V1) 66, (V1) 109
    of newborn, (ESG9) 14
Breasts
    assessment of, (V1) 394, (V2) 275p–279p
    characteristics of, (V1) 376–377
    photo of, (V1) 377f
Breast self-exam (BSE)
    in adolescence, (ESG9) 30b
    controversy about, (V1) 376–377,
        (V1) 1013, (ESG9) 31
    self-care and, (V1) 53
    teaching about, (V1) 789
    in young adult, (ESG9) 32
Breathing
    abnormal sounds from, (V1) 325, (V1) 380
    assessment of, (V1) 862, (V2) 860tb
    chest tube, monitoring, (V1) 882
    control of, (V1) 850–851
    deep, (V1) 875
    halitosis, (V1) 460
    mechanics of, (V1) 322–323
    normal sounds from, (V1) 379–380,
        (V1) 379f
    stimulus for, (V1) 322
Brevity, in communication, (V1) 341
Brewster, Mary, (V1) 9
Bricker's loop, (V1) 638
Bright, Mary Anne, (V1) 23
British Pharmacopoeia, (V1) 475
Bronchial asthma, (V1) 803
Bronchial breath sounds, (V1) 379, (V1) 379f
Bronchioles, (V1) 846f, (V1) 847
Bronchodilator, (V1) 884
Bronchospasm, (V1) 847
Bronchovesicular breath sounds, (V1) 379f,
        (V1) 380
Bronchus, (V1) 846–847, (V1) 846f
Broussat, Frederic and Mary Ann, (V1) 248
Bruise (contusion), (V1) 814, (V1) 815t
Bruit, (V1) 382, (V2) 289
Brushing teeth, (V1) 462, (V2) 406p–408p
Bruxism, (V1) 803
Buccal medication, (V1) 500
Buccal mucosa, (V1) 375
Buddha, (V1) 252f
Buddhism, (V1) 252
Buffer system, (V1) 895
Building the Future, (ESGV1) 13
Bulimia nervosa, (V1) 190, (ESG9) 29
Burnout, (V1) 564
Burns, (V1) 425
Butterfly needle, (V1) 906–907, (V1) 907f

C
Cable, (V1) 974
Caffeine, sleep and, (V1) 800
Calcium (Ca²⁺)
    deficiency, (V1) 737
    fluid and electrolyte balance, (V1) 904
    function and regulation of, (V1) 892t
    osteoporosis, (V1) 582
    recommended intake of, (V1) 894, (V1) 894t
Calcium channel blocking agent, (V1) 859
Callings, (V1) 249
Callus, (V1) 455
Calming, (V2) 964tb
Calorie, (V1) 591–592
Calorie-protein diet, (V1) 601

Calorie-restricted diet, (V1) 601
Calorimeter, (V1) 592
Calyx, (V1) 620
Campinha-Bacote culturally competent
        model of, (V1) 237
Canada's Food Guide for Healthy Eating,
        (V1) 587, (V1) 588f
Canada's Health Care Providers, (ESGV1) 13
Canada Health Act
    aim of, (ESGV1) 3–4
    dispute resolution, (ESGV1) 8
    federal government, role of, (ESGV1) 5–6
    home health care coverage, (ESGV1) 20
    legislation, (ESGV1) 6
    long-term care facility coverage, (ESGV1)
        19
    overview of, (ESG46 V2) 1
    principles of, (ESGV1) 4–5, (ESGV1) 4t
    services defined in, (ESGV1) 4
Canadian Commonwealth Conference (CCF),
        (ESG46 V1) 2
Canadian constitution, (ESGV1) 3
Canadian Federation of Nurses Unions,
        (ESGV1) 24
Canadian Formulary, (V1) 475
Canadian healthcare delivery system
    components of, (ESGV1) 17–18
    financial stability of, (ESGV1) 21–23
    governance and management of,
        (ESGV1) 5
    health human resources in, (ESGV1)
        13–17
    history of, (ESG46 V1) 1
    overview of, (ESG46 V2) 1
Canadian Institute of Health Information
        (CIHI), (ESGV1) 26
Canadian Narcotic Control Act, (V1) 477
Canadian Nurse, (V1) 18
Canadian Nurses Association (CNA)
    Canada Health Act, (ESGV1) 24
    code of ethics, (V1) 1059, (V1) 1060b
    definition of nursing, (V1) 11
    nursing process, (V1) 31
    professional standards for
        assessment, (V1) 39, (V1) 40b
        diagnosing, (V1) 57b
        planning outcomes, (V1) 83b
        standards of practice, (V1) 16, (V1) 18b
Canadian Nursing Advisory Committee
        (CNAC), (ESGV1) 26–27
Canadian Occupational Nurses Association,
        (ESGV1) 20
Cancer
    bone, (V1) 738
    cervical, (ESG9) 32
    lung, (V1) 857
    of middle adult, (ESG9) 34
    of oral cavity, (V1) 460–461
    research for cause of, (V1) 399
    signs of malignancy, (V1) 368
Cancer Care Manitoba Act, (ESGV1) 8
Cancer Program Act, (ESGV1) 8
Cane
    characteristics of, (V1) 758
    teaching patient to use, (V2) 719tb–720tb
    types of, (V1) 758f
Canker sore, (V1) 375
Cannula
    adding medication to IV bag/bottle, (V1)
        519, (V1) 519f
    for oxygen administration, (V2)
        819p–822-p

Capillary, (V1) 852
    hemangioma, (V2) 333
    refill test, (V2) 292
Caput succedaneum, (ESG9) 15
Car accident, (V1) 428–429
Carbohydrate (CHO)
    catabolism of, (V1) 308
    chemical structures of, (V1) 577
    as energy nutrient, (V1) 576t
    function of, (V1) 577
    types of, (V1) 577f
Carbon dioxide (CO₂)
    change in concentration, (V1) 322
    diffusion of, (V1) 850, (V1) 853
    measurement of, (V1) 326
    transportation of, (V1) 853
Carbon dioxide narcosis, (V1) 859
Carbonic acid (H₂CO₃), (V1) 895
Carbonic acid-sodium bicarbonate system,
        (V1) 895
Carbon monoxide
    oxygenation and, (V1) 861
    poisoning by, (V1) 424
Cardia ischemia, (V1) 860
Cardiac arrest
    DNR and DNAR orders, (V1) 273
    signs of, (V1) 885
Cardiac cycle, (V1) 852
Cardiac function, (V1) 328
Cardiac monitor, (V1) 864p, (V2)
        812p–814p
Cardiac muscle, (V1) 727
Cardiac output, (V1) 317, (V1) 328
Cardiac sphincter, (V1) 651
Cardiac standstill (asystole), (V1) 273
Cardiomyopathy, (V1) 860
Cardiopulmonary resuscitation (CPR)
    DNAR order, (V1) 273, (V1) 274f, (V1)
        275b, (V2) 158
    DNR order, (V1) 273, (V1) 274f
    one- and two-person, (V2) 855p–859p
    performance of, (V1) 885
Cardiorespiratory fitness, (V1) 1009
Cardiovascular depressant, (V1) 859
Cardiovascular disease (CVD)
    increasing surgical risk, (V1) 926b
Cardiovascular system
    abnormalities of, (V1) 860–861
    adaptation failure and, (V1) 562
    age-related changes for, (ESG9) 36t
    auscultation sites, (V1) 381f
    benefits of exercise, (V1) 734b
    at birth, (ESG9) 13
    cardiac cycle, (V1) 380
    cardiac landmarks, (V1) 380–381
    injury from exercise, (V1) 733
    pain and, (V1) 706
    regulating function of, (V1) 853–854
    structures of
        coronary arteries, (V1) 853
        heart, (V1) 851–852
        systemic and pulmonary blood vessels,
            (V1) 852–853
    of toddler, (ESG9) 19
Care
    effect of organization characteristics on
        quality of, (V1) 131
    end-of-life, (V1) 20
        barrier to communication, (V1) 282b
        competencies of, (V1) 271–272
        hospice care, (V1) 273–274
        palliative care, (V1) 272–273

Care (continued)
  expanded variety of settings for, (V1) 22
  for family of patient, (V1) 153
  guidelines for documenting, (V1) 301–302
  holistic, (V1) 28–29
  hygiene, (V1) 446
  postmortem, (V1) 285
  purpose for, (V1) 19–20
  recipients for, (V1) 19
  transpersonal, (V1) 153
Career, community nursing, (V1) 1027–1029
Caregiver
  role strain, (V1) 1039–1040
  See also Family; Nurse; Support system
Care plan
  charting summary, (V1) 297
  comprehensive, (V1) 85
    components of, (V1) 86f
    documents in, (V1) 85–86
    information in, (V1) 85
    nursing diagnosis standardized form,
        (V1) 88f
    Patient Care Protocol, (V1) 87f
    preprinted, standardized plans,
        (V1) 86–87, (V1) 89
  evaluation and revision of, (V1) 135–136
  failure to implement, malpractice,
      (V1) 1082
  goals and outcomes, (V1) 93
  growth and development of client, (V1) 165
  individualized, (V1) 89–90, (V1) 92
  information in, (V2) 44
  integrated, (V1) 89
  nursing, (V1) 91
  problem-oriented records, (V1) 290
  research-based, (V1) 28
  standardized
    adapting to patient needs, (V1) 89
    computer printout for, (V1) 88f
    individualizing, (V1) 92
  steps of, (V1) 82–85
  for stress urinary incontinence,
      (V1) 627–630
  student, (V1) 91–92
    individualized, (V1) 89, (V1) 91
    as learning activity, (V1) 91
    mind-mapping, (V1) 91–92
Caries, (V1) 460, (V1) 462, (ESG9) 17
Caring processes, (V2) 77
Carminative enema, (V1) 668–669
Carotid artery
  pulse rate assessment, (V1) 319,
      (V1) 319f, (V2) 205
  turbulence in, (V1) 382
Carotid stenosis, (V1) 382
Carpuject prefilled system, (V1) 508–509
Carrier, disease, (V1) 399
Cartilage, (V1) 376, (V1) 376f
Cartilage rings, (V1) 847
Case-based instruction, (V1) 36
Case manager, (V1) 13t
Catabolism
  of amino acid, (V1) 578
  energy release and, (V1) 577
  of fats and carbohydrates, (V1) 308
Cataplexy, (V1) 802
Cataract, (V1) 371, (V1) 685b
Catecholamine, (V1) 855
Categorical imperative, (V1) 1057
Catherization
  definition of, (V1) 640–641
  supplies for, (V1) 643, (V1) 643f

Catheter
  central venous, (V1) 616, (V1) 907–908
  external (condom) application, (V2)
      616p–618p
  indwelling, (V1) 632, (V1) 632f
  insertion of, (V1) 643, (V1) 645
  inside-the-needle, (V1) 906, (V1) 906f
  irrigation of, (V1) 644, (V1) 645, (V2)
      610p–612p
  midline peripheral, (V1) 907
  nontunneled central venous,
      (V1) 907–908
  over-the-needle, (V1) 906, (V1) 906f
  as risk factor for UTI, (V1) 636
  suctioning, (V1) 879f
  types of, (V1) 640–641, (V1) 641f,
      (V1) 643, (V1) 643f
  urinary, insertion of, (V2) 598p–609p
  urine specimen from, (V2) 620tb
Catheter embolus, (V1) 917t
Cation, (V1) 888
Caucasian
  statistics in nursing, (V1) 10t
  types of folk healers, (V1) 230t
Cause-and-effect relationship, avoiding,
      (V1) 195
Cavity, (V1) 460
CCC. See Clinical Care Classification
CDC. See Center for Disease Control (CDC)
C-delta fiber, (V1) 701–702, (V1) 702f,
      (V1) 703f
Cecum, (V1) 653
Celibacy, (V1) 778
Cell-mediated immunity, (V1) 404
Cellular-capillary membrane, (V1) 853
Cellular malfunction theory, (ESG9) 35
Cellulose, (V1) 577f
Celsius scale, (V1) 310
Census, (V1) 1021–1022, (V1) 1022f
Census tract, (V1) 1022, (V1) 1022f
Centenarians, (ESG9) 35
Center for Disease Control (CDC)
  sexually transmitted infection (STI),
      (V1) 778
  tier one: standard precautions, (V1) 410
  tier two: transmission-based precautions,
      (V1) 412
Center of gravity, (V1) 730, (V1) 730f
Centigrade scale, (V1) 310, (V1) 312, (V2) 219
Central chemoreceptor, (V1) 322
Central line, (V1) 907
Central nervous system (CNS)
  acupuncture and, (V1) 994
  disorder affecting mobility, (V1) 738
  pain modulation, (V1) 702, (V1) 703f
  restless leg syndrome (RLS), (V1) 801
Central sleep apnea (CSA), (V1) 802
Central venous access device (CVAD),
      (V1) 907–908, (V1) 909f
Central venous catheter (CVS)
  parenteral nutrition, (V1) 616
  types of, (V1) 907–908
Central vessels, (V1) 382, (V1) 382f
Cephalocaudal pattern of growth, (V1) 166,
      (ESG9) 3
Cerebellar function, (V1) 389–390
Cerebral cortex, (V1) 555
Cerebrospinal fluid (CSF), injection to,
      (V1) 939, (V1) 939f
Cerebrovascular accident (CVA), (V1) 64
Certification, (ESGV1) 9, (V1) 1075
Certified nursing assistant, (ESGV1) 17

Cerumen (wax)
  impaction of, (V1) 468
  protecting middle ear, (V1) 373
Cervical cancer, (ESG9) 32
Cervical lymph nodes, (V1) 376, (V1) 376f,
      (V2) 272
Chain of infection, (V1) 398, (V1) 399f
Change
  implementation of, (V1) 964
  integration of, (V1) 964–965
  management of, (V1) 963–964
  model of, (V1) 1007–1008
  resistance to, (V1) 963–964
  strategy to reduce resistance to,
      (V1) 965b
Change agent, (V1) 13t
Change-of-shift report, (V1) 299–300,
      (V2) 182
Channel, (V1) 340
Channels (meridians), (V1) 993
Charaka and Samhita, (V1) 4
Chart audit, (V1) 289
Charting
  assessment flow sheet, (V2) 187
  computerized, (V1) 298
  delegation of, (V1) 302
  intake and output (I&O), (V2) 188
  long-term care flow sheet, (V2) 186
  mechanics of, (V2) 183
  for minimizing malpractice, (V1) 1084
  pressure ulcers healing, (V1) 828f
  types of, (V1) 291–293
Charting by exception (CBE), (V1) 292–293,
      (V2) 178
Checklist
  for evaluation, (V2) 69–71
  example of, (V1) 295f
  for home safety, (V2) 379–380
  recording assessments and care, (V1) 294
Cheilosis, (V1) 460
Chelation therapy, (V1) 997
Chemical digestion, (V1) 651
Chemical name, (V1) 474
Chemical pain relief, (V1) 716–717
Chemicals, oxygenation and, (V1) 857
Chemical stimuli, (V1) 701
Chemical thermometer, (V1) 311, (V1) 312f,
      (V2) 201p
Chemoreceptor
  central and peripheral, (V1) 322
  function of, (V1) 850, (V1) 854
  locations for, (V1) 681
Chemotherapeutic effect, (V1) 488
Chemotherapy, sexual function and,
      (V1) 774t
Cheng, Nien, (V1) 175
Chest
  assessment of, (V1) 394p–395p,
      (V2) 280p–286p
  barrel chest, (V1) 379f
  drainage system, (V1) 881–882, (V1) 881f,
  excursion of, (V2) 283
  imaginary lines describing locations of,
      (V1) 377, (V1) 377f, (V1) 378,
      (V1) 378f
  landmarks of, (V1) 377, (V1) 377f,
      (V1) 378f
  movement of, (V1) 325–326
  percussion of, (V1) 875, (V1) 875f
  shape and size of, (V1) 378
  vibration of, (V1) 875, (V1) 875f
Chest physiotherapy, (V1) 875

Chest tube, *(V1)* 881–882, *(V2)* 850p–855p
Chi. *See* Qi
Child
    assessment of, *(V1)* 364, *(ESG9)* 26
    bowel elimination patterns, *(V1)* 655
    bruit, *(V2)* 289
    chest size and shape, *(V1)* 378
    Clark's rule, *(V2)* 522
    death of, *(V1)* 268
    depression in, *(V1)* 202
    development of task theory, *(ESG9)* 4t
    developmental *(ESG9)* 24–26
    diabetes mellitus, type II, *(ESG9)* 25
    drug therapy for, *(V1)* 487t
    fire death, *(V1)* 425
    fremitus of, *(V2)* 284
    gender identity, *(V1)* 767
    genu verum (bowlegs), *(V2)* 301
    grief and development, *(V1)* 267
    health problems, *(ESG9)* 25
    health promotion and screenings,
        (V1) 1010t
    heart sounds of, *(V2)* 290
    immunization schedule, *(ESG9)* 19f
    injection, administering, *(V1)* 512
    intervention for, *(ESG9)* 26
    liver of, *(V2)* 298
    lordosis, *(V2)* 301
    loss, dealing with, *(V1)* 285
    memory assessment of, *(V2)* 310
    milestones of, *(ESG9)* 25b
    nails of, *(V2)* 249
    nature versus nurture, *(V1)* 165
    nutritional needs, *(V1)* 595–596
    oral hygiene for, *(V1)* 462–463
    oral medication administration, *(V1)* 501
    oxygenation of, *(V1)* 855
    pain assessment, *(V1)* 704, *(V1)* 707
    pain scale, *(V1)* 707
    poisoning of, *(V1)* 422, *(V1)* 422b
    promotion of self-esteem to, *(V1)* 198
    rectal suppository administration,
        (V2) 475
    restless leg syndrome (RLS), *(V1)* 801
    safety of, *(V1)* 421
    same-gender friendships, *(ESG9)* 24f
    sensory stimulation needs, *(V1)* 682
    sexual development, *(V1)* 768–769
    skin of, *(V1)* 812
    sleep
        patterns of, *(V1)* 799
        requirements for, *(V1)* 795t
    stressors of, *(V1)* 552b
    suffocation and asphyxiation prevention,
        (V1) 427
    suicide of, *(V1)* 422
    teaching, *(V1)* 535
    teeth development, *(V1)* 459, *(V1)* 459f
    urinary elimination, *(V1)* 623
Child abuse, *(ESG9)* 17, *(ESG9)* 18p
Chiropractic adjustment
    as CAM therapy, *(V1)* 998
    for stress management, *(V1)* 570
Chlamydia, *(V1)* 778
Chloride (Cl⁻)
    function and regulation of, *(V1)* 893t
    recommended intake of, *(V1)* 894
Cholesterol
    chemical structure for, *(V1)* 579f
    importance of, *(V1)* 579
    skin breakdown, *(V1)* 813
Christian era, spirituality during, *(V1)* 246

Christian hospital, *(V1)* 4
Christianity, *(V1)* 5, *(V1)* 251
Christian Science, *(V1)* 251
Chromosome, *(V1)* 766f
Chromosome, X and Y, *(V1)* 766
Chronic grief, *(V1)* 268
Chronic illness, *(V1)* 180, *(ESG9)* 25
Chronic infection, *(V1)* 401
Chronic obstructive pulmonary disease
        (COPD)
    barrel chest, *(V1)* 378, *(V1)* 379f
    hypoventilation and, *(V1)* 326
    as sleep-provoked disorder, *(V1)* 803
Chronic pain
    depression and, *(V1)* 704
    duration of, *(V1)* 700
    outcomes and interventions for,
        (V2) 695
Chronic renal failure, *(V1)* 59
Chronic wound, *(V1)* 814, *(V1)* 815t
Church of Jesus Christ of Latter-Day Saints,
        (V1) 251
Chvostek's sign, assessment for, *(V2)* 903p
Chyme, *(V1)* 652
Cilia, *(V1)* 845
CINAHL (Cumulative Index to Nursing and
        Allied Health Literature), *(V1)* 161,
        (V2) 949
Circadian rhythm
    body temperature and, *(V1)* 310
    disorder of, *(V1)* 801
    sleep and, *(V1)* 795
Circulating nurse, *(V1)* 937
Circulation
    impaired, diagnoses for, *(V2)* 868
    of newborn, *(ESG9)* 13
    pressure ulcers and, *(V1)* 449,
        (V1) 456
    problems of, *(V1)* 872
    promoting, *(V1)* 883
    skin and, *(V1)* 448
    types of, *(V1)* 380
Circulatory system, *(V1)* 813
Circumcision
    as culture specific, *(V1)* 227
    of female, *(V1)* 772
    of male, *(V1)* 390
Circumduction
    assessment of, *(V2)* 305p–306p
    as movement, *(V2)* 727f
Circumference, body fat percentage, *(V1)* 603
Civil claim, *(V1)* 1080–1081
Civil law, *(V1)* 1077
Claims
    civil, *(V1)* 1080–1081
    damage, *(V1)* 1078
    malpractice, *(V1)* 1081–1083
Claims made insurance, *(V1)* 1089
Clarity, in communication, *(V1)* 341
Clark's rule for children, *(V2)* 522
Class, *(V1)* 71
Classification system
    describing nursing diagnoses, *(V1)* 71
    of elements, ideas or objects, *(V1)* 70
    in health care, *(V1)* 70–71
Clavicle, fracture of, *(ESG9)* 15
Clean-catch sample, *(V1)* 632, *(V1)* 645
Clean-contaminated wound, *(V1)* 816
Cleansing enema, *(V1)* 668, *(V2)* 663tb
Clean team, *(V1)* 937
Clean wound, *(V1)* 816
Clear liquid diet, *(V1)* 601

Client
    general survey, *(V1)* 365
    health status and expectations,
        perception of, *(V1)* 46
    honoring health/illness experience of,
        (V1) 182–183
    individual differences of, *(V1)* 28
    physical examination
        positioning for, *(V1)* 360, *(V1)* 361t–362t
        preparing for, *(V1)* 359–360
Client advocate, *(V1)* 13t
Client/family educator, *(V1)* 13t
Client profile, *(V1)* 86
Client record, *(V1)* 289–290, *(V2)* 178
Clinical Care Classification (CCC)
    components of, *(V2)* 1002
    diagnoses and interventions, *(V2)* 1002
    family and community outcomes, *(V1)* 99
    for home health and community care,
        (V1) 114–115
    for home health care diagnoses,
        (V1) 1040
    nursing diagnoses and, *(V1)* 71
    vocabulary
        for intervention, *(V2)* 53
        for outcome, *(V2)* 44
Clinical depression, *(V1)* 202
Clinical emotional psychiatric diagnosis,
        (V1) 195
Clinical judgment, *(V1)* 10
Clinical practice guidelines
    development of, *(V1)* 108
    on pressure ulcer formation, *(V1)* 109b
Clinical practice theory, *(V1)* 140, *(V1)* 145
Clinical problem, sources of, *(V1)* 158–159
Clinical reasoning, *(V1)* 28t
Clinical wisdom, *(V1)* 15
Clitoris, *(V1)* 764
Clock, 24-hour/military, *(V1)* 302, *(V1)* 302f
Clonus, *(V1)* 389, *(V1)* 740b
Closed questions, *(V1)* 47t
Closed system, *(V1)* 152, *(V1)* 615
Closed wound, *(V1)* 814
Clot, preventing, *(V1)* 884
Clubbing, *(V1)* 326, *(V1)* 370f
Cluster cue, *(V1)* 64
Coagulation disorder, *(V1)* 926b
Cocaine
    sexual function and, *(V1)* 774t
    teratogenic effect on fetus, *(ESG9)* 9
Code for Nurses, *(V1)* 16, *(V1)* 247
Code of Ethics, nursing
    American Nurses Association (ANA),
        (V1) 40, *(V1)* 1056, *(V1)* 1060b
    Canadian Nurses Association (CNA),
        (V1) 1060b
    guarantees of, *(V1)* 1076–1077
    purpose of, *(V1)* 1059
Cognitive-behavioral therapy, *(V1)* 711
Cognitive development
    of adolescence, *(ESG9)* 27
    age-related changes in, *(ESG9)* 36t
    of child, *(ESG9)* 24–25
    of elderly, *(ESG9)* 35
    of infant, *(ESG9)* 16–17
    of middle adult, *(ESG9)* 33
    of newborn, *(ESG9)* 15
    of preschooler, *(ESG9)* 22–23
    stages of, *(V1)* 534–535
    theory of, *(V1)* 167
    of toddler, *(ESG9)* 19–20
    of young adult, *(ESG9)* 31

Cognitive development theory
    overview of, (ESG9) 5
    stages of, (ESG9) 6t
Cognitive goal, (V1) 133t
Cognitive impairment
    communication and, (V1) 355, (V2) 226tb
    pain expression, (V1) 705
    self-care ability, (V1) 443
Cognitive learning, (V1) 530, (V1) 531t
Cognitive response, to stressors, (V1) 559b,
        (V1) 565
Cognitive restructuring, (V1) 571
Cohabitation, (V1) 210
Coitus, (V1) 777
Cold, applying to wound, (V2) 792tb
Cold compress
    for pain relief, (V1) 710
    for wounds, (V1) 842, (V1) 843
Colic, (ESG9) 17
Collaboration, discharge plan, (V1) 85
Collaborative intervention, (V1) 106
Collaborative problem
    care plan document, (V1) 85
    comparing to medical and nursing
            diagnoses, (V1) 60t
    diagnostic statement format for, (V1) 74t
    evaluation of, (V1) 135
    goals for, (V1) 96–97
    postoperative, (V1) 944, (V1) 945t–948t
    recognizing, (V1) 61
Collagen
    formation of, (V1) 813
    healing wound and, (V1) 817
Collective bargaining, (V1) 21
Colloid, (V1) 889
Colon
    Escherichia coli (E. coli), (V1) 635
    segments of, (V1) 653
Colonized wound, (V1) 814, (V1) 816
Color
    of nails, (V1) 369
    skin variations, (V1) 366, (V1) 367t
    statistics in nursing, (V1) 9, (V1) 10t
Color blindness, (V1) 372
Color change test, (V2) 292
Color vision, (V1) 372
Colostomy
    irrigation of, (V1) 663p, (V1) 672,
            (V2) 659p–662p
    loop, (V1) 659f
    purpose and location of, (V1) 658–659
    types of, (V1) 658f
Colostrum, (V2) 276
Coma, (V1) 270
Combustion, oxygenation and, (V1) 857
Comfort, (V1) 153
Comfort zone, (V1) 963
Commission on the Future of Health Care
        in Canada, (ESGV1) 20–21,
        (ESGV1) 27
Commodity distribution program, (V1) 608
Common law, (V1) 1072
Communication
    assessment of, (V1) 348–349, (V2)
            311p–312p
    barrier to end-of-life, (V1) 282b
    client record for, (V1) 289
    crying as, (ESG9) 15
    culture and, (V1) 242t, (V1) 243
    definition of, (V1) 338
    electronic forms of, (V1) 974–977
    etiology, (V1) 349

facilitating, (V1) 181–182
factors affecting, (V1) 343–345
health of, (V1) 1022–1023
hearing-impaired, (V2) 679tb
impaired cognition and consciousness,
        (V2) 226tb
impaired hearing or speech, (V1) 355
knowledge map for, (V2) 229
language barrier, (V1) 228, (V1) 244,
        (V2) 144tb
leadership and, (V1) 962
learning and, (V1) 534
levels of, (V1) 338–339
nonverbal, (V1) 49, (V1) 342–343,
        (V2) 225tb
oral, (V1) 289
outcome and intervention for impaired,
        (V2) 227
of pain, (V1) 705
patterns within family, (V1) 217
process of, (V1) 339–340, (V1) 339f
sensory deficit, (V2) 226tb
therapeutic
    for depression-related diagnoses,
            (V1) 206
    for dying and grieving, (V1) 282
    enhancing, (V1) 349–351
therapeutic relationship
    overview of, (V2) 219
    phases of, (V1) 346
    role of, (V1) 345–346
    verbal, (V1) 340–342
    visually impaired, (V2) 679tb
Communicator, (V1) 13t
Community
    assessment of, (V1) 1029
    components of, (V1) 1022
    healthcare services and, (V1) 1023
    safety hazards in, (V1) 428–429
    understanding, (V1) 1021
Community health
    classes and intervention, (V2) 993
    goals of, (V1) 99
    home health care versus, (V1) 1035
    public health versus, (V1) 1025f
Community nursing
    approaches to, (V1) 1025f
    career opportunities for, (V1) 1027–1029
    focus of, (V1) 1024–1025
    intervention, levels of, (V1) 1026–1027
    knowledge map of, (V2) 996
    overview of, (V2) 986
    pioneers of, (V1) 1025
    roles of, (V1) 1025–1026
Community special needs assessment,
        (V1) 44
Comorbidities, (V1) 27
Compensation
    process of, (V1) 895
    psychological defense mechanism,
            (V1) 560t
Compensatory justice, (V1) 1056–1057
Competence
    cultural, (V1) 44
    promotion in children, (V1) 198
Complaint
    in civil claim, (V1) 1081
    seeking health care, (V1) 46
Complementary and alternative medicine
        (CAM)
    in Canada, (ESGV1) 29
    categories of, (V1) 991–992, (V1) 992f

client history and current use of, (V1) 46
definition of, (V1) 22
for depression and anxiety, (V1) 207
effectiveness of, (V1) 989
end-of-life care, (V1) 272
enthusiasm for, (V1) 116
essential oils, (V1) 687
intercessory prayer, (V1) 259
for menopause, (V1) 789
most widely used in U.S., (V1) 992f
overview of, (V2) 960
practitioner qualifications, (V1) 1002
spiritual care, (V1) 257
statistics on American use of,
        (V1) 990–991
Complementary health care, (V1) 989
Complementary medicine, (V1) 235
Complementary modality, (V1) 989
Complement cascade
    as defense against infection, (V1) 402
    as method of destroying pathogens,
            (V1) 403
Complete bed bath, (V1) 450
Complete blood count (CBC), (V1) 902–903
Complete protein food, (V1) 578
Complex carbohydrate, (V1) 577
Complex etiology, (V1) 76
Complex thinking processes, (V1) 28t
Compliance, (V1) 328
Complicated grief, (V1) 268
Comprehensive assessment
    content of, (V1) 44
    definition of, (V1) 42
Comprehensive care plan, (V1) 83
Comprehensive data, gathering, (V1) 42
Comprehensiveness, (ESGV1) 4–5, (ESGV1) 4t
Comprehensive nursing care plan
    components of, (V1) 86f
    definition of, (V1) 85
    documents in, (V1) 85–86
    information in, (V1) 85, (V2) 44
    nursing diagnosis standardized form,
            (V1) 88f
    Patient Care Protocol, (V1) 87f
    preprinted, standardized plans,
            (V1) 86–87, (V1) 89
Comprehensive physical assessment,
        (V1) 357, (V1) 359
Compression device, (V1) 883–884
Compression stockings, (V1) 818
Compression test, manual, (V1) 383
Computed tomography (CT) scan, GI tract,
        (V2) 667–668
Computer
    automation decreasing errors, (V1) 980
    connectivity and, (V1) 974
    evidence-based practice and, (V1)
            977–978, (V1) 981
    literature searching skills, (V1) 982
    microchip for, (V1) 973f
    operations of, (V1) 973
Computer-assisted diagnosing, (V1) 68
Computer-assisted instruction (CAI), (V1) 546
Computer-based patient record, (V1) 978
Computer-generated intervention, (V1) 113,
        (V1) 113f
Computer information systems, (V1) 977b
Computerized care plan
    example of, (V1) 90f
    information in, (V2) 44
    process of, (V1) 91
    using NIC in, (V1) 114

Computerized charting, (V1) 298
Computerized dispensing system, (V1) 478, (V1) 478f
Computerized medical record, (V1) 978
Computerized tomography, (V2) 633
Computing, point-of-access, (V1) 979f
Concentration medication, (V1) 995
Concept, theory and, (V1) 141
Conception, (V1) 777, (ESG9) 8
Conceptual framework
    definition of, (V1) 142
    for informatics, (V1) 972–973
Conceptual model, (V1) 142
Concreteness, in therapeutic communication, (V1) 347
Concrete operation
    of child, (ESG9) 24–25
    of development, (V1) 534–535
Condom, (V1) 645, (V1) 790, (V2) 616p–618p
Conduct and Utilization of Research in Nursing project (CURN), (V1) 156
Conduction, (V1) 308
Conductive hearing loss, (V2) 264
Condyloid joint, (V1) 728t
Confidentiality
    maintaining, (V1) 1086
    research participant's right to, (V1) 158
Conflict
    reasons and levels of, (V1) 965
    "win-win" resolution, (V1) 965–966
Conflict resolution, (V1) 966
Confrontation, (V1) 266
Confrontation, in therapeutic communication, (V1) 347
Confused client, intervention, (V1) 696–697
Congenital abnormality, (V1) 737
Connectivity, types of, (V1) 974
Connotation, (V1) 340–341
Consciousness, reduced level, (V1) 355
Conscious sedation, (V1) 938
Consequentialism, (V1) 1057
Consequentialist, (V1) 1057
Constant fever, (V1) 314
Constipation
    characteristics of, (V1) 664
    foods causing, (V1) 677b
    management of, (V1) 667
    outcomes and interventions for, (V2) 669
    overview of, (V2) 636
    as postoperative collaborative problem, (V1) 947t
    as side effect of opioids, (V1) 713, (V1) 714b
Constitution Act of 1867, (ESGV1) 3
Constitutional law, (V1) 1071
Contact lenses
    care for, (V1) 466–467
    removing and care, (V2) 422p–423p
    storage of, (V1) 467f
Contact precautions, (V1) 412
Contaminated wound, (V1) 816
Contamination
    skin breakdown, (V1) 814
    wound and, (V1) 815, (V1) 816
Contemporary nursing practice
    caring for clients, (V1) 19–20
    end-of-life care, (V1) 20
    factors influencing
        trends in nursing and health care, (V1) 22–23
        trends in society, (V1) 21
    work settings, (V1) 20–21

Content
    learning and, (V1) 534
    of teaching, (V1) 540
Contextual awareness
    addressing, (V1) 29, (V1) 31
    definition of, (V1) 30t
    of evaluation, (V1) 136
    intervention selection, (V1) 111–112
    model of critical thinking, (V1) 31f
Continence, (V1) 43b
Continent ileostomy, (V1) 658, (V1) 658f
Continent urostomy, (V1) 638, (V1) 638f
Continuing education, (V1) 15
Continuum
    assessment for depression, (V1) 205f
    health-illness, (V1) 172, (V1) 172f
    Neuman, (V1) 172–173, (V1) 173f
Contraception
    adolescence and, (V1) 769
    method of, (V2) 736–737
    teaching about, (V1) 789
Contract law, (V1) 1078
Contracture, (V1) 739
Contralateral stimulation, (V1) 710
Control, external and internal locus of, (V1) 190
Controlled substance, (V1) 476, (V1) 477f
Controlling leadership, (V1) 954
Contusion (bruise), (V1) 814, (V1) 815t
Convalescence, (V1) 401
Convection, (V1) 308
Conversation, (V1) 351
Conversational dyspnea, (V1) 863
Conversion
    Fahrenheit and Centigrade scales, (V2) 219
    of medication, (V2) 520–521
    psychological defense mechanism, (V1) 560t
Coordination, (V1) 730
    assessment of, (V2) 303p
    expectations of, (V1) 126
COPD (chronic obstructive pulmonary disease), (V1) 326
Coping
    approaches to, (V1) 553
    with family illness or death, (V1) 219
    process within family, (V1) 217–218
    strategies for, (V1) 553
    See also Stress
Coping responses, (V1) 551
Copper, (V1) 813
Cordotomy, (V1) 718
Core temperature, (V1) 307
Cornea, (V1) 371
Corneal abrasion, (V1) 371
Corns, of feet, (V1) 455
Coronary artery, (V1) 853, (V1) 853f
Coronary artery disease, (V1) 803
Coronary circulation, (V1) 380
Coronary vessel, (V1) 853f
Correctional facility nursing, (V1) 1028
Cortex, of kidney, (V1) 619
Corticosteroid, (V1) 926b
Corticotropin-releasing hormone (CRH), (V1) 555
Cortisol
    effects of, (V1) 555
    function of, (V1) 556f
    release of, (V1) 855
Cosmetic surgery, (V1) 924

Cough
    assessment of, (V1) 862–863
    definition of, (V1) 326
    mobilizing secretions, (V1) 874
    teaching patient to, (V2) 918p–921p
Cough suppressant, (V1) 884
Coumadin (warfarin), (V1) 84
Counseling
    for depression-related diagnoses, (V1) 110
    for health promotion, (V1) 1016–1017
    providing, (V1) 1086
Counselor, (V1) 13t
Countershock phase, of stress, (V1) 555
Couple
    childless, (V1) 211
    gay and lesbian, (V1) 211
Courage, intellectual, (V1) 27
Court, laws and, (V1) 1072
CPR (Cardiopulmonary resuscitation), (V1) 273
CPT (Current Procedural Terminology), (V1) 71
Crack cocaine, (ESG9) 9
Crackles, (V1) 325
Cradle cap, (V1) 369
Cranial nerve
    assessment of, (V2) 312p–315p
    name, type and function, (V1) 389t
    origin of, (V1) 388f
Crawling reflex, (ESG9) 14, (ESG9) 14f
Creatinine
    as marker of protein metabolism, (V1) 605
    measuring levels of, (V1) 635
Creation (kapha), (V1) 992
Credentialing, (V1) 1075
Credibility, in communication, (V1) 341–342
Credible source
    inquiry of, (V1) 30t
    intervention selection, (V1) 111–112
    model of critical thinking, (V1) 31f
Crepitus, (V1) 385, (V1) 737, (V1) 826
Cricoid cartilage, (V1) 376, (V1) 376f
Crime, (V1) 1077
Crimean War, (V1) 3, (V1) 6
Criminal, as nurse, (V1) 7
Criminal law, (V1) 1077
Crisis
    adaptation failure and, (V1) 563
    intervention, (V1) 572
Crisis counseling, (V2) 550
Criteria
    definition of, (V1) 129
    reliability and validity of, (V1) 130
Critical pathways
    definition of, (V1) 108
    example of, (V1) 90f
    outcome-based plan of care, (V1) 89
Critical reflection, about assessment, (V1) 52–54
Critical thinking
    analyzing and interpreting data, (V1) 63–65
    attitude in, (V1) 27
    cased-based instruction fostering, (V1) 36
    definition of, (V1) 26, (V1) 26b
    evaluation of assessment, (V1) 52–54
    full-spectrum nursing and, (V1) 10, (V1) 33, (V1) 34–36
    importance of, (V1) 27–29
    model for, (V1) 29, (V1) 30t, (V1) 31, (V1) 31f

Critical thinking *(continued)*
   nursing process and, *(V1)* 33, *(V2)* 11, *(V2)* 19
   requirements of, *(V1)* 28–29
   skills in, *(V1)* 26–27
Critiquing, *(V1)* 70b
Cross-dresser, *(V1)* 767
Cross eyes, *(V1)* 685b
Cross-linking theory, *(ESG9)* 35
Crusaders, *(V1)* 8
Crushing wound, *(V1)* 815t
Crust, skin, *(V2)* 246
Crutches
   gaits for, *(V1)* 760–761, *(V1)* 760f
   teaching patient to use, *(V2)* 719tb–720tb
   types of, *(V1)* 759, *(V1)* 759f
Crying, communication of infant, *(ESG9)* 15
Crystalloid, *(V1)* 889
CT scan (computed tomography), GI Tract, *(V2)* 667–668
CUBAN, reports and, *(V1)* 300, *(V2)* 182
Cue
   cluster, *(V1)* 64
   recognizing, *(V1)* 63, *(V1)* 64b
   subjective and objective, *(V1)* 75
Cuff, blood pressure
   auscultatory gap, *(V1)* 333
   bladder size of, *(V1)* 332t, *(V2)* 214–215
   calculating proper inflation of, *(V1)* 333
   site to use, *(V1)* 331
   size of, *(V1)* 330, *(V1)* 331f
Cultural assessment
   information for, *(V1)* 238
   models and tools for, *(V1)* 239
   as special needs assessment, *(V1)* 44
Cultural assimilation, *(V1)* 227
Cultural awareness, *(V1)* 235
Cultural beliefs, of nursing, *(V1)* 10
Cultural competence
   achieving, *(V1)* 235–236
   barriers to care, *(V1)* 237–238
   Campinha-Bacote model of, *(V1)* 237
   Leininger's theory of, *(V1)* 147–148, *(V1)* 237
   LIVE and LEARN, *(V1)* 244
   Purnell's model for, *(V1)* 236–237, *(V1)* 236f
   in teaching, *(V1)* 536b
   theory of, *(V1)* 147–148
   Watson's theory, *(V1)* 153–154
Culturally sensitive care, *(V1)* 116
Cultural sensitivity, *(V1)* 235
Culture
   biological variations, assessment, *(V2)* 140tb
   communication and, *(V1)* 344
   definition and characteristics of, *(V1)* 223–224
   dying patient needs, *(V1)* 284
   as factor influencing hygiene practice, *(V1)* 442–443
   Giger and Davidhizar's assessment model, using, *(V2)* 143tb
   grieving process and, *(V1)* 268
   health and, *(V1)* 175, *(V1)* 1012
   health care system, view of, *(V1)* 28
   interview, *(V2)* 141tb
   knowledge map of, *(V2)* 146
   language barrier, *(V2)* 144tb
   learning and, *(V1)* 535
   North American healthcare system, *(V1)* 232, *(V1)* 233t

   of nursing, *(V1)* 232
   nutrition and, *(V1)* 599
   overview of, *(V2)* 130
   pain behavior, *(V1)* 704–705
   pain perception assessment, *(V2)* 142tb
   postmortem care, *(V1)* 285
   rituals of, *(V1)* 227
   sensory function and, *(V1)* 682–683
   sexuality and, *(V1)* 770–772
   urination and, *(V1)* 623
   values, beliefs and practices of, *(V1)* 227
Culture brokerage, *(V1)* 241
Culture specifics
   definition of, *(V1)* 227
   expectation of health care, *(V1)* 227–228
   influencing health, *(V1)* 228–230
Cumulative effect, *(V1)* 491
Cumulative Index to Nursing and Allied Health Literature (CINAHL), *(V1)* 161, *(V1)* 983, *(V2)* 949
Cunnilingus, *(V1)* 777
Cure, *(V1)* 260
Curiosity, intellectual, *(V1)* 27
CURN (Conduct and Utilization of Research in Nursing project), *(V1)* 156
Current Procedural Terminology (CPT), *(V1)* 71
Cushing's disease, *(V1)* 370, *(V2)* 252
Custom, North American healthcare system, *(V1)* 233t
Cutaneous pain, *(V1)* 699–700
Cutaneous stimulation, *(V1)* 710
Cutaneous ureterostomy, *(V1)* 638
CVA (cerebrovascular accident), *(V1)* 64
Cyanosis, *(V1)* 321, *(V1)* 367t, *(V1)* 449, *(V2)* 333
Cyclic feeding, *(V1)* 614–615
Cyst, *(V2)* 245
Cystitis, *(V1)* 635
Cystometry, *(V2)* 633
Cystoscopy, *(V2)* 633
Cytotoxic T cell, *(V1)* 404

D
Daily living. *See* Activities of daily living (ADLs)
Daily worksheet, *(V1)* 968
Damage claims, *(V1)* 1078
Damages, proof of, *(V1)* 1079
Dangling, *(V1)* 757
DAR (data, action, response) format, *(V2)* 178
Data
   analysis of, *(V1)* 68–69, *(V1)* 70b
   analyzing and interpreting, *(V1)* 63–65
   bias and stereotyping influencing interpretation of, *(V1)* 69
   biographical, *(V1)* 46
   collection as holistic, *(V1)* 50
   computer screen capture of assessment, *(V1)* 54f
   definition of, *(V1)* 972
   documentation of, *(V1)* 50, *(V1)* 52
   gathering during assessment, *(V1)* 42
   graphic flow sheet, *(V1)* 53f
   guidelines for recording, *(V1)* 52
   identifying gaps and inconsistencies, *(V1)* 64–65
   organization of, *(V1)* 50
   pulse rate assessment, *(V1)* 320–321
   reassessment, *(V1)* 132
   reflecting critically about, *(V1)* 52–53
   for respiratory assessment, *(V1)* 324
   significant, *(V1)* 63

   sources of, *(V1)* 41
   tools for recording, *(V1)* 52
   transformation to knowledge, *(V1)* 972f
   types of, *(V1)* 42t
   validation of, *(V1)* 49–50
Database
   admission nursing, *(V1)* 293
   entry, *(V1)* 984, *(V1)* 984b
   for literature, *(V1)* 983–985
   of nursing assessment findings, *(V1)* 39
   for problem-oriented records, *(V1)* 290
   types of, *(V1)* 984t
Data-gathering stage, *(V1)* 32
Data processing, *(V1)* 973
Date rape, *(V1)* 780
Deacon (deaconess)
   role as nurse, *(V1)* 9
Deacon (deaconess), as nurse, *(V1)* 4
Death
   anesthesia as risk for, *(V1)* 938
   by assisted suicide, *(V1)* 273, *(V1)* 275
   autopsy, *(V1)* 275
   definition of, *(V1)* 269
   by euthanasia, *(V1)* 275
   grief work facilitation, *(V1)* 282–283
   from high temperature, *(V1)* 315
   hypertension as cause of, *(V1)* 334
   impending, *(V1)* 177–178
   legal and ethical concerns, *(V1)* 273
   postmortem care, *(V2)* 169tb–170tb
   stages leading to, *(V1)* 270–271
   types of, *(V1)* 269
   Uniform Determination of Death Act, *(V1)* 270, *(V1)* 270b
Death anxiety, *(V1)* 203
Deciduous teeth, *(V1)* 459, *(V1)* 459f
Decisional conflict, *(V1)* 75
Decision making
   as complex thinking process, *(V1)* 28t
   conflict of, *(V1)* 203
   critical thinking, *(V1)* 30t, *(V1)* 31f
   ethics and, *(V1)* 1067–1068
   as NOC outcome, *(V1)* 98
Decline, of infection, *(V1)* 401
Decoding, *(V1)* 340
Decubitus ulcer
   cause of, *(V1)* 449
   guidelines for, *(V1)* 109b
Deduction, *(V1)* 143
Deductive reasoning
   comparing inductive reasoning, *(V1)* 143f
   definition of, *(V1)* 143
Deep breathing, *(V1)* 324, *(V2)* 918p–921p
Deep somatic pain, *(V1)* 700
Deep vein thrombosis, *(V1)* 84
Defamation, *(V1)* 1078
Defecation
   process and pattern of, *(V1)* 654
   promoting normal or regular, *(V1)* 665–666
Defendant
   in civil claim, *(V1)* 1081
   definition of, *(V1)* 1078
Defense mechanism, *(ESG9)* 5
   coping with anxiety, *(V1)* 200
   ego, *(V1)* 559–560
   ego employing, *(V1)* 167
   psychological, *(V1)* 560t–561t
Defervescence phase, *(V1)* 314
Deficient knowledge, *(V1)* 67
   goal/outcome statement for, *(V1)* 539–540
   as primary problem or etiology, *(V1)* 538, *(V1)* 539

Definition
  as component of theory, *(V1) 141–142*
  as meaning of NIC label, *(V1) 114*
Degenerative joint disease (Heberden's nodes), *(V2) 335*
Dehiscence, *(V1) 819–820, (V1) 820f, (V1) 947t*
Dehydration
  from exercise, *(V1) 734*
  hematocrit level and, *(V1) 328*
  hypovolemia and, *(V1) 896*
  prevention of, *(V1) 315*
  skin and, *(V1) 448*
Delayed grief, *(V1) 268*
Delayed primary closure, *(V1) 816, (V1) 817f*
Delegation, *(V1) 106*
  apical pulse assessment, *(V2) 208*
  apical-radial pulse assessment, *(V2) 210*
  beard and mustache care, *(V2) 418*
  bedside urine testing, *(V1) 634*
  blood pressure assessment, *(V2) 214*
  of charting, *(V1) 302*
  client safety intervention, *(V1) 439–440*
  contact lenses, removing and care for, *(V2) 422*
  decision-making grid, *(V2) 68*
  definition of, *(V1) 126*
  denture care, *(V2) 409*
  external (condom) application, *(V2) 616*
  fingerstick blood glucose levels, *(V2) 566*
  foot care, *(V2) 402*
  intake and output (I&O) records, *(V1) 294*
  intramuscular injection, locating sites for, *(V2) 493*
  leadership and, *(V1) 962–963*
  malpractice risk, *(V1) 1086*
  medication administration, *(V2) 450*
  nasal medication administration, *(V2) 465*
  nasogastric and nasoenteric tube insertion, *(V2) 567*
  nutritional assessment, *(V1) 606*
  occupied bed, making, *(V2) 427*
  ophthalmic medication administration, *(V2) 459*
  oral care, unconscious patient, *(V2) 411*
  oral medication administration, *(V2) 454*
  otic medication administration, *(V2) 463*
  of pain management, *(V1) 709b*
  parenteral medications, *(V2) 475, (V2) 479, (V2) 489, (V2) 496*
  perineal care, *(V2) 399*
  pulse measurement, *(V2) 203*
  rectal suppository administration, *(V2) 471*
  respiration assessment, *(V2) 212p–213p*
  rights of, *(V1) 126–128, (V2) 67*
  shampooing bedrest patient, *(V2) 414p–417p*
  skin breakdown, *(V1) 829*
  for time management, *(V1) 968*
  unoccupied bed, making, *(V2) 424*
  urinary catheter insertion, *(V2) 598*
  vaginal medication administration, *(V2) 468*
  of vital signs (VS), *(V1) 336*
Delta (δ), *(V1) 702, (V1) 713*
Delta wave, *(V1) 796, (V1) 796f*
Demands, as factor disrupting health, *(V1) 178, (V1) 181*
Dementia, *(ESG9) 37*

Democratic leadership, *(V1) 954*
Demonstration, *(V1) 544*
Denial
  coping with anxiety, *(V1) 200*
  ineffective, *(V1) 67, (V1) 203*
  psychological defense mechanism, *(V1) 560t*
Denotation, *(V1) 340–341*
Dental care
  assessment of teeth, *(V2) 270p*
  patient teaching, *(V2) 271*
Dental caries, *(V1) 460, (V1) 462, (ESG9) 17*
Dentures
  care for, *(V2) 409p–410p*
  care of, *(V1) 463*
  poorly fitted or loose, *(V1) 459*
Denver Developmental Screening Test (DDST), *(ESG9) 18*
Deontological framework, *(V1) 1057*
Deontology, *(V1) 1057–1058*
Department of Health and Human Services (DHHS)
  Healthy People 2010, *(V1) 1005, (V1) 1006b*
  rights of research participants, *(V1) 158*
Dependence, opioids, *(V1) 713*
Depersonalization, prevention of, *(V1) 197*
Depilatory, *(V1) 466*
Deposition, *(V1) 1081*
Depression
  altering etiology and relieving symptoms of, *(V1) 206*
  assessment continuum, *(V1) 205f*
  assessment of, *(V2) 305p–306p*
  cause of, *(V1) 201*
  chronic pain and, *(V1) 704*
  complementary and alternative medicine (CAM), *(V1) 207*
  criteria for, *(V1) 200–201*
  depressed affect, *(V1) 201f*
  Geriatric Depression Scale (GDS), *(ESG9) 38*
  goal/outcome statement, *(V1) 205*
  identification of, *(V2) 110tb*
  as movement, *(V1) 727f*
  nursing care for, *(V1) 204–205*
  outcomes and interventions, *(V2) 115*
  overview of, *(V2) 100*
  physical and behavioral problems of, *(V1) 205*
  respiratory, *(V1) 713*
  response to stressor, *(V1) 562*
  signs and symptoms of, *(V1) 201–202*
  sleep patterns, *(V1) 803*
  treatment of, *(V1) 202*
  truths and myths of, *(V1) 201t*
Depth, of breathing, *(V1) 324*
Dermis, *(V1) 447, (V1) 811, (ESG9) 14*
Descending colon, *(V1) 653*
Desire
  aging and, *(V1) 775b*
  as sexual response, *(V1) 775–776*
Desired outcome
  as goal, *(V1) 92*
  intervention flowing from, *(V1) 111t*
  nursing diagnosis and, *(V1) 94–95*
  review of, *(V1) 111*
Desquamates, *(V1) 447*
Destruction (vata), *(V1) 992*
Development
  applying concepts of, *(V1) 168*
  assessment of, *(ESG9) 39*

body temperature and, *(V1) 309*
bowel elimination patterns, *(V1) 655*
cognitive abilities, *(V1) 167*
communication and, *(V1) 343–344*
definition of, *(V1) 165, (ESG9) 2*
Erickson's stages of, *(V1) 167*
of family, *(V2) 125*
grief and, *(V1) 267*
as health factor, *(V1) 174*
hygiene practice, *(V1) 443*
infection, risk of, *(V1) 405*
learning and, *(V1) 534–535*
nutrition and, *(V1) 594–597*
overview of, *(V2) 84*
oxygenation and, *(V1) 854–855*
pain expression, *(V1) 704*
of personality, *(V1) 167*
principles of, *(V1) 166, (ESG9) 3*
self-concept and, *(V1) 189*
sensory function and, *(V1) 682*
sexuality
  of female, *(V1) 391f*
  of male, *(V1) 390f*
skin and, *(V1) 448*
stages of family, *(V1) 212t*
theory of, *(ESG9) 3*
urination and, *(V1) 623*
Developmental dysplasia of the hip (DDH, *(V1) 737*
Developmental stressor, *(V1) 551*
Developmental task theory, *(V1) 166, (ESG9) 3, (ESG9) 4t*
Developmental theories
  for family, *(V1) 213*
  types of, *(V1) 151, (V1) 166–168*
DEXA test, *(ESG9) 34*
DHEPD (Do Help Every Patient Deliberately), *(V1) 45b*
Diabetes
  diet for, *(V1) 601*
  eyes and, *(V1) 372*
  foot care and, *(V1) 457*
  maternal, *(ESG9) 12*
  sedentary lifestyle and, *(V1) 1009*
  as sleep-provoked disorder, *(V1) 803*
Diabetes mellitus (DM)
  acanthous nigrican, *(V2) 277*
  in child, *(ESG9) 25*
  surgical risk and, *(V1) 926b*
  uncontrolled, *(V1) 67*
  urinary tract infection (UTI) and, *(V1) 636*
  in young adult, *(ESG9) 32*
Diabetic ulcer, *(V1) 815t*
Diagnosis
  of abnormal pulse, *(V1) 321*
  activity and exercise, *(V1) 747*
  algorithm for determining type of, *(V1) 62f*
  analyzing and interpreting data, *(V1) 63–65*
  of anxiety, *(V1) 203*
  bowel incontinence, *(V1) 674*
  bowel-related problems, *(V1) 664*
  choosing label, *(V1) 72–73*
  circulation problems, *(V1) 872*
  Clinical Care Classification (CCC), *(V2) 1002*
  collaborative problems, *(V1) 76*
  for communication problems, *(V1) 349*
  community-based, *(V1) 1029*
  computer-assisted, *(V1) 68*

Diagnosis *(continued)*
  critiquing diagnostic reasoning process, *(V1) 70b*
  cultural factors as etiology, *(V1) 239–240*
  deficient knowledge, *(V1) 538*
  definition of, *(V1) 56–57*
  diagnostic statement, *(V1) 73, (V1) 74t, (V1) 75–76, (V1) 77–79*
  disturbed energy field, *(V1) 1001*
  for dying and grieving, *(V1) 276–277*
  of eye problems, *(V1) 466*
  for family health status, *(V1) 218*
  of feet problems, *(V1) 456*
  fluid, electrolyte and acid-base imbalance, *(V1) 903*
  full-spectrum nursing and, *(V1) 35*
  growth and development problems, *(ESG9) 39*
  of health, *(V1) 182*
  health promotion, *(V1) 182*
  home health care visit, *(V1) 1039–1040*
  hypertension, *(V1) 334*
  hypotension, *(V1) 334*
  hypothermia, *(V1) 316*
  impaired ventilation and gas exchange, *(V2) 867–868*
  of infection, *(V1) 407*
  intervention flowing from, *(V1) 110f*
  for intraoperative phase, *(V1) 940, (V2) 932–934*
  knowledge map of, *(V2) 43*
  linking assessment to remaining nursing processes, *(V1) 58f*
  for loss and grieving, *(V1) 276–277*
  medical versus nursing, *(V1) 59–61*
  medication-related, *(V1) 496, (V2) 524–525*
  model for, *(V1) 57f*
  nail problems, *(V1) 458*
  NANDA nursing diagnosis component, *(V1) 71–72*
  NANDA nursing taxonomy, *(V1) 71*
  NIC intervention linking to, *(V1) 115t*
  NOC outcomes linking to NANDA, *(V1) 97, (V1) 97b*
  nursing process and, *(V1) 31f, (V1) 32, (V1) 32f*
  nutrition-related problems, *(V1) 606*
  of oral cavity/mouth, *(V1) 461*
  origins of, *(V1) 58–59*
  outcome and intervention, *(V1) 77*
  overview of, *(V2) 33*
  overweight and obesity, *(V1) 609–610*
  oxygenation problems, *(V1) 872*
  pain, *(V1) 708, (V1) 721*
  postoperative, *(V1) 944, (V2) 935–938*
  preoperative, *(V1) 930–931, (V2) 930–931*
  professional standards for, *(V1) 57b*
  psychosocial, *(V1) 193–195*
  recognizing health problems, *(V1) 59–61, (V1) 77*
  review of, *(V1) 136*
  risk for falls, *(V1) 439*
  schools teaching, *(V1) 58*
  self-care deficit, *(V1) 64, (V1) 445*
  self-concept, *(V1) 195–196*
  sensory-perceptual problems, *(V1) 691–692*
  sexual problems, *(V1) 782–783*
  of skin problems, *(V1) 449, (V1) 831*
  sleep pattern disturbance, *(V1) 804–805*
  spirituality, *(V1) 256–258*
  status of, *(V1) 61*
  stress-related, *(V1) 566–567, (V1) 566b*
  stress urinary incontinence, *(V1) 627*
  for temperature/fever, *(V1) 315*
  terminology for, *(V1) 57, (V1) 58t*
  theoretical knowledge of, *(V1) 68*
  types of, *(V1) 61–63*
  for underweight and malnutrition, *(V1) 611*
  urinary elimination problems, *(V1) 635*
  verification of, *(V1) 70b*
  wellness, *(V1) 62f, (V1) 63, (V1) 75, (V1) 100, (V1) 1013–1015*
Diagnosis-related group (DRG), *(V1) 89*
Diagnostic and Statistical Manual (DSM-IV), *(V1) 70*
Diagnostic label
  addressing health problems, *(V1) 58–59*
  definition of, *(V1) 71–72*
Diagnostic reasoning
  analyzing and interpreting data, *(V1) 63–65*
  critiquing process of, *(V1) 70b*
  definition of, *(V1) 63, (V1) 63f*
  drawing conclusions about health status, *(V1) 63*
  process for, *(V1) 63f*
  reflecting critically about, *(V1) 68–69*
Diagnostic screening, preoperative, *(V1) 930*
Diagnostic statements
  critiquing, *(V1) 70b*
  examples of, *(V1) 74t*
  formats for, *(V1) 73, (V1) 75*
  guidelines for judging quality of, *(V1) 77–79*
  for nursing diagnosis, *(V1) 57*
  reflecting critically about, *(V1) 77*
  variations of, *(V1) 75–76*
  writing, *(V1) 69–70*
Diagnostic surgery, *(V1) 924*
Diagnostic terminology, *(V1) 71*
Diagnostic testing
  for infection, *(V1) 407*
  for nutritional status, *(V1) 604–605*
Diaphoresis, *(V1) 314*
Diaphragm, *(V1) 848*
Diarrhea
  characteristics of, *(V1) 664*
  foods causing and alleviating, *(V1) 677b*
  management of, *(V1) 666–667*
  outcomes and interventions for, *(V2) 669–670*
  overview of, *(V2) 636*
Diarthroses, *(V1) 726*
Diary, food, *(V1) 602*
Diastole, *(V1) 317, (V1) 380, (V1) 852*
Diastolic pressure, *(V1) 327*
Dickens, Charles, *(V1) 7*
Diet, *(V1) 600–601*
Dietary fat, *(V1) 580t*
Dietary fiber, *(V1) 577*
Dietary guidelines
  for Americans, *(V1) 587b*
  Dietary Reference Intake (DRI)
    minerals for adults, *(V1) 585t–586t*
    vitamins for adults, *(V1) 583t–584t*
  ostomy patients, *(V1) 677b*
  USDA, *(V1) 587*
Dietary Reference Intake (DRI)
  establishment of standards, *(V1) 582*
  minerals for adults, *(V1) 585t–586t*
  as revision for RDA, *(V1) 586*
  vitamins for adults, *(V1) 583t–584t*
Dietary therapy, *(V1) 997*
Dieting, *(V1) 599*
Diffusion
  definition of, *(V1) 850*
  process of, *(V1) 889, (V1) 889f, (V1) 890t*
Digital subscriber line (DSL), *(V1) 974*
Diglyceride, *(V1) 579b*
Dignity
  definition of, *(V1) 1052t*
  urination and, *(V1) 623*
Diminished breath sounds, *(V1) 380*
Diploma program, *(V1) 14*
Dipstick testing, *(V1) 633–634*
Direct auscultation, *(V1) 45, (V1) 363*
Direct-care intervention, *(V1) 105*
Direct care provider, *(V1) 13t*
Directive interview, *(V1) 47*
Directive leadership, *(V1) 954*
Direct measurement of BMR, *(V1) 592*
Direct percussion, *(V1) 360, (V2) 233t*
Direct-to-consumer marketing, *(V1) 21*
Disaster services nursing, *(V1) 1028*
Discharge planning
  at admission, *(V1) 293*
  charting, *(V1) 297*
  form for, *(V2) 49*
  process of, *(V1) 84–85*
Disciplinary procedure, *(V1) 1075*
Discipline, *(V1) 12*
Disclosure
  research participant's right to, *(V1) 158*
Discovery, *(V1) 1081*
Discrimination, *(V1) 237*
Disease
  blood pressure and, *(V1) 329*
  bowel diversion, cause for, *(V1) 657*
  diets modified for, *(V1) 601*
  health and, *(V1) 176*
  infection, risk of, *(V1) 406*
  joint mobility, *(V1) 737–738*
  mobility and activity, *(V1) 737*
  nutrition and, *(V1) 599*
  peristalsis and, *(V1) 657*
  pharmacokinetics and, *(V1) 488*
  pulse rate, *(V1) 318*
  respiration and, *(V1) 323*
  skin and, *(V1) 448, (V1) 812*
  stress, outcome to, *(V1) 553*
  urination and, *(V1) 625*
Disenfranchised grief, *(V2) 268–269*
Disengagement theory, *(ESG9) 35*
Disinfection, *(V1) 408*
Displacement
  coping with anxiety, *(V1) 200*
  psychological defense mechanism, *(V1) 560t*
Disposable chemical thermometer, *(V1) 311, (V1) 312f*
Disposable chest drainage system, *(V1) 881, (V1) 882f*
Dispute resolution, *(ESGV1) 8, (V1) 1081*
Dissaccharide, *(V1) 577, (V1) 577f*
Dissociation, *(V1) 560t*
Distance leaning, *(V1) 546*
Distance vision, *(V1) 371*
Distention, of abdomen, *(V1) 383*
Distraction, from pain, *(V1) 711*
Distress, *(V1) 551*
Distribution
  of drug in body, *(V1) 484*
  of drugs in children and adult, *(V1) 487t*
Distributive justice, *(V1) 1056–1057*

Disturbed Sleep Pattern, (V1) 83–84
Diuretic, (V1) 884
    classification of, (V1) 624b, (V1) 625
    increasing surgical risk, (V1) 926b
Diurnal variation, (V1) 329
Diversity, cultural, (V1) 44
Diverticulitis, (V1) 657
Diverticulosis, (V1) 657
Dix, Dorothea, (V1) 8
DNAR order, (V1) 273, (V1) 275b
DNR order, (V1) 273, (V1) 274f
Doctoral degree, (V1) 14, (V1) 155
Doctor of nursing science (DNS), (V1) 15
Doctor of philosophy (PhD), (V1) 15
Documentation
    abuse assessment, (V2) 91–92
    apical pulse assessment, (V2) 209
    apical-radial pulse assessment, (V2) 211
    beard and mustache care, (V2) 419
    bed bath, (V2) 395
    bed-monitoring device, (V2) 371
    blood pressure assessment, (V2) 217
    of care guidelines, (V1) 301–302
    clean-catch specimen, collecting, (V2) 597
    contact lenses, removing and care for,
        (V2) 423
    continuous bladder irrigation, (V2) 615
    definition of, (V1) 289
    durable power of attorney, (V1) 273
    external (condom) application, (V2) 618
    as final step of implementation, (V1) 128
    fingerstick blood glucose levels, (V2) 566
    foot care, (V2) 405
    forms for
        assessment flow sheet, (V2) 187
        intake and output (I&O), (V2) 188
        long-term care flow sheet, (V2) 186
    gastric and enteric tube feedings, (V2)
        576
    guidelines for, (V2) 183tb–184tb, (V2)
        1022tb
    of home health care visit, (V1) 1042–1043
    implications of, (V2) 20
    intermittent bladder and catheter
        irrigation, (V2) 612
    intermittent infusion administration,
        (V2) 512
    intramuscular injection administration,
        (V2) 500
    intravenous medication administration,
        (V2) 507
    knowledge map of, (V2) 190
    living will, (V1) 273
    lung chest assessment, (V2) 286
    medication administration, (V2) 453
    for minimizing malpractice, (V1) 1084
    nasogastric and nasoenteric tubes
        insertion of, (V2) 571
        removal of, (V2) 578
    nursing requirements for, (V1) 293
    ophthalmic medication administration,
        (V2) 462
    oral care for unconscious patient,
        (V2) 413
    overview of, (V2) 178
    of pain care plan, (V1) 720
    perineal care, (V2) 402
    pulse rate assessment, (V2) 207
    rectal suppository administration,
        (V2) 475
    respiration assessment, (V2) 213
    restraints, using, (V2) 374

    shampooing bedrest patient, (V2) 417
    shaving patient, (V2) 421
    skin assessment, (V2) 243
    subcutaneous medication administration,
        (V2) 492
    systems of, (V1) 290
    temperature assessment, (V2) 203
    urinary catheter insertion, (V2) 609
    vaginal medication administration,
        (V2) 470
Do Help Every Patient Deliberately
    (DHEPD), (V1) 45b
Domain, (V1) 71
Domestic violence
    as challenge to family health, (V1) 216
    nursing education for, (V1) 15
    sexuality, (V1) 772
    in young adult, (ESG9) 32
Dominance, male, (V1) 166
Dominant culture, (V1) 225
Donation, organ/tissue, (V1) 275–276
Donor card, organ/tissue, (V1) 275, (V1) 275f
Do not attempt resuscitation (DNAR) order,
    (V1) 273, (V1) 274f, (V1) 275b,
    (V2) 158
Do not resuscitate (DNR) order, (V1) 273,
    (V1) 274f
Dorsal horn, (V1) 702, (V1) 702f
Dorsalis artery, (V1) 319, (V1) 319f, (V2) 207
Dorsal recumbent position, (V1) 643, (V1) 752
Dorsogluteal muscle, (V1) 516–517
Dosage
    body surface area (BSA), (V2) 521
    changing needles, measurement,
        (V2) 516tb
    Clark's rule for children, (V2) 522
    conversion of, (V2) 520–521
    measurement and calculation of,
        (V1) 492, (V2) 518–522
    pediatric, (V2) 521–522
Dosha, (V1) 992
Double-barreled colostomy, (V1) 659
Double locking, (V1) 476
Double-lumen catheter, (V1) 641, (V1) 641f,
Douche, (V1) 504
Douching, (V1) 788
Douglas, Tommy, (ESG46 V1) 2
Drainage
    of airways, (V1) 879–880
    chest systems for, (V1) 881–882,
        (V1) 881f, (V1) 882f
    postural, (V2) 815p–818p
Dressing
    as activity of daily living (ADL), (V1) 43b
    application of, (V1) 837
        hydrocolloid, (V2) 779p–781p
        transparent film, (V2) 776p–778p
    removing and applying
        dry, (V2) 770p–771p
        wet-to-damp, (V2) 773p–776p
    securing, (V1) 840–841
    self-care deficit, (V2) 434
    taping, (V2) 786tb
    types of, (V1) 837–840, (V1) 840t
Drinking, binge, (ESG9) 28
Droplet precautions, (V2) 412
Droplet transmission, (V1) 400
Drowning, (V1) 427
Drowsiness, opioids and, (V1) 714b
Drug
    allergic reaction to, (V1) 490, (V1) 490t
    assessment of patient, (V1) 495

    biological half-life of, (V1) 486
    blood flow affecting absorption, (V1) 484
    classification of, (V1) 474, (V1) 475t
    definition of, (V1) 474
    distribution in body, (V1) 484
    dosage calculation, (V1) 492
    drawing up from ampule or vial,
        (V1) 509
    effectiveness of, (V1) 485–487
    ensuring safe administration of, (V1) 497
    excretion of, (V1) 485
    factors affecting absorption, (V1) 479,
        (V1) 483
    forms of, (V1) 479
    incompatibility of, (V1) 491
    interactions of, (V1) 491
    legal considerations, (V1) 476
    legislation, (V1) 476, (V1) 477t
    listings and directories, (V1) 474–476
    measurement systems for, (V1) 492
    metabolization of, (V1) 485
    mixing in same syringe, (V1) 510
    name of, (V1) 474
    packaging of, (V1) 477f
    patch for, (V1) 503f
    pH and ionization, (V1) 483–484
    primary effects of, (V1) 488
    quality and safety of, (V1) 474
    reconstitution of, (V1) 510
    rights of, (V1) 497–499
    secondary effects, (V1) 488–491
    sexuality and, (V1) 773–774
    similar-sounding names of, (V1) 497b
    syringe for administration of, (V1) 503f
    therapeutic range of, (V1) 486
    three checks, (V1) 497
    tolerance of, (V1) 491
    types, advantages, and route of adminis-
        tration, (V1) 480t–483t
Drug abuse
    in adolescence, (ESG9) 28
    definition of, (V1) 492
    as health risk factor, (V1) 175
    infection, risk of, (V1) 405
Drug allergy, (V1) 296
Drug dependence, (V1) 491
Drug Enforcement Agency, U.S. (DEA),
    (V1) 476
Drug misuse, (V1) 492
Dry heat, (V1) 843
Dry mouth, (V1) 686
Dry powder inhaler (DPI), (V1) 505
Dry skin, (V1) 449
DSL (digital subscriber line), (V1) 974
DSM-IV (Diagnostic and Statistical Manual),
    (V1) 70
Dual-earner family, (V1) 210, (V2) 118
Duodenal ulcer, (V1) 803
Duodenum, (V1) 652
Durable power of attorney, (V1) 273,
    (V1) 1073
Duration
    of action of drug, (V1) 485–487
    of exercise, (V1) 732
Duty to assess, (V1) 1081–1082
Duty to report, conflict, (V1) 1079
Dwarfism, (V1) 737
Dying
    assessment, (V1) 276
    care for, (V1) 283–284
    DNR and DNAR orders, (V1) 273
    guidelines for assessment, (V2) 171–172

Dying (continued)
  health and, (V1) 177–178
  helping family members with, (V1) 283
  helping family with, (V2) 167tb
  knowledge map for, (V2) 176
  Kübler-Ross stages of, (V1) 271b
  meeting needs of patient, (V1) 284–285
  overview of, (V2) 158
  patient care, (V2) 168tb–169tb
  stages of, (V1) 270
Dynamic self, (V1) 189
Dynorphins, (V1) 702
Dysfunctional grieving, (V1) 276, (V2) 173
Dysmenorrhea, (V1) 779
Dyspareunia, (V1) 780
Dysplasia of the hip, (V1) 737
Dyspnea, (V1) 325
Dysrhythmia
  categories of, (V1) 870–871
  of heartbeat, (V1) 320
  hypothermia and, (V1) 317
  oxygenation and, (V1) 860
Dyssomnia, (V1) 800–801
Dysuria, (V1) 633b

E
E. coli (Escherichia coli), (V1) 635, (V1) 778
Ears
  alignment of, (V1) 373f
  assessment of, (V1) 394, (V2) 261p–265p
  equilibrium, (V1) 374
  external and middle, (V1) 373
  hearing aids for, (V1) 468–469, (V1) 468f
  hearing deficits, (V1) 686b, (V1) 695,
      (V1) 696
  hearing impaired, (V1) 355, (V1) 685
  NOC outcomes and NIC interventions,
      (V2) 436
  otic irrigation, (V1) 695
  parts of, (V1) 372, (V1) 373f
  structures of, (V2) 262
Earwax, (V1) 373
Eating disorder, (V1) 596b, (V1) 611
Ecchymosis, (V1) 367t
Economy, (V1) 21, (V1) 230
Ectocervix, (V2) 328
Ectopy, (V1) 3
Ectropion, (V1) 371
Edema, (V1) 813
Education
  for bereaved person, (V1) 285
  client record for, (V1) 289
  continuing, (V1) 15
  credentialing, (V1) 1075
  as culture specific influencing health,
      (V1) 229
  entry-level, (V1) 12
  graduate nursing, (V1) 14–15
  health promotion through, (V1) 1017
  informal, (V1) 15
  in-service, (V1) 15
  licensing, (V1) 1074–1075
  practical and vocational nursing, (V1) 14
  providing and participating, (V1) 1086
  registered nursing, (V1) 14
  sexual knowledge, (V1) 772
  state-specific requirements, (V1) 15
  teaching diagnosis, (V1) 58
  using theories in, (V1) 145
Effective coping, (V1) 553
Effleurage, (V1) 998
Effort, breathing, (V1) 325

Egg crate mattress, (V1) 832, (V1) 832f
Ego, (V1) 167, (ESG9) 5
Ego defense mechanism, (V1) 559–560
Ejaculation, (V1) 765, (V1) 776
Elastic recoil, (V1) 848
Elbow ROM, (V1) 743t
Elderly
  abdomen of, (V2) 295
  assessment of, (ESG9) 37–38
  body fluid of, (V1) 888t
  bowel elimination problems, (V1) 655
  breasts of, (V2) 276
  chest of, (V2) 281p
  daily food requirement for, (V1) 597t
  developmental task theory, (ESG9) 4t
  development of, (ESG9) 35, (ESG9) 37
  ears of, (V2) 262
  eyes of, (V2) 258–259
  fire death, (V1) 425
  foot problems of, (V1) 455
  gag response, (V2) 271
  hair of, (V2) 248
  health problems, (ESG9) 37
  health promotion and screenings,
      (V1) 1011t
  health risk factors of, (V1) 214–215
  hearing loss, (V2) 264
  heart sounds of, (V2) 290
  injection, administering, (V1) 512
  intervention for, (ESG9) 38
  memory of, (V2) 310
  mouth of, (V2) 269–270
  nails of, (V2) 249
  nutritional needs, (V1) 596–597, (V1) 609
  oral medication administration, (V1)
      501–502
  oxygenation of, (V1) 855
  pain and, (V1) 704
  pain management, (V1) 719
  pain threshold, (V2) 297
  peripheral edema, (V2) 293
  rectal suppository administration, (V2) 475
  restless leg syndrome (RLS), (V1) 801
  safety of, (V1) 421
  sexuality, (V1) 769–770
  skin of, (V1) 812, (V2) 242
  sleep
    patterns of, (V1) 799
    requirements for, (V1) 795, (V1) 795t
  stressors of, (V1) 552b
  urinary elimination, (V1) 623
  urinary tract infection (UTI) and,
      (V1) 636
  vision of, (V2) 254
Elective surgery, (V1) 924
Electrical safety
  preventing hazards to, (V1) 433–434
  promoting, (V1) 426
Electrical storm, (V1) 431
Electrocardiogram (ECG)
  for irregular heart rhythm, (V1) 320
  monitoring, (V1) 869–870
  twelve-lead, (V1) 871, (V1) 871f
Electrode placement, (V1) 871, (V1) 871f
Electroencephalogram (EEG), (V1) 796
Electrolyte
  assessment of, (V1) 901, (V2) 906–908
  charges of, (V1) 888
  electrical charge of, (V1) 887
  history of, (V2) 905
  imbalance, (V1) 896, (V1) 897t–898t,
      (V1) 904

  movement of, (V1) 889
  oral supplements, (V1) 904
  outcomes and interventions for diagnoses,
      (V2) 909–911
  overview of, (V2) 871
  parenteral replacement, (V1) 905–906
  regulation of, (V1) 891, (V1) 893–894
  types and functions of, (V1) 892t–893t
Electronic blood pressure monitor, (V1) 330
Electronic health record (EHR)
  benefits of, (ESGV1) 12, (V1) 978–979
  ethical use of, (V1) 980–981
  example of, (V1) 978f
  overview of, (V2) 949
  standardized nursing language and,
      (V1) 979–980
Electronic infrared tympanic membrane ther-
      mometer, (V1) 310, (V1) 312–313,
      (V1) 312f
Electronic infusion-control device, (V1) 911
Electronic infusion pump, (V1) 896
Electronic mail (e-mail), (V1) 975
Electronic thermometer, (V1) 310, (V1) 312,
      (V1) 312f, (V2) 199
Element, (V1) 70
Elevation
  assessment of, (V2) 305p–306p
  as movement, (V1) 727f
E-mail (electronic mail), (V1) 975
Embolism, (V1) 946t
Embolus, (V1) 884
  as IV therapy complication, (V1) 917t
  as postoperative collaborative problem,
      (V1) 946t
Embryonic phase, (ESG9) 8
Emergency department (ED)
  assessment in, (V1) 42
  violence in, (V1) 437–438
Emergency Medical Treatment and Active
      Labor Act (EMTALA), (V1) 1072
Emergency surgery, (V1) 924
Emotion
  body temperature and, (V1) 309
  as factor increasing pain, (V1) 703–704
  response to stressor, (V1) 559b, (V1) 565
Emotional psychiatric diagnosis, (V1) 195
Emotional response, (V1) 59
Empathy, intellectual, (V1) 27
Empathy, in therapeutic communication,
      (V1) 346
Empirical data, (V1) 156
Employment
  of nurse, (V1) 6–7
  work settings, (V1) 20–21
Empowerment
  definition of, (V1) 960
  nursing intervention as, (V1) 1025
  sources of, (V1) 961–962
Encoding, (V1) 339
Endocervical smear, (V2) 328
Endocrine system
  adaptation failure and, (V1) 562
  age-related changes for, (ESG9) 36t
  exercise and, (V1) 734b
  pain and, (V1) 706
  response to alarm of stressor, (V1) 555
End-of-life care, (V1) 20
  barriers to communication during,
      (V1) 282b
  competencies of, (V1) 271–272
  hospice care, (V1) 272–273
  palliative care, (V1) 272

Endogenous analgesia system, *(V1) 702*
Endogenous nosocomial infection, *(V1) 401*
Endogenous opioids, *(V1) 702*
Endorphin, *(V1) 555*
Endotracheal airway, *(V1) 878–879,*
    (V2) 863tb
Endotracheal tube
    management of, *(V1) 878*
    placement of, *(V1) 878f*
    suctioning of, *(V2) 840p–845p*
    use of, *(V1) 878*
End-stage renal disease (ESRD), *(V1) 633b*
Enema
    administration of, *(V1) 662p,*
        (V1) 669–670, (V2) 646p–650p
        barium, *(V2) 667*
        cleansing, *(V1) 668, (V2) 647p–648p*
        oil-retention, *(V1) 668, (V2) 663tb*
        prepackaged, *(V2) 648p*
        return-flow, *(V1) 669, (V2) 663tb*
        solutions used in, *(V1) 669t*
        types of, *(V1) 668–669*
Energy
    calculating client's needs, *(V1) 593,*
        (V1) 593t
    of grieving, *(V1) 266*
    maintenance and mobility, *(V2) 724*
    qi, *(V1) 993, (V1) 994f*
    yin and yang, *(V1) 992*
Energy balance, *(V1) 591–592*
Energy nutrient, *(V1) 575, (V1) 576t*
Energy therapy, *(V1) 999–1000*
Enjoying, *(V1) 181, (V1) 182*
Enkephalins, *(V1) 702*
Enlightenment, *(V1) 252*
Enteral medication, *(V1) 500*
Enteral nutrition
    feeding schedules for, *(V1) 614*
    feeding systems, *(V1) 615*
    monitoring patient receiving, *(V2) 582tb*
    solutions for, *(V1) 615b*
Enteric-coated drug, *(V1) 479*
Enteric tube, feeding through,
    (V2) 572p–576p
Enterohepatic recirculation, *(V1) 485*
Entropion, *(V1) 371*
Entry, portal of, *(V1) 400*
Enuresis, *(V1) 803*
    management of, *(V1) 648*
    overview of, *(V1) 623, (V1) 637*
Environment
    assessment of, *(V1) 690*
    body temperature and, *(V1) 309*
    communication and, *(V1) 343*
    definition of, *(V1) 420*
    drug absorption, *(V1) 483–484*
    as factor of health, *(V1) 176*
    heat exchange, *(V1) 308*
    importance in care of patients, *(V1) 145*
    infection, risk of, *(V1) 406*
    learning and, *(V1) 533*
    loss adjustment, *(V1) 265, (V1) 266*
    for medical asepsis, *(V1) 408*
    mobility concerns, *(V1) 735, (V1) 737,*
        (V1) 741
    oxygenation and, *(V1) 855*
    of patient/client, *(V1) 469–470*
    pharmacokinetics and, *(V1) 488*
    physical examination preparation,
        (V1) 359–360
    pollution in, *(V1) 431*
    sleep and, *(V1) 800*

sterility of, *(V1) 414*
for surgical asepsis, *(V1) 413*
theory and, *(V1) 144*
urination and, *(V1) 623*
Environmental control
    culture care etiquette, *(V1) 242t*
    as culture specific influencing health,
        (V1) 229
Environmental hazards, *(V1) 420*
Environmental health, *(ESGV1) 7*
Environmental Protection Agency (EPA)
    dangers of mercury, *(V1) 312, (V1) 436*
    reducing solid waste, *(V1) 431*
Enzymatic debridement, *(V1) 836*
Enzyme, *(V1) 578*
Eosinophil, *(V1) 402, (V1) 403t*
Epidemiology, *(V1) 9*
Epidermis, *(V1) 447, (V1) 811, (ESG9) 14*
Epidural anesthesia, *(V1) 939, (V1) 939f*
Epidural catheter, care for, *(V2) 691tb*
Epiglottis, *(V1) 846, (V1) 846f*
Epinephrine
    function of, *(V1) 557f*
    increasing metabolism, *(V1) 307*
    production of, *(V1) 308*
Epithelial healing, *(V1) 816*
Epithelization, *(V1) 817*
Equianalgesia, *(V1) 716*
Equilibrium, *(V1) 374*
Equipment-related accident, *(V1) 433*
Equipment safety, *(V2) 1021tb*
Erectile dysfunction (ED)
    aging and, *(V1) 770*
    as arousal disorder, *(V1) 780*
Erickson, Erik, *(V1) 151, (V1) 166, (V1) 167,*
    (V1) 189
Erogenous zone, *(V1) 775*
Erosion, skin, *(V2) 246*
Error
    automation decreasing, *(V1) 980*
    medication-related, *(V1) 521,*
        (V1) 525–526
Erythema, *(V1) 367t, (V1) 448*
Eschar, *(V1) 822, (V1) 822f*
Eschatology, *(V1) 248*
Escherichia coli (E. coli), *(V1) 635, (V1) 778*
Esophagogastroduodenoscopy (EGD),
    (V2) 666
Esophagus, function of, *(V1) 651*
Essential amino acid, *(V1) 577, (V1) 578t*
Essential fatty acid, *(V1) 580*
Essential hypertension, *(V1) 334*
Essential nutrient, *(V1) 582*
Essential oils, *(V1) 687*
Essential patient goal, *(V1) 95–96*
Esteem, *(V1) 50, (V1) 67*
Estrogen, *(V1) 770*
Ethical agency, *(V1) 1048*
Ethical knowledge, *(V1) 29*
Ethics
    code of, *(V1) 40, (V1) 1056, (V1) 1059,*
        (V1) 1060b, (V1) 1076–1077
    compromising, *(V1) 1066–1067*
    decision-making, *(V1) 1063, (V1) 1068*
    definition of, *(V1) 1045–1046*
    feminist, *(V1) 1058*
    in health care, *(V1) 1062*
    knowledge map of, *(V2) 1005*
    MORAL model, *(V1) 1065–1066*
    morals and values relating to, *(V1) 1054*
    nursing, *(V1) 1047–1048*
    obligations in decisions, *(V1) 1067–1068*

    overview of, *(V2) 1005*
    problem solving, *(V1) 1065*
    professional guidelines, *(V1) 1059*
Ethics committee, *(V1) 1068–1069*
Ethics-of-care, *(V1) 1058–1059*
Ethnic group, *(V1) 225–226*
Ethnicity
    definition of, *(V1) 225–226*
    knowledge map of, *(V2) 146*
    nutrition and, *(V1) 599*
    statistics in nursing, *(V1) 10t*
    in United States, *(V1) 223f*
Ethnocentrism, *(V1) 224, (V1) 237*
Ethnocultural, *(V1) 227*
Etiology
    bowel-related problems, *(V1) 664*
    of communication diagnoses, *(V1) 349*
    complex, *(V1) 76*
    deficient knowledge as, *(V1) 538, (V1) 539*
    diagnostic statement, *(V1) 73, (V1) 74t,*
        (V1) 77–78
    identification of problem, *(V1) 66*
    impaired oxygenation, *(V1) 872–873*
    impaired skin integrity as, *(V1) 449*
    loss and grieving as, *(V1) 277*
    nutrition-related, *(V1) 606*
    overweight and obesity, *(V1) 610*
    self-concept as, *(V1) 195*
    sexual problems, *(V1) 782–783*
    sleep pattern disturbance, *(V1) 805*
    underweight and malnutrition, *(V1) 611*
    unknown, *(V1) 76*
    urinary retention, *(V1) 636*
Eupnea, *(V1) 324*
European American, folk healer, *(V1) 230t*
    healing system of, *(V1) 234t*
Eustress, *(V1) 551*
Euthanasia, *(V1) 275*
Evaluate, failure to, *(V1) 1083*
Evaluation
    abuse assessment, *(V2) 91*
    of anxiety, *(V1) 203*
    apical pulse assessment, *(V2) 209*
    apical-radial pulse assessment, *(V2) 211*
    beard and mustache care, *(V2) 419*
    bed bath, *(V2) 394*
    bed-monitoring device, *(V2) 370*
    blood pressure assessment, *(V2) 216*
    bowel incontinence, *(V1) 675*
    bowel-related problems, *(V1) 665*
    checklist for, *(V2) 69–71*
    clean-catch specimen, collecting, *(V2) 597*
    of collaborative problems, *(V1) 135*
    for communication problems, *(V1) 349*
    contact lenses, removing and care for,
        (V2) 423
    continuous bladder irrigation, *(V2) 615*
    for dying and grieving, *(V1) 277*
    of evidence, *(V1) 985*
    external (condom) application, *(V2) 618*
    eyes before medication administration,
        (V2) 461
    for family health status diagnoses,
        (V1) 218
    of feet problems, *(V1) 456*
    as final step of nursing process, *(V1) 128*
    fingerstick blood glucose levels, *(V2) 565*
    foot care, *(V2) 404*
    full-spectrum nursing and, *(V1) 36,*
        (V1) 128–129
    gastric and enteric tube feedings,
        (V2) 575

Evaluation (continued)
  hand washing, (V2) 345
  of health, (V1) 182
  health information web site,
    (V1) 985b–986b
  for home health care diagnoses,
    (V1) 1040
  hypertension, (V1) 334
  for hypotension, (V1) 334
  ineffective sexuality pattern, (V1) 786
  of infection, (V1) 407–408
  of integumentary problems, (V1) 449
  intermittent bladder and catheter irriga-
    tion, (V2) 612
  intermittent infusion administration,
    (V2) 512
  intradermal medication administration,
    (V2) 486–488
  intramuscular injection administration,
    (V2) 499
  Intravenous medication administration,
    (V2) 507
  knowledge map of, (V2) 72
  of learning, (V1) 547
  medication administration, (V2) 452
  model of, (V1) 121f
  nail care, (V1) 458
  nasal medication administration, (V2) 467
  nasogastric and nasoenteric tubes
    insertion, (V2) 571
  nasogastric and nasoenteric tubes
    removal, (V2) 578
  nursing process and, (V1) 32f, (V1) 33,
    (V1) 132
  nursing process model, (V1) 31f
  nutrition-related problems, (V1) 606–607
  oral care for unconscious patient,
    (V2) 413
  overview of, (V2) 62
  pain management, (V1) 720
  of patient progress, (V1) 132
  perineal care, (V2) 401
  pulse rate assessment, (V2) 207
  recording evaluative statement,
    (V1) 133–134
  rectal suppository administration, (V2) 475
  reflecting critically about, (V1) 136
  respiration assessment, (V2) 213
  restraints, using, (V2) 373
  shampooing bedrest patient, (V2) 417
  shaving patient, (V2) 421
  sleep pattern disturbance, (V1) 805
  for spirituality diagnoses, (V1) 258
  standards and criteria in, (V1) 129–130
  stress-related problems, (V1) 567
  stress urinary incontinence, (V1) 630
  subcutaneous medication administration,
    (V2) 491
  temperature, (V2) 202
  for temperature/fever diagnoses, (V1) 315
  types of, (V1) 130–131
  urinary catheter insertion, (V2) 608
  urinary elimination, (V1) 638
  vaginal medication administration,
    (V2) 470
  of vital signs (VS), (V1) 335–336
  for weight control, (V1) 610
Evaluation data, (V1) 132
Evaporation, heat loss and, (V1) 308
Eversion
  assessment of, (V2) 305p–306p
  as movement, (V1) 727f

Evidence-based medicine, (V1) 108
Evidence-based practice
  computers and, (V1) 977–978, (V1) 981
  goal of, (V1) 108
  informatics and, (V1) 981
  knowledge map of, (V2) 73
Evidence-Based Practice Center (EPC),
  (V1) 108
Evidence reports, (V1) 108
Evil eye, prevention of, (V1) 227
Evisceration, (V1) 820, (V1) 820f
  as postoperative collaborative problem,
    (V1) 948t
Evolution of nursing
  knowledge map of, (V2) 11
  overview of, (V2) 6
Exacerbation, (V1) 180
Excess Fluid Volume, (V1) 59
Excitement
  aging and, (V1) 775b
  as sexual response, (V1) 776
Exclusion, (V1) 1088
Excoriation, (V1) 449
Excoriation, skin, (V2) 246
Excretion, of drugs, (V1) 485, (V1) 487t
Excursion, of chest, (V2) 283
Exercise
  in bed, teaching patient to,
    (V2) 918p–921p
  benefits of, (V1) 732–733, (V1) 734b
  blood pressure and, (V1) 329
  body temperature and, (V1) 309
  bowel function and, (V1) 655–656
  defecation and, (V1) 666
  as defense of infection, (V1) 405
  guidelines for, (V1) 731–732
  health and, (V1) 174
  health promotion and, (V1) 1016
  history questions, (V2) 721
  importance of, (V1) 568
  Kegel, (V1) 647
  management of, (V2) 724
  overview of, (V2) 696
  oxygenation and, (V1) 857
  pelvic floor muscle, (V1) 647
  physical assessment of, (V2) 722–723
  physical conditioning for walking,
    (V2) 718tb
  program for, (V1) 733
  promoting, (V1) 748
  pulse rate, (V1) 318
  range of motion, (V1) 757
  respiration and, (V1) 323
  risks associated with, (V1) 733–734
  skin integrity, (V1) 814
  sleep and, (V1) 800
  for stress management, (V1) 570
  tests for intensity of, (V1) 732b
  types of, (V1) 731
  urination and, (V1) 623–624
Exhalation, (V1) 848, (V1) 848f
Exhaustion, (V1) 557
Exhaustion stage, of GAS, (V1) 555f, (V1) 557
Exit, portal of, (V1) 400
Exocrine glands, (V1) 485
Exogenous nosocomial infection, (V1) 401
Exophthalmos, (V1) 371
Expectation, identification of, (V1) 151
Expected outcome
  as goal, (V1) 92
  problem type and, (V1) 96t
  reflecting critically about, (V1) 100–102

Experience, nursing behavior factor, (V1) 68–69
Expertise, sharing and enhancing, (V1)
  961–962
Expert witness, (V1) 1080
Expiration, (V1) 323f
Expiratory reserve volume (ERV), (V1) 849
Extended family, (V1) 210
Extended healthcare services, (ESGV1) 4
Extension
  assessment of, (V2) 305p–306p
  as movement, (V1) 727f
External (condom) catheter, (V1) 645,
  (V2) 616p–618p
External ear, (V1) 372
External locus of control, (V1) 190
External loss, (V1) 264
External respiration, (V1) 322, (V1) 850
External rotation, (V1) 727f
External sphincter, (V1) 653, (V1) 654f
External stressor, (V1) 551
External urethral sphincter, (V1) 622
Extracellular fluid (ECF)
  as body fluid compartment, (V1) 887–888
  types of, (V2) 871
  water and, (V1) 582
Extraocular muscle (EOM), (V1) 372
Extravasation, (V1) 916t
Extrinsic factors, pressure ulcer, (V1) 821
Eyeglasses, care for, (V1) 466
Eyelid, abnormal findings, (V1) 371
Eyes
  abnormalities of, (V2) 334
  artificial, care for, (V1) 467–468,
    (V2) 430tb
  assessment of, (V1) 370, (V1) 394,
    (V1) 466, (V2) 253p–260p, (V2) 433
  care of, (V1) 466
  defense against infection, (V1) 402
  diagnosis of problems, (V1) 466
  external structures of, (V1) 370–372,
    (V1) 371f
  eyeglasses and contact lenses, (V1) 466
  eyelids, (V1) 370–371
  impaired vision, (V1) 355, (V1) 685
  internal structures of, (V1) 372
  mercury effect on, (V1) 436t
  movement of, (V1) 372
  NOC outcomes and NIC interventions,
    (V2) 436
  PERRLA, (V1) 371
  treatment for poisoning of, (V1) 424
  visual acuity of, (V1) 371–372
  visual deficits, (V1) 685b, (V1) 694–695,
    (V1) 696
  visual field, (V1) 372
Eye shield, (V1) 410f
Eyewitness, (V1) 1080

F
Face
  appearance of, (V1) 370
  assessment of, (V1) 393–394
Face mask, (V1) 410f, (V2) 819p–822p
Face-to-face conversation, (V1) 338
Facial expression, (V1) 342
Facsimile (fax), (V1) 975
FACT, for charting and documenting,
  (V1) 1084, (V2) 1022tb
Fact witness, (V1) 1080
Fahrenheit scale, (V1) 310, (V1) 312, (V2) 219
Fair-mindedness, (V1) 27
Faith, (V1) 248–249

Faith development
　overview of, *(ESG9) 8*
　stages of, *(ESG9) 9t*
　theory of, *(V1) 168*
Faithfulness, *(V1) 1055–1056*
Falls
　injury prevention from, *(V1) 433f*
　preventing injury from, *(V1) 425–426,*
　　(V1) 432–433
　risk assessment, *(V1) 438*
False imprisonment, *(V1) 1078*
Family
　assessment of, *(V2) 124tb*
　caring for, *(V1) 153*
　change in behavior or attitude of member
　　of, *(V1) 212*
　definition of, *(V1) 210*
　development of, *(V2) 125*
　of dying patient, *(V1) 283*
　health of, *(V1) 99, (V1) 218b*
　health risk factors of, *(V1) 213–216*
　homelessness, *(V1) 216*
　infectious disease and, *(V1) 215–216*
　intervention for, *(V1) 218, (V1) 219*
　loss of, *(V1) 265*
　mobility concerns, *(V1) 741*
　nursing care for, *(V1) 217–218*
　outcome statement, *(V1) 218*
　overview of, *(V2) 118*
　patient at home, preparing for, *(V1) 84*
　poverty and unemployment, *(V1) 215*
　pressure ulcer prevention, teaching,
　　(V1) 833
　promoting wellness, *(V1) 219*
　relationship as health factor, *(V1) 175*
　self-concept and, *(V1) 190*
　as special needs assessment, *(V1) 44*
　stages of development, *(V1) 212t*
　structural-functional approaches to,
　　(V1) 212–213
　structure of, *(V1) 210–211*
　teaching about pain, *(V1) 720*
　violence and neglect within, *(V1) 216*
Family care/health
　approaches to, *(V1) 211*
　intervention for, *(V2) 127*
　knowledge map of, *(V2) 129*
　outcome labels, *(V2) 126*
　theories for, *(V1) 211–213*
Family history, *(V1) 46, (V1) 328*
Family nursing, *(V2) 118*
Farsightedness, *(V1) 372, (V1) 685b*
Fat
　catabolism of, *(V1) 308*
　definition of, *(V1) 579*
　glycerides as true, *(V1) 579*
　types of, *(V1) 580t*
Fat-restricted diet, *(V1) 601*
Fat-soluble vitamin, *(V1) 581,*
　(V1) 583t
Fatty acid, *(V1) 580*
Fax (facsimile), *(V1) 975*
Fear
　definition of, *(V1) 199, (V1) 203*
　as an emotional response, *(V1) 59*
　response to stressor, *(V1) 559*
　of spiritual care, *(V1) 254–255*
Febrile episode, *(V1) 314*
Fecal impaction
　management of, *(V1) 667–668*
Fecal incontinent pouch, *(V1) 671*
Fecal occult blood test, *(V1) 661*

Feces, *(V1) 651*
　characteristics and variations of, *(V1) 660t*
　definition of, *(V1) 654*
　elimination of
　　diagnostic testing for, *(V1) 660–661*
　　overview of, *(V2) 636*
　　pattern assessment, *(V2) 636*
　　process of, *(V1) 654*
　fluid output, *(V1) 891*
　See also Stool
Federal government
　Canada Health Act, *(ESGV1) 5–6*
　health care funding, *(ESGV1) 10*
　Healthy Environment and Consumer
　　Safety, *(ESGV1) 7*
Federal law, *(V1) 1072–1074*
Feedback
　communication and, *(V1) 340*
　learning and, *(V1) 533*
　from patient about activity, *(V1) 123*
　of system, *(V1) 152*
Feeding, as ADL, *(V1) 43b*
Feeding methods
　enteral nutrition (tube feeding),
　　(V1) 613–616
　gastric and enteric tube, *(V2) 572p–576p*
　parenteral nutrition (central venous
　　catheter), *(V1) 616–617*
Feeding tube
　checking placement of, *(V1) 614, (V2) 581*
　types of, *(V1) 613–614*
Fellatio, *(V1) 777*
Felony, *(V1) 1077*
Female circumcision, *(V1) 772*
Female condom
　application of, *(V1) 790*
Female reproductive system, *(V1) 764,*
　(V1) 764f
Feminist ethics, *(V1) 1058*
Femoral artery
　pulse rate assessment, *(V1) 319,*
　　(V1) 319f, (V2) 206
Fencing reflex, *(ESG9) 14*
Fertilization, *(ESG9) 8*
Fetal alcohol syndrome, *(ESG9) 15*
Fetus, *(ESG9) 8, (ESG9) 9, (ESG9) 10t–11t*
Fever
　infection, defense against, *(V1) 402*
　nursing activities for, *(V1) 315*
　phases of, *(V1) 314*
　pulse rate, *(V1) 318*
　respiration and, *(V1) 323*
　skin breakdown, *(V1) 814*
　types of, *(V1) 314*
Fiber
　A-delta, *(V1) 701–702, (V1) 702f,*
　　(V1) 703f
　bowel function and, *(V1) 655–656*
　C-delta, *(V1) 701–702, (V1) 702f,*
　　(V1) 703f
　digestion of, *(V1) 577*
　high-fiber foods, *(V1) 655b*
Fiberoptic colonoscopy, *(V2) 666–667*
Fibroblast, *(V1) 817*
Fidelity, *(V1) 1055–1056*
"Fight or flight", *(V1) 555*
Filter needle, *(V1) 507*
Filter straw, of needle, *(V1) 507*
Filtrate, *(V1) 620*
Filtration
　glomerular, *(V1) 620*
　process of, *(V1) 889, (V1) 890t*

Final cause, *(V1) 1057*
Finances
　health and, *(V1) 176*
　hygiene practice and, *(V1) 443*
　oral problems and, *(V1) 459*
Finances, as factor of health, *(V1) 214,*
　(V1) 215
Fingers ROM, *(V1) 743t*
Fingerstick blood glucose level,
　(V2) 563p–566p
Fire
　prevention of, *(V1) 425–426,*
　　(V1) 433–434
　response in healthcare facility, *(V1) 434b*
Firearm safety, *(V1) 426*
First Conference on Nursing Diagnosis,
　(V1) 58
First-contact health service, *(ESGV1) 18*
First Nations, health services, *(ESGV1) 7*
First-pass effect, *(V1) 485*
Fissure, skin, *(V2) 246*
Fistula, *(V1) 820, (V1) 820f*
Fitness assessment, *(V1) 1009*
Fixed-pie myth, *(V1) 966*
Flaccidity, *(V1) 740b*
Flatus
　with bowel elimination, *(V1) 654*
　foods causing, *(V1) 677b*
　management of, *(V1) 670*
Flexibility
　assessment of, *(V1) 1009*
　Swedish massage and, *(V1) 998*
　training, *(V1) 731–732*
Flexible envisioning, *(V1) 183*
Flexion
　assessment of, *(V2) 305p–306p*
　as movement, *(V1) 727f*
Flora, normal, *(V1) 399*
Flossing teeth, *(V1) 462, (V2) 406p–408p*
Flow rate calculation, *(V1) 915*
flow sheet
　for assessment, *(V1) 294, (V2) 187*
　graphic, *(V1) 53f*
　long-term care, *(V2) 186*
Fluid
　assessment of, *(V2) 906–908*
　assessment of imbalance, *(V1) 901*
　defecation and, *(V1) 666*
　history of, *(V2) 905*
　hypervolemia and, *(V1) 896*
　hypovolemia and, *(V1) 896*
　imbalance prevention, *(V1) 904*
　intake
　　facilitating, *(V1) 905*
　　recommendations for, *(V1) 890–891*
　intake and output (I&O), *(V1) 902*
　outcomes and interventions for diagnoses,
　　(V2) 909–911
　overload as IV therapy complication,
　　(V1) 917t
　overview of, *(V2) 871*
　parenteral replacement, *(V1) 905–906*
　pharmacokinetics and, *(V1) 488*
　promoting normal urination, *(V1) 639*
　restriction, *(V1) 905*
　See also Body fluid
Fluid output, *(V1) 891*
Fluid volume deficit (hypovolemia), *(V1) 896*
Fluid volume excess (hypervolemia), *(V1) 896*
Fluoxetine (Prozac), *(V1) 788*
Flushing, of skin, *(V1) 367t*
Focus charting, *(V1) 292*

Focused assessment, *(V1) 42*
Focused physical assessment, *(V1) 359*
Foley catheter, *(V1) 632, (V1) 641*
Folic acid, *(ESG9) 12–13*
FOLK, *(V1) 49*
FOLK (active listening behavior), *(V1) 49*
Folk healer, *(V1) 230t, (V1) 235*
Folk medicine
   definition of, *(V1) 235*
   as indigenous health care system,
      (V1) 231
Follicular phase, *(V1) 764*
Follower
   definition of, *(V1) 958*
   effective skills for, *(V1) 959b*
Followership, *(V1) 958–959*
Fomite, *(V1) 400*
Fontanelles (soft spots), *(ESG9) 13,*
   (ESG9) 13f
Food
   assisting patient with, technique,
      (V2) 580
   high-fiber, *(V1) 655b*
   pulse rate, *(V1) 318*
   sleep and, *(V1) 800*
   unprocessed, *(V1) 997*
Food allergy, *(V1) 657*
Food and Drug Administration (FDA)
   fat substitutes, *(V1) 611*
   regulating drugs and medications,
      (V1) 476
   severe adverse reaction, *(V1) 489*
Food-borne pathogen, *(V1) 429*
Food diary, *(V1) 602*
Food Guide
   Canada, *(V1) 587, (V1) 588f*
   serving sizes, *(V1) 590t*
   USDA, *(V1) 587, (V1) 589f*
Food guides, *(V1) 582*
Food intolerance, *(V1) 657*
Food poisoning, *(V1) 429*
Food safety, *(V1) 430*
Food stamp program, *(V1) 608*
Foot
   assessment of, *(V1) 456, (V2) 432–433*
   care for, *(V2) 402p–405p*
   care of, *(V1) 455*
   deformity affecting mobility and activity,
      (V1) 737
   diabetic care of, *(V1) 457*
   diagnosis of problems, *(V1) 456*
   intervention/implementation, *(V1) 456*
   NOC outcomes and NIC interventions,
      (V2) 435
   odor of, *(V1) 456*
   outcome and evaluation of, *(V1) 456*
   problems of, *(V1) 455–456*
   range of motion, *(V1) 745t*
   self-care and, *(V1) 53*
Footboard, *(V1) 749, (V1) 750f*
Foot cradle, *(V1) 749*
Forearm support crutch, *(V1) 759*
Forgiveness, *(V1) 249*
Formalism, *(V1) 1057*
Formal operational stage, of development,
   (V1) 535, (ESG9) 27, (ESG9) 31
Formal planning, *(V1) 82*
Formulary, *(V1) 474, (V1) 475*
Fowler, James, *(V1) 168, (ESG9) 8*
Fowler's position, *(V1) 750, (V1) 750t,*
   (V1) 752
Fraction of inspired oxygen (F\text{IO}$_2$), *(V1) 869*

Fracture, *(V1) 738*
Framework
   concept of, *(V1) 50*
   conceptual, *(V1) 142*
   deontological, *(V1) 1057–1058*
   moral (philosophical), *(V1) 1057*
Framingham Study, *(V1) 139, (V1) 156*
France, Hôtel Dieu, *(V1) 4, (V1) 4f*
Fraud, *(V1) 1078–1079*
Fremitus, *(V2) 284*
French (Fr) scale, *(V1) 613*
French catheter, *(V1) 641*
Frequency
   of exercise, *(V1) 732*
   of urination, *(V1) 633b*
Freud, Anna, *(ESG9) 5*
Freud, Sigmund, *(V1) 166, (V1) 167, (ESG9) 5*
Friction
   pressure ulcers and, *(V1) 821*
   Swedish massage and, *(V1) 998*
Friction-reducing device, *(V1) 753–754*
Friendship, same-gender, *(ESG9) 24–25*
Fruitarian, *(V1) 598*
Full liquid diet, *(V1) 601*
Full-spectrum nursing, *(V1) 10, (V1) 15*
   definition of, *(V1) 33*
   importance of evaluation, *(V1) 128–129*
   informatics and, *(V1) 972–973*
   as jigsaw puzzle, *(V1) 140*
   model of, *(V1) 33, (V1) 34f, (V2) 11*
   then and now, *(V1) 3*
   understanding model of, *(V1) 34–36*
Full-thickness wound, *(V1) 816*
Function
   optimum level from patient, *(V1) 93*
   and role of nurse, *(V1) 13t*
Functional ability assessment, *(V1) 43, (V1) 47*
Functional Health Patterns, Gordon's,
   (V1) 51b
Functional residual capacity (FRC), *(V1) 849*
Fungus, *(V1) 857*
Fungus infection, *(V2) 334*

G
Gag response, in elderly, *(V2) 271*
Gait
   abnormalities of, *(V1) 385, (V2) 335*
   assessment of, *(V1) 746, (V2) 302p–303p*
   for crutches, *(V1) 760–761, (V1) 760f*
   as nonverbal communication,
      (V1) 342–343
Galactosemia, *(ESG9) 16*
Gaming, *(V1) 546*
Gamp, Sairy, *(V1) 7*
Gang rape, *(V1) 779*
Gang violence, *(V1) 216*
Gas. *See* Flatus
Gas exchange. *See* Respiration
Gas transport, *(V1) 322*
Gastric lipase, *(V1) 651*
Gastric secretions, decreased, *(V1) 609*
Gastric tube, feeding through,
   (V2) 572p–576p
Gastroenteritis, *(V1) 905–906*
Gastroesophageal reflux, *(V1) 609*
Gastroesophageal sphincter, *(V1) 651*
Gastrointestinal (GI) tract
   adaptation failure and, *(V1) 562*
   age-related changes for, *(ESG9) 36t*
   anatomical structures of, *(V1) 651–653*
   defense against infection, *(V1) 402*
   drug excretion, *(V1) 485*

   exercise and, *(V1) 734b*
   immobility, effects on, *(V1) 740*
   oral drugs, absorption of, *(V1) 485*
   stressor response, *(V1) 555–556*
   structure and function of, *(V1) 652f*
   studies of, *(V2) 665–668*
   surgery preparation, *(V1) 933*
Gastronomy medication, *(V1) 500*
Gate-control theory, *(V1) 702–703, (V1) 703f*
Gauge, *(V1) 507, (V1) 906*
Gauze dressing
   characteristics of, *(V1) 837*
   shapes and forms of, *(V1) 837f*
   types and use of, *(V1) 838t*
Gay couple, *(V1) 211*
Gay man, *(V1) 768*
Gender
   determination of, *(V1) 766*
   self-concept and, *(V1) 189*
Gender, as factor of health, *(V1) 173*
Gender identity, *(V1) 767, (V1) 770*
Gender role, *(V1) 766–767*
General adaptation syndrome (GAP)
   as response to stressors, *(V1) 554*
   stages of, *(V1) 555f*
      alarm, *(V1) 555–556*
      exhaustion or recovery, *(V1) 557*
      resistance, *(V1) 556–557*
General anesthesia, *(V1) 937–938, (V1) 938f*
General premise, *(V1) 143*
General survey
   aspects of, *(V1) 365*
   assessment of, *(V1) 393p, (V2) 234p,*
      (V2) 237p–240p
   documentation of, *(V1) 392–393*
General systems theory, *(V1) 212*
General weight guide, *(V1) 594*
Generativity, *(ESG9) 33*
Generic name, *(V1) 474*
Genetics
   as health factor, *(V1) 173*
   pharmacokinetics and, *(V1) 488*
Genetic theory, *(ESG9) 35*
Genital herpes, *(ESG9) 32*
Genital wart, *(V2) 336, (ESG9) 32*
Genital warts, *(V1) 778*
Genitourinary system
   abnormalities of, *(V2) 336*
   age-related changes for, *(ESG9) 36t*
   assessment of, *(V1) 390–391, (V1) 396p*
      female, *(V1) 390–391, (V2) 325p–330p*
      male, *(V1) 390, (V2) 321p–324p*
   defense against infection, *(V1) 402*
   genitalia, female, *(V1) 391f*
   immobility, effects on, *(V1) 740*
   pain and, *(V1) 706*
   sexual development
      female, *(V1) 391f*
      male, *(V1) 390f*
Genuineness, in therapeutic communication,
   (V1) 346–347
Genu varum (bowlegs), *(V2) 301*
Geopolitical boundary, *(V1) 1022, (V1) 1022f*
Geriatric Depression Scale (GDS), *(ESG9) 38*
Germ theory, *(V1) 145*
Gestational period, *(ESG9) 8*
Gesture, in communication, *(V1) 343*
Giger and Davidhizar's transcultural assess-
   ment model, *(V2) 143tb*
Gilligan, Carol, *(V1) 167, (ESG9) 8*
Gingiva, *(V1) 374, (V1) 459*
Gingival recession, *(V2) 334*

Gingivitis, (V1) 375, (V1) 460
Ginkgo biloba, (V1) 207
Ginseng, (V1) 207
Glass thermometer, (V1) 312, (V1) 312f, (V2) 199
Glaucoma, (V1) 685b
Gliding joint, (V1) 728t
Gliding joint ROM, (V1) 745t
Global assessment, (V1) 42
Globin, (V1) 605
Glomerular filtration rate, (V1) 620
Glomerulus, (V1) 620
Glossitis, (V1) 375, (V1) 460
Glucose, (V1) 519
Glucose intolerance, (V1) 609
Gluteal muscles, (V1) 757
Glycerides, (V1) 579, (V1) 579b
Glycogen, (V1) 577f
Goal
    for collaborative problem, (V1) 96–97
    comparing long-term and short-term, (V1) 93, (V1) 94t
    definition of, (V1) 92–93
    essential versus nonessential, (V1) 95–96
    formulation, (V1) 92
    health promotion, (V1) 182
    importance of, (V1) 93
    judge achievement of, (V1) 133
    for learning, (V1) 538–540
    nursing diagnosis and, (V1) 94–95
    reassessment of, (V1) 133t
    relating to nursing diagnosis, (V1) 95t
    sexual problems, (V2) 737
    types of, (V1) 132–133
    writing for groups, (V1) 99
Goal/expected outcome
    bowel incontinence, (V1) 673
    formulation of, (V1) 92
    for home health care diagnoses, (V1) 1040–1041
    ineffective sexuality pattern, (V1) 784
    intervention flowing from, (V1) 111t
    for nursing diagnosis, (V1) 96
    purpose of, (V1) 93
    reflecting critically about, (V1) 100–102
    stress urinary incontinence, (V1) 627
Goal statement
    activity and exercise, (V1) 747
    for aggregates, (V1) 1031
    for client safety, (V1) 439
    components of, (V1) 93–94, (V2) 44
    for eye care, (V1) 466
    for family, (V1) 218
    for feet problems, (V1) 456
    fluid and electrolyte balance, (V1) 903
    growth and development, (ESG9) 39
    health promotion, (V1) 1015–1016
    for hypothermia, (V1) 316
    for integumentary problems, (V1) 449
    for intraoperative phase, (V1) 941
    medication-related, (V1) 496
    nail care, (V1) 458
    normal bowel patterns, (V1) 665
    nutrition-related problems, (V1) 606–607
    for oral cavity/mouth problems, (V1) 461
    pain relief, (V1) 709
    for psychosocial diagnosis, (V1) 203
    for pulse status, (V1) 321
    reflecting cultural sensitivity, (V1) 240
    for self-care deficit, (V1) 446
    for sensory perception, (V1) 692

    skin integrity and wound healing, (V1) 831
    sleep promotion, (V1) 805
    stress-related problems, (V1) 567
    for underweight and malnutrition, (V1) 611
    for urinary elimination, (V1) 638
    for weight control, (V1) 610
Gonorrhea, (V1) 778, (ESG9) 12
Good Samaritan law, (V1) 1074, (V1) 1087
Gordon's Functional Health Patterns, (V1) 51b
Government, nurses in, (ESGV1) 24
Grace and Grit, (V1) 175
Gram, (V2) 518
Grand theory, (V1) 145
Granulation, (V1) 817, (V1) 817f
Granulation tissue, (V1) 816, (V1) 817
Graphesthesia, (V1) 389
Graphic flow sheet, (V1) 53f
Graphic record, (V1) 294
Grasp reflex, (ESG9) 14
Graves' disease, (V1) 370
Gravity feeding, (V1) 614
Gravity flow, (V1) 911
Gravity, line and center of, (V1) 730, (V1) 730f
Grief
    anticipatory or dysfunctional, (V1) 195
    definition of, (V1) 265
    diagnosis, (V1) 276–277
    education for, (V1) 285
    facilitating work for, (V1) 282–283
    factors affecting, (V1) 266
    knowledge map for, (V2) 176
    Kübler-Ross stages of, (V1) 271b
    overview of, (V2) 158
    reactions to, (V1) 269t
    stages of, (V1) 265–266
    theory about, (V1) 145
    types of, (V1) 268–269
Grieving
    communication for, (V2) 166tb
    standard outcomes and interventions, (V2) 173–174
Grooming
    general survey of client, (V1) 365–366
    self-care deficit, (V1) 445, (V2) 434
    shaving as part of, (V1) 465
Gross hearing ability, (V1) 373
Group
    characteristics of a successful, (V1) 348b
    discussion as format for learning/teaching, (V1) 544
Group communication, (V1) 339, (V1) 347–348
Growth
    applying concepts of, (V1) 168
    assessment of, (ESG9) 39
    definition of, (V1) 165, (ESG9) 2
    overview of, (V2) 84
    principles of, (V1) 166, (ESG9) 3
    theory of, (ESG9) 3
Guaiac test, (V1) 661
Guided imagery, (V2) 966tb
Gulf War, (V1) 9
Gun safety, (V1) 426
Gustatory deficit
    intervention for, (V1) 696
    safety and health measures, (V1) 696
Gynecomastia, (V2) 276

H
H_2 receptor antagonist, (V1) 935t
Habit, North American healthcare system, (V1) 233t
Hahnemann, Dr. Samuel, (V1) 994
Hair
    abnormalities of, (V2) 334
    assessment of, (V1) 369, (V1) 393p, (V2) 433
    care of, (V1) 465
    cells of, (V1) 680
    combs and brushes for, (V1) 465f
    NOC outcomes and NIC interventions, (V2) 436
    shampooing, (V1) 465–466, (V2) 414p–417p
Half-and-half nails, (V2) 334
Halitosis, (V1) 460
Hall, Justice Emmett, (ESG46 V1) 3
Hand-held nebulizer, (V1) 505
Hand-hygiene antiseptic agents, (V1) 411t
Handmaiden, nurse as, (V1) 5–7
Hand ROM, (V1) 743t
Hand washing
    infection transmission and, (V1) 409f
    medical asepsis and, (V1) 408–410
    procedure for, (V1) 410p, (V2) 344p–345p
    surgical, (V1) 414p, (V2) 349p–351p
Hardiness, (V1) 180
Haustra, (V1) 653
Haustral churning, (V1) 653
Havighurst, Robert, (V1) 166, (ESG9) 3
Hay fever, (V1) 856
Head assessment, (V1) 370, (V2) 251p–252p
Head lice, (V1) 369
Head-to-toe approach, (V1) 359–360
Healing
    definition of, (V1) 558
    presence of, (V1) 185
    pressure ulcer, charting of, (V1) 828f
    timing for, (V1) 814
    of wound, (V1) 816–817, (V1) 818f
Healing modality, of CAM, (V1) 991
Healing systems, (V1) 234t
Health
    aboriginal, (ESGV1) 7
    activities promoting, (V1) 567–568
    affecting self-care ability, (V1) 443
    assessment
        definition of, (V1) 357
        overview of, (V2) 230
    beliefs
        cultural and personal, (V1) 1012–1013
        of family, (V1) 217
        system of, (V1) 231
    birth, problems at, (ESG9) 15
    Canada legislation, (ESGV1) 6, (ESGV1) 6t
    client perception of status and expectations, (V1) 46
    concepts of, (V1) 171
    drawing conclusions about status of, (V1) 63f, (V1) 65
    environmental, (ESGV1) 7
    experts view on, (V1) 171b
    factors disrupting
        competing demands, (V1) 178
        imbalance, (V1) 178–179
        impending death, (V1) 177–178
        injury, (V1) 176
        isolation, (V1) 179
        loss, (V1) 177
        mental illness, (V1) 177

Health *(continued)*
    pain, *(V1) 177*
    physical disease, *(V1) 176*
    the unknown, *(V1) 178*
    factors influencing
        biological, *(V1) 173–174*
        culture, *(V1) 175*
        environment, *(V1) 176*
        family relationships, *(V1) 175*
        finances, *(V1) 176*
        lifestyle choices, *(V1) 174–175*
        meaningful work, *(V1) 174*
        nutrition, *(V1) 174*
        physical activity, *(V1) 174*
        religion and spirituality, *(V1) 175–176*
        sleep and rest, *(V1) 174*
    grid, *(V1) 172f*
    history, *(V1) 238–239*
    images of, *(V1) 170*
    impaired adjustment to change in, *(V1) 195*
    as individual experience, *(V1) 171*
    ineffective maintenance of, *(V1) 196*
    infant problems, *(ESG9) 17–18*
    nursing process to promote, *(V1) 181–182*
    overview of, *(V2) 94*
    problem, definition of, *(V1) 59*
    products and food, *(ESGV1) 7*
    public
        community health versus, *(V1) 1025f*
        goals of, *(V1) 99*
        nursing, *(V1) 1024*
        population and, *(ESGV1) 7*
    public achievements of, *(V1) 1024b*
    screenings for, *(V1) 1010t–1011t, (V1) 1013, (V1) 1014b*
    sensory perceptual, *(V1) 693*
    sexuality and, *(V1) 773*
    skin and, *(V1) 447–448*
    smoking cessation and, *(V1) 858b*
    as surgical risk factor, *(V1) 925*
    theory and, *(V1) 144*
    Watson's theory, *(V1) 144*
    WHO definition of, *(V1) 19*
Health Act of 1996, *(ESGV1) 8*
Health Authorities Act, *(ESGV1) 8*
Health care
    abbreviations used in, *(V2) 185*
    automation decreasing errors in, *(V1) 980*
    culture of, *(V1) 175*
    economic climate of, *(V1) 960*
    ethical issues in, *(V1) 1062*
    federal government, role of, *(ESGV1) 3–4*
    indigenous versus professional, *(V1) 231*
    integrative, *(V1) 989*
    payment for, *(ESG46 V2) 1*
        individual, *(ESGV1) 11*
        private funding, *(ESGV1) 9*
        public funding, *(ESGV1) 9–10*
        taxation, *(ESGV1) 9*
    primary care in Canada, *(ESGV1) 19b*
    reason for seeking, *(V1) 46*
    role of consumer in, *(V1) 21*
    teams for, *(ESGV1) 21*
    technology for, *(V1) 23*
    trends in, *(V1) 22–23*
Healthcare delivery system
    development of, *(ESG46 V1) 3*
    factors affecting
        demographics, *(ESGV1) 11–12*
        technology, *(ESGV1) 12–13*

overview of, *(ESG46 V2) 1*
public administration of, *(ESGV1) 4*
quality issues in, *(ESGV1) 25*
Healthcare institution
    home health care, *(ESGV1) 20*
    hospital, *(ESGV1) 19*
    long-term care facility, *(ESGV1) 19*
    medication policies and procedures, *(V1) 476*
    power of physician in, *(V1) 6*
    primary care, *(ESGV1) 18–19*
    response to fire in, *(V1) 434b*
    safety hazards in, *(V1) 432–433*
    violence in, *(V1) 437–438*
Healthcare policy
    Canadian healthcare delivery system, *(ESGV1) 21*
    influence of nurses on, *(V1) 23*
    nursing's role in, *(ESGV1) 24–25*
Healthcare professional
    Canada employment of, *(ESGV1) 17–18*
    nurse as, *(ESGV1) 13–17*
Healthcare proxy, *(V1) 273*
The Health Care Quality Improvement Act of 1986 (HCQIA), *(V1) 1072*
Healthcare reform, Canada, *(ESGV1) 18*
Healthcare workers
    bloodborne pathogen exposure, *(V1) 416–417*
    hazards to, *(V1) 437–438*
    infection control for, *(V1) 416*
    vocabulary for, *(V1) 340*
Health-illness continuum, *(V1) 172, (V1) 172f*
Health information web site, *(V1) 985b–986b*
Health Insurance Portability and Accountability Act (HIPAA), *(V1) 981, (V1) 1073*
Health promotion
    activity, *(V1) 19*
    assessment, *(V1) 1009, (V1) 1012–1013*
    education for, *(V1) 1017*
    health protection versus, *(V1) 1004–1005*
    Healthy People 2010, *(V1) 1005*
    intervention, *(V1) 109*
    knowledge map for, *(V2) 983*
    life span of, *(V1) 1008, (V1) 1010t–1011t*
    lifestyle and risk assessment, *(V2) 976–978*
    nurse's role in, *(V1) 1015*
    outcome for, *(V1) 1015–1016, (V2) 979*
    overview of, *(V2) 970*
    Pender's Health promotion model (HPM), *(V1) 1006, (V1) 1007f*
    physical fitness assessment, *(V2) 975–976*
    programs for, *(V1) 1008–1009*
    role modeling, *(V1) 1016*
    steps for, *(V1) 1009*
    theory on, *(V1) 145*
    transtheoretical model of change, *(V1) 1007–1008*
    wellness diagnosis, *(V1) 1013–1015*
    Wheel of Wellness, *(V1) 1006, (V1) 1007f*
Health protection
    health promotion versus, *(V1) 1004–1005*
    levels of, *(V1) 1005*
Health restoration activity, *(V1) 19–20*
Health risk appraisal (HRA), *(V1) 1012*
Healthy Environment and Consumer Safety, *(ESGV1) 7*
Healthy People 2010
    focus areas of, *(V1) 1006b*
    goals of, *(V1) 1015*
    for health protection, *(V1) 1005*

Hearing
    assessment of, *(V1) 373–374, (V1) 394, (V2) 261p–265p*
    bedside assessment of, *(V2) 681*
    conductive and sensorineural loss of, *(V2) 264*
    deficits of, *(V1) 686b, (V1) 695, (V1) 696*
    impaired, *(V1) 355, (V1) 685b*
    sensory perceptual health, *(V1) 693*
    types of tests for, *(V1) 374*
Hearing aids, *(V1) 468–469, (V1) 468f, (V2) 431tb*
Heart
    assessment of, *(V1) 395p, (V2) 287p–293p*
    autonomic nervous system, *(V1) 853*
    ECG for monitoring, *(V1) 869*
    hypovolemia and, *(V1) 896*
    immobility, effects on, *(V1) 739*
    inspection and palpation of, *(V1) 381*
    locations for assessment of, *(V1) 381t*
    sedentary lifestyle and disease of, *(V1) 1009*
    sounds from, *(V1) 381–382*
    structures of, *(V1) 851–852, (V1) 851f*
    valve abnormalities, *(V1) 860*
Heart attack
    anesthesia as risk for, *(V1) 938*
    during exercise, *(V1) 733*
Heart failure
    as cause of hypotension, *(V1) 333*
    oxygenation and, *(V1) 860*
Heart-lung death, *(V1) 269*
Heat
    body and environment exchange, *(V1) 308*
    body producing, *(V1) 308*
    inhibition of production of, *(V1) 307*
    local application of, *(V2) 791tb*
    vasodilation, *(V1) 856*
Heat exhaustion, exercise and, *(V1) 734*
Heating pad
    for pain relief, *(V1) 710*
    for wounds, *(V1) 842–843*
Heaves, *(V1) 381*
Heberden's nodes (degenerative joint disease), *(V2) 335*
Height-weight table, *(V1) 594*
Heimlich maneuver
    on adult, *(V2) 376p–377p*
    definition of, *(V1) 427*
    on infant or child, *(V2) 375p–376p*
Helper T cell, *(V1) 403, (V1) 404*
Hematocrit, *(V1) 328*
Hematoma, *(V1) 819, (V1) 916t*
Hematuria, *(V1) 633b*
Heme, *(V1) 605*
Hemiplegia, *(V1) 740b*
Hemoccult test, *(V1) 661*
Hemodilution, *(V1) 896*
Hemoglobin
    as marker of protein metabolism, *(V1) 605*
    respiration and, *(V1) 323*
Hemorrhage
    as cause of hypotension, *(V1) 333*
    as postoperative collaborative problem, *(V1) 946t*
    of wound, *(V1) 819*
Hemorrhoids, *(V1) 392, (V1) 653*
Hemostasis, *(V1) 816, (V1) 818f, (V1) 819*
Henderson, Virginia, *(V1) 11, (V1) 146, (V1) 146b*

Henry Street Settlement, (V1) 9
Heparin
    administration of, (V1) 515
    blood clots prevention, (V1) 154
    subcutaneous administration, (V2) 518tb
Hepatotoxicity, (V1) 713
Heraclitus, (V1) 165, (ESG9) 2
Herb
    client history and current use of, (V1) 46
    pros and cons of, (V1) 997t
Herbal
    sleep aid, (V1) 808
    therapy, (V1) 997
Heritage consistency, (V1) 239
Hermaphrodite, (V1) 767
Hernia, (V1) 390
Heroin, (ESG9) 9
Herpes simplex, (V2) 333, (ESG9) 32
Herpes vulvovaginitis, (V2) 336
Heterosexual, (V1) 767, (V1) 768
Heterosexuality, (V1) 768
Hierarchy of needs, Maslow's, (V1) 50,
        (V1) 66–67, (V1) 150–151, (V1) 150f
    overview of, (V2) 100
    resistance to change, (V1) 963
High-density lipoprotein (HDL), (V1) 580
Higher-brain death, (V1) 269
High-fiber food, (V1) 655b
High-Fowler's position, (V1) 752
Hillman, James, (V1) 202
Hinduism, (V1) 4, (V1) 252
Hinge joint, (V1) 728t, (V1) 745t
HIPAA (Health Insurance Portability and
        Accountability Act), (V1) 981,
        (V1) 1073
Hippocrates, (V1) 994
Hip ROM, (V1) 744t–745t
Hirsutism, (V1) 369
Hispanic Americans
    gender role, (V1) 771
Hispanic/Latino, (V1) 226
    healing system of, (V1) 234t
    statistics in nursing, (V1) 10t
    types of folk healers, (V1) 230t
Histamine, (V1) 701
History
    of client, (V1) 46, (V1) 406
    images of nursing throughout
        angel of mercy, (V1) 4–5
        battle-ax, (V1) 7
        Caucasian woman, (V1) 9–10
        handmaiden, (V1) 5–7
        military image, (V1) 8–9
        naughty nurse, (V1) 7–8
        nursing and religion, (V1) 4–5
    of nursing research, (V1) 154
HIV. See Human immunodeficiency
        syndrome
Hive, (V2) 245
Holism, (V1) 988–989, (V1) 990
Holistic belief system, (V1) 231–232
Holistic care, (V1) 28–29
    standardized language and, (V1) 115–116
    Watson's theory, (V1) 152–153
Holistic Health and Healing, (V1) 23
Holistic health care
    beliefs of, (V1) 989
    knowledge map for, (V2) 969
    overview of, (V2) 960
    techniques for, (V2) 964tb–967tb
Holistic nursing, (V1) 139, (V1) 991
Holistic patient, (V1) 990

Holistic theory, (V1) 991
Holmes-Rahe readjustment scale, (V2) 551
Home health care
    abuse, prevention and intervention for,
        (V2) 92
    advantages and disadvantages,
        (V1) 1034–1035
    apical pulse assessment, (V2) 209
    apical-radial pulse assessment, (V2) 211
    bed bath, (V2) 394–395
    blood pressure assessment, (V2) 217
    Canadian health coverage for,
        (ESGV1) 20
    clean-catch specimen, collecting, (V2) 597
    Clinical Care Classification (CCC),
        (V1) 1040
    community health versus, (V1) 1035
    continuous bladder irrigation, (V2) 615
    definition of, (V1) 1033
    discharge plan for, (V1) 84
    enteral and parenteral feedings, (V1) 616
    external (condom) application, (V2) 618
    fingerstick blood glucose levels, (V2) 566
    food safety, (V1) 430
    foot care, (V2) 405
    future of, (V1) 1037
    gastric and enteric tube feedings,
        (V2) 576
    goals of, (V1) 1034
    home hospice care versus, (V1) 1036
    infection control, (V1) 409, (V1)
        1041–1042
    informatics in, (V1) 975
    intermittent bladder and catheter
        irrigation, (V2) 612
    intermittent infusion administration,
        (V2) 512
    intramuscular injection administration,
        (V2) 499
    Intravenous medication administration,
        (V2) 507
    knowledge map for, (V2) 1004
    lung disease risk factors, (V2) 285
    management of incontinence, (V1) 646
    medication administration, (V2) 452
    mobility concerns, (V1) 741
    nasogastric and nasoenteric tubes
        insertion, (V2) 571
    nasogastric and nasoenteric tubes
        removal, (V2) 578
    needles and syringes, reusing, (V1) 514
    nursing bag, (V1) 1038f
    nursing visit
        before, (V1) 1038
        during, (V1) 1038–1042, (V1) 1039f
        after, (V1) 1042–1043
        conducting, (V2) 1001
    ophthalmic medication administration,
        (V2) 462
    oral care for unconscious patient,
        (V2) 413
    overview of, (V2) 997
    peak flow meter, (V1) 870, (V1) 870f
    perineal care, (V2) 401
    personal protective equipment, (V2) 348
    poisoning, preventing and treating,
        (V1) 423–424
    preoperative assessment of surgical
        client, (V1) 927
    preventing injury from fire, (V1) 426
    professionals providing, (V1) 1035–1036
    pulse rate assessment, (V2) 207

    referring clients to, (V1) 1038
    reimbursement, (V1) 1037–1038
    respiration assessment, (V2) 213
    restraints, using, (V2) 374
    safety considerations, (V2) 1001–1002
    self-monitoring of blood pressure,
        (V1) 332
    sensory deficit-safety and health
        measures, (V1) 696
    shampooing bedrest patient, (V2) 417
    showers and baths, (V1) 453
    skin assessment, (V2) 243
    sterile gloves, applying, (V2) 356
    subcutaneous medication administration,
        (V2) 491–492
    temperature assessment, (V1) 314,
        (V2) 202
    urinary catheter insertion, (V2) 608
Home Health Care Classification. See Clinical
        Care Classification (CCC)
Home hospice care, (V1) 1036
Homelessness, (V1) 216
Homeopathy, (V1) 994–995
Home safety assessment, (V1) 438
Home safety checklist, (V2) 379–380
Homosexual, (V1) 768
Homosexuality, (V1) 768, (V1) 772
Honoring personhood, (V1) 153
Hope
    as core issue of spirituality, (V1) 249
Hopelessness
    cause of, (V1) 196
    diagnosis of, (V1) 205
    goal/outcome statement, (V1) 206
    outcomes and interventions for, (V2) 173
Hordeolum, (V2) 334
Hormone
    body temperature and, (V1) 309
    regulation of, (V1) 891
    thyroid, (V1) 308
Hormone replacement therapy (HRT),
        (V1) 788–789
Hospice care
    home health care versus, (V1) 1036
    purpose of, (V1) 272–273, (V2) 158
Hospital
    care of patient bedding, (V1) 470
    Christian, (V1) 4
    Hôtel Dieu, (V1) 4, (V1) 4f
    military, (V1) 8
    municipal authorities taking over, (V1) 7
    nursing outside of, (V1) 22
    physician power in, (V1) 6
    program management, (ESGV1) 21
    reduced number in Canada, (ESGV1) 19
Hospitaler
    image of, (V1) 8f
    orders of, (V1) 8
    providing nursing care, (V1) 9
Hospital Insurance and Diagnostic Services
        Act, (ESG46 V1) 3
Hospitalization, Canadian rate of,
        (ESGV1) 19
Host, susceptible, (V1) 400
Hostility, (V1) 562
Hôtel Dieu, (V1) 4, (V1) 4f
Houlihan, Hot Lips, (V1) 7
Household system
    apothecary and metric equivalents,
        (V2) 521
    for medication dosage, (V1) 492, (V2) 519
Human development. See Development

Human immunodeficiency syndrome (HIV)
   as disability, *(V1) 1072–1073*
   as family health challenge, *(V1) 215–216*
   as latent infection, *(V1) 401*
   nursing education for, *(V1) 15*
Human papillomavirus infection (HPV),
   (V1) 778
Human relations-oriented management,
   (V1) 955–956
Human response, *(V1) 59*
Humidifier, *(V1) 875*
Humidity, *(V1) 308*
Humility, intellectual, *(V1) 27*
Humor, *(V1) 342*
   effectiveness of, *(V1) 996*
   as holistic therapy, *(V2) 965tb*
   for pain relief, *(V1) 711*
Humoral immunity, *(V1) 402–403, (V1) 403f*
Hydration
   bowel function and, *(V1) 655–656*
   maintaining, *(V1) 875*
   skin and, *(V1) 813*
   urination and, *(V1) 623–624*
Hydrocephalus, *(V1) 370*
Hydrochloric acid (HCl), *(V1) 651, (V1) 895*
Hydrocolloid dressing, *(V1) 839*
Hydrodensitometry, *(V1) 604*
Hydrogel dressing, *(V1) 839*
Hydrogen ion (pH), *(V1) 322*
Hydrometer, *(V1) 634*
Hydrostatic pressure, *(V1) 889*
Hydrotherapy, *(V1) 836*
Hygiene
   assessment of, *(V1) 444, (V2) 432–433*
   factors influencing, *(V1) 442–443*
   general survey of client, *(V1) 365*
   NOC outcomes and NIC interventions,
      (V2) 435–436
   oral, *(V1) 459*
   overview of, *(V2) 384*
   procedures for, *(V1) 451p–452p*
   promoting host defense of infection,
      (V1) 405
   promoting normal urination, *(V1) 640*
   self-care deficit, *(V2) 434*
   types of scheduled care, *(V1) 446*
Hyperactive bowel sounds, *(V1) 384,*
   (V1) 659
Hyperalgesia, *(V1) 702*
Hyperbaric oxygen therapy (HBOT),
   (V1) 819
Hypercalcemia, *(V1) 898t*
Hypercapnia, *(V1) 859*
Hypercarbia, *(V1) 859, (V1) 869*
Hypercoagulability, *(V1) 884*
Hyperemia, *(V1) 558, (V1) 826*
Hyperglycemia, *(V1) 605*
Hyperkalemia, *(V1) 897t*
Hypermagnesemia, *(V1) 898t*
Hypernatremia, *(V1) 897t*
Hyperopia, *(V1) 372, (V1) 685b*
Hyperperistalsis, *(V2) 295*
Hyperphosphatemia, *(V1) 898t*
Hyperplasia, *(V1) 459–460*
Hyperpyrexia, *(V1) 314*
Hypersomnia, *(V1) 801*
Hypertension
   definition of, *(V1) 334*
   eyes and, *(V1) 372*
   in middle adults, *(ESG9) 33*
   obesity and, *(V1) 857*
   overview of, *(V2) 191*

Hyperthermia
   from exercise, *(V1) 734*
   malignant, *(V1) 938*
   nursing activities for, *(V1) 315*
Hyperthyroidism
   basal metabolic rate and, *(V1) 308*
   sleep patterns, *(V1) 803*
   thyroid enlargement and, *(V1) 376*
Hypertonic fluid, *(V1) 906*
Hypertonic solution, *(V1) 889*
Hypertrophy, *(V1) 625, (V1) 740b*
Hyperventilation, *(V1) 326, (V1) 848*
Hypervolemia (fluid volume excess), *(V1) 896*
Hypnosis
   for disturbed energy field, *(V1) 1002*
   for pain relief, *(V1) 711*
   use of, *(V1) 996*
Hypnotics, *(V1) 800*
Hypoactive bowel sounds, *(V1) 384, (V1) 659*
Hypoactive sexual desire, *(V1) 780*
Hypocalcemia, *(V1) 897t*
Hypocapnia, *(V1) 326, (V1) 859*
Hypocarbia, *(V1) 859, (V1) 869*
Hypochondrias, *(V1) 563*
Hypoglycemia, *(V1) 605*
Hypokalemia, *(V1) 897t*
Hypomagnesemia, *(V1) 898t*
Hypometabolic state, *(V1) 861*
Hyponatremia, *(V1) 897t*
Hypoperistalsis, *(V2) 295*
Hypophosphatemia, *(V1) 898t*
Hypotension, *(V1) 333*
Hypothalamus
   corticotropin-releasing hormone (CRH),
      (V1) 555
   regulating body temperature, *(V1) 307*
Hypothermia
   artificial, *(V1) 856*
   definition of, *(V1) 316*
   from exercise, *(V1) 734*
Hypothesis, *(V1) 157*
Hypothetical thinking, *(ESG9) 8*
Hypothyroidism, *(ESG9) 16*
   basal metabolic rate and, *(V1) 308*
   facial appearance and, *(V1) 370*
   sleep patterns, *(V1) 803*
   thyroid enlargement and, *(V1) 376*
Hypotonic fluid, *(V1) 906*
Hypotonic solution, *(V1) 889*
Hypoventilation, *(V1) 326, (V1) 848*
Hypovolemia, *(V1) 315, (V1) 946t*
Hypovolemia (fluid volume deficit), *(V1) 896*
Hypoxemia, *(V1) 848*
Hypoxia
   definition of, *(V1) 848*
   oxygenation and, *(V1) 859*
   signs of, *(V1) 326, (V1) 370f*

I

Ibuprofen
   chemical name for, *(V1) 474*
   for menstrual pain, *(V1) 788*
   for pain relief, *(V1) 712*
*ICD-10 (International Classification of
   Disease), (V1) 70*
ICNP (International Classification for Nurs-
   ing Practice), *(V1) 71*
Icteric sclera, *(V1) 371*
Id, *(V1) 167, (ESG9) 5*
Idea, classification of, *(V1) 70*
Ideal body image, *(V1) 190*
Identification, *(V1) 560t*

Identity
   gender, *(V1) 767, (V1) 770*
   personal, *(V1) 191–192*
Idiosyncratic reaction, *(V1) 491*
Ileal conduit, *(V1) 638, (V1) 638f*
Ileal loop, *(V1) 638*
Ileocecal valve, *(V1) 653*
Ileostomy, *(V1) 657–658, (V1) 658f*
Ileum, *(V1) 652*
Ileus, *(V1) 947t*
Illicit drugs, *(V1) 492, (V1) 858*
Illness
   end-of-life care, *(V1) 271–272*
   examples of chronic, *(V1) 180b*
   hospice care for, *(V1) 272–273*
   hypertension as cause of, *(V1) 334*
   as individual experience, *(V1) 171*
   medical view of, *(V1) 171*
   nature of, *(V1) 180*
   overview of, *(V2) 94*
   palliative care for, *(V1) 272*
   present history of, *(V1) 46*
   prevention of, *(V1) 19*
   sensory function and, *(V1) 683*
   sexuality and, *(V1) 773*
   sleep/rest and, *(V1) 794, (V1) 794f,*
      (V1) 800
   as stage of infection, *(V1) 401*
   stages of, *(V1) 179–180*
Imagery technique
   effectiveness of, *(V1) 995–996*
   as holistic therapy, *(V2) 966tb*
   for pain relief, *(V1) 711*
   for stress management, *(V1) 570*
Imaging technique, for body mass, *(V1) 604*
Imbalance, as factor disrupting health,
   (V1) 178–179
Immigrant, *(V1) 227*
Immobility
   effects of, *(V1) 739–740*
   hazards of, *(V1) 739*
   management of, *(V2) 724*
   skin breakdown, *(V1) 812*
Immobilization, pain relief and, *(V1) 710–711*
Immune response, *(V1) 855*
Immune system, *(V1) 562*
Immunity
   active, *(V1) 405*
   cell-mediated, *(V1) 404*
   humoral, *(V1) 402–403, (V1) 403f*
   passive, *(V1) 404*
   specific, *(V1) 402*
Immunization
   of child, *(ESG9) 26*
   of infant, *(ESG9) 18*
   promoting host defense of infection,
      (V1) 405
   respiratory function, preventing disease,
      (V1) 873
   schedule for, *(ESG9) 19f*
   smallpox, *(V1) 1030*
   tetanus, *(V1) 826*
Immunoglobins (Ig), *(V1) 403, (V1) 403–404*
Impaired nursing practice, *(V1) 1049,*
   (V1) 1087
Impaired Skin Integrity, *(V1) 60*
Implementation
   for abnormal pulse, *(V1) 321*
   as action phase of nursing process,
      (V1) 121
   activity and exercise, *(V1) 747*
   bowel-related problems, *(V1) 665*

client participation and adherence, (V1) 125–126
for communication problems, (V1) 349
coordination of care, (V1) 126
cultural sensitivity in, (V1) 240–241
documentation of, (V1) 128
doing or delegating, (V1) 125–128
eye care, (V1) 466
fluid and electrolyte balance, (V1) 903–904
full-spectrum nursing and, (V1) 35–36
of health care, (V1) 182
for hypertension, (V1) 335
for hypothermia, (V1) 316
for infection, (V1) 408
for integumentary problems, (V1) 450
for intraoperative phase, (V1) 941
knowledge and skills needed, (V1) 125
knowledge map of, (V2) 72
medication-related, (V1) 496
nail care, (V1) 458
nursing process and, (V1) 31f, (V1) 32–33, (V1) 32f, (V1) 121
for oral cavity/mouth problems, (V1) 461
overview of, (V2) 62
of pain relief, (V1) 709
perioperative care, (V1) 931
preparation for, (V1) 121–123, (V1) 125
professional standards for, (V1) 122b
reflecting critically about, (V1) 128
review of, (V1) 136
for self-care deficit, (V1) 446
sensory-perceptual problems, (V1) 692
sleep promotion, (V1) 805
for spirituality diagnoses, (V1) 259
for temperature/fever diagnoses, (V1) 315
for weight control, (V1) 610
Impotence, (V1) 780
Imprisonment, false, (V1) 1078
Incentive spirometry
for high-risk pneumonia and atelectasis, (V1) 949, (V1) 949f
teaching and assisting with, (V1) 874
teaching patient about, (V1) 950
Incident report, (V1) 298, (V1) 1084–1085
Incisional wound, (V1) 815t
Incomplete protein food, (V1) 578
Incontinence, (V1) 637–638, (V1) 646
Incubation, infection and, (V1) 401
Independent intervention, (V1) 105
Indian healthcare, as early nursing, (V1) 4
Indicator, NOC outcome component, (V1) 97, (V1) 98–99
Indigenous healthcare system, (V1) 231
Indirect auscultation, (V1) 45, (V1) 363
Indirect calculation, of BMR, (V1) 592
Indirect-care intervention, (V1) 105
Indirect percussion, (V1) 360, (V2) 233t
Individualized nursing care plan, (V1) 89–90, (V1) 92
Induction, (V1) 143
Inductive reasoning
comparing to deductive reasoning, (V1) 143f
definition of, (V1) 143
Indwelling catheter
example of, (V1) 632f
patient care, (V1) 644f, (V2) 623tb–624tb
removal of, (V1) 644, (V1) 646, (V2) 625tb
supplies for, (V1) 643f
for urine measurement, (V1) 632, (V1) 641

Ineffective breastfeeding, (V1) 66, (V1) 109
Ineffective coping, (V1) 553
Ineffective denial
myocardial infarction, (V1) 89
outcomes and interventions for, (V2) 173
Ineffective sexuality pattern
care map for, (V1) 787
nursing care plan, (V1) 784–786
Ineffective thermoregulation, (V1) 315
Infant
abdomen of, (V2) 294
adaptation, (ESG9) 5
assessment of, (ESG9) 18
baby-bottle tooth decay, (V1) 459
bowel elimination patterns, (V1) 655
breathing rhythm of, (V1) 325–326
breathing sounds of, (V2) 285
car seat for, (V1) 428f
chest of, (V2) 281p
cradle cap in, (V1) 369
developmental task theory, (ESG9) 4t
development of, (ESG9) 16–17
failure to thrive, (ESG9) 17
hair of, (V2) 248
health problems, (ESG9) 17–18
health promotion and screenings, (V1) 1010t
heart sounds of, (V2) 290
injection, administering, (V1) 512
intervention for, (ESG9) 18
milestones of, (ESG9) 17b
modification of assessment for, (V1) 363
neck of, (V2) 282
nutritional needs, (V1) 594–595
osteogenesis imperfecta (OA), (V1) 737
oxygenation of, (V1) 854
pain and, (V1) 704
safety of, (V1) 421
sensory stimulation needs, (V1) 682
sexual development, (V1) 768
skin of, (V1) 812
sleep requirement, (V1) 795, (V1) 795t
suffocation and asphyxiation prevention, (V1) 427
teeth development, (V1) 459, (V1) 459f
urinary elimination, (V1) 623
Infected wound, (V1) 816
Infection
air travel as cause of, (V1) 400
antimicrobial spectrum/hand/hygiene antiseptic agents, (V1) 411t
assessment of, (V1) 406–407
body's defense against
primary, (V1) 401–402
secondary, (V1) 402
tertiary, (V1) 402–404
control of, (V1) 409, (V1) 841, (V1) 1041–1042
definition of, (V1) 399
diagnostic testing for, (V1) 407
exogenous and endogenous nosocomial, (V1) 401
factors increasing risk of, (V1) 405–406
head of, (V2) 251
increasing surgical risk, (V1) 926b
as IV therapy complication, (V1) 917t
local or system, (V1) 401
medical asepsis, (V1) 408–410
mode of transmission, (V1) 400
outbreak of, (V1) 398
outcome and evaluation of, (V1) 407–408
overview of, (V2) 337

protection for healthcare workers, (V1) 416
protective isolation, (V1) 412–413
of pulmonary system, (V1) 860
reservoir as source of, (V1) 399
role of nurse for control of, (V1) 417
sexually transmitted, (V1) 778–779
skin breakdown, (V1) 814
stages of, (V1) 401
standard precautions, (V1) 410
transmission-based precautions, (V1) 412
upper respiratory, (V1) 854–855
of wound, (V1) 819
Infectious agent, (V1) 398–399
Infectious disease
as challenge to family health, (V1) 215–216
germ theory of, (V1) 145
mortality and, (V1) 5
outbreak of, (V1) 398, (V1) 417
Infectious microorganism, (ESG9) 15
Inference
of data, (V1) 70b
making, (V1) 65–66
Infertility, (ESG9) 32
Infibulation, (V1) 772
Infiltration, (V1) 916t
Inflammation
agents causing, (V1) 558b
as defense against infection, (V1) 402
as method of destroying pathogens, (V1) 403
of penis (balanitis), (V1) 780
response to stressor, (V1) 557–558
signs and symptoms of, (V1) 402
urinary retention and, (V1) 636
of wound, (V1) 816, (V1) 818f
Inflammatory phase of healing, (V1) 816, (V1) 818f
Inflammatory response, (V1) 855
Influenza immunization, (V1) 873
Informal negotiation, (V1) 966
Informal planning, (V1) 82
Informatics
definition of, (V1) 972
evidence-based practice and, (V1) 981
knowledge map for, (V2) 959
overview of, (V2) 949
role in nursing, (V1) 977
standardized minimum data set, (ESGV1) 12–13
Information, defining, (V1) 972
Information-literate person, (V1) 982b
Information processing, (V1) 973
Informed consent
for minimizing malpractice, (V1) 1085–1086
from study participants, (V1) 158
for surgery, (V1) 931–932
Infusion
intermittent, (V1) 519–520, (V1) 525p
intravenous (IV) fluid, (V1) 154
large-volume, adding medication to, (V1) 519
pump-controlled, (V1) 614
Infusion kit, (V1) 909, (V1) 909f
Infusion pump, (V1) 911
Ingrown toenail, (V1) 456
Inhalation, (V1) 848, (V1) 848f
Inhaler, types of, (V1) 505, (V1) 505f
Initial assessment, (V1) 42, (V1) 45f
Initial planning, (V1) 83

Injectable penicillin, (V1) 5
Injection
    angles for, (V1) 513f
    charting site of, (V1) 296
    types of
        intradermal, (V1) 512–513
        subcutaneous, (V1) 513–515
        Z-track technique, (V1) 516, (V1) 525p
Injury
    bowel diversion, cause for, (V1) 657
    from electrical storm, (V1) 431
    from fire, (V1) 425–426
    from firearm, (V1) 426
    health and, (V1) 176
    medication-related, (V1) 496
    from motor vehicle accident,
        (V1) 428–429
    risk factors for, (V1) 421, (V1) 422t
Inner ear, (V1) 372
Input, (V1) 152
Inquiry
    about evaluation, (V1) 136
    based on credible sources, (V1) 30t
    intervention selection, (V1) 112
    model of critical thinking, (V1) 31f
IN SAD CAGES, depression and, (V2) 110
Insensible loss, (V1) 308
In-service education, (V1) 15
Inside-the needle catheter, (V1) 906,
        (V1) 906f
Insomnia, (V1) 801
Inspection
    of abdomen, (V1) 383
    of client for physical examination,
        (V1) 360
    for physical assessment, (V2) 230t
    physical assessment technique, (V1) 44
Inspiration
    diaphragm contracting, (V1) 323f
    gaining knowledge by, (V1) 155
Inspiratory capacity (IC), (V1) 849
Inspiratory reserve volume (IRV), (V1) 849
Instillation, (V1) 503
Instinctual drives, (V1) 166–167,
        (ESG9) 5
Institute of Medicine (IOM)
    fluid intake recommendation, (V1) 891
    Quality of Health Care in America,
        (ESGV1) 25
Institutional Review Board (IRB), (V1) 158
Instruction format, (V1) 544–547
Instrumental activities of daily living (IADLs),
        (V1) 741, (ESG9) 37–38
Insulin
    administration of, (V1) 514–515
    mixing in same syringe, (V2) 517tb
Insulin syringe, (V1) 508, (V1) 508f
Insurance
    liability, (V1) 1088–1089
    for physician's services, (ESG46 V1) 3
    private, for health care funding,
        (ESGV1) 10
    universal hospital, (ESG46 V1) 2
Insured health care services, (ESGV1) 4
Insured persons, (ESGV1) 4
Intake and output (I&O) record, (V1) 294,
        (V2) 188
Integrated care pathways, (ESGV1) 21
Integrated plans of care (IPOC), (V1) 89,
        (V1) 297
Integrative health care, (V1) 989
Integrity, (V1) 1052t

Integumentary system
    age-related changes for, (ESG9) 36t
    exercise and, (V1) 734b
    immobility, effects on, (V1) 740
    parts of, (V1) 366, (V1) 447
    skin color variation, (V1) 366, (V1) 367t
Intellectualization, (V1) 560t
Intellectual skills, (V1) 27
Intensity
    of anxiety, (V1) 199
    of exercise, (V1) 732
Intentional tort, (V1) 1078
Intercessory prayer, (V1) 259
Intercostal retraction, (V1) 325–326
Interdependent intervention, (V1) 106
Intermittent evaluation, (V1) 131
Intermittent feeding, (V1) 615
Intermittent fever, (V1) 314
Intermittent infusion
    administration of, (V1) 525p,
        (V2) 508p–512p
        piggyback setup, (V2) 510p
        tandem setup, (V2) 511p
        volume-control infusion setup,
            (V2) 509p
    overview of, (V1) 519–520
Intermittent injection, (V1) 154
Intermittent self-catherization, (V1) 641
Internal influence, (V1) 190
Internal locus of control, (V1) 190
Internal loss, (V1) 265
Internal respiration, (V1) 322, (V1) 850
Internal rotation, (V1) 727f
Internal sphincter, (V1) 653, (V1) 654f
Internal stressor, (V1) 551
Internal urethral sphincter, (V1) 622
International Classification for Nursing
        Practice (ICNP), (V1) 71
International Classification of Disease
        (ICD-10), (V1) 70
International Council of Nurses (ICN),
        (V1) 1059
International Council of Nursing (ICN)
    definition of nursing, (V1) 11
    ensuring quality in nursing, (V1) 18
International nursing, (V1) 1029
Internet
    connectivity and, (V1) 974
    health information web site, evaluating,
        (V1) 985b–986b
    image of nurse, (V1) 7
    nursing education, (V1) 15
Interpersonal communication, (V1) 338–339
Interpersonal relations, theory of, (V1) 146
Interpersonal role conflict, (V1) 191
Interpretation
    of communication, (V1) 340
    of data, (V1) 70b
Interpreter, (V1) 244
Interrole conflict, (V1) 191
Intersexed, (V1) 767
Interstitial fluid, (V1) 888, (V1) 888f
Intertarsal joint ROM, (V1) 745t–746t
Intervention
    for abnormal pulse, (V1) 321
    activity and exercise, (V1) 747, (V2) 724
    of adolescence health, (ESG9) 29–31
    for anxiety, (V1) 258–259
    bowel diversion, (V1) 672
    bowel incontinence, (V1) 674–675
    bowel-related problems, (V1) 665,
        (V2) 669–670

child health, (ESG9) 26
    for client safety, (V1) 439–440
    Clinical Care Classification (CCC),
        (V2) 1002
    for communication problems, (V1) 349
    community-based diagnosis, (V1) 1031
    for community health, (V2) 993
    computer-generated, (V1) 113
    coughing, enhancing, (V1) 874–875
    crisis intervention guidelines, (V2) 550
    critical pathways for, (V1) 89
    cultural sensitivity in, (V1) 240–241
    deriving from nursing diagnosis, (V1) 95t
    disturbed energy field, (V1) 1001–1002
    for dying and grieving, (V1) 277,
        (V1) 282–283
    for elderly health, (ESG9) 38
    elimination of, (V1) 104–105
    as empowerment, (V1) 1025
    equipment related accidents, preventing,
        (V1) 433
    etiology suggesting, (V1) 95
    eye care, (V1) 466
    factors influencing patient response to,
        (V1) 28
    for family health status diagnoses,
        (V1) 218–219, (V2) 127
    fire and electrical hazards, preventing,
        (V1) 433–434
    flowing from nursing diagnosis, (V1) 110f
    for fluid and electrolyte diagnoses,
        (V2) 909–911
    fluid, electrolyte and acid-base
        imbalance, (V1) 903–904
    growth and development problems,
        (ESG9) 39–40
    guide in selecting, (V1) 106
    for health care, (V1) 182
    for health knowledge, (V2) 537
    for health promotion, (V1) 1016
    for health protection, (V1) 1005
    for home health care diagnoses,
        (V1) 1041
    for hypertension, (V1) 335
    for hypotension, (V1) 334
    for hypothermia, (V1) 316
    identifying and choosing, (V1) 111–112
    immobility management, (V2) 724
    impaired swallowing, (V2) 580
    impaired verbal communication, (V2) 227
    individualizing standardized, (V1) 112
    ineffective sexuality pattern,
        (V1) 785–786
    for infant health, (ESG9) 18
    for infection, (V1) 408
    injury prevention from
        electrical storm, (V1) 431
        falls, (V1) 425–426, (V1) 432–433,
            (V1) 433f
        fires, (V1) 425
    for integumentary problems, (V1) 450
    for intraoperative phase, (V1) 941,
        (V2) 932–934
    knowledge map of, (V2) 61
    locating appropriate NIC, (V1) 114
    loss and grieving, (V2) 173–174
    medication-related, (V1) 496,
        (V2) 524–525
    of middle adult health, (ESG9) 34
    model of, (V1) 105f
    nail care, (V1) 458
    neonate transitioning, (ESG9) 16

nursing
  interview, (V1) 100–102
  levels of care, (V1) 1026–1027
  orders, (V1) 116–118
  reflecting direct and indirect care,
    (V1) 105
nutrition-related problems, (V2) 588
Omaha System categories and targets,
    (V2) 994
for oral cavity/mouth problems, (V1) 461
overview of, (V2) 53
for oxygenation diagnoses, (V1) 873–876,
    (V2) 869
for pain, (V1) 709, (V1) 721, (V2) 695
perioperative care, (V1) 931
PICC line, (V1) 907
planning, (V1) 32, (V1) 32f, (V1) 35
postoperative collaborative problems,
    (V1) 948
for postoperative diagnoses, (V2) 935–938
prenatal care, (ESG9) 12–13
for preoperative diagnoses, (V2) 930–931
of preschooler, (ESG9) 24
prevention and treatment of carbon
    monoxide poisoning,
    (V1) 424–425
  food poisoning, (V1) 429
  poisoning, (V1) 422–424
  scalds and burns, (V1) 425
  vector-borne pathogen, (V1) 429–430
prevention of
  mercury poisoning, (V1) 436
  motor vehicle accidents, (V1) 428–429
  suffocation and asphyxiation, (V1) 427
problem status influencing, (V1) 109
process for generating and selecting,
    (V1) 109–112
professional standards for, (V1) 107b
progress notes for, (V1) 296
promoting firearm safety, (V1) 426–427
reasoning and reflection, (V1) 27
reducing pollution, (V1) 430–431
reflecting critically about, (V1) 118
relating to outcome, (V1) 77, (V1) 135
research influencing, (V1) 106–108
review of, (V1) 136
safety problems, (V2) 382
for self-care deficit, (V1) 446
self-care deficit, (V2) 434
self-concept, selected nursing activities
    for, (V2) 113
sensory-perceptual problems, (V1) 692,
    (V2) 682
sexual problems, (V2) 738
for skin and wound diagnoses,
    (V2) 795–796
sleep diagnoses, (V2) 752
sleep pattern disturbance, (V1) 805
for spirituality diagnoses, (V1) 257,
    (V1) 258
standardized language for home health
    and community care, (V1) 114–116
stress-related problems, (V2) 554
stress urinary incontinence, (V1) 628–630
for temperature/fever diagnoses,
    (V1) 315
theory influencing, (V1) 106
of toddler, (ESG9) 21
types of, (V1) 105–106
for urinary incontinence, (V1) 646–648
urinary problems, (V2) 634
using restraints safely, (V1) 434–436

using standardized language for, (V1) 113
visual deficits, (V1) 694–695
vital signs, abnormal, (V2) 218
for weight control, (V1) 610
for wellness diagnoses, (V2) 980–981
writing rationales, (V1) 91
  See also Nursing Intervention Classifica-
    tion (NIC)
of young adult health, (ESG9) 32
Intervention model, (ESGV1) 9
Interview
  assessment of memory during, (V1) 54
  closing, (V1) 49
  components of health history, (V1) 46–47
  conducting, (V1) 48–49
  for data collection, (V2) 20
  preparing for, (V1) 47–48
  reflecting critically about, (V1) 53
  types of, (V1) 47
Intestine
  large, (V1) 653
  small, (V1) 652–653
Intimate distance, (V1) 343–344
Intolerance
  food, (V1) 657
  glucose, (V1) 609
Intonation, (V1) 341
Intracellular fluid (ICF)
  as body fluid compartment, (V1) 887–888
  distribution in body, (V1) 888f
  overview of, (V2) 871
  water and, (V1) 582
Intractable pain, (V1) 700–701
Intradermal injection
  administration of, (V1) 524p,
    (V2) 486p–488p
  overview of, (V1) 512–513
Intramuscular injection
  administration of, (V1) 524p–525p,
    (V2) 496p–500p
  of opioids, (V1) 715
  sites, locating, (V2) 493p–495p
  sites for, (V1) 515–517
Intraoperative phase
  diagnoses, outcomes, and interventions
    for, (V2) 932–934
  intraoperative team, (V1) 936–937
  questionnaire, (V2) 928
  safety measures, (V1) 942
Intraoperative team, (V1) 936–937
Intrapersonal communication, (V1) 338
Intraspinal analgesia, (V1) 715–716
Intrauterine development, (ESG9) 8
Intravascular fluid, (V1) 888, (V1) 888f
Intravenous (IV) fluid infusion, (V1) 154
  adding medication to, (V2) 500p–502p,
    (V2) 500p–502p
  changing solution, tubing and dressing,
    (V2) 888p–892p
  complications of, (V1) 916t–917t,
    (V1) 916t–917t
  discontinuing, (V1) 154, (V1) 918
  equipment and supplies for, (V1) 908–910
  flow rate, regulation of, (V2) 882p–884p
  hypervolemia and, (V1) 896
  piggyback setup, (V2) 510p
  procedures for, (V1) 912p–914p,
    (V1) 912p–914p
  regulating and maintaining, (V1) 911
  site selection for, (V1) 910
  solution, tubing and dressing, changing,
    (V1) 915

tandem setup, (V2) 511p
venipuncture for, (V1) 911
Intravenous administration
  changing solution, tubing and dressing,
    (V2) 888p–892p
  discontinuing, (V2) 895p–897p
  fluid and electrolyte replacement,
    (V1) 905–906
  IV pump, setting up and using,
    (V2) 885p–887p
  of opioids, (V1) 715
  primary line to heparin or saline lock,
    (V2) 893p–895p
  solutions for, (V1) 906
Intravenous medication
  adding to, (V1) 525p
  complication from, (V1) 519f
  overview of, (V1) 518–519
Intravenous pyelogram (IVP), (V2) 633
Intrinsic factors, pressure ulcer, (V1) 821
Introspection, (V1) 254
Intubation, (V1) 879
Intuit citizens, health services, (ESGV1) 7
Intuition, gaining knowledge by, (V1) 155
Invasion of privacy, (V1) 1079
Inversion
  assessment of, (V2) 305p–306p
  as movement, (V1) 727f
Involvement, active, (V1) 532
Ionization, (V1) 483–484
Ionized drug molecule, (V1) 484
IPOC (Integrated plans of care), (V1) 89
Iron
  deficiency of, (V1) 582
  needs for ovo-lacto vegetarian, (V1) 598
  peristalsis and, (V1) 656
  restless leg syndrome (RLS), (V1) 801
  total iron-binding capacity test (TIBC),
    (V1) 605
Irrigation
  of catheter and bladder, (V1) 644,
    (V1) 645
  continuous bladder, (V2) 613p–615p
  definition of, (V1) 503
  intermittent bladder and catheter,
    procedure, (V2) 610p–612p
  otic, (V1) 695
Irritable bowel syndrome (IBS), (V1) 655
Ischemia, (V1) 317, (V1) 826
Ishihara cards, (V1) 372, (V2) 255
Islam, (V1) 251–252
Isokinetic exercise, (V1) 731
Isolation
  as cause of depression, (V1) 201, (V1) 201t
  as factor disrupting health, (V1) 179
  intimacy versus, (V1) 167
  protective (reverse), (V1) 412–413
  psychological needs of patients in,
    (V1) 413
  transmission-based, (V1) 413
Isometric exercise, (V1) 731
Isotonic, (V1) 889
Isotonic exercise, (V1) 731
Isotonic fluid, (V1) 906
IV infusion
  equipment and supplies for,
    (V1) 908–910, (V1) 909f
  site selection for, (V1) 910
  venipuncture for, (V1) 911
IV KCI replacement, (V1) 3
IV pump, setting up and using,
    (V2) 885p–887p

IV push medication
  administration of, *(V1) 525p,*
    (V2) 503p–504p
    IV lock, no extension tubing,
      (V2) 505p–506p
    IV lock, with extension tubing,
      (V2) 506p–507p
    running primary IV line,
      (V2) 504p–505p
  overview of, *(V1) 519*
IV therapy
  access device, *(V1) 906f*
  for fluid and electrolyte replacement,
    (V1) 905–906

J

JAREL spiritual well-being scale, *(V1) 256*
Jaundice, *(ESG9) 15*
  as cause skin color variation, *(V1) 367t*
  example of, *(V2) 333*
  skin and, *(V1) 448*
Jehovah's Witness, *(V1) 251*
Jejunostomy tube, *(V1) 613–614*
Jejunum, *(V1) 652*
Jewish faith, *(V1) 251*
Johnson's behavioral system model, *(V1) 152*
Joint
  classification of, *(V1) 726*
  degenerative disease of, *(V2) 335*
  disease affecting mobility, *(V1) 737–738*
  range of motion, *(V1) 742t–746t*
Joint Commission on Accreditation of
    Healthcare Organizations (JCAHO)
  accreditation, *(V1) 1075*
  normal blood pressure, *(V1) 327*
  patient misidentification/wrong-site
    surgery, *(V1) 935*
  patient safety goals, *(V1) 432b*
  professional standards for assessment,
    (V1) 39
  requiring special needs assessment, *(V1) 43*
  responsibilities of teaching, *(V1) 529*
  reviewing client records, *(V1) 289*
  standards of care, *(V1) 1076*
  use of restraints, *(V1) 435–436*
Joint mobility, *(V1) 385, (V1) 385f*
Journal, articles in, *(V1) 161*
Judaism, *(V1) 250*
Judgment
  clinical, *(V1) 10*
  evaluation of data collection, *(V1) 52–54*
Jugular vein, *(V1) 382*
Jugular venous distention (JVD), *(V1) 382*
Justice, types of, *(V1) 1056–1057*

K

Kapha (creation), *(V1) 992*
Kappa (κ), *(V1) 702, (V1) 713*
Kardex, *(V1) 92, (V1) 297*
Karnofsky Performance Scale, *(V1) 44*
Katz Index of ADL scale, *(V1) 43*
Kava, *(V1) 207*
KCI replacement, *(V1) 3*
Kegel exercise, *(V1) 647*
Keloid, *(V2) 246*
Keratinocyte, *(V1) 811*
Keratogenous cyst, *(V2) 245*
Kidney
  at birth, *(ESG9) 13*
  cross-section of, *(V1) 620f*
  drug excretion, *(V1) 485*
  function of, *(V1) 619–620*

glomerular filtration, *(V1) 620*
indicators of functioning level, *(V1) 605*
infection of (pyelonephritis), *(V1) 636*
plasma bicarbonate regulation, *(V1) 895*
tubular reabsorption, *(V1) 620–621*
tubular secretion, *(V1) 621*
urine formation, *(V1) 620–621*
Kidney stone, *(V1) 636*
Killer T cell, *(V1) 404*
Kilocalorie (kcal), *(V1) 591–592*
Kinesthesia, *(V1) 688b, (V2) 681*
Kinesthetic sense, *(V1) 688b*
King's interacting systems framework, *(V1) 152*
Kinsey, Alfred C., *(V1) 767*
Kith, *(V1) 211*
Klein, Fritz, *(V1) 767*
Knee ROM, *(V1) 745t*
Knights of St. John, *(V1) 8*
Knights of St. Lazarus, *(V1) 8*
Knowledge
  data transformation to, *(V1) 972f*
  deficient, *(V1) 67, (V1) 195, (V1) 538*
  formation of, *(V1) 972*
  hygiene practice, *(V1) 443*
  methods of gaining, *(V1) 155–156*
  personal integration of, *(V1) 15*
  types of, *(V1) 29*
Kock pouch, *(V1) 638, (V1) 658, (V1) 658f*
Kohlberg, Lawrence, *(V1) 167, (V1) 1046,
    (ESG9) 7*
Kohlberg's moral development theory, *(V1)
    151, (V1) 167, (V1) 1046, (V1) 1046t*
Kokopelli, *(V1) 253f*
Kolcaba, Dr. Katherine, *(V1) 145*
Koran (Qu'ran), *(V1) 251*
Korean War, *(V1) 9*
Korotkoff, Nicolai, *(V1) 331*
Korotkoff sound, *(V1) 331, (V1) 331f,
    (V1) 333, (V2) 215–216*
Kosher food, *(V1) 251*
Kreiger, Delores, *(V1) 999*
Kübler-Ross, Dr. Elizabeth
  psychology of dying, *(V1) 271*
  stages of dying and grief, *(V1) 271b*
Kunz, Dora, *(V1) 999*
Kyphosis, *(V1) 378, (V1) 385, (V2) 281p,
    (V2) 282, (V2) 335*

L

Labeling
  appropriate for problem, *(V1) 72*
  diagnostic, *(V1) 58–59*
  family care/health, *(V2) 126*
  from mental illness, *(V1) 177*
  NANDA, *(V1) 76*
    for anxiety, *(V1) 203*
    for communication problems, *(V1) 349*
    community-based diagnosis, *(V1) 1029*
    eye problems, *(V1) 466*
    for family health status diagnoses,
      (V1) 218
    growth and development problems,
      (ESG9) 39
    impaired skin integrity, *(V1) 449*
    impaired swallowing, *(V1) 608*
    nutrition-related problems, *(V1) 606*
    overweight and obesity, *(V1) 609–610*
    for pain, *(V1) 708*
    safety problems, *(V1) 439*
    for self-concept, *(V1) 195–196*
    sexual problems, *(V1) 782–783*
    sleep pattern disturbance, *(V1) 805*

for spirituality diagnoses, *(V1) 256–258*
for wellness diagnoses, *(V1) 538*
wellness diagnoses, *(V1) 1013–1015*
Nursing Intervention Classification (NIC),
    (V1) 114, (V2) 993–994
Omaha System, (V2) 991, (V2) 993–994
and ranking of problems, *(V1) 68*
Labia majora, *(V1) 764*
Labia minora, *(V1) 764*
Laboratory study, stool specimen, *(V1) 661*
Laceration, *(V1) 815t*
Lactated Ringer's solution, *(V1) 519*
Lactation, *(V1) 597–598*
Lacto-vegetarian, *(V1) 598*
"Lady of the Lamp", *(V1) 7f*
Laissez-faire leadership, *(V1) 954*
The Lalonde Report, *(ESGV1) 28*
Landmarks
  cardiac, *(V1) 380–381*
  of chest, *(V1) 377, (V1) 377f, (V1) 378f*
Langerhans cells, *(V1) 811*
Language
  as barrier
    to communication, *(V1) 244*
    to culturally competent care, *(V1) 238*
  development in toddler, *(ESG9) 20*
  for nursing, *(V2) 957–958*
  pain translation, *(V1) 705b*
  patronizing, *(V1) 354*
  Spanish words and phrases, *(V2) 225*
  standardized nursing language
    computer care systems, *(V1) 114*
    definition of, *(V1) 69–70*
    holistic care and, *(V1) 115–116*
    planning
      interventions/implementations,
        (V1) 113
    purpose of, *(V1) 70*
    writing diagnostic statements,
      (V1) 69–70
Large intestine
  segments of, *(V1) 653*
  view of, *(V1) 653f*
Laryngospasm, *(V1) 846*
Larynx, *(V1) 846, (V1) 846f*
Late entry, *(V1) 302*
Latent infection, *(V1) 401*
Lateral position, *(V1) 751t, (V1) 752*
Lateral recumbent position, *(V1) 752*
Latino. See Hispanic/Latino
Law
  advanced directive, *(V1) 273*
  autopsy requirement, *(V1) 275*
  civil, *(V1) 1078*
  contract, *(V1) 1078*
  criminal, *(V1) 1077*
  as culture specific influencing health,
    (V1) 229
  definition of, *(V1) 1071*
  for drug quality and safety, *(V1) 477t*
  overview of, *(V2) 1016*
  regulating drugs and medications,
    (V1) 476
  reporting patient changes to primary
    provider, *(V1) 299*
  safe harbor, *(V1) 1088*
  sources of, *(V1) 1071–1072*
  tort, *(V1) 1078*
  See also Legal issues
Lawsuit, nursing, *(V1) 1082b*
Lawton Instrumental Activities of Daily
    Living, *(V1) 43–44, (V2) 26*

Laxative
  peristalsis and, (V1) 656
  types of, (V1) 667b
  use of, (V1) 668
Leader
  challenges of, (V1) 959
  effective, (V1) 953
  job skills for, (V1) 957b
  mentors and preceptors, (V1) 957–958
  nurse as, (V1) 13t
  qualities and behaviors of, (V1) 955t
  SWOT analysis plan, (V1) 957t
Leadership
  communication and, (V1) 962
  definition of, (V1) 953
  delegation and, (V1) 962–963
  influencing response to change, (V1) 965
  knowledge map for, (V2) 948
  overview of, (V2) 942
  types of, (V1) 954
Leadership theory, (V1) 953
Lead poisoning, (V1) 422
Learning
  adult, principles of, (V1) 535b
  assessment, (V1) 537
  assessment of, (V2) 536
  barriers to, (V1) 536, (V1) 537b
  Bloom's domains of, (V1) 531t
  deficient knowledge, (V1) 538–540
  definition of, (V1) 529
  documentation of, (V1) 547
  domains of, (V1) 529–530, (V1) 539t
  evaluation of, (V1) 547
  factors affecting, (V1) 531–533
  instruction format, (V1) 544–547
  knowledge map of, (V2) 539
  materials for, (V1) 540
  outcome of, (V1) 538–540
  overview of, (V2) 527
  scheduling sessions for, (V1) 533,
    (V1) 540
Lecture, (V1) 541–543, (V1) 544
Legal issues
  federal law, (V1) 1072–1074
  knowledge map for, (V2) 1024tb
  in nursing practice, (V1) 1089
  overview of, (V2) 1016
  practice guidelines, (V1) 1076–1077
  standards of practice, (V1) 1075–1076
  state law, (V1) 1074–1075
  See also Law
Legal requirements. See Law
Legislation
  for drug quality and safety, (V1) 477t
  for drug regulation, (V1) 476
  health, in Canada, (ESGV1) 6,
    (ESGV1) 6t
  health service delivery system,
    (ESGV1) 8
  omnibus, (ESGV1) 9
  professional, (ESGV1) 8–9
Legislature, (V1) 1071
Leininger, Madeleine
  cultural competence theory, (V1) 147–148,
    (V1) 237
  photo of, (V1) 147f
Length, of needle, (V1) 507
Lens opacities, (V1) 371
Lesbian couple, (V1) 211
Lesbian woman, (V1) 768
Lesion, of skin, (V1) 368, (V2) 244–247,
  (V2) 333

Leukemia, (V1) 857
Leukoplakia, (V1) 375, (V2) 334
Levoy, Gregg, (V1) 249
Lewis, C S., (V1) 177, (V1) 249
Liability
  insurance for, (V1) 1088–1089
  malpractice, (V1) 1079
  vicarious, (V1) 1080
Libel, (V1) 1078
Libido
  aging and, (V1) 775b
  as level of desire, (V1) 775
  low, (V1) 780
Lice, head, (V1) 369
Lice (pediculosis), (V1) 369, (V2) 334
Licensed practical nurse (LPN)
  in Canada, (ESGV1) 17
  education for, (V1) 14
  RN delegating patient care activities to,
    (V1) 126
  weekly summary report, (V1) 299
Licensed vocational nurse (LVN)
  education for, (V1) 14
  RN delegating patient care activities to,
    (V1) 126
  weekly summary report, (V1) 299
Licensing, (V1) 1074–1075
Licensure, (ESGV1) 9
Life
  attaining health, (V1) 185
  uncertainties of, (V1) 183
  using critical thinking in, (V1) 27
Life and Death in Shanghai, (V1) 175
Life-changing event
  Holmes-Rahe readjustment scale,
    (V2) 551
  stress and, (V1) 1012
Life span
  bowel elimination patterns, (V1) 655
  development, (ESG9) 3
  growth and development
    definition of, (V1) 165
    principles of, (V1) 166
    theories of, (V1) 166–168
  health promotion throughout, (V1) 1009,
    (V1) 1010t–1011t
  intervention for, (V2) 127
  overview of, (V2) 84
  stressors throughout, (V1) 552b
Lifestyle
  assessment of, (V2) 976–978
  blood pressure and, (V1) 328
  change in, (V1) 1017–1018
  death due to, (V1) 1005
  as health factor, (V1) 174–175, (V1) 184
  health promotion and, (V1) 1016
  health risk appraisal (HRA), (V1) 1012
  mobility and activity, (V1) 735
  nutrition and, (V1) 598
  oxygenation and, (V1) 856
  promoting host defense of infection,
    (V1) 404–405
  sensory function and, (V1) 683
  sexuality, (V1) 772
  sleep and, (V1) 799–800
  as surgical risk factor, (V1) 925
  for urinary incontinence, (V1) 647
Life support, (V1) 273
Lifts, (V1) 381
Ligament, (V1) 726
Line of gravity, (V1) 730, (V1) 730f
Linoleic acid (omega-6), (V1) 580

Lipid
  chemical structure for, (V1) 579f
  definition of, (V1) 579
  as energy nutrient, (V1) 576t
  function of, (V1) 581
  types of, (V1) 579, (V1) 579b
Lipoprotein
  components of, (V1) 579
  types of, (V1) 580
Liquid diet, (V1) 601
Liquid effluent, (V1) 657
Liquid medication, (V1) 500
Liquid oxygen unit, (V1) 876, (V1) 877f
Listening, (V1) 153
Listserv
  as electronic mailing list, (V1) 975–976
  for nurses, (V1) 976b
  relaying messages by, (V1) 976f
List serves, (V1) 546
Liter, (V2) 518
Literacy, (V1) 535–536
Literature
  databases for, (V1) 983–985
  using computer to search, (V1) 982
Litigation, civil claim, (V1) 1080–1081
LIVE and LEARN, (V1) 244
Liver
  disease of, (V1) 926b
  drug excretion, (V1) 485
  indicators of functioning level, (V1) 605
Liver mortis, (V1) 285
Living will, (V1) 273, (V1) 1073
Local adaptation syndrome, (V1) 557
Local anesthesia, (V1) 717, (V1) 938
Local effects, of drug, (V1) 479
Local infection, (V1) 401
Logic, (ESG9) 8
Logical reasoning
  gaining knowledge by, (V1) 155
  purpose of, (V1) 143
Logrolling, (V1) 753
Long-term care
  documentation of, (V1) 299
  form for, (V2) 186
Long-term care facility
  Canadian health coverage for,
    (ESGV1) 19
  intermediate care services, (V1) 299
  using admission forms, (V1) 293–294
Long-term goal, (V1) 93, (V1) 967
Long-term memory, (ESG9) 35
Loop-acting diuretics, (V1) 624b
Loop colostomy, (V1) 659, (V1) 659f
Lordosis, (V1) 385, (V2) 301, (V2) 335
Loss
  assessment, (V1) 276
  definition of, (V1) 264
  diagnosis, (V1) 276–277
  disrupting health, (V1) 177
  guidelines for assessment, (V2) 171–172
  knowledge map for, (V2) 176
  overview of, (V2) 158
  of potential in child death, (V1) 268
  standard outcomes and interventions,
    (V2) 173–174
  types of, (V1) 264–265
  of water, (V1) 308
  See also Grief
Love
  as core issue of spirituality, (V1) 249
  as hierarchy of need, (V1) 50, (V1) 67,
    (V1) 150, (V1) 150f

Love (continued)
  promotion in children, (V1) 198
Low-density lipoprotein (LDL), (V1) 580
Lower airway, (V1) 846
Low-income family, (V1) 215
Low libido, (V1) 780
Lubricant, (V1) 780
Luer-Lok, (V1) 507, (V1) 508f
Lumen, (V1) 613
Lung cancer, (V1) 857
Lung compliance, (V1) 848
Lung receptor, (V1) 851
Lungs
  abnormal sounds from, (V2) 286
  assessment of, (V1) 394p–395p, (V2) 280p–286p
  drug excretion, (V1) 485
  fluid output, (V1) 891
  immobility, effects on, (V1) 739
  recollapse of, (V1) 882
  reexpansion of, (V1) 882
  restoring pH levels, (V1) 895
  structures of, (V1) 847
  volume and capacity of, (V1) 849
Luteal hormone (LH), (V1) 764
Luteal phase, (V1) 764
Lymph node
  cervical, (V1) 376, (V1) 376f
  clavicular and axillae, (V2) 278–279
Lymphocyte
  function of, (V1) 403t
  as marker of protein metabolism, (V1) 605
  specific immunity and, (V1) 402

M
Maceration, (V1) 813–814
Macromineral (major), (V1) 581
Macrophage, (V1) 402
Macula lutea, (V1) 685b
Macular degeneration, (V1) 685b
Macule, (V2) 244
Magico-religious system, (V1) 231
Magic spell, (V1) 4
Magnesium (Mg²⁺)
  deficiency of, (V1) 582
  function and regulation of, (V1) 892t
  recommended intake of, (V1) 894
Magnetic resonance imaging (MRI), GI tract, (V2) 667
Magnetism, (V1) 1000
Magnet therapy, (V1) 1000
Mainstream bronchus, (V1) 846–847
Major depressive disorder, (V1) 200, (V2) 110
Major mineral (macromineral), (V1) 581
Major surgery, (V1) 924
Maladaptive behavior, (V1) 568
Maladaptive coping, (V1) 553
Male chauvinism, (V1) 238
Male condom, (V1) 790
Male reproductive system, (V1) 764–765, (V1) 766f
Malignant hyperthermia, (V1) 938
Malignant lesion, ABCDE, (V1) 368, (V2) 242
Malingering, (V1) 563
Malnutrition
  NOC outcomes and NIC interventions, (V2) 589
  nursing processes for, (V1) 611–612
  signs of, (V1) 604

Malpractice
  avoiding, (V2) 1021tb–1022tb
  claims, types of, (V1) 1081–1083
  elements of, (V1) 1079
  insurance for, (V1) 1088–1089
  minimizing risk of, (V1) 1084
    informed consent, (V1) 1085
    medication and treatment errors, (V1) 1083–1084
    nursing process, using, (V1) 1083
    professional standards of care, (V1) 1083
    report and document, (V1) 1084
  witness, nurse as, (V1) 1080
Maltreatment, family, (V1) 216
Man
  in female-dominated fields, (V1) 10
  fluid intake recommendation, (V1) 891
  genitourinary system of, (V1) 390, (V1) 390f
  as nurse, (V1) 9–10, (V1) 10f
  risk factors for UTI, (V1) 636
  sexual health history, (V2) 734–735
  sexual response cycle of, (V1) 774–776
  urinary incontinence (UI), (V1) 637
Man's Search for Meaning, (V1) 174
Management
  definition of, (V1) 955
  types of, (V1) 955–956
Manager
  activities of effective, (V1) 956
  challenges of, (V1) 959
  definition of, (V1) 955
  job skills for, (V1) 957b
  mentors and preceptors, (V1) 957–958
  nurse as, (V1) 13t
  qualities of effective, (V1) 956
  SWOT analysis plan, (V1) 957t
Mandatory reporting laws, (V1) 1074
Mandatory retirement, (ESG9) 35, (ESG9) 37
Manipulative therapy, (V1) 998
Manometer, (V1) 329–330, (V1) 330f
Mantra (sound), (V1) 995
Manual compression test, (V1) 383
Marketing, direct-to-consumer, (V1) 21
Marriage, (V1) 770–772
Martin Chuzzlewitt, (V1) 7
Masked grief, (V1) 268
Maslow, Abraham, (V1) 188
Maslow's hierarchy of needs, (V1) 50, (V1) 66–67, (V1) 150–151, (V1) 150f
  application of theory, (V1) 151
  overview of, (V2) 100
  resistance to change, (V1) 963
Massage
  back, (V1) 455, (V1) 806p, (V2) 748p–750p
  as holistic therapy, (V2) 966tb
  for pain relief, (V1) 710
  for stress management, (V1) 570
  types of, (V1) 998–999
Master's degree, (V1) 14, (V1) 15, (V1) 155
Mastication, (V1) 651
Mastitis, (V2) 276
Masturbation, (V1) 777
Mattress overlay, (V1) 832
Maturation phase of healing, (V1) 817, (V1) 818f
Maximum effect, of drug, (V1) 486f
McCaffery, Margo, (V1) 699
McLellan, Anne, (ESGV1) 8
Mead, Margaret, (V1) 189
Meals, (V2) 580tb
Meaning
  denotative and connotative, (V1) 340–341
  holistic concept and, (V1) 991

Meaningful work, as factor of health, (V1) 174
Measurement
  anthropometric, (V1) 602
  apothecary system, (V1) 492, (V2) 518–519
  circumference for body composition, (V2) 579tb
  criteria for, (V1) 57b, (V1) 83b
  household system, (V2) 519
  metric system, (V1) 492, (V2) 518
  skinfold, (V1) 602–603
  tricep skinfold, (V2) 579tb
  urine concentration, (V1) 634f
  urine output, (V1) 626, (V1) 632
Measurement scale
  Fahrenheit and centigrade, (V1) 310, (V1) 312
  Nursing Outcomes Classification (NOC), (V1) 97, (V1) 98–99, (V2) 50
Measures, intervention, (V1) 105
Mechanical aid
  walking, (V1) 758–761
Mechanical debridement, (V1) 836
Mechanical digestion, (V1) 651
Mechanical lift, (V1) 755–756, (V1) 756f
Mechanical soft diet, (V1) 601
Mechanical stimuli, (V1) 701
Mechanical ventilator
  general anesthesia and, (V1) 938, (V1) 938f
  patient care, (V1) 880–881, (V2) 846p–849p
Mechanism, defense, (V1) 167
Mechanistic nursing, (V1) 139, (V1) 146
Mechanoreceptor
  locations for, (V1) 680
Meconium, (V1) 655, (ESG9) 14
Mediastinum, (V1) 847
Mediation
  in civil claim, (V1) 1081
Medicaid
  home health care and, (V1) 1037
Medical asepsis
  examples of, (V1) 408–413
  overview of, (V2) 337
Medical Care Act, (ESG46 V1) 3
Medical diagnosis
  comparing to nursing diagnosis and collaborative problems, (V1) 60t
  recognizing, (V1) 59–60
Medical framework, (V1) 50
Medical history, (V1) 46
Medical order
  care plan document, (V1) 85
  individualizing, (V1) 106
Medical treatment, (V1) 460
Medicare, (V1) 1038
Medicated enema, (V1) 669
Medication
  abbreviations used in, (V2) 522–524
  adding to intravenous fluids, procedure, (V2) 500–501
  adding to IV bag/bottle, (V2) 501p
  allergic reaction to, (V1) 490, (V1) 490t
  antipyretic, (V1) 314–315
  assessment of patient, (V1) 495
  associated with urinary retention, (V1) 625b
  biological half-life of, (V1) 486
  blood flow affecting absorption, (V1) 484
  blood pressure and, (V1) 329

buccal and sublingual, *(V1) 500*
causing nausea, *(V1) 600b*
changing needles, measurement, *(V2) 516tb*
charting assessment, *(V1) 296*
charting patient refusal of, *(V1) 296*
for children, *(V1) 501*
Clark's rule for children, *(V2) 522*
client history and current use of, *(V1) 46*
diagnoses, outcomes, interventions of administration, *(V2) 524–525*
distribution in body, *(V1) 484*
diuretic interaction, *(V1) 624b*
documentation of, *(V1) 499f*
dosage calculation, *(V1) 492, (V2) 520–521*
double locking, *(V1) 476*
drawing from ampule, *(V2) 475p–476p*
drawing from vial, *(V2) 476p–478p*
drawing up from ampule or vial, *(V1) 509, (V1) 523p*
effectiveness of, *(V1) 485–487*
effect on taste, *(V1) 686b*
for elderly, *(V1) 501–502*
ensuring safe administration of, *(V1) 497*
enteral, *(V1) 500*
enteral tube
    administration of, *(V2) 456p–457p*
errors and malpractice, *(V1) 1083–1084*
excretion of, *(V1) 485*
as factor for oral problems, *(V1) 459*
factors affecting absorption, *(V1) 479, (V1) 483*
forms of, *(V1) 479*
gastronomy, *(V1) 500*
guidelines for, *(V2) 450–453*
height and weight for dosage, *(V1) 365–366*
heparin, *(V1) 515*
increasing surgical risk, *(V1) 926b*
infection, risk of, *(V1) 406*
injectable
    administration of, *(V1) 511–512*
    preparation of, *(V1) 508*
insulin, *(V1) 514–515*
interactions of, *(V1) 491*
intermittent infusion administration, *(V1) 525p, (V2) 508p–512p*
    overview of, *(V1) 519–520*
    piggyback setup, *(V2) 510p*
    tandem set, *(V2) 511p*
    volume-control setup, *(V2) 509p*
intradermal, *(V2) 486p–488p*
    administration of, *(V1) 524p*
    overview of, *(V1) 512–513*
intramuscular, *(V2) 496p–500p*
    administration of, *(V1) 524p–525p*
    sites for, *(V1) 515–517, (V2) 493–495*
intravenous
    administration of, *(V1) 525p*
    complications from, *(V1) 519f*
    overview of, *(V1) 518–519*
IV push, *(V1) 525p, (V2) 503p–504p, (V2) 504p–505p*
    IV lock, no extension tubing, *(V2) 505p–506p*
    IV lock, with extension tubing, *(V2) 506p–507p*
    overview of, *(V1) 519*
large-volume infusion, adding to, *(V1) 519*

measurement systems for, *(V1) 492*
    apothecary, *(V2) 518–519*
    household, *(V2) 519*
    metric, *(V2) 518*
metabolization of, *(V1) 485*
mixing in same syringe, *(V1) 510, (V1) 523p, (V2) 479p–482p*
mydriatics, *(V1) 371*
nasal
    administration of, *(V1) 522p, (V2) 465p–467p*
    overview of, *(V1) 504*
nasogastric, *(V1) 500*
ophthalmic
    administration of, *(V1) 522p, (V2) 459p–462p*
    overview of, *(V1) 503*
oral, *(V1) 522*
    administration of, *(V2) 454p–458p*
    overview of, *(V1) 499–502*
organizer for, *(V1) 423f*
otic
    administration of, *(V1) 522p, (V2) 463p–464p*
    overview of, *(V1) 503–504*
overview for administration of, *(V2) 438*
oxygenation and, *(V1) 858*
package inserts, *(V1) 475*
parenteral, *(V1) 505, (V1) 508*
patch for, *(V1) 503f*
patient responsibility for, *(V1) 294*
pediatric dosage, *(V2) 521–522*
peristalsis and, *(V1) 656*
pH and ionization, *(V1) 483–484*
prefilled unit-dose system, *(V2) 514tb*
preoperative, *(V1) 935t*
preparing and drawing up, *(V2) 474p–478p*
primary effects of, *(V1) 488*
pulse rate, *(V1) 318*
recapping needles, *(V1) 511, (V1) 523p*
reconstitution of, *(V1) 510, (V2) 515tb*
rectal
    overview of, *(V1) 504*
    suppositories, *(V1) 523p, (V2) 471p–473p*
respiration and, *(V1) 323*
respiratory inhalation
    overview of, *(V1) 504–505*
rights of, *(V1) 497–499*
schedules for, *(V1) 296*
secondary effects, *(V1) 488–491*
sensory function and, *(V1) 683*
sexuality and, *(V1) 773–774*
similar-sounding names of, *(V1) 497b*
skin, application, *(V2) 513tb*
skin integrity impairment, *(V1) 813*
sleep and, *(V1) 800, (V1) 807–808*
subcutaneous, *(V2) 489p–492p*
    administration of, *(V1) 524p*
    overview of, *(V1) 513–515*
    sites for, *(V1) 513f*
surgery preparation, *(V1) 934*
as surgical risk factor, *(V1) 925*
syringe for administration of, *(V1) 503f*
systems for storing and distributing, *(V1) 477–478*
teratogenic effect on fetus, *(ESG9) 12*
therapeutic range of, *(V1) 486*
three checks, *(V1) 497*
tolerance of, *(V1) 491*
topical (lotions, creams, ointments), *(V1) 502*

transdermal, *(V1) 502*
types, advantages, and route of administration, *(V1) 480t–483t*
urination and, *(V1) 625b*
vaginal
    administration of, *(V1) 523p, (V2) 467p–470p*
    overview of, *(V1) 504*
Z-track technique, *(V1) 516, (V1) 525p*
Medication administration record (MAR), *(V1) 296*
Medication error, *(V1) 521, (V1) 525–526*
Medication order
    abbreviations used in, *(V1) 493, (V1) 493b*
    communication of, *(V1) 494*
    elements of, *(V1) 492–493*
    steps for correcting, *(V1) 494*
    types of, *(V1) 494*
Medication records
    inpatient facility, *(V1) 296*
    outpatient facility, *(V1) 294, (V1) 296*
Medicine
    physicians, role of, *(V1) 5–6*
    study of the ethical problems in, *(V1) 270*
Meditation
    effects of, *(V1) 995*
    facilitating, *(V2) 965tb*
    for stress management, *(V1) 570*
MEDLINE, *(V1) 971, (V1) 983, (V2) 949*
Medulla, of kidney, *(V1) 619*
Medulla oblongata, *(V1) 322*
Meet the Parents, *(V1) 10*
Melanin, *(V1) 447, (V1) 811*
Melanocyte, *(V1) 811*
Melatonin, *(V1) 808*
Memory
    assessment of, *(V2) 310*
    loss in elderly, *(ESG9) 35*
    during nursing interview, *(V1) 54*
Memory T cell, *(V1) 404*
Menarche. *See* Menstruation
Menopause, *(V1) 770*
    complementary and alternative medicine (CAM), *(V1) 789*
    teaching about, *(V1) 788–789*
Menstrual phase, *(V1) 764*
Menstruation
    age of onset, *(ESG9) 27*
    dysmenorrhea, *(V1) 779*
    gestation calculation and, *(ESG9) 8*
    onset of, *(V1) 769*
    phases of, *(V1) 764, (V1) 765f*
    premenstrual syndrome (PMS), *(V1) 779*
    teaching about, *(V1) 788*
Mental health
    exercise and, *(V1) 734b*
    health care delivery system and, *(ESGV1) 20–21*
Mental Health Act, *(ESGV1) 8*
Mental illness
    affecting self-care ability, *(V1) 443*
    health and, *(V1) 177*
    sexuality and, *(V1) 773*
Mental state
    assessment of, *(V1) 690, (V2) 320p*
    general survey of client, *(V1) 365*
    as surgical risk factor, *(V1) 925*
Mentor, *(V1) 957–958, (V1) 958b*
Mercury
    characteristics of, *(V1) 436*
    dangers of, *(V1) 312*
    health effects of, *(V1) 436t*

Mercury manometer, *(V1) 329–330*
Meridians (channels), *(V1) 993*
Message
    definition of, *(V1) 340*
    restating, clarifying and validating, *(V1) 350*
Meta-analysis, *(V1) 154*
Metabolic acidosis, *(V1) 898, (V1) 900t*
Metabolic alkalosis, *(V1) 898, (V1) 900t*
Metabolism
    creating heat, *(V1) 309–310*
    definition of, *(V1) 485*
    of drugs in children and adult, *(V1) 487t*
    epinephrine increasing, *(V1) 307*
    heat and cold effects on, *(V1) 856*
    immobility, effects on, *(V1) 739–740*
    importance of vitamins for, *(V1) 581*
    of protein, *(V1) 578*
    stressor response, *(V1) 555–556*
    types of, *(V1) 575, (V1) 577*
Meter, *(V2) 518*
Metered-dose inhaler, *(V1) 505, (V1) 506*
Methamphetamine
    sexual function and, *(V1) 774t*
    teratogenic effect on fetus, *(ESG9) 9*
Metric scale, *(V1) 310*
Metric system, *(V1) 492*
    apothecary and household equivalents, *(V2) 521*
    conversion of, *(V2) 520–521*
    for medication dosage, *(V2) 518*
Microcephaly, *(V1) 370*
Microchip, *(V1) 973, (V1) 973f*
Microcomputer, *(V1) 973f*
Micronutrient, *(V1) 581–582*
Microorganisms
    mutation of, *(V1) 399*
Microsleep, *(V1) 801*
Microvilli, *(V1) 653*
Micturition, *(V1) 622*
Middle ear, *(V1) 372*
Middle-income family, *(V1) 215*
Midlife changes, *(V1) 214*
Midlife crisis, *(ESG9) 33*
Midline peripheral catheter, *(V1) 907*
Mid-range theory, *(V1) 145*
Mild anxiety, *(V1) 199*
Military
    Florence Nightingale nursing, *(V1) 3, (V1) 145*
    image of nurse, *(V1) 8–9*
    injectable penicillin, use of, *(V1) 5*
    nurses serving during war, *(V1) 9*
Military hospital, *(V1) 8*
Military time, *(V1) 302, (V1) 302f*
Milliequivalents (mEq), *(V1) 492, (V1) 888*
Milligram, *(V1) 888*
Mind-body intervention/therapy, *(V1) 995–996*
Mindfulness meditation, *(V1) 995*
Mind-mapping, *(V1) 91–92*
Mineral, *(V1) 581*
    adult dietary reference intake (DRI), *(V1) 585t–586t*
    supplementation, *(V1) 607*
Mini Mental Stat Exam (MMSE), *(ESG9) 38*
Minimization, *(V1) 560t*
Minimum Data Set for Residential Assessment and Care Screening (MDS), *(V1) 299*
Minimum effective concentration, of drug, *(V1) 485–487, (V1) 486f*

Minority group, *(V1) 225*
Minor surgery, *(V1) 924*
Miosis, *(V1) 371*
Miracle, *(V1) 260, (V1) 262*
Misdemeanor, *(V1) 1077*
Misplaced breath sounds, *(V1) 380*
Mixed apnea, *(V1) 802*
Mnemonic
    for observing, *(V1) 45b*
Mobility
    as activity of daily living (ADL), *(V1) 43b*
    affecting self-care ability, *(V1) 443*
    assessment of, *(V1) 740–747*
    disease affecting joint, *(V1) 737–738*
    factors affecting, *(V1) 735, (V1) 737–739*
    physiology of
        muscles, *(V1) 726–728*
        nervous system, *(V1) 728*
        skeletal system, *(V1) 725–726*
    positioning devices, *(V1) 749–750*
Modality, *(V1) 989*
Mode
    of exercise, *(V1) 732*
    of transmission, *(V1) 400*
Model
    definition of, *(V1) 142*
Model care plan, *(V1) 89*
Model of care
    nursing, *(ESGV1) 21–22*
    provision for, *(ESGV1) 21*
Model of Change, *(V1) 1007–1008*
Modem, *(V1) 974*
Moderate anxiety, *(V1) 199–200*
Modulation, of pain, *(V1) 702–703*
Moist heat, *(V1) 842–843*
Moisture
    pressure ulcers and, *(V1) 821*
    in skin, *(V1) 367*
Mold, *(V1) 857*
Moltmann, Jurgen, *(V1) 171b*
Money. See Finances
Monocytes, *(V1) 402, (V1) 403t*
Monogamy, serial, *(V1) 769*
Monoglyceride, *(V1) 579b*
Monosaccharide, *(V1) 577*
Monounsaturated fat, *(V1) 580, (V1) 580t*
Mons pubis, *(V1) 764*
Montgomery straps, *(V1) 841f, (V1) 841t*
Mood disorder, *(V2) 110*
Moral agency, *(V1) 1048*
Moral behavior, *(V1) 1045*
Moral development theory, *(V1) 151*
    overview of, *(ESG9) 7–8*
    three-stage approach to, *(V1) 167, (V1) 1046t*
Moral distress, *(V1) 1048*
Moral framework, *(V1) 1057*
MORAL model, *(V1) 1065–1066, (V2) 1005, (V2) 1013tb*
Moral outrage, *(V1) 1048–1049*
Moral principles, *(V1) 1054*
Morals
    decision-making factors, *(V1) 1050–1051*
    development of, *(V1) 1046–1047*
    modern theory of, *(V1) 1045*
    values and ethics relating to, *(V1) 1054*
Mormonism, *(V1) 251*
Moro reflex, *(ESG9) 14*
Morphine, *(V1) 717t*
    teratogenic effect on fetus, *(ESG9) 9*
Morse Fall Scale, *(V1) 438*

Mortality
    decreased rate of, *(V1) 9*
    infectious disease and, *(V1) 5*
Morula, *(ESG9) 8*
Mosquito, *(V1) 429–430*
Motivation
    learning and, *(V1) 531–532*
Motor cortex, *(V1) 851*
Motor development
    of infant, *(ESG9) 16*
    of preschooler, *(ESG9) 22*
    of toddler, *(ESG9) 19*
Motor function, *(V1) 389–390*
Motor vehicle accident, *(V1) 428–429, (ESG9) 28*
Motrin
    for menstrual pain, *(V1) 788*
    for pain relief, *(V1) 712*
Mourning, *(V1) 265*
Mouth
    abnormal findings of, *(V1) 375*
    abnormalities of, *(V2) 334*
    assessment of, *(V1) 394, (V1) 461, (V2) 268p–271p*
    defense against infection, *(V1) 402*
    function of, *(V1) 651*
    hygiene of, *(V1) 459*
    NOC outcomes and NIC interventions, *(V2) 435*
    problems of, *(V1) 460–461*
    risk factors for problems, *(V1) 459–460*
    self-care deficit, *(V1) 461*
    structures of, *(V1) 374–375, (V1) 374f, (V2) 271*
    teeth development, *(V1) 459, (V1) 459f*
    treatment of poisoning by, *(V1) 424*
    vocalization, *(V1) 375*
Movement
    assessment of, *(V2) 302p–303p*
    bed, patient out of, *(V1) 754–756*
    bed-bound patient, *(V1) 750–754*
    of chest and abdomen, *(V1) 325–326*
    of musculoskeletal system, *(V1) 385*
    overview of, *(V2) 696*
    physiology of
        muscles, *(V1) 726–728*
        nervous system, *(V1) 728*
        skeletal system, *(V1) 725–726*
    terms to describe, *(V1) 727f*
MRI (magnetic resonance imaging), GI tract, *(V2) 667*
Mu (μ), *(V1) 702, (V1) 713*
Mu agonist, *(V1) 713*
Mucolytic agent, *(V1) 884*
Multidisciplinary treatment, *(V1) 85*
Municipal authorities, *(V1) 7*
Murmur, heart, *(V1) 381, (V1) 382, (V2) 291*
Muscle
    deltoid, *(V1) 517, (V1) 517f*
    dorsogluteal, *(V1) 516–517*
    function of, *(V1) 385, (V1) 727–728*
    immobility, effects on, *(V1) 739*
    mass, of child, *(ESG9) 24*
    problems of, *(V1) 740b*
    rectus femoris, *(V1) 517*
    strength assessment, *(V1) 385, (V2) 307*
    types of, *(V1) 726–727*
    vastus lateralis muscle, *(V1) 517, (V1) 517f*
    ventrogluteal, *(V1) 516, (V1) 516f*
Muscular fitness, *(V1) 1009*

Musculoskeletal system
  abnormalities of, *(V2)* 335
  adaptation failure and, *(V1)* 562
  age-related changes for, *(ESG9)* 36t
  assessment of, *(V1)* 384–385, *(V1)* 395p,
    (V2) 300p–307p
  exercise and, *(V1)* 734b
  injury from exercise, *(V1)* 733
  pain and, *(V1)* 706
  stressor response, *(V1)* 555–556
Music therapy, *(V1)* 1002
Muslim faith, *(V1)* 251–252
Mustache care, *(V1)* 465, *(V2)* 418p–419p
Mydrias, *(V1)* 371
Mydriatics, *(V1)* 371
Myocardial infarction, *(V1)* 89, *(V1)* 91
Myofascial release, *(V1)* 999
Myopia, *(V1)* 371, *(V1)* 685b
Myotonia, *(V1)* 776
Myxedema, *(V1)* 370

N
Nails
  abnormalities of, *(V2)* 334
  assessment of, *(V1)* 369, *(V1)* 393p,
    (V1) 458, *(V2)* 249p, *(V2)* 433
  characteristics of, *(V1)* 457
  NOC outcomes and NIC interventions,
    (V2) 435
  plate angel of, *(V1)* 370f
NANDA
  classification system of, *(V1)* 71
  components of nursing diagnosis,
    (V1) 71–72
  diagnostic labels, *(V1)* 59
  NOC outcomes linking to, *(V1)* 97, *(V1)* 97b
  Taxonomy II, (V1) 71
NANDA diagnosis
  anxiety-related, *(V2)* 114
  depression-related, *(V2)* 115
  descriptors for, *(V2)* 41
  labeling, *(V2)* 33
  safety problems, *(V2)* 381–382
NANDA label
  adding words to, *(V1)* 76
  for anxiety, *(V1)* 203
  for communication problems, *(V1)* 349
  community-based diagnosis, *(V1)* 1029
  criteria for choosing, *(V1)* 77
  criticism of, *(V1)* 79
  descriptors for, *(V2)* 41
  for diagnosis, *(V2)* 33
  eye problems, *(V1)* 466
  for family health status diagnoses, *(V1)* 218
  growth and development problems,
    (ESG9) 39
  impaired skin integrity, *(V1)* 449
  impaired swallowing, *(V1)* 608
  nutrition-related problems, *(V1)* 606
  overweight and obesity, *(V1)* 609–610
  for pain, *(V1)* 708
  parts of, *(V1)* 76
  safety problems, *(V1)* 439
  sexual problems, *(V1)* 782–783
  sleep pattern disturbance, *(V1)* 805
  for spirituality diagnoses, *(V1)* 256–258,
    (V2) 147
  for wellness diagnoses, *(V1)* 538,
    (V1) 1013–1015
NANDA/NIC/NOC linkages book, *(V1)* 97–98
NANDA Nursing Diagnosis Taxonomy II,
  (V1) 51b

NANDA Taxonomy II, (V1) 71, *(V2)* 39–40
Nanotechnology, *(V1)* 973
Narcolepsy, *(V1)* 802
Narcotics, packaging of, *(V1)* 477f
Narrative charting, *(V1)* 291
Narrow-mindedness, *(V1)* 27
Nasal administration, opioids, *(V1)* 714–715
Nasal decongestant, *(V1)* 884
Nasal medication
  administration of, *(V1)* 522p,
    (V2) 465p–467p
  overview of, *(V1)* 504
Nasal passage, *(V1)* 846
Nasoenteric (NE) tube
  for enteric feedings, *(V1)* 613
  insertion of, *(V2)* 567p–571p
  removal of, *(V2)* 577p–578p
Nasogastric medication, *(V1)* 500
Nasogastric tube (NG), *(V1)* 613f
  bowel sounds and, *(V1)* 383
  for enteric feedings, *(V1)* 613–614
  insertion of, *(V1)* 612p, *(V2)* 567p–571p
  removal of, *(V2)* 577p–578p
Nasopharyngeal airway
  example of, *(V1)* 878f
  insertion of, *(V2)* 863tb
  suctioning of, *(V1)* 879–880,
    (V2) 831p–834p
  use of, *(V1)* 878
Nasotracheal tube
  endotracheal airways and, *(V1)* 878
  suctioning of, *(V1)* 880, *(V2)* 835p–839p
National Association for Home Care (NAHC),
  (V1) 1033
National Center for Complementary and
  Alternative Medicine, *(V1)* 22,
  (V1) 235, *(V1)* 989
National Center for Health Statistics
  (NCHS), *(V1)* 990–991
National Center for Injury Prevention and
  Control (NCIPC), *(ESG9)* 32
National Council Licensure Exam (NCLEX),
  (V1) 14, *(V1)* 16
National Council of State Boards, *(V1)* 39
National Council on Aging, *(V1)* 770
National economy, *(V1)* 21
National Electronic Disease Surveillance
  (NEDSS), *(V1)* 971
National Formulary (NF), *(V1)* 474, *(V1)* 475
National Health Council, *(ESGV1)* 26
National High Blood Pressure Education
  Program, *(V1)* 327
National Institute for Health, *(V1)* 971
National Institute of Allergy and Infectious
  Disease (NIAID), *(V1)* 657
National Institute of Health
  healthcare outside traditional health care
    system, *(V1)* 22
  identifying research themes and
    priorities, *(V1)* 155
  National Center for Complementary and
    Alternative Medicine, *(V1)* 22,
    (V1) 235
National Institute of Nursing Research
  (NINR), *(V1)* 155
National Institute of Occupational Safety and
  Health (NIOSH), *(V1)* 511
National Labor Relations Act of 1935,
  (V1) 1073–1074
National League for Nursing (NLN), *(V1)* 18
National school lunch and breakfast
  program, *(V1)* 608

National Standards for Culturally and
  Linguistically Appropriate Services
  (CLAS), *(V1)* 244
National Steering Committee on Patient
  Safety, *(ESGV1)* 25–26
National Student Nurses Association
  (NSNA), *(V1)* 18
Native American
  healing system of, *(V1)* 234t
  kokopelli, *(V1)* 253f
  religion of, *(V1)* 253
  statistics in nursing, *(V1)* 10t
  types of folk healers, *(V1)* 230t
Nature
  definition of, *(V1)* 165
  nurture versus, *(ESG9)* 2–3
Naturopathy, *(V1)* 995, *(V1)* 997
Naughty nurse, *(V1)* 7–8
Nausea
  medications causing, *(V1)* 600b
  peristalsis and, *(V1)* 657
  as postoperative collaborative problem,
    (V1) 946t
  as side effect of opioids, *(V1)* 714b
NCLEX-PN exam, *(V1)* 14, *(V1)* 16
Nearsightedness, *(V1)* 371, *(V1)* 685b
Near vision, *(V1)* 372
Nebulizer
  function of, *(V1)* 875
  types of, *(V1)* 505f
Neck
  anterior and posterior triangles of,
    (V1) 376f
  assessment of, *(V1)* 394, *(V2)* 272p–274p
  components of, *(V1)* 375–376
  parts of anterior, *(V1)* 376f
  range of motion, *(V1)* 742t
  structures of, *(V2)* 274
Needle
  characteristics of, *(V1)* 507
  dead space, *(V1)* 510
  recapping, *(V1)* 511, *(V1)* 524p,
    (V2) 483p–485p
  transfer, *(V1)* 519
Needle aspiration, *(V1)* 829, *(V1)* 829p,
  (V2) 763p–765p
Needlestick injury, *(V1)* 437, *(V1)* 510–511,
  (V2) 378
Needlestick Safety and Prevention Act,
  (V1) 907
Needs
  adapting standarized care plan to
    patient, *(V1)* 89
  addressed by nursing care, *(V1)* 146,
    (V1) 146b
  of dying patient, *(V1)* 284–285
  Maslow's hierarchy of, *(V1)* 50,
    (V1) 66–67, *(V1)* 150–151,
    (V1) 150f, *(V2)* 100
  resistance to change, *(V1)* 963
Negative nitrogen balance, *(V1)* 578
Negative pressure ventilator, *(V1)* 880
Negligence
  malpractice and, *(V1)* 1079, *(V1)* 1081
  vicarious liability, *(V1)* 1080
Negotiation
  in civil claim, *(V1)* 1081
  informal, *(V1)* 966
Nephron, *(V1)* 620
Nephropathy, *(V1)* 633b
Nephrotoxic, *(V1)* 623–626, *(V1)* 633b
Nerve block, *(V1)* 716–717, *(V1)* 938–939

Nerve fiber, (V1) 322
Nerve impulse, generation of, (V1) 374
Nervous system, (V1) 728
    age-related changes for, (ESG9) 36t
    autonomic, (V1) 322
Neuman, Betty
    health as energy, (V1) 1004
    health continuum, (V1) 172–173,
        (V1) 173f
Neuman system model, (V1) 152
Neural tube defect, (ESG9) 12–13
Neurectomy, (V1) 718
Neurogenic bladder, (V1) 625
Neuroleptic, (V1) 935t
Neurological disorder, (V1) 926b
Neurological problems, (V1) 636
Neurological system
    age-related changes for, (ESG9) 36t
    assessment of, (V1) 385, (V1) 395p–396p
    cerebral function, (V1) 386
    cranial nerve function, (V1) 387, (V1) 389
    cranial nerve origin, (V1) 388f
Neuromuscular system, (ESG9) 14
Neuropathic pain, (V1) 700
Neurotransmitters, (V1) 702
Neutralization
    as method of destroying pathogens,
        (V1) 403
Neutrophil, (V1) 403t
Nevi, (V1) 368
Nevus flammeus (port-wine stain), (V2) 333
Newborn
    body fluid of, (V1) 888t
    breasts of, (V2) 276
    head of, (V2) 251
    length of, (ESG9) 13f
    nails of, (V2) 249
    oxygenation of, (V1) 854
    skin of, (V2) 242
    skull, sutures and fontanelles of,
        (ESG9) 13f
    sleep requirement, (V1) 795, (V1) 795t
Newborns' and Mothers' Health Protection
    Act of 1996 (NMHPA), (V1) 1073
New Brunswick Mental Health Act,
    (ESGV1) 8
Newman, Margaret, (V1) 991
NIC intervention
    bathing, (V1) 114b
    linking to NANDA diagnosis, risk for
        aspiration, (V1) 115t
    locating appropriate, (V1) 114
    for psychosocial diagnosis, (V1) 196
Nicotine
    sleep and, (V1) 800
    teratogenic effect on fetus, (ESG9) 9
Nightingale, Florence, (V1) 145
    clean environment theory, (V1) 145
    community-based nursing, (V1) 1025
    contributions of, (V1) 6
    contributions to epidemiology, (V1) 9
    defining health, (V1) 171b
    holistic nursing and, (V1) 991
    as "Lady of the Lamp", (V1) 6
    modern nursing founder, (V1) 6
    nursing research and, (V1) 154
    nursing soldiers, (V1) 3
    photo of, (V1) 7f
The Nightingales, (V1) 7
Nightmare, (V1) 803
Night terrors, (V1) 803
Nirvana, Jehovah's Witness, (V1) 252

Nit, (V1) 369
Nitrogen balance, (V1) 578
NOC. See Nursing Outcomes Classification
    (NOC)
Nocebo effect, (V1) 990
Nociceptive pain, (V1) 700
Nociceptors, (V1) 700, (V1) 702f
Nocturia, (V1) 633b
Nocturnal enuresis, (V1) 623, (V1) 637
Nocturnal frequency, (V1) 623
Nodule, (V2) 245
Noise level, (V1) 469–470
Noise pollution, (V1) 431
Nonadherence, (V1) 496
Non-benzodiazepines, (V1) 807
Noncompliance, (V1) 60, (V1) 496
Nondirective interview, (V1) 47
Nondirective leadership, (V1) 954
Nonelectrolyte, (V1) 887
Nonessential amino acid, (V1) 577, (V1) 578t
Nonessential fatty acid, (V1) 580
Nongovernmental agency (NGO), (ESGV1) 21
Nonionized drug molecule, (V1) 484
Non-Luer-Lok, (V1) 507, (V1) 508f
Nonmaleficence, (V1) 1055
Nonopioid analgesic, (V1) 712–713, (V1) 712b
Nonpharmacological pain relief, (V1) 709–711
Nonprescription drug, (V1) 474
Nonproprietary name, (V1) 474
Non-rapid eye movement (NREM) sleep,
    (V1) 796–798
Nonselective debridement, (V1) 836
Nonshivering thermogenesis, (V1) 308
nonsteroidal anti-inflammatory drugs
    (NSAIDs)
    increasing surgical risk, (V1) 926b
    for menstrual pain, (V1) 788
    for pain relief, (V1) 712–713
    peristalsis and, (V1) 656
Nontunneled central venous catheter,
    (V1) 907–908, (V1) 908f
Nonverbal communication, (V1) 49,
    (V1) 342–343
Norepinephrine
    function of, (V1) 557f
    production of, (V1) 308
Norm, identification of, (V1) 151
Normal anxiety, (V1) 199
Normal flora, (V1) 399
North American healthcare system, (V1) 232,
    (V1) 233t
North American Nursing Diagnosis
    Association. See NANDA
Norton scale, (V1) 823, (V1) 825f
Nose
    assessment of, (V1) 394, (V2) 266p–268p
    care of, (V1) 468
    characteristics of, (V1) 374
    impaired smell, (V1) 686–687
    treatment for inhaled poisons, (V1) 424
Nosocomial infection
    decreased rate of, (V1) 9
    exogenous and endogenous, (V1) 401
    transmission of, (V1) 398
Novice, nurse as, (V1) 140
Novice-to-expert theory, (V1) 147
NPO diet, (V1) 601, (V1) 608
NSAIDs (nonsteroidal anti-inflammatory
    drugs)
    for menstrual pain, (V1) 788
    for pain relief, (V1) 712–713
    peristalsis, (V1) 656

Nuclear family, traditional, (V1) 210, (V2) 118
Numerical rating scale (NRS), for pain,
    (V2) 693
Nuremberg Code, (V1) 158
Nurse
    acquiring clinical skill and judgment,
        (V1) 15
    bloodborne pathogen exposure, (V1)
        416–417
    Caucasian woman as, (V1) 9–10
    complex critical thinking processes,
        (V1) 27–29
    criminal as, (V1) 7
    diagnosis and treatment of medical
        problems, (V1) 59
    duty to report, (V1) 1079
    early role of, (V1) 5
    effect of touch on, (V1) 688b
    employment status of, (V1) 6–7
    empowerment of, (V1) 961–962
    enhancing therapeutic communication,
        (V1) 349–351
    ethical problems, sources of,
        (V1) 1049–1050
    Florence Nightingale as, (V1) 3
    forming union, (V1) 7
    grief and loss, (V1) 286
    healing presence of, (V2) 94
    health promotion, role in, (V1) 1015
    honoring health/illness experience of
        client, (V1) 182–183
    impaired functioning of, (V1) 1049,
        (V1) 1087
    importance of health of, (V1) 185
    infection control, (V1) 417
    infectious disease, exposure to, (V1) 5
    influence on healthcare policy, (V1) 23
    interview process, (V1) 46–49
    intrapersonal communication, (V1) 338
    knowledge, types of, (V1) 29
    legal safeguards for, (V1) 1087–1089
    listservs for, (V1) 976b
    meals, assisting patient, (V1) 609
    naughty, (V1) 7–8
    as operative personnel, (V1) 936–937
    race and ethnicity of, (V1) 10t
    reasons for not using research, (V1) 161
    responding to patient pain, (V1) 705
    role and function of, (V1) 13t
    self-care for, (V1) 1002
    sexual behavior, inappropriate, (V1)
        790–791
    theories and, (V1) 144–145, (V1) 149–152
    therapeutic communication barriers,
        (V1) 351–354
    as warrior against disease, (V1) 9,
        (V1) 9f
    as witness, (V1) 1080
    workforce in U.S., (V1) 960
    working with diverse population,
        (V1) 254
Nurse anesthetist (CRNA), (V1) 937
Nurse-patient relationship, (V1) 8
Nurse practice act, (V1) 476, (V1) 1074
Nurse practitioner, (ESGV1) 16
Nurse Ratched, (V1) 7
Nurses' Associated Alumnae of the United
    States and Canada, (V1) 16
Nurse theorist, (V1) 148t–149t
Nursing
    action as intervention, (V1) 105
    activities of, (V1) 6t

code of ethics, organizational, (V1) 1059
community-oriented, (V1) 1024–1025
computer information systems and,
    (V1) 977b
credentialing, (V1) 1075
culture of, (V1) 232
definition of, (V1) 11–14
    International Council of Nurses (ICN),
        (V1) 11
    Nurses Association, (V1) 11
entry-level education, (V1) 12
evolution of
    knowledge map, (V2) 11
    overview, (V2) 6
full-spectrum, (V1) 10, (V1) 15
    concepts of model for, (V1) 33
    definition of, (V1) 33
    importance of evaluation, (V1) 128–129
    as jigsaw puzzle, (V1) 140
    then and now, (V1) 3
growing role outside hospital, (V1) 22
hazards to, (V1) 437–438
history, images throughout, (V2) 6
    angel of mercy, (V1) 4–5
    battle-ax, (V1) 7
    Caucasian woman, (V1) 9–10
    handmaiden, (V1) 5–7
    military image, (V1) 8–9
    naughty nurse, (V1) 7–8
holistic, (V1) 991
informatics and, (V1) 977
judging effectiveness of, (V1) 92
knowledge map of, (V2) 11
labor market, (V1) 960
language for, (V2) 957–958
laws and regulations guiding
    federal law, (V1) 1072–1074
    practice guidelines, (V1) 1076–1077
    standards of practice, (V1) 1075–1076
    state law, (V1) 1074–1075
lawsuit, (V1) 1082b
licensing, (V1) 1074–1075
model of care, (ESG46 V2) 1
organizations for, (V1) 16–18
perioperative, (V1) 923
preoperative, (V1) 923
as a profession, (V1) 12–14
regulation of, (V1) 16–19
requirements of documentation, (V1) 293
standards of practice, (V1) 16, (V1) 17t
stereotyping, (V2) 6
strategies for culturally competent care,
    (V1) 241–243
teams, (ESGV1) 21
then and now, (V1) 3
values of, (V1) 16b, (V1) 232
Nursing: Scope and Standards of Practice,
    (V1) 1061
Nursing: Social Policy Statement, (V1) 58
Nursing activity
    bowel incontinence, (V1) 674–675
    for client safety, (V1) 439
    for depression-related diagnoses, (V1) 206
    disturbed energy field, (V1) 1001
    for dying and grieving, (V1) 277, (V1)
        282–283
    exercise and, (V1) 748
    for family health status diagnoses,
        (V1) 219
    foot care, (V1) 456–457
    for health promotion, (V1) 1016–1017
    for hypertension, (V1) 335

for hypotension, (V1) 334
for hypothermia, (V1) 316–317
ineffective sexuality pattern,
    (V1) 785–786
knowledge and ability to perform,
    (V1) 122
medication-related, (V1) 497
nail care, (V1) 458
nutrition-related problems, (V1) 607
for oral cavity/mouth problems, (V1) 461
organization of work, (V1) 123
oxygenation, (V1) 873
for pain relief, (V1) 709
preparing patient for, (V1) 123, (V1) 125
for psychosocial diagnosis, (V1) 196–198
for sexual problems, (V1) 783, (V2) 738
skin integrity and wound healing, (V1)
    831–833
for sleep pattern disturbance,
    (V1) 805–808
stress-related problems, (V1) 567
stress urinary incontinence, (V1) 628–630
for temperature/fever diagnoses,
    (V1) 315–316
for underweight and malnutrition,
    (V1) 611
for weight control, (V1) 610
wound drains, maintaining, (V1) 835–836
Nursing aid, (V2) 22–23
Nursing assistant, (ESGV1) 17
Nursing care, (V1) 19
Nursing care plan, (V1) 92
    comprehensive
        components of, (V1) 86f
        documents in, (V1) 85–86
        information in, (V1) 85
        nursing diagnosis standardized form,
            (V1) 88f
        Patient Care Protocol, (V1) 87f
        preprinted, standardized plans,
            (V1) 86–87, (V1) 89
    individualized, (V1) 89–90
    information in, (V2) 44
    special discharge or teaching plans,
        (V1) 91
    standardized
        adapting to patient needs, (V1) 89
        computer printout for, (V1) 88f
        individualizing, (V1) 92
    theoretical knowledge, (V1) 183–184
Nursing database, (V1) 42
Nursing diagnosis, (V1) 89
    of abnormal pulse, (V1) 321
    activity and exercise, (V1) 747
    actual, (V1) 61–62
    algorithm for determining type of,
        (V1) 62f
    analyzing and interpreting data,
        (V1) 63–65
    of anxiety, (V1) 203
    bowel incontinence, (V1) 674
    bowel-related problems, (V1) 664
    care plan document, (V1) 85
    choosing label, (V1) 72–73
    circulation problems, (V1) 872
    collaborative problems, (V1) 76
    community-based, (V1) 1029
    comparing to goals, (V1) 95t
    comparing to medical diagnosis and
        collaborative problems, (V1) 60t
    components of NANDA nursing
        diagnosis, (V1) 71–72

critiquing diagnostic reasoning process,
    (V1) 70b
cultural bias and, (V1) 240b
cultural factors as etiology, (V1) 239–240
deficient knowledge, (V1) 538
definition of, (V1) 57
diagnostic statement, (V1) 73, (V1) 74t,
    (V1) 75–76, (V1) 77–79
disturbed energy field, (V1) 1001
for dying and grieving, (V1) 276–277
of eye problems, (V1) 466
for family health status, (V1) 218
of feet problems, (V1) 456
first conference on, (V1) 58
fluid, electrolyte and acid-base
    imbalance, (V1) 903
Goal/expected outcome for, (V1) 96
growth and development problems,
    (ESG9) 39
of health, (V1) 182
home health care visit, (V1) 1039–1040
hypertension, (V1) 334
hypotension, (V1) 334
for hypothermia, (V1) 316
individualized care plan, (V1) 89
of infection, (V1) 407
intervention flowing from, (V1) 110f
intraoperative, (V1) 940
medication-related, (V1) 496
nail problems, (V1) 458
NANDA descriptors, (V2) 41
NANDA nursing taxonomy, (V1) 71
NIC intervention linking to, (V1) 115t
NOC outcomes linking to NANDA,
    (V1) 97, (V1) 97b
nutrition-related problems, (V1) 606
of oral cavity/mouth, (V1) 461
outcome and intervention, (V1) 77
overview of, (V2) 33
overweight and obesity, (V1) 609–610
oxygenation problems, (V1) 872
pain, (V1) 708, (V1) 721
postoperative collaborative problems,
    (V1) 944
for preoperative client, (V1) 930–931
psychosocial, (V1) 193–194, (V1) 193–195,
    (V1) 194t
recognizing, (V1) 59, (V1) 77
review of, (V1) 110–111, (V1) 136
risk for falls, (V1) 439
self-care deficit, (V1) 445
self-concept
    guidelines for, (V1) 195–196
    outcomes, standardized and individual-
        ized, (V2) 112
sensory-perceptual problems,
    (V1) 691–692
sexual problems, (V1) 782–783
of skin breakdown, (V1) 831
of skin problems, (V1) 449, (V1) 831
sleep pattern disturbance, (V1)
    804–805
status of, (V1) 61
stress-related, (V1) 566–567, (V1) 566b
stress urinary incontinence, (V1) 627
for temperature/fever, (V1) 315
urinary elimination problems, (V1) 635
wellness, (V1) 1013–1015
Nursing Diagnosis Taxonomy II, NANDA,
    (V1) 51b
Nursing doctorate (ND), (V1) 14
Nursing drug handbooks, (V1) 475

Nursing ethics
  definition of, (V1) 1047
  studying, (V1) 1047–1048
Nursing informatics
  definition of, (V1) 971–972
  knowledge map for, (V2) 959
  overview of, (V2) 949
  standardized minimum data set, (ESGV1) 12–13
Nursing intervention
  elimination of, (V1) 104–105
  guide in selecting, (V1) 106
  independent intervention, (V1) 105
  model of, (V1) 105f
  problem status influencing, (V1) 109
  reflecting critically about, (V1) 118
  types of, (V1) 105–106
  using standardized language for, (V1) 113
Nursing Intervention Classification (NIC)
  for abnormal pulse, (V1) 321
  activity and exercise, (V1) 747, (V2) 724
  for anxiety, (V2) 114
  bowel incontinence, (V1) 674
  bowel-related problems, (V1) 665, (V2) 669–670
  for client safety, (V1) 439
  for communication problems, (V1) 349
  community-based diagnosis, (V1) 1031
  components of, (V1) 114
  computerized care plans, (V1) 114
  for depression, (V2) 115
  development of, (V1) 113
  disturbed energy field, (V1) 1001–1002
  for family health status diagnoses, (V1) 218–219, (V2) 127
  feeding, (V1) 609
  for feet problems, (V1) 456
  for fluid and electrolyte diagnoses, (V2) 909–911
  fluid, electrolyte and acid-base imbalance, (V1) 903–904
  growth and development problems, (ESG9) 39–40
  for health knowledge, (V2) 537
  health promotion, (V1) 1016
  for home health care diagnoses, (V1) 1041
  hygiene problems, (V2) 435–436
  for hypertension, (V1) 335
  for hypothermia, (V1) 316
  immobility management, (V2) 724
  impaired verbal communication, (V2) 227
  ineffective sexuality pattern, (V1) 785–786
  for integumentary problems, (V1) 450
  for intraoperative phase, (V2) 932–934
  labels for, (V2) 993–994
  loss and grieving, (V2) 173–174
  medication-related, (V1) 496, (V2) 524–525
  nail care, (V1) 458
  nutrition-related problems, (V1) 607–608, (V2) 588
  for oral cavity/mouth problems, (V1) 461
  oxygenation, (V1) 873
  for oxygenation diagnoses, (V2) 869
  for pain diagnoses, (V2) 695
  for pain relief, (V1) 709
  perioperative care, (V1) 931
  for postoperative diagnoses, (V1) 948, (V2) 935–938
  for preoperative diagnoses, (V2) 930–931

for psychosocial diagnosis, (V1) 196
safety problems, (V2) 382
for self-care deficit, (V1) 446, (V2) 434
self-concept, selected nursing activities for, (V2) 113
sensory-perceptual problems, (V1) 692, (V2) 682
sexual problems, (V2) 738
for skin and wound diagnoses, (V2) 795–796
sleep diagnoses, (V2) 752
sleep pattern disturbance, (V1) 805
for spirituality diagnoses, (V1) 258, (V2) 153tb–154tb
stress-related problems, (V1) 567, (V2) 554
stress urinary incontinence, (V1) 627
for underweight and malnutrition, (V1) 611
urinary problems, (V2) 634
vital signs, abnormal, (V2) 218
vocabulary for intervention, (V2) 53
for weight control, (V1) 610
for wellness diagnoses, (V2) 980–981
Nursing knowledge
  full-spectrum nursing and, (V1) 33–36
  types of, (V1) 29
Nursing model, (V1) 50
Nursing orders
  components of, (V1) 116–118
  creation and persecution of, (V1) 5
  post-Reformation period, (V1) 246–247
  reflecting critically about, (V1) 118
  writing to individualizing medical order, (V1) 106
Nursing Outcomes Classification (NOC), (V1) 97–98
  activity and exercise, (V1) 747
  for anxiety, (V2) 114
  bowel incontinence, (V1) 673
  bowel-related problems, (V1) 665, (V2) 669–670
  for client safety, (V1) 439
  for communication problems, (V1) 349
  community-based diagnosis, (V1) 1031
  components of, (V1) 97–98
  deficient knowledge, (V1) 539
  defining goal and outcome, (V1) 92–93
  definition of, (V1) 97
  for depression-related diagnoses, (V1) 205–206, (V2) 115
  disturbed energy field, (V1) 1001
  for dying and grieving, (V1) 277
  energy maintenance and mobility, (V2) 724
  for family health, (V1) 218, (V2) 126
  for feet problems, (V1) 456
  for fluid and electrolyte diagnoses, (V1) 903, (V2) 909–911
  growth and development problems, (ESG9) 39
  for health knowledge, (V2) 537
  for health promotion, (V1) 1015, (V2) 979
  for home health care diagnoses, (V1) 1040–1041
  hygiene problems, (V2) 435–436
  for hypertension, (V1) 334–335
  for hypothermia, (V1) 316
  impaired verbal communication, (V2) 227
  ineffective sexuality pattern, (V1) 784
  for integumentary problems, (V1) 449

for intraoperative phase, (V2) 932–934
loss and grieving, (V2) 173–174
measurement scale, (V2) 50
medication-related, (V1) 496, (V2) 524–525
nail care, (V1) 458
nutrition-related problems, (V1) 606–607, (V2) 588
for oral cavity/mouth problems, (V1) 461
for oxygenation diagnoses, (V1) 873, (V2) 869
for pain diagnoses, (V2) 695
for pain relief, (V1) 709
postoperative collaborative problems, (V1) 944, (V1) 948
for postoperative diagnoses, (V2) 935–938
for preoperative diagnoses, (V2) 930–931
preoperative phase, (V1) 931
for psychosocial diagnosis, (V1) 196
for pulse status, (V1) 321
safety problems, (V2) 381–382
for self-care deficit, (V1) 44–446
self-care deficit, (V2) 434
self-concept, standardized and individualized, (V2) 112
sensory-perceptual problems, (V1) 692, (V2) 682
sexual problems, (V2) 737
for skin and wound diagnoses, (V2) 795–796
sleep diagnoses, (V2) 752
sleep promotion, (V1) 805
for spirituality diagnoses, (V1) 258
stress-related problems, (V1) 567, (V2) 554
stress urinary incontinence, (V1) 627
for temperature/fever diagnoses, (V1) 315
for underweight and malnutrition, (V1) 611
urinary elimination, (V1) 638
using with computerized care plan, (V1) 99
vital signs, abnormal, (V2) 218
vocabulary for outcome, (V2) 44
for weight control, (V1) 610
writing aggregate goals, (V2) 992
Nursing Practice, Taxonomy of, (V1) 51b
Nursing process
  assessment
    of adolescence, (ESG9) 29
    of anxiety, (V1) 202–203
    at birth, (ESG9) 15–16
    of blood pressure, (V1) 329–331, (V1) 333
    bowel elimination patterns, (V1) 659
    of child, (ESG9) 26
    collaborative care and, (V1) 39
    of communication problems, (V1) 348–349
    community-based, (V1) 1029
    computer screen capture of data, (V1) 54f
    concepts of models for structuring, (V1) 51b
    critical reflection about, (V1) 52–54
    cultural, (V1) 238–239
    definition of, (V1) 38
    delegation of, (V1) 39–41
    documentation of data, (V1) 50, (V1) 52
    for dying and grieving, (V1) 276
    of elderly, (ESG9) 37–38
    eyes, (V1) 466

for family health status diagnoses, *(V1) 217–218*
feet problems, *(V1) 456*
fever, *(V1) 314–315*
fluid, electrolyte and acid-base imbalance, *(V1) 901*
graphic flow sheet, *(V1) 53f*
growth and development, *(ESG9) 39*
guidelines for recording data, *(V1) 52*
of health, *(V1) 181*
health promotion, *(V1) 1009, (V1) 1012–1013*
holistic, *(V1) 1001*
home health care visit, *(V1) 1039*
hygiene, *(V1) 444*
impaired oxygenation, *(V1) 861–863*
of infant, *(ESG9) 18*
for infection, *(V1) 406–407*
intraoperative/postoperative surgery phase, *(V1) 927, (V1) 928f–929f*
knowledge map of, *(V2) 32*
learning, *(V1) 537*
medication-related, *(V1) 495*
of middle adult, *(ESG9) 34*
mobility and activity, *(V1) 740–747*
nursing interview, *(V1) 46–49*
nutrition-related problems, *(V1) 602–605*
observation, *(V1) 44, (V1) 45b*
oral cavity/mouth, *(V1) 461*
organization of data, *(V1) 50*
pain, *(V1) 707–708*
pain management, *(V1) 720–721*
postoperative nursing care, *(V1) 943–944*
pregnancy, *(ESG9) 12*
preoperative, *(V1) 940*
of preschooler, *(ESG9) 23–24*
professional standards defining, *(V1) 40b*
professional standards organizations defining, *(V1) 39*
psychosocial, *(V1) 192–193*
of pulse, *(V1) 318–321*
relating to other phases of, *(V1) 38*
of respiration, *(V1) 324–326*
risk for falls, *(V1) 438*
self-concept and self-esteem, *(V1) 193*
sensory perception, *(V1) 689–690*
sexual health, *(V1) 781*
skin, *(V1) 448–449, (V1) 823, (V1) 825*
sleep patterns, *(V1) 804*
spiritual, *(V1) 256*
techniques for physical, *(V1) 44–45*
temperature, *(V1) 310–314*
of toddler, *(ESG9) 21*
tools for recording data, *(V1) 52*
types of, *(V1) 42–44*
urinary elimination, *(V1) 626*
validation of data, *(V1) 49–50*
wounds, *(V1) 825–826, (V1) 829*
of young adult, *(ESG9) 32*
critical thinking, *(V1) 33*
as cyclical process, *(V1) 33*
definition of, *(V1) 31*
diagnosis
    of abnormal pulse, *(V1) 321*
    activity and exercise, *(V1) 747*
    analyzing and interpreting data, *(V1) 63–65*
    of anxiety, *(V1) 203*
    bowel incontinence, *(V1) 674*

bowel-related problems, *(V1) 664*
choosing label, *(V1) 72–73*
circulation problems, *(V1) 872*
collaborative problems, *(V1) 76*
community-based, *(V1) 1029*
components of NANDA nursing diagnosis, *(V1) 71–72*
critiquing diagnostic reasoning process, *(V1) 70b*
cultural factors as etiology, *(V1) 239–240*
deficient knowledge, *(V1) 538*
definition of, *(V1) 56–57*
diagnostic reasoning, *(V1) 63–69*
diagnostic statements, *(V1) 74t, (V1) 77–79*
disturbed energy field, *(V1) 1001*
for dying and grieving, *(V1) 276–277*
eyes, *(V1) 466*
for family health status, *(V1) 218*
feet problems, *(V1) 456*
fluid, electrolyte and acid-base imbalance, *(V1) 903*
formats for diagnostic statements, *(V1) 73, (V1) 75–76*
growth and development problems, *(ESG9) 39*
of health, *(V1) 182*
home health care visit, *(V1) 1039–1040*
hypertension, *(V1) 334*
for hypotension, *(V1) 334*
for hypothermia, *(V1) 316*
of infection, *(V1) 407*
intraoperative, *(V1) 940*
knowledge map of, *(V2) 43*
medication-related, *(V1) 496*
nails, *(V1) 458*
NANDA Nursing taxonomy of diagnostic terminology, *(V1) 71*
nutrition-related problems, *(V1) 606*
oral cavity/mouth, *(V1) 461*
origins of, *(V1) 58–59*
overview of, *(V2) 33*
overweight and obesity, *(V1) 609–610*
pain, *(V1) 708, (V1) 721*
postoperative problems, *(V1) 944*
for preoperative client, *(V1) 930–931*
professional standards for, *(V1) 57b*
psychosocial, *(V1) 193–195*
recognizing health problems, *(V1) 59–61*
relating to outcome and intervention, *(V1) 77*
risk for falls, *(V1) 439*
self-care deficit, *(V1) 445*
self-concept, *(V1) 195–196*
sensory-perceptual problems, *(V1) 691–692*
sexual problems, *(V1) 782–783*
of skin breakdown, *(V1) 831*
of skin problems, *(V1) 449, (V1) 831*
sleep pattern disturbance, *(V1) 804–805*
spiritual, *(V1) 256*
stress-related, *(V1) 566–567, (V1) 566b*
stress urinary incontinence, *(V1) 627*
for temperature/fever, *(V1) 315*
terminology for, *(V1) 57, (V1) 58t*
types of, *(V1) 61–63*
for underweight and malnutrition, *(V1) 611*
urinary elimination problems, *(V1) 635*
wellness, *(V1) 1013–1015*

evaluation
    of anxiety, *(V1) 203*
    bowel incontinence, *(V1) 675*
    bowel-related problems, *(V1) 665*
    for communication problems, *(V1) 349*
    for dying and grieving, *(V1) 277*
    for family health status diagnoses, *(V1) 218*
    as final step, *(V1) 128*
    full-spectrum nursing and, *(V1) 128–129*
    of health, *(V1) 182*
    for home health care diagnoses, *(V1) 1040*
    of hypertension, *(V1) 334–335*
    for hypotension, *(V1) 334*
    for hypothermia, *(V1) 316*
    intraoperative phase, *(V1) 940*
    knowledge map of, *(V2) 72*
    model of, *(V1) 121f*
    nutrition-related problems, *(V1) 606–607*
    overview of, *(V2) 62*
    oxygenation, *(V1) 873*
    pain management, *(V1) 720*
    of patient progress, *(V1) 132–135*
    recording evaluative statement, *(V1) 133–134*
    reflecting critically about, *(V1) 136*
    relating to other phases of nursing process, *(V1) 132*
    sleep pattern disturbance, *(V1) 805*
    for spirituality diagnoses, *(V1) 258*
    stress-related problems, *(V1) 607*
    stress urinary incontinence, *(V1) 630*
    for temperature/fever diagnoses, *(V1) 315*
    types of, *(V1) 130–131*
    for underweight and malnutrition, *(V1) 611*
    urinary elimination, *(V1) 638*
    using standards and criteria in, *(V1) 129–130*
    for weight control, *(V1) 610*
focus of, *(V2) 20*
full-spectrum nursing and, *(V1) 33, (V1) 34–36*
implementation
    knowledge map of, *(V2) 72*
    overview of, *(V2) 62*
for minimizing malpractice, *(V1) 1083*
model of, *(V1) 31f,*
phases of, *(V1) 31f, (V1) 32f, (V2) 11*
planning interventions/implementations
    for abnormal pulse, *(V1) 321*
    as action phase, *(V1) 121*
    activity and exercise, *(V1) 747*
    of adolescence health, *(ESG9) 29–31*
    for anxiety, *(V1) 258–259*
    bowel incontinence, *(V1) 674–675*
    bowel-related problems, *(V1) 665*
    carbon monoxide poisoning, *(V1) 425*
    child health, *(ESG9) 26*
    for communication problems, *(V1) 349*
    computer-generated, *(V1) 113*
    cultural sensitivity in, *(V1) 240–241*
    disturbed energy field, *(V1) 1001–1002*
    documentation of, *(V1) 128*
    doing or delegating, *(V1) 125–128*
    for dying and grieving, *(V1) 277*
    for elderly, *(ESG9) 38*
    electrical storm, *(V1) 431*

Nursing process (continued)
  equipment-related accident, (V1) 433
  eye care, (V1) 466
  falls, (V1) 425–426, (V1) 432–433,
    (V1) 433f
  for family health status diagnoses,
    (V1) 218–219
  feet problems, (V1) 456
  fire and electrical hazards,
    (V1) 433–434
  firearm safety, (V1) 426–427
  food poisoning, (V1) 429
  growth and development problems,
    (ESG9) 39–40
  guide in selecting, (V1) 106
  of health care, (V1) 182
  for health care, (V1) 182
  health promotion, (V1) 1016
  for home health care diagnoses,
    (V1) 1041
  for hypertension, (V1) 335
  for hypotension, (V1) 334
  for hypothermia, (V1) 316
  individualizing standardized, (V1) 112
  for infant health, (ESG9) 18
  for infection, (V1) 408
  injury from fires, (V1) 425–426
  for integumentary problems, (V1) 450
  for intraoperative phase, (V1) 941
  medication-related, (V1) 496
  mercury poisoning, (V1) 436
  of middle adult health, (ESG9) 34
  model of, (V1) 105f, (V1) 121f
  motor vehicle accidents, (V1) 428–429
  nail care, (V1) 458
  neonate transitioning, (ESG9) 16
  Nursing Intervention Classification
    (NIC), (V1) 113–114
  nursing interview, (V1) 100–102
  nursing orders, (V1) 116–118
  nutrition-related problems, (V1) 607
  oral cavity/mouth, (V1) 461
  overview of, (V2) 53, (V2) 61
  oxygenation, (V1) 873–876
  for pain relief, (V1) 709
  perioperative care, (V1) 931
  poisoning, (V1) 422–424
  postoperative, (V1) 948
  prenatal care, (ESG9) 12–13
  preparation for, (V1) 121–123, (V1) 125
  problem status influencing, (V1) 109
  process for generating and selecting,
    (V1) 109–112
  professional standards for, (V1) 107b,
    (V1) 122b
  reducing pollution, (V1) 430–431
  reflecting critically about, (V1) 118,
    (V1) 128
  relating to other phases of nursing
    process, (V1) 121
  research influencing choice of,
    (V1) 106–108
  scalds and burns, (V1) 425
  for self-care deficit, (V1) 446
  sensory-perceptual problems, (V1) 692
  sleep pattern disturbance, (V1) 805
  for spirituality diagnoses, (V1) 258
  standardized language for home health
    and community care, (V1) 114–116
  stress-related, (V1) 567
  stress urinary incontinence,
    (V1) 628–630

  suffocation and asphyxiation, (V1) 427
  for temperature/fever diagnoses,
    (V1) 315
  theory influencing choice of, (V1) 106
  for toddler health, (ESG9) 21
  types of, (V1) 105–106
  for underweight and malnutrition,
    (V1) 611
  using restraints safely, (V1) 434–436
  using standardized language for,
    (V1) 113
  vector-borne pathogen, (V1) 429–430
  water-borne pathogen, (V1) 430
  for weight control, (V1) 610
  planning outcomes
    activity and exercise, (V1) 747
    of anxiety, (V1) 203
    bowel-related problems, (V1) 665
    client safety, (V1) 439
    for communication problems, (V1) 349
    community-based diagnosis, (V1) 1031
    comparing long-term and short-term,
      (V1) 93, (V1) 94t
    comparing nursing diagnosis and goals,
      (V1) 94–97, (V1) 95t
    components of goal statement,
      (V1) 93–94
    components of nursing care plan,
      (V1) 86f
    comprehensive nursing care plan,
      (V1) 85–89
    computerized care plan, (V1) 91
    cultural sensitivity in, (V1) 240
    deriving goals and interventions from
      diagnosis, (V1) 95t
    disturbed energy field, (V1) 1001
    for dying and grieving, (V1) 277
    expected outcome for problem types,
      (V1) 96t
    for family health status diagnoses,
      (V1) 218
    feet problems, (V1) 456
    fluid, electrolyte and acid-base imbal-
      ance, (V1) 903
    growth and development, (ESG9) 39
    of health, (V1) 182
    health promotion, (V1) 1015
    for home health care diagnoses,
      (V1) 1040–1041
    for hypertension, (V1) 334–335
    for hypotension, (V1) 334
    for hypothermia, (V1) 316
    individualized care plan, (V1) 89,
      (V1) 91
    of infection, (V1) 407–408
    for integumentary problems, (V1) 449
    knowledge map of, (V2) 52
    for learning, (V1) 538–540
    medication-related, (V1) 496
    nail care, (V1) 458
  Nursing Outcomes Classification
    (NOC), (V1) 97–99
  nutrition-related problems, (V1)
    606–607
  oral cavity/mouth, (V1) 461
  overview of, (V2) 43, (V2) 44
  oxygenation, (V1) 873
  for pain relief, (V1) 709, (V1) 721
  Patient Care Protocol, (V1) 87f
  patient goals/outcomes, (V1) 92
  postoperative problems, (V1) 944,
    (V1) 948

  preoperative phase, (V1) 931
  professional standards for, 83b
  psychosocial, (V1) 196
  for pulse, (V1) 321
  purpose of goal statement, (V1) 93
  reflecting critically about expected
    outcomes/goals, (V1) 100–102
  self-care deficit, (V1) 446
  self-concept and self-esteem, (V1) 196
  sensory function, (V1) 466
  sexual problems, (V1) 783
  sleep promotion, (V1) 805
  special discharge or teaching plan,
    (V1) 91
  for special teaching plan, (V1) 100
  for spirituality diagnoses, (V1) 258
  standardized care plan, (V1) 88f,
    (V1) 89
  stress-related problems, (V1) 567
  student care plan, (V1) 91
  for temperature/fever diagnoses,
    (V1) 315
  types of planning, (V1) 82–85
  for underweight and malnutrition,
    (V1) 611
  urinary elimination, (V1) 638
  for weight control, (V1) 610
  writing goals for groups, (V1) 99
  writing goals for wellness diagnosis,
    (V1) 100
  writing individualized care plan,
    (V1) 92
  to promote health, (V1) 181–182
  purpose of, (V1) 32
  strategies for culturally competent care,
    (V1) 242t
  as systemic problem-solving process,
    (V2) 11
  thinking critically about, (V2) 11,
    (V2) 19
  for underweight and malnutrition,
    (V1) 611
  for urinary elimination, (V1) 639
Nursing research
  analyzing, (V1) 159
  Conduct and Utilization of Research
    in Nursing project (CURN),
    (V1) 156
  definition of, (V1) 154
  development of priorities for, (V1)
    154–155
  education for, (V1) 155
  finding articles, (V1) 161
  history of, (V1) 154
  online sources for, (V1) 982–983
  problem areas for, (V1) 158–159
  process of, (V1) 157
  utilization of, (V1) 161
Nursing science, doctor of, (V1) 15
Nursing-sensitive outcome, (V1) 92
The Nursing Strategy for Canada,
  (ESGV1) 24
Nursing telepractice, (ESGV1) 12
Nursing theory
  components of, (V1) 144f
  concepts of, (V1) 144
  importance of, (V1) 139
  knowledge map of, (V2) 81
  overview of, (V2) 73
Nurture
  definition of, (V1) 165
  nature versus, (ESG9) 2–3

Nutrient
  carbohydrates, *(V1) 577*, *(V1) 577f*
  energy, *(V1) 575*, *(V1) 576t*
  fetus and, *(ESG9) 9*
  lipid, *(V1) 579–581*
  micronutrient, *(V1) 579–581*
  protein, *(V1) 577–579*
  supplementation, *(V1) 607*
  water as essential, *(V1) 582*
Nutrition
  assessment of, *(V1) 602*, *(V1) 612*
  bowel function and, *(V1) 655–656*
  Canada's Food Guide for Healthy Eating,
    (V1) 587, *(V1) 588f*
  daily food requirement for elderly,
    (V1) 597t
  defecation and, *(V1) 666*
  definition of, *(V1) 575*
  developmental stage and, *(V1) 594–597*
  diagnostic testing for, *(V1) 604–605*
  dietary guidelines for Americans, *(V1)*
    587b
  Dietary Reference Intake (DRI), *(V1) 582*,
    (V1) 586
  dieting for weight loss, *(V1) 599*
  disease and, *(V1) 599*
  eating disorder, warning signs of,
    (V1) 596b
  energy balance, *(V1) 591–592*
  enteral, *(V1) 613–616*
  as factor for oral problems, *(V1) 459*
  functional limitation affecting,
    (V1) 599–600
  as health factor, *(V1) 174*
  health promotion and, *(V1) 1016*
  impaired status, *(V2) 584*
  importance of, *(V1) 567–568*
  on limited budget, *(V1) 608*
  minerals: DRI, *(V1) 585t–586t*
  mobility and activity, *(V1) 735*
  NOC outcomes and NIC interventions,
    (V2) 588
  overview of, *(V2) 557*
  oxygenation and, *(V1) 857*
  parenteral, *(V1) 616–617*
  physical examination for status,
    (V2) 586–587
  poorly fitted or loose dentures, *(V1) 459*
  during pregnancy and lactation, *(V1)*
    597–598
  prenatal care and, *(ESG9) 12–13*
  problem assessment, *(V2) 584–585*
  as problem or etiology, *(V1) 606*
  promoting host defense of infection,
    (V1) 404–405
  promoting normal urination, *(V1) 639*
  serving sizes, *(V1) 591f*
  skin and, *(V1) 447*, *(V1) 813*, *(V1) 814*,
    (V1) 832
  sources of information on, *(V1) 582*
  special needs, *(V1) 608–609*
  supplementation, *(V1) 607*
  surgery preparation, *(V1) 932–933*
  urination and, *(V1) 623–624*
  USDA Food Guide Pyramid, *(V1) 587*,
    (V1) 589f
  vegetarian diet pyramid, *(V1) 591t*
  vitamins: DRI, *(V1) 583t–584t*
Nutritional assessment, *(V1) 43*, *(V1) 1013*,
  (V2) 583–585
Nutritional disorder, *(V1) 926b*
Nutritional supplements, *(V1) 46*

Nutrition Facts panel, *(V1) 591*, *(V1) 592f*
Nutritive enema, *(V1) 669*

O
OASIS, *(V1) 299*, *(V2) 178*
OASIS data set, *(V1) 1043*
Obesity
  in adolescence, *(ESG9) 29*
  atherosclerosis, *(V1) 857*
  blood pressure and, *(V1) 329*
  BMI of, *(V1) 609*
  hypertension, *(V1) 857*
  NOC outcomes and NIC interventions,
    (V2) 589
  oxygenation and, *(V1) 857*
  skin and, *(V1) 812*
  in young adult, *(ESG9) 32*
Object, classification of, *(V1) 70*
Objective cue, *(V1) 75*
Objective data, *(V1) 42t*
  definition of, *(V2) 20*
  of nail care, *(V1) 458*
  of skin assessment, *(V1) 448–449*
Objectivity, *(V1) 156*
Oblique position, *(V1) 752*, *(V1) 752f*
Observation
  of body language, *(V1) 350–351*
  definition of, *(V1) 44*
  mnemonic for, *(V1) 45b*
Observation intervention, *(V1) 109*
Obstruction, *(V1) 636*
Obstructive sleep apnea (OSA), *(V1) 802*
Occult blood, testing stool, *(V2) 640p–643p*
Occupational health nursing, *(ESGV1) 20*,
  (V1) 1027
Occupational Safety and Health
  Administration
  needleless system, *(V1) 907*
  personal protective equipment,
    (V1) 410
  preventing needlestick injury, *(V1) 437*
  recapping needles, *(V1) 511*
Occurrence report
  as agency report, *(V1) 298*
  events requiring, *(V1) 298b*
Occurrence-type insurance, *(V1) 1089*
Office of Minority Health (OMH), *(V1) 244*
Official name, *(V1) 474*
Oil, *(V1) 579*
Oil-retention enema, *(V1) 668*, *(V2) 663tb*
Olfaction, *(V1) 363*
Olfactory deficit
  intervention for, *(V1) 695–696*
  safety and health measures, *(V1) 696*
Oliguria, *(V1) 633b*
Omaha System, *(V1) 71*, *(V1) 113*
  family and community outcomes, *(V1) 99*
  for home health and community care,
    (V1) 115
  intervention categories and targets,
    (V2) 994
  problem labels for, *(V2) 991*
  problem rating scale, *(V2) 992*
  vocabulary
    for intervention, *(V2) 53*
    for outcome, *(V2) 44*
  writing aggregate goals, *(V2) 992*
Omega-3 fatty acid (alpha-linoleic),
  (V1) 580
Omega-6 fatty acid (linoleic), *(V1) 580*
Omnibus legislation, *(ESGV1) 9*
One-bottle system, *(V1) 881*, *(V1) 881f*

One Flew Over the Cuckoo's Nest, *(V1) 7*
One-on-one instruction, *(V1) 544*
Ongoing assessment, *(V1) 42*, *(V1) 359*
  content and methods of, *(V1) 45f*
  continued focus on care, *(V1) 84*
Ongoing evaluation, *(V1) 131*
Ongoing group, *(V1) 347*
Ongoing planning, *(V1) 83–84*
Onset of action, *(V1) 485–487*
Onychomycosis, *(V1) 369*
Open-ended questions, *(V1) 47t*
Open system, *(V1) 152*, *(V1) 615*
Open wound, *(V1) 814*
Operative field, creating, *(V2) 927tb*
Operative suite, transfer to, *(V1) 936*
Ophthalmic medication
  administration of, *(V1) 522p*, *(V2)*
    459p–462p
  overview of, *(V1) 503*
Opioid analgesic
  acupuncture and, *(V1) 994*
  administration of, *(V1) 714–716*
  equianalgesic doses of, *(V1) 717t*
  increasing surgical risk, *(V1) 926b*
  oxygenation and, *(V1) 858*
  as preoperative medication, *(V1) 935t*
  sexual function and, *(V1) 774t*
  side effects of, *(V1) 713–716*, *(V1) 714b*
Opposition
  assessment of, *(V2) 305p–306p*
  as movement, *(V1) 727f*
Oral administration, opioids, *(V1) 714*
Oral cavity
  abnormal findings of, *(V1) 375*
  assessment of, *(V1) 394p*, *(V1) 461*,
    (V2) 433
  defense against infection, *(V1) 402*
  problems of, *(V1) 460–461*
  risk factors for problems, *(V1) 459–460*
  self-care deficit, *(V1) 461*
  structures of, *(V1) 459–460*
  teeth development, *(V1) 459*, *(V1) 459f*
  treatment of poisoning by, *(V1) 424*
  vocalization, *(V1) 375*
Oral communication, *(V1) 289*
Oral-genital stimulation, *(V1) 777*
Oral hygiene, *(V1) 459*
Oral malignancy, *(V1) 460–461*
Oral medication
  administration of, *(V1) 522p*, *(V2)*
    454p–458p
  overview of, *(V1) 499–502*
Oral mucosa, *(V1) 459*
Oral reporting, *(V1) 299*, *(V2) 182tb*
Oral sex
  in adolescence, *(V1) 769*
  reasons for, *(V1) 777*
Oral stage, *(ESG9) 17*
Oral temperature, *(V1) 313*, *(V2) 199p*
Order
  physician, *(V1) 302–303*
  telephone and verbal, *(V1) 300–301*,
    (V2) 183
Orem's Self-Care Model, *(V1) 51b*
Organization
  of data, *(V1) 50*
  for nursing, *(V1) 17–18*
  preparing supplies and equipment, *(V1) 123*
  specialty, *(V1) 17–18*
  time-sequenced work plan, *(V1) 123*
Organ/tissue donation, *(V1) 275–276*
Organ/tissue donor card, *(V1) 275f*

Orgasm
    aging and, (V1) 775b
    as sexual response, (V1) 776
    sexual response cycle of, (V1) 774f
Orgasmic disorder, (V1) 780–781
Oropharyngeal airway
    example of, (V1) 878f
    insertion of, (V2) 862tb
    suctioning of, (V1) 879–880, (V2)
        831p–834p
    use of, (V1) 878
Oropharynx
    abnormalities of, (V2) 334
    assessment of, (V1) 394, (V2) 268p–271p
    structures of, (V1) 375
Orotracheal tube
    endotracheal airways and, (V1) 878
    placement of, (V1) 878f
    suctioning of, (V1) 880, (V2) 835p–839p
Orthodox Jews, (V1) 251
Orthopnea, (V1) 325, (V1) 863
Orthopneic position, (V1) 752, (V1) 752f
Orthostatic hypotension, (V1) 333, (V1) 739
Osmol, (V1) 889
Osmolality, (V1) 889
Osmosis, (V1) 889, (V1) 889f, (V1) 890t
Osmotic pressure, (V1) 890
Ossicles, (V1) 372
Osteoarthritis (OA), (V1) 737
Osteoblast, (V1) 726
Osteoclast, (V1) 726
Osteogenesis imperfecta (OA), (V1) 737
Osteomyelitis, (V1) 738
Osteopath (DO), (V1) 999
Osteopathy, (V1) 999
Osteoporosis
    bone integrity and, (V1) 738
    changing chest size and shape, (V1) 378,
        (V2) 281p
    overview of, (ESG9) 37
    statistics of, (V1) 894
Ostomy
    bowel diversion, (V1) 657
    dietary changes with, (V1) 677b
    living with, (V1) 672
    urinary diversion, (V1) 638
Ostomy appliance, (V1) 663p, (V2) 654p–658p
Otic irrigation, (V1) 695, (V2) 676p–678p
Otic medication
    administration of, (V1) 522p,
        (V2) 463p–464p
    overview of, (V1) 503–504
Otitis externa, (V1) 373
Otitis media, (V1) 373
Otoscope, (V1) 372
Outcome
    achieving, (V1) 33
    of anxiety, (V1) 203
    bowel-related problems, (V1) 665,
        (V2) 669–670
    for communication problems, (V1) 349
    comparing long-term and short-term, (V1)
        93, (V1) 94t
    components of nursing care plan,
        (V1) 86f
    comprehensive nursing care plan,
        (V1) 85–89
    computerized care plan, (V1) 91
    critical pathways for, (V1) 89
    cultural sensitivity in, (V1) 240
    definition of, (V1) 92–93
    desired, (V1) 92, (V1) 94–95

disturbed energy field, (V1) 1001
energy maintenance and mobility,
    (V2) 724
for family health status diagnoses,
    (V1) 218
for fluid and electrolyte diagnoses,
    (V2) 909–911
of health, (V1) 182
health beliefs and, (V1) 1012–1013
for health knowledge, (V2) 537
for home health care diagnoses, (V1)
    1040–1041
hypotension, (V1) 334
impaired verbal communication, (V2) 227
individualized care plan, (V1) 89, (V1) 91
of infection, (V1) 407–408
for intraoperative phase, (V2) 932–934
knowledge map of, (V2) 52
for learning, (V1) 538–540
loss and grieving, (V2) 173–174
medication-related, (V2) 524–525
NOC linking to NANDA diagnosis,
    (V1) 97, (V1) 97b
Nursing Outcomes Classification (NOC),
    (V1) 97–99
nutrition-related problems, (V2) 588
Omaha System problem rating scale,
    (V2) 992
overview of, (V2) 44
for oxygenation diagnoses, (V2) 869
for pain diagnoses, (V2) 695
pain relief, (V1) 721
Patient Care Protocol, (V1) 87f
planning, (V1) 32, (V1) 32f, (V1) 35
for postoperative diagnoses, (V2) 935–938
for preoperative diagnoses, (V2) 930–931
preoperative phase, (V1) 931
for problem types, (V1) 96t
professional standards for, (V1) 83b
psychosocial, (V1) 196
reflecting critically about, (V1) 100–102
relating to intervention, (V1) 77, (V1) 135
review of, (V1) 132, (V1) 136
safety problems, (V2) 381–382
self-care deficit, (V2) 434
self-concept
    self-esteem and, (V1) 196
    standardized and individualized,
        (V2) 112
sensory-perceptual problems, (V2) 682
sexual problems, (V1) 783, (V2) 737
for skin and wound diagnoses,
    (V2) 795–796
sleep diagnoses, (V2) 752
special discharge, (V1) 91
for special teaching plan, (V1) 91,
    (V1) 100
for spirituality diagnoses, (V1) 258
standardized care plan, (V1) 88f, (V1) 89
stress-related problems, (V1) 553,
    (V1) 567, (V2) 554
student care plan, (V1) 91
for temperature/fever diagnoses, (V1) 315
types of, (V1) 82–85, (V1) 92
using standardized terminology for,
    (V1) 97
vital signs, abnormal, (V2) 218
Outcome and Assessment Information Set
    (OASIS), (V1) 299, (V2) 178
Outcome label
    as component of NOC outcome, (V1) 97
    family health, (V2) 126

Outcomes evaluation, (V1) 131
Outcome statement
    activity and exercise, (V1) 747
    for aggregates, (V1) 1031
    for client safety, (V1) 439
    on family health
    for feet problems, (V1) 456
    fluid and electrolyte balance, (V1) 903
    growth and development problems,
        (ESG9) 39
    health promotion, (V1) 1015
    for hypothermia, (V1) 316
    for integumentary problems, (V1) 449
    for intraoperative phase, (V1) 941
    medication-related, (V1) 496
    nail care, (V1) 458
    normal bowel patterns, (V1) 665
    nutrition-related problems, (V1) 606–607
    for oral cavity/mouth problems, (V1) 461
    pain relief, (V1) 709
    for psychosocial diagnosis, (V1) 203
    for pulse status, (V1) 321
    reflecting cultural sensitivity, (V1) 240
    for self-care deficit, (V1) 446
    for sensory perception, (V1) 692
    skin integrity and wound healing,
        (V1) 831
    sleep promotion, (V1) 805
    stress-related problems, (V1) 567
    for underweight and malnutrition,
        (V1) 611
    for urinary elimination, (V1) 638
    for weight control, (V1) 610
Output, (V1) 152
Ova, (V1) 764
Overhydration, (V1) 896
Over-the-counter (OTC) drug, (V1) 474
Over-the-counter remedy, (V1) 231
Over-the-needle catheter, (V1) 906, (V1) 906f
Overweight, (V1) 609
    NOC outcomes and NIC interventions,
        (V2) 589
    oxygenation and, (V1) 857
    skin and, (V1) 812
Ovo-lacto vegetarian, (V1) 598
Ovulation, (V1) 764
Oxygen (O$_2$)
    cannula, face mask or face tent adminis-
        tration of, (V2) 819p–822p
    change in concentration, (V1) 322
    concentrator, (V1) 876
    delivery methods, (V2) 823–825
    demand for, illness, (V1) 861
    diffusion of, (V1) 850
    flow meter, (V1) 877
    hazards of, (V1) 877
    measurement of, (V1) 326
    supplying therapy, (V1) 876–877
    therapy safety precautions, (V2) 862tb
    transportation of, (V1) 853
Oxygenation
    anemia and carbon monoxide, (V1) 861
    arterial blood gas (ABG) and, (V2) 866
    assessment of, (V1) 305, (V1) 862
    clinical signs of, (V1) 326
    definition of, (V1) 848
    diagnostic testing for, (V1) 868–869
    factors influencing, (V1) 854–859
    outcomes and interventions for diagnoses,
        (V2) 869
    overview of, (V2) 798
    questions for risk assessment, (V2) 864

testing for, *(V2) 865*
tracheostomy care, *(V2) 825p–830p*
Oxygen saturation, *(V1) 326*
Oxygen tank, *(V1) 876, (V1) 876f*

P

Pacing, in communication, *(V1) 341*
Packaged bath, *(V1) 452–453,*
    (V2) 397p–398p
Paeu d'orange, *(V2) 276*
Paget's disease, *(V1) 737*
Pain
    adaptation failure and, *(V1) 563*
    affecting self-care ability, *(V1) 443*
    assessment of, *(V1) 43, (V1) 239,*
        (V1) 707, (V1) 707b
    association of nurse with, *(V1) 7*
    blood pressure and, *(V1) 329*
    care map for, *(V1) 722*
    cause of, *(V1) 700*
    chemical relief, *(V1) 716–717*
    definition of, *(V1) 699*
    in differing languages, *(V1) 705b*
    disrupting health, *(V1) 177*
    documentation of, *(V1) 720*
    duration of, *(V1) 700*
    factors influencing, *(V1) 703–705*
    history of, *(V2) 692*
    holistic comfort, *(V1) 145*
    from loss or grieving, *(V1) 265*
    misconceptions about, *(V1) 718, (V1) 718t*
    modulation of, *(V1) 702–703*
    nonpharmacological relief, *(V1) 709–711*
    nonverbal signs of, *(V1) 705, (V1)*
        707–708, (V2) 692
    nursing care for, *(V1) 720–721*
    origin of, *(V1) 699–700*
    outcomes and interventions for, *(V2) 695*
    perception of, *(V1) 702*
    pharmacokinetics and, *(V1) 488*
    pharmacological relief
        nonopioid analgesics, *(V1) 712–713*
        opioid analgesics, *(V1) 713–716*
    proposed vital sign (VS), *(V1) 305*
    quality of, *(V1) 701*
    reaction to, *(V1) 705, (V1) 706b*
    reflex response to stressor, *(V1) 557*
    relief with placebo, *(V1) 719–720*
    respiration and, *(V1) 323*
    scales for, *(V2) 692–693*
    sleep and, *(V1) 803*
    surgical interruption for, *(V1) 718*
    threshold, *(V1) 702*
    tolerance of, *(V1) 702*
    transduction of, *(V1) 701*
    transmission of, *(V1) 701–702*
    types of, *(V1) 700f*
Pain fiber, *(V1) 702, (V1) 702f*
Pain management
    delegation of, *(V1) 709b*
    in elderly, *(V1) 719*
    overview of, *(V2) 684*
Pain scale, *(V1) 708, (V2) 692–693*
Palate, hard and soft, *(V1) 375*
Palliative care, *(V1) 272*
Palliative effect, *(V1) 488*
Palliative surgery, *(V1) 924*
Pallor, *(V1) 321, (V1) 367t, (V1) 448*
Palmar grasp reflex, *(ESG9) 14f*
Palpation
    of abdomen, *(V1) 384*
    of client for physical examination, *(V1) 360*

for physical assessment, *(V2) 230t*
physical assessment technique, *(V1) 45*
pulse rate assessment, *(V1) 318*
using with auscultation, *(V1) 333*
Panic anxiety, *(V1) 200*
Paper thermometer, *(V1) 312f*
Papule, *(V2) 244*
Paradigm, *(V1) 142*
Paradoxical sleep, *(V1) 798*
Paralytic ileus, *(V1) 656*
Paranasal sinuses, *(V1) 374f*
Paraplegia, *(V1) 740b*
Parasomnia, *(V1) 801–803*
Parenteral medication
    administration of, *(V1) 505*
    delegation of, *(V2) 475, (V2) 479*
    injection, administering, *(V1) 511–512*
    needles and syringes for, *(V1) 507–509,*
        (V1) 507f
    types of, *(V1) 506*
Parenteral nutrition
    definition of, *(V1) 616–617*
    monitoring patient receiving, *(V2) 582tb*
    subclavian vein as site for, *(V1) 616f*
Parent-infant attachment, *(ESG9) 16*
Paresis, *(V1) 740b*
Paresthesia, *(V1) 740b*
Parish nursing, *(V1) 1027–1028*
Paronychia, *(V1) 370, (V2) 334*
Parotitis, *(V1) 375*
Paroxysmal nocturnal dyspnea (PND),
    (V1) 863
Partial bath, *(V1) 450*
Partial parenteral nutrition, *(V1) 616*
Partial pressure of carbon dioxide (PCO_2),
    (V1) 869
Partial pressure of oxygen (PO_2), *(V1) 869*
Partial pressure of oxygen in arterial blood
    (PaO_2), *(V1) 322*
Partial-thickness wound, *(V1) 816*
Participant, rights in research study, *(V1) 158*
Participative leadership, *(V1) 954*
Passive approach to resistance, *(V1) 964*
Passive euthanasia, *(V1) 275*
Passive immunity, *(V1) 403f*
Passive range of motion (PROM), *(V1) 385,*
    (V1) 757
Passive relaxation, *(V1) 570*
Passive resistance, *(V1) 964*
Passive transport system, *(V1) 889*
Passwords, EHR ethics and, *(V1) 980*
Paternalism, *(V1) 1055*
Pathogen
    bloodborne, *(V1) 416–417*
    as cause of disease, *(V1) 399*
    definition of, *(V1) 429*
    food-borne, *(V1) 429*
    vector-borne, *(V1) 429–430*
    water-borne, *(V1) 430*
Pathophysiology, *(V1) 59*
Patient
    activity, feedback from, *(V1) 123*
    admitting to nursing unit, *(V1) 185p,*
        (V2) 98p
    assessment of vital signs (VS), *(V1) 305*
    barriers to therapeutic communication,
        (V1) 351–354
    bias and stereotyping of, *(V1) 69*
    bowel diversion, care for, *(V1) 671–672*
    care summary, *(V1) 297*
    conclusions about health status,
        (V1) 65–66

death of, *(V1) 269*
dying, care for, *(V1) 283–284*
end-of-life care, *(V1) 271–273*
enhancing therapeutic communication,
    (V1) 349–351
environment of, *(V1) 469–470*
evaluation of progress, *(V1) 132*
improving appetite of, *(V1) 612–613*
individual differences of, *(V1) 33*
indwelling catheter, care for, *(V1) 644f*
meals, assisting with, *(V1) 609*
misidentification of, *(V1) 935*
planning goals/outcome
    comparing long-term and short-term,
        (V1) 93, (V1) 94t
    components of statement, *(V1) 93–94*
    definition of, *(V1) 92–93*
    essential versus nonessential,
        (V1) 95–96
    expected outcome for problem types,
        (V1) 96t
    formulation of, *(V1) 92*
    purpose of statement, *(V1) 93*
    relating to nursing diagnosis,
        (V1) 94–95, (V1) 95t
praying with, *(V2) 154tb–155tb*
preparing for nursing interview, *(V1) 48*
pressure ulcer prevention, teaching,
    (V1) 833
refusal of medication, *(V1) 296*
responsibility of taking medication,
    (V1) 294
safety of, *(V1) 432b, (V1) 434, (V1) 1086*
stages of dying, *(V1) 270–271*
steering committee for safety of, *(ESGV1)*
    25–26
surgery, preparing room after, *(V2) 927tb*
teaching about pain, *(V1) 720*
teaching about vital signs (VS), *(V1) 336*
urinary diversion, care for, *(V1) 649*
viewing problems with, *(V1) 66*
Patient's Bill of Rights, *(V1) 21, 529, (V1)*
    1061, (V1) 1072
Patient advocacy, *(V1) 1068–1069*
Patient benefit model, *(V1) 1068*
Patient Care Partnership, *(V1) 529, (V1)*
    1061–1062, (V1) 1061b, (V1) 1077
Patient care plan, *(V1) 85*
Patient-controlled analgesia pump
    connection of, *(V1) 716, (V2) 688p–691p*
    for opioids, *(V1) 715*
Patient database, *(V1) 42*
Patient Self-Determination Act (PSDA),
    (V1) 273, (V1) 1073
Patient situation, *(V1) 34–36*
Pattern, growth and development, *(V1) 166,*
    (ESG9) 3
Peak action, of drug, *(V1) 485–487*
Peak expiratory flow rate (PEFR), *(V1) 869,*
    (V1) 870f
Peak flow, monitoring, *(V1) 869*
Peak flow meter, *(V1) 870f*
Peak level, of drug, *(V1) 486*
Pedal pulse, *(V1) 319*
Pediatric dosage, *(V2) 521–522*
Pediculosis (lice), *(V1) 369, (V2) 334*
Peer review, *(V1) 982*
Peers
    importance to child, *(ESG9) 25*
    self-concept and, *(V1) 190*
Pelvic floor muscle exercise (PFME),
    (V1) 647

Pelvic inflammatory disease (PID)
  douching and, *(V1) 789*
  as STI, *(V1) 778*
Pender, Nola, *(V1) 145*
Pender's Health promotion model (HPM), *(V1) 1006, (V1) 1007f*
Penetrating wound, *(V1) 815t, (V1) 816*
Penicillin, injectable, *(V1) 5*
Penis
  function of, *(V1) 765*
  inflammation of (balanitis), *(V1) 780*
Penrose drain, *(V1) 835*
Peplau, Hildegard
  levels of anxiety, *(V1) 199–200*
  theory of interpersonal relations, *(V1) 146*
Pepsin, *(V1) 651*
Perceived body image, *(V1) 190*
Perceived loss, *(V1) 264*
Perception, *(V1) 681, (V1) 702f*
Percussion
  of abdomen, *(V1) 384*
  of client for physical examination, *(V1) 360, (V1) 363*
  performance of, *(V2) 815p–818p*
  for physical assessment, *(V2) 230t, (V2) 233t*
  physical assessment technique, *(V1) 45*
Percutaneous electrical stimulation (PENS), *(V1) 710*
Percutaneous gastrostomy tube (PEG)
  for enteric feedings, *(V1) 613–614*
  example of, *(V1) 614f*
Performance. *See* Role performance
Perfusion, *(V1) 848*
Pericardium, *(V1) 851*
Perineal care, *(V1) 450*
  procedure for, *(V2) 399p–402p*
  sitz bath for, *(V1) 843f*
Perineum, *(V1) 450*
Periodic table, *(V1) 70*
Periodontal disease, *(V1) 459, (V1) 460, (V1) 462*
Perioperative nursing, *(V1) 923*
Perioperative Nursing Data Set (PNDS), *(V1) 71*
Peripheral access device, *(V1) 906, (V1) 906f*
Peripheral chemoreceptor, *(V1) 322*
Peripheral edema, *(V2) 293*
Peripheral intravenous infusion
  initiation of, *(V1) 912p, (V2) 877p–881p*
  lock for, *(V1) 907*
  sites for, *(V1) 910*
  venipuncture for, *(V1) 911*
Peripheral intravenous lock, *(V1) 907f, (V1) 918*
Peripherally inserted central catheter (PICC line), *(V1) 907–908, (V1) 908f*
Peripheral nervous system, *(V1) 702, (V1) 703f*
Peripheral pulse, *(V1) 311f, (V2) 203p*
Peripheral resistence, *(V1) 328*
Peripheral vasodilation, *(V1) 307*
Peripheral vessels, *(V1) 382–383*
Peripheral vision, *(V1) 372*
Peristalsis
  esophagus and, *(V1) 651*
  high-fiber foods promoting, *(V1) 655–656*
  large intestine and, *(V1) 653*
  medication and procedures affecting, *(V1) 656–657*
  nutrition and, *(V1) 609*

Peristaltic wave, *(V2) 295*
Permanent bowel diversion, *(V1) 657*
Permanent teeth, *(V1) 459, (V1) 459f*
Permissive leadership, *(V1) 954*
Peroxidase, *(V1) 661*
PERRLA charting, *(V1) 371*
Persecution, nurses and, *(V1) 5*
Perseverance, intellectual, *(V1) 27*
Persistent vegetative state (PVS), *(V1) 270*
Person
  as concept of theory, *(V1) 144*
  responding to stressor, *(V1) 554*
  as sample in research study, *(V1) 157*
  standards of research, *(V1) 158*
Personal appearance, *(V1) 343*
Personal bias, *(V1) 28*
Personal identity
  of adolescence, *(ESG9) 27–28*
  assessment of, *(V2) 108*
  as component of self-concept, *(V1) 191–192*
  disturbed, *(V1) 195*
Personality
  age-related changes for, *(ESG9) 36t*
  sensory function and, *(V1) 683*
Personal knowledge, *(V1) 29*
Personal presence, *(V1) 153*
Personal protective equipment (PPE)
  donning and removal of, *(V1) 414, (V2) 346p–348p*
  face masks and eye shields, *(V1) 410f*
  requirements for health care workers, *(V1) 410*
Personal space
  communication and, *(V1) 343–344*
  culture care etiquette, *(V1) 242t*
  as culture specific influencing health, *(V1) 228*
Personal time inventory, *(V1) 967*
Personal values, *(V1) 227–228, (V1) 1051–1053*
Personhood, honoring, *(V1) 153*
PES format (problem, etiology, and symptom), *(V1) 75*
Petechiae, *(V1) 367t, (V2) 333*
Petrissage, *(V1) 998*
Pet therapy, *(V1) 1002*
Pew Commission, *(V1) 529*
pH
  acid-base balance, *(V1) 895*
  drug absorption, *(V1) 483–484*
  range scale, *(V1) 899f*
  of urine, *(V1) 903*
Phagocyte, *(V1) 314*
Phagocytosis, *(V1) 402, (V1) 403, (V1) 816*
Phantom pain, *(V1) 700*
Pharmacist, *(V1) 475*
Pharmacodynamics, *(V1) 488*
Pharmacokinetics
  definition of, *(V1) 478, (V1) 479f*
  factors affecting, *(V1) 487–488*
  overview of, *(V2) 438*
Pharmacological pain relief, *(V1) 712–716*
Pharmacology
  definition of, *(V1) 474*
  texts, *(V1) 475*
Pharmacopoeia, *(V1) 474, (V1) 475*
Pharynx, *(V1) 846*
Phenazopyridine hydrochloride (Pyridium), *(V1) 625*
Phenomena, *(V1) 141*
Phenylketonuria (PKU), *(ESG9) 16*

Philosophical framework, *(V1) 1057*
Philosophy
  as culture specific influencing health, *(V1) 229*
  doctor of, *(V1) 15*
Phimosis, *(V1) 780*
Phlebitis, *(V1) 916t*
Phonation, *(V1) 375*
Phosphate ($PO_4{}^-$)
  function and regulation of, *(V1) 893t*
  recommended intake of, *(V1) 894*
Phosphate system, *(V1) 895*
Phospholipid, *(V1) 579, (V1) 579b*
Photoreceptor, *(V1) 681*
Physical assessment, *(V1) 741–746*
  for biocultural variations, *(V1) 239*
  for bowel elimination, *(V1) 659*
  comprehensive, *(V1) 357, (V1) 359*
  focused, *(V1) 359*
  for infection, *(V1) 406–407*
  reflecting critically about, *(V1) 53–54*
  techniques for, *(V1) 44–45*
  of urinary system, *(V1) 626*
Physical conditioning, *(V1) 757*
Physical dependence, opioids, *(V1) 713*
Physical development
  of adolescence, *(ESG9) 27*
  of child, *(ESG9) 24*
  of elderly, *(ESG9) 35*
  of infant, *(ESG9) 16*
  of middle adult, *(ESG9) 33*
  of preschooler, *(ESG9) 21–22*
  of toddler, *(ESG9) 19*
  of young adult, *(ESG9) 31*
Physical examination
  of abdomen, *(V1) 383–384*
  of cardiovascular system
    cardiac auscultation sites, *(V1) 381f*
    cardiac cycle, *(V1) 380*
    cardiac landmarks, *(V1) 380–381*
    heart murmur, *(V1) 382*
    heart sounds, *(V1) 381–382*
    inspection and palpation of heart, *(V1) 381*
    locations for heart assessment, *(V1) 381t*
  of chest
    barrel chest, *(V1) 379f*
    imaginary lines describing locations of, *(V1) 377–378, (V1) 377f–378f*
    landmarks of, *(V1) 377, (V1) 377f–378f*
    shape and size of, *(V1) 378*
  documentation of findings, *(V1) 392–393*
  of ears
    alignment of, *(V1) 373f*
    examining external and middle, *(V1) 373*
    maintaining equilibrium, *(V1) 374*
    parts of, *(V1) 372, (V1) 373f*
  equipment needed, *(V2) 235–236*
  of eyes
    external structures of, *(V1) 370–372, (V1) 371f*
    eyelids, *(V1) 370–371*
    internal structures of, *(V1) 372*
    movement of, *(V1) 372*
    visual acuity of, *(V1) 371–372*
  of genitourinary system
    anus, rectum, and prostate, *(V1) 391f*
    female, *(V1) 390–391*

female sexual development, *(V1) 391f*
male, *(V1) 390, (V1) 390f*
of hair, *(V1) 369*
for health promotion, *(V1) 1009*
of mouth and oropharynx
abnormal findings of, *(V1) 375*
structures of, *(V1) 374–375, (V1) 374f*
vocalization, *(V1) 375*
of musculoskeletal system, *(V1) 384–385*
of nails, *(V1) 369*
of neck
anterior and posterior triangles of, *(V1) 376f*
components of, *(V1) 375–376*
parts of anterior, *(V1) 376f*
of neurological system
assessment of, *(V1) 385*
cerebral function, *(V1) 386*
cranial nerve function, *(V1) 387, (V1) 389*
of nose, *(V1) 374*
nutrition-focused, *(V2) 586–587*
overview of, *(V2) 230*
positioning client for, *(V1) 361t–362t*
positioning the client, *(V1) 360*
preparation for, *(V1) 359*
purpose of, *(V1) 357*
skills needed, *(V1) 360, (V1) 363*
of skin
cancer, ABCDE, *(V1) 368*
characteristics of, *(V1) 366–368*
color variations, *(V1) 366, (V1) 367t*
lesions of, *(V1) 368*
of skull and face, *(V1) 370*
summary of, *(V1) 393p–396p*
tests for nutritional status, *(V1) 604*
of vascular system, *(V1) 382*
Physical fitness assessment, *(V1) 1009, (V2) 975–976*
Physical loss, *(V1) 264*
Physical response, *(V1) 59*
Physician
Canada employment of, *(ESGV1) 17*
insurance for services, *(ESG46 V1) 3*
nurse as handmaiden to, *(V1) 5–7*
power of, *(V1) 6*
public funding for, *(ESGV1) 20*
Physician's Desk Reference (PDR), *(V1) 475*
Physician's order, *(V1) 493*
Physician anesthesiologist, *(V1) 937*
Physician order, *(V1) 302–303*
Physiological need
of dying, *(V2) 168tb*
as hierarchy of need, *(V1) 50*
maintaining life, *(V1) 150, (V1) 150f*
survival and stimulation, *(V1) 67*
Physiological response, *(V1) 706b*
Physiological stage, of dying, *(V1) 270–271*
Physiological stressors, *(V1) 552*
Piaget, Jean, *(V1) 166–167, (ESG9) 5*
PIE charting, *(V1) 292*
Piggyback setup, IV infusion, *(V1) 520, (V1) 520f, (V2) 510p*
Pillow, *(V1) 749*
Piloerection, *(V1) 307*
Pilot study, *(V1) 157*
Pinworm
testing for, *(V2) 663tb*
Pinworm testing, *(V1) 661*
Pitta (preservation), *(V1) 992*
Pivot joint, *(V1) 728t*
Placebo, *(V1) 488, (V1) 719–720*

Placebo effect, *(V1) 488*
Placebo response, *(V1) 990*
Placenta, *(ESG9) 9*
"Plain old telephone service" (POTS), *(V1) 974*
Plaintiff
in civil claims, *(V1) 1080–1081*
definition of, *(V1) 1078*
Plan, failure to, *(V1) 1082*
Planning
computerized, *(V1) 91*
definition of, *(V1) 82*
full-spectrum nursing and, *(V1) 35*
nursing process and, *(V1) 32, (V1) 32f*
nursing process model, *(V1) 31f*
patient goals/outcomes, *(V1) 92*
relating to other phases of nursing process, *(V1) 82–83*
special discharge or teaching, *(V1) 91*
types of, *(V1) 82–84*
Plan of care
failure to implement, malpractice, *(V1) 1082*
integrated, *(V1) 297*
for problem-oriented records, *(V1) 290*
Plantar wart, *(V1) 456*
Plaque, *(V1) 460*
Plasma
formation of, *(V1) 605*
transfusion of, *(V1) 919*
Plasma osmolality, *(V1) 891*
Plateau
aging and, *(V1) 775b*
as sexual response, *(V1) 776*
Platelet
transfusion of, *(V1) 919–920*
wound healing, *(V1) 816*
Platelet-derived growth factor, *(V1) 819*
pleading, *(V1) 1081*
Pleura, *(V1) 847*
Pleural space, *(V1) 847*
Plexor, *(V2) 233*
Plexus, *(V1) 716–717*
PLISSIT model, *(V1) 788–789*
PNDS (Perioperative Nursing Data), (V1) 71
Pneumatic compression device, *(V1) 883*
Pneumonia, *(V1) 873–874, (V1) 945t*
Pneumothorax, *(V1) 908*
Podiatrist, *(V1) 458*
Point-of-access computing, *(V1) 979f*
Point of insertion, muscle, *(V1) 727*
Point of maximal impulse (PMI), *(V1) 381*
Point of origin, muscle, *(V1) 727*
Poisoning, *(V1) 422*
carbon monoxide, *(V1) 424–425*
food, *(V1) 429*
mercury, *(V1) 312, (V1) 436, (V1) 436t*
prevention and treatment of, *(V1) 422–424*
Police powers, *(V1) 1071*
Policy, *(V1) 87*
Policy development, nursing's role in, *(ESGV1) 24–25*
Politics, *(V2) 229*
Pollution, *(V1) 430–431*
Polygamy, *(V1) 771–772*
Polypharmacy, *(ESG9) 37*
Polysaccharide, *(V1) 577*
Polysaturated fatty acid, *(V1) 580*
Polyunsaturated fat, *(V1) 580t*
Polyuria, *(V1) 633b*
Pons, *(V1) 322*

Popliteal artery, *(V1) 319, (V1) 319f, (V2) 206*
Population, *(V1) 157*
census of, *(V1) 1021–1022, (V1) 1022f*
definition of, *(V1) 1021*
health in Canada, *(ESGV1) 28*
learning and, *(V1) 534*
vulnerability of, *(V1) 225, (V1) 1023*
Population-based care, *(V1) 1035*
Portability, *(ESGV1) 4t, (ESGV1) 5*
Portal of entry, *(V1) 400*
Portal of exit, *(V1) 400*
Port-wine stain (nevus flammeus), *(V2) 333*
Position
assisting client for normal urination, *(V1) 639*
blood pressure and, *(V1) 329*
of client for physical examination, *(V1) 360, (V1) 361t–362t*
dorsal recumbent, *(V1) 643, (V1) 644f*
promoting normal defecation, *(V1) 665*
respiration and, *(V1) 318, (V1) 323*
scheduled changes in, *(V1) 832b*
for sexual intercourse, *(V1) 777*
Sims', *(V1) 392, (V1) 644*
types of, *(V1) 750–752*
for ventilation, *(V1) 874*
Positioning
devices for, *(V1) 749–750*
for mobility and activity, *(V1) 748*
of surgery patient, *(V1) 941–942*
techniques for, *(V1) 750–752*
Positive inotrope, *(V1) 884*
Positive nitrogen balance, *(V1) 578*
Positive pressure ventilator, *(V1) 880*
Positive self-talk, *(V1) 571*
Possible nursing diagnosis, *(V1) 62, (V1) 62f*
Postanesthesia care unit (PACU)
nursing care for, *(V1) 943*
transfer patient to, *(V1) 942*
Posterior tibial artery, *(V1) 319f, (V2) 207*
Posterior triangle, *(V1) 376*
Postmortem care, *(V1) 285, (V2) 169tb–170tb*
Postoperative phase, *(V1) 942, (V2) 935–938*
Postoperative transsexual, *(V1) 767*
Post-Reformation period, *(V1) 246–247*
Post-traumatic stress disorder, *(V1) 564*
Postural draining, *(V2) 815p–818p*
Postural hypotension, *(V1) 333*
Posture, *(V1) 342–343, (V1) 729*
Post-void residual volume, *(V1) 640*
Potassium (K$^+$)
diuretics, *(V1) 624b*
fluid and electrolyte balance, *(V1) 904*
function and regulation of, *(V1) 892t*
recommended intake of, *(V1) 893–894*
Potassium chloride (KCl), *(V1) 3*
POTS ("plain old telephone service"), *(V1) 974*
Poverty, *(V1) 215*
as factor influencing hygiene practice, *(V1) 443*
nutrition and, *(V1) 608, (V1) 609*
sexuality, *(V1) 772*
Power
definition of, *(V1) 960*
of nurse, *(V1) 8*
of physician, *(V1) 6*
sources of, *(V1) 960–961*
Powerlessness
diagnosis of, *(V1) 205*
goal/outcome statement, *(V1) 206*
outcomes and interventions for, *(V2) 173*

Power of attorney, durable, (V1) 273, (V1) 1073
Practical knowledge, (V1) 29, (V1) 152
Practical nursing
    education for, (V1) 14
Practice
    definition of, (V1) 227
    of North American healthcare system, (V1) 233t
    using theories in, (V1) 145
Practice guidelines, (V1) 1076–1077
Practice theory, (V1) 145
Prayer
    as CAM modality, (V1) 995
    intercessory, (V1) 259
    with patient, (V2) 154tb–155tb
    for spiritual care, (V1) 259–260
    treating patient with, (V1) 4
    types of, (V1) 260
Pre-albumin, (V1) 605
Precautions
    contact, droplet, and airborne, (V1) 412
    standard, (V1) 410, (V1) 411b
    transmission-based, (V1) 412
Preceptor, (V1) 957–958, (V1) 958b
Preconceptual phase, (ESG9) 19–20
Precordium, (V1) 381
Predicted outcome, (V1) 92
Preexisting condition
    increasing surgical risk, (V1) 926b
    pregnancy and, (ESG9) 12
    as surgical risk factor, (V1) 925
Prefilled unit-dose system, (V1) 508–509, (V1) 509f, (V2) 514tb
Pregnancy
    in adolescence, (V1) 769
    assessment during, (ESG9) 12
    baseline weight, establishing, (ESG9) 12f
    breasts during, (V2) 276
    as factor for oral problems, (V1) 459
    nutritional needs, (V1) 597–598
    oxygenation during, (V1) 856–857
    peristalsis and, (V1) 657
    pharmacokinetics and, (V1) 487–488
Prehypertension, (V1) 334
Prejudice
    as barrier to culturally competent care, (V1) 237
    justification of, (V1) 27
Premature birth, (ESG9) 12–13
Premature ejaculation, (V1) 780
Premature infant, (V1) 854
Premenstrual syndrome (PMS), (V1) 779, (V1) 788
Prenatal visits, (ESG9) 12
Preoperational stage, (V1) 534
Preoperative assessment form, AORN, (V1) 928f–929f
Preoperative nursing, (V1) 923
Preoperative stage
    assessment of patient, (V2) 928
    diagnoses, outcomes, and interventions for, (V2) 930–931
    nursing care during, (V1) 923
Preoperative transsexual, (V1) 767
Presbyopia, (V1) 372, 685b
Preschooler
    assessment of, (ESG9) 23–24
    development of, (ESG9) 21–23
    health problems, (ESG9) 23

health promotion and screenings, (V1) 1010t
    intervention for, (ESG9) 21
    modification of assessment for, (V1) 364
    nutritional needs, (V1) 595
    oxygenation of, (V1) 855
    poisoning of, (V1) 422, (V1) 422b
    safety of, (V1) 421
    sexual development, (V1) 768
    sleep requirement, (V1) 795t
    suffocation and asphyxiation prevention, (V1) 427
Prescription, (V1) 493, (V1) 493f
Prescription drug, (V1) 474
Presence, personal, (V1) 153
Preservation (pitta), (V1) 992
President's Challenge, (V1) 1016
Pressure ulcer
    assessment of, (V1) 826
    Braden scale, (V1) 823, (V1) 824f
    cause of, (V1) 449
    charting healing process, (V1) 828f
    development of, (V1) 820–821, (V1) 821f,
    of foot, (V1) 456
    guidelines for, (V1) 109b
    Norton scale, (V1) 823, (V1) 825f
    prevention of, (V1) 831
    PUSH tool, (V1) 827f
    sites for, (V1) 821, (V1) 821f,
    stages of, (V1) 822, (V1) 822f
    as type of wound, (V1) 815t
Pretrial motion, (V1) 1081
Prevention intervention, (V1) 109
Preventive Services Task Force, (V1) 1013
Priest, as nurse, (V1) 4
Primary care, (ESGV1) 18–19, (ESGV1) 19b
Primary defense, infection, (V1) 401–402
Primary effects, (V1) 488
Primary health care, (ESGV1) 18–19, (ESGV1) 19b
Primary hypertension, (V1) 334
Primary infection, (V1) 401
Primary intention healing, (V1) 816, (V1) 817f
Primary skin lesion, (V1) 368
Principle of utility, (V1) 1057
Printed material, as format for learning/teaching, (V1) 545
Prion, (V1) 413
Priority
    documentation of, (V1) 68
    patient choosing problem as, (V1) 67–68
    of patient problems, (V1) 70b
Privacy
    bowel elimination, (V1) 655
    invasion of, (V1) 1079
    maintaining, (V1) 1086
    during nursing interview, (V1) 48
    promoting normal defecation, (V1) 665
    promoting normal urination, (V1) 639
    research participant's right to, (V1) 158
    urination and, (V1) 623
Privacy rule. See HIPPA
PRN (pro re nata) medication, (V1) 296
PRN order, (V1) 494
Problem
    collaborative, (V1) 76
    deficient knowledge as, (V1) 538
    diagnostic statement, (V1) 73, (V1) 74t, (V1) 77–79
    expected outcome for, (V1) 96t
    future consequences of, (V1) 67

    labeling and ranking, (V1) 68
    loss and grieving as, (V1) 276
    nutrition-related, (V1) 606
    patient perceived priority of, (V1) 67–68
    prioritizing, (V1) 66
    self-concept as, (V1) 195
    sleep pattern as, (V1) 804
    status influencing intervention, (V1) 109
    status of, (V1) 135
    urgency of, (V1) 67
Problem etiology, (V1) 66
Problem list
    example of, (V1) 291f
    for problem-oriented records, (V1) 290
Problem-oriented record (POR), (V1) 290
Problem solving, (V1) 10, (V1) 28t
Procedural justice, (V1) 1057
Procedure
    abdomen assessment, (V2) 293p–299p
    abuse assessment, (V2) 89p–92p
    admitting patient to nursing unit, (V1) 185p, (V2) 98p
    ambulation of patient, (V1) 755p
    antiembolism stockings, applying, (V1) 934p, (V2) 920p–924p
    apical pulse assessment, (V2) 208p–209p
    apical-radial pulse assessment, (V1) 311f, (V2) 210p–211p
    arterial blood gas (ABG), interpreting, (V2) 904p
    arterial oxygen saturation, monitoring, (V2) 809p–811p
    back massage, (V1) 806p
    bathing
        bed bath, (V2) 384p–395p
        packaged bath, (V2) 397p–398p
        towel bath, (V2) 396p–397p
    beard and mustache care, (V2) 418p–419p
    bed, moving patient, (V1) 754p–755p
    bed-monitoring device, using, (V2) 369p–371p
    bed-monitoring device and restraints, (V1) 434p–436p
    bedpan, placing and removing, (V1) 662p, (V2) 643p–645p
    blood pressure assessment, (V1) 311f, (V2) 214p–217p
    blood transfusion, (V2) 898p–903p
    breast and axillae assessment, (V2) 275p–279p
    cardiac monitor, application and care of, (V1) 864p
    cardiopulmonary resuscitation (CPR), (V1) 867p, (V2) 855p–859p
    changing IV solution, tubing and dressing, (V2) 888p–892p
    changing ostomy appliance, (V1) 663p
    chemical strip temperature, (V2) 201p
    chest and lung assessment, (V2) 280p–286p
    chest tube, patient care, (V1) 867p, (V2) 850p–855p
    clean-catch sample, (V1) 645p
    clean-catch specimen, collecting, (V2) 595p–597p
    colostomy, irrigation of, (V1) 663p, (V2) 659p–662p
    connecting PCA pump, (V1) 716
    contact lenses, removing and care for, (V2) 422p–423p
    continuous bladder irrigation, (V2) 613p–615p

coughing, deep breathing, moving in bed, leg exercises, (V1) 934p, (V2) 918p–921p

dangling patient at side of bed, (V2) 709p

denture care, (V2) 409p–410p

discontinuing, (V2) 895p–897p

drawing medication up from ampule, (V2) 475p–476p

drawing medication up from vial, (V2) 476p–478p

dressings
    dry, (V2) 770p–771p
    hydrocolloid, (V2) 779p–781p
    transparent film, (V2) 776p–778p
    wet-to-damp, (V2) 773p–776p

ear assessment, (V2) 261p–265p

endotracheal tube suctioning, (V2) 840p–845p

enema administration, (V1) 662p, (V2) 646p–650p
    cleansing, (V2) 647p–648p
    prepackaged, (V2) 648p

enteral tube, administering medication, (V2) 456p–457p

expectorated specimen, (V1) 864p

eye assessment, (V2) 253p–260p

fingerstick blood glucose levels, (V1) 612p, (V2) 563p–566p

foot care, (V2) 402p–405p

gastric and enteric tube feedings, (V2) 572p–576p

general survey of client, (V2) 234p, (V2) 237p–240p

hand washing, (V1) 410f, (V2) 344p–345p, (V2) 349p–351p

head assessment, (V2) 251p–252p

hearing assessment, (V2) 261p–265p

heart and vascular system assessment, (V2) 287p–293p

Heimlich maneuver
    on adult, (V2) 376p–377p
    on infant or child, (V2) 375p–376p

hygiene, (V1) 451p–452p

infection, risk of, (V1) 406p

intermittent bladder and catheter irrigation, (V2) 610p–612p

intermittent infusion administration, (V2) 508p–512p
    piggyback setup, (V2) 510p
    tandem setup, (V2) 511p
    volume-control setup, (V2) 509p

interpretation of, (V1) 87

intradermal medication administration, (V2) 486p–488p

intramuscular injection, locating sites for, (V2) 493p–495p

intramuscular injection administration, (V2) 496p–500p

IV flow rate, regulation of, (V2) 882p–884p

IV fluid infusion, (V1) 912p–914p

IV pump, setting up and using, (V2) 885p–887p

IV push, running primary IV line, (V2) 504p–505p

IV push medication, (V2) 503p–504p
    IV lock, no extension tubing, (V2) 505p–506p
    IV lock, with extension tubing, (V2) 506p–507p

mechanical ventilator, caring for patient, (V1) 867p, (V2) 846p–849p

medical and surgical asepsis, (V1) 414p

medication to intravenous fluid, (V2) 500p–501p

mixing medication using same syringe, (V2) 479p–482p

monitoring pulse oximetry, (V1) 864p

mouth and oropharynx assessment, (V2) 268p–271p

musculoskeletal system assessment, (V2) 300p–307p

nasal medication administration, (V2) 465p–467p

nasogastric and nasoenteric tubes, (V1) 612p

nasogastric and nasoenteric tubes removal, (V2) 577p–578p

nasopharyngeal suctioning, (V1) 865p, (V2) 831p–834p

nasotracheal suctioning, (V1) 865p–866p, (V2) 835p–839p

neck assessment, (V2) 272p–274p

needle aspiration, wound, (V1) 829p

nose and sinus assessment, (V2) 266p–268p

occult blood, testing stool for, (V2) 640p–643p

occupied bed, making, (V2) 427p–428p

ophthalmic medication administration, (V2) 459p–462p

oral care, unconscious patient, (V2) 411p–413p

oral medication administration, (V2) 454p–458p

oral temperature, (V2) 199p

oropharyngeal suctioning, (V1) 865p, (V2) 831p–834p

orotracheal suctioning, (V1) 865p–866p, (V2) 835p–839p

ostomy appliance, changing, (V2) 654p–658p

otic irrigation, (V1) 695, (V2) 676p–678p

otic medication administration, (V2) 463p–464p

oxygen, administration of, (V1) 865p

patient-controlled analgesia pump, (V2) 688p–691p

percussion, vibration and postural drainage, (V1) 864p–865p

perineal care, (V2) 399p–402p

peripheral intravenous infusion, initiating, (V1) 912p, (V2) 877p–881p

peripheral pulse assessment, (V2) 203p–207p

peristalsis and, (V1) 656–657

physical examination summary, (V1) 393p–396p

positioning patient in bed, (V2) 699p–704p
    logrolling, (V2) 703p–704p
    moving and turning, (V2) 699p–702p

PPE, donning and removal of, (V2) 346p–348p

preparing and drawing up medication, (V2) 474p–478p

primary line to heparin or saline lock, (V2) 893p–895p

pulse oximetry, monitoring, (V2) 809p–811p

recapping needle, one-handed, (V2) 483p–485p

rectal suppository administration, (V2) 471p–473p

rectal temperature, (V2) 200p

respiration assessment, (V2) 212p–213p

restraints, using, (V2) 371p–374p

sensory-neurological system assessment
    arousal and orientation, (V2) 309p
    communication, (V2) 311p–312p
    cranial nerve function, (V2) 312p–315p
    judgment, (V2) 311p
    memory, (V2) 310p
    memory state, (V2) 320p
    modifications, (V2) 308p
    reflexes, (V2) 317p–319p
    sensations, (V2) 315p–317p
    thought process and abstract thinking, (V2) 310p–311p

sequential compression device (SCD), applying, (V1) 934p, (V2) 924p–926p

shampooing bedrest patient, (V2) 414p–417p

for skin assessment, (V2) 239p–243p

specimen by suction, (V1) 864p

sputum specimen collection, (V2) 803p–808p
    expectorated, (V2) 805p
    suctioned, (V2) 806p–807p

sterile field, preparing and maintaining, (V2) 357p–359p

sterile gown and gloves (closed method), (V2) 352p–354p

stool
    removing digitally, (V1) 662p–663p, (V2) 650p–653p
    testing for occult blood, (V1) 662p

subcutaneous medication administration, (V2) 489p–492p

surgical hand washing, (V2) 349p–351p

teeth, brushing and flossing, (V2) 406p–408p

temperature assessment, (V2) 198p–199p

tracheostomy care, (V1) 865p, (V2) 825p–830p

tracheostomy or endotracheal suctioning, (V1) 866p

tracheostomy suctioning, (V2) 840p–845p

transferring from bed, (V2) 704p–711p
    to chair, (V2) 709p–710p
    to stretcher, (V2) 706p–708p

Trousseau's and Chvostek's signs, (V2) 903p

tympanic temperature, (V2) 202p

unoccupied bed, making, (V2) 424p–426p

urinary catheter insertion, (V2) 598p–599p
    indwelling, (V2) 603p–607p
    straight, (V2) 599p–603p

vaginal medication administration, (V2) 467p–470p

vital signs assessment, (V1) 311f

wound, (V1) 830p

wound culture, (V1) 829p
    by needle aspiration, (V2) 763p–765p
    by swab, (V2) 759p–762p

wound irrigation, (V1) 829p, (V2) 766p–769p

Process
    of community, (V1) 1022
    definition of, (V1) 339

Process evaluation, (V1) 131

Process recording, (V1) 347

Procurement surgery, (V1) 924

Prodromal stage, (V1) 401

Productive cough, (V1) 862
Profession, criteria for, (V1) 12
Professional healthcare system, (V1) 231
Professional standards
    for assessment, (V1) 39, (V1) 40b
    for diagnosis, (V1) 57b
    for implementation, (V1) 122b
    for minimizing malpractice, (V1) 1083
    for planning intervention, (V1) 107b
    for planning outcomes, (V1) 83b
    recording evaluative statement,
        (V1) 133–134
Professional values
    behaviors and, (V1) 1052t
    personal values and, (V1) 1051–1053
Progesterone, (V1) 770
Programmed instruction, (V1) 545
Progressive relaxation, (V1) 570
Progress notes
    documentation of intervention, (V1) 296
    for problem-oriented records, (V1) 290
Projection, (V1) 561t
Proliferative phase of healing, (V1) 817,
        (V1) 818f
Pronation
    assessment of, (V2) 305p–306p
    as movement, (V1) 727f
Prone position, (V1) 751t, (V1) 752
Propionic acid (ibuprofen), (V1) 474
Proposition, theory and, (V1) 142
Proprietary name, (V1) 474
Proprioception, (V1) 389–390, (V1) 689b
Proprioceptor
    detecting stretch in muscles, (V1) 689
    locations for, (V1) 681
Pro re nata (PRN) medication, (V1) 296
Prostaglandins, (V1) 314, (V1) 701
Prostate, (V1) 392, (V1) 622
Prostate-specific antigen (PSA), (V1) 1013
Prosthesis, (V1) 934–935
Prosthetic eye, (V1) 467–468, (V1) 468f
Protective isolation, (V1) 412–413, (V2) 342tb
Protein
    amino acid, (V1) 577
    complete and incomplete, (V1) 578
    as energy nutrient, (V1) 576t
    function of, (V1) 578–579
    markers of metabolism of, (V1) 605
    metabolism of, (V1) 578
    needs for ovo-lacto vegetarian, (V1) 598
    skin maintenance, (V1) 813
    storage of, (V1) 605
Protein-binding, of drug, (V1) 484
Protein-calorie malnutrition, (V1) 599
Protein-controlled diet, (V1) 601
Protein system, (V1) 895
Proteinuria, (V1) 633b
Protocol, therapeutic action, (V1) 87
Protraction, (V1) 727f
Provincial/territorial jurisdiction
    healthcare funding, (ESGV1) 10
    healthcare insurance administration,
        (ESGV1) 4, (ESGV1) 4t
    legislation and, (ESGV1) 8
    responsibility of, (ESGV1) 7–8
Proximodistal pattern of development,
        (V1) 166
Prozac (fluoxetine), (V1) 788
Pruritus, (V1) 449, (V1) 714b
Pseudomonas aeruginosa, (V1) 819
Psoriasis, (V2) 246
Psychiatric nurse, (ESGV1) 16–17

Psychoanalytic theory, (V1) 166–167,
        (ESG9) 5
Psychogenic pain, (V1) 700
Psychological abuse, (V2) 90
Psychological dependence, opioids, (V1) 713
Psychological factors, (V1) 488
Psychological integrity, threat to, (V1) 167
Psychological loss, (V1) 264
Psychological need, (V2) 168tb–169tb
Psychological response
    immobility and, (V1) 740
    to pain, (V1) 706b
Psychological stage, of dying, (V1) 271
Psychological stressor, (V1) 552
Psychomotor goal, (V1) 133t
Psychomotor learning, (V1) 530, (V1) 531t
Psychosexual development
    overview of, (ESG9) 5
    stages of, (ESG9) 6t
Psychosis, (V1) 200
Psychosocial assessment
    categories of, (V1) 192–193
    as special needs assessment, (V1) 44
Psychosocial development, (ESG9) 20–21
    of adolescence, (ESG9) 27–28
    of child, (ESG9) 25
    of elderly, (ESG9) 35, (ESG9) 37
    factors of, (V1) 187
    of infant, (ESG9) 17
    of middle adult, (ESG9) 33
    of newborn, (ESG9) 15
    of preschooler, (ESG9) 23
    of young adult, (ESG9) 31, (ESG9) 31–32
Psychosocial development theory, (V1) 151,
        (V1) 189
    overview of, (V2) 100
    stages of, (V1) 167, (ESG9) 7
Psychosocial diagnosis, (V1) 193–194,
        (V1) 194t
Psychosocial health
    knowledge map of, (V2) 117
    overview of, (V2) 100
    self-concept as aspect of, (V1) 188–189
Psychosocial illness
    anxiety
        coping with, (V1) 200
        definition of, (V1) 199
        levels of, (V1) 199–200
        nursing assessment of, (V1) 202–203
        nursing diagnosis of, (V1) 203
        planning
            interventions/implementations,
                (V1) 204
        planning outcomes/evaluation of,
                (V1) 203
    depression
        assessment continuum, (V1) 205f
        cause of, (V1) 201
        criteria for, (V1) 200–201
        depressed affect, (V1) 201f
        nursing assessment of, (V1) 204–205
        nursing diagnosis of, (V1) 205
        physical and behavioral problems of,
                (V1) 205
        planning outcomes/evaluation of,
                (V1) 205–206
        signs and symptoms of, (V1) 201–202
        treatment of, (V1) 202
        truths and myths of, (V1) 201t
    overview of, (V2) 100
Psychosocial outcome, (V1) 196
Psychosocial theory, (V1) 188

Pterygium, (V1) 371, (V2) 334
Ptosis, (V1) 365, (V1) 371
Ptyalin, (V1) 651
Puberty, (ESG9) 24
    onset of, (ESG9) 27
    skin during, (V1) 812
Public department nursing, (V1) 1028
Public distance, (V1) 343–344
Public health
    community health versus, (V1) 1025f
    concerns in Canada, (ESGV1) 20
    goals of, (V1) 99
    population and, (ESGV1) 7
Public health nursing, (V1) 1024, (V2) 986
Public speaking, (V1) 339
PubMed, (V1) 21
Pulmonary allergen, (V1) 856
Pulmonary circulation, (V1) 380
Pulmonary embolism
    as postoperative collaborative problem,
        (V1) 945t
Pulmonary embolus, (V1) 860
Pulmonary hypertension, (V1) 860
Pulmonary system
    abnormalities of, (V1) 860
    components of
        airway, (V1) 845–847
        lungs, (V1) 847
    function of
        pulmonary ventilation, (V1) 848–849
Pulmonary ventilation,
        (V1) 322–323
    process of, (V1) 848–849
Pulse
    assessment of, (V1) 311f
    definition of, (V1) 317
    documentation of, (V1) 320–321
    equipment for assessment, (V1) 318–319
    production and regulation of, (V1) 317
    respiration and, (V1) 323
    sites for measurement of, (V1) 319,
        (V1) 319f
    as vital sign (VS), (V1) 305
Pulse deficit, (V1) 319–320
Pulse oximeter, (V1) 326
Pulse oximetry, (V1) 305, (V1) 326
    accurate readings, (V2) 861tb
    equipment for, (V1) 867f
    monitoring, (V1) 864p, (V2) 809p–811p
    performance of, (V1) 867p
Pulse pressure, (V1) 327
Pulse rate
    delegation of, (V2) 203–207
    factors influencing, (V1) 317–318
    normal for adults, (V1) 317
    overview of, (V2) 191
    traditional Chinese medicine (TCM),
        (V1) 993
Pulse volume, (V1) 320–321
Pump-controlled infusion, (V1) 614
Puncture wound, (V1) 815t
Pupil, (V1) 371
Pureed diet, (V1) 601
Purnell model for cultural competence, (V1)
        236–237, (V1) 236f, (V1) 239
Purosaguineous exudate, (V1) 819
Purulent exudate, (V1) 819
Push, IV
    administration of, (V1) 525p, (V2)
        503p–504p
    IV lock, no extension tubing, (V2)
        505p–506p

IV lock, with extension tubing, (V2) 506p–507p
running primary IV line, (V2) 504p–505p
overview of, (V1) 519
Pustule, (V2) 245
P wave, (V1) 870
Pyelonephritis, (V1) 636
Pyogenic bacteria, (V1) 819
Pyorrhea, (V1) 459, (V1) 460
Pyramid
USDA, (V1) 587, (V1) 589f
vegetarian, (V1) 591f
Pyrexia, (V1) 314
Pyrogen, (V1) 314
Pyuria, (V1) 633b

Q

Qi (energy), (V1) 993, (V1) 994f
Qigong, (V1) 999
QRS complex, (V1) 870
Qu'ran (Koran), (V1) 251
Quadriceps
drills for, (V1) 757
Quadriplegia, (V1) 740b
Qualitative research
comparing to quantitative research, (V1) 157t
overview of, (V2) 73
purpose of, (V1) 156
Quality
of pulse, (V1) 320
of transformational leadership, (V1) 955t
Quality assurance (QA)
client record for, (V1) 289
Quality assurance (QA) program, (V1) 136
Quality of care
effect of organization characteristics on, (V1) 131
in healthcare setting, (V1) 136
Quantitative research
comparing to qualitative research, (V1) 157t
overview of, (V2) 73
purpose of, (V1) 156
Quasi-International torts, (V1) 1078
Questions
closed and open-ended, (V1) 47t
Quickening, (ESG9) 8

R

Race
blood pressure and, (V1) 329
categories of, (V1) 226
definition of, (V1) 226
statistics in nursing, (V1) 9, (V1) 10t
in United States, (V1) 223f
Racism, (V1) 237
Radial artery, (V1) 319, (V1) 319f, (V2) 204
Radiating pain, (V1) 700
Radiation, (V1) 857
as factor for heat loss, (V1) 308
injury from, (V1) 437
Radiographic verification, of feeding tube, (V1) 614
Rahe, Richard, (V1) 1012
Ramayana, (V1) 252
Rando, Theresa
phases of grieving, (V1) 266
theories of grief, a comparison, (V1) 266t
Range of motion (ROM), (V1) 385
assessment of, (V2) 305p–306p
exercises for, (V1) 757

of joints, (V1) 742t–746t
performing passive, (V2) 717tb
Rape, (V1) 779–780
Rapid eye movement (REM) sleep, (V1) 796, (V1) 798
Rastafarianism, (V1) 253
Ratched, Nurse, (V1) 7
Rate
pulse, (V1) 317–318
of respiration, (V1) 324, (V1) 325t
Rationale, (V1) 91
Rationalization, (V1) 561t
Reaction formation, (V1) 561t
Reactive hyperemia, (V1) 826
Readiness, learning, (V1) 532
Reading, analytic, (V1) 159–161
Reanastomosis, (V1) 657
Reasoning
clinical, (V1) 28t
determining intervention, (V1) 27
logical, (V1) 143, (V1) 155
Reassessment data, (V1) 132
Rebound effect, (V1) 504
Receiver, (V1) 340
Reception, (V1) 680–681
Receptor site, (V1) 702
Recommended Dietary Allowance (RDA), (V1) 586
Reconstructive surgery, (V1) 924
Record
of client/patient, (V1) 289–290
computerized, (V1) 298
graphic, (V1) 294
intake and output (I&O), (V1) 294
medication, (V1) 294
source-oriented and problem-oriented, (V1) 290
Recovery
adaptation to stressor, (V1) 557
from anesthesia and surgery, (V1) 942–949, (V1) 944b
as final stage of illness, (V1) 180
Recovery stage, of GAS, (V1) 555f, (V1) 557
Rectal medication
overview of, (V1) 504
suppositories, (V1) 522p, (V2) 471p–473p
Rectal temperature, (V1) 313, (V2) 200p
Rectal tube, inserting, (V2) 664tb
Rectum, (V1) 653
assessment of, (V1) 396p, (V2) 330p–331p
examination of, (V1) 392
opioid administration, (V1) 715
Rectus femoris muscle, (V1) 517
Red blood cell transfusion, (V1) 919
Red-Yellow-Black (RYB) Color Code, (V1) 833, (V1) 833t
Reeve, Christopher, (V1) 176, (V1) 191
Refereed journal, (V1) 159
Referred pain, (V1) 700, (V1) 700f
Reflection
about assessment, (V1) 52–54
about evaluation, (V1) 136
about expected outcomes/goals, (V1) 100–102
about implementation, (V1) 128
about interventions, (V1) 118
Reflective skepticism, (V1) 30t, (V1) 31
about evaluation, (V1) 136
intervention selection, (V1) 112
model of critical thinking, (V1) 31f

Reflex
assessment of, (V2) 317p–319p
at birth, (ESG9) 14
of infant, (ESG9) 14f
of newborn, (ESG9) 16
Reflexology
as CAM therapy, (V1) 999
for stress management, (V1) 571
Reflux, (V1) 621
Refractometer, (V1) 634, (V1) 634f
Refractory period, (V1) 776
Regeneration, (V1) 558
Regenerative healing, (V1) 816
Regional anesthesia, (V1) 938
Regional health authority, (ESGV1) 21
Registered nurse (RN)
in Canada
demographics and supply, (ESGV1) 13
education of, (ESGV1) 15–16
employment of, (ESGV1) 14t–16t, (ESGV1) 15, (ESGV1) 16f
delegation of patient care activities, (V1) 126
education pathways for, (V1) 14
Registered nurse first assistant (RNFA), (V1) 937
Registered practical nurse (RPN), (ESGV1) 17
Registered psychiatric nurse, (ESGV1) 16–17
Registration, (ESGV1) 9
Regression, (V1) 561t
Regulation, health care professionals, (ESGV1) 8
Rehabilitation facility, (V1) 84
Reiki
as CAM therapy, (V1) 999
for stress management, (V1) 570
Reimbursement, insurance company for, (V1) 289
Relapsing fever, (V1) 314
Related factor, (V1) 72
Relationship
communication and, (V1) 344
loss of, (V1) 265
negative intimate, (V1) 779
Relationship focus, (V1) 954
Relaxation
as holistic therapy, (V2) 967tb
promoting, (V1) 806
as stress management technique, (V1) 570
Swedish massage and, (V1) 998
Reliable
criteria as, (V1) 130
research as, (V1) 160
Religion
comparing to spirituality, (V1) 247t
as culture specific influencing health, (V1) 229
definition of, (V1) 226
as factor influencing hygiene practice, (V1) 442–443
health and, (V1) 175–176
map of, (V1) 247–248
nursing and, (V1) 4–5
nutrition and, (V1) 599
sexuality and, (V1) 772
types of, (V1) 250–253
Religious groups
nursing, role in development of, (V2) 6
in society and nursing, (V1) 5

Remedy, (V1) 231
Remission, (V1) 180
Remittent fever, (V1) 314
REM sleep behavior disorder, (V1) 803
Renaissance period, (V1) 7
Renal biopsy, (V2) 633
Renal calculi, (V1) 625, (V1) 739
Renal disease
    end stage, (V1) 633b
    increasing surgical risk, (V1) 926b
Renal disease, end-stage, (V1) 896
Renal failure, (V1) 947t
Renal function, (V1) 605
Renal pelvis, (V1) 619–620
Renin, (V1) 891
Renin-angiotensin system, (V1) 891
Repetition, learning, (V1) 533
Reporting, (V1) 289
    knowledge map of, (V2) 190
    overview of, (V2) 178
    regulation, mandatory, (V1) 1087
Repression
    psychological defense mechanism,
        (V1) 561t
    sexual, (V1) 166
Reproductive system
    external female genitalia, (V1) 391f
    female genitourinary system, (V1)
        390–391
    female organs for, (V1) 764, (V1) 764f
    female sexual development, (V1) 391f
    male genitourinary system, (V1) 390
    male organs for, (V1) 764–765, (V1) 766f
    male sexual development, (V1) 390f
    menstrual cycle, (V1) 764, (V1) 765f
Rescue Remedy, (V1) 994–995
Research
    analytic reading, (V1) 159–161
    analyzing, (V1) 159
    categories of design, (V1) 156
    client record for, (V1) 289
    Conduct and Utilization of Research in
        Nursing project (CURN), (V1) 156
    definition of, (V1) 154
    development of priorities for,
        (V1) 154–155
    discovery of pathogens, (V1) 399
    finding articles, (V1) 161
    history of, (V1) 154
    identifying clinical problems in, (V1) 158
    influencing choice of intervention,
        (V1) 106–108
    knowledge map of, (V2) 81
    online sources for, (V1) 982–983
    overview of, (V2) 73
    problem areas for, (V1) 158–159
    process of, (V1) 157
    rights of participants/subjects in,
        (V1) 158
    using theories in, (V1) 145
    utilization of, (V1) 161
Research-based care plan, (V1) 28
Research consumer, (V1) 13t
Reservoir, infection, (V1) 399
Residual volume (RV), (V1) 849
Resistance stage, of GAS, (V1) 555f,
    (V1) 556–557
Resistance to change, (V1) 963–964
Resistance training, (V1) 732
Resolution
    aging and, (V1) 775b
    alternative dispute, (V1) 1081

to conflict, (V1) 966
    dispute, (ESGV1) 8
    as sexual response, (V1) 776
    "win-win", (V1) 965–966
Respect, in therapeutic communication,
    (V1) 346
Respecting, (V1) 182
Respiration
    assessment of, (V2) 212p–213p
    at birth, (ESG9) 13
    chest tube, monitoring, (V1) 882
    impaired, diagnoses for, (V2) 867–868
    overview of, (V2) 191
    of toddler, (ESG9) 19
Respiration (gas exchange)
    alterations in, (V1) 326
    assessment of, (V1) 311f, (V1) 863
    definition of, (V1) 322, (V1) 848
    equipment for assessment, (V1) 324
    factors influencing, (V1) 323
    internal and external, (V1) 850
    neuromuscular abnormalities, (V1) 860
    normal for adults, (V1) 306t
    normal rate of, (V1) 322
    oxygenation, (V1) 305, (V1) 326
    problems with, (V1) 872
    rates and rhythm, (V1) 325t
    regulation of, (V1) 322
    as vital sign (VS), (V1) 305
Respiratory (pulmonary) arrest, (V1) 885
Respiratory acidosis, (V1) 898, (V1) 900t
Respiratory alkalosis, (V1) 898, (V1) 900t
Respiratory anti-inflammatory agent, (V1) 884
Respiratory center, (V1) 322
Respiratory depressant
    oxygenation and, (V1) 858, (V1) 859
Respiratory depression, (V1) 714b
    as side effect of opioids, (V1) 713
Respiratory disorder, (V1) 926b
Respiratory distress, of newborn, (ESG9) 15
Respiratory distress syndrome (RDS), (V1) 854
Respiratory effort, (V1) 325
Respiratory failure, (V1) 273
Respiratory infection, (V1) 857
Respiratory inhalations, (V1) 504–505
Respiratory rate, (V1) 324
Respiratory system
    adaptation failure and, (V1) 562–563
    age-related changes for, (ESG9) 36t
    anterior view of, (V1) 846f
    benefits of exercise, (V1) 734b
    pain and, (V1) 706
Respiratory tree, (V1) 401
Response-based model of stress, (V1) 553,
    (V1) 554
Resposition
    assessment of, (V2) 305p–306p
    as movement, (V1) 727f
Rest
    definition of, (V1) 793
    illness and, (V1) 794, (V1) 794f, (V1) 800
    importance of, (V1) 568
    overview of, (V2) 741
    promoting host defense of infection,
        (V1) 405
Restitution, (V1) 561t
Restless leg syndrome (RLS), (V1) 801
Restorative effect, (V1) 488
Restraint
    definition of, (V1) 434
    using, (V1) 435p, (V2) 371p–374p
    using safely, (V1) 434–436

Resuscitation
    CPR (Cardiopulmonary resuscitation),
        (V1) 273
    DNR and DNAR orders, (V1) 273
Retention catheter, (V1) 632, (V1) 641
Retention enema, (V1) 668–669
Reticular activating system (RAS), (V1) 681,
    (V1) 796, (V1) 796f
Reticular formation, (V1) 796, (V1) 796f
Retirement, mandatory, (ESG9) 35, (ESG9) 37
Retraction
    intercostal and substernal, (V1) 325–326
    as movement, (V1) 727f
    respiratory effort and, (V1) 863
Retrograde ejaculation, (V1) 781
Retrograde pyelogram, (V2) 633
Retroperitoneal, (V1) 619
Return demonstration, (V1) 544
Return-flow enema, (V1) 669
    administration of, (V2) 663tb
Reverse isolation, (V1) 412–413
Rheumatoid arthritis (RA), (V1) 737
Rhizotomy, (V1) 718
Rhonchi, (V1) 325
Rhythm
    of pulse, (V1) 320
    of respiration, (V1) 324–325, (V1) 325t
Ribbon dressing, (V1) 839
Rigdon, Dr. Imogene, (V1) 145
Rights
    of delegation, (V1) 126–128, (V2) 67
    for medications administration,
        (V1) 497–499
    of teaching, (V1) 530b
Rigor mortis, (V1) 285
Ringworm, (V2) 333
Rinne test, (V1) 374
Risk factor, (V1) 72
Risk nursing diagnosis, (V1) 62, (V1) 62f
Risk-taking behavior, (V1) 214
Ritual
    of North American Healthcare System,
        (V1) 233t
    practiced by cultures, (V1) 227
Rogers, Martha, (V1) 991
Role, (V1) 13t
    of client influencing health care, (V1) 28
    communication and, (V1) 344
Role modeling, (V1) 546, (V1) 1016
Role performance
    assessment of, (V2) 108
    as component of self-concept, (V1) 191
    facilitating enhancement, (V1) 198
    ineffective, (V1) 195
Role-playing, (V1) 545–546
Role strain, (V1) 191, (V2) 173
Roller bandage, application of, (V1) 842
Roman Catholicism, (V1) 251
Roman Empire, (V1) 8
Romberg test, (V1) 374
Room air, (V1) 869
Rooting, (ESG9) 14
Rotation
    assessment of, (V2) 305p–306p
    as movement, (V1) 727f
Routine urinalysis (UA), (V1) 633–634
Roy Adaptation Model, (V1) 51b

S

Sacraments, (V1) 251
Saddle joint, (V1) 728t, (V1) 745t
Safe harbor law, (V1) 1088

Safety
assessment of, (V1) 438
assessment of home for, (V1) 438
automation decreasing errors, (V1) 980
delegating interventions for, (V1) 439–440
diagnosis of risk for falls, (V1) 439
equipment and, (V2) 1021tb
factors affecting, (V1) 421
food, (V1) 430
hazards in the community, (V1) 428–429
hazards in the home, (V1) 422
as hierarchy of need, (V1) 50, (V1) 67
home health visit, (V2) 1001–1002
individual risk factors, (V1) 421, (V1) 422t
intervention/implementation, (V1) 439
for intraoperative phase, (V1) 942
NANDA diagnoses and NOC outcomes for problems, (V2) 381–382
NIC intervention for problems, (V2) 382
nursing activities for, (V1) 439
outcome and evaluation of, (V1) 439
overview of, (V2) 361
oxygen therapy precautions, (V2) 862tb
of patient, (V1) 1086
physical and emotional, (V1) 150, (V1) 150f
protocol for research participants, (V1) 158
psychological, (V1) 964
sleepwalking and, (V1) 807
steering committee for patient, (ESGV1) 25–26
using restraints, (V1) 434
Safety assessment scale (SAS), (V1) 438–439
Saline
adding medication to, (V1) 519
blood clots prevention, (V1) 154
Salivary amylase, (V1) 651
SAMe, (V1) 207
Same-gender friendship, (ESG9) 24f
Sample, research, (V1) 157
Sandbag, (V1) 750
Sanger, Margaret, (V1) 1025
Sanguineous exudate, (V1) 819
Sanitation
proper measure of, (V1) 9
as source of pathogens, (V1) 430
SARS (Severe acute respiratory syndrome), (V1) 215
Saskatchewan Commission on Medicare, (ESGV1) 27–28
Saskatchewan Health Quality Council, (ESGV1) 26
Saskatchewan Vital Statistics Act, (ESGV1) 8
Saturated fat, (V1) 580, (V1) 580t
Saturated fatty acid, (V1) 580
Saturation, (V1) 580
Scalding, (V1) 425
Scale
Borg Rate of Perceived Exertion, (V1) 732b
Braden, (V1) 823, (V1) 824f
French (Fr), (V1) 613
Geriatric Depression Scale (GDS), (ESG9) 38
Holmes-Rahe readjustment scale, (V2) 551
JAREL spiritual well-being, (V1) 256
Karnofsky Performance Scale, (V1) 44
Katz Index of ADL, (V1) 43

Lawton Instrumental Activities of Daily Living, (V1) 43–44
Morse Fall Scale, (V1) 438
Norton, (V1) 823, (V1) 825f
Omaha System problem rating, (V2) 992
pain, (V1) 707–708, (V2) 692–693
Safety assessment scale (SAS), (V1) 438–439
sedation rating, (V2) 694
for temperature measurement, (V1) 310, (V1) 312
Scales, skin, (V2) 246
Scalp, characteristics, (V1) 369, (V2) 248
Scalp vein needle, (V1) 906–907, (V1) 907f
Scar, skin, (V2) 246
Scheduled medications, (V1) 296
Scheduling, teaching sessions, (V1) 533
School-age child. See Child
School nursing, (V1) 1027
Schwartz, Morrie, (V1) 175, (V1) 189
Science of Human Caring, (V1) 139
Scientific inquiry, (V1) 156
Scientific management, (V1) 955
Scientific medical health system, (V1) 231
Scientific method
characteristics of, (V1) 156, (V1) 156t
methods of gaining knowledge, (V1) 155–156
Sclera, (V1) 371
Scleroderma, (V1) 368
Scoliosis, (V1) 378, (V1) 385, (V2) 282, (ESG9) 26
example of, (V2) 335
mobility and activity, (V1) 737
Scoot sheet, (V1) 753, (V1) 753f
Scrub nurse, (V1) 937
Sebaceous glands, (V1) 447
Seborrheic keratosis, (V2) 244
Secondary defense, infection, (V1) 402
Secondary effect, (V1) 488–491
Secondary hypertension, (V1) 334
Secondary infection, (V1) 401
Secondary intention healing, (V1) 816, (V1) 817f
Secondary skin lesion, (V1) 368
Secretion, mobilizing, (V1) 875
Security
as hierarchy of need, (V1) 50, (V1) 67
physical and emotional, (V1) 150, (V1) 150f
promotion in children, (V1) 198
Sedation rating scale, (V2) 694
Selective serotonin reuptake-inhibiting drugs (SSRIs), (V1) 788
Self
changing perception of, (V1) 571
dynamic, (V1) 189
loss of aspects of, (V1) 265
therapeutic use of, (V1) 346
transcendence, (V1) 150f, (V1) 151
Self-actualization
growth and cognitive needs, (V1) 151
as hierarchy of need, (V1) 50, (V1) 67, (V1) 150f
theory of, (V1) 188
Self-administration, of medication, (V1) 478
Self-assessment
teaching, (V1) 53
Self-care
assessment of abilities, (V1) 444
in Canada, (ESGV1) 29

classification of ability, (V1) 445b
exercising, (V1) 733
fluid and electrolyte balance, (V1) 904
foot care, (V1) 457
health status affecting, (V1) 443
helping children deal with loss, (V1) 285
hypertension, (V1) 336
incentive spirometry, (V1) 950
laxative use, (V1) 668
maintaining proper posture, (V1) 729
nail care, (V1) 457
for nurses, (V1) 1002
nutrition on limited budget, (V1) 608
oral hygiene, (V1) 462–463
oral medication administration, (V1) 501
Orem's Self-Care Model, (V1) 51b
pelvic floor muscle exercise (PFME), (V1) 647
preventing back injury, (V1) 748
preventing UTI, (V1) 639
self-medication, (V1) 518
sensory perceptual health, (V1) 693
teaching, (V1) 53
upper respiratory infection, preventing, (V1) 1017
using a condom, (V1) 790
using metered-dose inhaler (MDI), (V1) 506
Self-care deficit, (V1) 64
feeding, (V1) 609
standardized outcomes and interventions for, (V2) 434
toileting, (V1) 664
Self-concept
assessment of, (V1) 193, (V2) 108tb
components of
body image, (V1) 190–191
personal identity, (V1) 191–192
role performance, (V1) 191
self-esteem, (V1) 192
definition of, (V1) 188–189
diagnoses of, (V1) 195
as etiology, (V1) 195–196
factors affecting, (V1) 189–190
formation of, (V1) 189
knowledge map of, (V2) 117
outcomes of, (V1) 196
overview of, (V2) 100
as problem, (V1) 195
promotion of, (V1) 197
Self-correction, (V1) 156
Self-determination, right to, (V1) 158
Self-esteem
assessment of, (V1) 193, (V2) 108
chronic low, (V1) 195
as component of self-concept, (V1) 192
determination of, (V1) 192f
as hierarchy of need, (V1) 50, (V1) 67, (V1) 150, (V1) 150f
inventory of, (V2) 109tb
outcome of, (V1) 196
promotion in children, (V1) 198
promotion of, (V1) 197
Self-help group, (V1) 347–348
Self-identity, (V1) 190
Self-instruction, (V1) 546
Self knowledge, (V1) 68
Self-permanence, (V1) 190
Self-talk, (V1) 338, (V1) 571
Self-transcendence, (V1) 188

Self-treatment remedy, (V1) 231
Selye, Hans, (V1) 151
    general adaptation syndrome (GAP), (V1) 554–557, (V1) 555f
    life stress review, (V1) 1012
    response-based model, (V1) 553
Semi-Fowler's position, (V1) 752
Semi-vegetarian, (V1) 598
Sender, (V1) 339
Sensation
    assessment of, (V2) 315p–317p
    diminished, (V1) 813
    responding to, (V1) 682
Senses, (V1) 44
Sensorimotor phase, (ESG9) 16, (ESG9) 19–20
Sensorineural hearing loss, (V2) 264
Sensoristasis, (V1) 684
Sensory aid, (V1) 690
Sensory deficit, (V1) 685
    caring for clients
        auditory, (V1) 695
        confused, (V1) 696–697
        gustatory, (V1) 696
        olfactory, (V1) 695–696
        tactile, (V1) 696
        unconscious, (V1) 697
        visual, (V1) 694–695
    safety and health measures, (V1) 696
Sensory deprivation
    overview of, (V2) 672
    prevention of, (V1) 692–694
    risk factors for, (V1) 684
    signs of, (V1) 684b
Sensory experience, (V1) 680
Sensory function, (V1) 389
    affecting self-care ability, (V1) 443
    age-related changes for, (ESG9) 36t
    assessment of, (V1) 395p–396p, (V1) 689–690
    bedside assessment of, (V2) 681
    changes with age, (V1) 683t
    factors affecting, (V1) 682–683
    outcome and evaluation of, (V1) 466
    promoting optimal, (V1) 692
Sensory-neurological system, (V2) 308p–320p
Sensory overload
    overview of, (V2) 672
    prevention of, (V1) 694
    risk factors for, (V1) 684–685
    signs of, (V1) 684b
Sensory perception
    assessment of, (V1) 689–690, (V2) 680–681
    outcomes and interventions for, (V2) 682
    overview of, (V2) 672
Septicemia, (V1) 401, (V1) 917t
Sequential compression device (SCD), (V1) 883
    application of, (V1) 934p, (V2) 924p–926p
    for high-risk thrombophlebitis, (V1) 948, (V1) 948f
Sequential muscle relaxation (SMR), (V1) 711
Serial monogamy, (V1) 769
Serosanguineous drainage, (V1) 819
Serous exudate, (V1) 819
Sertraline (Zoloft), (V1) 788
Serum electrolytes, (V1) 902
Serum osmolality, (V1) 902
Serum protein, (V1) 605
Settling in, (V1) 181–182
Seventh Day Adventist hospital system, (V1) 5

Severe acute respiratory syndrome (SARS), (ESGV1) 7, (V1) 215
Severe adverse reaction, (V1) 489
Severe anxiety, (V1) 200
Severe hypothermia, (V1) 316
A Severe Mercy, (V1) 183
Sewage, (V1) 9
Sex, (V1) 770
    in adolescence, (ESG9) 28
    blood pressure and, (V1) 328
    communication and, (V1) 343
    pharmacokinetics and, (V1) 487
    pulse rate, (V1) 318
    of young adult, (ESG9) 32
Sexism, (V1) 237
Sexual abuse, (V2) 89
Sexual assault, (V1) 779–780
Sexual assault nurse examiner (SANE), (V1) 780
Sexual dysfunction, (V1) 196
    cause of, (V1) 782–783
    intervention and nursing activities for, (V2) 738
    outcomes and goals for, (V2) 737
Sexual expression
    alternate forms of, (V1) 778
    forms of, (V1) 776–778
Sexual harassment, (V1) 779, (V1) 791, (V1) 1087
Sexual health
    assessment of, (V1) 781
    definition of, (V1) 774
    history of, (V2) 733tb, (V2) 734–735
    overview of, (V2) 726
    teaching about, (V1) 783, (V1) 788
Sexual identity, (V1) 765
Sexual intercourse
    painful, (V1) 780
    types of, (V1) 777–778
Sexual intimacy, (V1) 770, (V1) 770f
Sexuality
    definition of, (V1) 765
    development of
        by age, (V1) 768–770
        female, (V1) 390–391, (V1) 391f,
        male, (V1) 390, (V1) 390f
    exploration of, (V1) 769
    factors affecting, (V1) 770–774
    ineffective patterns of, (V1) 196
    infection, risk of, (V1) 406
    knowledge map for, (V2) 740
    medication and, (V1) 773–774, (V1) 774t
    problems affecting, (V1) 778
    as risk factor for UTI, (V1) 636
Sexually transmitted infection (STI)
    prevention of, (V1) 777
    from rape, (V1) 780
    symptoms and treatment of, (V1) 778–779
    teaching about, (V1) 789
Sexual orientation, (V1) 767–768
Sexual repression, (V1) 166
Sexual response cycle
    aging and, (V1) 775b
    disorders of, (V1) 780–781
    stages of, (V1) 774
Sexual therapy, (V1) 788–789
Shaken-baby syndrome, (ESG9) 17
Shallow breathing, (V1) 324
Shampooing, bedrest patient, (V2) 414p–417p
Sharp debridement, (V1) 836
Shaving, (V1) 465–466, (V2) 420p–421p

Shearing, pressure ulcer, (V1) 821
Shiatsu massage, (V1) 999
Shock phase, of stress, (V1) 555
Short-term goal, (V1) 93, (V1) 967
Short-term group, (V1) 347
Short-term memory, (ESG9) 35
Shoulder ROM, (V1) 742t–743t
Shower, (V1) 453, (V2) 429tb
Sickle-cell disease, (ESG9) 16
Side effects
    of diuretics, (V1) 624b
    of medication, (V1) 488–489
Side-lying position, (V1) 644f
Siderail, (V1) 434, (V1) 749
SIGECAPS, depression and, (V2) 110
Sigma (σ), (V1) 702, (V1) 713
Sigma Theta Tau International (STTI), (V1) 18
Sigmoid colon, (V1) 653
Sigmoidoscopy, (V2) 666
Significant data, (V1) 63
Sikhism, (V1) 252
Silence, in communication, (V1) 351
Simple carbohydrate, (V1) 577
Sims' position, (V1) 751t, (V1) 752
    for catherization of woman, (V1) 644
    for rectal exam of man, (V1) 392
Simulation, as format for learning/teaching, (V1) 545
Single-lumen catheter, (V1) 641, (V1) 641f
Single order, (V1) 494
Single-parent family, (V1) 210, (V1) 215, (V2) 118
Sinoatrial (SA) node, (V1) 852
Sinus
    assessment of, (V1) 394, (V2) 266p–268p
    paranasal, (V1) 374f
Situational stressor, (V1) 551–552
Situational theory, (V1) 954
Skeletal muscles
    creating heat, (V1) 309–310
    function of, (V1) 726
Skeletal system, (V1) 725–726
Skepticism, reflective. See Reflective skepticism
Skilled nursing facility, (V1) 84
Skilled nursing services, (V1) 1034, (V1) 1034b
Skills
    in critical thinking, (V1) 26–27
    development of, (V1) 166
Skin
    of abdomen, (V1) 383
    assessment of, (V1) 393p, (V1) 448–449, (V1) 823b, (V1) 825, (V2) 239p–243p, (V2) 432
    at birth, (ESG9) 14
    care of, (V1) 831–832
    characteristics of, (V1) 366–368
    color variations, (V1) 366, (V1) 367t, (V2) 333
    defense against infection, (V1) 401
    dry, (V1) 449
    factors affecting, (V1) 447–448, (V1) 811–814
    fluid output, (V1) 891
    function of, (V1) 447
    hemorrhoids, (V1) 392
    impaired integrity of, (V1) 449
    impaired tactile perception, (V1) 687
    lesions of, (V1) 368, (V2) 244–247
    lotions, creams and ointments, (V1) 502

medication, application, *(V2) 513tb*
medication affecting, *(V1) 813–814*
mercury effect on, *(V1) 436t*
moisture on, *(V1) 813–814*
NOC outcomes and NIC interventions, *(V2) 435*
outcomes and interventions for diagnoses, *(V2) 795–796*
overview of, *(V2) 754*
perineal care, *(V1) 646*
self-care and, *(V1) 53*
structure of, *(V1) 447, (V1) 811, (V1) 812f*
surgery preparation, *(V1) 933, (V1) 941*
treatment for poisoning, of, *(V1) 424*
tuberculin test, reading, *(V2) 866*
tuberculosis screening, *(V1) 874*
turgor of, *(V1) 813*
variations by age, *(V1) 812*
Skin cancer, ABCDE, *(V1) 368*
Skin elasticity, *(V1) 813*
Skinfold measurement, *(V1) 602–603, (V2) 579tb*
Skin tag, *(V1) 368*
Skull, *(ESG9) 13f*
assessment of, *(V1) 393–394*
infant
bones of, *(ESG9) 13*
shape of, *(V1) 370*
Slander, *(V1) 1078*
Sleep
"Back to Sleep" campaign, *(ESG9) 18f*
circadian rhythms influencing, *(V1) 795*
cycles of, *(V1) 798*
definition of, *(V1) 793–794*
deprivation of, *(V1) 801*
diary of, *(V2) 752*
disorder of, *(V1) 800–801*
factors affecting, *(V1) 799–800*
as health factor, *(V1) 174*
health promotion and, *(V1) 1016*
history and diary, *(V1) 804*
history of, *(V2) 751*
hygiene, *(V1) 807*
illness and, *(V1) 794, (V1) 794f, (V1) 800*
importance of, *(V1) 568*
medication for, *(V1) 807–808*
outcomes and interventions for diagnoses, *(V2) 752*
overview of, *(V2) 741*
patterns of, *(V1) 804, (ESG9) 16*
physiology of, *(V1) 795*
promoting host defense of infection, *(V1) 405*
prone position, *(ESG9) 18*
purpose of, *(V1) 794*
quality of, *(V1) 799–800*
regulation of, *(V1) 796, (V1) 796f*
requirements for, *(V1) 794–795, (V1) 795t*
stages of, *(V1) 796–798, (V1) 797t*
Sleep apnea, *(V1) 801–802, (V1) 857*
Sleep-provoked disorder, *(V1) 803*
Sleeptalking, *(V1) 803*
Sleep-wake cycle
disorder of, *(V1) 801*
time zone affecting, *(V1) 795*
Sleepwalking (somnambulism), *(V1) 802–803*
Slough, *(V1) 825*
Slow-wave sleep (SWS), *(V1) 797*
Small-group communication, *(V1) 339*
Small intestine
segments of, *(V1) 652–653*
view of, *(V1) 652f*

Smallpox vaccination, *(V1) 1030*
Smell
bedside assessment of, *(V2) 681*
impaired, *(V1) 686–687*
olfactory deficit, *(V1) 695–696*
Smoking
adolescence and, *(ESG9) 29*
as cause of home fire, *(V1) 425*
cessation of, *(V1) 858b*
as health risk factor, *(V1) 174*
infection, risk of, *(V1) 405*
oral problems and, *(V1) 460*
oxygenation and, *(V1) 857–858*
respiration and, *(V1) 323*
skin integrity, *(V1) 814*
sleep and, *(V1) 800*
teratogenic effect on fetus, *(ESG9) 9*
Smooth muscle, *(V1) 726–727*
Snellen chart, *(V1) 371–372*
Snoring, *(V1) 802*
SOAP charting, *(V1) 291–292, (V2) 178*
Social distance, *(V1) 343–344*
Social functioning, *(V1) 189*
Social history, *(V1) 46*
Social identity, *(V1) 190*
Social interaction, impaired, *(V1) 196*
Socialization, *(V1) 15, (V1) 227*
Social justice, *(V1) 1052t*
Social justice model, *(V1) 1068*
Social organization
culture care etiquette, *(V1) 242t*
as culture specific influencing health, *(V1) 229*
Social Union Framework Agreement (SUFA), *(ESGV1) 8*
Societal trends, *(V1) 21*
Socioeconomic status
as cause of depression, *(V1) 201, (V1) 201t*
communication and, *(V1) 344*
self-concept and, *(V1) 189–190*
Sodium (Na⁺)
function and regulation of, *(V1) 892t*
recommended intake of, *(V1) 893*
restricted diet, *(V1) 601*
Sodium bicarbonate (NaHCO₃⁻), *(V1) 895*
Sodomy, *(V1) 778*
Soft diet, mechanical, *(V1) 601*
Soft spots (fontanelles), *(ESG9) 13, (ESG9) 13f*
Soldiers. *See* Military
Solid waste, reduction of, *(V1) 431*
Solubility, of drug, *(V1) 479*
Solute, *(V1) 887*
Solution
determining, *(V1) 985*
for enema, *(V1) 669t*
for enteral nutrition, *(V1) 615b*
hypotonic and hypertonic, *(V1) 889*
for intravenous (IV) administration, *(V1) 906*
Lactated Ringer's, *(V1) 519*
Somatic nervous system, *(V1) 728*
Somatization
adaptation failure and, *(V1) 563*
Somatoform disorder
adaptation failure and, *(V1) 563*
Somnambulism (sleepwalking), *(V1) 802–803*
Sound vibration, *(V1) 374*
Source-oriented record, *(V1) 290*
Spacity, *(V1) 740b*
Spanish words and phrases, *(V2) 219*

Special needs assessment, *(V1) 43*
Specific deduction, *(V1) 143*
Specific gravity, *(V1) 622, (V1) 634*
of urine, *(V1) 903*
of urine, measurement, *(V2) 622tb*
Specific immunity, *(V1) 402*
Specimen, sputum
expectorated, *(V1) 864p*
obtaining by suction, *(V1) 864p*
Speculum examination, *(V1) 391, (V2) 328–329*
Speech
general survey of client, *(V1) 365*
impaired, *(V1) 355*
Sphincter, *(V1) 653, (V1) 654f*
Sphygmomanometer, *(V1) 329, (V2) 214–215*
Spina bifida, *(ESG9) 12*
Spinal alterations, *(V1) 378, (V1) 385*
Spinal anesthesia, *(V1) 939, (V1) 939f*
Spinal cord, *(V1) 702*
Spine
curves of, *(V1) 729, (V1) 729f*
deformity assessment, *(V2) 301*
SPIRIT, as assessment tool, *(V1) 256*
Spiritual assessment, *(V1) 256*
Spiritual care
barriers to, *(V1) 254–255*
as concept of Watson's theory, *(V1) 153*
history of, *(V1) 246*
intervention, *(V1) 116, (V1) 257*
making referrals, *(V1) 259*
nursing activities for, *(V1) 258*
prayer, *(V1) 259–260*
Spiritual development theory, *(V1) 168*
overview of, *(ESG9) 8*
stages of, *(ESG9) 9t*
Spiritual distress, *(V1) 256–257, (V1) 259*
Spiritual healing, *(V1) 260*
Spiritual health assessment, *(V1) 44*
Spiritual intervention, *(V1) 258–259*
Spirituality
addressing for dying patient, *(V1) 284*
affecting health, *(V1) 249–250*
assessment guidelines and tools, *(V2) 151–152*
comparing to religion, *(V1) 247t*
core issues of, *(V1) 248–249*
diagnoses, *(V1) 256–258*
differences in, *(V1) 255*
as factor influencing hygiene practice, *(V1) 442–443*
grieving process and, *(V1) 268*
health and, *(V1) 175–176*
holism and, *(V1) 990*
journey of, *(V1) 248*
knowledge map for, *(V2) 157*
lack of awareness, *(V1) 254–255*
NIC interventions and activities, *(V2) 153tb–154tb*
nursing and, *(V1) 5*
overview of, *(V2) 147*
providing postmortem care, *(V1) 285*
as support system, *(V1) 572*
Spiritual Literacy: Reading the Sacred in Everyday Life, (V1) 248
Spirometry, *(V1) 849*
Splints, *(V1) 750*
Sports massage, *(V1) 999*
Sprain, *(V1) 738*
Sputum
assessment of, *(V1) 862–863*
specimen collection, *(V2) 803p–808p*

Sputum *(continued)*
    expectorated, *(V2) 805p*
    suctioned, *(V2) 806p–807p*
St. John's wort, *(V1) 207*
Stagnation, *(ESG9) 33*
Standardized (model) nursing care plan
    adapting to patient needs, *(V1) 89*
    computer printout for, *(V1) 88f*
    individualizing, *(V1) 92*
Standardized nursing language
    computer care systems, *(V1) 114*
    definition of, *(V1) 69–70*
    for electronic health record (EHR),
        (V1) 979–980
    holistic care and, *(V1) 115–116*
    planning interventions/implementations,
        (V1) 113
    purpose of, *(V1) 70*
    writing diagnostic statements, *(V1) 69–70*
Standard precautions, *(V1) 410, (V1) 411b,*
        (V2) 341tb
Standards, *(V1) 582*
Standards of care, *(V1) 1075*
Standards of practice, *(V1) 1075–1076*
    American Nurses Association (ANA),
        (V1) 17t
    Canadian Nurses Association (CNA),
        (V1) 18b
    nursing governed by, *(V1) 16*
Standards of Professional Performance,
        (V1) 1061b, (V1) 1076b
Standard syringe, *(V1) 508, (V1) 508f*
Standard written orders, *(V1) 494*
Standing assist device, *(V1) 756, (V1) 756f*
Standing order, *(V1) 494*
Staples, *(V2) 783tb*
Starch, *(V1) 577f*
Startle reflex, *(ESG9) 14*
Stasis ulcer, *(V2) 246*
Stat, *(V1) 296*
State board of registered nursing (BRN)
    continuing education requirements, *(V1) 15*
    responsibilities of, *(V1) 16*
State law, *(V1) 1074–1075*
Statement, theory and, *(V1) 142*
Stat medication, *(V1) 296*
STAT order, *(V1) 494*
Status, community, *(V1) 1022*
Statute, *(V1) 1071*
Statutory rape, *(V1) 779–780*
Stepfamily, *(V1) 210*
Stepping reflex, *(ESG9) 14, (ESG9) 14f*
Stereognosis, *(V1) 389*
Stereotyping
    as barrier to culturally competent care,
        (V1) 237
    as barrier to therapeutic communication,
        (V1) 353–354
    definition of, *(V1) 69*
    of man as nurse, *(V1) 9, (V1) 10f*
    of nurse, *(V1) 4–10, (V2) 6*
Sterile, *(V1) 413–416*
    attire, *(V1) 414–415*
    fields, *(V1) 416*
    technique, *(V1) 415–416*
Sterile field
    creation of, *(V1) 937*
    preparing and maintaining, *(V2)*
        357p–359p
Sterile gloves
    applying, closed method, *(V2) 352p–354p*
    applying, open method, *(V2) 355p–356p*

Sterile gown
    donning, closed method, *(V2) 352p–354p*
Sterile team, *(V1) 937*
Sterile technique, *(V2) 343tb*
Sterility
    retrograde ejaculation, *(V1) 781*
    sexually transmitted infection (STI),
        (V1) 778
Sterilization, *(V1) 408*
Steri-Strips (adhesive strips), *(V1) 818,*
        (V2) 782tb
Sterols, *(V1) 579, (V1) 579b*
Stertor, *(V1) 325*
Stigma, of mental illness, *(V1) 177*
Stiller, Ben, *(V1) 10*
Still Me, (V1) 176, (V1) 191
Stimulant
    sexual function and, *(V1) 774t*
Stimulus, *(V1) 680*
Stock supply, *(V1) 478*
Stoma
    assessment of, *(V1) 671–672*
    bowel elimination from, *(V1) 657*
    color of, *(V1) 671f*
    urinary elimination from, *(V1) 638*
    view of, *(V1) 638f*
Stomach, function of, *(V1) 651*
Stomatitis, *(V1) 375, (V1) 460*
Stool
    handling specimen of, *(V1) 661*
    occult blood, testing for, *(V2)*
        640p–643p
    removing digitally, *(V1) 662p–663p,*
        (V1) 670, (V2) 650p–653p
    traditional Chinese medicine (TCM),
        (V1) 993
    See also Feces
Storm, electrical, *(V1) 431*
Strabismus, *(V1) 685b*
Straight catheter, *(V1) 641, (V1) 641f,*
        (V1) 643f
Strain, *(V1) 738*
Strategy, *(V1) 105*
Stratum corneum, *(V1) 811*
Stratum germinativum, *(V1) 811*
Street drugs, *(V1) 492*
Stress, *(V1) 565*
    adaptation versus disease, *(V1) 553–554*
    assessment of, *(V1) 564–565*
    assessment questions, *(V2) 552–553*
    blood pressure and, *(V1) 329*
    body temperature and, *(V1) 309*
    coping approaches to, *(V1) 553*
    definition of, *(V1) 551*
    diagnosis associated with, *(V1) 566b*
    emotional response to, *(V1) 565*
    "fight or flight", *(V1) 555*
    irritable bowel syndrome, *(V1) 655*
    knowledge map of, *(V2) 556*
    life-changing events and, *(V1) 1012*
    management techniques, *(V1) 570*
    mobility and activity, *(V1) 735*
    outcomes and interventions for diagnoses,
        (V2) 554
    overview of, *(V2) 542*
    oxygenation and, *(V1) 855*
    peristalsis and, *(V1) 656*
    physiological responses to, *(V1) 565,*
        (V1) 565b
    psychological responses to, *(V1) 558–562,*
        (V1) 559b, (V1) 565
    pulse rate, *(V1) 318*

    reduction for promoting host defense of
        infection, *(V1) 405*
    Rescue Remedy for, *(V1) 994–995*
    respiration and, *(V1) 323*
    response-based model of, *(V1) 552–554*
    sensory function and, *(V1) 683*
    shock and countershock phase of,
        (V1) 555
    spiritual response to, *(V1) 562*
    in workplace, *(V1) 572*
Stress and adaptation theory, *(V1) 151*
Stressor
    changing perception of, *(V1) 571*
    coping approaches to, *(V1) 553*
    definition of, *(V1) 551*
    general adaptation syndrome (GAP),
        (V1) 554–557, (V1) 555f
    physiological responses to, *(V1) 565b*
    response to, *(V1) 554*
    types of, *(V1) 551–552*
Stress urinary incontinence
    care map for, *(V1) 631*
    nursing care plan for, *(V1) 627–630*
Striae, *(V1) 368*
Stridor, *(V1) 325, (V1) 863*
Stroke, *(V1) 938*
Stroke volume, *(V1) 317*
Structural-functional theory, *(V1) 212–213*
Structure, community, *(V1) 1022*
Structure evaluation, *(V1) 131*
Student, liability insurance, *(V1) 1089*
Student care plan
    individualized, *(V1) 89, (V1) 91*
    as learning activity, *(V1) 91*
    mind-mapping, *(V1) 91–92*
Study of the Ethical Problems in Medicine,
        (V1) 270
Subconjunctival hemorrhage, *(V1) 371,*
        (V2) 334
Subculture, *(V1) 225*
Subcutaneous injection
    administration of, *(V1) 524p, (V2)*
        489p–492p
    of opioids, *(V1) 715*
    overview of, *(V1) 513–515*
    sites for, *(V1) 513f*
Subcutaneous layer, of skin, *(V1) 811*
Subject, rights in research study,
        (V1) 158
Subjective cue, *(V1) 75*
Subjective data, *(V1) 42t*
    definition of, *(V2) 20*
    of nail care, *(V1) 458*
    of skin assessment, *(V1) 448*
Sublimation, *(V1) 561t*
Sublingual medication, *(V1) 500*
Subluxation, *(V1) 998*
Subscriber, *(V1) 976*
Substance abuse
    in adolescence, *(ESG9) 28*
    drug-addicted baby, *(ESG9) 15*
    infection, risk of, *(V1) 405*
    oxygenation and, *(V1) 858*
    pain management with, *(V1) 719*
    in workplace, *(V1) 1088b*
Substance P, *(V1) 702*
Substernal retraction, *(V1) 325–326*
Substitutive effect, *(V1) 488*
Subsystem, *(V1) 151–152, (V1) 212*
Sucking reflex, *(ESG9) 14*
Sudden infant death syndrome (SIDS),
        (ESG9) 9

Suffocation, *(V1) 427*
Suicide
  assisted, *(V1) 273, (V1) 275*
  of child or adolescent, *(V1) 422,*
    (ESG9) 28
  diagnosis of risk for, *(V1) 205*
  goal/outcome statement, *(V1) 206*
Sunlight, bilirubin and, *(ESG9) 15*
Superego, *(V1) 167, (ESG9) 5*
Superficial pain, *(V1) 699–700*
Superficial reflexes, *(V1) 389*
Superficial vein, *(V1) 910f*
Superficial wound, *(V1) 816*
Superinfection, *(V1) 406*
Supination
  assessment of, *(V2) 305p–306p*
  as movement, *(V1) 727f*
Supine position, *(V1) 751t, (V1) 752*
Supplemental food program for women,
    infants and children (WIC),
    (V1) 608
Supplements
  client history and current use of, *(V1) 46*
Supportive effect, *(V1) 488*
Support system
  assessment of, *(V1) 565–566, (V1) 690*
  as factor of stress outcome, *(V1) 553–554*
  family as, *(V1) 175*
  identifying and using, *(V1) 572*
  teaching about pain, *(V1) 720*
Suppository, *(V2) 471p–473p*
Suppressor T cell, *(V1) 404*
Suprapubic catheter, *(V1) 643, (V1) 643f*
Suprasystem, *(V1) 212*
Surface temperature, *(V1) 307*
Surfactant, *(V1) 847*
Surgery
  attire for, *(V1) 414–415*
  classification of, *(V1) 924*
  informed consent for, *(V1) 931–932*
  intraoperative phase of, *(V1) 936*
  operative team, *(V1) 936–937*
  pain conduction pathway, *(V1) 718*
  peristalsis and, *(V1) 656–657*
  positioning of patient, *(V1) 941–942*
  preoperative phase, *(V1) 923*
  preoperative screening tests, *(V2) 929*
  preparing patient physically for, *(V1)*
    932–935
  recovery from, *(V1) 942–949*
  risk factors for, *(V1) 924–925*
  room preparation after, *(V2) 927tb*
  skin preparation, *(V1) 933, (V1) 941*
  sterile fields, *(V1) 416*
  sterile technique, *(V1) 415–416*
  urination and, *(V1) 625*
  for wound closure, *(V1) 818*
Surgical asepsis, *(V1) 413*
Surgical glue, of wound, *(V1) 818*
Surgical hand washing, *(V1) 414p,*
    (V2) 349p–351p
Surgical scrub, *(V1) 413*
Surgical staples, of wound, *(V1) 818*
Surgical unit
  postoperative nursing care, *(V1) 943*
Survey, general
  aspects of, *(V1) 365*
  assessment of, *(V1) 393p*
  documentation of, *(V1) 392–393*
Susceptible host, *(V1) 400*
Sustained fever, *(V1) 314*
Sustained-release drug, *(V1) 479*

Sutures
  of newborn skull, *(ESG9) 13, (ESG9) 13f*
  removal of, *(V2) 783tb*
  for wound closure, *(V1) 818*
Swabbing, of wound, *(V1) 829*
Swallowing, impaired, *(V2) 580*
Swallowing reflex, *(ESG9) 14*
Sweat glands, *(V1) 447*
Sweating, *(V1) 307*
Swedish massage
  strokes of, *(V1) 998*
Sympathectomy, *(V1) 718*
Sympathetic nervous system
  cardiovascular disease, *(V1) 855*
  response to alarm of stressor, *(V1) 556*
Symptom
  sleep pattern as, *(V1) 805*
  as stage of illness behavior, *(V1) 179–180*
Synarthroses, *(V1) 726*
Syndactylism, *(V1) 737*
Syndrome nursing diagnosis, *(V1) 62–63,*
    (V1) 62f, (V1) 75
Synergistic drug relationship, *(V1) 491*
Synovial fluid, *(V1) 726*
Synovial joint
  characteristics of, *(V1) 726*
  types of, *(V1) 728t*
Syphilitic chancre, *(V2) 336*
Syringe
  disposal of, *(V1) 511f*
  mixing medication using same,
    (V1) 510, (V2) 479p–482p,
    (V2) 517tb
  needless connector, *(V1) 511f*
  safety, *(V1) 511f*
  types of, *(V1) 507–509, (V1) 508f*
System
  concept of, *(V1) 151*
  elements of, *(V1) 152*
Systemic circulation, *(V1) 380*
Systemic effect, *(V1) 479*
Systemic infection, *(V1) 401*
System theory, *(V1) 151–152*
Systole, *(V1) 317, (V1) 380, (V1) 852*
Systolic pressure, *(V1) 326–327*

T
T'ai Chi, *(V1) 999, (V1) 1000f*
Tachycardia, *(V1) 320*
Tachypnea, *(V1) 324*
Tactile deficit, *(V1) 813*
  intervention for, *(V1) 696*
  safety and health measures, *(V1) 696*
Tactile perception
  bedside assessment of, *(V2) 681*
  impaired, *(V1) 687*
Taenia coli, *(V1) 653*
Take-home toxin, *(V1) 428*
Talk test, *(V1) 732b*
Tandem set, IV infusion, *(V2) 511p*
Tandem setup, IV infusion, *(V1) 520,*
    (V1) 520f
Tanner staging, *(V2) 324, (ESG9) 27t*
Tanning, skin integrity and, *(V1) 814*
Tape, *(V1) 840, (V1) 840f*
Taped report, *(V1) 300*
Tapotement, *(V1) 998*
Target area, blood flow to, *(V1) 484*
Target heart rate, *(V1) 732b*
Task focus, *(V1) 954*
Task Force on Community Preventive
    Services, *(V1) 1018*

Task group, *(V1) 347*
Task model, *(ESGV1) 9*
Task-relationship theory, *(V1) 954*
Taste
  bedside assessment of, *(V2) 681*
  effect of medicine on, *(V1) 686b*
  impaired, *(V1) 686*
  olfactory deficit, *(V1) 695–696*
  sensory perceptual health, *(V1) 693*
Tattoo, *(V1) 814*
Taxonomy
  components of NANDA nursing
    diagnosis, *(V1) 71–72*
  definition of, *(V1) 70–71*
  of diagnostic terminology, *(V1) 71*
Taxonomy II, *(V1) 71, (V2) 39–40*
Taxonomy of Nursing Practice
    (NANDA/NOC/NIC), *(V1) 51b*
T cell lymphocyte, *(V1) 402*
  function of, *(V1) 403t*
Teaching
  abdomen care, *(V2) 299*
  abuse, prevention and intervention
    for, *(V2) 92*
  adult learning, principles of, *(V1) 535b*
  apical pulse assessment, *(V2) 209*
  apical-radial pulse assessment, *(V2) 211*
  approaches to, *(V1) 534*
  assessment of learner, *(V1) 537*
  barriers to, *(V1) 536, (V1) 537b*
  bed bath, *(V2) 394*
  bed-monitoring device, *(V2) 370*
  blood pressure assessment, *(V2) 216*
  Bloom's domains of learning, *(V1) 531t*
  breast self-examination, *(V2) 279*
  clean-catch specimen, collecting, *(V2) 597*
  contact lenses, removing and care for,
    (V2) 423
  coughing, deep breathing, moving in
    bed, leg exercises, *(V1) 934p,*
    (V2) 918p–921p
  culturally competent, *(V1) 536b*
  deficient knowledge, *(V1) 538–540*
  definition of, *(V1) 529*
  dental care, *(V2) 271*
  documentation of, *(V1) 547*
  domains of learning, *(V1) 529–530,*
    (V1) 539t
  evaluation of learning, *(V1) 547*
  factors affecting learning, *(V1) 531–533*
  fingerstick blood glucose levels, *(V2) 565*
  foot care, *(V2) 404*
  gastric and enteric tube feedings, *(V2) 575*
  importance of, *(V1) 528*
  incentive spirometry, *(V1) 874*
  intermittent infusion administration,
    (V2) 512
  intradermal medication administration,
    (V2) 486–488
  Intravenous medication administration,
    (V2) 507
  knowledge map of, *(V2) 539*
  learners, *(V1) 528–529*
  learning assessment guidelines and tools,
    (V2) 536
  lung disease risk factors, *(V2) 285*
  materials for, *(V1) 540*
  medication administration, *(V2) 452*
  medications producing sleep, *(V1) 807*
  nasal medication administration, *(V2) 467*
  nasogastric and nasoenteric tubes
    insertion, *(V2) 571*

Teaching (continued)
  nasogastric and nasoenteric tubes removal, (V2) 578
  ophthalmic medication administration, (V2) 461–462
  oral care for unconscious patient, (V2) 413
  outcome of, (V1) 538–540
  overview of, (V2) 527
  perineal care, (V2) 401
  postoperative, (V1) 948–949
  preoperative, (V1) 932, (V1) 933b
  pressure ulcers prevention, (V1) 833
  protective isolation, maintaining, (V2) 342tb
  pulse rate assessment, (V2) 207
  rectal suppository administration, (V2) 475
  respiration assessment, (V2) 213
  responsibilities of, (V1) 529
  restraints, reason for using, (V2) 374
  rights of, (V1) 530b
  scheduling sessions for, (V1) 533, (V1) 540
  sexual health, (V1) 783, (V1) 788–789
  shampooing bedrest patient, (V2) 417
  skin assessment, (V2) 243
  sleep hygiene, (V1) 807
  strategies for, (V1) 540, (V1) 544–547
  subcutaneous medication administration, (V2) 491
  temperature assessment, (V2) 202
Teaching plan, (V1) 91
  creation of, (V1) 540
  example of, (V1) 541–543
  outcome for special, (V1) 100
Team nursing, (ESGV1) 21
Technique
  accurate blood pressure assessment, (V2) 217tb
  advocacy guidelines, (V2) 1013tb
  angry patients, (V2) 549tb
  artificial eye, care for, (V2) 430tb
  aspiration, prevention of, (V2) 861tb
  auscultation, performance of, (V2) 234t
  autogenic training, (V2) 964tb
  bandage application, (V2) 788tb–790tb
  binder application, (V2) 786tb–788tb
  biological variations, assessment of, (V2) 140tb
  body mechanics, principles of, (V2) 716tb
  breathing assessment, (V2) 860tb
  for calming patient, (V2) 964tb
  closed-wound drainage system, emptying, (V2) 785tb
  cold application, (V2) 792tb
  communication
    hearing-impaired, (V2) 679tb
    with language barrier, (V2) 144tb
    visually impaired, (V2) 679tb
  crisis intervention guidelines, (V2) 550
  cultural information, obtaining, (V2) 141tb
  depression, identification for referral, (V2) 110tb
  dipstick testing of urine, (V2) 621tb
  documentation guidelines, (V2) 183tb–184tb, (V2) 1022tb
  dressings, taping, (V2) 786tb
  dying, patient care, (V2) 168tb–169tb
  endotracheal airway, patient care, (V2) 863tb

  enteral nutrition (tube feeding), monitoring, (V2) 582tb
  epidural catheter, care for, (V2) 691tb
  equipment safety, (V2) 10021tb
  family, assessment of, (V2) 124tb
  feeding tube placement, (V2) 581tb
  Giger and Davidhizar's transcultural assessment model, (V2) 143tb
  grieving, communicating with, (V2) 166tb
  guided imagery, (V2) 966tb
  hearing aids, care for, (V2) 431tb
  heat application, (V2) 791tb
  helping family with dying patient, (V2) 167tb
  heparin, administering subcutaneously, (V2) 518tb
  humor, (V2) 965tb
  impaired swallowing, intervention for, (V2) 580
  indwelling catheter
    care for, (V2) 623tb–624tb
    removal of, (V2) 625tb
  malpractice, avoiding, (V2) 1021tb–1022tb
  massage, (V2) 966tb
  meals, assisting patient, (V2) 580
  measuring circumference for body composition, (V2) 579tb
  measuring dosage, changing needles, (V2) 516tb
  meditation, (V2) 965tb
  mixing medication using same syringe, (V2) 517tb
  MORAL model, (V2) 1013tb
  nasopharyngeal airway, insertion of, (V2) 863tb
  nonverbal communication, (V2) 225tb
  operative field, creating, (V2) 927tb
  oral reporting, (V2) 182tb
  orders, telephone and oral, (V2) 182tb
  oropharyngeal airway, insertion of, (V2) 862tb
  oxygen therapy safety precautions, (V2) 862tb
  pain perception assessment, cultural groups, (V2) 142tb
  parenteral nutrition, monitoring patient, (V2) 582tb
  percussion, (V2) 233t
  physical conditioning for walking, (V2) 718tb
  pinworm testing, (V2) 663tb
  postmortem care, (V2) 169tb–170tb
  prefilled unit-dose system, (V2) 514tb
  range of motion (ROM), passive, (V2) 717tb
  reconstitution of medication, (V2) 515tb
  rectal tube, (V2) 664tb
  relaxation therapy, (V2) 967tb
  room preparation after surgery, (V2) 927tb
  self-concept, assessment of problems, (V2) 108tb
  self-esteem inventory, performing, (V2) 109tb
  sensory deficits, communication with client, (V2) 226tb
  sexual health history, (V2) 733tb
  shower or tub, assisting with, (V2) 429tb
  skin, application to, (V2) 513tb
  Spanish words and phrases, (V2) 225tb
  specific gravity of urine measurement, (V2) 622tb

  spiritual diagnosis, NIC interventions and activities, (V2) 153tb–154tb
  standard precautions, following, (V2) 341tb
  for sterile technique, (V2) 343tb
  Steri-Strips, placing, (V2) 782tb
  sutures and staples, removing, (V2) 783tb
  therapeutic touch, (V2) 967tb
  transmission-based precautions, following, (V2) 342tb
  tricep skinfold measuring, (V2) 579tb
  trochanter roll, making, (V2) 717tb
  twenty-four hour specimen, (V2) 620tb
  urinary diversion, (V2) 628tb
  urinary incontinence (UI), (V2) 626tb–627tb
  urine measurement, indwelling catheter, (V2) 619tb
  urine specimen from catheter, (V2) 620tb
  urine specimen, measuring and obtaining, (V2) 619tb
  walking aids
    instruction for using, (V2) 719tb–720tb
    sizing, (V2) 718tb
  wound drain, shortening, (V2) 784tb
Technology
  advances in, (V1) 23
  as culture specific influencing health, (V1) 229
  healthcare delivery factor, (ESGV1) 12
Teeth
  assessment of, (V1) 375
  brushing and flossing, (V1) 462, (V2) 406p–408p
  development of, (V1) 459, (V1) 459f
  eruption in infant, (ESG9) 16
  unconscious patient, care of, (V2) 411p–413p
Telehealth, (ESGV1) 12, (V1) 976–977, (V1) 976f
Teleology, (V1) 1057
Telephone
  counseling by, (V1) 1017
  as electronic communication source, (V1) 974–975
  medical orders by, (V1) 300–301, (V1) 494
Temperature
  assessment of, (V1) 311f
  assessment procedure, (V2) 198–199
  axillary, (V2) 201p
  benefits of fever, (V1) 314–315
  chemical strip method, (V2) 201p
  dangers of extreme, (V1) 315
  equipment for, (V1) 312–313
  factors influencing, (V1) 309–310
  hypovolemia and, (V1) 896
  normal for adults, (V1) 306t
  oral, (V2) 199p
  overview of, (V2) 191
  of patient's room, (V1) 469
  ranges for normal and altered, (V1) 307f
  rectal, (V2) 200p
  risk for imbalanced, (V1) 315
  sites for measurement of, (V1) 313–314
  of skin, (V1) 367
  thermometer for assessment of, (V1) 310f
  tympanic membrane, (V2) 202p
  variations of, (V1) 307
  as vital sign (VS), (V1) 305
  water maintaining, (V1) 582
Temple, (V1) 4

Temporal pulse, *(V2) 206p*
Temporary bowel diversion, *(V1) 657*
Temporomandibular joint (TMJ) syndrome, *(V1) 370*
Tendon, *(V1) 726*
Tension pneumothorax, *(V1) 882*
Tenting, of skin, *(V1) 368*
Teratogen, *(ESG9) 9*
Terminal evaluation, *(V1) 131*
Terminology
    client understanding of, *(V1) 49*
    diagnosis, *(V1) 57, (V1) 58t*
    NANDA taxonomy of diagnostic, *(V1) 71*
    Nursing Outcomes Classification (NOC), *(V1) 92, (V1) 97*
    standardized nursing language, *(V1) 69–70*
Territoriality, *(V1) 344*
Tertiary defense, infection, *(V1) 402–404*
Tertiary intention healing, *(V1) 816, (V1) 817f*
Testicular self-exam (TSE), *(ESG9) 31*
    in adolescence, *(ESG9) 31b*
    self-care and, *(V1) 53*
    in young adult, *(ESG9) 32–33*
Testosterone, *(V1) 770*
Tetanus-prone wound, *(V1) 826*
Teutonic Knights, *(V1) 8*
Texture
    of hair, *(V1) 369*
    of nails, *(V1) 369*
    of skin, *(V1) 368*
Theology, *(V1) 247*
Theoretical framework, *(V1) 142*
Theoretical knowledge, *(V1) 29*
    of diagnosis, *(V1) 68*
    recognizing cues, *(V1) 63*
Theorist
    caring, *(V1) 146–147*
    nursing
        Florence Nightingale, *(V1) 145*
        Hildegard Peplau, *(V1) 146*
        Virginia Henderson, *(V1) 146*
Theory
    components of, *(V1) 141–142*
    definition of, *(V1) 141*
    development of, *(V1) 143*
    for family care, *(V1) 211–213*
    of grief, a comparison, *(V1) 266t*
    influencing choice of intervention, *(V1) 106*
    nurses using, *(V1) 144–145*
    nursing
        components of, *(V1) 144f*
        concepts of, *(V1) 144*
    practical knowledge about, *(V1) 152*
    trait, *(V1) 953*
Theory X, *(V1) 955–956*
Theory Y, *(V1) 955–956*
Therapeutic bath, *(V1) 454*
Therapeutic communication
    barriers to, *(V1) 351–354*
    characteristics of, *(V1) 346–347*
    as client-centered, *(V1) 346*
    for depression-related diagnoses, *(V1) 206*
    for dying and grieving, *(V1) 282*
    enhancement of, *(V1) 349–351*
    grief work, facilitating, *(V2) 158*
    overview of, *(V2) 219*
Therapeutic effect, *(V1) 488*
Therapeutic level, of drug, *(V1) 486*
Therapeutic range, of drug, *(V1) 486*

Therapeutic relationship
    communication
        overview of, *(V2) 219*
        role of, *(V1) 345–346*
    phases of, *(V1) 346*
Therapeutic touch (TT)
    benefits of, *(V1) 999*
    centering and healing, *(V1) 1000b*
    as holistic therapy, *(V2) 967tb*
    for pain relief, *(V1) 711*
    for stress management, *(V1) 570*
Therapy, CAM, *(V1) 47*
Therapy group, *(V1) 348*
Thermal stimuli, *(V1) 701*
Thermogenesis, *(V1) 308*
Thermometer
    electronic and tympanic, *(V1) 310*
    glass, *(V1) 310f*
    types of, *(V1) 312–313, (V1) 312f*
Thermoreceptor, *(V1) 681*
Thermoregulation, *(ESG9) 13*
    definition of, *(V1) 307*
    ineffective, *(V1) 315*
Thermostat, of body, *(V1) 314*
Theta wave, *(V1) 796, (V1) 796f*
Thiazide diuretics, *(V1) 624b*
Thinking
    clinical, *(V1) 10*
    complex, *(V1) 28t*
    independent, *(V1) 27*
Thinking skills, *(V1) 27*
Thoracic cavity, *(V1) 323f*
Three-bottle system, *(V1) 881, (V1) 881f,*
Thrill, *(V1) 381*
Thrombophlebitis
    as IV therapy complication, *(V1) 917t*
    as postoperative collaborative problem, *(V1) 946t*
    SCD for, *(V1) 948, (V1) 948f*
Thrombosis, *(V1) 917t*
Thrombus, *(V1) 884*
Throughput, *(V1) 152*
Thrush, *(V1) 375*
Thumb ROM, *(V1) 743t–744t*
Thyroid cartilage, *(V1) 376, (V1) 376f*
Thyroid gland, *(V1) 376*
Thyroid hormone, *(V1) 891*
Thyroid-stimulation hormone (TSH), *(V1) 555*
Thyroxine, *(V1) 308*
Tidal volume (V_T), *(V1) 324, 849*
Time inventory, personal, *(V1) 967*
Time management
    components of, *(V1) 969t*
    importance of, *(V1) 568*
    knowledge map for, *(V2) 948*
    overview of, *(V2) 942*
    setting goals for, *(V1) 967*
    work organization, *(V1) 967–968*
    work smarter, not harder, *(V1) 968b*
Time orientation
    culture care etiquette, *(V1) 242t*
    as culture specific influencing health, *(V1) 228*
Time-release drug, *(V1) 479*
Time-sequenced work plan, *(V1) 123*
Timing
    24-hour/military, *(V1) 302*
    communication process, *(V1) 341*
    learning and, *(V1) 532*
    pharmacokinetics and, *(V1) 488*

promoting normal defecation, *(V1) 666*
    urination and, *(V1) 623*
Tinea pedis, *(V1) 455–456*
Tissue biopsy
    of wound, *(V1) 829*
Tissue oxygenation, *(V1) 899*
Tissue protein, *(V1) 605*
TMJ (temporomandibular joint) syndrome, *(V1) 370*
Tobacco
    oxygenation and, *(V1) 857*
Toddler
    abdomen of, *(V2) 294*
    assessment of, *(ESG9) 21*
    baby-bottle tooth decay, *(V1) 459*
    body fluid of, *(V1) 888t*
    bowel elimination patterns, *(V1) 655*
    development of, *(ESG9) 19–21*
    health problems, *(ESG9) 21*
    health promotion and screenings, *(V1) 1010t*
    intervention for, *(ESG9) 21*
    milestones of, *(ESG9) 20b*
    modification of assessment for, *(V1) 363–364*
    nutritional needs, *(V1) 595*
    oxygenation of, *(V1) 854*
    poisoning of, *(V1) 422, (V1) 422b*
    safety of, *(V1) 421*
    sexual development, *(V1) 768*
    sleep requirement, *(V1) 795, (V1) 795t*
    suffocation and asphyxiation prevention, *(V1) 427*
    teeth development, *(V1) 459, (V1) 459f*
Toenail, ingrown, *(V1) 456*
Toes ROM, *(V1) 745t–746t*
Toileting
    as activity of daily living (ADL), *(V1) 43b*
    facilitating routines, *(V1) 639*
    self-care deficit, *(V1) 445, (V2) 434*
    of toddler, *(ESG9) 19*
Tolerance
    of opioids, *(V1) 713*
    of pain, *(V1) 702*
Tone, high- and low-pitched, *(V1) 373–374*
Tongue
    abnormal findings of, *(V1) 375*
    geographic, *(V1) 375f*
Tonicity, *(V1) 889*
Tonic neck reflex, *(ESG9) 14, (ESG9) 14f*
Tonsils
    of children, *(V2) 271*
    enlargement of, *(V2) 334*
Topical anesthesia, *(V1) 717, (V1) 938*
Topical medication, *(V1) 502–504*
Tort law, *(V1) 1078*
Torturer, nurse as, *(V1) 7*
Total colectomy with ileaoanal reservoir, *(V1) 658, (V1) 658f*
Total iron-binding capacity test (TIBC), *(V1) 605*
Total parenteral nutrition (TPN), *(V1) 616*
Total Urinary Incontinence, *(V1) 64*
Touch
    in communication, *(V1) 343*
    effect on nurses, *(V1) 688b*
    impaired perception of, *(V1) 687*
    as sexual expression, *(V1) 777*
Towel bath, *(V1) 452, (V2) 396p–397p*
Toxic reaction, *(V1) 489*
Toxin, take-home, *(V1) 428*
Trace mineral, *(V1) 581*

Trachea, (V1) 846, (V1) 846f
Tracheal rings, (V1) 376, (V1) 376f
Tracheostomy
    care for, (V2) 825p–830p
    oxygen delivery, (V1) 877
    suctioning of, (V2) 840p–845p
    using ventilator with, (V1) 880
Tracheostomy tube, (V1) 878
Trade name, (V1) 474
Traditional Chinese medicine (TCM)
    as alternative medical system, (V1)
        992–993
    as complementary and alternative
        medicine (CAM), (V1) 235
    defining health, (V1) 171b
Trait, (V1) 953
Trait theory, (V1) 953
Tranquilizer, (V1) 926b
Transcellular fluid, (V1) 888, (V1) 888f
Transcendence of self, (V1) 151
Transcutaneous electrical nerve stimulation
        (TENS), (V1) 703
Transcutaneous electrical nerve stimulator
        (TENS), (V1) 710
Transdermal administration, opioids,
        (V1) 715
Transdermal medication, (V1) 502, (V2) 513tb
Transduction, (V1) 701
Trans-fatty acid, (V1) 580, (V1) 580t
Transfer belt, (V1) 756, (V1) 756f
Transfer board, (V1) 755, (V1) 755f
Transfer cannula, (V1) 519, (V1) 519f
Transfer from bed/chair, (V1) 43b
Transfer needle, (V1) 519
Transfer report, (V2) 182
Transferrin, (V1) 605
Transfer roller sheet, (V1) 753, (V1) 753f
Transformation, (V1) 972f
Transformational leadership
    ability of, (V1) 955
    qualities and behaviors of, (V1) 955t
Transformation theory, (V1) 954–955
Transfusion, (V1) 914p
Transgendered, (V1) 767
Transition, (ESG9) 33
Translator, (V1) 244, (V1) 355
Transmission, mode of, (V1) 400
Transmission-based isolation, (V1) 413
Transmission-based precautions, (V1) 412,
        (V2) 342tb
Transparent film dressing, (V1) 838t,
        (V1) 839f
Transpersonal caring, (V1) 153
Transplant surgery, (V1) 924
Transsexual, (V1) 767
Transtheoretical model of change,
        (V1) 1007–1008
Transtracheal catheter, (V1) 880
Transverse colon, (V1) 653
Transvestite, (V1) 767
Trapeze bar, (V1) 749, (V1) 749f
Trauma
    bowel diversion, cause for, (V1) 657
    musculoskeletal system and, (V1) 738
Treatment, errors and malpractice,
        (V1) 1083–1084
Tremor, (V1) 740b
Trends
    in nursing and health care, (V1) 22–23
    in society, (V1) 21
Trial, civil, (V1) 1081
Trial and error, (V1) 155

Triangle, anterior and posterior, (V1) 376
Tricep, skinfold measurement, (V2) 579tb
Tricyclic antidepressants, (V1) 808
Triglyceride
    chemical structure for, (V1) 579f
    as type of lipid, (V1) 579b
Triple-lumen catheter, (V1) 641, (V1) 641f
Trochanter roll, (V1) 750
Trochanter roll, making, (V2) 717tb
Trough level, of drug, (V1) 486
Trousseau's sign, assessment for, (V2) 903p
True fat, (V1) 579
Trunk ROM, (V1) 746t
Trust
    establishing with patient, (V1) 183–184,
        (V1) 350
    faith and, (V1) 249
    mistrust versus, (V1) 167
Tub bath, (V1) 453–454, (V2) 429tb
Tuberculin skin test, reading, (V2) 866
Tuberculin syringe, (V1) 508, (V1) 508f
Tuberculosis (TB)
    community surveillance for, (V1) 1024
    nurse fighting monster of, (V1) 9, (V1) 9f
    return of, (V1) 216
    testing for, (V1) 868
Tubex prefilled system, (V1) 508–509
Tubman, Harriet, (V1) 8
Tuesdays with Morrie, (V1) 174
Tuning fork, (V1) 372–374
Tunneled central venous catheter,
        (V1) 908, (V1) 908f
Tunnel wound, (V1) 815t
Turgor, of skin, (V1) 368
T wave, (V1) 870
Twelve-lead electrocardiogram, (V1) 871,
        (V1) 871f,
Twenty-four hour
    clock, (V1) 302, (V1) 302f
    recall, (V1) 602
    urine specimen, (V2) 620tb
Two-bottle system, (V1) 881, (V1) 881f
Tylenol
    for fever, (V1) 314
    for pain relief, (V1) 712
Tympanic membrane (TM)
    characteristics of, (V1) 373
    rupture of, (V1) 468
Tympanic temperature, (V1) 314, (V2) 202p
Tympanic thermometer, (V1) 310, (V1) 312,
        (V1) 312f
Type II diabetes mellitus (DM), (V1) 59–60,
        (V1) 67
    in child, (ESG9) 25
    in young adult, (ESG9) 32

U
U.S. Constitution, (V1) 1071
U.S. Department of Health and Human
        Services (U.S. DHHS)
    Healthy People 2010, (V1) 1005,
        (V1) 1006b
    rights of research participants,
        (V1) 158
U.S. Drug Enforcement Agency (DEA),
        (V1) 476
U.S. Preventive Services Task Force,
        (V1) 1013
U.S. Public Health Service (USPHS),
        (V1) 99
Ulcer
    duodenal, (V1) 803

pressure
    assessment of, (V1) 823, (V1) 826
    Braden scale, (V1) 823, (V1) 824f
    cause of, (V1) 449
    development of, (V1) 820–821, (V1) 821f
    of foot, (V1) 456
    guidelines for, (V1) 109b
    Norton scale, (V1) 823, (V1) 825f
    PUSH tool, (V1) 827f
    sites for, (V1) 821, (V1) 821f
    stages of, (V1) 822f
    staging of, (V1) 822
    stasis, (V2) 246
    types of, (V1) 815t
Ultrasonic nebulizer, (V1) 505
Ultrasonography (ultrasound)
    of gastrointestinal tract, (V2) 667
    of urinary system, (V2) 633
Umbrella, (ESGV1) 9
Unauthorized practice, (V1) 1087
Uncomplicated grief, (V1) 268
Unconscious mind, (ESG9) 5
Unconscious patient
    communication and, (V2) 226tb
    communication with, (V1) 167
    eye care for, (V1) 466
    intervention for, (V1) 697
    oral care, (V2) 411p–413p
    oral care of, (V1) 167
Underground Railroad, (V1) 8
Underwater weighing, for body composition,
        (V1) 604
Underweight
    NOC outcomes and NIC interventions,
        (V2) 589
    nursing processes for, (V1) 611–612
Unemployment, (V1) 215
Uniform Anatomical Gift Act, (V1) 275,
        (V1) 276b
Uniform Determination of Death Act,
        (V1) 270, (V1) 270b, (V2) 158
Unionization, Canadian healthcare providers,
        (ESGV1) 9
Unit, as drug measurement, (V1) 492
Unit-dose system, (V1) 478
United Nations Children's Fund, (V1) 772
United States
    dietary guidelines for, (V1) 587b
    racial and ethnic makeup, (V1) 223f
    sexuality, (V1) 771
United States Adopted Name Council (USAN
        Council), (V1) 474
United States Bureau of Census,
        (V1) 1021–1022, (V1) 1022f
United States Pharmacopeia (USP),
        (V1) 474–475
Unit standards of care, (V1) 87–88
Universal hospital insurance, (ESG46 V1) 2
Universality, (ESGV1) 4t, (ESGV1) 5
Universal precautions. See standard
        precautions
University of Notre Dame, (V1) 5
Unknown etiology, (V1) 76
Unlicensed assistive personnel (UAP),
        (V1) 22–23
    client care activities, (V1) 963b
    client safety intervention, (V1) 439–440
    hygiene care, (V1) 336, (V1) 446–447
    pain management, (V1) 709b
    RN delegating patient care activities to,
        (V1) 126
    vital signs, (V1) 336

Unsaturated fat, *(V1) 580*
Unsaturated fatty acid, *(V1) 580*
Upmanship, *(V1) 254*
Upper airway, *(V1) 846*
Upper respiratory infection
  increasing surgical risk, *(V1) 926b*
  prevention of, *(V1) 874, (V1) 1017*
Upper respiratory infection (URI), *(V1)
  854–855*
Urea, *(V1) 605*
Ureter
  infection of (pyelonephritis), *(V1) 636*
  transporting urine, *(V1) 621*
Urethra
  infection of (urethritis), *(V1) 635*
  transporting urine, *(V1) 622*
Urethritis, *(V1) 635*
Urgency, of urination, *(V1) 633b*
Urgent surgery, *(V1) 924*
Urinalysis
  routine, *(V1) 633–634*
  variations and expected findings,
    (V2) 631–632
Urinalysis, routine, *(V1) 903*
Urinary catherization, *(V1) 640*
Urinary catheter
  insertion of, *(V2) 598p–609p*
    indwelling, *(V2) 603p–607p*
    straight, *(V2) 599p–603p*
Urinary diversion
  caring for patient with, *(V1) 649,
    (V2) 628tb*
  conditions requiring, *(V1) 638*
  ileal conduit as, *(V1) 638f*
Urinary elimination, *(V1) 622–626*
  assessment of, *(V2) 630*
  history questions, *(V2) 629*
  overview of, *(V2) 591*
  surgery preparation, *(V1) 933–934*
Urinary incontinence (UI)
  management of, *(V1) 646,
    (V2) 626tb–627tb*
  treatment for, *(V1) 648*
  types of, *(V1) 637–638*
Urinary meatus, *(V1) 622*
Urinary retention
  etiology of, *(V1) 636*
  management of, *(V1) 640*
  medications associated with, *(V1) 625b*
  as postoperative collaborative problem,
    (V1) 947t
Urinary system, *(V1) 643f*
  bladder, *(V1) 621–622*
  diuretics, *(V1) 624b*
  exercise and, *(V1) 734b*
  kidney function, *(V1) 619–620*
  Nursing Intervention Classification (NIC),
    (V2) 634
  organs of, *(V1) 619, (V1) 620f*
  penis function, *(V1) 765*
  physical assessment of, *(V1) 626*
  stressor response, *(V1) 555–556*
  stress urinary incontinence care map,
    (V1) 631
  stress urinary incontinence care plan,
    (V1) 627–630
  studies of, *(V1) 635, (V2) 633*
  ureter function, *(V1) 620*
  urethra function, *(V1) 622*
  urinary tract infection (UTI)
    cause of, *(V1) 622, (V1) 635*
    diagnosis and treatment of, *(V1) 636*

prevention of, *(V1) 636, (V1) 640*
  risk factors for, *(V1) 636*
Urinary tract infection (UTI)
  cause of, *(V1) 622, (V1) 635*
  diagnosis and treatment of, *(V1) 636*
  as postoperative collaborative problem,
    (V1) 947t
  prevention of, *(V1) 636, (V1) 640*
  risk factors for, *(V1) 636*
Urination, *(V1) 622*
  factors affecting, *(V1) 623–626*
  patterns of, *(V1) 622*
Urine
  acidic versus alkaline, *(V1) 646*
  characteristics of, *(V1) 622*
  clean-catch specimen, *(V2) 595p–597p*
  dipstick testing, *(V2) 621tb*
  fluid output, *(V1) 891*
  formation of, *(V1) 620, (V1) 621f*
  hypervolemia and, *(V1) 896*
  measuring
    concentration of, *(V1) 634f*
    from indwelling catheter, *(V2) 619tb*
    obtaining specimen and, *(V2) 619tb*
    output, *(V1) 626, (V1) 632*
  methods for collecting specimen, *(V1)
    632, (V1) 633f*
  of newborn skull, *(ESG9) 13*
  routine urinalysis, *(V1) 633–634*
  specific gravity, measurement, *(V2) 622tb*
  specimen from catheter, *(V2) 620tb*
  testing kit, *(V1) 634f*
  traditional Chinese medicine (TCM),
    (V1) 993
  transportation of, *(V1) 621*
  twenty-four hour specimen, *(V2) 620tb*
Urine osmolality, *(V1) 902*
Urinometer, *(V1) 634*
Urostomy, *(V1) 638*
USDA dietary guidelines, *(V1) 587*
USDA Food Guide Pyramid, *(V1) 587,
  (V1) 589f*
Utilitarianism, *(V1) 1057*
Utility, principle of, *(V1) 1057*
Utilization
  Conduct and Utilization of Research in
    Nursing project (CURN), *(V1) 156*
  of nursing research, *(V1) 161*

V
Vaccination, *(V1) 216*
  of infant, *(ESG9) 18*
  promoting host defense of infection,
    (V1) 405
  schedule for, *(ESG9) 19f*
  smallpox, *(V1) 1030*
Vacuum-assisted wound closure, *(V1) 818*
Vagina, *(V1) 764*
Vaginal birth, *(ESG9) 13*
Vaginal medication
  administration of, *(V1) 522p,
    (V2) 467p–470p*
  overview of, *(V1) 504*
Vaginismus, *(V1) 780*
Validation
  of criteria, *(V1) 130*
  of data, *(V1) 49–50*
Validation theory, *(V1) 151*
Validity, research, *(V1) 160*
Valsalva maneuver, *(V1) 654*
Values
  affecting nurse behavior, *(V1) 68–69*

clarification of, *(V1) 1062–1063,
  (V1) 1063f*
  definition of, *(V1) 1051*
  in differing cultures, *(V1) 227*
  modes of transmission, *(V1) 1053t*
  morals and ethics relating to, *(V1) 1054*
  neutrality of, *(V1) 1053–1054*
  in nursing, *(V1) 16b*
  overview of, *(V2) 1005*
Value set, *(V1) 1051*
Value system, *(V1) 1051*
Vanauken, Sheldon, *(V1) 183*
Variable, *(V1) 157*
Varicosities, *(V1) 383, (V2) 293*
Vascular access device, *(V1) 906–908*
Vascular collapse, *(V1) 315*
Vascular system, *(V1) 382*
  assessment of, *(V1) 395p, (V2) 287p–293p*
  autonomic nervous system, *(V1) 853–854*
Vasocongestion, *(V1) 776*
Vasoconstriction, *(V1) 307, (V1) 314*
Vasodilation, *(V1) 307, (V1) 856*
Vasodilator, *(V1) 884*
Vastus lateralis muscle, *(V1) 517, (V1) 517f*
Vata (destruction), *(V1) 992*
Vector, *(V1) 400*
  types of, *(V1) 429*
Vector-borne pathogen, *(V1) 429–430*
Vedas, *(V1) 4, (V1) 252*
Vegan, *(V1) 598*
Vegetarianism
  food pyramid, *(V1) 591f*
  nutrition and, *(V1) 598*
Vein, *(V1) 382, (V1) 852*
Venipuncture
  performance of, *(V1) 911*
  site selection for, *(V1) 910*
Venous return, *(V1) 883*
Venous star, *(V2) 333*
Venous stasis ulcer, *(V1) 815t*
Venous system, *(V1) 382*
Ventilation, *(V1) 469, (V1) 848*
  deep breathing, *(V1) 874*
  impaired, diagnoses for, *(V2) 867–868*
  position for maximum, *(V1) 874*
  problems with, *(V1) 872*
Ventilator
  mechanical, *(V1) 880–881, (V2)
    846p–849p*
  tracheostomy, using with, *(V1) 880*
Ventricles, *(V1) 851*
Ventrogluteal muscle, *(V1) 516, (V1) 516f*
Venule, *(V1) 852*
Veracity, *(V1) 1056*
Verbal communication
  definition of, *(V1) 340*
  types of, *(V1) 340–342*
Verbal orders, *(V1) 301, (V1) 494*
Verification
  of data, *(V1) 49–50*
  of problem with patient, *(V1) 66*
Vernix caseosa, *(V1) 812*
Vesicle (blister), *(V2) 244, (V2) 333*
Vesicular breath sounds, *(V1) 379f, (V1) 380*
Vestigial organ, *(V1) 653*
Vial, drawing medication up from, *(V1) 509,
  (V1) 523p, (V2) 476p–478p*
Vibration, *(V1) 998, (V2) 815p–818p*
Vicarious liability, *(V1) 1080*
Videoconferencing, *(V1) 975, (V1) 975f*
Vietnam War, *(V1) 9*
Villi, *(V1) 652–653*

Violence
  as challenge to family health, (V1) 216
  in health care facility, (V1) 437–438
  in young adult, (ESG9) 32
Virchow's triad, (V1) 739
Virginity, (V1) 769
Visceral pain, (V1) 700
Viscosity, (V1) 328
Vision
  bedside assessment of, (V2) 681
  deficits of, (V1) 685b, (V1) 694–696
  distance, near and color, (V1) 371–372
  impaired, (V1) 355, (V1) 685
  sensory perceptual health, (V1) 693
Vision test, (V2) 255
Visual acuity, (V1) 371, (ESG9) 19
Visual analogue scale (VAS), for pain,
    (V2) 692
Visual deficit
  safety and health measures for,
      (V1) 696
  types of, (V1) 685b
Visual field, (V1) 372
Visualization
  effectiveness of, (V1) 995–996
  for stress management, (V1) 570
  as study for GI tract, (V1) 660–661
Vital capacity (VC), (V1) 849
Vital signs (VS)
  abnormal, outcome and intervention,
      (V2) 218
  of adolescence, (ESG9) 27
  for adults, (V1) 306t
  definition of, (V1) 305
  delegation of, (V1) 336
  evaluation of, (V1) 335–336
  fluid, electrolyte and acid-base
      imbalance, (V1) 901
  general survey of client, (V1) 365
  hypervolemia and, (V1) 896
  measuring and recording of, (V1) 306
  of newborn, (ESG9) 16
  normal for adults, (V1) 306t
  overview of, (V2) 191
  pain as fifth, (V1) 707
Vital Statistics Act, (ESGV1) 8
Vitamin
  adult dietary reference intake (DRI),
      (V1) 583t–584t
  mixed reviews on, (V1) 997
  supplementation, (V1) 607
  types of, (V1) 581
Vitamin B$_{12}$, (V1) 598
Vitamin D
  deficiency, (V1) 737
  formation of, (V1) 447
  needs for ovo-lacto vegetarian, (V1) 599
Vitiligo, (V2) 333
Vocabulary, healthcare workers, (V1) 340
Vocalization, (V1) 375
Voiding, (V1) 622
Voiding reflex center, (V1) 622
Volume-control infusion set, (V1) 520–521,
    (V1) 521f,, (V1) 911, (V2) 509p
Vomiting
  peristalsis and, (V1) 657
  as postoperative collaborative problem,
      (V1) 946t
  as side effect of opioids, (V1) 714b
Voodoo, (V1) 231, (V1) 231f
Vulnerable population, (V1) 225
Vulva, (V1) 764

W
Waist ROM, (V1) 746t
Wald, Lillian, (V1) 9
Walker
  teaching patient to use, (V2) 719tb–720tb
  types of, (V1) 759, (V1) 759f
Walking
  aids for, (V1) 758
    instruction for using, (V2) 719tb–720tb
    sizing, (V2) 718tb
  assisting with, (V1) 757, (V1) 758f
  for musculoskeletal assessment, (V1) 385
  physical conditioning for, (V2) 718tb
Warfarin (Coumadin), (V1) 84
Wart
  genital, (V2) 336
  plantar, (V1) 456
Water
  drowning in, (V1) 427
  as essential nutrient, (V1) 582
  hypovolemia and, (V1) 896
  loss of, (V1) 308
  osmosis of, (V1) 889, (V1) 889f
  pollution in, (V1) 431
  safe drinking, (V1) 9
Water-borne pathogen, (V1) 430
Water-soluble vitamin, (V1) 581,
    (V1) 583t–584t
Watson, Dr. Jean
  defining health, (V1) 171b
  health, elements of, (V1) 1004
  holistic nursing and, (V1) 991
  photo of, (V1) 140f
  Science of Human Caring, (V1) 139–140
Watson's theory
  caring processes, (V2) 77
  concepts of, (V1) 152–154
  in education, (V1) 145
  improving health, (V1) 144
Wear-and-tear theory, (ESG9) 35
Weber test, (V1) 374
WebMed, (V1) 21
Web sites, (V1) 546
Weight
  baseline for pregnancy, (ESG9) 12f
  fluid status, monitoring for, (V1) 902
  hypovolemia and, (V1) 896
  obesity, (V1) 609
  overweight and obesity, (V1) 329
  pharmacokinetics and, (V1) 487
  standards of, (V1) 594
  underweight and undernutrition,
      (V1) 611
Weight Watchers, (V1) 1018
Weil, Andrew, (V1) 989
Wellness
  as balancing act, (V1) 184
  definition of, (V1) 171, (V1) 1004
  environment nourishing, (V1) 176
  envisioning, (V1) 183
  health and, (V1) 174
  intervention for, (V2) 980–981
  intervention for diagnoses of, (V1) 538
  promotion in family, (V1) 219
  as special needs assessment, (V1) 44
  Wheel of Wellness, (V1) 1006, (V1) 1007f
Wellness diagnosis
  algorithm for, (V1) 62f
  health status, (V1) 63
  one-part statement, (V1) 75
  writing goals for, (V1) 100
Wellness intervention, (V1) 116

West Nile virus, (V1) 215
Wheal, (V2) 245
Wheel of Wellness, (V1) 1006, (V1) 1007f
Wheezing, (V1) 325, (V1) 863
Whirlpool treatment, (V1) 836
Whistleblower, (V1) 1049
Whistleblowing, (V1) 1048–1049
White blood cell, (V1) 403t
Whitman, Walt, (V1) 8
Whole blood transfusion, (V1) 919
Whole-brain death, (V1) 269
Whopping cough, (V1) 326
Wilber, Ken, (V1) 175
Wilber, Treya Killam, (V1) 176
Will, living, (V1) 273
Windshield survey, (V1) 1029
Wired communication, (V1) 974
Wireless communication, (V1) 974
Wisdom, (V1) 972–973
Wisdom, clinical, (V1) 15
Wisdom teeth, (V1) 459
Witness, nurse as, (V1) 1080
Woman
  fluid intake recommendation, (V1) 891
  genitourinary system of, (V1) 390–391,
      (V1) 391f
  maturation status of, (V2) 330
  nutrition during pregnancy, (V1)
      597–598
  risk factors for UTI, (V1) 636
  sexual health history, (V2) 734–735
  sexual response cycle of, (V1) 774–776
  as sexy, mindless nurse, (V1) 7
  skin of, (V1) 812
  statistics as nurse, (V1) 9–10
  urinary incontinence (UI), (V1) 637
Women's movement, (V1) 21
Worden, William
  theories of grief, a comparison, (V1) 266t
  theory of grief, (V1) 265–266
Work
  as health factor, (V1) 174
  organization of, (V1) 968
Workplace
  quality of, (ESGV1) 26
  substance abuse in, (V1) 1088b
Work-related social support group, (V1) 348
Worksheet, daily, (V1) 968
World Health Organization (WHO)
  analgesic selection, (V1) 712, (V1) 712f
  defining health, (V1) 19, (V1) 171b,
      (V1) 1004
  female circumcision, (V1) 772
  sexual health, (V1) 774
  sexuality, (V1) 765
World War I, (V1) 9
World War II
  injectable penicillin, use of, (V1) 5
  nurses serving in, (V1) 9
Wound
  assessment of, (V1) 823b, (V1) 825–826,
      (V2) 793
  bandage application, (V2) 788tb–790tb
  binder application, (V2) 786tb–788tb
  chronic, (V1) 815t
  classification of, (V1) 814, (V1) 816,
      (V1) 833, (V1) 833t
  cleansing, (V1) 833, (V1) 835
  closure of, (V1) 818
  collaborative treatments, (V1)
      818–819
  complications of healing, (V1) 819

culture of, *(V1) 829*
   by needle aspiration, *(V2) 763p–765p*
   by swab, *(V2) 759p–762p*
debriding, *(V1) 836–837*
delay in healing, *(V1) 813*
drain
   emptying closed-wound, *(V2) 785tb*
   shortening, *(V2) 784tb*
   types of, *(V1) 835*
drainage of, *(V1) 819*
dressings, *(V1) 829p, (V1) 837–841*
   dry, *(V2) 770p–771p*
   hydrocolloid, *(V2) 779p–781p*
   taping, *(V2) 786tb*
   transparent film, *(V2) 776p–778p*
   wet-to-damp, *(V2) 773p–776p*
healing process and stages, *(V1) 816–817,*
   (V1) 818f
heat application, *(V2) 791tb*
infection of, *(V1) 841, (V1) 925t, (V1) 948t*
irrigation of, *(V1) 829p, (V1) 835,*
   (V2) 766p–769p

outcomes and interventions for diagnoses,
   (V2) 795–796
overview of, *(V2) 754*
Steri-Strips (adhesive strips), *(V1) 818*
supporting and immobilizing
   bandage, *(V1) 842*
   binder, *(V1) 841*
as surgical risk factor, *(V1) 925*
sutures and staples, removing,
   (V2) 783tb
testing for, *(V2) 794*
types of, *(V1) 815t*
Wrist ROM, *(V1) 743t*
Writing
   discharge plans, *(V1) 84*
   goals for groups, *(V1) 99*
   nursing care plan, *(V1) 85*
   nursing orders, *(V1) 106, (V1) 116–118*
   process for individualized nursing care
     plan, *(V1) 92*
   rationales, *(V1) 91*
   wellness diagnosis goals, *(V1) 100*

Written order, *(V1) 494*
Wrong-Baker FACES paint rating scale,
   (V2) 693
Wrong-site surgery, *(V1) 935*

X
X chromosome, *(V1) 766, (V1) 766f*
Xerostomia, *(V1) 686*

Y
Y chromosome, *(V1) 766, (V1) 766f*
Yoga, *(V1) 996, (V1) 996f*
Youth violence, *(V1) 216*

Z
Zinc
   collagen formation, *(V1) 813*
   needs for ovo-lacto vegetarian,
     (V1) 599
Zoloft (sertraline), *(V1) 788*
Z-track technique, *(V1) 516, (V1) 525p*

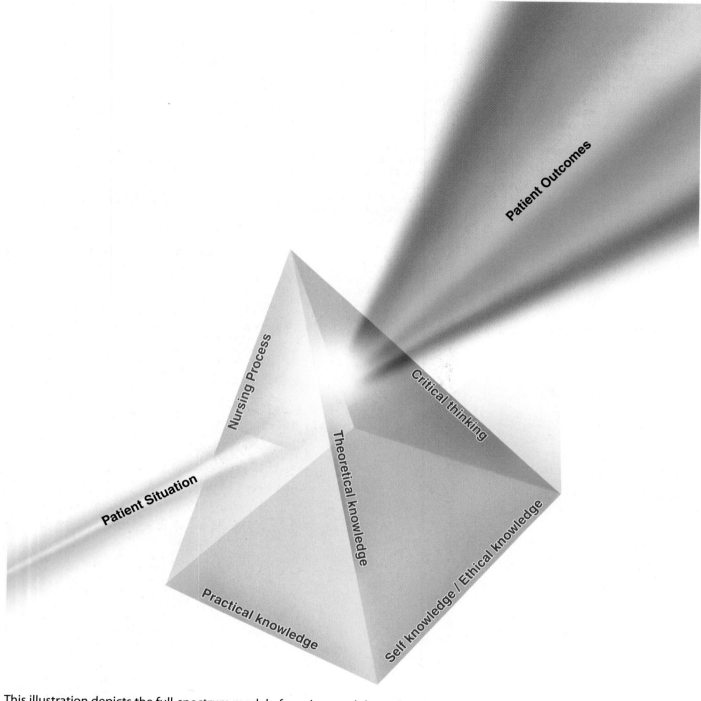

This illustration depicts the full-spectrum model of nursing used throughout this learning package. A full-spectrum nurse uses critical thinking and the nursing process to apply various types of knowledge (theoretical, practical, ethical, and self-knowledge) to the patient situation to bring about desired health outcomes. Truly, thinking and doing.